Saunders

Q&A REVIEW FOR

NCLEX-PN

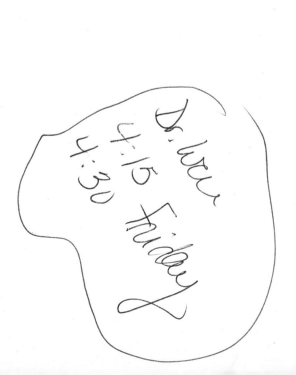

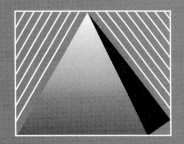

SAUNDERS
Q & A
REVIEW FOR
NCLEX-PN

LINDA ANNE SILVESTRI, MSN, RN

Assistant Professor of Nursing,
Salve Regina University,
Newport, Rhode Island;
President, Nursing Reviews, Inc., and
Professional Nursing Seminars, Inc.,
Charlestown, Rhode Island

SECOND EDITION

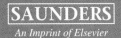

An Imprint of Elsevier

SAUNDERS

An Imprint of Elsevier

The Curtis Center
Independence Square West
Philadelphia, Pennsylvania 19106

NOTICE

Pharmacology is an ever-changing field. Standard safety precautions must be followed, but as new research and clinical experience broaden our knowledge, changes in treatment and drug therapy may become necessary or appropriate. Readers are advised to check the most current product information provided by the manufacturer of each drug to be administered to verify the recommended dose, the method and duration of administration, and contraindications. It is the responsibility of the treating appropriately licensed health care provider, relying on experience and knowledge of the patient, to determine dosages and the best treatment for each individual patient. Neither the publisher nor the editor assumes any liability for any injury and/or damage to persons or property arising from this publication.

Previous edition copyrighted 2000 by W.B. Saunders Company

Library of Congress Cataloging-in-Publication Data
Silvestri, Linda Anne.
 Saunders Q&A review for NCLEX-PN / Linda Anne Silvestri.– 2nd ed.
   p. ; cm.
 Includes bibliographical references.
 ISBN 0-7216-9716-X
   1. Practical nursing–Examinations, questions, etc. I. Title: Saunders Q & A review for NCLEX-PN.
II. Title: Saunders Q and A review for NCLEX-PN. III. Title: Q&A review for NCLEX-PN. IV. Title.
   [DNLM: 1. Nursing, Practical–Examination Questions. WY 18.2 S587sc 2004]
   RT62.S53 2004
   610.73'076–dc22

                                                                        2003057289

Executive Editor: Loren S. Wilson
Senior Developmental Editor: Michele D. Hayden
Production Services Manager: Patricia Tannian
Project Manager: Sharon Corell
Design Manager: Gail Morey Hudson
Cover Design: Dianne Ricks

Printed in the United States of America

Last digit is the print number: 9 8 7 6 5 4 3

In memory of
Jo Ann Farwell Meehan, LPN
Your love of life,
your dedication to family, and
your contributions to nursing
will live with us forever.

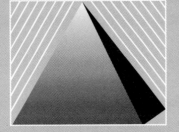

About the Author

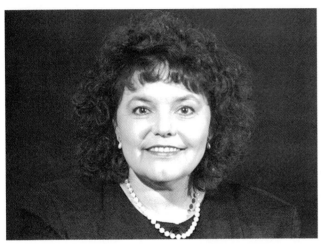

PHOTO BY Laurent W. Valliere

Linda Anne Silvestri received her diploma in nursing at Cooley Dickinson Hospital School of Nursing in Northampton, Massachusetts. After completion of her course of study, she worked in acute medical-surgical units, the intensive care unit, the emergency department, pediatric units, and other acute care units at Baystate Medical Center in Springfield, Massachusetts. She later received an associate's degree from Holyoke Community College in Holyoke, Massachusetts, and then received her bachelor of science degree in nursing from American International College in Springfield, Massachusetts.

A native of Springfield, Massachusetts, Linda began her teaching career as an instructor of medical-surgical nursing and leadership-management nursing at Baystate Medical Center School of Nursing in 1981. In 1985 she earned her master of science degree in nursing from Anna Maria College, Paxton, Massachusetts, with a dual major in nursing management and patient education.

Linda relocated to Rhode Island in 1989 and began teaching advanced medical-surgical nursing and psychiatric nursing to RN and LPN students at the Community College of Rhode Island. While she was teaching at the Community College of Rhode Island, a group of students approached Linda, asking her to help them prepare for the NCLEX. On the basis of her experience as a nursing educator and as an NCLEX item writer, she developed a comprehensive review course to prepare nursing graduates for the NCLEX examination.

Linda began teaching medical-surgical nursing at Salve Regina University in Newport, Rhode Island, in 1994. She also prepares nursing students at Salve Regina University for the NCLEX-RN examination. Linda is a member of Sigma Theta Tau.

In 1991 Linda established Professional Nursing Seminars, Inc., and in 2000, she established Nursing Reviews, Inc. Both companies are dedicated to conducting NCLEX-RN and NCLEX-PN review courses and assisting nursing graduates to achieve their goals of becoming registered nurses or licensed practical or vocational nurses.

Today Linda Silvestri's companies conduct NCLEX review courses throughout New England. She is the successful author of numerous NCLEX-RN and NCLEX-PN review products, including *Saunders Comprehensive Review for NCLEX-RN, Saunders Q&A Review for NCLEX-RN, Saunders Computerized Review for NCLEX-RN, Saunders Instructor's Resource Package for NCLEX-RN, Saunders Comprehensive Review for NCLEX-PN, Saunders Q&A Review for NCLEX-PN,* and *Saunders Instructor's Resource Package for NCLEX-PN.*

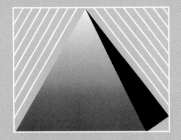

Contributors

Jo Ann Meehan, LPN
Florida Community College at Jacksonville
Jacksonville, Florida

Jo Ann Barnes Mullaney, PhD, RN, CS
Professor of Nursing, Salve Regina University
Newport, Rhode Island

Laurent W. Valliere, BS
Vice President, Professional Nursing Seminars, Inc.
Charlestown, Rhode Island

The author and publisher would also like to acknowledge the following individuals for contributions to the first edition of this book:

Nancy Diane Blasdell, MSN, RN
Visiting Lecturer, University of Massachusetts, Dartmouth
Dartmouth, Massachusetts

Jean DeCoffe, MSN, RN
Assistant Professor, Curry College
Boston, Massachusetts;
Doctoral Student, University of Massachusetts, Lowell
Lowell, Massachusetts

Kathleen Anne Fiato, RNC
Clinical Instructor
Questar III – Rensselaer School of Practical Nursing
Troy, New York;
Owner, Nursing Education and Consulting Services
Nassau, New York

Debbie Jean Fitzgerald, MSN, RN
Program Leader
Health Occupations for Norfolk Public Schools
Norfolk, Virginia

Mary Ann Hogan, MSN, RN, CS
Clinical Assistant Professor
University of Massachusetts
Amherst, Massachusetts

Deborah Keller, MSN, RN
Director, Allied Health Programs, EHOVE Career Center
EHOVE School of Practical Nursing
Milan, Ohio

Roberta P. Ramont, MS, RN
Vocational Nursing Instructor
North Orange County Regional Occupational Program
Anaheim, California

Lyndi C. Shadbolt, MS, RN
Assistant Professor of Nursing
Amarillo College
Amarillo, Texas

Ruth Sieperman, MN, NNP
Nursing Faculty, Scottsdale Community College
Scottsdale, Arizona
Neonatal Nurse Practitioner, Phoenix Children's Hospital
Phoenix, Arizona

Lucy White, DNS
Program Chair, Practical Nursing
Ivy Tech State College
Greencastle, Indiana

REVIEWERS

Dolores Cotton, MS, RN
Practical Nursing Coordinator
Meridian Technology Center
Stillwater, Oklahoma

Cecilia Jane Maier, MS, RN, CCRN
Assistant Professor
Mount Carmel College of Nursing
Columbus, Ohio

Pat Recek, MSN, RN
Department Chair
Austin Community College
Vocational Nursing Program
Austin, Texas

STUDENT REVIEWERS

Kristin Alberti
Salve Regina University
Newport, Rhode Island

Joanna Bort
Salve Regina University
Newport, Rhode Island

Sara Cabral
Salve Regina University
Newport, Rhode Island

April Oland Childs
Salve Regina University
Newport, Rhode Island

Danielle Darisse
Salve Regina University
Newport, Rhode Island

Jody DelliSante
Salve Regina University
Newport, Rhode Island

Danielle DeMelis
Salve Regina University
Newport, Rhode Island

Margaret Eldridge
Salve Regina University
Newport, Rhode Island

Kristen K. Foti
Salve Regina University
Newport, Rhode Island

Stephanie Hall
Salve Regina University
Newport, Rhode Island

Rebecca Hormanski
Salve Regina University
Newport, Rhode Island

Moira Houlihan
Salve Regina University
Newport, Rhode Island

Kristin Long
Salve Regina University
Newport, Rhode Island

Paul Lovely
Salve Regina University
Newport, Rhode Island

Nicole Mackin
Salve Regina University
Newport, Rhode Island

Lisa Mattson
Salve Regina University
Newport, Rhode Island

Kristin Roy
Salve Regina University
Newport, Rhode Island

Tonya Scharn
Salve Regina University
Newport, Rhode Island

Shandrea Silva
Salve Regina University
Newport, Rhode Island

Lindsay Stokes
Salve Regina University
Newport, Rhode Island

Kelly Sullivan
University of Rhode Island
Kingston, Rhode Island

Cristyna Vanasse
Salve Regina University
Newport, Rhode Island

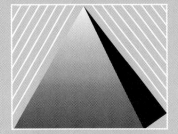

Preface

*"Success is climbing a mountain,
facing the challenge of obstacles, and
reaching the top of the mountain."*
Linda Anne Silvestri, MSN, RN

Welcome to Saunders Pyramid to Success!

The *Saunders Q&A Review for NCLEX-PN* is one of a series of products designed to assist you in achieving your goal of becoming a licensed practical or vocational nurse. The *Saunders Q&A Review for NCLEX-PN* provides you with 3000 practice NCLEX-PN test questions based on the 2002 NCLEX-PN test plan.

The new 2002 test plan for NCLEX-PN identifies a framework based on *Client Needs*. These Client Needs categories include Safe, Effective Care Environment; Physiological Integrity; Psychosocial Integrity; and Health Promotion and Maintenance. *Integrated Concepts and Processes* are also identified as a component of the test plan. These include Caring, Clinical Problem Solving Process (Nursing Process), Communication and Documentation, Cultural Awareness, Self-Care, and Teaching and Learning. This book has been uniquely designed and includes chapters that describe each specific component of the 2002 NCLEX-PN Test Plan framework and chapters that contain practice questions specific to each component.

CAT NCLEX-PN TEST PREPARATION

This book begins with information regarding NCLEX-PN preparation. Chapter 1 addresses all of the information related to the 2002 NCLEX-PN test plan and the testing procedures related to the examination. This chapter answers all of the questions that you may have about the testing procedures. Chapter 2 discusses the NCLEX-PN from a nonacademic view and emphasizes a holistic approach for your individual test preparation. This chapter identifies the components of a structured study plan and pattern, anxiety-reducing techniques, and personal focus issues.

Nursing students want to hear what other students have to say about their experiences with NCLEX-PN.

Students seek a view of what it is really like to take this examination. Chapter 3 is written by a nursing student who took this examination. This chapter addresses the issue of what NCLEX-PN is all about, and includes the student's "story of success."

Chapter 4, "Test-Taking Strategies," includes all of the important strategies that will assist in teaching you how to read a question, how not to read into a question, and how to use the process of elimination and various other methods to select the correct response from the options presented.

Client Needs

Chapters 5 to 9 address the 2002 NCLEX-PN test plan component *Client Needs*. Chapter 5 describes each category of *Client Needs* as identified by the test plan and lists the subcategories of each category, the percentage of test questions for each category, and some of the content included on NCLEX-PN. Chapters 6 to 9 contain practice test questions related specifically to each category of *Client Needs*. Chapter 6 contains questions related to Safe, Effective Care Environment; Chapter 7 contains Health Promotion and Maintenance questions; Chapter 8 contains Psychosocial Integrity questions; and Chapter 9 contains the Physiological Integrity questions.

Integrated Concepts and Processes

Chapters 10 and 11 address *Integrated Concepts and Processes* as identified in the test plan for NCLEX-PN. Chapter 10 describes each *Integrated Concept and Process*. Chapter 11 contains practice test questions related specifically to each *Integrated Concept and Process*, including Caring, Clinical Problem Solving Process (Nursing Process), Communication and Documentation, Cultural Awareness, Self-Care, and Teaching and Learning.

Comprehensive Test

A comprehensive test is included at the end of this book. It consists of 85 practice questions representative of the components of the 2002 test plan framework for NCLEX-PN.

SPECIAL FEATURES OF THE BOOK

Book Design

The book is designed with a unique two-column format. The left column presents the practice questions and options, and the right column provides the corresponding answers, rationales, test-taking strategies, and references. The two-column format makes the review easier because you do not have to flip through pages in search of answers and rationales.

Practice Questions

While you are preparing for the NCLEX-PN, it is crucial that you review practice test questions. This book contains more than 1500 practice questions in NCLEX format, including multiple-choice and the new alternate items. The accompanying software includes all the multiple-choice questions from the book, plus an additional 1500 questions, for a total of more than 3000 test questions.

Answer Sections for Practice Questions

Each practice question is followed by the correct answer, rationale, test-taking strategy, question categories, and a reference source. The structure of the answer section is unique and provides the following information for every question.

Rationale: The rationale provides you with significant information about both correct and incorrect options.

Test-Taking Strategy: The test-taking strategy provides you with the logic for selecting the correct option and assists you in selecting an answer to a question on which you must guess. Specific suggestions for review are identified in the test-taking strategy.

Question Categories: Each question is identified based on the categories used by the NCLEX-PN test plan. Additional content area categories are provided with each question to assist you in identifying areas in need of review. The categories identified with each question include Level of Cognitive Ability, Client Needs, Integrated Concept and Process, and the specific nursing Content Area. All categories are identified by their full names so that you do not need to memorize codes or abbreviations.

Reference Source: The reference source, including a page number, is provided so that you can easily find the information that you need to review in your undergraduate nursing textbooks.

NCLEX-PN REVIEW SOFTWARE

Packaged in this book you will find an NCLEX-PN review CD-ROM. This software contains more than 3000 questions, 1500 from the book and 1500 additional questions, including image alternate test items. This Windows- and Macintosh-compatible program offers three testing modes for review of the questions.

Quiz: Ten randomly chosen questions on the Client Needs, Integrated Concept/Process, or specific Content Area. Results are given and review of the answer, rationale, and test-taking strategy is provided after you answer all 10 questions.

Study: All questions on Client Needs, Integrated Concept/Process, or specific Content Area. The answer, rationale, and test-taking strategy appear after you answer each question.

Examination: One hundred randomly chosen questions from the entire pool of 3000 questions, chosen according to Client Needs, Integrated Concept/Process, or specific Content Area. Results are given and review is provided after you answer all 100 questions.

The CD-ROM allows you to customize your review and determine your areas of strength and weakness. It also provides you with a wealth of practice test questions while at the same time simulating the NCLEX-PN experience on computer.

HOW TO USE THIS BOOK

Saunders Q&A Review for NCLEX-PN is especially designed to help you with your successful journey to the peak of the Pyramid to Success, becoming a licensed practical or vocational nurse. As you begin your journey through this book, you will be introduced to all of the important points regarding the CAT NCLEX-PN examination, the process of testing, and the unique and special tips regarding how to prepare yourself for this important examination. Read the chapter from the nursing graduate who passed NCLEX-PN, and consider what this graduate has to say about the examination. The test-taking strategy chapter will provide you with important strategies that will guide you in selecting the correct option or assist you in guessing the answer. Read this chapter and practice these strategies as you proceed through your journey with this book.

Once you have completed reading the introductory components of this book, it is time to begin the practice questions. As you read through each question and select an answer, be sure to read the rationale and the test-taking strategy. The rationale provides you with the significant information about both the correct and incorrect options, and the test-taking strategy provides you with the logic for selecting the correct option. The strategy also identifies the content area that you should review if you had difficulty with the question. Use the reference source provided so that you can easily find the information that you need to review.

As you work your way through *Saunders Q&A Review for NCLEX-PN* to identify your areas of strength and weakness, you can return to the companion book, *Saunders Comprehensive Review for NCLEX-PN*, to focus your study on these areas. The companion book and its accompanying CD-ROM provide you with a comprehensive review of all areas of the nursing content reflected in the 2002 CAT NCLEX-PN test plan. The final component of the Saunders Pyramid to Success is *Saunders Instructor's Resource Package for NCLEX-PN*. This manual and CD-ROM accompany the Saunders program of NCLEX-PN review products. Be sure to ask your nursing program director and nursing faculty about the CD-ROM and its use for a review course or a self-paced review in your school's computer laboratory.

Good luck with your journey through the Pyramid to Success! I wish you continued success throughout your new career as a Licensed Practical or Vocational Nurse!

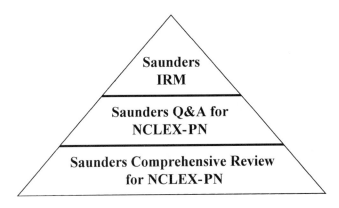

ACKNOWLEDGMENTS

There are many individuals who in their own way have contributed to my success in making my professional dreams become a reality.

First, I want to acknowledge my parents, who opened my door of opportunity in education. I thank my mother, Frances Mary, for all of her love, support, and assistance as I continuously worked to achieve my professional goals. I thank my father, Arnold Lawrence, who always provided insightful words of encouragement. My memories of his love and support will always remain in my heart.

I also thank my sister, Dianne Elodia, my brother, Lawrence Peter, and my niece, Gina Marie, who were continuously supportive, giving, and helpful during my research and preparation of this publication.

I sincerely thank Mary Ann Hogan, MSN, RN, who has always encouraged and supported me through my professional endeavors. Her numerous contributions to this publication are reflections of her dedication to the profession of nursing and to nursing students.

A very special thank you to Sarah Miller, my assistant. She provided continuous support and dedication to my work both in the NCLEX review courses and in preparing the second edition of this book.

I want to thank all of my nursing students at the Community College of Rhode Island in Warwick for approaching me in 1991 and persuading me to assist them in preparing to take the NCLEX examination. Their enthusiasm and inspiration led to the commencement of my professional endeavors in conducting NCLEX review courses for nursing students. I also thank the numerous nursing students who have attended my review courses for their willingness to share their needs and ideas. Their input has added a special uniqueness to this publication.

I thank all of the contributors, who provided practice questions that are contained in this publication, and the many faculty and student reviewers of this publication. A special thank you to Dr. JoAnn Mullaney from Salve Regina University in Newport, Rhode Island, for her numerous and expert contributions to this publication and to Jo Ann Meehan, LPN, for providing a chapter to this publication about her experiences with NCLEX-PN.

I wish to acknowledge all of the nursing faculty who taught in my NCLEX review courses. Their commitment, dedication, and expertise has assisted nursing students in achieving success with the NCLEX examination. In addition, I want to acknowledge Laurent W. Valliere for his contribution to this publication, for teaching in my NCLEX review courses, and for his commitment and dedication in assisting my nursing students to prepare for NCLEX from a non-academic point of view.

I sincerely acknowledge and thank two very important individuals from Elsevier. I thank Loren Wilson, Executive Editor, for all of her assistance throughout the preparation of this edition and for her continuous enthusiasm, support, and expert professional guidance. I thank Shelly Hayden, Senior Developmental Editor, for her continuous assistance and for keeping me on track. Her expert organizational skills maintained order for all of the work that I submitted for manuscript production. I also thank Jennifer A. Jost, Editorial Assistant, for assisting in facilitating the publication of this book.

I want to acknowledge all of the staff at Elsevier for their tremendous assistance throughout the preparation and production of this publication. A special thank you to all of them.

I thank all of the special people in the production department: Sharon Corell, Project Manager, whose consistent editing assisted in finalizing this publication; Trish Tannian, Publishing Services Manager; and Gail Morey Hudson, Book Design Manager. I sincerely thank Bob Boehringer, Marking Manager from the Nursing Marketing Department, whose support, hard work, and special creativity assisted with this publication.

I would also like to acknowledge Patricia Mieg, Educational Sales Representative, who encouraged me to submit my ideas and initial work to the W.B. Saunders Company and initiated my meeting with Maura Connor, my former Senior Acquisitions Editor. I want to thank Maura for her professional direction that led me to success as I initially created the *Saunders Pyramid to Success* products.

I thank Salve Regina University for the opportunity to educate nursing students in the baccalaureate nursing program and for its support during my research and writing of this publication. I would like to especially acknowledge Dr. Louise Murdock, Chairperson of the Department of Nursing at Salve Regina University, for her continuous support, academic mentoring, and astute vision about the profession of nursing.

I wish to acknowledge the University of Rhode Island, College of Nursing, for providing me with the opportunity for professional growth in my nursing education. I also wish to acknowledge the Community College of Rhode Island, which provided me the opportunity to educate nursing students in the Associate Degree of Nursing Program, and give a special thank you to Patricia Miller, MSN, RN, and Michelina McClellan, MS, RN, from Baystate Medical Center, School of Nursing, in Springfield, Massachusetts, who were my very first mentors in nursing education.

Lastly, a very special thank you to all my nursing students: you light up my life, and your hearts and minds will shape the future of the profession of nursing!

Linda Anne Silvestri, MSN, RN

To All Future Licensed Practical and Vocational Nurses:

Congratulations to you!

Whether you are a nursing student in a nursing program completing your studies, or a graduate preparing to take the NCLEX-PN examination, you should be very proud and pleased with yourself on your many accomplishments. I know that you are working very hard to become successful and that you have proved to yourself that you indeed can achieve your goals.

I have been teaching nursing students for many years and have been conducting NCLEX review courses since 1991. Preparing to take an examination can be an anxiety-producing experience. A component of achieving success in examinations is possessing the knowledge and experience needed to answer a question correctly. An additional component of achieving success in this examination is to become comfortable and confident in the ability to face the challenge of a question and to answer the question correctly. In my experience in working with students, I have found that students definitely benefit from review of practice questions. The more questions, answers, and rationales with which a student can practice, the more proficient the student becomes with test-taking strategies and the ability to answer a question correctly. One of the things that you should realize is that when you take an examination consisting of multiple-choice questions, the answer is right there in front of you. You should use your nursing knowledge and skills and become proficient in the strategy involved in reading a question and specifically identifying what the question is asking you. Your knowledge, your experience, and the incorporation of test-taking strategies will lead you to success. Consistent practice with test questions will assist you in becoming comfortable, confident, and proficient with answering the questions correctly.

I am excited and pleased to be able to provide you with the second editions of *Saunders Pyramid to Success* products. These products will prepare you for your most important professional goal, becoming a licensed practical or vocational nurse. *Saunders Pyramid to Success* products provide you with everything that you need to prepare for NCLEX-PN. These products include material that is required for examination preparation for all nursing students regardless of educational background, specific strengths, areas in need of improvement, or clinical experience during the nursing program.

Saunders Q&A Review for NCLEX-PN is designed to provide you with questions specifically representative of the components of the 2002 NCLEX-PN test plan. The framework for the test plan focuses on *Client Needs* and *Integrated Concepts and Processes*. Therefore chapters representative of this framework are included in this book.

So let's get started and begin our journey through the Pyramid To Success, and welcome to the wonderful profession of nursing!

Sincerely,

Linda Anne Silvestri MSN, RN

Linda Anne Silvestri MSN, RN

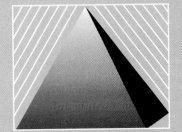

Contents

SAUNDERS
Q&A REVIEW FOR
NCLEX-PN

NCLEX-PN Preparation

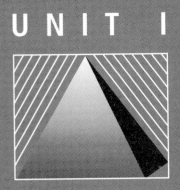

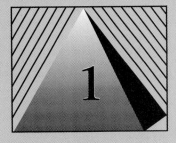

NCLEX-PN

THE PYRAMID TO SUCCESS

Welcome to *Saunders Q&A Review for NCLEX-PN*, the second component of the Pyramid to Success!

At this time, you have completed your first path toward the peak of the Pyramid with the Saunders Comprehensive Review for NCLEX-PN. Now it is time to continue that journey to become a Licensed Practical/Vocational Nurse with the *Saunders Q&A Review for NCLEX-PN*!

As you begin your journey through this book, you will be introduced to all of the important points regarding the NCLEX-PN examination, the process of testing, and the unique and special tips regarding how to prepare yourself for this very important examination. You will read what a nursing graduate who passed NCLEX-PN has to say about the examination. All of those important test-taking strategies are detailed. These details will guide you in selecting the correct option or in making a logical guess when you are unsure of the correct answer.

Saunders Q&A Review for NCLEX-PN contains 3000 NCLEX-PN–style practice questions. The chapters have been developed to provide a description of the components of the NCLEX-PN test plan, including the Client Needs and the Integrated Concepts and Processes. In addition, chapters have been prepared to contain practice questions specific to each category of Client Needs and the Integrated Concepts and Processes. In each chapter that contains practice questions, a rationale, test-taking strategy, and reference source containing the page number are provided with each question. Each question is coded on the basis of the Level of Cognitive Ability, Client Needs category, Integrated Concept and Process, and the content area being tested. The rationale provides you with significant information regarding both the correct and incorrect options. The test-taking strategy provides you with the logical path to selecting the correct option and identifies the content area to review, if necessary. The reference source and page number provide easy access to the information that you need to review.

Let's continue with our journey through The Pyramid to Success!

THE EXAMINATION PROCESS

An important step in the Pyramid to Success is to become as familiar as possible with the examination process. The challenge of this examination can arouse significant anxiety. Knowing what the examination is all about and knowing what you will encounter during the process of testing will help alleviate fear and anxiety. The information contained in this chapter addresses the procedures related to the development of the NCLEX-PN Test Plan, the components of the Test Plan, and the answers to the questions most commonly asked by nursing students and graduates preparing to take the NCLEX-PN. The information related to the development of the NCLEX-PN Test Plan, the components of the Test Plan, and the testing procedures was adapted from *Test Plan for the National Council Licensure Examination for Practical/Vocational Nurses*, National Council of State Boards of Nursing, Chicago, 2001, and *The NCLEX Process: Serving as an Anchor for the NCLEX Examination*, National Council of State Boards of Nursing, Chicago, 2000.

DEVELOPMENT OF THE TEST PLAN

As an initial step in the test development process, the National Council of State Boards of Nursing considers the legal scope of nursing practice as governed by state laws and regulations, including the Nurse Practice Act. The National Council uses these laws to define the areas of NCLEX-PN that will assess the competence of candidates for nurse licensure.

The National Council of State Boards of Nursing also conducts a Practice Analysis study to determine the framework for the Test Plan for NCLEX-PN. Since nursing practice continues to change, this study is conducted every 3 years. The results of this study, most recently conducted in 2000, provided the structure for the new Test Plan implemented in April of 2002.

PRACTICE ANALYSIS STUDY

The participants of this study include newly licensed practical and vocational nurses. The participants are provided a list of nursing activities and are asked about the frequency of performing these specific activities, their impact on maintaining client safety, and the setting where the activities were performed. The analysis of the data obtained from this study guides the development of a framework for entry-level nurse performance that incorporates specific client needs and the concepts and processes fundamental to the practice of nursing. The NCLEX-PN Test Plan is derived from this framework.

THE TEST PLAN

The content of NCLEX-PN reflects the activities that an entry-level practical and vocational nurse must be able to perform to provide clients with safe and effective nursing care. The questions are written to address the Levels of Cognitive Ability, Client Needs, and Integrated Concepts and Processes as identified in the Test Plan.

Levels of Cognitive Ability

The NCLEX-PN examination consists primarily of multiple-choice questions written at the cognitive levels of knowledge, comprehension, application, and analysis (Box 1-1).

Client Needs

In the new Test Plan implemented in April 2002, the National Council of State Boards of Nursing identifies a test plan framework based on *Client Needs*. This framework was selected on the basis of the findings in the Practice Analysis study. Additionally, Client Needs provide a structure for defining nursing actions and competencies across all settings for all clients and meet requirements specified by state laws and statutes. The National Council of State Boards of Nursing identifies four major categories of Client Needs. These categories are further divided into subcategories, and the percentage of test questions in each subcategory is identified. Table 1-1 identifies these categories and subcategories and the associated percentage of test questions. Refer to Chapter 5 for a detailed description of the categories of Client Needs and the NCLEX-PN examination.

Integrated Concepts and Processes

The National Council of State Boards of Nursing has identified six concepts and processes that are fundamental to the practice of nursing. These concepts and processes are a component of the Test Plan and are incorporated throughout the major categories of Client Needs. Box 1-2 identifies these six concepts and processes. Refer to Chapter 10 for a detailed description of the Integrated Concepts and Processes and the NCLEX-PN examination.

BOX 1-1

Level of Cognitive Ability

A pregnant client is positive for the human immunodeficiency virus (HIV). Based on this information, the nurse recognizes that:
1. The client has the herpes simplex virus
2. HIV antibodies are detected on the enzyme-linked immunosorbent assay (ELISA) test
3. The newborn will develop this disease after birth
4. This client has contacted an airborne disease

Answer: 2
Level of Cognitive Ability: Comprehension
The nurse must understand the significance of a positive HIV test and the implications associated with a positive HIV pregnant client in order to answer this question correctly. Diagnosis depends on serological studies to detect HIV antibodies. The most commonly used test is the enzyme-linked immunosorbent assay (ELISA) test.

TABLE 1-1

Client Needs and the Percentage of Test Questions

SAFE, EFFECTIVE CARE ENVIRONMENT	
Coordinated Care	6%-12%
Safety and Infection Control	7%-13%
HEALTH PROMOTION AND MAINTENANCE	
Growth and Development Through the Life Span	4%-10%
Prevention and Early Detection of Disease	4%-10%
PSYCHOSOCIAL INTEGRITY	
Coping and Adaptation	6%-12%
Psychosocial Adaptation	4%-10%
PHYSIOLOGICAL INTEGRITY	
Basic Care and Comfort	10%-16%
Pharmacological Therapies	5%-11%
Reduction of Risk Potential	11%-17%
Physiological Adaptation	13%-19%

From National Council of State Boards of Nursing (eds.) (2001). *Test Plan for the National Council Licensure Examination for Practical/Vocational Nurses.* Chicago: Author.

CAT NCLEX-PN

The term NCLEX-PN stands for National Council Licensure Examination for Practical and Vocational Nurses. The term CAT stands for Computerized Adaptive Testing. CAT NCLEX-PN is a computer-administered examination that the nursing graduate must take and pass to practice as a practical and vocational nurse. This examination measures the test candidate's knowledge, skills, and abilities required to perform safely and competently as a newly licensed, entry-level practical and vocational nurse.

COMPUTERIZED ADAPTIVE TESTING (CAT)

The CAT system provides each candidate with a unique examination experience, because the examination adapts to each test taker's skill level. The CAT examination is assembled interactively as the candidate answers the questions. All of the test questions are stored in a large test bank and are categorized on the basis of the test plan structure and the level of difficulty of the question. With the CAT method of testing, an examination is created and tailored to test the candidate's knowledge and skills while fulfilling test plan requirements. In this way, the candidate will not waste time answering questions that are far above or below his or her competency level.

When a candidate answers a question on CAT NCLEX-PN, the computer will calculate a competency skill estimate based on the answer that the candidate selected. If the candidate selected a correct answer to a question, the computer scans the test bank and selects a more difficult question. If the candidate selected an incorrect answer, the computer scans the test bank and selects an easier question. This process continues until the Test Plan requirements are met and a reliable pass or fail decision is made.

THE PROCESS OF REGISTRATION

The initial step in the registration process is to have each candidate apply to the State Board of Nursing in the state in which he or she intends to obtain licensure. (The addresses, telephone numbers, and web sites, if available, of Boards of Nursing in all states and territories of the United States are provided at the end of this chapter.) The candidate should obtain information from the Board of Nursing regarding the specific registration process, because the process may vary from state to state. It is very important that the candidate follow the registration instructions and complete the registration forms precisely and accurately. Registration forms not properly completed, or not accompanied by the proper fees in the required method of payment, will be returned to the candidate and will delay testing. The initial fee for the application process may vary from state to state. Each Board of Nursing will set its initial license fee according to its own needs. The registration forms will identify the registration and testing service fees. When the Board of Nursing receives the completed registration form, the candidate's eligibility is determined, on the basis of the criteria established by the Board, and the Board authorizes his or her admission to the examination.

Once eligibility to test has been determined by the Board of Nursing in the jurisdiction in which licensure is requested, the valid NCLEX registration is processed and an Authorization to Test form will be sent to the candidate. The candidate cannot make an appointment until the Board of Nursing declares eligibility and an Authorization to Test form is received. The Authorization to Test form will provide a candidate identification number and an authorization number; these numbers will be needed to make an appointment with the testing center.

SPECIAL TESTING CIRCUMSTANCES

A candidate who is requesting special accommodations should contact the Board of Nursing before submitting a registration form. The Board of Nursing will provide the candidate with the procedures for the request. The Board of Nursing must authorize special testing accommodations. Following Board of Nursing approval, the National Council of State Boards reviews the requested accommodations to ensure that the proposed modification does not affect the psychometric properties of NCLEX or cause a security risk. The National Council of State Boards must also approve the accommodations.

MAKING AN APPOINTMENT TO TEST

The CAT NCLEX-PN examination is administered on a year-round basis. Each candidate will be provided with a list of testing centers and the telephone numbers of these centers. The candidate must note the expiration date on the Authorization to Test form and must schedule and make an appointment before this expiration date. The candidate may take the examination at any approved testing center and does not have to test in the same jurisdiction in which licensure is sought. An eligible candidate taking NCLEX for the first time will be offered an appointment date within 30 days of the telephone call to the testing center. Repeat candidates will be offered an appointment date within 45 days of the telephone call to the testing center. A confirmation notice will not be sent to the candidate; therefore it is important that the candidate note the date and time of the appointment. When the testing center is called, it is also important to verify the address and the directions to the testing center.

CANCELING OR RESCHEDULING AN APPOINTMENT

If for any reason the candidate must cancel or reschedule the appointment to take the examination, he or she must remember that the scheduling change must be made before noon, 2 business days before the scheduled appointment. The original appointment must be canceled before a new appointment can be scheduled.

LATE ARRIVALS TO THE TEST CENTER

It is important that the candidate arrive at the testing center 30 minutes before the examination is scheduled. Candidates arriving late for the scheduled testing appointment may be required to forfeit the NCLEX appointment. If it is necessary for the appointment to be forfeited, the candidate will need to reregister for the examination and pay an additional fee. The Board of Nursing will be notified that the candidate will not test. A few days before the scheduled date of testing, the candidate should take the time to drive to the testing center to determine its exact location, the length of time required to arrive at that destination, and any potential obstacles that might cause a delay, such as road construction, traffic, or parking sites.

THE TESTING CENTER

The testing center is designed to ensure complete security of the testing process. Strict candidate identification requirements have been established. To be admitted to the testing center, the candidate must bring the Authorization to Test form, along with two forms of identification. Both forms of identification must be signed by the candidate, and one must contain the candidate's photograph. The photograph identification must bear the same name as that stated on the Authorization to Test form. Examples of acceptable forms of identification will be included in the information received with the Authorization to Test form. The candidate will be required to sign in and out on the test center log form. Each candidate will be thumbprinted and photographed at the test center, and the photograph will accompany the NCLEX results to confirm the candidate's identity. Personal belongings are not allowed in the testing room. Secure storage will be provided for the candidate; however, storage space is limited, so the candidate must plan accordingly. In addition, the testing center will not assume responsibility for the candidate's personal belongings. The waiting areas are generally small; therefore friends or family members who accompany candidates are not permitted to wait in the testing center while candidates are taking the NCLEX-PN.

Once the candidate has completed the admission process and a brief orientation, the proctor will escort the candidate to the assigned computer. The candidate will be seated at an individual table area with an appropriate work space that includes computer equipment, appropriate lighting, scratch paper, and a pencil. Unauthorized scratch paper may not be brought into or removed from the testing room. Eating, drinking, and smoking are not allowed in the testing room. A video camera is located in the testing room, and all test sessions are videotaped with full sound and motion.

Candidates should keep two forms of identification with them at all times. Candidates cannot leave the testing room without the permission of the proctor. If a candidate leaves the testing room for any reason, he or she will be required to show two forms of identification and provide a fingerprint to be readmitted. Candidates must follow the directions given by the test center staff and must remain seated during the test, except when authorized to leave. If a candidate believes that there is a problem with the computer, needs more scratch paper, or needs the proctor for any reason, he or she must raise a hand to notify the proctor.

THE COMPUTER

Computer experience is not needed to take the CAT NCLEX-PN examination. A keyboard tutorial is administered to all test takers at the start of the examination. In addition, a proctor is present to assist in explaining the use of the computer to ensure the candidate's full understanding of how to proceed.

CAT NCLEX-PN TEST QUESTIONS

The examination is composed of individual (stand-alone) test questions. In other words, this examination does not present a case situation followed by several test questions that relate to that case situation. With an individual (stand-alone) test question, you can expect that the question will appear on the left-hand side of the screen, with the four options on the right-hand side of the screen, or the question appears across the top of the screen with the four options below (Box 1-3).

The test questions will be primarily multiple-choice (question and four options) questions. There may also be questions that display a visual, fill-in-the-blank

BOX 1-3

Appearance of an Individual (Stand Alone) Test Question on the Computer Screen

The most appropriate method for feeding an infant with a cleft lip or palate is with the infant('s):
1. Head in an upright position
2. In a lying position
3. In a side-lying position
4. Prone

A client is admitted to the hospital with a diagnosis of myasthenia gravis. Pyridostigmine (Mestinon) is prescribed for the client. The nurse monitors the client knowing that an adverse effect of this medication is:
1. Muscle cramps
2. Mouth ulcers
3. Depression
4. Unexplained weight gain

questions, or multiple-response questions. Movement through the examination, including the selection of answers, will require use of the computer mouse. For example, you may be presented with a visual that displays an adult client's thorax. In this visual, you may be asked to "point and click" (using the computer mouse) on the area where the stethoscope would be placed to take an apical pulse rate. A drop-down calculator is available on the computer for use during the examination.

When a test question is presented on the computer screen, it must be answered or the examination will not move on. This means that you will not be able to skip questions, go back and review questions, or go back and change answers. Students preparing for CAT NCLEX-PN become anxious and frustrated because questions cannot be skipped and returned to at a later time during the examination process. Remember, in a CAT examination, once an answer is recorded, all subsequent questions administered depend, to an extent, on the answer selected for that question. Skipping questions and returning to them later are not compatible with the logical methodology of a computerized adaptive test. Recall the number of times you may have changed a correct answer to an incorrect one on a pencil-and-paper nursing examination during your nursing education. The inability to skip questions or go back to change previous answers will not be a disadvantage to you. Actually, you will not fall into that trap of changing a correct answer to an incorrect one with CAT.

There is no penalty for guessing on CAT NCLEX-PN. Remember, the answer to the question will be right in front of you. If you need to guess, use your nursing knowledge to its fullest extent, as well as all of the test-taking strategies provided to you in Chapter 4 of this book.

TESTING TIME

The maximum testing time is 5 hours. This time period includes the tutorial, sample questions, and all rest breaks. There is no minimum amount of examination time. A preprogrammed optional break can be taken after 2 testing hours, and a second preprogrammed optional break can be taken at the end of 3.5 hours of testing. You must leave the testing room during breaks. All breaks count against testing time.

LENGTH OF THE EXAMINATION

The minimum number of questions that you will need to answer to meet adequate testing in each area of the test plan is 85. Of these 85 questions, 70 will be real (scored) questions and 15 will be tryout (unscored) questions. The maximum number of questions in the test is 205. Fifteen of the total number of questions that you need to answer will be tryout (unscored) questions.

The tryout questions are questions that may be presented as scored questions on future NCLEX-PN examinations. These tryout questions are not identified as such. In other words, you do not know which questions are the tryout (unscored) questions.

COMPLETING THE EXAM

Once the examination is completed, the candidate will complete a brief computer-delivered questionnaire about the testing experience. After this questionnaire is completed, the test proctor will collect all scratch paper, sign the candidate out, and permit the candidate to leave.

PROCESSING RESULTS

When a candidate completes the examination, the examination is transmitted electronically to the data center for scoring. The results are then transmitted to the Board of Nursing in the state in which the candidate applied for licensure. The Board of Nursing will mail the results to the candidate. In some states, results may be obtained from the Board of Nursing web site. Additionally, some states may allow results to be given via a telephone service through the National Council of State Boards. Telephone results usually require a fee.

INTERSTATE ENDORSEMENT

Since the CAT NCLEX-PN is a national examination, the candidate can apply to take the examination in any state. Once licensure is received, the practical or vocational nurse can apply for Interstate Endorsement. The procedures and requirements for Interstate Endorsement may vary from state to state, and these procedures can be obtained from the State Board of Nursing in the state in which endorsement is sought.

ADDITIONAL INFORMATION REGARDING NCLEX-PN

Additional information regarding the NCLEX-PN examination can be obtained from the National Council of State Boards of Nursing, Inc., 111 East Wacker Drive, Suite 2900, Chicago, Illinois 60601. The telephone number for the testing service is (866) 293-9600 or (312) 525-3750. The web site is: http://www.ncsbn.org.

STATE BOARDS OF NURSING

Alabama Board of Nursing
770 Washington Avenue
RSA Plaza, Ste 250
Montgomery, AL 36130-3900
Phone: (334) 242-4060
FAX: (334) 242-4360
Web Site: http://www.abn.state.al.us/

Alaska Board of Nursing
Div. of Occupational Licensing
3601 C Street, Suite 722
Anchorage, AK 99503
Phone: (907) 269-8161
FAX: (907) 269-8196
Web Site: http://www.dced.state.ak.us/occ/pnur.htm

American Samoa Health Services
Regulatory Board
LBJ Tropical Medical Center
Pago Pago, AS 96799
Phone: (684) 633-1222
FAX: (684) 633-1869

Arizona State Board of Nursing
1651 E. Morten Avenue, Suite 210
Phoenix, AZ 85020
Phone: (602) 331-8111
FAX: (602) 906-9365
Web Site: http://www.azboardofnursing.org/

Arkansas State Board of Nursing
University Tower Building
1123 S. University, Suite 800
Little Rock, AR 72204-1619
Phone: (501) 686-2700
FAX: (501) 686-2714
Web Site: http://www.state.ar.us/nurse

California Board of Vocational Nurse
and Psychiatric Technician Examiners
2535 Capitol Oaks Drive, Suite 205
Sacramento, CA 95833
Phone: (916) 263-7800
FAX: (916) 263-7859
Web Site: http://www.bvnpt.ca.gov/

Colorado Board of Nursing
1560 Broadway, Suite 880
Denver, CO 80202
Phone: (303) 894-2430
FAX: (303) 894-2821
Web Site: http://www.dora.state.co.us/nursing/

Connecticut Board of Examiners for Nursing
Dept. of Public Health
410 Capitol Avenue, MS# 13PHO
P.O. Box 340308
Hartford, CT 06134-0328
Phone: (860) 509-7624
FAX: (860) 509-7553
Web Site: http://www.state.ct.us/dph/

Delaware Board of Nursing
861 Silver Lake Blvd
Cannon Building, Suite 203
Dover, DE 19904
Phone: (302) 739-4522
FAX: (302) 739-2711
Web Site:
http://www.professionallicensing.state.de.us/
boards/nursing/index.shtml

District of Columbia Board of Nursing
Department of Health
825 N. Capitol Street, N.E., 2nd Floor
Room 2224
Washington, DC 20002
Phone: (202) 442-4778
FAX: (202) 442-9431
Web Site: http://www.dchealth.dc.gov

Florida Board of Nursing
Capital Circle Officer Center
4052 Bald Cypress Way
Rm 120
Tallahassee, FL 32399-3252
Phone: (850) 488-0595
Web Site: http://www.doh.state.fl.us/mqa/

Georgia State Board of Licensed
Practical Nurses
237 Coliseum Drive
Macon, GA 31217-3858
Phone: (478) 207-1300
FAX: (478) 207-1633
Web Site: http://www.sos.state.ga.us/ebd-lpn/

Guam Board of Nurse Examiners
P.O. Box 2816
1304 East Sunset Boulevard
Barrgada, GU 96913
Phone: (671) 475-0251
FAX: (671) 477-4733

Hawaii Board of Nursing
Professional & Vocational Licensing Division
P.O. Box 3469
Honolulu, HI 96801
Phone: (808) 586-3000
FAX: (808) 586-2689
Web Site:
http://www.state.hi.us/dcca/pvl/areas_nurse.html

Idaho Board of Nursing
280 N. 8th Street, Suite 210
P.O. Box 83720
Boise, ID 83720
Phone: (208) 334-3110
FAX: (208) 334-3262
Web Site:
http://www.state.id.us/ibn/ibnhome.htm

Illinois Department of Professional Regulation
James R. Thompson Center
100 West Randolph, Suite 9-300
Chicago, IL 60601
Phone: (312) 814-2715
FAX: (312) 814-3145
Web Site: http://www.dpr.state.il.us/

Illinois Department of Professional Regulation
320 W. Washington St.
3rd Floor
Springfield, IL 62786
Phone: (217) 782-8556
FAX: (217) 782-7645
Web Site: http://www.dpr.state.il.us/

Indiana State Board of Nursing
Health Professions Bureau
402 W. Washington Street, Room W041
Indianapolis, IN 46204
Phone: (317) 232-2960
FAX: (317) 233-4236
Web Site: http://www.state.in.us/hpb/boards/isbn/

Iowa Board of Nursing
River Point Business Park
400 S.W. 8th Street
Suite B
Des Moines, IA 50309-4685
Phone: (515) 281-3255
FAX: (515) 281-4825
Web Site:
http://www.state.ia.us/government/nursing/

Kansas State Board of Nursing
Landon State Office Building
900 S.W. Jackson, Suite 551-S
Topeka, KS 66612
Phone: (785) 296-4929
FAX: (785) 296-3929
Web Site: http://www.ksbn.org

Kentucky Board of Nursing
312 Whittington Parkway, Suite 300
Louisville, KY 40222
Phone: (502) 329-7000
FAX: (502) 329-7011
Web Site: http://www.kbn.state.ky.us/

Louisiana State Board of Practical
Nurse Examiners
3421 N. Causeway Boulevard, Suite 203
Metairie, LA 70002
Phone: (504) 838-5791
FAX: (504) 838-5279
Web Site: http://www.lsbpne.com/

Maine State Board of Nursing
158 State House Station
Augusta, ME 04333
Phone: (207) 287-1133
FAX: (207) 287-1149
Web Site:
http://www.state.me.us/boardofnursing

Maryland Board of Nursing
4140 Patterson Avenue
Baltimore, MD 21215
Phone: (410) 585-1900
FAX: (410) 358-3530
Web Site: http://www.mbon.org

Massachusetts Board of Registration
in Nursing
Commonwealth of Massachusetts
239 Causeway Street
Boston, MA 02114
Phone: (617) 727-9961
FAX: (617) 727-1630
Web Site: http://www.state.ma.us/reg/boards/rn/

Michigan CIS/Office of Health Services
Ottawa Towers North
611 W. Ottawa, 4th Floor
Lansing, MI 48933
Phone: (517) 373-9102
FAX: (517) 373-2179
Web Site:
http://www.cis.state.mi.us/bhser/genover.htm

Minnesota Board of Nursing
2829 University Avenue SE
Suite 500
Minneapolis, MN 55414
Phone: (612) 617-2270
FAX: (612) 617-2190
Web Site: http://www.nursingboard.state.mn.us/

Mississippi Board of Nursing
1935 Lakeland Drive, Suite B
Jackson, MS 39216-5014
Phone: (601) 987-4188
FAX: (601) 364-2352
Web Site: http://www.msbn.state.ms.us/

Missouri State Board of Nursing
3605 Missouri Blvd.
P.O. Box 656
Jefferson City, MO 65102-0656
Phone: (573) 751-0681
FAX: (573) 751-0075
Web Site:
http://www.ecodev.state.mo.us/pr/nursing/

Montana State Board of Nursing
301 South Park
PO Box 200513
Helena, MT 59620-0513
Phone: (406) 841-2340
FAX: (406) 841-2343
Web Site:
http://www.discoveringmontana.com/dli/bsd/license/
bsd_boards/nur_board/board_page.htm

Northern Mariana Islands
Commonwealth Board of Nurse Examiners
PO Box 501458
Saipan, MP 96950
Phone: (670) 664-4810
FAX: (670) 664-4813

Nebraska Health and Human Services System
Dept. of Regulation & Licensure, Nursing Section
301 Centennial Mall South
Lincoln, NE 68509-4986
Phone: (402) 471-4376
FAX: (402) 471-3577

Nursing and Nursing Support Web Site:
http://www.hhs.state.ne.us/crl/nursing/
nursingindex.htm

Nevada State Board of Nursing
License Certification and Education
4330 S. Valley View Blvd.
Suite 106
Las Vegas, NV 89103
Phone: (702) 486-5800
FAX: (702)) 486-5803
Web Site: http://www.nursingboard.state.nv.us

New Hampshire Board of Nursing
P.O. Box 3898
78 Regional Drive, BLDG B
Concord, NH 03302
Phone: (603) 271-2323
FAX: (603) 271-6605
Web Site: http://www.state.nh.us/nursing/

New Jersey Board of Nursing
P.O. Box 45010
124 Halsey Street, 6th Floor
Newark, NJ 07101
Phone: (973) 504-6586
FAX: (973) 648-3481
Web Site: http://www.state.nj.us/lps/ca/medical.htm

New Mexico Board of Nursing
4206 Louisiana Boulevard, NE
Suite A
Albuquerque, NM 87109
Phone: (505) 841-8340
FAX: (505) 841-8347
Web Site: http://www.state.nm.us/clients/nursing

New York State Board of Nursing
Education Bldg.
89 Washington Avenue
2nd Floor West Wing
Albany, NY 12234
Phone: (518) 474-3817 Ext. 120
FAX: (518) 474-3706
Web Site: http://www.nysed.gov/prof/nurse.htm

North Carolina Board of Nursing
3724 National Drive, Suite 201
Raleigh, NC 27612
Phone: (919) 782-3211
FAX: (919) 781-9461
Web Site: http://www.ncbon.com/

North Dakota Board of Nursing
919 South 7th Street, Suite 504
Bismarck, ND 58504

Phone: (701) 328-9777
FAX: (701) 328-9785
Web Site: http://www.ndbon.org/

Ohio Board of Nursing
17 South High Street, Suite 400
Columbus, OH 43215-3413
Phone: (614) 466-3947
FAX: (614) 466-0388
Web Site: http://www.state.oh.us/nur/

Oklahoma Board of Nursing
2915 N. Classen Boulevard, Suite 524
Oklahoma City, OK 73106
Phone: (405) 962-1800
FAX: (405) 962-1821
Web Site:
http://www.youroklahoma.com/nursing

Oregon State Board of Nursing
800 NE Oregon Street, Box 25
Suite 465
Portland, OR 97232
Phone: (503) 731-4745
FAX: (503) 731-4755
Web Site: http://www.osbn.state.or.us/

Pennsylvania State Board of Nursing
124 Pine Street
Harrisburg, PA 17101
Phone: (717) 783-7142
FAX: (717) 783-0822
Web Site:
http://www.dos.state.pa.us/bpoa/nurbd/mainpage.htm

Commonwealth of Puerto Rico
Board of Nurse Examiners
800 Roberto H. Todd Avenue
Room 202, Stop 18
Santurce, PR 00908
Phone: (787) 725-7506
FAX: (787) 725-7903

Rhode Island Board of Nurse
Registration and Nursing Education
105 Cannon Building
Three Capitol Hill
Providence, RI 02908
Phone: (401) 222-5700
FAX: (401) 222-3352
Web Site: http://www.health.state.ri.us

South Carolina State Board of Nursing
110 Centerview Drive
Suite 202
Columbia, SC 29210

Phone: (803) 896-4550
FAX: (803) 896-4525
Web Site:
http://www.llr.state.sc.us/pol/nursing

South Dakota Board of Nursing
4300 South Louise Ave., Suite C-1
Sioux Falls, SD 57106-3124
Phone: (605) 362-2760
FAX: (605) 362-2768
Web Site: http://www.state.sd.us/dcr/nursing/

Tennessee State Board of Nursing
426 Fifth Avenue North
1st Floor -Cordell Hull Building
Nashville, TN 37247
Phone: (615) 532-5166
FAX: (615) 741-7899
Web Site: http://www.state.tn.us/health

Texas Board of Vocational Nurse Examiners
William P. Hobby Building, Tower 3
333 Guadalupe Street, Suite 3-400
Austin, TX 78701
Phone: (512) 305-8100
FAX: (512) 305-8101
Web Site: http://www.bvne.state.tx.us/

Utah State Board of Nursing
Heber M. Wells Bldg., 4th Floor
160 East 300 South
Salt Lake City, UT 84111
Phone: (801) 530-6628
FAX: (801) 530-6511
Web Site: http://www.commerce.state.ut.us/

Vermont State Board of Nursing
109 State Street
Montpelier, VT 05609-1106
Phone: (802) 828-2396
FAX: (802) 828-2484
Web Site:
http://vtprofessionals.org/oprl/nurses/

Virgin Islands Board of Nurse Licensure
Veterans Drive Station
St. Thomas, VI 00803
Phone: (340) 776-7397
FAX: (340) 777-4003

Virginia Board of Nursing
6606 W. Broad Street, 4th Floor
Richmond, VA 23230
Phone: (804) 662-9909
FAX: (804) 662-9512
Web Site: http://www.dhp.state.va.us/

Washington State Nursing Care Quality
Assurance Commission
Department of Health
1300 Quince Street SE
Olympia, WA 98504-7864
Phone: (360) 236-4700
FAX: (360) 236-4738
Web Site: http://www.doh.wa.gov/nursing/

West Virginia Board of Examiners
for Licensed Practical Nurses
101 Dee Drive
Charleston, WV 25311
Phone: (304) 558-3572
FAX: (304) 558-4367
Web Site: http://www.lpnboard.state.wv.us/

Wisconsin Department of Regulation
and Licensing
1400 E. Washington Avenue
P.O. Box 8935
Madison, WI 53708
Phone: (608) 266-0145
FAX: (608) 261-7083
Web Site: http://www.drl.state.wi.us/

Wyoming State Board of Nursing
2020 Carey Avenue, Suite 110
Cheyenne, WY 82002
Phone: (307) 777-7601
FAX: (307) 777-3519
Web Site: http://nursing.state.wy.us/

REFERENCES

de Wit, S. (2001). *Fundamental concepts and skills for nursing.* Philadelphia: W.B. Saunders.

Hodgson, B., & Kizior, R. (2003). *Saunders nursing drug handbook 2003.* Philadelphia: W.B. Saunders.

National Council of State Boards of Nursing (eds.) (2001). *Test Plan for the National Council Licensure Examination for Practical/Vocational Nurses.* Chicago: Author.

National Council of State Boards of Nursing (eds.) (2000). *The NCLEX Process: Serving as an Anchor for the NCLEX Examination.* Chicago: Author.

National Council of State Boards of Nursing. Web Site: http://www.ncsbn.org

Potter, P., & Perry, A. (2001). *Fundamentals of nursing* (5th ed.). St. Louis: Mosby,

Riley, J. (2000). *Communication in nursing* (4th ed.). St. Louis: Mosby.

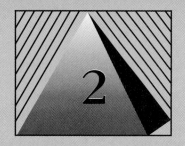

Profiles to Success

LAURENT W. VALLIERE, BS

Preparing to take the NCLEX-PN examination can produce a great deal of anxiety. You may be thinking that NCLEX-PN is the most important examination that you will ever have to take, and that it reflects the culmination of everything that you have worked so hard for. NCLEX-PN is an important examination because receiving that nursing license means that you can begin your career as a Licensed Practical or Vocational Nurse. Important to your success on NCLEX-PN is that you expel all thoughts that allow this examination to appear overwhelming and intimidating. Such thoughts will take complete control over your destiny.

Nursing students may have difficulty in developing a plan to prepare for the NCLEX-PN examination. The most important component in developing such a plan is to identify the profile that has guided you to the achievements and successes during your nursing education. It is important to begin your venture by reflecting on all of the challenges that you experienced during your nursing education. Take some time to focus on the thoughts, preparations, and emotions that you experienced before taking an examination during your nursing program. Examine the successful study methods that you used in preparing for these examinations both academically and from the perspective of how you managed the anxiety that accompanies the experience of facing an examination.

These factors are very important considerations in preparing for the NCLEX-PN examination. The reason that these factors are so critical to your continued success is that you have established a pattern of successful study habits that has and will continue to bring you success in test taking. Allow yourself a moment to reflect. Your study habits were successful or you would not be at the point of preparing for the NCLEX-PN examination.

Each individual requires his or her own methods of preparing for an examination. Graduates who have taken the NCLEX-PN examination will probably share their experiences and methods of preparing for this challenge with you. It is very helpful to listen to what they may tell you. These graduates will provide you with important strategies that they have used. Learn from their experience but never lose sight of the fact that this examination is all about you. Your personality and what you as an individual require in terms of preparation are most important.

Reflect on those methods and strategies that worked for you throughout your nursing program. Do not think that you need to develop new methods and strategies in preparing for the NCLEX-PN examination. Continue with the study habits that work for you. Take some time to reflect on these strategies, write them down on a large blank card, sign your name to this card, and place LPN or LVN after your name. Post the card with your name and the letters LPN or LVN in a place where you will see it every morning of every day. Commit to your own special strategies. These strategies reflect your profile and personality. These profiles will lead you through the pathway to success!

A frequent concern of graduates preparing for the NCLEX-PN examination relates to deciding whether they should study alone or become a part of a study group. Examining your profile will easily direct you to make the right decision. Reflect on what has worked for you throughout your nursing program as you prepared for examinations. Remember, your needs are most important. Address your own needs and do not become pressured by peers who are encouraging you to join a study group if this is not your normal pattern for study. Remember, additional pressure is not what you need at this important time of your life.

Graduates preparing for the NCLEX-PN examination frequently inquire about the best method of preparing for this examination. First, remember that you are prepared. In fact, you began preparing for this examination on the first day that you entered your nursing program.

The task that you are faced with is to review, in a comprehensive manner, all of the nursing content that you learned in your nursing program. It can become terribly overwhelming to look at your bookshelf overflowing with the nursing books that you studied during nursing school, and your challenge becomes monumental when you look at the boxes of nursing lecture notes that you have accumulated. It is unrealistic to even consider that you could read all of those nursing books and lecture notes again in preparation for the NCLEX-PN examination. These books and lecture notes should be used as a reference source, if needed, during your preparation for NCLEX-PN. *Saunders Comprehensive Review for NCLEX-PN* has identified for you all of the important nursing content areas relevant to the examination. As you study using the *Saunders Comprehensive Review for NCLEX-PN*, you should note those areas that may be unfamiliar or unclear. Be sure that you take the time to become familiar with these areas that need further review. Now, progress through the Pyramid to Success and test your knowledge in *Saunders Q&A Review for NCLEX-PN*. You may identify nursing content areas that still require further review. Take the time to review, as you are guided to do in this book.

Your profile to success requires that you develop realistic time goals to prepare for the NCLEX-PN examination. It is necessary that you take time to examine your life and all of the commitments that you may have. These commitments may include family, work, and friends. As you develop your goals, remember to plan time for fun and exercise. To achieve success, you require a balance of both work time and recreational time. If you do not plan for some recreational time, you will become frustrated and perhaps even angry. These negative feelings will block your ability to focus and concentrate. Remember, you need time for you.

As you develop your goals, consider all of your life commitments. Goal development may be a relatively easy process because you have probably been juggling your life commitments ever since you entered nursing school. Remember that your goal is to identify a daily time frame and time period for you to use in reviewing and preparing for the NCLEX-PN examination. Open your calendar and identify those days in which life commitments will not allow you to spend this time preparing. Block those days off and do not consider them as a part of your review time. Review your normal day. Identify the time that is best for you in terms of your ability to concentrate and focus, so that you can accomplish the most in your identified time frame. Be sure that you consider a time that is quiet and free of distractions. Many individuals find that the morning hours provide the most productive hours, whereas others may find the afternoon and evening hours most productive. Remember, this examination is all about you, so select the time period that will be most conducive to your needs.

The place of study is also very important. Select a place that is quiet and comfortable for study and where you normally do your studying and preparing. Some individuals prefer to study at home in their own environment, and if this is your normal pattern, be sure that you are able to free yourself of distractions during your scheduled preparation time. If you are not able to free yourself of distractions, you may consider spending your preparation time at a library. Reflect on what worked best for you during your nursing program in selecting your place of study.

Selecting the amount of daily preparation time has frequently been a dilemma for many graduates preparing for NCLEX-PN. It is very important to set a realistic time period that can be adhered to on a daily basis. Set a time frame that can be achieved and that will provide you with quality time. If you set a time frame that is not realistic and cannot be achieved every day, you will begin to become frustrated. This frustration will begin to block your journey toward the peak of the Pyramid to Success. The best suggestion is to spend at least two hours daily for NCLEX-PN preparation. Two hours is a realistic time period both in terms of quality time and achievability. You may find that after two hours your ability to focus and concentrate will diminish. You may, however, find that on some days you are able to spend more than the scheduled two hours, and if you can—and if you feel your ability to concentrate and focus is still present—then do so.

Discipline and perseverance will automatically bring control. Control will provide you with the momentum that will sweep you to the peak of the Pyramid to Success. Discipline yourself to spend time preparing for the NCLEX-PN examination every day. Daily preparation is very important because it maintains a consistent pattern and keeps you in synchrony with the mind flow needed on the day that you are scheduled to take the NCLEX-PN examination. Some days you may think about skipping your scheduled preparation time because you are not in the mood for study or you just don't feel like studying. On these days, practice discipline and persevere. Stand yourself up, shake off those thoughts of skipping a day of preparation, take a deep breath, and get the oxygen flowing throughout your body. Look in the mirror, smile, and say to yourself, "This time is for me and I can do this!" Look at your card that displays your name with LPN or LVN after it, and get yourself to that special study place. Remember, discipline and perseverance will bring control and ultimately success!

In the profile to success, academic preparation directs the path to the peak of the Pyramid to Success. There are, however, additional factors that will influence successful achievement to the peak. These factors include your ability to control anxiety, physical stamina, rest and relaxation, self-confidence, and the belief in yourself that you will achieve success on the NCLEX-PN examination. You need to take time to think about these important factors and incorporate these factors into your daily preparation schedule. Anxiety is a common concern among individuals preparing to take the NCLEX-PN examination. Some anxiety is a normal feeling and will keep your senses sharp and alert. A great deal of anxiety, however, can block your process of thinking and distract your ability to focus and concentrate. You have already practiced the task of controlling anxiety when you took examinations in nursing school. Now you need to continue with this practice and incorporate this control on a daily basis. Each day, before beginning your scheduled preparation time, sit in your quiet special study place, close your eyes, and take a slow deep breath. Fill your body with oxygen, hold your breathe to a count of four, then exhale slowly through your mouth. Continue with this exercise and repeat it four to six times. This exercise will relieve your mind of any unnecessary chatter and will deliver oxygen to all of your body tissues and to your brain. On the day you are scheduled to take the NCLEX-PN examination, following the necessary pretesting procedures, you will be escorted to your test computer. Practice this exercise before beginning the examination. Use this exercise during the examination if you feel yourself becoming anxious or distracted or are having difficulty focusing and concentrating. Remember, breathing will move that oxygen to your brain and assist you in regaining control!

Physical stamina is a necessary component of readiness for NCLEX-PN. Plan to incorporate a balance of exercise with adequate rest and relaxation time in your preparation schedule. It is important that you maintain healthy eating habits. Begin to practice these healthy habits now if you haven't already done so. There are a few points to keep in mind each day as you plan your daily meals. Three balanced meals are important, including snacks, such as fruits, between meals. Remember that food items that contain fat will slow you down, and food items that contain caffeine will cause nervousness and sometimes shakiness. These food items should be avoided. Carbohydrate-type foods can work best to supply you with your energy needs. Remember that your brain can work like a muscle and requires carbohydrates. Additionally, don't forget to include your needed fruits and vegetables.

If you are not a breakfast eater, work on changing that habit. Practice this habit now, as you are preparing for NCLEX-PN. Attempt to provide your brain with energy in the morning with some form of carbohydrate food. It will make a difference. On the day you are scheduled to take the NCLEX-PN examination, feed your brain by eating a healthy breakfast. Additionally, on this very important day, bring some form of snack, such as a bagel or fruit, for break time and feed your brain again so that you will have the energy to concentrate, focus, and complete your examination.

Adequate rest, relaxation, and exercise are important in your preparation process. Many graduates preparing for the NCLEX-PN examination have difficulty sleeping, particularly the night before the examination. Begin now to develop methods that will assist in relaxing your body and mind and allow you to obtain a restful sleep. You may already have a particular method developed to help you sleep. If not, it may be helpful to try the breathing exercise while you lie in bed to assist in eliminating any mind chatter that is present. It is also helpful to visualize your favorite and most peaceful place while you do these breathing exercises. Graduates have also shared that listening to quiet music and relaxation tapes has assisted in helping them to relax and sleep. Begin to practice some of these helpful methods now, while you are preparing for the NCLEX-PN examination. Identify those that work best for you. The night before your scheduled examination is an important one. Spend time having some fun, get to bed early, and incorporate the relaxation method that you have been utilizing to help you sleep.

Confidence and the belief that you have the ability to achieve success will help you reach your goals. Reflect on your profile maintained during your nursing education. Your confidence and belief in yourself, along with your academic achievements, have brought you to the status of a graduate from a nursing program. Now you are facing one more important challenge. Can you meet this challenge successfully? Yes, you can! There is no reason to think otherwise if you have taken all of the necessary steps to ensure that profile to success.

Each morning, place your feet on the floor, stand tall, take a deep breath, and believe. Take both hands and brush any negatives that you may be feeling off of you. Look at your card that bears your name with the letters LPN or LVN after it, and tell yourself that "Yes, I can, I believe!"

Believe in yourself, and you will reach the peak of the Pyramid to Success!

Congratulations! I wish you continued success in your career as a Licensed Practical or Vocational Nurse!

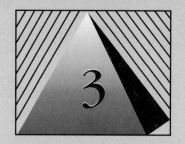

The NCLEX-PN Examination: From a Student's Perspective

JO ANN MEEHAN, LPN

It had been a long and stressful final semester. On the final day of classes I sat in the parking lot looking up at the banner that read "Congratulations Practical Nursing Students." At this point I became full of emotion, and my release was apparent by the tears that flowed from my weary, yet determined eyes. The tears were a definition of all of the long hours dedicated to study and client care. With all that I had accomplished in reaching graduation, I realized that there was one more challenge before me: the NCLEX-PN examination. With all my accomplishments, the classes, the clinicals, graduating from the LPN program, and the pinning ceremony, all of this was meaningless unless I passed this examination.

How was I to prepare for this examination? It was apparent that I needed a plan of action. I needed to think the problem through. I remembered what someone had mentioned to me about removing yourself to a place of peace and quiet to give yourself the freedom of uninhibited thought. I followed that valuable advice.

The first item to be dealt with was how to study and what worked best for me. Then I had to fit the study schedule into a busy family life. How many hours per day was quality study time for me? Should I study in the morning or late evening? Where was I going to study, at home or at the library? Was I going to study from my classroom notes and course textbooks?

With all these questions to be answered, I took out my notebook and started the process of deciding my best path to success. This was not an easy task. It took me several days of working through some tough decisions to complete the needed plan of action.

The next step was to present the plan to my family. What would I do if one or all did not support my study needs? The answer came to me without any delay. I had worked too hard and too long. My path was determined and I would succeed! My presentation to my family went well and all understood that I needed this schedule to succeed, and then my plan began to unfold.

I purchased a review book and balanced the review book with my classroom notes to study. The practice CD-ROM helped give me confidence that I could manage the computer test. I adhered to my study schedule diligently. The plan worked well for my family because I did not deviate from it. A synchronous flow was established, and it began to become as natural as the sun rising in the morning. I was in control.

Reality shock came the day that I received my notice to make an appointment. My immediate thought was, I will never be ready. I do not have enough time to prepare. I knew I needed to regain control. I took a few deep breaths and calmed myself down. I took that time to review what I had done to this point. I had a plan and it was in place and working. Nothing needed to change. I would continue with my study schedule. I knew I was on schedule to meet the examination date. I was back in control!

I decided it would be good for me to take a test drive to the site where the NCLEX-PN examination would be given. Just the thought of driving there made me nervous. At this point I knew I needed to make the trip. I arrived at the testing facility and sat in the parking lot. I found myself naturally taking deep breaths to control my anxiety. A thousand things ran through my mind. I decided it would help if I walked into the facility. Maybe this would help calm some of my anxiety. On the day of the examination, I found that this little trip had been very helpful. I had been here before and the unexpected was already in the past. It helped to diminish my anxiety significantly.

The day before the exam I stopped all study. I gave myself a day of rest and enjoyment. I knew from previous experience that I needed to be fresh and alert the day of the examination. I treated myself very well that day and got to bed at a reasonable hour to ensure I was well rested. The day of the examination came and I was determined to stay in control. I woke up that morning and took a deep breath. I had prepared well for this day and I would succeed. I knew I was scared and that this was an important day in my life. I tried to stay positive and focused. Every time my nerves began to overwhelm me I took deep breaths to regain composure.

I arrived at the testing facility and promised myself I would stay focused. My anxiety level was up but at the same time I knew I had prepared well both academically and personally. "Take the deep breaths and stay in control," I repeated to myself. The pretest preparation was accomplished smoothly, and the first question came up on the computer screen. I took a deep breath, answered the first question, and realized I was prepared to meet the challenge. When the screen on the computer displayed a message that I completed the examination, I felt relieved yet anxious. Now I knew that I had to wait for the results.

Waiting for the results was a challenge all to itself. The time seemed to go by slowly, and then the envelope arrived. I had been told over and over that a thin envelope is good, a thin envelope is good. And it was a thin envelope. I took one more deep breath and nervously opened the envelope. Jo Ann Meehan, Licensed Practical Nurse. I sat there and the emotion overcame me and the tears of success flowed steadily down my cheeks.

My best suggestion to you is to prepare yourself for this very important examination. You have worked hard up to this point and need to persevere and proceed toward success. Develop your own plan and stick to it. Let everyone close to you know what your plan is. Spend 2 hours every day reviewing and preparing for this examination, and be sure to select an appropriate time of day and place to ensure that you will not be distracted. Purchase a review book. Practice answering as many review questions as you can. This will help you perfect your test-taking abilities and will help identify the nursing areas that you need to review. Be confident and believe in yourself!

To all of you who read this and use this book to help you succeed, I can tell you that dedication, proper planning, self-control, and a positive attitude will help guide you to your goal of becoming a Licensed Practical Nurse.

Congratulations to you! I wish you continued success in your new career as a Licensed Practical Nurse!

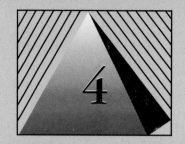

Test-Taking Strategies

I. Pyramid To Success (Box 4-1)
II. How To Avoid Reading Into The Question
   A. Pyramid Points
      1. Identify the case situation from the stem of the question
      2. Identify what the question is asking
      3. Look for the key words
      4. Read every option
      5. Use the process of elimination
      6. As you read the question, avoid asking yourself "What if...?"
   B. The Case Situation (Box 4-2)
      1. The case situation provides you with the information about a clinical health problem and the information that you need to consider in answering the question
      2. Read all of the information and every word in the case situation
   C. The Stem of the Question (Box 4-2)
      1. The stem of the question follows the case situation and asks something specific about the case situation
      2. Read the stem carefully, and specifically identify exactly what is being asked
   D. The Options (Box 4-2)
      1. The options are all of the answers, and you must select one
      2. Read every option carefully and reread the stem of the question to be sure that you understand what is being asked
      3. Use the process of elimination
      4. Once you have eliminated two incorrect options, reread the stem of the question again to identify specifically what the question is asking before selecting the correct option

III. Key Words (Box 4-3)
   A. Key words focus your attention on critical ideas in the case situation, the stem, and in the options
   B. Key words are important to identify because they will assist in eliminating the incorrect options (Box 4-4)
   C. Some of the key words may indicate that all of the options are correct, and that it will be necessary to prioritize in order to select the correct option
IV. The Client Of The Question
   A. Identify the client of the question
   B. The client is the person who is the focus of the question
   C. It is important to remember that the client of the question may not necessarily be the person with the health problem; in the test question, the client may be a relative, friend, spouse, significant other, or another member of the health care team
   D. After identifying the client of the question, select the option that relates to and most directly addresses that client
V. The Issue Of The Question (Box 4-5)
   A. Identify the issue of the question
   B. The issue of the question is the specific subject content that the question is asking about
   C. Identifying the issue of the question will assist in eliminating the incorrect options and direct you to selecting the correct option
   D. The issue of the question can include
      1. A medication or intravenous (IV) therapy
      2. A side effect of a medication
      3. An adverse or toxic effect of a medication
      4. A treatment or procedure

BOX 4-1

Pyramid to Success

Read the question and every option thoroughly and carefully!

Ask yourself, "What is the question specifically asking?"

Be alert to key words and true and false response stems!

Eliminate the incorrect options!

Use all of your nursing knowledge, your clinical experiences, and your test-taking skills and strategies to answer the question!

BOX 4-2

Case Situation, Stem, and Options

Case Situation: A nurse assisting in the care of a client with myocardial infarction is helping the client fill out the diet menu request form.

Stem: The nurse recommends that the client select which of the following beverages from the menu?

Options:
1. Fruit juice
2. Cola
3. Coffee
4. Tea

Answer: 1

BOX 4-3

Common Key Words

Early or late
Best
First
Initial
Immediately
Most likely or least likely
Most appropriate or least appropriate
On the day of
After several days

BOX 4-4

Key Words to Eliminate Incorrect Options

Noting the key words in each of these situations will assist in directing you to select the correct option:

▲ Which of the following is an *early* sign of shock?

▲ Which of the following is a *late sign* of shock?

▲ *On the day of surgery*, following a transurethral resection of the prostate (TURP), a nurse notes that the client's urine is bright red. Which of the following nursing actions is *most appropriate?*

▲ *After several days*, following a transurethral resection of the prostate (TURP), a nurse notes that the client's urine is bright red. Which of the following nursing actions is *most appropriate?*

▲ The *early* signs of shock are quite different from the *late* signs of shock!

▲ Bright red urine might be expected *on the day of* surgery following a TURP, but would not be expected *after several days!*

BOX 4-5

The Issue of the Question

A client with a brain lesion is receiving acetazolamide (Diamox). The nurse knows that the *purpose* of this medication for this client is to:
1. Prevent hyperthermia
2. Prevent hypertension
3. Decrease cerebrospinal fluid production
4. Maintain an adequate blood pressure for cerebral perfusion

Answer: 3

Test-Taking Strategy: Focus on the issue, the purpose of the medication for a client with a brain lesion. Use your nursing knowledge, clinical experiences, and test-taking skills and strategies to answer the question. Recalling that acetazolamide is a carbonic anhydrase inhibitor, and is used in the client with or at risk for increased intracranial pressure to decrease cerebrospinal fluid production will direct you to the correct option. The other options are not actions of this medication.

5. A complication of a health care problem, treatment, or procedure
6. A specific nursing action
VI. True or False Response Stems
   A. True Response Stem (Box 4-6)
      1. True response stems use key words that ask you to select an option that is true regarding the case situation in the question
      2. Common key words used in a true response stem
         a. Most or most appropriate
         b. Most likely
         c. Most helpful
         d. Best
         e. Best judgment
         f. Initial
         g. First
         h. Chief
         i. Immediate
   B. False Response Stem (Box 4-7)
      1. False response stems use key words that ask you to select an option that is NOT true regarding the case situation in the question
      2. Common key words used in a false response stem
         a. Least likely
         b. Need for further instructions or education
         c. Lowest priority
         d. Incorrect
         e. Unsafe
         f. Except, not, avoid

BOX 4-6

True Response Stem

A client with suspected meningitis is being scheduled for diagnostic tests. The nurse knows that which of the following diagnostic tests will *most likely* be used to confirm the diagnosis?
1. Serum electrolytes
2. Electromyography
3. White blood cell count
4. Lumbar puncture

Answer: 4

Test-Taking Strategy: This question identifies an example of a true response stem. Note the key words *most likely* and *confirm*. Focus on the diagnosis presented in the question and the associated pathophysiology to assist in directing you to option 4. Remember, meningitis is an acute or chronic inflammation of the meninges and the cerebrospinal fluid. The key diagnostic test used in meningitis is the lumbar puncture. A white blood cell count and serum electrolytes test may also be performed. Electromyography is not a key diagnostic test.

BOX 4-7

False Response Stem

Cortisone (Cortone) is prescribed for a client with adrenal insufficiency. The nurse reinforces instructions to the client regarding the medication. Which of the following statements if made by the client would indicate a *need for further instruction*?
1. "I will eat a good breakfast every day."
2. "I will avoid people with colds."
3. "I will limit my sodium intake."
4. "I will stop the medication when I feel better."

Answer: 4

Test-Taking Strategy: This question identifies an example of a false response stem. Note the key words *need for further instruction*. These key words indicate that you should select an option that identifies an incorrect client statement. Glucocorticoids should not be abruptly discontinued to prevent acute adrenal insufficiency. You should easily be able to eliminate options 1, 2, and 3 remembering that the client should not stop these medications, or in fact, any medication without physician approval.

VII. Questions That Require Prioritizing
  A. Identify the key words in the question that indicate the need to prioritize
  B. Common key words
    1. Initial
    2. Essential
    3. Vital
    4. Immediate
    5. Highest
    6. Best
    7. Most
    8. Priority

  C. Use Maslow's Hierarchy of Needs theory as a guide to prioritize (Box 4-8)
    1. Physiological needs come FIRST; select an option that addresses a physiological need
    2. When a physiological need is not addressed in the question or noted in one of the options, safety needs receive priority; select an option that addresses safety
  D. ABCs: Airway, Breathing, and Circulation (Box 4-9)
    1. Use the ABCs when selecting an option
    2. Remember the order of priority: airway, breathing, and circulation

BOX 4-8

Prioritizing: Maslow's Hierarchy of Needs Theory

A nurse is assigned to care for a client experiencing dystocia. When assisting in planning care, the nurse would consider the *highest* priority to be frequent:
1. Explanations to family members about what is happening in this situation
2. Comfort measures, change of position, and touch
3. Reinforcement of breathing techniques learned in childbirth preparatory classes
4. Monitoring for changes in the physical condition of the mother and fetus

Answer: 4

Test-Taking Strategy: All the options are correct and would be implemented during the care of the client. Use Maslow's Hierarchy of Needs theory to prioritize, remembering that physiological needs come first. Using this guideline will direct you to option 4. Also, note that option 4 is the only option that addresses both the mother and the fetus.

BOX 4-9

Prioritizing: Use of the ABCs

A nurse is assisting in the care of a client who received morphine sulfate for pain relief. When reviewing the plan of care for the client, the nurse understands that which of the following is the *priority* action?
1. Monitoring the urinary output
2. Monitoring the temperature
3. Monitoring mental status
4. Monitoring the respirations

Answer: 4

Test Taking Strategy: Note the key word *priority*. Use the ABCs—airway, breathing, and circulation—as a guide to direct you to the correct option. Recall that morphine sulfate is a narcotic analgesic and suppresses the respiratory reflex. The correct option addresses airway.

TABLE 4-1

Steps of the Nursing Process (Clinical Problem-Solving Process)

Data Collection	Follow the steps of the nursing process to select an option.
Planning	The first step of the nursing process is data collection
Implementation	When the question asks you what the nurse's initial, first, or most appropriate action is, select the option that
Evaluation	relates to data collection relative to the client.

E. Nursing Process (Clinical Problem Solving Process) (Table 4-1)
   1. Guidelines
      a. Use the steps of the Nursing Process to prioritize
      b. Remember that data collection is the first step in the Nursing Process
      c. When you are asked to select your first and initial nursing action, follow the steps of the Nursing Process to select the correct option
      d. If an option contains the concept of data collection, select that option
   2. Data Collection (Box 4-10)
      a. Data collection questions will address the process of gathering subjective and objective data relative to the client, communicating and documenting information gained in data collection, and contributing to the formulation of nursing diagnoses
      b. Remember that data collection is the first step in the nursing process
      c. When you are asked a question regarding your initial or first nursing action, select the option that addresses the process of data collection
      d. If a data collection action is not one of the options, follow the steps of the nursing process as your guide to select your initial or first action
      e. When answering questions that focus on data collection, look for key words in the options that reflect the collection of data relative to the client (Box 4-11)
   3. Planning (Box 4-12)
      a. Planning questions will require providing input into plan development, assisting in the formulation of the goals of

BOX 4-11

Data Collection: Key Words

Check
Collect
Determine
Find out
Gather
Identify
Monitor
Observe
Obtain information
Recognize

BOX 4-10

Nursing Process: Data Collection

A nurse is reinforcing the prescribed dietary measures with a client with diabetes mellitus. The client expresses frustration in learning the dietary regimen. The nurse would *initially*:
1. *Identify* the cause of the frustration
2. Continue with the dietary instructions
3. Notify the registered nurse
4. Tell the client that the diet needs to be followed

Answer: 1
Test-Taking Strategy: Use the steps of the nursing process. Data Collection is the first step. Of the four options presented, the only option that reflects the process of collecting data is option 1. Options 2, 3, and 4 identify the implementation step of the nursing process. The initial action is to identify the cause of the frustration.

BOX 4-12

Nursing Process: Planning

A nurse is assisting in developing a *dietary plan* for a client with a diagnosis of hypoparathyroidism. The nurse *plans* to include which of the following items on a list of foods that are acceptable to eat?
1. Fish
2. Cereals
3. Vegetables
4. Meat and poultry

Answer: 3
Test-Taking Strategy: Planning questions require providing input into plan development, assisting in the formulation of the goals of care, and assisting in the development of a plan of care. The client with hypoparathyroidism should increase calcium intake but restrict the amount of phosphorus in the diet. The client should limit meat, poultry, fish, eggs, cheese, and cereals. Vegetables should be encouraged in the diet. Recalling these concepts will direct you to option 3.

care, and assisting in the development of a plan of care

b. Remember that this is a nursing examination and the answer to the question most likely involves something that is included in the nursing care plan, rather than the medical plan

4. Implementation (Box 4-13)

a. This exam is about NURSING, so focus on the nursing action rather than on the medical action, unless the question is asking you what prescribed medical action is anticipated

b. Implementation questions address the process of assisting with organizing and managing care, providing care to achieve established goals, and communicating and documenting nursing interventions thoroughly and accurately

c. On NCLEX-PN, the only client that you need to be concerned about is the client in the question that you are answering

d. When you are answering a question, remember that this client is your only assigned client

e. Answer the question as if the situation were textbook and ideal and the nurse had all the time and resources needed and readily available at the client's bedside

5. Evaluation (Box 4-14)

a. Evaluation questions focus on comparing the actual outcomes of care with the expected outcomes, and communicating and documenting findings

b. These questions focus on assisting in determining the client's response to care, and identifying factors that may interfere with implementation of the plan of care

c. In an evaluation question, be alert to false response stems because they are frequently used in evaluation-type questions

d. The question may ask for the client's statement that indicates either *accurate* or *inaccurate* information regarding the issue of the question

VIII. Client Needs

A. Safe, Effective Care Environment

1. These questions address the provision of providing nursing care, collaborating with other health care team members to ensure effective client care, and protecting clients, significant others, and health care personnel from environmental hazards

2. Be alert to safety needs addressed in a question, and remember the importance of hand washing, call bells, bed positioning, and the appropriate use of side rails

B. Health Promotion and Maintenance

1. These questions address the provision that the nurse provides and assists in directing nursing care to promote and maintain health

2. Content addressed in these questions relates to assisting the client and significant others through the normal expected stages of growth and development, and assisting the client and significant others to develop health practices that promote wellness and to recognize alterations in health care status

---

BOX 4-13

Nursing Process: Implementation

A nurse is assisting in the care of a client with angina pectoris who begins to experience chest pain. The nurse administers a sublingual nitroglycerin (Nitrostat) tablet as prescribed, but the pain is unrelieved. The nurse should take which of the following actions *next*?
1. Contact the physician
2. Call the client's family
3. Administer another nitroglycerin tablet
4. Reposition the client

Answer: 3
Test-Taking Strategy: Implementation questions address the process of organizing and managing care. This question also requires that you prioritize the nursing actions. Note the key word *next* in the stem of the question. Recalling that the nurse would administer nitroglycerin times three to relieve chest pain will assist in directing you to option 3.

BOX 4-14

Nursing Process: Evaluation

A client with multiple sclerosis has been taking oxybutynin (Ditropan). The nurse *determines the degree of effectiveness* of the medication by asking the client about changes in:
1. Extent of muscle spasms
2. Level of fatigue
3. Bowel movements
4. Patterns of urination

Answer: 4
Test-Taking Strategy: This is an evaluation question. Note the key words *determines the degree of effectiveness*. Oxybutynin is an antispasmodic used to relieve symptoms of urinary urgency, frequency, nocturia, and incontinence in clients with uninhibited or reflex neurogenic bladder. Recalling that this medication is used to treat bladder dysfunction will easily direct you to option 4.

3. Use Teaching/Learning theory if the question addresses client education, remembering the nurse's role to facilitate the acquisition of knowledge, skills, and attitudes that lead to a change in behavior

4. Be alert to false response stems in questions that address health promotion and maintenance

C. Psychosocial Integrity

1. These questions address the provision that the nurse promotes and supports the emotional, mental, and social well-being of the client and significant others

2. Content addressed in these questions relates to promoting the client's or significant others' ability to cope, adapt, or problem solve in situations such as illnesses, disabilities, or stressful events

3. Content also includes the nurse's role in recognizing and providing care for clients with maladaptive behavior, and assisting with behavior management of the client with an acute or chronic mental illness or a cognitive psychosocial disturbance

4. Communication Questions (Table 4-2)

   a. Identify the use of therapeutic communication techniques

   b. Use of therapeutic communication techniques indicates a *correct* option

   c. Use of nontherapeutic communication techniques indicates an *incorrect* option

   d. Always focus on the client's feelings first; if an option reflects the client's feelings, select that option as the answer to the question (Box 4-15)

D. Physiological Integrity

1. These questions address the provision that the nurse provides comfort and helps the client perform activities of daily living, provides care related to the administration of medications, and monitors clients receiving parenteral therapies

2. These questions also address the nurse's ability to reduce the client's potential for developing complications or health problems related to treatments, procedures, or existing conditions, and the nurse's role in providing care to clients with acute, chronic, or life-threatening physical health conditions

3. Use Maslow's Hierarchy of Needs theory and remember that physiological needs are a priority and are addressed first

4. Use the ABCs—airway, breathing, and circulation—and the steps of the nursing process when selecting an option addressing physiological integrity

IX. Pyramid Points (Box 4-16)

A. Unfamiliar Content

1. Answer questions by using your nursing knowledge, clinical experiences, and test-taking skills and strategies

2. If the content of the question is unfamiliar and you are unable to answer the question by using your nursing knowledge, look for a global option, similar distracters, or similar words, behaviors, thoughts, or feelings in the question and in one of the options

B. Global Option (Box 4-17)

1. When more than one option appears to be correct, look for a global option

2. A global option is a general statement and may include the ideas of the other options within it

C. Similar Distracters

1. If you don't know the answer, try looking for similar distracters

2. Remember that there is only *one* correct option

TABLE 4-2

Communication Tools and Blocks

Tools	Blocks
Being silent	Giving advice
Offering self for assistance	Showing approval/disapproval
Showing empathy	Using clichés and false reassurance
Focusing	Requesting an explanation "Why?"
Restatement	Devaluing client feelings
Validation/clarification	Being defensive
Giving information	Focusing on inappropriate issues or persons
Dealing with the here and now	Placing the client's issues on "hold"
Always focus on the client's feelings FIRST!	
If an option reflects the client's feelings, select that option!	

BOX 4-15

Focusing on the Client's Feelings

A mother says to the nurse, "I am afraid that my child might have another febrile seizure." Which response by the nurse is most therapeutic?
1. "Why worry about something that you cannot control?"
2. "Most children will never experience a second seizure."
3. "Tell me what frightens you the most about seizures."
4. "Acetaminophen (Tylenol) can prevent another seizure from occurring."

Answer: 3

Test Taking Strategy: Option 3 is the only option that addresses the client's feelings and concerns. Option 1 blocks communication because it states that the mother should not worry. Options 2 and 4 are incorrect because the nurse is giving false assurance that a seizure will not reoccur or can be prevented in this child.

BOX 4-16

Pyramid Points

▲ If the question asks for an immediate action or response, all options may be correct; therefore, base your selection on priorities.

▲ Reword a difficult question, but if you do so, be careful not to change the intent of the question.

▲ Relate the situation to something that you are familiar with and try to visualize the client as you go through the case situation and the question.

▲ If there are words in the case situation or stem of the question that are unfamiliar, try to figure out the meaning in terms of the context of the sentence or break down the word and use medical terminology skills.

▲ If one option includes qualifiers such as *generally, usually, tends to, possibly,* or *may,* and other options do not, select that option.

▲ Absolute terminology such as *always, never, all, every, none, must,* and *only* tend to make an option incorrect.

▲ With medication calculations, talk yourself through each step and be sure the answer makes sense; recheck the calculation before selecting an option, particularly if the answer seems like an unusual dosage.

▲ Remember, the only client you need to be concerned about is the one in the question you are answering, and answer the question as if the situation were ideal and the nurse had all the time and resources readily available at the client's bedside.

▲ Pace yourself, concentrate, and focus on one item at a time; if you find yourself becoming distracted, take a few minutes to breathe deeply and then refocus.

SMILE!
BELIEF!
CONFIDENCE!
CONTROL!
SUCCESS!

BOX 4-17

Global Option

A nurse is assisting in caring for a client with a head injury. The nurse monitors which of the following as the most critical index of this client's central nervous system function?
1. Temperature
2. Ability to speak
3. Blood pressure
4. Level of consciousness

Answer: 4

Test-Taking Strategy: Note the key words *most critical* in the stem of the question. Focusing on the issue of the question, a neurological problem, will assist in directing you to option 4. Also, option 4 is the global option.

3. If two options say the same thing or include the same idea, then *neither of these options* can be correct

4. The answer to the question is the option that is different

D. Similar Words, Behaviors, Thoughts, or Feelings

1. If you do not know the answer, look for a similar word, behavior, thought, or feeling used in the case situation or the stem of the question and in one of the options

2. If you find a word, behavior, thought, or feeling that is used in the case situation or the stem of the question and is repeated in one of the options, that option *may* be the correct one

E. Pharmacology Questions

1. If you are familiar with the medication, use nursing knowledge to answer the question

2. Remember that the question will identify both the generic name and trade name of the medication

3. If the case situation identifies a diagnosis, then you can make a relationship between the medication and the diagnosis; for example, you can determine that cyclophosphamide (Cytoxan) is an antineoplastic medication if the question refers to a client with breast cancer who is taking this particular medication

4. Try to determine the classification of the medication being addressed to assist in answering the question; identifying the classification will assist in determining a medication action and/or side effects (Cardizem is a cardiac medication)

5. Use medical terminology and break the name of the medication into parts; for

example, Lopressor can be broken down into *Lo* and *pressor*, meaning lowering the blood pressure

6. Look at the prefix and/or suffix of the medication name; for example, "ase" indicates a thrombolytic, "sone" indicates a corticosteroid; "line" indicates a bronchodilator, and "lol" indicates a beta-blocker

7. General principles to remember
   a. Clients are instructed to avoid alcohol with medications
   b. Capsules and sustained-released medications are not to be crushed
   c. The nurse never adjusts or changes the client's medication dosage and never discontinues a medication
   d. Medications are never administered if the order is difficult to read, is unclear, or identifies a medication dose that is not a normal one

REFERENCES

deWit, S. (2001). *Fundamental concepts and skills for nursing*. Philadelphia: W.B. Saunders.

Hill, S., & Howlett, H. (2001). *Success in practical/vocational nursing* (4th ed.). Philadelphia: W.B. Saunders.

Hodgson, B., & Kizior, R. (2003). *Saunders nursing drug handbook 2003*. Philadelphia: W.B. Saunders.

National Council of State Boards of Nursing (eds.) (2001). *Test Plan for the National Council Licensure Examination for Practical/Vocational Nurses*. Chicago: Author.

Potter, P., & Perry, A. (2001). *Fundamentals of nursing* (5th ed.). St Louis: Mosby.

Riley, J. (2000). *Communication in nursing* (4th ed.). St Louis: Mosby.

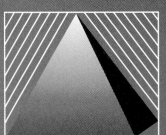

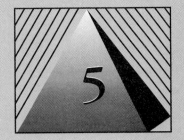

Client Needs and the NCLEX-PN Test Plan

CLIENT NEEDS

In the new Test Plan implemented in April 2002, the National Council of State Boards of Nursing has identified a test plan framework based on *Client Needs*. This framework was selected based on the analysis of the findings in a practice analysis study of newly licensed practical or vocational nurses in the United States. This study identified the nursing activities performed by these entry-level nurses. Also, the Client Needs categories identified by the National Council of State Boards of Nursing provide a structure for defining nursing actions and competencies across all settings for all clients. The National Council of State Boards of Nursing identifies four major categories of Client Needs. These categories are further divided into subcategories, and the percentage of test questions in each subcategory is identified. (Table 5-1)

SAFE, EFFECTIVE CARE ENVIRONMENT

The Safe, Effective Care Environment category addresses content related to the nurse's role in providing nursing care and collaborating with other health care team members to promote the achievement of client outcomes and to protect family or clients, significant others, and other health care personnel from environmental hazards. The Safe, Effective Care Environment category includes two subcategories: Coordinated Care, and Safety and Infection Control. The National Council of State Boards of Nursing identifies nursing content related to the subcategories of this Client Needs category (Box 5-1). Coordinated Care (6% to 12%) addresses content related to promoting effective client care through collaboration with other health care team members. Safety and Infection Control (7% to 13%) addresses content that tests the knowledge, skills, and ability required to protect clients and health care

personnel from environmental hazards (Box 5-2). Refer to Chapter 6 for practice questions that reflect this Client Needs category.

HEALTH PROMOTION AND MAINTENANCE

The Health Promotion and Maintenance category addresses content related to the nurse's role in providing and assisting in directing nursing care and in promoting and maintaining client health. The Health Promotion and Maintenance category includes two subcategories: Growth and Development Through the Life Span, and the Prevention and Early Detection of Disease. The National Council of State Boards of Nursing identifies nursing content related to the subcategories of this Client Needs category (Box 5-3). Growth and Development Through the Life Span (4% to 10%) addresses content that tests the knowledge, skills, and ability required to assist the client and significant others through the normal, expected stages of growth and development from conception through advanced old age. Prevention and Early Detection of Disease (4% to 10%) addresses content that tests the knowledge, skills, and ability required to assist clients to recognize alterations in health and to develop health practices that promote and support wellness (Box 5-4). Refer to Chapter 7 for practice questions reflective of this Client Needs category.

PSYCHOSOCIAL INTEGRITY

The Psychosocial Integrity category addresses content related to the nurse's role in providing nursing care that promotes and supports the emotional, mental, and social well-being of the client and significant others. The Psychosocial Integrity category includes two subcategories: Coping and Adaptation, and Psychosocial Adaptation.

TABLE 5-1

Client Needs and the Percentage of Test Questions

Safe, Effective Care Environment	Percentage (%)
Coordinated Care	6%-12%
Safety and Infection Control	7%-13%
HEALTH PROMOTION AND MAINTENANCE	
Growth and Development Through the Life Span	4%-10%
Prevention and Early Detection of Disease	4%-10%
PSYCHOSOCIAL INTEGRITY	
Coping and Adaptation	6%-12%
Psychosocial Adaptation	4%-10%
PHYSIOLOGICAL INTEGRITY	
Basic Care and Comfort	10%-16%
Pharmacological Therapies	5%-11%
Reduction of Risk Potential	11%-17%
Physiological Adaptation	13%-19%

From National Council of State Boards of Nursing (eds.) (2001). *Test Plan for the National Council Licensure Examination for Practical/Vocational Nurses*. Chicago: Author.

BOX 5-1

NCLEX-PN

CONTENT: SAFE, EFFECTIVE CARE ENVIRONMENT
COORDINATED CARE
Advance directives
Advocacy
Client care assignments
Client rights
Concepts of management and supervision
Confidentiality
Consultation with members of the health care team
Continuity of care
Continuous quality improvement
Establishing priorities
Ethical practice
Incident/irregular occurrence/variance reports
Informed consent
Legal responsibilities
Referral processes
Resource management

SAFETY AND INFECTION CONTROL
Accident/error prevention
Disaster planning
Handling hazardous and infectious materials
Medical and surgical asepsis
Standard (universal) and other precautions
Use of restraints

From National Council of State Boards of Nursing (eds.) (2001). *Test Plan for the National Council Licensure Examination for Practical/Vocational Nurses*. Chicago: Author.

BOX 5-2

Safe, Effective Care Environment Questions

COORDINATED CARE
A nurse is planning client care assignments. Which activity is least appropriate for the nursing assistant?
1. Feeding a client who is profoundly developmentally disabled
2. Obtaining frequent oral temperatures on a client
3. Ambulating a client
4. Collecting a urine specimen

Answer: 1
Rationale: This question addresses the subcategory, Coordinated Care, in the Client Needs category of Safe, Effective Care Environment, and specifically addresses content related to client care assignments. An activity that is assigned to a health care team member must be done consistent with the individual's level of expertise and licensure or lack of licensure. In this case, the least appropriate activity for a nursing assistant would be to feed a profoundly developmentally disabled client. The client is likely to have difficulty eating and has a high potential for complications, such as choking and aspiration. The remaining three options do not include situations to indicate that these activities carry any risk.

SAFETY AND INFECTION CONTROL
A nurse has given a subcutaneous injection to the client with acquired immunodeficiency syndrome (AIDS). The nurse disposes of the used needle and syringe by:
1. Recapping the needle and discarding the syringe in the disposal unit
2. Placing the uncapped needle and syringe in a labeled, rigid plastic container
3. Breaking the needle before discarding it
4. Placing the uncapped needle and syringe in a labeled cardboard box

Answer: 2
Rationale: This question addresses the subcategory, Safety and Infection Control, in the Client Needs category of Safe, Effective Care Environment, and specifically addresses content related to Standard (Universal) Precautions. Universal Precautions include specific guidelines for handling of needles. Needles should not be recapped, bent, broken, or cut after use. They should be disposed of in a labeled, impermeable container specific for this purpose. Needles should not be discarded in cardboard boxes, because cardboard boxes are not impervious. Needles should never be left lying around after use.

BOX 5-3

NCLEX-PN Content: Health Promotion and Maintenance

GROWTH AND DEVELOPMENT THROUGH THE LIFE SPAN
Aging process
Antepartum, intrapartum, and postpartum periods
Developmental stages and transitions
Expected body image changes
Family interaction patterns
Family planning
Human sexuality
Newborn

PREVENTION AND EARLY DETECTION OF DISEASE
Data collection techniques
Disease prevention
Health promotion programs
Health screening
Immunizations
Lifestyle choices

From National Council of State Boards of Nursing (eds.) (2001). *Test Plan for the National Council Licensure Examination for Practical/Vocational Nurses.* Chicago: Author.

BOX 5-4

Health Promotion and Maintenance Questions

GROWTH AND DEVELOPMENT THROUGH THE LIFE SPAN
A nurse is reinforcing instructions to a client in the third trimester of pregnancy regarding measures to relieve heartburn. The nurse tells the client to:
1. Eat fatty foods only once a day in the morning
2. Avoid milk and hot tea
3. Eat small, frequent meals
4. Use antacids that contain sodium

Answer: 3
Rationale: This question addresses the subcategory, Growth and Development Through the Life Span in the Client Needs category of Health Promotion and Maintenance, and addresses the antepartum period. Measures to provide relief of heartburn include small frequent meals, avoiding fatty and fried foods, coffee, and cigarettes. Mild antacids can be used if they do not contain aspirin or sodium and if prescribed by the health care provider. Frequent sips of milk, hot tea, or water are helpful. Gum is also helpful in the relief of heartburn.

PREVENTION AND EARLY DETECTION OF DISEASE
A client with atherosclerosis asks the nurse about dietary modifications to lower the risk of heart disease. The nurse encourages the client to eat which of the following foods that will lower this risk?
1. Baked chicken with skin
2. Fresh cantaloupe
3. Broiled cheeseburger
4. Mashed potato with gravy

Answer: 2
Rationale: This question addresses the subcategory, Prevention and Early Detection of Disease in the Client Needs category of Health Promotion and Maintenance, and addresses disease prevention. To lower the risk of heart disease, the diet should be low in saturated fat with the appropriate number of total calories. The diet should include fewer red meats and more white meat, with the skin removed. Dairy products used should be low in fat, and foods with high amounts of empty calories should be avoided. Fresh fruits and vegetables are naturally low in fat.

The National Council of State Boards of Nursing identifies nursing content related to the subcategories of this Client Needs category (Box 5-5). Coping and Adaptation (6% to 12%) addresses content that tests the knowledge, skills, and ability required to promote the client and/or significant others' ability to cope, adapt, and/or problem solve situations related to illnesses, disabilities, or stressful events. Psychosocial Adaptation (4% to 10%) addresses content that tests the knowledge, skills, and ability required to participate in recognizing and providing care for clients with maladaptive behavior and to assist with behavior management of clients with acute or chronic mental illness and psychosocial disturbances. Box 5-6 provides questions addressing these subcategories. Refer to Chapter 8 for practice questions reflective of this Client Needs category.

PHYSIOLOGICAL INTEGRITY

The Physiological Integrity category addresses content related to the nurse's role in providing care and comfort to promote physical health and well-being, reduce the client's risk potential, and assist in managing the client's health alterations. The Physiological Integrity category includes four subcategories: Basic Care and Comfort, Pharmacological Therapies, Reduction of Risk Potential, and Physiological Adaptation. The National Council of State Boards of Nursing identifies nursing content related to the subcategories of this Client Needs

---

NCLEX-PN Content: Psychosocial Integrity

COPING AND ADAPTATION
Behavior management
Coping mechanisms
End of life issues
Grief and loss
Mental health concepts
Religious and spiritual influences on health
Sensory/perceptual alterations
Situational role changes
Stress management
Support systems

Therapeutic communication
Unexpected body image changes

PSYCHOSOCIAL ADAPTATION
Abuse and neglect
Behavioral interventions
Chemical dependency
Crisis intervention
Mental illness concepts
Suicide
Therapeutic environment

From National Council of State Boards of Nursing (eds.) (2001). *Test Plan for the National Council Licensure Examination for Practical/Vocational Nurses.* Chicago: Author.

BOX 5-6

Psychosocial Integrity Questions

COPING AND ADAPTATION
A stillborn was delivered in the birthing suite a few hours ago. After the birth, the family has remained together, holding and touching the baby. Which statement by the nurse would further assist them in their initial period of grief?
1. "Don't worry, there is nothing you could do to prevent this from happening."
2. "We need to take the baby from you now so that you can get some sleep."
3. "What have you named your lovely baby?"
4. "We will see to it that you have an early discharge so that you don't have to be reminded of this experience."

Answer: 3
Rationale: This question addresses the subcategory, Coping and Adaptation in the Client Needs category of Psychosocial Integrity, and addresses content related to grief and loss. The nurse should explore measures that assist the family to create a memory of the baby so that the existence of the child is confirmed and the parents can complete the grieving process. Option 3 addresses this issue and also demonstrates a caring and empathetic response. Option 1, 2, and 4 are blocks to communication and devalue the parents' feelings.

PSYCHOSOCIAL ADAPTATION
A nurse is assisting in planning care for a client being admitted to the nursing unit who attempted suicide. Which of the following priority nursing interventions will the nurse include in the plan of care?
1. Check the whereabouts of the client every 15 minutes
2. Suicide precautions with 30 minute checks
3. One-to-one suicide precautions
4. Ask that the client report suicidal thoughts immediately

Answer: 3
Rationale: This question addresses the subcategory, Psychosocial Adaptation in the Client Needs category of Psychosocial Integrity, and addresses content related to suicide. One-to-one suicide precautions are required for the client who has attempted suicide. Options 1 and 2 may be appropriate but not at the present time considering the situation. Option 4 may also be an appropriate nursing intervention, but the priority is stated in option 3. The best option is constant supervision so that the nurse may intervene as needed if the client attempts to cause harm to self.

---

category (Box 5-7). Basic Care and Comfort (10% to 16%) addresses content that tests the knowledge, skills, and ability required to provide comfort and assistance in the performance of activities of daily living. Pharmacological Therapies (5% to 11%) addresses content that tests the knowledge, skills, and ability required to administer medications and monitor clients receiving parenteral therapies. Reduction of Risk Potential (11% to 17%) addresses content that tests the knowledge, skills, and ability required to reduce the likelihood

that clients will develop complications or health problems related to existing conditions, treatments, or procedures. Physiological Adaptation (13% to 19%) addresses content that tests the knowledge, skills, and ability required to participate in providing care to clients with acute, chronic, or life-threatening physical health conditions. Box 5-8 provides practice questions addressing these subcategories. Refer to Chapter 9 for practice questions reflective of this Client Needs category.

BOX 5-7

NCLEX-PN Content: Physiological Integrity

BASIC CARE AND COMFORT
Assistive devices
Elimination
Mobility and immobility
Nonpharmacological pain interventions
Nutrition and oral hydration
Palliative care
Personal hygiene
Rest and sleep

PHARMACOLOGICAL THERAPIES
Adverse effects
Expected effects
Medication administration
Pharmacological actions
Pharmacological agents
Side effects

REDUCTION OF RISK POTENTIAL
Diagnostic tests
Laboratory values
Potential for alterations in body systems
Potential for complications of diagnostic tests, procedures, surgery, and health alterations
Therapeutic procedures

PHYSIOLOGICAL ADAPTATION
Alterations in body systems
Basic pathophysiology
Fluid and electrolyte imbalances
Medical emergencies
Radiation therapy
Respiratory care
Unexpected responses to therapies

From National Council of State Boards of Nursing (eds.) (2001). *Test Plan for the National Council Licensure Examination for Practical/Vocational Nurses.* Chicago: Author.

BOX 5-8

Physiological Integrity Questions

BASIC CARE AND COMFORT
A client has been taught to use a walker to aid in mobility following internal fixation of a hip fracture. The nurse determines that the client is using the walker incorrectly if the client:
1. Holds the walker using the hand grips
2. Leans forward slightly when advancing the walker
3. Advances the walker with reciprocal motion
4. Supports body weight on the hands while advancing the weaker leg

Answer: 3
Rationale: This question addresses the subcategory, Basic Care and Comfort in the Client Needs category of Physiological Integrity, and addresses content related to the use of an assistive device. The client should use the walker by placing the hands on the hand grips for stability. The client lifts the walker to advance it, and leans forward slightly while moving it. The client walks into the walker, supporting the body weight on the hands while moving the weaker leg. A disadvantage of the walker is that it does not allow for reciprocal walking motion. If the client were to try to use reciprocal motion with a walker, the walker would advance forward one side at a time as the client walks; thus the client would not be supporting the weaker leg with the walker during ambulation.

PHARMACOLOGICAL THERAPIES
A nurse is caring for a client who received an allogenic liver transplant. The client is receiving tacrolimus (Prograf) daily. Which of the following indicates to the nurse that the client is experiencing an adverse effect of the medication?
1. A decrease in urine output
2. Hypotension
3. Profuse sweating
4. Photophobia

Answer: 1
Rationale: This question addresses the subcategory, Pharmacological Therapies in the Client Needs category of Physiological Integrity, and addresses content related to the adverse effect of a medication. Tacrolimus (Prograf) is an immunosuppressant medication used in the prophylaxis of organ rejection in clients receiving allogenic liver transplants. Frequent side effects include headache, tremor, insomnia, paresthesia, diarrhea, nausea, constipation, vomiting, abdominal pain, and hypertension. Adverse and toxic effects include nephrotoxicity and pleural effusion. Nephrotoxicity is characterized by an increasing serum creatinine level and a decrease in urine output.

REDUCTION OF RISK POTENTIAL
A nurse is caring for the client who is going to have an arthrogram using a contrast medium. Which of the following information would be of highest priority?
1. Client allergy to iodine or shellfish
2. Ability of the client to remain still during the procedure
3. Whether the client has any remaining questions about the procedure
4. Whether the client wishes to void before the procedure

Answer: 1
Rationale: This question addresses the subcategory, Reduction of Risk Potential in the Client Needs category of Physiological Integrity, and addresses a potential complication of a diagnostic test. Because of the risk of allergy to contrast dye, the nurse places highest priority on determining whether the client has an allergy to iodine or shellfish. The nurse also reinforces information about the test, tells the client about the need to remain still during the procedure, and encourages the client to void before the procedure for comfort.

BOX 5-8—cont'd

Physiological Integrity Questions—cont'd

PHYSIOLOGICAL ADAPTATION

A pregnant client tells a nurse that she felt wetness on her peri-pad and that she found some clear fluid. The nurse immediately inspects the perineum and notes the presence of the umbilical cord. The nurse's immediate action is to:

1. Notify the registered nurse
2. Monitor fetal heart rate
3. Transfer the client to the delivery room
4. Place the client in Trendelenburg's position

Answer: 4

Rationale: This question addresses the subcategory, Physiological Adaptation in the Client Needs category of Physiological Integrity, and addresses an acute and life-threatening physical health condition. On inspection of the perineum, if the umbilical cord is noted, the nurse immediately places the client into Trendelenburg's position while pushing the presenting part upward to relieve the cord compression. This position is maintained and the registered nurse is notified who will then contact the physician. The nurse monitors the fetal heart rate. The client is transferred to the delivery room when prescribed by the physician.

REFERENCES

Burroughs, A., & Leifer, G. (2002). *Maternity nursing* (8th ed.). Philadelphia: W.B. Saunders.

deWit, S. (2001). *Fundamental concepts and skills for nursing.* Philadelphia: W.B. Saunders.

Hill, S., & Bauer, B. (2002). *Mental health nursing.* Philadelphia: W.B. Saunders.

Hodgson, B., & Kizior, R. (2003). *Saunders nursing drug handbook 2001.* Philadelphia: W.B. Saunders.

National Council of State Boards of Nursing (eds.) (2001). *Test Plan for the National Council Licensure Examination for Practical/Vocational Nurses.* Chicago: Author.

National Council of State Boards of Nursing (eds.) (2000). *The NCLEX Process: serving as an Anchor for the NCLEX Examination.* Chicago: Author.

National Council of State Boards of Nursing. Web Site: http://www.ncsbn.org/files/boards/boardscontact.asp

Potter, P., & Perry, A. (2001). *Fundamentals of nursing* (5th ed.). St. Louis: Mosby.

Riley, J. (2000). *Communication in nursing* (4th ed.). St. Louis: Mosby.

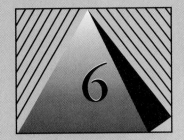

Safe, Effective Care Environment

1. A nurse employed in a long-term care facility has planned a get-together for clients and their families to celebrate the birthday of a client who is 100 years old. During the party, the nurse takes pictures of some of the clients and plans to develop the pictures and submit the pictures to the local newspaper. Which of the following client rights has the nurse violated?

1. Invasion of privacy
2. False imprisonment
3. Assault
4. Battery

Answer: 1

Rationale: Invasion of privacy takes place when an individual's private affairs are unreasonably invaded. Taking photographs of a client is an example of such a violation. Telling the client that he or she cannot leave the hospital constitutes an example of false imprisonment. Threatening to place a client in restraints is an example of an assault. Performing a procedure without consent is an example of battery.

Test-Taking Strategy: Use the process of elimination. The key words are *takes pictures*. Focus on the situation identified in the question to assist in directing you to the correct option. If you had difficulty with this question, review those situations that include invasion of privacy.

Level of Cognitive Ability: Comprehension
Client Needs: Safe, Effective Care Environment
Integrated Concept/Process: Nursing Process/Implementation
Content Area: Fundamental Skills

Reference:
Brent, N. (2002). *Nurses and the law* (2nd ed.). Philadelphia: W.B. Saunders, p. 122.

---

2. A nurse overhears a client ask the physician if the results of a biopsy indicated cancer. The physician tells the client that the results have not returned, when in fact the physician is aware that the results of the biopsy indicated the presence of malignancy. The nurse is upset that the physician has not shared the results with the client and tells another nurse that the physician has lied to the client and that this physician probably lies to all of the clients. Which

Answer: 2

Rationale: Defamation takes place when something untrue is said (slander) or written (libel) about a person resulting in injury to that person's good name and reputation. An assault occurs when a person puts another person in fear of a harmful or an offensive contact. Negligence involves the actions of professionals that fall below the standard of care for a specific professional group. Although the physician may be aware of the biopsy results, the physician decides when it is best to share such a diagnosis with the client.

Test-Taking Strategy: Use the process of elimination. You should easily eliminate options 3 and 4 first recalling the definitions of

legal tort has the nurse violated by this statement?

1   Libel
2   Slander
3   Assault
4   Negligence

these items. Recalling that slander constitutes verbal defamation will direct you to option 2 from the remaining options. If you had difficulty with this question, review the torts identified in each option.

Level of Cognitive Ability: Comprehension
Client Needs: Safe, Effective Care Environment
Integrated Concept/Process: Nursing Process/Implementation
Content Area: Fundamental Skills

Reference:
Brent, N. (2002). *Nurses and the law* (2nd ed.). Philadelphia: W.B. Saunders, p. 121.

---

3. A nurse employed in a long-term care facility is preparing to administer medications to an assigned client and notes that the order for furosemide (Lasix) is higher than the recommended dosage. The nurse calls the physician to clarify the order and asks the physician to prescribe a dosage within the recommended range. The physician refuses to change the order and instructs the nurse to administer the dose as prescribed. Which of the following actions would the nurse take?

1   Discontinue the order
2   Administer the dose as prescribed
3   Call the state medical board and report the physician
4   Contact the nursing supervisor

Answer: 4
Rationale: If the physician writes an order that requires clarification, it is the nurse's responsibility to contact the physician for clarification. If there is no resolution regarding the order because the order remains as it was written after talking with the physician, or because the physician cannot be located, the nurse should then contact the nurse manager or supervisor for further clarification as to what the next step should be. Under no circumstances should the nurse proceed to carry out the order until clarification is obtained. Option 1 is not within the scope of nursing practice. Option 3 is a premature action.

Test-Taking Strategy: Use the process of elimination. Eliminate option 2 first because this is an unsafe action. Eliminate option 1 next because this action is outside the scope of nursing practice. Option 3 is premature and should be eliminated. Additionally, the nurse should follow the organizational chain of command and seek assistance from the nursing supervisor. Review nursing responsibilities related to physician's orders if you had difficulty with this question.

Level of Cognitive Ability: Application
Client Needs: Safe, Effective Care Environment
Integrated Concept/Process: Nursing Process/Implementation
Content Area: Fundamental Skills

Reference:
Potter, P., & Perry, A. (2001). *Fundamentals of nursing* (5th ed.). St. Louis: Mosby, p. 899.

---

4. The nurse is administering medications to a client and administers a dose of methyldopa (Aldomet) 250 mg PO instead of the prescribed 125 mg dose. The nurse discovers the error when documenting that the medication has been administered. Which of the following is not an appropriate nursing action regarding the incident?

Answer: 4
Rationale: An incident report needs to be completed whenever an unusual incident occurs. The incident report is confidential and privileged information, and should not be copied, placed in the chart, or have any reference made to it in the client's record. A complete entry in the client's record should be made concerning the incident. The incident report is not a substitute for such an entry. The client's blood pressure should be monitored because this medication is an antihypertensive. The physician is notified.

1 Monitor the client's blood pressure
2 Document a complete entry in the client's record concerning the incident
3 Complete an incident report
4 Make a copy of the incident report for the physician

Test-Taking Strategy: Use the process of elimination. Note the key word *not*. Knowing that this medication is an antihypertensive will assist in eliminating option 1. Knowledge that an incident report needs to be completed when a medication error occurs will assist in eliminating option 3. Recalling that incident reports should not be copied will direct you to option 4 from the remaining options. Review nursing responsibilities related to incident reports if you had difficulty with this question.

Level of Cognitive Ability: Application
Client Needs: Safe, Effective Care Environment
Integrated Concept/Process: Nursing Process/Implementation
Content Area: Fundamental Skills

Reference:
Potter, P., & Perry, A. (2001). *Fundamentals of nursing* (5th ed.). St. Louis: Mosby, p. 521.

---

5. A new nurse graduate asks another licensed practical nurse (LPN) about the need to obtain professional liability insurance. The most appropriate response by the LPN is:
1 "The hospital insurance covers your actions."
2 "It is very expensive and you really don't need it since the hospital covers you."
3 "Nurses should have their own malpractice insurance."
4 "Lawsuits are filed against physicians and the hospital so you are safe not to obtain it."

Answer: 3
Rationale: Nurses need their own liability insurance for protection against malpractice lawsuits. Nurses erroneously assume that they are protected by an agency's professional liability policies. Usually when a nurse is sued, the employer is also sued for the nurse's actions or inactions. Even though this is the norm, nurses are encouraged to have their own malpractice insurance.

Test-Taking Strategy: Use the process of elimination. Note that the issue of the question relates to "obtaining professional liability insurance." This issue should easily direct you to option 3. Also, note the similarity between options 1, 2, and 4 in that they all refer to not obtaining the malpractice insurance. Review liability related to malpractice insurance if you had difficulty with this question.

Level of Cognitive Ability: Application
Client Needs: Safe, Effective Care Environment
Integrated Concept/Process: Nursing Process/Implementation
Content Area: Fundamental Skills

Reference:
Potter, P., & Perry, A. (2001). *Fundamentals of nursing* (5th ed.). St. Louis: Mosby, p. 427.

---

6. A licensed practical nurse witnesses an accident in which a victim was hit by a car. The nurse stops at the scene of the accident and administers safe care to the victim, who sustained a compound fracture of the femur. The victim is hospitalized and later develops sepsis as a result of the fractured femur. The victim files suit against the nurse who pro-

Answer: 2
Rationale: A Good Samaritan law is passed by the state legislature to encourage nurses and other health care providers to provide care to a person when an accident, emergency, or injury occurs, without fear of being sued for the care provided. Called immunity from suit, this protection usually applies only if all of the conditions of the law are met, such as the health care provider receives no compensation for the care provided, and the care given is not willfully and wantonly negligent.

vided care at the scene of the accident. Which of the following most accurately describes the nurse's immunity from this suit?

1   The Good Samaritan Law will not protect the nurse

2   The Good Samaritan Law will protect the nurse if the care given at the scene was not negligent

3   The Good Samaritan Law always provides immunity from suit even if the nurse accepted compensation for the care provided

4   The Good Samaritan Law protects lay persons and not professional health care providers

Test-Taking Strategy: Focus on the information in the question and use the process of elimination. Options 1 and 4 are similar and incorrect statements and can be eliminated first. Eliminate option 3 next because it is incorrect and there is no information in the question that the nurse accepted compensation for the care provided. Review the Good Samaritan Law if you had difficulty with this question.

Level of Cognitive Ability: Comprehension
Client Needs: Safe, Effective Care Environment
Integrated Concept/Process: Nursing Process/Implementation
Content Area: Fundamental Skills

Reference:
Potter, P., & Perry, A. (2001). *Fundamentals of nursing* (5th ed.). St. Louis: Mosby, p. 429.

---

7. A nurse working in a long-term care facility responds after hearing someone calling "Help, the bed is on fire!" On entering the room, the nurse finds an older client slapping at the flames on the bedspread with a pillow. Both hands have been burned. Which of the following actions should the nurse take first?

1   Remove the client from the room
2   Close the door to the room
3   Pull the nearest fire alarm
4   Run to get the nearest fire extinguisher

Answer: 1
Rationale: In a fire emergency, the steps to follow use the acronym *RACE*. The first step is to remove the victim. The next steps are: activate the alarm, contain the fire, and then extinguish as needed. This is a universal standard that may be applied to any type of fire emergency. Option 1 is correct because it removes the victim from the area. Option 3 would be the next step (alarm). The fire is next contained (option 2) and then extinguished (option 4).

Test-Taking Strategy: Use the process of elimination. Note that the question contains the key word *first*. With this in mind, sequence the activities using the *RACE* acronym. This will direct you to option 1. Review fire safety, if you had difficulty with this question.

Level of Cognitive Ability: Application
Client Needs: Safe, Effective Care Environment
Integrated Concept/Process: Nursing Process/Implementation
Content Area: Fundamental Skills

Reference:
Potter, P., & Perry, A. (2001). *Fundamentals of nursing* (5th ed.). St. Louis: Mosby, p. 1044.

---

8. An adult client is brought to the emergency room by ambulance after being hit by a car. The client is unconscious and is in shock. A perforated spleen is suspected and emergency surgery is required immediately to save the client's life. There are no family members present but the nurse finds identification on the client. In regard to informed consent for the surgical procedure, the nurse understands that which of the following is the best nursing action?

1   Call a family member to obtain telephone consent before the surgical procedure

Answer: 2
Rationale: Generally there are only two instances in which the informed consent of an adult client is not needed. One instance is when an emergency is present and delaying treatment for the purpose of obtaining informed consent would result in injury or death to the client. The second instance is when the client waives the right to give informed consent.

Test-Taking Strategy: Use the process of elimination. Option 3 can be easily eliminated first. Next, note the key words *surgery is required immediately*. Options 1 and 4 would delay treatment and should be eliminated. Review the issues surrounding informed consent if you had difficulty with this question.

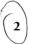

2 Transport the client to the operating room immediately

3 Ask the hospital chaplain to sign the consent form

4 Call the nursing supervisor to initiate a court order for the surgical procedure

Level of Cognitive Ability: Comprehension
Client Needs: Safe, Effective Care Environment
Integrated Concept/Process: Nursing Process/Implementation
Content Area: Fundamental Skills

Reference:
Potter, P., & Perry, A. (2001). *Fundamentals of nursing* (5th ed.). St. Louis: Mosby, p. 431.

---

9. A nurse is asked to check the corneal reflex on an unconscious client. The nurse would use which of the following as the safest stimulus to touch the client's cornea?

1 Wisp of cotton
2 Sterile drop of saline
3 Sterile glove
4 Tip of a 1-mL syringe

Answer: 2
Rationale: The client who is unconscious is at great risk of corneal abrasion. The safest way to test the corneal reflex is by using a drop of sterile saline. Options 1, 3, and 4 can cause injury to the cornea.

Test-Taking Strategy: Use the process of elimination. Remember that options that are similar are not likely to be correct. In this case, each of the incorrect options is a solid substance, and the correct option is a liquid. Review the method for checking the corneal reflex if you had difficulty with this question.

Level of Cognitive Ability: Application
Client Needs: Safe, Effective Care Environment
Integrated Concept/Process: Nursing Process/Implementation
Content Area: Adult Health/Neurological

Reference:
Potter, P., & Perry, A. (2001). *Fundamentals of nursing* (5th ed.). St. Louis: Mosby, p. 182.

---

10. A client tells the nurse that he or she has seen many articles in the health care section of the newspaper about case management. The client asks the nurse what this means. To provide the client with accurate information, the nurse tells the client which of the following?

1 "A single case manager plans the care for all of the clients in the nursing unit."

2 "One nurse takes care of one client and is responsible for that client."

3 "One nurse supervises all of the other employees when they care for clients."

4 "It represents an interdisciplinary health care delivery system."

Answer: 4
Rationale: Case management represents an interdisciplinary health care delivery system to promote appropriate use of hospital personnel and material resources to maximize hospital revenues while providing for optimal outcome of care. Case management manages client care by managing the client care environment. Options 1, 2, and 3 are incorrect descriptions.

Test-Taking Strategy: Use the process of elimination. Note the similarity in options 1, 2, and 3 in that they all address a single individual managing the client care environment. Review the basic characteristics of case management if you had difficulty with this question.

Level of Cognitive Ability: Application
Client Needs: Safe, Effective Care Environment
Integrated Concept/Process: Nursing Process/Implementation
Content Area: Fundamental Skills

Reference:
Potter, P., & Perry, A. (2001). *Fundamentals of nursing* (5th ed.). St. Louis: Mosby, p. 71.

11. A client is scheduled for a bone marrow aspiration. The nurse plans to bring which of the following skin cleansing agents to the bedside before this procedure for skin cleansing to prevent infection as a result of the procedure?
1   Soap and water
2   Povidone-iodine
3   Hydrogen peroxide
4   Alcohol swabs

Answer: 2
Rationale: Before bone marrow aspiration, the needle insertion site is cleansed with an antiseptic solution such as povidone-iodine. This helps reduce the number of bacteria on the skin and decreases the risk of infection from the procedure. The other options are incorrect.

Test-Taking Strategy: Use the process of elimination and knowledge of general asepsis and topical cleansing agents to answer this question. Recalling that this procedure is invasive will assist in directing you to the correct option. Review this procedure if you had difficulty with this question.

Level of Cognitive Ability: Application
Client Needs: Safe, Effective Care Environment
Integrated Concept/Process: Nursing Process/Planning
Content Area: Fundamental Skills

Reference:
deWit, S. (2001). *Fundamental concepts and skills for nursing.* Philadelphia: W.B. Saunders, p. 421.

---

12. A nurse arrives to work on the day shift and is assigned to care for a client with terminal cancer. The nurse notes that the client has been receiving a narcotic analgesic every 3 hours for pain. When entering the client's room, the client states "I am so glad that you are here. The medicine never works when the nurse who cared for me last night gives me the medicine." The nurse has previously observed this same occurrence with both this client and other clients and suspects that the night nurse is substance impaired. Which of the following actions will the nurse take?
1   Call the night nurse who gave the medication and discuss the situation with the nurse
2   Report the information to a supervisor
3   Call the impaired nurse organization and report the nurse
4   Report the information to the police

Answer: 2
Rationale: Nurse practice acts require reporting the suspicion of impaired nurses. The Board of Nursing has jurisdiction over the practice of nursing and may develop plans for treatment and supervision. This suspicion should be reported to the nursing supervisor who will then report to the Board of Nursing. Option 1 is incorrect and may cause a conflict. Option 3 and 4 are premature actions.

Test-Taking Strategy: Use the process of elimination. Remember to follow the channel of organizational structure to report situations such as this one. By reporting the information, the nurse alerts the institution of the potential problem and sets the stage for further investigation and appropriate action. Review nursing actions when substance abuse in the workplace is suspected if you had difficulty with this question.

Level of Cognitive Ability: Application
Client Needs: Safe, Effective Care Environment
Integrated Concept/Process: Nursing Process/Implementation
Content Area: Fundamental Skills

Reference:
Potter, P., & Perry, A. (2001). *Fundamentals of nursing* (5th ed.). St. Louis: Mosby, p. 386.

---

13. A client is to receive 1000 mL of 5% dextrose, 125 mL per hour. The drop factor is 10 drops per mL. The nurse adjusts the flow rate at how many drops per minute?
1   10 drops
2   18 drops

Answer: 3
Rationale: The first step is to determine how many hours the intravenous (IV) solution will last. This requires simple division of the total volume of mL to be infused (1000 mL) by the total mL per hour (125 mL), which is 8 hours. Then convert hours to minutes (8 hours = 480 minutes). Next, use the formula to calculate the flow rate.

3   21 drops
4   30 drops

Formula:

$$\frac{\text{Total volume in mL} \times \text{drop factor}}{\text{Time in minutes}} = \text{Flow rate in drops per minute}$$

$$\frac{1000 \text{ mL} \times 10 \text{ drops}}{480 \text{ minutes}} = \frac{10{,}000}{480} = 20.8 \text{ or } 21 \text{ drops per minute}$$

Test-Taking Strategy: Use the formula for IV drop rates when calculating these IV problems. Remember that you need to convert hours to minutes. Be careful with the multiplication and division. Using the formula carefully will direct you to the correct option. Review this formula if you had difficulty with this question.

Level of Cognitive Ability: Application
Client Needs: Safe, Effective Care Environment
Integrated Concept/Process: Nursing Process/Implementation
Content Area: Fundamental Skills

Reference:
deWit, S. (2001). *Fundamental concepts and skills for nursing.* Philadelphia: W.B. Saunders, p. 723.

---

14. A physician prescribes 1000 mL of normal saline to be infused over 12 hours. The drop factor is 15 drops per mL. The nurse adjusts the flow rate to how many drops per minute?
   1   15 drops
   2   18 drops
   3   21 drops
   4   28 drops

Answer: 3
Rationale: Use the formula for calculating intravenous (IV) drop rates.

Formula:

$$\frac{\text{Total volume in mL} \times \text{drop factor}}{\text{Time in minutes}} = \text{Flow rate in drops per minute}$$

$$\frac{1000 \text{ mL} \times 15 \text{ drops}}{720 \text{ minutes}} = \frac{15000}{720} = 20.8 \text{ or } 21 \text{ drops per minute}$$

Test-Taking Strategy: Use the formula for IV drop rates when calculating these IV problems. Remember to convert hours to minutes. Be careful with the multiplication and division. Using the formula carefully will direct you to the correct option. Review this formula if you had difficulty with this question.

Level of Cognitive Ability: Application
Client Needs: Safe, Effective Care Environment
Integrated Concept/Process: Nursing Process/Implementation
Content Area: Fundamental Skills

Reference:
deWit, S. (2001). *Fundamental concepts and skills for nursing.* Philadelphia: W.B. Saunders, p. 723.

15. An adolescent asks a nurse about the procedure to become an organ donor. The nurse most accurately tells the adolescent that:

1   An individual who is at least 16 years of age can sign papers to become a donor
2   Written consent is never required to become a donor
3   The family is responsible for making the decision about organ donation at the time of death
4   A donor must be 18 years or older to provide consent

Answer: 4

Rationale: Any person 18 years of age or older may become an organ donor by indicating his or her consent in writing. In the absence of appropriate documentation, a family member or legal guardian may authorize donation of the decedent's organs.

Test-Taking Strategy: Use the process of elimination. Noting that two of the options address an age provides a clue that one of these options may be correct. In this case, it is best to select the higher age. If you had difficulty with this question, review the procedure for organ donation.

Level of Cognitive Ability: Application
Client Needs: Safe, Effective Care Environment
Integrated Concept/Process: Nursing Process/Implementation
Content Area: Fundamental Skills

Reference:
deWit, S. (2001). *Fundamental concepts and skills for nursing.* Philadelphia: W.B. Saunders, p. 194.

---

16. A nurse employed at a medical unit of a local hospital arrives at work and is told to report (float) to the pediatric unit for the day because several pediatric admissions occurred during the night and the pediatric unit needs assistance in caring for the children. The nurse has never worked in the pediatric unit and is anxious about floating to this area. Which of the following is the most appropriate nursing action?

1   Call the nursing supervisor
2   Refuse to float to the pediatric unit
3   Report to the pediatric unit and identify tasks that can be safely performed
4   Ask another nurse to float to the pediatric unit

Answer: 3

Rationale: Floating is an acceptable legal practice used by hospitals to solve their understaffing problems. Legally, a nurse cannot refuse to float unless a union contract guarantees that nurses can work only in a specified area or the nurse can prove the lack of knowledge for the performance of assigned tasks. When encountered with this situation, the nurse should set priorities and identify potential areas of harm to the client. A nurse cannot refuse an assignment and should not ask another nurse to perform an assignment. The supervisor would be called if the nurse is asked to perform a task that could not be safely performed.

Test-Taking Strategy: Use the process of elimination. Note the key words *most appropriate.* This may indicate that more than one option may be correct. Options 2 and 4 can be eliminated first because a nurse cannot refuse an assignment or ask someone else to perform an assignment. From the remaining options, it is premature to call the nursing supervisor. Option 3 is the most appropriate action. Review nursing responsibilities related to floating if you had difficulty with this question.

Level of Cognitive Ability: Application
Client Needs: Safe, Effective Care Environment
Integrated Concept/Process: Nursing Process/Implementation
Content Area: Fundamental Skills

Reference:
Potter, P., & Perry, A. (2001). *Fundamentals of nursing* (5th ed.). St. Louis: Mosby, p. 435.

17. A 22-year-old client who was struck by a car while jogging is brought to the emergency room by the ambulance team. The client is unconscious and a ruptured spleen is suspected. Emergency measures are instituted but are unsuccessful. The client's fiancée is with the client and tells the nurse that the client is an organ donor. In anticipation that the client's eyes will be donated, which of the following would the nurse plan to implement initially?
  1 Call the National Eye Bank to confirm that the client is a donor
  2 Position the deceased supine and place dry sterile dressings over the eyes
  3 Close the deceased client's eyes and place wet saline gauze pads and an ice pack on the eyes
  4 Ask the fiancée to obtain the client's will from the lawyer

Answer: 3
Rationale: When a corneal donation is anticipated, the clients eyes are closed and gauze pads wet with saline are placed over them with a small ice pack. Within 2 to 4 hours the eyes are enucleated. The cornea is usually transplanted within 24 to 48 hours. The head of the bed should also be elevated. Options 2 and 4 are incorrect actions. Option 1 is not an initial action.

Test-Taking Strategy: Use the process of elimination. Note that the issue is donation of the eyes. This should assist you in eliminating options 1 and 4. Knowing how to care for the eyes of a deceased organ donor will lead you to option 3. Review this procedure if you had difficulty with the question.

Level of Cognitive Ability: Application
Client Needs: Safe, Effective Care Environment
Integrated Concept/Process: Nursing Process/Implementation
Content Area: Fundamental Skills

Reference:
Potter, P., & Perry, A. (2001). *Fundamentals of nursing* (5th ed.). St. Louis: Mosby, p. 636.

---

18. A client with metastatic bladder cancer is admitted to the hospital for chemotherapy. A nurse is asked to collect data from the client. During collection of the data, the client tells the nurse that a living will was prepared 2 years ago and asks if this document is still effective. The most appropriate nursing response is which of the following?
  1 "Yes, because it can't be changed once it is written."
  2 "You will have to discuss the issue with your lawyer."
  3 "A living will should be reviewed yearly with your physician."
  4 "Living wills are valid for 6 months."

Answer: 3
Rationale: The client should discuss the living will with the physician, and it should be reviewed annually to ensure that it contains the client's current wishes and desires. Options 1 and 4 are inaccurate. Option 2 is not the most appropriate response and places the client's question on hold.

Test-Taking Strategy: Use the process of elimination. Option 1 and 4 are incorrect. Although changing a living will would require consultation with a lawyer, the most appropriate and accurate nursing response would be to inform the client that the living will should be reviewed annually. Review procedures related to living wills if you had difficulty with this question.

Level of Cognitive Ability: Application
Client Needs: Safe, Effective Care Environment
Integrated Concept/Process: Nursing Process/Implementation
Content Area: Fundamental Skills

Reference:
Potter, P., & Perry, A. (2001). *Fundamentals of nursing* (5th ed.). St. Louis: Mosby, p. 437.

---

19. A client was brought to the emergency room 2 weeks ago after an episode of acute anginal pain. The client was hospitalized and diagnostic studies were performed. After treatment, the client was discharged. The client is readmitted to the hospital and tells the nurse that a living will was prepared during the last hospital

Answer: 4
Rationale: Copies of a living will should be kept with the medical record, at the physician's office, and in the home of the client. A copy will also be retained in the lawyer's office. These documents are not maintained in emergency room files.

Test-Taking Strategy: Note the key word *not* and use the process of elimination. It would seem reasonable that a physician would

admission. The nurse would not expect a copy of this document to be located in which of the following?

1   In the client's home
2   In the physician's office
3   In the medical record at the hospital
4   In the hospital emergency room files

keep a copy of this document in the medical files. The client would certainly have a copy in the home because this document identifies the client's wishes. It would also seem reasonable that a copy would be maintained in the client's medical record to provide guidance to care providers if a situation arose during hospitalization requiring referral to this document. It is not realistic for an emergency room to maintain such documents in their files. Review procedures related to living wills if you had difficulty with this question.

Level of Cognitive Ability: Comprehension
Client Needs: Safe, Effective Care Environment
Integrated Concept/Process: Nursing Process/Data Collection
Content Area: Fundamental Skills

Reference:
Potter, P., & Perry, A. (2001). *Fundamentals of nursing* (5th ed.). St. Louis: Mosby, p. 437.

---

20. A licensed practical nurse (LPN) is preparing to suction a client with a diagnosis of acquired immunodeficiency syndrome (AIDS). The LPN would gather which of the following supplies to perform this procedure safely?

1   Gloves, mask, and protective eyewear
2   Gloves, gown, and mask
3   Gown, mask, and protective eyewear
4   Gloves, gown, and protective eyewear

Answer: 1
Rationale: Standard (Universal) Precautions include the use of gloves whenever there is actual or potential contact with blood or body fluids. During suctioning, the nurse wears gloves, a mask, and protective eyewear or a face shield. Impervious gowns are worn in those instances when it is anticipated that there will be contact with a large amount of body fluid or blood.

Test-Taking Strategy: Use the process of elimination. Note that the issue is suctioning, so expect airborne secretions with this procedure. Basic knowledge of Standard (Universal) Precautions would direct you to an option that includes mask, protective eyewear, and gloves. The only option that contains these three items is option 1. Review these precautions if you had difficulty with this question.

Level of Cognitive Ability: Application
Client Needs: Safe, Effective Care Environment
Integrated Concept/Process: Nursing Process/Implementation
Content Area: Fundamental Skills

Reference:
Potter, P., & Perry, A. (2001). *Fundamentals of nursing* (5th ed.). St. Louis: Mosby, p. 859.

---

21. A licensed practical nurse (LPN) employed in a long-term care facility is observing a nursing assistant ambulating a client with right-sided weakness. The LPN would determine that the nursing assistant was performing the procedure safely if the LPN observed the nursing assistant:

1   Standing behind the client
2   Standing in front of the client

Answer: 4
Rationale: When walking with a client, the nurse should stand on the client's affected side. The nurse should position the free hand on the client's shoulder so that the client can be pulled toward the nurse in the event that the client falls forward. The client should be instructed to look up and outward rather than at his or her feet. Options 1, 2, and 3 are incorrect.

3 Standing on the left side of the client

4 Standing on the right side of the client

Test-Taking Strategy: Use the process of elimination. Note the key words *right-sided* in the question. This will assist in eliminating option 3. Eliminate options 1 and 2 because neither position places the nurse in a strategic position should the client lose balance and begin to fall forward or backward. Recalling that support is needed on a client's affected side will direct you to the correct option. Review this procedure if you had difficulty with this question.

Level of Cognitive Ability: Comprehension
Client Needs: Safe, Effective Care Environment
Integrated Concept/Process: Nursing Process/Data Collection
Content Area: Fundamental Skills

Reference:
Potter, P., & Perry, A. (2001). *Fundamentals of nursing* (5th ed.). St. Louis: Mosby, p. 1539.

---

22. A nurse is caring for a client who is receiving a dose of an intramuscular antibiotic. The nurse enters the client's room to administer the prescribed antibiotic, and the client tells the nurse that the medication burns and that he or she does not want the medication to be given. The nurse tells the client that the medication is necessary and administers the medication. Which of the following can the client legally charge as a result of the nursing action?
1 Assault
2 Battery
3 Negligence
4 Invasion of privacy

Answer: 2
Rationale: An assault occurs when a person puts another person in fear of a harmful or offensive contact. For this intentional tort to be actionable the victim must be aware of the threat of harmful or offensive contact. Battery is the actual contact with one's body. Negligence involves actions below the standards of care. Invasion of privacy occurs when the individual's private affairs are unreasonably invaded. In this situation, the nurse can be charged with battery because the nurse administers a medication that the client has refused.

Test-Taking Strategy: Use the process of elimination. Note that the client refuses the medication and the nurse administers the medication regardless of the client's request. This should easily direct you to option 2. If you had difficulty with this question, review the descriptions associated with the terms in each option.

Level of Cognitive Ability: Comprehension
Client Needs: Safe, Effective Care Environment
Integrated Concept/Process: Nursing Process/Implementation
Content Area: Fundamental Skills

Reference:
Potter, P., & Perry, A. (2001). *Fundamentals of nursing* (5th ed.). St. Louis: Mosby, p. 425.

---

23. A licensed practical nurse (LPN) is reinforcing teaching done by a registered nurse (RN) to parents of a child with celiac disease. The LPN reminds the parents to do which of the following to ensure that the diet is safe based on the child's physical needs?
1 Keep the intake of fresh starchy vegetables to a minimum

Answer: 3
Rationale: Gluten is added to many foods such as hydrolyzed vegetable protein derived from cereal grains. Grains are also frequently added to processed foods as thickening or fillers. Because of this, it is important to read food labels. Gluten is found primarily in the grains of wheat and rye. Rice, corn, and other vegetables are acceptable in a gluten-free diet. Many pasta products contain gluten and should be avoided.

2   Serve pasta dishes instead of cereals with grain
3   Read food labels carefully to avoid hidden sources of gluten
4   Restrict corn and rice in the diet

Test-Taking Strategy: Use the process of elimination. Begin to answer this question by recalling that a gluten-free diet is indicated to manage celiac disease. Also recall which foods are high in gluten. Choose correctly by selecting the most global option. If you had difficulty with this question, review celiac disease and which foods are safe to eat.

Level of Cognitive Ability: Application
Client Needs: Safe, Effective Care Environment
Integrated Concept/Process: Teaching/Learning
Content Area: Child Health

Reference:
Wong, D., & Hockenberry-Eaton, M. (2001). *Wong's essentials of pediatric nursing* (6th ed.). St. Louis: Mosby, p. 927.

---

24. A nurse notes that a child who has been diagnosed with intussusception has a formed brown bowel movement. The nurse should do which of the following at once to ensure that a safe plan of care is implemented for the child?
    1   Ask the child about any increase in abdominal pain
    2   Prepare the child for hydrostatic reduction
    3   Report the passage of the normal stool to the registered nurse (RN)
    4   Warn the child and his or her parents that surgery is imminent

Answer: 3
Rationale: Passage of a formed brown bowel movement usually indicates that an intussusception has reduced itself. The nurse immediately reports this data to the RN, who will in turn report it to the physician. This finding may change the course of the plan of care. Increased abdominal pain is not expected because the child's gastrointestinal tract is more functional. The finding does not indicate the need for immediate surgery.

Test-Taking Strategy: Use the process of elimination. Recalling that the passage of a normal stool may indicate that an intussusception is resolving or has resolved will direct you to option 3. If you had difficulty with this question, review care to the child with intussusception.

Level of Cognitive Ability: Application
Client Needs: Safe, Effective Care Environment
Integrated Concept/Process: Nursing Process/Implementation
Content Area: Child Health

Reference:
Wong, D., & Hockenberry-Eaton, M. (2001). *Wong's essentials of pediatric nursing* (6th ed.). St. Louis: Mosby, p. 923.

---

25. A psychotic client is belligerent and agitated, making aggressive gestures and pacing in the hallway. To ensure a save environment, which of the following is the nurse's highest priority?
    1   Provide comfort and consolation to the other clients on the unit
    2   Assist other staff in restraining the client
    3   Provide safety for the client and other clients on the unit
    4   Ask the client politely to calm down and regain control over his or her behavior

Answer: 3
Rationale: A psychotic client who is out of control may require seclusion to ensure the safety of the client and other clients in the unit. The correct option is the only one that addresses the safety needs of both the client and others. Options 1 and 2 do not provide for the client's safety needs or rights, respectively. Option 4 may be ineffective and does not address the safety needs of others in the unit.

Test-Taking Strategy: The issue of the question is safety (note the key words *belligerent, agitated,* and *aggressive*) Use the process of elimination and Maslow's Hierarchy of Needs theory to prioritize. Option 3 is the global option and addresses the safety of all. Review care to the psychotic client if you had difficulty with this question.

Level of Cognitive Ability: Application
Client Needs: Safe, Effective Care Environment
Integrated Concept/Process: Nursing Process/Implementation
Content Area: Mental Health

Reference:
Hill, S., & Bauer, B. (2000). *Mental health nursing.* Philadelphia: W.B. Saunders, p. 296.

---

26. A client with Bell's palsy is scheduled for a magnetic resonance imaging (MRI). The nurse should implement which of the following standard orders to ensure a safe environment in preparation for this test?
1 Shave the groin for insertion of a femoral catheter
2 Apply metal-tipped electrodes on the client's chest
3 Ensure that the client stays NPO for 6 hours beforehand
4 Remove all objects containing metal from the client

Answer: 4
Rationale: An MRI uses magnetic fields to produce a diagnostic image. All metal objects such as rings, bracelets, hairpins, and watches should be removed. The client's history should also be reviewed to determine if the client has any internal metallic devices such as orthopedic hardware, pacemakers, and shrapnel. A femoral catheter is not inserted. For an abdominal MRI, the client is usually NPO, but this is not necessary for an MRI of the head. Option 2 is also incorrect.

Test-Taking Strategy: Use the process of elimination. Note the physiological location as it relates to the client's diagnosis. Recalling that metallic objects cannot be in place during an MRI and focusing on the client's diagnosis will direct you to option 4. If you are unfamiliar with client preparation for an MRI, review this content.

Level of Cognitive Ability: Application
Client Needs: Safe, Effective Care Environment
Integrated Concept/Process: Nursing Process/Implementation
Content Area: Adult Health/Neurological

Reference:
deWit, S. (2001). *Fundamental concepts and skills for nursing.* Philadelphia: W.B. Saunders, p. 424.

---

27. A nurse assisting in the care of a client who has been in a coma for more than a year is told by the physician to stop the tube feeding that is providing sustenance to the client. The nurse, who is aware of the legal basis needed for carrying out the order, first determines whether which of the following requirements has been met?
1 Authorization by the family to discontinue the treatment
2 Institutional Ethics Committee approval
3 A court order to discontinue the treatment
4 A written order by the physician to remove the tube

Answer: 1
Rationale: The family or a legal guardian can make treatment decisions, generally in collaboration with physicians, other health care workers, and other trusted advisors. The nurse first checks for family authorization to discontinue the treatment. Next, option 4 would be appropriate. Although options 2 and 3 may be necessary in some situations, these options are not the first actions in this situation.

Test-Taking Strategy: Use the process of elimination. Note the key word *first*. This tells you that the correct option is determined according to a proper sequence of action. Recalling that the family or legal guardian can make decisions about discontinuing treatment will direct you to option 1. Review legal principles surrounding end-of-life decisions if you had difficulty with this question.

Level of Cognitive Ability: Application
Client Needs: Safe, Effective Care Environment

Integrated Concept/Process: Nursing Process/Implementation
Content Area: Fundamental Skills

Reference:
Brent, N. (2002) *Nurses and the law* (2nd ed.). Philadelphia: W.B. Saunders, p. 241.

---

28. A nurse who is assisting a physician with insertion of a Miller-Abbott tube would do which of the following to ensure a safe environment and decrease the client's risk of aspiration?

1 Place the client in a high-Fowler's position

2 Instruct the client to bear down if there is an urge to gag

3 Assist with inserting the tube with the balloon inflated

4 Ask the client to cough when the tube reaches the nasopharynx

Answer: 1
Rationale: A Miller-Abbott tube is a nasoenteric tube used to correct a bowel obstruction and decompress the intestine. A high-Fowler position decreases the risk of aspiration if vomiting occurs. A physician inserts the tube with the balloon deflated in a manner similar to that used with a nasogastric tube. The client usually sips water to facilitate passage of the tube through the nasopharynx and esophagus. Options 2, 3, and 4 are incorrect actions.

Test-Taking Strategy: Use the process of elimination. The issue of the question is decreasing the risk of aspiration during insertion of a Miller-Abbott tube. Eliminate option 3 first because a tube could not be inserted with the balloon inflated. Next eliminate options 2 and 4 because coughing and bearing down will not facilitate passage of the tube. Review the procedure for insertion of nasoenteric tubes if you had difficulty with this question.

Level of Cognitive Ability: Application
Client Needs: Safe, Effective Care Environment
Integrated Concept/Process: Nursing Process/Implementation
Content Area: Adult Health/Gastrointestinal

Reference:
Ignatavicius, D., & Workman, M. (2002). *Medical-surgical nursing: critical thinking for collaborative care* (4th ed.). Philadelphia: W.B. Saunders, p. 1228.

---

29. A nurse who is assisting in the care of a client with cancer is following medication orders to manage the cancer pain. Which of the following strategies outlined in the care plan would the nurse follow to ensure adequate and safe pain control?

1 Rely entirely on prescription and over-the-counter medications for pain relief

2 Ensure that the client is kept at a low baseline pain level to avoid sedation or addiction

3 Try multiple simultaneous medications for maximum pain relief effect

4 Start with low medication doses and gradually increase to a dose that relieves pain without exceeding the maximal daily dose

Answer: 4
Rationale: The most appropriate approach is to begin with low doses and increase as needed to maintain a dose that relieves the pain. Option 1 ignores the benefits of other options that may relieve pain such as massage, therapeutic touch, or music. Keeping the client at a baseline level of pain is inappropriate practice. Multiple medication interventions do not guarantee effectiveness and can also be unsafe.

Test-Taking Strategy: Use the process of elimination. Begin to answer this question by eliminating options 1 and 3 because they contain the words "entirely" and "multiple." Choose correctly between the remaining options using basic principles of pain management. Review these principles if you had difficulty with this question.

Level of Cognitive Ability: Application
Client Needs: Safe, Effective Care Environment
Integrated Concept/Process: Nursing Process/Implementation
Content Area: Adult Health/Oncology

Reference:
Ignatavicius, D., & Workman, M. (2002). *Medical-surgical: critical thinking for collaborative care* (4th ed.). Philadelphia: W.B. Saunders, p. 77.

---

30. A licensed practical nurse (LPN) is reinforcing instructions given by a registered nurse (RN) to a client about how to take medications after discharge from the hospital. The LPN should use which of the following approaches to best ensure safe administration of medication in the home?

1 Tell the client to double up on medications if a dose has been missed
2 Count the number of pills remaining in the prescription bottle once a week
3 Show the client the proper way to take prescribed medications
4 Allow the client to verbalize and demonstrate correct administration procedure

Answer: 4

Rationale: The most effective method of teaching to ensure safe self-administration of medications in the home setting is to have the client verbalize and also demonstrate how to take medications. This ensures that the client has both the knowledge and the physical ability to comply with medication therapy. Option 3 is useful early in the teaching or learning process, but is not the best method because it does not allow for the client to demonstrate his or her own ability. Option 1 is incorrect because it is a dangerous and incorrect statement. Option 2 is unrealistic and does not enhance self-care.

Test-Taking Strategy: Use the process of elimination. Begin to answer the question by eliminating options 1 and 2 first. From the remaining options, select the one that most globally addresses the full abilities needed by the client when discharged. Review teaching and learning principles if you had difficulty with this question.

Level of Cognitive Ability: Application
Client Needs: Safe, Effective Care Environment
Integrated Concept/Process: Teaching/Learning
Content Area: Fundamental Skills

Reference:
Potter, P., & Perry, A. (2001). *Fundamentals of nursing* (5th ed.). St. Louis: Mosby, p. 486.

---

31. A 45-year-old client with ventricular dysrhythmias noted on Holter monitoring is scheduled for electrophysiology (EP) studies. The nurse would include which of the following pieces of information when reinforcing teaching to provide accurate information to the client about this procedure?

1 It is a noninvasive test to determine whether the current antidysrhythmic medications are working
2 It is important to continue to take your medications on the morning of the test
3 A special wire will be used to produce the dysrhythmias that cause the signs and symptoms
4 The sedative medications used during the procedure will cause total amnesia of the test

Answer: 3

Rationale: EP studies examine the heart's electrical system and determine the cause and origin of a client's dysrhythmias. The client should be taught this is an invasive procedure in which a special wire is introduced into the heart to produce dysrhythmias. The client should be NPO for 6 to 8 hours before the studies, and all antidysrhythmic medications should be held for at least 24 hours before the test. Heavy sedation is avoided because the client's verbal response to the rhythm changes are important.

Test-Taking Strategy: The issue of the question is knowledge of the purpose and procedure of EP studies as they apply to client teaching. Review this procedure if you had difficulty with this question.

Level of Cognitive Ability: Application
Client Needs: Safe, Effective Care Environment
Integrated Concept/Process: Nursing Process/Implementation
Content Area: Adult Health/Cardiovascular

Reference:
Ignatavicius, D., & Workman, M. (2002). *Medical-surgical nursing: critical thinking for collaborative care* (4th ed.). Philadelphia: W.B. Saunders, p. 646.

32. A client with thrombophlebitis is being treated with heparin sodium (Liquaemin) therapy. The registered nurse (RN) asks the licensed practical nurse (LPN) to check the medication supply to ensure that the antidote for this therapy is available. The nurse checks the medication supply for which medication?
1 Streptokinase (Streptase)
2 Phytonadione (vitamin K)
3 Aminocaproic acid (Amicar)
4 Protamine sulfate

Answer: 4
Rationale: Protamine sulfate is the antidote for heparin sodium. Streptokinase is a thrombolytic agent used to dissolve blood clots. Vitamin K is the antidote for warfarin (Coumadin). Amicar is an antifibrinolytic used to prevent the breakdown of clots already formed.

Test-Taking Strategy: Specific knowledge of the antidote to heparin is needed to answer this question correctly. Review common antidotes if you had difficulty with this question.

Level of Cognitive Ability: Application
Client Needs: Safe, Effective Care Environment
Integrated Concept/Process: Nursing Process/Implementation
Content Area: Pharmacology

Reference:
Hodgson, B., & Kizior, R. (2003). *Saunders nursing drug handbook 2003.* Philadelphia: W.B. Saunders, p. 944.

33. A nurse who is assisting in the care of a client with cardiomyopathy would give careful attention to which of the following to ensure client safety?
1 Administering vasodilator medications
2 Taking measures to prevent orthostatic changes when the client stands
3 Conducting a thorough pain assessment
4 Telling the client about the importance of avoiding over-the-counter medications

Answer: 2
Rationale: Orthostatic changes can occur in the client with cardiomyopathy as a result of impaired venous return. These changes could lead to dizziness and client falls. Vasodilators should not be administered. There is no mention of pain in the question, and pain may not directly affect safety in this situation. Option 4 is an accurate statement but is not directly related to the issue of safety.

Test-Taking Strategy: The issue of the question is a nursing measure that will protect the client's safety. Use the process of elimination. The only logical option is the one that deals with prevention of orthostatic changes that can occur with cardiomyopathy. Review care to the client with cardiomyopathy if you had difficulty with this question.

Level of Cognitive Ability: Application
Client Needs: Safe, Effective Care Environment
Integrated Concept/Process: Nursing Process/Implementation
Content Area: Adult Health/Cardiovascular

Reference:
Ignatavicius, D., & Workman, M. (2002). *Medical-surgical: critical thinking for collaborative care* (4th ed.). Philadelphia: W.B. Saunders, p. 724.

34. A licensed practical nurse (LPN) is reinforcing teaching done by the registered nurse (RN) with a client who has been diagnosed with endocarditis. The LPN

Answer: 2
Rationale: Clients with endocarditis are at risk for developing thrombi along the walls of the heart, which could become emboli leading to stroke. For this reason, clients with endocarditis are

explains that it is important for this client to use an electric razor rather than a straight razor for shaving because of which of the following?

1 Straight razors harbor too many microorganisms
2 Any cuts or skin injury should be avoided while taking anticoagulants
3 The client is at higher risk for infection from any nick or cut
4 An electric razor can be sanitized more easily

treated with anticoagulant therapy to prevent thrombus formation. Clients on anticoagulants should implement measures to prevent injury and subsequent bleeding. The other options are incorrect because infection rather than bleeding is their primary focus.

Test-Taking Strategy: Use the process of elimination and recall that the client with endocarditis is on anticoagulant therapy. Remember that similar options are not likely to be correct. With this in mind, you could eliminate each of the incorrect options because they deal with infection rather than bleeding. Review care to the client with endocarditis if you had difficulty with this question.

Level of Cognitive Ability: Application
Client Needs: Safe, Effective Care Environment.
Integrated Concept/Process: Teaching/Learning
Content Area: Adult Health/Cardiovascular

Reference:
Ignatavicius, D., & Workman, M. (2002). *Medical-surgical nursing: critical thinking for collaborative care* (4th ed.). Philadelphia: W.B. Saunders, p. 719.

---

35. A licensed practical nurse (LPN) is assisting a registered nurse (RN) in caring for a client who just underwent cardiac catheterization using the femoral artery approach. The nurse would avoid taking which of the following actions in caring for this client because it is unsafe?

1 Ask the client to wiggle the toes when collecting data about neurovascular status
2 Resume prescribed medications
3 Have the client sit upright for a meal
4 Encourage the client to drink extra fluids

Answer: 3
Rationale: For 6 hours after cardiac catheterization using the femoral approach, the client should not bend or hyperextend the affected leg to avoid blood vessel occlusion or hemorrhage. This means that having the client sit upright would be contraindicated. The precatheterization medications are generally resumed after the procedure. Asking the client to wiggle the toes to determine neurovascular status is acceptable and should be done because vascular status could be impaired if a hematoma or thrombus were developing. Fluids should be increased to aid in eliminating the contrast medium through the kidneys.

Test-Taking Strategy: Use the process of elimination. Note the key words *avoid* and *unsafe*. Use knowledge of postcatheterization care and keep in mind that the femoral access site was used. Review postcardiac catheterization care if you had difficulty with this question.

Level of Cognitive Ability: Application
Client Needs: Safe, Effective Care Environment
Integrated Concept/Process: Nursing Process/Implementation
Content Area: Adult Health/Cardiovascular

Reference:
deWit, S. (2001). *Fundamental concepts and skills for nursing.* Philadelphia: W.B. Saunders, p. 426.

---

36. A nurse is delivering a meal tray to a client with heart failure. The nurse would remove which of the following items from the tray before bringing it to the client's bedside because the food item

Answer: 1
Rationale: Clients with heart failure should monitor and restrict sodium intake. Saltine crackers are high in sodium and should be avoided. Green beans and sherbet are low in sodium. Baked chicken would contain only physiologic saline

would be unsafe for the client to consume?

1   Saltine crackers
2   Sherbet
3   Green beans
4   Baked chicken

because it is an animal product and would not have to be avoided by the client.

Test-Taking Strategy: The issue of the question is knowing that a client with heart failure should eat a low sodium diet. From this point, use the process of elimination to select the food that is highest in sodium. Review foods that are high in sodium if you had difficulty with this question.

Level of Cognitive Ability: Application
Client Needs: Safe, Effective Care Environment
Integrated Concept/Process: Nursing Process/Implementation
Content Area: Adult Health/Cardiovascular

Reference:
Williams, S. (2001) *Basic nutrition & diet therapy* (11th ed.). St. Louis: Mosby, p. 364.

---

37. An older client with diabetes mellitus is vomiting because of gastroenteritis. The nurse should do which of the following to maintain oral intake to safely minimize the risk of dehydration?

1   Encourage the client to drink up to 8 to 12 ounces of fluid every hour while awake
2   Restrict the client to clear liquids for at least 3 days to allow for bowel rest
3   Give only sips of water until the client is able to tolerate solid foods
4   Withhold all food and fluids until vomiting has ceased for at least 8 hours

Answer: 1
Rationale: Small amounts of fluid may be tolerated even when vomiting is present. The client should be offered up to 8 to 12 ounces of liquid containing both glucose and electrolytes hourly. The diet should be advanced to a regular diet as soon as it is tolerated and should include a minimum of 100 to 150 grams of carbohydrates daily. Options 2, 3, and 4 are incorrect actions.

Test-Taking Strategy: Use the process of elimination. Begin to answer this question by eliminating options 3 and 4 because of the absolute words *only* and *all.* Choose correctly from the remaining options knowing that a 3-day time frame is excessive. Review measures to minimize dehydration if you had difficulty with this question.

Level of Cognitive Ability: Application
Client Needs: Safe, Effective Care Environment
Integrated Concept/Process: Nursing Process/Implementation
Content Area: Adult Health/Gastrointestinal

Reference:
deWit, S. (2001). *Fundamental concepts and skills for nursing.* Philadelphia: W.B. Saunders, p. 454.

---

38. A client who does not have an artificial airway has a new order for a sputum culture. The nurse should avoid doing which of the following to obtain a suitable specimen?

1   Ask the client to rinse the mouth before expectoration
2   Have the client take deep breaths before coughing
3   Place the culture container lid face down on the bedside table
4   Obtain the specimen early in the morning

Answer: 3
Rationale: The lid would be contaminated if it is placed face down on the bedside table, which could lead to inaccurate test results. The client should rinse the mouth or brush the teeth before specimen collection to avoid contaminating the specimen. The client should take deep breaths before expectoration for best sputum production. The specimen is optimally obtained early in the morning, because sputum has a longer amount of time to collect in the airways during sleep.

Test-Taking Strategy: Use the process of elimination. The key word is *avoid.* This tells you that the correct option is an incorrect nursing action. Use knowledge of the principles of aseptic technique to choose correctly. Review these principles if you had difficulty with this question.

Level of Cognitive Ability: Application
Client Needs: Safe, Effective Care Environment
Integrated Concept/Process: Nursing Process/Implementation
Content Area: Fundamental Skills

Reference:
deWit, S. (2001). *Fundamental concepts and skills for nursing.* Philadelphia: W.B. Saunders, p. 229.

---

39. A nurse is implementing measures to prevent the spread of infection to other clients. The nurse understands that which of the following is the best way to prevent the spread of infection?
1 Read the policy and procedure manual before performing treatments
2 Use proper hand washing techniques
3 Use sterile technique with all procedures
4 Never stop in the middle of performing a procedure

Answer: 2
Rationale: Proper hand washing is the best way to prevent the spread of infection. Reading the policy and procedure manual does not guarantee that infection will not spread. All procedures do not require sterile technique. It may be necessary in some situations to stop in the middle of performing a procedure, but option 4 is not the best way to prevent the spread of infection.

Test-Taking Strategy: Focus on the issue of the question and use the process of elimination. Recalling the basic principles related to preventing infection will direct you to option 2. Review these basic principles if you had difficulty with this question.

Level of Cognitive Ability: Comprehension
Client Needs: Safe, Effective Care Environment
Integrated Concept/Process: Nursing Process/Implementation
Content Area: Fundamental Skills

Reference:
Potter, P., & Perry, A. (2001). *Fundamentals of nursing* (5th ed.). St. Louis: Mosby, p. 854.

---

40. A nurse is carrying out an order to obtain a sputum sample, which must be obtained using the saline inhalation method. The nurse guides the client in using the nebulizer safely and effectively by encouraging the client to do the following:
1 Keep the lips closed lightly over the seal
2 Keep the lips closely tightly over the seal
3 Alternate one vapor breath with one breath from room air
4 Hold the nebulizer under the nose

Answer: 1
Rationale: Inhaling vaporized saline is an effective means to assist a client to cough productively because the vapor condenses on respiratory mucosa, stimulating the cough reflex and the expectoration of secretions. The nurse tells the client to close the mouth lightly over the mouthpiece. It is not necessary to form a tight seal. The client inhales vaporized saline with each breath until coughing results. The nebulizer is not held under the nose.

Test-Taking Strategy: To answer this question accurately, you must be familiar with this procedure and its purpose. Visualizing this procedure will direct you to option 1. Review this procedure if you had difficulty with this question.

Level of Cognitive Ability: Application
Client Needs: Safe, Effective Care Environment
Integrated Concept/Process: Nursing Process/Implementation
Content Area: Adult Health/Respiratory

Reference:
Potter, P., & Perry, A. (2001). *Fundamentals of nursing* (5th ed.). St. Louis: Mosby, p. 1154.

---

41. A client has a tracheostomy with a nondisposable inner cannula. After completing tracheostomy care, the nurse reinserts the inner cannula into the tracheostomy tube immediately after doing which of the following?

  1 Tapping it dry lightly against a sterile surface

  2 Drying it with a sterile cotton ball

  3 Suctioning the airway

  4 Rinsing it in sterile water

Answer: 1

Rationale: The nurse reinserts the inner cannula immediately after tapping it dry against a sterile surface. Once inserted, it is turned clockwise to lock it into place. It should not be dried with a cotton ball, which could leave cotton particles on the cannula. The client's airway is suctioned before doing tracheostomy care. Rinsing in sterile water is done before tapping it dry.

Test-Taking Strategy: The wording of the question tells you that there is a particular time sequence that must be followed in completing the steps of the procedure. Use the process of elimination to reason that the step that would be done "immediately before" reinsertion would be a course of action related to drying the tube. Review the procedure for tracheotomy care if you had difficulty with this question.

Level of Cognitive Ability: Application
Client Needs: Safe, Effective Care Environment
Integrated Concept/Process: Nursing Process/Implementation
Content Area: Adult Health/Respiratory

Reference:
Ignatavicius, D., & Workman, M. (2002). *Medical-surgical nursing: critical thinking for collaborative care* (4th ed.). Philadelphia: W.B. Saunders, p. 503.

---

42. A nurse is assisting in the care of a client with a nasogastric (NG) tube. The nurse understands that which of the following would be the most potentially hazardous method for checking tube placement when giving care to the client?

  1 Submerging the NG tube in water to check for bubbling

  2 Instilling 10 to 20 mL of air into the NG tube while auscultating over the stomach

  3 Aspirating the NG tube with a 50 mL syringe for gastric contents

  4 Measuring the pH of gastric aspirate

Answer: 1

Rationale: The most potentially hazardous method for checking NG tube placement is to submerge the end of the tube in water to observe for bubbling. This could put the client at risk for aspiration if the client breathed in fluid while the tube was in the lungs. Each of the other methods described is acceptable. The best method of determining tube placement is to verify by x-ray.

Test-Taking Strategy: Use the process of elimination. The key words are *most potentially hazardous*. This tells you that the correct answer is an option that puts the client at risk for possible injury. Evaluate each of the options noting that the correct option puts the client at risk, in this case for aspiration. Review this procedure if you had difficulty with this question.

Level of Cognitive Ability: Comprehension
Client Needs: Safe, Effective Care Environment
Integrated Concept/Process: Nursing Process/Implementation
Content Area: Adult Health/Respiratory

Reference:
Ignatavicius, D., & Workman, M. (2002). *Medical-surgical nursing: critical thinking for collaborative care* (4th ed.). Philadelphia: W.B. Saunders, p. 1210.

43. An elderly client who has not been hospitalized previously is extremely anxious after hospital admission. To provide a safe environment for the client and minimize the stress of hospitalization, the nurse would do which of the following?
1 Keep visitors to the minimum number possible
2 Keep the door open and room lights on at all times
3 Admit the client to a room far away from the nurse's station
4 Allow the client to have as many choices related to care as possible

Answer: 4
Rationale: Several general interventions will reduce the hospitalized client's level of stress. These include acknowledging the client's feelings, offering information, providing social support, and letting the client have control over choices related to care. Options 1 and 3 could increase anxiety, whereas option 2 could add to the disruption created by the hospitalization and interfere with the client's sleep pattern.

Test-Taking Strategy: Use the process of elimination. The key words are *safe*, and *minimize the stress*. This tells you that the correct option is one that calms the client's feelings of fear and anxiety after he or she is suddenly placed in a foreign environment. Use general principles related to safety and stress reduction to answer the question and review these principles if you had difficulty with this question.

Level of Cognitive Ability: Application
Client Needs: Safe, Effective Care Environment
Integrated Concept/Process: Nursing Process/Implementation
Content Area: Adult Health/Cardiovascular

Reference:
Ignatavicius, D., & Workman, M. (2002). *Medical-surgical nursing: critical thinking for collaborative care* (4th ed.). Philadelphia: W.B. Saunders, p. 1242.

44. A prenatal client who has acquired the sexually transmitted virus *Condyloma acuminatum* (human papilloma virus) asks the nurse to explain again the treatment for the infection. The nurse would reinforce additional information about which of the following treatments with this client?
1 Cytotoxic medications
2 Interferon therapy
3 Laser therapy
4 No therapy is available

Answer: 3
Rationale: For the pregnant client, laser therapy is the most effective method of destroying the virus. This therapy is localized, while medications (which are considered toxic to the fetus) would have a systemic effect. The primary neonatal effect of the virus is respiratory or laryngeal papillomatosis, although the exact route of perinatal transmission is unknown. Options 1, 2, and 4 are incorrect.

Test-Taking Strategy: Using the process of elimination, begin by eliminating option 4. Remember that options that are similar are not likely to be correct. With this in mind, eliminate options 1 and 2 next because they are both medications. If you had difficulty with this question, review care of the prenatal client with *Condyloma acuminatum* infection.

Level of Cognitive Ability: Application
Client Needs: Safe, Effective Care Environment
Integrated Concept/Process: Nursing Process/Implementation
Content Area: Maternity

Reference:
McKinney, E., Ashwill, J., Murray, S. et al. (2000). *Maternal-child nursing.* Philadelphia: W.B. Saunders, p. 799.

45. A nurse is assisting in the care of a client in labor who has a history of sickle cell anemia. Knowing that the client has a high risk for sickling crisis during labor, the nurse should give priority to implementing which of the following safe nursing actions to prevent a crisis from occurring?
1 Maintain strict hand washing technique
2 Remind the client not to bear down for more than 3 seconds
3 Give the client reassurance and encouragement
4 Ensure that the client uses oxygen during labor

Answer: 4
Rationale: Administering oxygen as needed is an effective intervention to prevent sickle cell crisis during labor. During the labor process the client is at high risk for being unable to meet the oxygen demands of labor and unable to prevent sickling. Option 1 is a safe nursing action, but does nothing to prevent sickling crisis. Option 2 is not realistic and would not prevent sickling crisis. Option 3 is another generally helpful nursing measure, but again is not related to prevention of sickling crisis.

Test-Taking Strategy: The issue of the question is a safe nursing action that will help prevent sickling crisis. Use the ABCs: airway, breathing, and circulation. Note that the question contains the key word *priority*. Select the option that addresses the issue of the question and supports the client's airway. Review measures to prevent sickle cell crisis if you had difficulty with this question.

Level of Cognitive Ability: Application
Client Needs: Safe, Effective Care Environment
Integrated Concept/Process: Nursing Process/Implementation
Content Area: Maternity

Reference:
McKinney, E., Ashwill, J., Murray, S. et al. (2000). *Maternal-child nursing.* Philadelphia: W.B. Saunders, p. 1297.

46. A client who is admitted to the labor and delivery unit in active labor has active genital herpes lesions present in the genital tract. The licensed practical nurse should reinforce teaching done by the registered nurse about which of the following immediate plans for the client?
1 Preparation for spontaneous vaginal delivery
2 Imminent artificial rupture of the membranes
3 Preparation for a cesarean delivery
4 Placement on protective isolation

Answer: 3
Rationale: Cesarean delivery reduces the risk of neonatal infection with a mother in labor who has either herpetic genital tract lesions or ruptured membranes. Options 1 and 2 would expose the fetus to the virus. Standard (Universal) Precautions are necessary, not protective isolation.

Test-Taking Strategy: Use the process of elimination and note the key words *lesions present in the genital tract*. Use knowledge of the labor process and disease transmission to reason that the infant should not be born vaginally. This would help you to eliminate option 1. Eliminate option 2 next knowing that this could also expose the fetus to the virus. Eliminate option 4 knowing that Standard (Universal) Precautions are needed, while protective isolation is not. Review care to the client with active genital herpes lesions if you had difficulty with this question.

Level of Cognitive Ability: Application
Client Needs: Safe, Effective Care Environment
Integrated Concept/Process: Teaching/Learning
Content Area: Maternity

Reference:
McKinney, E., Ashwill, J., Murray, S. et al. (2000). *Maternal-child nursing.* Philadelphia: W.B. Saunders, p. 468.

47. A client with possible renal disease is scheduled to undergo diagnostic testing by intravenous pyelogram (IVP). To ensure client safety, the nurse would be certain to collect data from this client about a history of which of the following?
1 Allergy to shellfish or iodine
2 Family incidence of renal disease
3 Frequent and chronic antibiotic use
4 Long-term use of diuretic medications

Answer: 1

Rationale: A client undergoing diagnostic testing that uses a contrast medium, such as IVP, should be questioned about allergy to shellfish, seafood, or iodine. This would identify a potential allergic reaction to the contrast dye that may be used in this test. The other items are useful as part of the general health history, but are not as critical as the allergy determination.

Test-Taking Strategy: Use the process of elimination. Note the key words *to ensure client safety*. This implies that more than one or all options may be correct, but that one of them is most important for the client's safety. Eliminate options 3 and 4 first because they both collect data about prior medication therapy. Choose correctly between the remaining options using knowledge of the IVP procedure. Review preprocedure care for an IVP if you had difficulty with this question.

Level of Cognitive Ability: Application
Client Needs: Safe, Effective Care Environment
Integrated Concept/Process: Nursing Process/Data Collection
Content Area: Adult Health/Renal

Reference:
Ignatavicius, D., & Workman, M. (2002). *Medical-surgical nursing: critical thinking for collaborative care* (4th ed.). Philadelphia: W.B. Saunders, p. 737.

48. A nurse has an order to insert an indwelling bladder catheter. The nurse would avoid doing which of the following while safely completing this procedure?
1 Inflate the balloon with 4 to 5 mL more than the stated balloon capacity
2 Place the bag lower than bladder level, with no kinks in the tubing
3 Inflate the balloon to test patency before catheter insertion
4 Advance the catheter just until urine appears in the catheter tubing

Answer: 4

Rationale: The nurse should advance the catheter 1 to 2 inches beyond the point where urine flow begins. This ensures that the balloon is placed entirely in the bladder before it is inflated. Each of the other options represents correct procedure.

Test-Taking Strategy: Use the process of elimination. Note the key word *avoid*. With this in mind, eliminate options 2 and 3 first because they are most obviously correct. Choose correctly between options 1 and 4 knowing that either the catheter is advanced 1 to 2 inches after urine appears, or that extra fluid is needed to fill the lumen connecting the external port and the balloon near the tip of the catheter. Review this procedure if you had difficulty with this question.

Level of Cognitive Ability: Application
Client Needs: Safe, Effective Care Environment
Integrated Concept/Process: Nursing Process/Implementation
Content Area: Adult Health/Renal

Reference:
Perry, A., & Potter, P. (2002). *Clinical nursing skills & techniques* (5th ed). St. Louis; Mosby, p. 733.

49. A nurse is carrying out an order for a 24-hour urine collection for a client with a suspected renal disorder. Which of the following actions would the nurse avoid to ensure proper collection technique?
1 Refrigerate the container or place it on ice
2 Ask the client to void at the end time, and add this specimen to the container
3 Ask the client to void at the start time, and place this specimen in the container
4 Save all voidings after the first one in the 24-hour period

Answer: 3
Rationale: To collect a 24-hour urine specimen, the nurse should ask the client to void at the beginning of the collection period, and discard the urine sample. This is done because the urine in that voiding has been in the bladder for an unknown period of time. All subsequent voided urine is saved in a container, which is placed on ice or refrigerated. The nurse should ask the client to void at the finish time, and add this sample to the collection. The nurse then labels the container, places it on fresh ice, and sends it to the laboratory immediately.

Test-Taking Strategy: Note the key word *avoid*. The issue of the question is proper collection technique for a 24-hour urine specimen. Use your knowledge of this basic procedure to answer the question. If you had difficulty with this question, review this procedure.

Level of Cognitive Ability: Application
Client Needs: Safe, Effective Care Environment
Integrated Concept/Process: Nursing Process/Implementation
Content Area: Adult Health/Renal

Reference:
Potter, P., & Perry, A. (2001). *Fundamentals of nursing* (5th ed.). St. Louis: Mosby, p. 863.

50. A licensed practical nurse (LPN) who is assisting a registered nurse (RN) in caring for a client in active labor would do which of the following to best prevent fetal heart rate decelerations?
1 Measure maternal and fetal vital signs every 30 minutes
2 Begin preparations for a cesarean delivery
3 Suggest asking the physician about the advisability of an oxytocin (Pitocin) drip
4 Encourage upright or side-lying maternal positions

Answer: 4
Rationale: Side-lying and upright positions such as walking, standing, and squatting can improve venous return and encourage effective uterine activity, which in turn will reduce the likelihood of fetal heart rate decelerations. Cesarean delivery will not prevent decelerations. Oxytocin could aggravate fetal heart rate decelerations because of increased uterine activity and decreased uteroplacental perfusion. Measuring vital signs every 30 minutes will do nothing to prevent decelerations.

Test-Taking Strategy: Use the process of elimination and note the key word *prevent*. Eliminate each of the incorrect options because they do not have an immediate effect on the physiological status of the mother and the fetus. Remember that side-lying and upright positions will encourage effective uterine activity and provide a safe environment. Review measures to prevent fetal heart rate decelerations if you had difficulty with this question.

Level of Cognitive Ability: Application
Client Needs: Safe, Effective Care Environment
Integrated Concept/Process: Nursing Process/Implementation
Content Area: Maternity

Reference:
Burroughs, A., & Leifer, G. (2002). *Maternity nursing* (8th ed.). Philadelphia: W.B. Saunders, p. 83.

51. A nurse employed in a clinic is assisting in the care of a client with diabetes mellitus who is 36 weeks pregnant. The results of three previous weekly nonstress tests have been reactive. This week the test was nonreactive after 40 minutes. The nurse should anticipate that orders will be given for which of the following to safely monitor this client?

1   A follow-up appointment in 3 days to repeat the nonstress test
2   A contraction stress test
3   Admission to the hospital for immediate induction of labor
4   Admission to the hospital for continuous fetal monitoring

Answer: 2

Rationale: A nonreactive test requires further follow-up evaluation, indicating the need for a contraction stress test. To send the client home for 3 days could place the fetus in jeopardy. Hospitalizing the client for either induction of labor or continuous fetal monitoring are premature without further diagnostic test data.

Test-Taking Strategy: Use the process of elimination. Begin to answer this question by eliminating options 3 and 4 because they are unnecessary at this time. Choose correctly between the remaining options by selecting the one that provides follow-up evaluation. Review the meanings of nonstress test results if you had difficulty with this question.

Level of Cognitive Ability: Comprehension
Client Needs: Safe, Effective Care Environment
Integrated Concept/Process: Nursing Process/Planning
Content Area: Maternity

Reference:
McKinney, E., Ashwill, J., Murray, S. et al. (2000). *Maternal-child nursing.* Philadelphia: W.B. Saunders, p. 343.

---

52. A nurse who begins to administer medications to a client via a nasogastric feeding tube suspects that the tube has become clogged. The nurse should take which of the following safe actions first?

1   Flush with a carbonated liquid, such as cola
2   Prepare to remove and replace the tube
3   Flush the tube with warm water
4   Aspirate the tube

Answer: 4

Rationale: The nurse should first attempt to unclog the feeding tube by aspirating it. If this does not work, the nurse should try to flush the tube with warm water. Carbonated liquids such as cola may also be used, but only if agency policy identifies it as acceptable. Replacement of the tube is the last step if others are unsuccessful.

Test-Taking Strategy: Use the process of elimination and note the key word *first*. Focusing on this key word and noting the word *clogged* will direct you to option 4. Review these interventions if you had difficulty with this question.

Level of Cognitive Ability: Application
Client Needs: Safe, Effective Care Environment
Integrated Concept/Process: Nursing Process/Implementation
Content Area: Fundamental Skills

Reference:
deWit, S. (2001). *Fundamental concepts and skills for nursing.* Philadelphia: W.B. Saunders, p. 495.

---

53. A client with depression who was admitted to the psychiatric unit the previous day suddenly begins smiling and stating that the current episode of depression has lifted. The client continues to be talkative and engages in conversation with other clients on the unit. The licensed practical nurse (LPN) consults with the registered

Answer: 2

Rationale: A depressed client hospitalized for only one day is unlikely to have a dramatic cure. A sudden elevation in mood probably indicates that the client has decided to harm himself or herself. An increase in the level of suicide precaution is indicated to keep the client safe. The other options are not indicated (option 1) or could place the client at increased risk (options 3 and 4).

nurse knowing that which of the following changes should be made to the client's treatment plan?

1   Allow increased "in room" activities
2   Increase the level of suicide precautions
3   Allow the client to spend time off the unit
4   Reduce the dosage of antidepressant medication

Test-Taking Strategy: Use the process of elimination. Each of the incorrect options supports the client's idea that the depression has resolved. Keeping in mind that safety is of the utmost importance, eliminate each of the incorrect options. If this question was difficult, review care of the depressed client.

Level of Cognitive Ability: Comprehension
Client Needs: Safe, Effective Care Environment
Integrated Concept/Process: Nursing Process/Planning
Content Area: Mental Health

Reference:
Varcarolis, E. (2002). *Foundations of psychiatric mental health nursing* (4th ed.). Philadelphia: W.B. Saunders, p. 461.

---

54. A nurse who is assisting in the care of suicidal clients in a psychiatric nursing unit would plan to implement special precautions at which of the following times of increased risk?

1   8 AM to 2 PM
2   Shift change
3   Day shift
4   Weekdays

Answer: 2
Rationale: During the change of shifts, fewer staff members may be available to observe clients. The staff in a psychiatric nursing unit should increase precautions during shift change for clients identified as suicidal. Other times of increased risk for suicides are weekends (not weekdays), and the night shift (not day shift).

Test-Taking Strategy: Use the process of elimination. Remember that options that are similar are not likely to be correct. With this in mind, eliminate options 1 and 3 first. Choose between the remaining options by selecting the time when fewer staff members would be available to observe clients. Review care of the client at risk for suicide if you had difficulty with this question.

Level of Cognitive Ability: Application
Client Needs: Safe, Effective Care Environment
Integrated Concept/Process: Nursing Process/Planning
Content Area: Mental Health

Reference:
Varcarolis, E. (2002). *Foundations of psychiatric mental health nursing* (4th ed.). Philadelphia: W.B. Saunders, p. 648.

---

55. A nurse is assisting in the admission of a postoperative client from the postanesthesia care unit to the surgical nursing unit. The nurse should do which of the following for the safety of the client?

1   Put the bed rails up after moving the client from the stretcher
2   Ask the client to slide from the stretcher to the bed
3   Move the client rapidly from the stretcher to the bed
4   Uncover the client before transferring him or her from the stretcher to the bed

Answer: 1
Rationale: Because the client may still be experiencing residual effects of anesthesia, the nurse should raise the side rails after transferring the client from the stretcher to the bed. It is not realistic to ask the client to slide from the stretcher to the bed because of the effects of anesthesia and postoperative pain. Hurried movements and rapid changes in position should be avoided since these predispose the client to hypotension. During the transfer of the client after surgery, the nurse should avoid exposing the client because of potential heat loss, respiratory infection, and shock.

Test-Taking Strategy: Use the process of elimination. Begin to answer this question by eliminating options 3 and 4 first because they are not standard nursing interventions. Choose between the remaining options knowing that the issue of the question is client safety, and the only option that addresses safety is option 1. Review care of the postoperative client if you had difficulty with this question.

Level of Cognitive Ability: Application
Client Needs: Safe, Effective Care Environment
Integrated Concept/Process: Nursing Process/Implementation
Content Area: Fundamental Skills

Reference:
Ignatavicius, D., & Workman, M. (2002). *Medical-surgical: critical thinking for collaborative care* (4th ed.). Philadelphia: W.B. Saunders, p. 286.

---

56. A nurse is caring for a child with a fever. The nurse implements which safe action when giving this child a tepid tub bath?

1 Add cool water slowly to the warmer bath water
2 Let the child soak in the tub for 10 minutes
3 Add isopropyl alcohol to the bath water
4 Warm the water to the same body temperature of the child

Answer: 1
Rationale: Cool water should be added to an already warm bath because this will cause the water temperature to slowly drop. The child will be able to gradually adjust to the changing water temperature and will not experience chilling. The child should be in a tepid tub bath for 20 to 30 minutes to achieve maximum results. Alcohol is toxic and contraindicated for tepid sponge or tub baths. To achieve the best cooling results for the child with a fever, the water temperature should be at least 2 degrees lower than the child's body temperature.

Test-Taking Strategy: Use the process of elimination. Begin to answer this question by eliminating option 4 because this would not lower the child's temperature. Eliminate option 3 next knowing that isopropyl alcohol should not be used. To choose correctly between the remaining options, you must be familiar with either the time frames indicated to lower temperature for a tepid bath or the proper methods for cooling the bath water. Review measures for hyperthermia if you had difficulty with this question.

Level of Cognitive Ability: Application
Client Needs: Safe, Effective Care Environment
Integrated Concept/Process: Nursing Process/Implementation
Content Area: Child Health

Reference:
Schulte, E., Price, D., & Gwin, J. (2001). *Thompson's pediatric nursing* (8th ed.). Philadelphia: W.B. Saunders, p. 352.

---

57. A nurse is assisting in the care of a child who underwent surgical repair of a cleft lip the previous day. The nurse would implement which safe nursing intervention when caring for the surgical incision?

1 Rinse the incision with sterile water after using diluted peroxide
2 Remove the Logan bar carefully to clean the incision
3 Clean the incision only if serous exudate forms

Answer: 1
Rationale: The incision should be rinsed with sterile water when it is cleaned with a solution other than water or saline. The Logan bar is intended to maintain integrity of the suture line; removing the Logan bar on the first postoperative day is incorrect because removal would increase tension on the surgical incision. The incision is cleaned after every feeding and when serous exudate forms. The incision should be dabbed and not rubbed to maintain its integrity.

Test-Taking Strategy: Use the process of elimination. Eliminate option 2 first recalling that the Logan bar maintains integrity of

4 Rub the incision gently with a sterile cotton-tipped swab

the suture line. Next eliminate option 3 because of the word *only* and option 4 because of the word *rub*. Review care of a child after surgical repair of a cleft lip if you had difficulty with this question.

Level of Cognitive Ability: Application
Client Needs: Safe, Effective Care Environment
Integrated Concept/Process: Nursing Process/Implementation
Content Area: Child Health

Reference:
Schulte, E. Price, D., & Gwin, J. (2001). *Thompson's pediatric nursing* (8th ed.). Philadelphia: W.B. Saunders, p. 91.

---

58. A nurse is assigned to care for an older client who has been identified as a victim of physical abuse. In planning care for this client, the nurse's priority is focused toward:

1 Referring the abusing family member for treatment
2 Adhering to the mandatory abuse reporting laws
3 Encouraging the client to file charges against the abuser
4 Removing the client from any immediate danger

Answer: 4
Rationale: Whenever the abused client remains in the abusive environment, priority must be placed on determining whether the person is in any immediate danger. If so, emergency action must be taken to remove him or her from the abusing situation. Options 1 and 2 may be appropriate interventions but are not the priority. Option 3 is not an appropriate intervention at this time and may produce increased fear and anxiety in the client.

Test-Taking Strategy: Use the process of elimination and eliminate option 3 first because this action may produce increased fear and anxiety in the client. Use Maslow's Hierarchy of Needs theory to select from the remaining options remembering that if a physiological need is not present, then safety is the priority. This should direct you to option 4, the only option that directly addresses client safety. Review care to the victim of abuse if you had difficulty with this question.

Level of Cognitive Ability: Application
Client Needs: Safe, Effective Care Environment
Integrated Concept/Process: Nursing Process/Planning
Content Area: Mental Health

Reference:
Lueckenotte, A. (2002). *Gerontologic nursing* (2nd ed.). St. Louis: Mosby, p. 37.

---

59. A nurse assists in developing a plan of care for a client who will be hospitalized for insertion of an internal cervical radiation implant. Which of the following will the nurse suggest to include in the client's plan of care?

1 Place the client in a private room near the nurses' station
2 Place a radiation sign on the door of the client's room
3 Reinsert the implant into the vagina immediately if it becomes dislodged

Answer: 2
Rationale: The client's room should be marked with appropriate signs stating the presence of radiation. The client should be placed in a private room at the end of the hall because this location provides less chance of radiation exposure to others. A lead container and long-handled forceps should be kept in the client's room at all times during internal radiation therapy. If the implant becomes dislodged, the nurse should pick up the implant with long-handled forceps and place it in the lead container. The nurse does not reinsert it. Visiting time is limited to 30 minutes per visit.

Test-Taking Strategy: Use the process of elimination and knowledge about the precaution and care of a client with a radiation

4 Limit visiting time to 60 minutes per visit

implant to answer the question. Eliminate option 4 because of the lengthy time frame for visits. Eliminate option 1 because of the words *near the nurses' station*. Knowing that it is not within the scope of nursing practice to reinsert an implant will assist in eliminating option 3. Review these precautions if you had difficulty with this question.

Level of Cognitive Ability: Application
Client Needs: Safe, Effective Care Environment
Integrated Concept/Process: Nursing Process/Planning
Content Area: Adult Health/Oncology

Reference:
Black, J., Hawks, J., & Keene, A. (2001). *Medical-surgical nursing: clinical management for positive outcomes* (6th ed.). Philadelphia: W.B. Saunders, p. 378.

---

60. A nurse is observing a nursing assistant talking to a client who is hearing impaired. The nurse would intervene if which of the following were performed by the nursing assistant during communication with the client?
1 The nursing assistant is facing the client when speaking
2 The nursing assistant is speaking clearly to the client
3 The nursing assistant is speaking directly into the impaired ear
4 The nursing assistant is speaking in a normal tone

Answer: 3
Rationale: When communicating with a hearing-impaired client, the nurse should speak in a normal tone to the client and should not shout. The nurse should talk directly to the client while facing the client and speak clearly. If the client does not seem to understand what is said, the nurse should express the statement differently. Moving closer to the client and toward the better ear may improve communication, but the nurse should avoid talking directly into the impaired ear.

Test-Taking Strategy: Use the process of elimination and knowledge regarding effective communication techniques for the hearing impaired to answer this question. Noting the key words *would intervene* will direct you to option 3. If you had difficulty with this question, review these techniques.

Level of Cognitive Ability: Application
Client Needs: Safe, Effective Care Environment
Integrated Concept/Process: Nursing Process/Implementation
Content Area: Adult Health/Ear

Reference:
deWit, S. (2001). *Fundamental concepts and skills for nursing*. Philadelphia: W.B. Saunders, p. 93.

---

61. Ultraviolet (UVL) light therapy is prescribed in the treatment plan for a client with psoriasis. The nurse reinforces instructions to the client regarding safety measures related to the therapy. Which of the following statements if made by the client indicates a need for further instructions?
1 "I should wear eye goggles during the treatment."
2 "Each treatment will last 30 minutes."
3 "I will cover my face with a loosely applied covering."

Answer: 2
Rationale: Safety precautions are required during UVL therapy. Most UVL treatments require the person to stand in a light treatment chamber for up to 15 minutes. It is best to expose only those areas requiring treatment to the UVL. Placing protective wrap-around goggles prevents exposure of the eyes to UVL. The face should be shielded with a loosely applied cloth if it is unaffected. Direct contact with the light bulbs of the treatment unit should be avoided to prevent burning of the skin.

Test-Taking Strategy: Use the process of elimination. Note the key words *indicates a need for further instructions*. Note that option 2 addresses a time frame of 30 minutes, which is an extensive time

4 "I will expose only the area requiring treatment."

period for exposure to UVL. If you had difficulty with this question, review client instructions for UVL treatments.

Level of Cognitive Ability: Comprehension
Client Needs: Safe, Effective Care Environment
Integrated Concept/Process: Teaching/Learning
Content Area: Adult Health/Integumentary

Reference:
Black, J., Hawks, J., & Keene, A. (2001). *Medical-surgical nursing: clinical management for positive outcomes* (6th ed.). Philadelphia: W.B. Saunders, p. 1293.

---

62. A nurse is assigned to care for a client who sustained a burn injury. The nurse reviews the physician's orders and would question the registered nurse about which of the following?
1 Administer morphine sulfate intramuscularly every 3 hours PRN for pain
2 Maintain the nasogastric tube to intermittent suction
3 Monitor urine output hourly
4 Monitor weight daily

Answer: 1
Rationale: Oral, subcutaneous, and intramuscular routes for administering medications are contraindicated in the burned client because of the poor absorption factor. When fluid balance is stabilized, oral narcotic agents can be used. Options 2, 3, and 4 are all appropriate interventions for the client with a burn.

Test-Taking Strategy: Use the process of elimination. Read each option carefully and think about the physiology that occurs in the client with a burn. Recalling that poor absorption will occur with medications administered by the oral, subcutaneous, or intramuscular routes will direct you to option 1. Review pain management for the burned client if you had difficulty with this question.

Level of Cognitive Ability: Application
Client Needs: Safe, Effective Care Environment
Integrated Concept/Process: Nursing Process/Implementation
Content Area: Adult Health/Integumentary

Reference:
Black, J., Hawks, J., & Keene, A. (2001). *Medical-surgical nursing: clinical management for positive outcomes* (6th ed.). Philadelphia: W.B. Saunders, p. 1343.

---

63. A nurse is caring for an older client who had a hip pinned after being fractured. In planning nursing care, the nurse would avoid which of the following to minimize the chance for further injury?
1 Keeping the call bell in reach
2 Answering the call bell promptly
3 Leaving the side rails down
4 Ensuring that the nightlight is working

Answer: 3
Rationale: Safe nursing actions intended to prevent injury to the client include keeping the side rails up, keeping the bed in low position, and providing a call bell that is within the client's reach. Responding promptly to the client's use of the call light minimizes the chance that the client will try to get up alone, which could result in a fall. Nightlights are built into the lighting systems of most facilities, and these bulbs should be routinely checked to ensure that they are working.

Test-Taking Strategy: Use the process of elimination and note the key word *avoid*. Because options 1 and 2 are standard safety measures, they are eliminated first as possible choices. Use of a nightlight would help prevent falls, which is also helpful, and can also be eliminated. Review safety measures if you had difficulty with this question.

Level of Cognitive Ability: Application
Client Needs: Safe, Effective Care Environment
Integrated Concept/Process: Nursing Process/Implementation
Content Area: Adult Health/Musculoskeletal

Reference:
Potter, P., & Perry, A. (2001). *Fundamentals of nursing* (5th ed.). St. Louis: Mosby, p. 1035.

---

64. A nurse has reinforced instructions to a parent regarding the safe methods to prevent Lyme disease. Which of the following statements if made by a parent would indicate the need for additional instruction?
1   "We should avoid the use of insect repellents because they will attract the ticks."
2   "Wearing long-sleeved tops and long pants is important."
3   "We should wear hats when we go on our hiking trip."
4   "We should wear closed shoes and socks that can be pulled up over the pants."

Answer: 1
Rationale: To prevent Lyme disease, individuals should be instructed to use an insect repellent on the skin and clothes in areas where ticks are likely to be found. Long-sleeved tops and long pants, closed shoes, and a hat or cap should be worn. If possible, heavily wooded areas or areas with thick underbrush should be avoided. Socks can be pulled up and over pant legs to prevent ticks from entering under clothing.

Test-Taking Strategy: Note the key words *need for additional instructions*. Use the process of elimination noting that option 1 uses the word *avoid*. Reading carefully will assist in directing you to this option. If you had difficulty with this question, review measures to prevent contact with ticks.

Level of Cognitive Ability: Comprehension
Client Needs: Safe, Effective Care Environment
Integrated Concept/Process: Teaching/Learning
Content Area: Adult Health/Integumentary

Reference:
Black, J., Hawks, J., & Keene, A. (2001). *Medical-surgical nursing: clinical management for positive outcomes* (6th ed.). Philadelphia: W.B. Saunders, p. 1829.

---

65. A client with paraplegia has a risk for injury related to spasticity of leg muscles. The nurse avoids which of the following actions that would be least helpful in dealing with this problem?
1   Using restraints to immobilize the limbs
2   Administering a prn order for a muscle relaxant
3   Removing potentially harmful objects placed near the client
4   Performing range of motion exercises with the affected limbs

Answer: 1
Rationale: Using limb restraints will not alleviate spasticity and could harm the client. Their use should be avoided. Use of muscle relaxants may be helpful if the spasms cause discomfort to the client or pose a risk to the client's safety. Removing potentially harmful objects is a good basic safety measure. Range of motion exercises are beneficial in stretching muscles, which may diminish spasticity.

Test-Taking Strategy: Use the process of elimination and note the key words *least helpful*. The wording of the question guides you to look for a response that is potentially harmful to the client. This will direct you to option 1. If this question was difficult, review the care of the client with limb spasticity.

Level of Cognitive Ability: Application
Client Needs: Safe, Effective Care Environment
Integrated Concept/Process: Nursing Process/Implementation
Content Area: Adult Health/Neurological

Reference:
Black, J., Hawks, J., & Keene, A. (2001). *Medical-surgical nursing: clinical management for positive outcomes* (6th ed.). Philadelphia: W.B. Saunders, p. 2050.

66. A client is admitted to the hospital with severe hypoparathyroidism. The nurse would do which of the following activities to promote client safety?
1 Use a waist restraint continuously
2 Institute seizure precautions
3 Keep the room slightly cool
4 Keep the head of bed lowered

Answer: 2
Rationale: Hypoparathyroidism results from insufficient parathyroid hormone, leading to low serum calcium levels. Hypocalcemia can cause tetany, which if untreated can lead to seizures. The nurse should institute seizure precautions to maintain a safe environment. The other options do nothing to help this health problem or promote a safe environment for this client.

Test-Taking Strategy: Use the process of elimination and note the key words *hypoparathyroidism* and *client safety*. Answer this question by recalling the complications of low calcium levels, which are tetany and ultimately seizures. With this in mind, eliminate each of the incorrect options. Review the complications associated with hypoparathyroidism if you had difficulty with this question.

Level of Cognitive Ability: Application
Client Needs: Safe, Effective Care Environment
Integrated Concept/Process: Nursing Process/Implementation
Content Area: Adult Health/Endocrine

Reference:
Black, J., Hawks, J., & Keene, A. (2001). *Medical-surgical nursing: clinical management for positive outcomes* (6th ed.). Philadelphia: W.B. Saunders, p. 1114.

67. A nurse is assisting in preparing a plan of care for a client being admitted to the hospital for insertion of a cervical radiation implant. Which of the following would the nurse suggest for this client following insertion of the implant?
1 Out of bed in a chair only
2 Elevate the head of the bed 45 degrees
3 Maintain bed rest
4 Maintain the client in the side-lying position

Answer: 3
Rationale: The client with a cervical radiation implant should be maintained on bed rest in the dorsal position to prevent movement of the radiation source. The head of the bed is elevated to a maximum of 10 to 15 degrees for comfort. Turning the client on the side is avoided. If turning is absolutely necessary, a pillow is placed between the knees and, with the body in straight alignment, the client is logrolled.

Test-Taking Strategy: Use the process of elimination. To answer the question, consider the anatomical location of the implant and the risk of dislodgement. Options 1, 2, and 4 can cause dislodgement of the implant. If you had difficulty with this question, review care to the client with a radiation implant.

Level of Cognitive Ability: Application
Client Needs: Safe, Effective Care Environment
Integrated Concept/Process: Nursing Process/Planning
Content Area: Adult Health/Oncology

Reference:
Black, J., Hawks, J., & Keene, A. (2001). *Medical-surgical nursing: clinical management for positive outcomes* (6th ed.). Philadelphia: W.B. Saunders, p. 378.

68. A nurse is assigned to care for a client who has returned to the nursing unit after an oral cholecystogram. At this point in time, the nurse would question which of the following physician's orders in the medical record?

1   Maintain a clear liquid status for 72 hours
2   Monitor the client for abdominal discomfort
3   Monitor the client's hydration status
4   Assess for nausea and vomiting

Answer: 1

Rationale: The client should be able to resume the usual diet once the nurse is assured that the client's gastrointestinal (GI) function is normal. It is not necessary to keep the client on clear liquids for 72 hours after the procedure. The nurse would monitor the client for complaints of GI discomfort and nausea and vomiting. The nurse would also assess the client's hydration status as part of routine care for the client undergoing a GI diagnostic test.

Test-Taking Strategy: Use the process of elimination. Note the key words *at this point* and *question*. This tells you that the correct option is one that would have been needed before the procedure, but is no longer necessary. Note that options 2, 3, and 4 are assessments that are appropriate after this procedure; option 1 is an intervention that is not necessary at this time. Review postprocedure care after an oral cholecystogram if you had difficulty with this question.

Level of Cognitive Ability: Application
Client Needs: Safe, Effective Care Environment
Integrated Concept/Process: Nursing Process/Implementation
Content Area: Adult Health/Gastrointestinal

Reference:
Black, J., Hawks, J., & Keene, A. (2001). *Medical-surgical nursing: clinical management for positive outcomes* (6th ed.). Philadelphia: W.B. Saunders, p. 1085.

69. A nurse employed in a physician's office is asked to check the client for the results of the Purified Protein Derivative (PPD) implanted 72 hours previously. The nurse reads the PPD as measuring 11 mm induration in diameter. Which of the following actions would the nurse take next?

1   Document the normal finding in the client's record
2   Ask the client for permission to repeat the test
3   Notify the physician
4   Tell the client to make an appointment with a pulmonologist

Answer: 3

Rationale: An area of induration that measures 10 mm or more is considered a positive reading. The nurse who observes a positive PPD reading notifies the physician immediately. The physician would then order a chest x-ray to determine whether the client has clinically active tuberculosis (TB) or old, healed lesions. A sputum culture would then be done to confirm a diagnosis of active TB. Option 1 is incorrect because the reading is not a normal finding. Option 2 is incorrect because the test results are positive. The physician, not a nurse, would request a consultation with a pulmonologist.

Test-Taking Strategy: Use the process of elimination. Note the key word *next*. Begin to answer this question by eliminating option 1 as incorrect. Option 4 is eliminated next because it is not a nursing responsibility to obtain physician consultations. Knowing that the results indicate a positive test will assist in directing you to option 3. Review this test if you had difficulty with this question.

Level of Cognitive Ability: Application
Client Needs: Safe, Effective Care Environment
Integrated Concept/Process: Nursing Process/Implementation
Content Area: Adult Health/Respiratory

Reference:
Black, J., Hawks, J., & Keene, A. (2001). *Medical-surgical nursing: clinical management for positive outcomes* (6th ed.). Philadelphia: W.B. Saunders, p. 1719.

70. A nurse reinforced information about the disease and recuperation to the client diagnosed with tuberculosis. The nurse evaluates that the client understands the information presented if the client states that it is possible to return to work when:

1   The PPD and chest x-ray are negative
2   A sputum culture and a PPD test are negative
3   Three sputum cultures are negative
4   Five sputum cultures are negative

Answer: 3

Rationale: The client must have sputum cultures performed every 2 to 4 weeks after initiation of antituberculosis medication therapy. The client may return to work when the results of three sputum cultures are negative because the client is considered noninfectious at that point. One negative sputum culture is not sufficient and five negative cultures are unnecessary.

Test-Taking Strategy: Use the process of elimination. Knowing that a positive PPD never reverts to negative helps you to eliminate options 1 and 2. From the remaining options, it is necessary to know that three negative sputum cultures are required. If this question was difficult, review the teaching points related to this infectious disease.

Level of Cognitive Ability: Comprehension
Client Needs: Safe, Effective Care Environment
Integrated Concept/Process: Nursing Process/Evaluation
Content Area: Adult Health/Respiratory

Reference:
Black, J., Hawks, J., & Keene, A. (2001). *Medical-surgical nursing: clinical management for positive outcomes* (6th ed.). Philadelphia: W.B. Saunders, p. 1720.

---

71. A registered nurse (RN) tells a licensed practical nurse (LPN) that a client who is suspected of having tuberculosis (TB) is being admitted to the hospital. The LPN is asked to prepare a room for the client. The LPN prepares the room knowing that this client's room must have:

1   Venting to the roof and ultraviolet light
2   Venting to the outside, 6 air exchanges per hour, and ultraviolet light
3   Ultraviolet light and 3 air exchanges per hour
4   Ten air exchanges per hour and venting to the roof

Answer: 2

Rationale: The client must be admitted to a private room that has at least six air exchanges per hour and negative pressure in relation to surrounding areas. The room should be vented to the outside and have ultraviolet lights installed. Options 1, 3, and 4 are inaccurate.

Test-Taking Strategy: Begin to answer this question by recalling the specific requirements of physical facilities that are used in the care of clients with TB. Knowing that ultraviolet light is required helps you to eliminate option 4. The correct option is the only one that addresses all of the room requirements. Review these protective requirements if you had difficulty with this question.

Level of Cognitive Ability: Application
Client Needs: Safe, Effective Care Environment
Integrated Concept/Process: Nursing Process/Planning
Content Area: Adult Health/Respiratory

Reference:
Black, J., Hawks, J., & Keene, A. (2001). *Medical-surgical nursing: clinical management for positive outcomes* (6th ed.). Philadelphia: W.B. Saunders, p. 1722.

---

72. A nurse is planning to give an injection to a client with acquired immunodeficiency syndrome (AIDS). The nurse plans to do which of the following after giving the injection?

Answer: 3

Rationale: Standard (Universal) Precautions include specific guidelines for handling of sharps. Needles should not be recapped, bent, broken, or cut after use. They should be disposed of in a labeled, impermeable container that is specifically used

1   Break the needle and discard it
2   Place the uncapped needle and syringe in a labeled cardboard box
3   Place the uncapped needle and syringe in a labeled, rigid plastic container
4   Recap the needle and discard the syringe in a disposal unit

for this purpose. Needles should not be discarded in cardboard boxes because they could puncture the cardboard, causing needle-stick injury. Needles should always be properly discarded after use.

Test-Taking Strategy: Use the process of elimination. Recalling that needles should never be broken or recapped will assist in eliminating options 1 and 4. Noting that option 2 identifies a container that could be punctured by the needle will assist in eliminating this option. If this question was difficult, review these principles.

Level of Cognitive Ability: Application
Client Needs: Safe, Effective Care Environment
Integrated Concept/Process: Nursing Process/Implementation
Content Area: Adult Health/Respiratory

Reference:
Potter, P., & Perry, A. (2001). *Fundamentals of nursing* (5th ed.). St. Louis: Mosby, p. 859.

---

73. A licensed practical nurse (LPN) is asked to prepare a room for a child who will be admitted to the pediatric unit with a diagnosis of tonic-clonic seizures. The LPN prepares the room and plans to place which of the following items at the bedside?
1   Suction apparatus and an airway
2   A tracheotomy set and oxygen
3   An emergency cart and padded side rails
4   An endotracheal tube and an airway

Answer: 1
Rationale: Tonic-clonic seizures cause tightening of all body muscles followed by tremors. An obstructed airway and increased oral secretions are the major complications during and after a seizure. Suction apparatus and an airway are helpful to prevent choking and cyanosis. Options 2, 3, and 4 are incorrect. Inserting a tracheostomy or endotracheal tube is not done. It is not necessary to have an emergency cart at the bedside, but a cart should be available in the treatment room or in the nursing unit.

Test-Taking Strategy: Use the process of elimination. Recalling that tonic-clonic seizures produce excessive oral secretions and airway obstruction will assist in selecting the correct option. If you had difficulty with this question, review the plan of care associated with seizure precautions.

Level of Cognitive Ability: Application
Client Needs: Safe, Effective Care Environment
Integrated Concept/Process: Nursing Process/Planning
Content Area: Child Health

Reference:
Schulte, E., Price, D., & Gwin, J. (2001). *Thompson's pediatric nursing* (8th ed.). Philadelphia: W.B. Saunders, p. 223.

---

74. An extremely angry and aggressive client in the mental health inpatient unit has been placed in restraints. When working with this client, the nurse should suggest removal of the restraints when the client:
1   Initiates no aggressive acts for an hour after the release of two leg restraints

Answer: 1
Rationale: The best indicator that the client's behavior is under control is when the client refrains from aggression after being partially released from the restraints. Restraints are initially placed around the waist, wrists, and ankles. The ankle restraints are removed first, one at a time, at regular intervals. The wrist and waist restraints are removed together when the client continues to exhibit nonaggressive behavior.

2 Has been sedated and is still experiencing its effects

3 Divulges all of the reasons for the aggressive behavior

4 Apologizes and tells the nurse that it will not happen again

Test-Taking Strategy: To answer this question accurately, you must be familiar with the legal and ethical issues involving restraints as they are used with aggressive mental illness. Review this protocol or procedure if you had difficulty with this question.

Level of Cognitive Ability: Application
Client Needs: Safe, Effective Care Environment
Integrated Concept/Process: Nursing Process/Implementation
Content Area: Mental Health

Reference:
Varcarolis, E. (2002). *Foundations of psychiatric mental health nursing* (4th ed.). Philadelphia: W.B. Saunders, p. 175.

---

75. A client who has been admitted to the mental health unit with obsessive-compulsive disorder repeatedly cleans the bathroom fixtures. The client has become enraged and has started to bite and kick the roommate for occupying the bathroom. Which of the following actions should the nurse take first?

1 Provide a safe environment for both clients

2 Notify the risk management department

3 Physically restrain the client

4 Administer a medication to provide chemical restraint

Answer: 1
Rationale: The first action of the nurse is to provide an environment that is safe for both clients. This may take a variety of forms, depending on the individual circumstance, agency protocols, and written physician orders. Seclusion, chemical restraint, and physical restraint are used only when alternative and less restrictive measures are not effective in controlling the client's behavior.

Test-Taking Strategy: Use Maslow's Hierarchy of Needs theory to answer this question. Physiological and safety needs come first. In this instance, the correct answer is the option that is the most global and meets the needs of both clients identified in the question. Review care to the client who is physically aggressive if you had difficulty with this question.

Level of Cognitive Ability: Application
Client Needs: Safe, Effective Care Environment
Integrated Concept/Process: Nursing Process/Implementation
Content Area: Mental Health

Reference:
Varcarolis, E. (2002). *Foundations of psychiatric mental health nursing* (4th ed.). Philadelphia: W.B. Saunders, p. 379.

---

76. A physician orders a 12-lead electrocardiogram (ECG) to be performed on a client. The client is concerned about the safety of the test, and the nurse provides information to the client. Which of the following would indicate that the client understands the test?

1 "I cannot breathe while the ECG is running."

2 "When the ECG begins, I must take a deep breath."

3 "I should lie still while the ECG is being done."

4 "If I move when the ECG begins I will be shocked."

Answer: 3
Rationale: Good contact between the skin and electrodes is necessary to obtain a clear 12-lead ECG printout. Therefore the electrodes are placed on the flat surfaces of the skin just above the ankles and wrists. Movement may cause a disruption in that contact. The client does not have to hold the breath or take a deep breath during the procedure. The client should be reassured that the procedure will not produce a shock.

Test-Taking Strategy: Use the process of elimination. While a 12-lead ECG is being done, it is best if the client does not move the extremities. This will aid in obtaining a clear ECG. Options 1, 2, and 4 are inappropriate statements. Review the procedure for obtaining an ECG if you had difficulty with this question.

Level of Cognitive Ability: Comprehension
Client Needs: Safe Effective Care Environment
Integrated Concept/Process: Nursing Process/Evaluation
Content Area: Adult Health/Cardiovascular

Reference:
Ignatavicius, D., & Workman, M. (2002). *Medical-surgical: critical thinking for collaborative care* (4th ed.). Philadelphia: W.B. Saunders, p. 657.

---

77. A nurse is assisting in planning the discharge of a client with chronic anxiety. The nurse assists in selecting the goals that will promote a safe environment at home. The most appropriate maintenance goal should focus on which of the following?

1   Continuing contact with a crisis counselor
2   Identifying anxiety producing situations
3   Ignoring feelings of anxiety
4   Eliminating all anxiety from daily situations

Answer: 2

Rationale: Recognizing situations that produce anxiety allows the client to prepare to cope with anxiety or avoid a specific stimulus. Counselors will not be available for all anxiety-producing situations, and this option does not encourage the development of internal strengths. Ignoring feelings will not resolve anxiety. It is impossible to eliminate all anxiety from daily situations.

Test-Taking Strategy: Use the process of elimination. Eliminate option 4 first because of the word *all*. Eliminate option 3 next because feelings should not be ignored. From the remaining options, select option 2 instead of option 1 because option 2 is more client centered and provides preparation for the client to deal with anxiety should it occur. Review goals for the client with chronic anxiety if you had difficulty with this question.

Level of Cognitive Ability: Application
Client Needs: Safe, Effective Care Environment
Integrated Concept/Process: Nursing Process/Planning
Content Area: Mental Health

Reference:
Varcarolis, E. (2002). *Foundations of psychiatric mental health nursing* (4th ed.). Philadelphia: W.B. Saunders, p. 325.

---

78. A nurse is planning to reinforce instructions to a client with chronic vertigo about safety measures to prevent worsening of symptoms or injury. The nurse plans to tell the client that it is important to:

1   Drive at times when the client does not feel dizzy
2   Go to the bedroom and lie down when vertigo is experienced
3   Remove throw rugs and clutter in the home
4   Turn the head slowly when spoken to

Answer: 3

Rationale: The client with chronic vertigo should avoid driving and using public transportation. The sudden movements involved in each could precipitate an attack. To further prevent vertigo attacks, the client should change position slowly and should turn the entire body, not just the head, when spoken to. If vertigo does occur, the client should immediately sit down or grasp the nearest piece of stable furniture. The client should maintain a clutter-free home with throw rugs removed because the effort of regaining balance after slipping could trigger vertigo.

Test-Taking Strategy: Use the process of elimination. Begin to answer this question by eliminating options 1 and 2 first because they put the client at greatest risk of injury secondary to vertigo. Option 3 is a safer intervention than option 4. Review safety measures for the client with chronic vertigo if you had difficulty with this question.

Level of Cognitive Ability: Application
Client Needs: Safe, Effective Care Environment
Integrated Concept/Process: Self-Care
Content Area: Adult Health/Neurological

Reference:
Ignatavicius, D., & Workman, M. (2002). *Medical-surgical nursing: critical thinking for collaborative care* (4th ed.). Philadelphia: W.B. Saunders, p. 1068.

---

79. A nurse is assigned to care for a client with Parkinson's disease who has recently begun taking L-dopa (levodopa). Which of the following is most important to check before ambulating the client?
1 Assistive devices used by the client
2 The degree of intention tremors exhibited by the client
3 The client's history of falls
4 The client's postural (orthostatic) vital signs

Answer: 4
Rationale: Clients with Parkinson's disease are at risk for postural (orthostatic) hypotension from the disease. This problem worsens when L-dopa is introduced because the medication can also cause postural hypotension, thus increasing the client's risk for falls. Although knowledge of the client's use of assistive devices and history of falls is helpful, it is not the most important piece of data based on the information in this question. Clients with Parkinson's disease generally have resting rather than intention tremors.

Test-Taking Strategy: Use the process of elimination and focus on the issue, the most important piece of data before ambulation for the client on L-dopa. Postural hypotension presents the greatest safety risk to the client. Review safety measures for the client with Parkinson's disease if you had difficulty with this question.

Level of Cognitive Ability: Comprehension
Client Needs: Safe, Effective Care Environment
Integrated Concept/Process: Nursing Process/Data Collection
Content Area: Pharmacology

Reference:
Hodgson, B., & Kizior, R. (2003). *Saunders nursing drug handbook 2003.* Philadelphia: W.B. Saunders, p. 169.

---

80. A nurse is giving a bed bath to a client who is on strict bed rest. To safely increase venous return, the nurse bathes the client's extremities by using:
1 Long, firm strokes from distal to proximal areas
2 Firm, circular strokes from proximal to distal areas
3 Short, patting strokes from distal to proximal areas
4 Smooth, light strokes back and forth from proximal to distal areas

Answer: 1
Rationale: Long, firm strokes in the direction of venous flow promote venous return when the extremities are bathed. Circular strokes are used on the face. Short, patting strokes and light strokes are not as comfortable for the client and do not promote venous return.

Test-Taking Strategy: Use the process of elimination. Eliminate options 2 and 4 first because a stroke from proximal to distal will not promote venous return. Select option 1 rather than option 3 because long, firm strokes will promote venous return and client comfort. Review this procedure if you had difficulty with this question.

Level of Cognitive Ability: Application
Client Needs: Safe, Effective Care Environment
Integrated Concept/Process: Nursing Process/Implementation
Content Area: Fundamental Skills

Reference:
deWit, S. (2001). *Fundamental concepts and skills for nursing.* Philadelphia: W.B. Saunders, p. 296.

81. A nurse is preparing to give an intramuscular (IM) injection that is irritating to the subcutaneous tissues. The drug reference recommends that it be given using the Z-track technique. Which of the following procedural steps would cause tracking the medication through the subcutaneous tissues?
1   Preparing a 0.2-mL air lock in the syringe after drawing up the medication
2   Massaging the site after injecting the medication
3   Attaching a new sterile needle to the syringe after drawing up the medication
4   Retracting the skin to the side before piercing the skin with the needle

Answer: 2

Rationale: The Z-track variation of the standard IM technique is used to administer IM medications that are highly irritating to subcutaneous and skin tissues. Attaching a new sterile needle is done so that the new needle will not have any medication adhering to the outside that could be irritating to the tissues. Preparing an air lock keeps the needle clean of medication on insertion and, as the air is injected behind the medication, will provide a seal at the point of insertion to prevent tracking of the medication. Retracting the skin provides a seal over the injected medication to prevent tracking through the subcutaneous tissues. The site should not be massaged because this can lead to tissue irritation.

Test-Taking Strategy: Use the process of elimination and focus on the issue, tracking the medication. Options 1, 3, and 4 are procedural steps for Z-track injection. Option 2 is incorrect because Z-track injections are not massaged because this could lead to tracking and tissue irritation. Review this procedure for administering medications if you had difficulty with this question.

Level of Cognitive Ability: Application
Client Needs: Safe, Effective Care Environment
Integrated Concept/Process: Nursing Process/Implementation
Content Area: Fundamental Skills

Reference:
deWit, S. (2001). *Fundamental concepts and skills for nursing.* Philadelphia: W.B. Saunders, p. 708.

82. A nurse is preparing to transfer an average-sized client with right-sided hemiplegia from the bed to the wheelchair. The client is able to support weight on the unaffected side. The nurse plans to use the hemiplegic transfer technique. The client is sitting upright in bed with the legs dangling over the side. For the safest transfer, where should the wheelchair be positioned?
1   Near the client's right leg
2   Next to either leg
3   As space in the room permits
4   Near the client's left leg

Answer: 4

Rationale: Although space in the room is an important consideration for placement of the wheelchair for a transfer, when the client has an affected lower extremity, movement should always occur toward the client's unaffected (strong) side. For example, if the client's right leg is affected, and the client is sitting on the edge of the bed, the wheelchair is positioned next to the client's left side. This wheelchair position allows the client to use the unaffected leg effectively and safely.

Test-Taking Strategy: Use the process of elimination and focus on the issue, the safest transfer for the client. Although option 3 is a consideration for wheelchair position, it is not the safest answer. Option 4 will provide the safest transfer because positioning the wheelchair next to the client's unaffected leg allows the client to use the stronger leg more effectively for a safe transfer. Review transfer techniques if you had difficulty with this question.

Level of Cognitive Ability: Application
Client Needs: Safe, Effective Care Environment
Integrated Concept/Process: Nursing Process/Implementation
Content Area: Fundamental Skills

Reference:
deWit, S. (2001). *Fundamental concepts and skills for nursing.* Philadelphia: W.B. Saunders, p. 273.

83. A nurse is preparing to suction a client's tracheostomy. To ideally promote deep breathing and coughing, in which position should the client be safely placed?
1 Supine position
2 Lateral position
3 High-Fowler's position
4 Semi-Fowler's position

Answer: 4
Rationale: If it is not contraindicated, before suctioning a tracheostomy, the client is placed in semi-Fowler's position to promote deep breathing, maximum lung expansion, and productive coughing. With the client in this position, gravity pulls downward on the diaphragm, which allows greater chest expansion and lung volume. Options 1 and 2 would not provide maximum lung expansion. The high-Fowler's position would not allow for easy visualization of the tracheotomy or easy access of the suction catheter.

Test-Taking Strategy: Use the process of elimination. You can easily eliminate options 1 and 2 first because they are similar. From the remaining options, eliminate option 3 because the high-Fowler's position would not allow for easy visualization of the tracheotomy or easy access of the suction catheter. Review this procedure if you had difficulty with this question.

Level of Cognitive Ability: Application
Client Needs: Safe, Effective Care Environment
Integrated Concept/Process: Nursing Process/Implementation
Content Area: Fundamental Skills

Reference:
deWit, S. (2001). *Fundamental concepts and skills for nursing.* Philadelphia: W.B. Saunders, p. 537.

84. The pregnant client is at full term. The fetal heart rate (FHR) is being monitored for a baseline rate. The nurse is satisfied with the results and tells the client that the baby is safe and that the baby's heart rate is within normal limits. The nurse bases this interpretation on which of the following data?
1 FHR of 90 beats per minute
2 FHR of 140 beats per minute
3 FHR of 80 beats per minute
4 FHR of 170 beats per minute

Answer: 2
Rationale: The average FHR at term is 140 beats per minute. The normal range is 110 to 160 beats per minute; therefore option 2 is the only correct option.

Test-Taking Strategy: Knowledge of the normal fetal heart rate is required to answer this question. Review this content if you had difficulty with this question.

Level of Cognitive Ability: Comprehension
Client Needs: Safe, Effective Care Environment
Integrated Concept/Process: Nursing Process/Data Collection
Content Area: Maternity

Reference:
Burroughs, A., & Leifer, G. (2002). *Maternity nursing* (8th ed.). Philadelphia: W.B. Saunders, p. 83.

85. A nurse is caring for a client with a grave clinical condition who is a potential organ donor. The nurse reviews the client's medical record and would identify a contraindication to organ donation if which of the following were documented in the client's record?
1 Allergy to penicillin-type antibiotics
2 Age of 38 years

Answer: 3
Rationale: A potential organ donor must meet age eligibility requirements, which vary by organ. For example, age must not exceed 65 (kidney donation), 55 (pancreas and liver), or 40 (heart) years old. The client should be free of communicable disease, such as human immunodeficiency virus or hepatitis, and the involved organ may not be diseased. Another contraindication to transplant is malignancy, with the exception of noninvolved skin and cornea.

3   Hepatitis B infection
4   Negative rapid plasma reagin (RPR) laboratory result

Test-Taking Strategy: Use the process of elimination. The key word is *contraindication*. With this in mind, eliminate option 2 first. Because allergies are not part of the decision-making criteria, eliminate option 1 next. Option 4 indicates an absence of syphilis (a communicable disease), which leaves option 3 (hepatitis B) as the correct option. Review the contraindications to organ donation if you had difficulty with this question.

Level of Cognitive Ability: Comprehension
Client Needs: Safe, Effective Care Environment
Integrated Concept/Process: Nursing Process/Data Collection
Content Area: Fundamental Skills

Reference:
Black, J., Hawks, J., & Keene, A. (2001). *Medical-surgical nursing: clinical management for positive outcomes* (6th ed.). Philadelphia: W.B. Saunders, p. 2219.

---

86. A nurse is assigned to care for a client with cervical cancer. The client has an internal radiation implant. Which of the following required items would the nurse ensure is kept in the client's room during this treatment?
1   A bedside commode
2   A lead shield
3   Long handled forceps and a lead container
4   A number 16 Foley catheter

Answer: 3
Rationale: In the case of dislodgement of an internal radiation implant, the radioactive source is never touched with the bare hands. It is retrieved with long-handled forceps and placed in the lead container kept in the client's room. In many situations, the client has a Foley catheter inserted and is on bed rest during treatment to prevent dislodgement. A lead shield, although one may be in the room, is not the required item. Nurses wear a dosimeter badge while in the client's room to measure the exposure to radiation.

Test-Taking Strategy: Use the process of elimination. Eliminate options 1 and 4 because they are similar and relate to urinary output. From the remaining options, select option 3 instead of option 2, keeping in mind the risk of dislodgement that can occur. Review these guidelines if you had difficulty with this question.

Level of Cognitive Ability: Application
Client Needs: Safe, Effective Care Environment
Integrated Concept/Process: Nursing Process/Implementation
Content Area: Fundamental Skills

Reference:
Black, J., Hawks, J., & Keene, A. (2001). *Medical-surgical nursing: clinical management for positive outcomes* (6th ed.). Philadelphia: W.B. Saunders, p. 995.

---

87. A client who suffered a severe head injury has had vigorous treatment to control cerebral edema. Brain death has now been determined. The nurse assigned to assist in caring for the client prepares to carry out which of the following orders to maintain viability of the kidneys before organ donation?

Answer: 2
Rationale: Perfusion to the kidney is affected by blood pressure, which is in turn affected by blood vessel tone and fluid volume. Therefore the client who was previously dehydrated to control intracranial pressure is now in need of rehydration to maintain perfusion to the kidneys. The nurse prepares to infuse IV fluids as ordered and to continue monitoring urine output.

1   Monitoring of temperature
2   Administration of intravenous (IV) fluids
3   Checking respirations
4   Frequent range of motion to extremities

Test-Taking Strategy: Use the process of elimination. Note the key words in the question that are *maintain viability.* This implies an action orientation, guiding you to look for options that are interventions rather than data collection. With this in mind, you would eliminate options 1 and 3 first. You would choose the correct of the remaining two options by comparing their benefit to the kidneys. Review the interventions related to care of the potential kidney donor if you had difficulty with this question.

Level of Cognitive Ability: Application
Client Needs: Safe, Effective Care Environment
Integrated Concept/Process: Nursing Process/Implementation
Content Area: Fundamental Skills

Reference:
Black, J., Hawks, J., & Keene, A. (2001). *Medical-surgical nursing: clinical management for positive outcomes* (6th ed.). Philadelphia: W.B. Saunders, p. 2219.

---

88. A nurse is assisting in the emergency room of a small local hospital when a client with multiple gunshot wounds arrives by ambulance. The nurse is asked to care for the client's personal belongings, which may be needed as legal evidence. Which of the following actions by the nurse is contraindicated in the proper handling of legal evidence?
1   Cut clothing along seams, avoiding bullet holes
2   Initiate a chain of custody log
3   Place personal belongings in a labeled, sealed paper bag
4   Give the clothing and wallet to the family

Answer: 4
Rationale: Basic rules for handling evidence include limiting the number of people with access to the evidence, initiating a chain of custody log to track handling and movement of evidence, and careful removal of clothing to avoid destroying evidence. This usually includes cutting clothes along seams, avoiding areas where there are obvious holes or tears. Potential evidence is never released to the family to take home.

Test-Taking Strategy: Use the process of elimination. The key word is *contraindicated.* You should easily be directed to option 4 because giving these belongings to the family may be jeopardizing evidence. If this question was difficult, review these principles.

Level of Cognitive Ability: Application
Client Needs: Safe, Effective Care Environment
Integrated Concept/Process: Nursing Process/Implementation
Content Area: Fundamental Skills

Reference:
Black, J., Hawks, J., & Keene, A. (2001). *Medical-surgical nursing: clinical management for positive outcomes* (6th ed.). Philadelphia: W.B. Saunders, p. 2263.

---

89. A nurse working on a medical nursing unit during an external disaster is called to assist with the care of clients coming into the emergency room. The nurse is asked to assist the triage nurse. Using principles of prioritizing, the nurse initiates care for a client with which of the following injuries first?
1   Bright red bleeding from a neck wound
2   Penetrating abdominal injury

Answer: 1
Rationale: The client with arterial bleeding from a neck wound is in immediate need of treatment to save the client's life. According to the triage process, the client in this classification would be issued a red tag. The client with a penetrating abdominal injury would be tagged yellow and classified as "delayed," requiring intervention within 30 to 60 minutes. A green or "minimal" designation would be given to the client with a fractured tibia; this client requires intervention but can provide self-care if needed. A designation of "expectant" and color code of "black" would be applied to the client with massive injuries and a minimal chance

3 Fractured tibia
4 Open severe head injury in a deep coma

of survival. These clients are given supportive care and pain management, but are given definitive treatment last.

Test-Taking Strategy: Use the process of elimination. To answer this question accurately, you must be able to apply principles of prioritizing to the clients identified in the options. Eliminate options 2 and 3 first because they are least in need of immediate care. Select between options 1 and 4 by determining which client has the better chance of a positive outcome from intervention. Review the principles of prioritizing if you had difficulty with this question.

Level of Cognitive Ability: Application
Client Needs: Safe, Effective Care Environment
Integrated Concept/Process: Nursing Process/Implementation
Content Area: Fundamental Skills

Reference:
Potter, P., & Perry, A. (2001). *Fundamentals of nursing* (5th ed.). St. Louis: Mosby, p. 74.

---

90. A nurse is orienting a nursing assistant to the clinical nursing unit. The nurse would intervene if the nursing assistant did which of the following during a routine hand washing procedure?
1 Kept the hands lower than the elbows
2 Used 3 to 5 mL of soap from the dispenser
3 Washed continuously for 10 to 15 seconds
4 Dried the hands from the forearm down to the fingers

Answer: 4
Rationale: Proper hand washing procedure involves wetting the hands and wrists and keeping the hands lower than the forearms so water flows toward the fingertips. The nurse uses 3 to 5 mL of soap and scrubs for 10 to 15 seconds using a rubbing and circular motion. The hands are rinsed and then dried, moving from the fingers to the forearms. The paper towel is then discarded, and a second one is used to turn off the faucet to avoid hand contamination.

Test-Taking Strategy: Use the process of elimination and note the key word *intervene*. Visualize each option and use basic principles of asepsis to answer this question. Review this fundamental nursing procedure if you had difficulty with this question.

Level of Cognitive Ability: Application
Client Needs: Safe, Effective Care Environment
Integrated Concept/Process: Nursing Process/Implementation
Content Area: Fundamental Skills

Reference:
Potter, P., & Perry, A. (2001). *Fundamentals of nursing* (5th ed.). St. Louis: Mosby, p. 854.

---

91. A client who is immunosuppressed is being admitted to the hospital on neutropenic precautions. The nurse assigned to care for the client plans to ensure that which of the following does not occur in the care of the client?
1 Placing a mask on the client if the client leaves the room

Answer: 3
Rationale: The client who is on neutropenic precautions is immunosuppressed and therefore is admitted to a single room on the nursing unit. A sign indicating that neutropenic precautions have been initiated should be placed on the door to the client's room. Sources of standing water and fresh flowers should be removed to decrease the microorganism count. The client should wear a mask for protection from exposure to microorganisms whenever he or she leaves the room.

2 Removal of a vase with fresh flowers left by a previous client

3 Admitting the client to a semiprivate room

4 Placing a neutropenic precautions sign on the door to the room

Test-Taking Strategy: Use the process of elimination. Note the key words *does not occur*. Knowing that neutropenic precautions are instituted when the client is at risk for infection because of impaired immune function will direct you to option 3. Review this type of infection control precaution if you had difficulty with this question.

Level of Cognitive Ability: Application
Client Needs: Safe, Effective Care Environment
Integrated Concept/Process: Nursing Process/Planning
Content Area: Adult Health/Oncology

Reference:
Black, J., Hawks, J., & Keene, A. (2001). *Medical-surgical nursing: clinical management for positive outcomes* (6th ed.). Philadelphia: W.B. Saunders, p. 392.

---

92. A client who received a dose of chemotherapy 12 hours ago is incontinent of urine while in bed. The nurse safely wears which of the following when cleaning the client?
1 Mask and gloves
2 Gown and gloves
3 Mask, gown, and gloves
4 Gown, gloves, and eyewear

Answer: 2
Rationale: The client who has received chemotherapy will have antineoplastic agents or their metabolites in body fluids and excreta for 48 hours. For this reason, the nurse should wear protection for likely sources of contamination. In this instance, the nurse should wear gloves and a gown to protect the hands and uniform from contamination.

Test-Taking Strategy: Use the process of elimination. Begin to answer this question by reasoning that the potential source of contamination in this situation is the client's urine. Since urine present on the hospital gown and bedclothes is not likely to splash, you can eliminate the options identifying a mask or eyewear. This leaves option 2 as the correct answer. Review these guidelines if you had difficulty with this question.

Level of Cognitive Ability: Application
Client Needs: Safe, Effective Care Environment
Integrated Concept/Process: Nursing Process/Implementation
Content Area: Adult Health/Oncology

Reference:
Black, J., Hawks, J., & Keene, A. (2001). *Medical-surgical nursing: clinical management for positive outcomes* (6th ed.). Philadelphia: W.B. Saunders, p. 388.

---

93. A clinic nurse is providing instructions to a mother of a child who was diagnosed with mumps. The mother is concerned about her other children and asks the nurse how the infection is transmitted. The nurse informs the mother that mumps is transmitted by:
1 Airborne droplets
2 Fecal oral route
3 Through contact with body sweat
4 Through contact with tears

Answer: 1
Rationale: Mumps is transmitted via airborne droplets, salivary secretions, and possibly the urine. Options 2, 3, and 4 are incorrect.

Test-Taking Strategy: Use the process of elimination. Knowing how mumps is transmitted is necessary to answer this question. Review the transmission route of this infectious disease if you had difficulty with this question.

Level of Cognitive Ability: Application
Client Needs: Safe, Effective Care Environment

Integrated Concept/Process: Teaching/Learning
Content Area: Child Health

Reference:
Wong, D., & Hockenberry-Eaton, M. (2001). *Wong's essentials of pediatric nursing* (6th ed.). St. Louis: Mosby, p. 460.

---

94. A nurse is assisting in preparing a client scheduled for a bone marrow aspiration. The client asks the nurse if the procedure will be painful. To provide the client with accurate information, the nurse should incorporate which of the following in a response to the client?
1   There is no pain from the procedure at all
2   The procedure is painful, but the client will be under anesthesia
3   A local anesthetic is used, but there is some pain during aspiration
4   The procedure is very painful, but the client will be heavily medicated beforehand

Answer: 3
Rationale: A local anesthetic is used to anesthetize the skin and subcutaneous tissue to minimize tissue discomfort with needle insertion. The client will feel some pain briefly when the sample is aspirated out of the marrow. Options 1, 2, and 4 are not true statements.

Test-Taking Strategy: Use the process of elimination. Recalling that the procedure may be performed at the bedside will assist in eliminating options 2 and 4. Knowing that the procedure is invasive will assist in eliminating option 1. Review this diagnostic test if you had difficulty with this question.

Level of Cognitive Ability: Application
Client Needs: Safe, Effective Care Environment
Integrated Concept/Process: Nursing Process/Implementation
Content Area: Fundamental Skills

Reference:
deWit, S. (2001). *Fundamental concepts and skills for nursing.* Philadelphia: W.B. Saunders, p. 421.

---

95. A nurse is preparing to assist a client from the bed to chair by using a hydraulic lift. The nurse would do which of the following to move the client safely with this device?
1   Have three staff members available to assist
2   Position the client in the center of the sling
3   Have the client grasp the chains attaching the sling to the lift
4   Lower the client rapidly once positioned over the chair

Answer: 2
Rationale: One person may operate a hydraulic lift. The client is positioned in the center of the sling, which is then attached to chains or straps that connect the sling to the lift. The client's hands and arms are crossed over the chest, and the client is raised from the bed into a sitting position. The lift raises the client off the mattress and lowers the client slowly once the sling is positioned over the chair.

Test-Taking Strategy: Use the process of elimination. Visualizing this procedure will assist in directing you to option 2. Review this procedure if you had difficulty with this question.

Level of Cognitive Ability: Application
Client Needs: Safe, Effective Care Environment
Integrated Concept/Process: Nursing Process/Implementation
Content Area: Fundamental Skills

Reference:
Potter, P., & Perry, A. (2001). *Fundamentals of nursing* (5th ed.). St. Louis: Mosby, p. 1534.

---

96. A older client in a long-term care facility is at risk for injury because of confusion. The client's gait is stable. Which of the fol-

Answer: 4
Rationale: If the client is confused and has a stable gait, the least intrusive method of restraint is the use of an alarm activating

lowing methods of restraint if prescribed would be best used by the nurse to prevent injury to the client?

1   Vest restraint
2   Waist restraint
3   Chair with a locking lap tray
4   Alarm-activating bracelet

bracelet, or "wandering bracelet." This allows the client to move about the residence freely while preventing the client from leaving the premises.

Test-Taking Strategy: Use the process of elimination and knowledge of the various restraint methods, and the ethical and legal consequences of restraint, to eliminate each of the incorrect options. The words *stable gait* will also guide your selection. Review the guidelines related to the use of restraints if you had difficulty with this question.

Level of Cognitive Ability: Application
Client Needs: Safe, Effective Care Environment
Integrated Concept/Process: Nursing Process/Implementation
Content Area: Fundamental Skills

Reference:
Potter, P., & Perry, A. (2001). *Fundamentals of nursing* (5th ed.). St. Louis: Mosby, p. 1038.

---

97. A nurse is suctioning the airway of a client with a tracheostomy. To safely perform the procedure, the nurse does which of the following?

1   Turns on wall suction to 190 mmHg
2   Inserts the catheter until coughing or resistance is felt
3   Withdraws the catheter while continuously suctioning
4   Reenters the catheter into the tracheostomy after suctioning the mouth

Answer: 2
Rationale: The wall suction unit is maintained between 120 and 180 mmHg of pressure. This allows adequate removal of secretions while protecting the airway from trauma. The nurse inserts the catheter until resistance is felt, and then withdraws it 1 cm to move away from mucosa. The nurse suctions intermittently and does not reenter the tracheostomy after suctioning the client's mouth.

Test-Taking Strategy: Use the process of elimination. Visualizing this procedure will assist in directing you to option 2. Review this procedure if you had difficulty with this question.

Level of Cognitive Ability: Application
Client Needs: Safe, Effective Care Environment
Integrated Concept/Process: Nursing Process/Implementation
Content Area: Adult Health/Respiratory

Reference:
Potter, P., & Perry, A. (2001). *Fundamentals of nursing* (5th ed.). St. Louis: Mosby, p. 1164.

---

98. Furosemide (Lasix) 40 mg PO has been prescribed for a client. The nurse administers furosemide 80 mg to the client at 10:00 AM. After discovering the error, the nurse completes an incident report. Which of the following would the nurse document on this report?

1   Lasix 80 mg was given to the client instead of 40 mg
2   The wrong dose of medication was given to the client at 10:00 AM
3   I meant to give 40 mg of Lasix but I was rushed to get to another client

Answer: 4
Rationale: When filing an incident report, the nurse should state the facts clearly. The nurse would not record assumptions, opinions, judgments, or conclusions about what occurred.

Test-Taking Strategy: Read the occurrence as stated in the question. Using the process of elimination, select the option that clearly and most directly states what has occurred. Option 1 is eliminated first because it contains unnecessary information. Option 2 is incorrect because it assigns blame to the nurse. Option 3 provides a judgment. Option 4 clearly and simply states the occurrence. Review the documentation guidelines associated with completing incident reports if you had difficulty with this question.

who needed me and I gave the wrong dose

4 Lasix 80 mg administered at 10:00 AM

Level of Cognitive Ability: Application
Client Needs: Safe, Effective Care Environment
Integrated Concept/Process: Communication and Documentation
Content Area: Fundamental Skills

Reference:
Potter, P., & Perry, A. (2001). *Fundamentals of nursing* (5th ed.). St. Louis: Mosby, p. 440.

---

99. A nurse employed in a long-term care facility assists a nursing assistant in completing an incident report for a client who was found sitting on the floor. After completion of the report, which of the following would the nurse avoid?
1 Document in the nurses' notes that an incident report was filed
2 Forward the incident report to the nursing director's office
3 Ask the unit secretary to call the physician
4 Notify the nursing supervisor

Answer: 1
Rationale: Nurses are advised not to document the filing of an incident report in the nurses' notes. Information in the medical record can be considered evidence, and the record can be obtained by subpoena if a lawsuit is filed. Incident reports inform the facility's administration of the incident so that risk management personnel can consider changes to prevent similar occurrences in the future. Incident reports also alert the facility's insurance company to a potential claim and the need for further investigation. Options 2, 3, and 4 are accurate interventions.

Test-Taking Strategy: Use the process of elimination. Note the word *avoid*. Options 2, 3, and 4 all relate to notification of individuals or departments. Option 1 relates to inappropriate documentation. Review the guidelines for completion of incident reports if you had difficulty with this question.

Level of Cognitive Ability: Application
Client Needs: Safe, Effective Care Environment
Integrated Concept/Process: Nursing Process/Implementation
Content Area: Fundamental Skills

Reference:
Potter, P., & Perry, A. (2001). *Fundamentals of nursing* (5th ed.). St. Louis: Mosby, p. 521.

---

100. A physician is visiting a client in the nursing unit and is called to another nursing unit to assess a client in extreme pain. The physician states to the nurse, "I'm in a hurry. Can you write the order to decrease the atenolol (Tenormin) to 25 mg daily?" Which of the following is the most appropriate nursing action?
1 Write the order as stated
2 Call the nursing supervisor to write the order
3 Ask the physician to return to the nursing unit to write the order
4 Inform the client of the change of medication

Answer: 3
Rationale: Nurses are not to accept verbal orders from the physician because of the risks of error. Although the client will be informed of the change in the treatment plan, this is not the most appropriate action at this time. The physician should write the new order.

Test-Taking Strategy: Use the process of elimination. Recalling that verbal orders are not acceptable will assist in selecting the correct option. Options 1 and 2 are similar; therefore eliminate these options. Option 4 is appropriate for a later time. Option 3 clearly identifies the nurse's responsibility in this situation. Review these principles if you had difficulty with this question.

Level of Cognitive Ability: Application
Client Needs: Safe, Effective Care Environment
Integrated Concept/Process: Nursing Process/Implementation
Content Area: Fundamental Skills

Reference:
Potter, P., & Perry, A. (2001). *Fundamentals of nursing* (5th ed.). St. Louis: Mosby, p. 899.

---

101. A nurse is preparing a client for a gallium scan. Which of the following should the nurse plan to include in preprocedure instructions to the client?

1   All metal objects must be removed

2   The client must not be allergic to iodine

3   There is no need for signed consent

4   There is absolutely no pain involved

Answer: 1

Rationale: A gallium scan uses an intravenous injection of the radioisotope gallium citrate. Tumors and inflammations take up the gallium, as do many organs. The scan is often used to differentiate a tumor from a pulmonary embolus when x-ray findings are unclear. There is no iodine involved, but there is local pain at the injection site. Serial scans are completed at 24, 48, and 72 hours. The client must remove all metal for the procedure. A signed consent is necessary for injection of the radioisotope.

Test-Taking Strategy: Use the process of elimination. Recall that gallium is a radioisotope. With this in mind, you may eliminate options 2 and 3. You would choose option 1 instead of option 4 by recalling that the substance may cause discomfort during injection. Review preprocedure preparation if you had difficulty with this question.

Level of Cognitive Ability: Application
Client Needs: Safe, Effective Care Environment
Integrated Concept/Process: Nursing Process/Implementation
Content Area: Adult Health/Respiratory

Reference:
Black, J., Hawks, J., & Keene, A. (2001). *Medical-surgical nursing: clinical management for positive outcomes* (6th ed.). Philadelphia: W.B. Saunders, p. 1645.

---

102. A nurse has prepared the client for an intravenous pyelogram. The nurse evaluates that the client is knowledgeable about the procedure if the client states to report which of the following sensations immediately?

1   Nausea

2   Difficulty breathing

3   Warm flushed feeling in the body

4   Salty taste in the mouth

Answer: 2

Rationale: Intravenous pyelography is a contrast study of the kidneys to determine a variety of disorders of the kidneys, ureters, and bladder. Normal sensations during injection of the iodine-based radiopaque dye includes a warm flushed feeling, salty taste in the mouth, and transient nausea. Difficulty breathing, wheezing, hives, or itching signals an allergic response and should be reported immediately. This complication is prevented by inquiring about allergies to iodine or shellfish before the procedure.

Test-Taking Strategy: Use the process of elimination. To answer this question correctly, it is necessary to know that this diagnostic test involves injection of an iodine-based contrast medium. Differentiate between the normal expectations and the symptom that would indicate a reaction. With this in mind, you can eliminate each of the incorrect options. Review this diagnostic test if you had difficulty with this question.

Level of Cognitive Ability: Comprehension
Client Needs: Safe, Effective Care Environment
Integrated Concept/Process: Nursing Process/Evaluation
Content Area: Adult Health/Renal

Reference:
Black, J., Hawks, J., & Keene, A. (2001). *Medical-surgical nursing: clinical manage-ment for positive outcomes* (6th ed.). Philadelphia: W.B. Saunders, p. 758.

---

103. A nurse is using a mercury glass ther-mometer to take a client's temperature. The nurse shakes down the thermometer and drops it on the floor. Which of the following actions will the nurse take?
1   Carefully wipe up the spill to avoid getting cut from the glass
2   Use a mop and dust pan to clean up the spill, avoiding contact with the glass and mercury
3   Notify the Environmental Services Department of the spill
4   Call the housekeeping department to clean up the spill and broken glass

Answer: 3
Rationale: Mercury is a hazardous material. Accidental breakage of a mercury-in-glass thermometer is a health hazard to the client, nurse, or other health care workers. Mercury droplets are not to be touched. If a breakage or spill occurs, the Environmental Services Department is called and a mercury spill kit is used to clean up the spill.

Test-Taking Strategy: Use the process of elimination. Remembering that mercury is a hazardous material will assist in eliminating options 1, 2, and 4. Review the principles associated with mercury spills if you had difficulty with this question.

Level of Cognitive Ability: Application
Client Needs: Safe, Effective Care Environment
Integrated Concept/Process: Nursing Process/Implementation
Content Area: Fundamental Skills

Reference:
Potter, P., & Perry, A. (2001). *Fundamentals of nursing* (5th ed.). St. Louis: Mosby, p. 685.

---

104. A client with a bone infection is sched-uled to have an indium imaging scan. The client asks the nurse to explain how the procedure is done. The nurse pro-vides accurate information by basing the response on the understanding that:
1   Indium is injected into the blood-stream and collects in normal bone but not in infected areas
2   Indium is injected into the blood-stream and highlights the vascular supply to the bone
3   A sample of the client's leukocytes is tagged with indium and will sub-sequently accumulate in infected bone
4   A sample of the client's red blood cells is tagged with indium and will highlight normal bone

Answer: 3
Rationale: A sample of the client's blood is collected and the leukocytes are tagged with indium. The leukocytes are then rein-jected into the client. They accumulate in infected areas of bone and can be detected with scanning. No special preparation or aftercare is necessary.

Test-Taking Strategy: Use the process of elimination and focus on the information in the question. Note that the client has a bone infection. With any type of infection, leukocytes migrate to the area. This will direct you to option 3. Review the procedure involved with this test if you had difficulty with this question.

Level of Cognitive Ability: Comprehension
Client Needs: Safe, Effective Care Environment
Integrated Concept/Process: Nursing Process/Implementation
Content Area: Fundamental Skills

Reference:
Black, J., Hawks, J., & Keene, A. (2001). *Medical-surgical nursing: clinical manage-ment for positive outcomes* (6th ed.). Philadelphia: W.B. Saunders, p. 548.

---

105. A client in the nursing unit has an order for dextroamphetamine sulfate (Dexedrine) 25 mg PO daily. The nurse

Answer: 2
Rationale: Dextroamphetamine sulfate is a central nervous system (CNS) stimulant. Caffeine is a stimulant also and should be

plans to collaborate with the dietitian to limit the amount of which of the following items on the client's dietary trays?

1   Starch
2   Caffeine
3   Protein
4   Fat

limited in the client taking this medication. The client should be taught to limit his or her own caffeine intake as well.

Test-Taking Strategy: Use the process of elimination and recall that this medication is a CNS stimulant. Next, evaluate each of the options to determine the additive stimulation each provides. Knowing that caffeine is also a stimulant will direct you to option 2. Review this medication if you had difficulty with this question.

Level of Cognitive Ability: Application
Client Needs: Safe, Effective Care Environment
Integrated Concept/Process: Nursing Process/Implementation
Content Area: Pharmacology

Reference:
Hodgson, B., & Kizior, R. (2003). *Saunders nursing drug handbook 2003.* Philadelphia: W.B. Saunders, p. 332.

---

106. A hospitalized client with hypertension is receiving captopril (Capoten). To ensure client safety, the nurse would make certain that the client does which of the following specific to this medication?

1   Eat foods that are high in potassium
2   Take in sufficient amounts of high fiber foods
3   Sit up and stand slowly while on this medication
4   Drink plenty of water while on this medication

Answer: 3

Rationale: Orthostatic hypotension is a concern for clients taking antihypertensive medications. Clients are advised to avoid standing in one position for lengthy amounts of time, change positions slowly, and avoid extreme warmth (showers, bath, weather). Clients are also taught to recognize the symptoms of orthostatic hypotension, including dizziness, light-headedness, weakness, and syncope.

Test-Taking Strategy: Use the process of elimination and note the client's diagnosis. Recalling that captopril is an antihypertensive will assist in directing you to option 3. Remember that orthostatic hypotension is a potential concern with all types of antihypertensives. Review this medication if you had difficulty with this question.

Level of Cognitive Ability: Application
Client Needs: Safe, Effective Care Environment
Integrated Concept/Process: Teaching/Learning
Content Area: Adult Health/Cardiovascular

Reference:
Hodgson, B., & Kizior, R. (2003). *Saunders nursing drug handbook 2003.* Philadelphia: W.B. Saunders, p. 165.

---

107. A nurse is assisting in planning care for the client who is scheduled for admission to the nursing unit after femoral-popliteal bypass grafting. The nurse understands that which of the following would impair circulation to the affected extremity?

1   Sheepskin
2   Bed cradle
3   Lightweight blanket
4   Elastic wraps

Answer: 4

Rationale: Use of sheepskin, a bed cradle, and lightweight blankets can promote warmth to the extremity and protect it from harm. Elastic wraps, if ordered, would be used when the client is out of bed to reduce edema, but they could impair circulation and wound healing. Frequently the surgical limb is left unwrapped for monitoring and is not covered by elastic wraps or pneumatic boots. These may be placed on the alternate extremity.

Test-Taking Strategy: Use the process of elimination and recall that the surgical limb needs frequent monitoring, warmth, and protection. Remembering this concept will direct you to option 4. Review care to the client following femoral-popliteal bypass grafting if you had difficulty with this question.

Level of Cognitive Ability: Comprehension
Client Needs: Safe, Effective Care Environment
Integrated Concept/Process: Nursing Process/Planning
Content Area: Adult Health/Cardiovascular

Reference:
Black, J., Hawks, J., & Keene, A. (2001). *Medical-surgical nursing: clinical management for positive outcomes* (6th ed.). Philadelphia: W.B. Saunders, p. 1407.

---

108. A nurse is changing a dressing on a venous stasis ulcer that is clean and has a growing bed of granulation tissue. The nurse would safeguard wound integrity by avoiding the use of which of the following dressing materials?
1 Wet-to-dry saline dressing
2 Wet-to-wet saline dressing
3 Hydrocolloid dressing
4 Vaseline gauze dressing

Answer: 1
Rationale: The use of wet-to-dry saline dressings provides a mechanical debridement, whereby both devitalized and viable tissue are removed. This method should not be used on a clean, granulating wound. Granulation tissue in a venous stasis ulcer is protected through the use of wet-to-wet saline dressings, Vaseline gauze, or moist occlusive dressings such as hydrocolloid dressings as prescribed.

Test-Taking Strategy: Use the process of elimination and note the key word *avoiding*. Note that the wound is clean with granulation tissue (which needs protection). Next, compare the options. Note that options 2, 3, and 4 all have one thing in common—continuous moisture. This will direct you to option 1 because it is the only dressing that could disrupt this healing tissue. Review the principles related to wound care if you had difficulty with this question.

Level of Cognitive Ability: Application
Client Needs: Safe, Effective Care Environment
Integrated Concept/Process: Nursing Process/Implementation
Content Area: Fundamental Skills

Reference:
Black, J., Hawks, J., & Keene, A. (2001). *Medical-surgical nursing: clinical management for positive outcomes* (6th ed.). Philadelphia: W.B. Saunders, p. 1429. ·

---

109. A licensed practical nurse (LPN) is assisting in caring for an older client being admitted to the nursing unit who has severe digitalis toxicity from accidental ingestion of a week's supply of the medication. The registered nurse (RN) asks the LPN to check the medication supply to see if the antidote for digitalis toxicity is available. The LPN checks the medication supply for which medication?

Answer: 1
Rationale: Digoxin immune fab is an antidote for severe digitalis toxicity. It contains an antibody produced in sheep, which antigenically binds any unbound digitalis in the serum and removes it. It also binds the digoxin reentering the bloodstream from the tissues, which is then excreted by the kidneys. Potassium chloride and furosemide are other medications commonly used in conjunction with digoxin for cardiac conditions. Protamine sulfate is the antidote for heparin.

1   Digoxin immune fab (Digibind)
2   Potassium chloride (K-Dur)
3   Protamine sulfate
4   Furosemide (Lasix)

Test-Taking Strategy: Use the process of elimination. Note the relationship between the name of the medication in the question and the correct option. Review this antidote if you had difficulty with this question.

Level of Cognitive Ability: Application
Client Needs: Safe, Effective Care Environment
Integrated Concept/Process: Nursing Process/Implementation
Content Area: Pharmacology

Reference:
Hodgson, B., & Kizior, R. (2003). *Saunders nursing drug handbook 2003.* Philadelphia: W.B. Saunders, p. 350.

---

110. A client receiving lisinopril (Prinivil) has a white blood cell (WBC) count of 3800 mm^3. The nurse would most appropriately plan to do which of the following in the care of this client?
1   Follow aseptic technique diligently
2   Request asking for prophylactic antibiotics from the physician
3   Place the client on respiratory isolation
4   Use antibacterial soap when bathing the client

Answer: 1
Rationale: The client taking an angiotensin-converting enzyme (ACE) inhibitor such as lisinopril is at risk of developing neutropenia. These clients require the use of strict aseptic technique by the nurse. The client should also be taught to report signs and symptoms of infection, such as sore throat and fever, to the physician. The WBC count with differential may be monitored monthly for up to 6 months in clients deemed at risk. Options 2, 3, and 4 are not specific to the information in the question.

Test-Taking Strategy: Use the process of elimination. Noting that the WBC count is low and that a low count places the client at risk for infection will direct you to option 1. Review this medication and the associated nursing interventions if you had difficulty with this question.

Level of Cognitive Ability: Application
Client Needs: Safe, Effective Care Environment
Integrated Concept/Process: Nursing Process/Planning
Content Area: Pharmacology

Reference:
Hodgson, B., & Kizior, R. (2003). *Saunders nursing drug handbook 2003.* Philadelphia: W.B. Saunders, p. 668.

---

111. A client with obsessive-compulsive disorder spends many hours during the day and night washing his or her hands. When initially planning for a safe environment, the nurse allows the client to continue this behavior because:
1   It relieves the client's anxiety
2   It decreases the chance of infection
3   It gives the client a feeling of self-control
4   It increases self-esteem

Answer: 1
Rationale: The compulsive act provides immediate relief from anxiety and is used to cope with stress, conflict, or pain. Although the client may feel the need to increase self-esteem, that is not the primary goal. Options 2, 3, and 4 are incorrect.

Test-Taking Strategy: Use the process of elimination. Recalling that the behavior associated with compulsive disorders relieves anxiety will direct you to option 1. Review this disorder if you had difficulty with this question.

Level of Cognitive Ability: Comprehension
Client Needs: Safe, Effective Care Environment
Integrated Concept/Process: Nursing Process/Planning
Content Area: Mental Health

Reference:
Varcarolis, E. (2002). *Foundations of psychiatric mental health nursing* (4th ed.). Philadelphia: W.B. Saunders, p. 379.

---

112. A client is scheduled to undergo cardiac catheterization for the first time. Which of the following points would the nurse plan to include in preprocedure teaching to provide the client with accurate information?

1   The procedure is performed in the operating room

2   The client may feel fatigue and have various aches because it is necessary to lie quietly on a hard x-ray table for approximately 4 hours

3   The client may feel certain sensations at various points during the procedure, such as a fluttery feeling, a flushed warm feeling, a desire to cough, or palpitations

4   The initial catheter insertion is quite painful; after that, there is little or no pain

Answer: 3

Rationale: During preprocedure teaching, the client should be told that the procedure is done in a darkened cardiac catheterization room and that ECG leads are attached to the limbs. A local anesthetic is used so there is little to no pain with catheter insertion. The x-ray table is hard and may be tilted periodically. The procedure may take up to 2 hours, and the client may feel various sensations with catheter passage and dye injection.

Test-Taking Strategy: Use the process of elimination. Eliminate option 1 because this procedure is not done in the operating room. Eliminate option 2 because *4 hours* is too long of a time frame and option 4 because the procedure is not *quite painful.* Review the client preparation for this procedure if you had difficulty with this question.

Level of Cognitive Ability: Application
Client Needs: Safe, Effective Care Environment
Integrated Concept/Process: Nursing Process/Planning
Content Area: Adult Health/Cardiovascular

Reference:
Black, J., Hawks, J., & Keene, A. (2001). *Medical-surgical nursing: clinical management for positive outcomes* (6th ed.). Philadelphia: W.B. Saunders, p. 1475.

---

113. A nurse is inserting an indwelling Foley catheter. When the nurse inflates the balloon, the client immediately complains of pain. The most appropriate nursing action would be to:

1   Tell the client that the discomfort will pass

2   Withdraw 1 mL from the balloon of the catheter

3   Deflate the balloon and inserts it further into the bladder

4   Call the physician

Answer: 3

Rationale: The appropriate procedure if the client complains of pain after the balloon is inflated is to deflate the balloon and insert it further into the bladder. If the client complains of pain, the balloon is most likely positioned in the urethra. Options 1 and 2 are incorrect actions. It is not necessary to call the physician.

Test-Taking Strategy: Focus on the data in the question. Visualizing this procedure and thinking about the anatomy of the urinary system will direct you to option 3. Review this procedure if you had difficulty with this question.

Level of Cognitive Ability: Application
Client Needs: Safe, Effective Care Environment
Integrated Concept/Process: Nursing Process/Implementation
Content Area: Fundamental Skills

Reference:
Perry, A., & Potter, A. (2002). *Clinical nursing skills & techniques* (5th ed.). St. Louis: Mosby, p. 411.

114. A nurse is caring for a client who is scheduled to have an arthrogram using a contrast dye. Which of the following data collected by the nurse would be of highest priority?
1   Allergy to iodine or shellfish
2   Ability of the client to remain still during the procedure
3   Whether the client has any remaining questions about the procedure
4   Whether the client wishes to void before the procedure

Answer: 1
Rationale: Because of the risk of allergy to contrast dye, the nurse places highest priority on determining whether the client has an allergy to iodine or shellfish. The nurse also reinforces information about the test, tells the client about the need to remain still during the procedure, and encourages the client to void before the procedure for comfort.

Test-Taking Strategy: Use the process of elimination. Note that this question asks which option is of "highest priority." This tells you that more than one or all of the options are correct (in fact, they all are). Although options 2, 3, and 4 all are important, only option 1 is related to a medical risk. The consequence of a possible allergic reaction makes this the correct option. Review this diagnostic test if you had difficulty with this question.

Level of Cognitive Ability: Comprehension
Client Needs: Safe, Effective Care Environment
Integrated Concept/Process: Nursing Process/Data Collection
Content Area: Adult Health/Musculoskeletal

Reference:
Black, J., Hawks, J., & Keene, A. (2001). *Medical-surgical nursing: clinical management for positive outcomes* (6th ed.). Philadelphia: W.B. Saunders, p. 546.

---

115. A client with a possible rib fracture has never had a chest x-ray. The nurse would plan to tell the client which of the following about the procedure?
1   The x-rays stimulate a great deal of pain
2   It is necessary to remove jewelry and any other metal objects
3   The client will be asked to breathe in and out during the x-ray
4   The x-ray technologist will stand next to the client during the x-ray

Answer: 2
Rationale: An x-ray is a photographic image of a part of the body on a special film, which is used to diagnose a wide variety of conditions. The x-ray itself is painless and any discomfort would arise from repositioning a painful body part for filming. The nurse may want to premedicate a client as prescribed who is at risk for pain. Any radiopaque objects such as jewelry or other metal must be removed. The client is asked to breathe in deeply and then hold the breath while the chest x-ray is taken. To minimize risk of radiation exposure, the x-ray technologist stands in a separate area protected by a lead wall. The client also wears a lead shield over the gonads.

Test-Taking Strategy: Use the process of elimination. Noting that the client is scheduled to have an x-ray will assist in eliminating options 1 and 4. Of the remaining options, eliminate option 3 because the client will be asked to hold the breath and remain still during the x-ray. Review this procedure if you had difficulty with this question.

Level of Cognitive Ability: Application
Client Needs: Safe, Effective Care Environment
Integrated Concept/Process: Nursing Process/Planning
Content Area: Adult Health/Musculoskeletal

Reference:
deWit, S. (2001). *Fundamental concepts and skills for nursing.* Philadelphia: W.B. Saunders, p. 423.

116. A nurse is reinforcing discharge instructions for a client with a spinal cord injury. To provide for a safe environment regarding home care, which of the following would be the priority?
  1 What the physician has indicated needs to be taught
  2 Follow-up laboratory and diagnostic tests
  3 Assisting the client to deal with long-term care placement
  4 Including the significant others in the teaching session

Answer: 4
Rationale: Involving the client's significant others in discharge teaching is a priority for the client with a spinal cord injury because the client will need the support of the significant others. Knowledge and understanding of what to expect will help both the client and significant others deal with the limitations. A physician's order is not necessary for providing instructions; this is an independent nursing action. Laboratory and diagnostic testing are inappropriate discharge instructions for this client. Long-term placement is not the only environment for clients with a spinal cord injury.

Test-Taking Strategy: Use the process of elimination. Eliminate option 3 first because long-term placement is not the only discharge option. Eliminate option 1 next; although the physician's orders should be addressed, teaching is an independent nursing action. From the remaining options, consider the client's diagnosis. Home care and support will be needed. This will direct you to option 4. Review care to the client with a spinal cord injury and the teaching and learning principles if you had difficulty with this question.

Level of Cognitive Ability: Application
Client Needs: Safe, Effective Care Environment
Integrated Concept/Process: Teaching/Learning
Content Area: Adult Health/Neurological

Reference:
Black, J., Hawks, J., & Keene, A. (2001). *Medical-surgical nursing: clinical management for positive outcomes* (6th ed.). Philadelphia: W.B. Saunders, p. 2066.

117. A nurse is asked to assist in applying electrocardiogram (ECG) electrodes to a diaphoretic client. The nurse would do which of the following to keep the electrodes from coming loose?
  1 Secure the electrodes with adhesive tape
  2 Place clear, transparent dressings over the electrodes
  3 Apply lanolin to the skin before applying the electrodes
  4 Apply tincture of benzoin to the skin before applying the electrodes

Answer: 4
Rationale: Tincture of benzoin is commonly used with a diaphoretic client to help the electrodes adhere to the skin. Placing adhesive tape or a clear dressing over the electrodes will not help the adhesive gel of the actual electrode make better contact with the diaphoretic skin. Lanolin or any other lotion makes the skin slippery and prevents good initial adherence.

Test-Taking Strategy: Use the process of elimination. Focusing on the issue—keeping the electrodes from coming loose—will assist in eliminating option 3. Note that options 1 and 2 are similar: they both provide an external form of providing security of the electrodes. Only option 4 addresses direct contact with the skin. Review this procedure if you had difficulty with this question.

Level of Cognitive Ability: Application
Client Needs: Safe, Effective Care Environment
Integrated Concept/Process: Nursing Process/Implementation
Content Area: Adult Health/Cardiovascular

Reference:
Black, J., Hawks, J., & Keene, A. (2001). *Medical-surgical nursing: clinical management for positive outcomes* (6th ed.). Philadelphia: W.B. Saunders, p. 1466.

118. A nurse observes a client wringing his hands and looking frightened. The client reports feeling out of control. Which approach by the nurse is most appropriate to maintain a safe environment?

1 Administer the ordered prn anxiety medication immediately

2 Move the client to a quiet room and talk about his or her feelings

3 Isolate the client in a "time-out" room

4 Observe the client in an ongoing manner but do not intervene

Answer: 2

Rationale: The anxiety symptoms demonstrated by this client require some form of intervention. Moving the client decreases environmental stimulus. Talking gives the nurse an opportunity to identify the cause of these feelings and to identify appropriate interventions. Isolation is appropriate if the client is a danger to self or others. There is no indication in the question that the client poses a threat to others. Medication is used only when other non-invasive approaches have been unsuccessful.

Test-Taking Strategy: Use the process of elimination. Note the key word *frightened*. Eliminate options 1 and 4 first, recalling that an intervention is necessary and that medication is used only when other noninvasive approaches have been unsuccessful. From the remaining options, select option 2 instead of option 3 because it addresses the client's feelings. Review care to the client with anxiety if you had difficulty with this question.

Level of Cognitive Ability: Application
Client Needs: Safe, Effective Care Environment
Integrated Concept/Process: Nursing Process/Implementation
Content Area: Mental Health

Reference:
Varcarolis, E. (2002). *Foundations of psychiatric mental health nursing* (4th ed.). Philadelphia: W.B. Saunders, p. 286.

119. A client has Buck's extension traction applied to the right leg. The nurse would perform which of the following interventions to prevent complications of the device?

1 Massage the skin of the right leg with lotion every 8 hours

2 Give pin care once a shift

3 Inspect the skin on the right leg at least once every 8 hours

4 Release the weights on the right leg for range of motion exercises daily

Answer: 3

Rationale: Buck's extension traction is a type of skin traction. The nurse inspects the skin of the limb in traction at least once every 8 hours for irritation or inflammation. Massaging the skin with lotion is not indicated. The nurse never releases the weights of traction unless specifically ordered by the physician. There are no pins to care for with skin traction.

Test-Taking Strategy: Use the process of elimination. Knowledge of Buck's extension traction allows you to eliminate options 2 and 4 easily. There are no pins, and the nurse never removes weights without a specific order to do so. Because the apparatus and traction would have to be removed to apply lotion, the answer is to inspect the skin. Also note that option 3 addresses the first step of the nursing process, data collection. Review care to the client in Buck's extension traction if you had difficulty with this question.

Level of Cognitive Ability: Application
Client Needs: Safe, Effective Care Environment
Integrated Concept/Process: Nursing Process/Implementation
Content Area: Adult Health/Musculoskeletal

Reference:
Black, J., Hawks, J., & Keene, A. (2001). *Medical-surgical nursing: clinical management for positive outcomes* (6th ed.). Philadelphia: W.B. Saunders, p. 607.

120. A client with urolithiasis is scheduled for extracorporeal shock wave lithotripsy. The nurse checks to ensure that which of the following are in place or maintained before sending the client for the procedure?
1   Signed informed consent, clear liquid restriction
2   Signed informed consent, NPO status
3   Clear liquid restriction, Foley catheter
4   IV line, Foley catheter

Answer: 2
Rationale: Extracorporeal shock wave lithotripsy is done under regional or general anesthesia. The client must sign an informed consent and be NPO for the procedure. The client requires an IV line for the procedure as well. A Foley catheter is not needed.

Test-Taking Strategy: Use the process of elimination. Begin to answer this question by eliminating options 3 and 4 because the client must sign an informed consent for this procedure. From the remaining options, it is necessary to know that premedication is needed for this procedure. With this in mind, you would realize that the client must be NPO. Review the preprocedure preparation if you had difficulty with this question.

Level of Cognitive Ability: Application
Client Needs: Safe, Effective Care Environment
Integrated Concept/Process: Nursing Process/Implementation
Content Area: Adult Health/Renal

Reference:
Black, J., Hawks, J., & Keene, A. (2001). *Medical-surgical nursing: clinical management for positive outcomes* (6th ed.). Philadelphia: W.B. Saunders, p. 827.

---

121. A nurse is assisting at a code and the physician is preparing to defibrillate this client. Which of the following items need not be removed from the bedside before the client is defibrillated?
1   Back board
2   Oxygen
3   Nitroglycerin patch
4   Ventilator

Answer: 1
Rationale: Flammable materials (oxygen and metal devices or liquids, which are capable of carrying electricity) are removed from the client and bed before discharging the paddles of the defibrillator. The nitroglycerin patch may have a metal backing and should be removed. A ventilator delivers oxygen to the client. The backboard is needed to resume cardiopulmonary resuscitation (CPR) immediately if defibrillation is unsuccessful.

Test-Taking Strategy: Use the process of elimination. Options 2 and 4 are similar and are eliminated first. From the remaining options, remember that the nitroglycerin patch may have a metallic backing and should be removed. Review the principles of CPR if you had difficulty with this question.

Level of Cognitive Ability: Application
Client Needs: Safe, Effective Care Environment
Integrated Concept/Process: Nursing Process/Implementation
Content Area: Adult Health/Cardiovascular

Reference:
Black, J., Hawks, J., & Keene, A. (2001). *Medical-surgical nursing: clinical management for positive outcomes* (6th ed.). Philadelphia: W.B. Saunders, p. 1567.

---

122. A licensed practical nurse (LPN) is reinforcing the discharge instructions provided by the registered nurse (RN) for an adult client who is a victim of family violence. The LPN plans to include:

Answer: 3
Rationale: Assisting the victim of family violence with a specific plan for removing himself or herself from the abuser (safe-havens, hot lines, etc.) is essential. An abused person is usually reluctant to call the police. Teaching the victim to fight back (as in

1 Instructions to call the police the next time the abuse occurs
2 Exploration of the pros and cons of remaining with the abusive family member
3 Specific information regarding "safe havens" or shelters in the client's neighborhood
4 Specific information about self-defense classes

the use of self-defense) is not appropriate when dealing with a violent person. Option 2 is an inappropriate intervention.

Test-Taking Strategy: Use Maslow's Hierarchy of Needs theory to recall that safety is the priority when a physiological condition is not present. Option 3 addresses safety. Review care to the client who is a victim of abuse if you had difficulty with this question.

Level of Cognitive Ability: Application
Client Needs: Safe, Effective Care Environment
Integrated Concept/Process: Nursing Process/Planning
Content Area: Mental Health

Reference:
Varcarolis, E. (2002). *Foundations of psychiatric mental health nursing* (4th ed.). Philadelphia: W.B. Saunders, p. 701.

---

123. A nurse is caring for a client with new application of a plaster leg cast. The nurse would take which action to prevent the development of compartment syndrome?
1 Elevate the limb and apply ice to the affected leg
2 Elevate and cover the limb with bath blankets
3 Place the leg in a slightly dependent position and apply ice
4 Keep the affected leg horizontal and apply heat

Answer: 1
Rationale: Compartment syndrome is prevented by controlling edema. Elevation and application of ice optimally achieve this. Options 2, 3, and 4 are incorrect.

Test-Taking Strategy: Use the process of elimination. Knowing that edema is controlled or prevented with limb elevation helps you to eliminate options 3 and 4. From the remaining options, think about the effects of ice versus bath blankets. Ice further controls edema, whereas bath blankets produce heat and prevent air circulation needed for the cast to dry. This will direct you to option 1. Review measures to prevent compartment syndrome if you had difficulty with this question.

Level of Cognitive Ability: Application
Client Needs: Safe, Effective Care Environment
Integrated Concept/Process: Nursing Process/Implementation
Content Area: Adult Health/Musculoskeletal

Reference:
Black, J., Hawks, J., & Keene, A. (2001). *Medical-surgical nursing: clinical management for positive outcomes* (6th ed.). Philadelphia: W.B. Saunders, p. 605.

---

124. An 8-year-old child is admitted to the hospital. The child has a recent history of sexual abuse by an adult family member. The child is withdrawn and appears frightened. The licensed practical nurse (LPN) is assigned to assist in caring for the child. Which of the following describes the best plan for the initial nursing encounter to convey concern and support?
1 Introduce yourself, explain your role, and ask the child to act out the sexual encounter with the abuser through the use of art therapy

Answer: 4
Rationale: The initial role of the nurse working with an abused victim is to establish trust. This is accomplished by providing a nonthreatening, stable, and safe environment. Establishing trust takes time. Victims of sexual abuse may exhibit fear and anxiety because of the recent incident. In addition, they may fear further abuse. When initiating contact with a child victim of sexual abuse who demonstrates fear of others, it is best to convey a willingness to spend time, and move slowly to initiate activities that may be perceived as threatening. Once rapport is established, the nurse may explore the child's feelings or use various therapeutic modalities to encourage a recounting of the offensive experience.

2 Introduce yourself, then ask the child to express how he or she feels about the events leading up to this admission
3 Introduce yourself and explain to the child that he or she is safe in the hospital
4 Introduce yourself and tell the child that the nurse would like to sit with him or her for awhile

Test-Taking Strategy: Use the process of elimination. Option 4 explains how to establish trust during an initial encounter by spending time with the child in a nonthreatening atmosphere. Options 1 and 2 may be implemented once trust and rapport are established. Option 3 may be appropriate but does not convey concern and support by the nurse. Review care to the child who is a victim of abuse if you had difficulty with this question.

Level of Cognitive Ability: Application
Client Needs: Safe, Effective Care Environment
Integrated Concept/Process: Nursing Process/Implementation
Content Area: Child Health

Reference:
Varcarolis, E. (2002). *Foundations of psychiatric mental health nursing* (4th ed.). Philadelphia: W.B. Saunders, p. 697.

---

125. A physician is about to defibrillate a client with ventricular fibrillation and says in a loud voice, "CLEAR!" The nurse immediately does which the following?
1 Shuts off the IV infusion going into the client's arm
2 Removes the back board
3 Steps away from the bed
4 Places the conductive gel pads for defibrillation on the client's chest

Answer: 3
Rationale: For the safety of all personnel, everyone must stand back and be clear of all contact with the client and the client's bed when the defibrillator paddles are being discharged. It is the primary responsibility of the person using the defibrillator paddles to communicate the "clear" message loudly enough for all to hear and to ensure everyone's compliance. All personnel must immediately comply with this command. The gel pads should have been placed on the client's chest before the defibrillator paddles were applied. The backboard is left in place for resuming cardiopulmonary resuscitation if necessary. Shutting off the IV infusion has no useful purpose.

Test-Taking Strategy: Use the process of elimination and focus on the issue of the question. Stepping back from the bed prevents the nurse from being defibrillated along with the client. Review safety measure related to defibrillation if you had difficulty with this question.

Level of Cognitive Ability: Application
Client Needs: Safe, Effective Care Environment
Integrated Concept/Process: Nursing Process/Implementation
Content Area: Adult Health/Cardiovascular

Reference:
Black, J., Hawks, J., & Keene, A. (2001). *Medical-surgical nursing: clinical management for positive outcomes* (6th ed.). Philadelphia: W.B. Saunders, p. 1566.

---

126. A client with chronic renal failure has an indwelling catheter in the abdomen that is used for peritoneal dialysis. The client spills water on the dressing while bathing. The licensed practical nurse reports the occurrence to the registered nurse (RN) and plans

Answer: 2
Rationale: Clients with peritoneal dialysis catheters are at high risk for infection. Because bacteria can reach the catheter insertion site more easily through a wet dressing, the nurse ensures that the dressing is kept dry at all times. In this circumstance, reinforcing the dressing is not a safe practice to prevent infection. Flushing the catheter is not indicated. Scrubbing the catheter with

to immediately assist with which of the following?
1   Reinforcing the dressing
2   Changing the dressing
3   Flushing the peritoneal dialysis catheter
4   Scrubbing the catheter with povidone iodine

povidone iodine is done at the time of connection or disconnection of peritoneal dialysis by the RN.

Test-Taking Strategy: Use the process of elimination. The issue of the question is that the dressing is wet. The correct option would focus on the dressing, not the catheter. This eliminates options 3 and 4. Knowing that it is better to change a wet dressing than reinforce it, you would choose option 2 as the correct option. Review the principles of asepsis if you had difficulty with this question.

Level of Cognitive Ability: Application
Client Needs: Safe, Effective Care Environment
Integrated Concept/Process: Nursing Process/Planning
Content Area: Adult Health/Renal

Reference:
Black, J., Hawks, J., & Keene, A. (2001). *Medical-surgical nursing: clinical management for positive outcomes* (6th ed.). Philadelphia: W.B. Saunders, p. 889.

---

127. A client diagnosed with tuberculosis (TB) is scheduled for an x-ray. Which of the following nursing interventions would be appropriate for the nurse to perform when sending the client to the x-ray department?
1   Apply a mask to the client
2   Apply a mask and gown to the client
3   Apply a mask, gown, and gloves to the client
4   Notify the x-ray department so the personnel will know to wear masks when the client arrives

Answer: 1
Rationale: Clients known or suspected of having tuberculosis should wear a mask when they are out of their room. A high efficiency particulate air (HEPA) respirator (mask) is worn by the nurse when caring for the client with tuberculosis. Gown and gloves are not needed for the client.

Test-Taking Strategy: Use the process of elimination. The issue relates to the times the client is out of his or her room. Common sense tells you that it would be impossible for everyone outside of the client's room to wear a mask; therefore eliminate option 4. Remember that the route of transmission of TB is airborne. Recalling this concept will eliminate options 2 and 3. Review the transmission associated with TB if you had difficulty with this question.

Level of Cognitive Ability: Application
Client Needs: Safe, Effective Care Environment
Integrated Concept/Process: Nursing Process/Implementation
Content Area: Adult Health/Respiratory

Reference:
Black, J., Hawks, J., & Keene, A. (2001). *Medical-surgical nursing: clinical management for positive outcomes* (6th ed.). Philadelphia: W.B. Saunders, p. 1722.

---

128. A nurse is caring for a client on contact isolation. After the nursing care has been performed, which protective item worn during client care would the nurse remove first when leaving the room?
1   Gloves
2   Mask
3   Eye wear
4   Gown

Answer: 3
Rationale: The nurse would remove eye wear (goggles) first. The nurse then unties the gown at the waist, removes one glove by grasping the cuff and pulling the glove inside out over the hand, and discards the glove. With the ungloved hand, the nurse tucks the finger inside the cuff of the remaining glove and pulls it off, inside out. The nurse unties the mask strings next and drops the mask into the trash receptacle. Then the nurse unties the neck strings of the gown and allows the gown to fall from the shoulders.

The nurse removes the hands from the sleeves, without touching the outside of the gown, holds the gown inside at the shoulder seams and folds it inside out, and discards it in the laundry bag. The nurse then washes the hands.

Test-Taking Strategy: Using knowledge of Universal Precautions and the methods to prevent contamination, attempt to visualize the correct process of removing contaminated clothing and items after caring for a client. This visualization should direct you to the correct option. Review this procedure if you had difficulty with this question.

Level of Cognitive Ability: Application
Client Needs: Safe, Effective Care Environment
Integrated Concept/Process: Nursing Process/Implementation
Content Area: Fundamental Skills

Reference:
Potter, P., & Perry, A. (2001). *Fundamentals of nursing* (5th ed.). St. Louis: Mosby, p. 859.

---

129. In planning safe activities for the depressed client during the early stages of hospitalization, the nurse most appropriately:
1. Provides an activity that is quiet and solitary in nature to avoid increased fatigue, such as working on a puzzle or reading a book
2. Plans nothing until the client asks to participate in milieu
3. Offers the client a menu of daily activities and insists that the client participates in all of them
4. Provides a structured daily program of activities and encourages the client to participate

Answer: 4
Rationale: A depressed person is often withdrawn. Also, the person experiences difficulty concentrating, loss of interest or pleasure, low energy, fatigue, feelings of worthlessness, and poor self-esteem. The plan of care should provide successful experiences in a stimulating yet structured environment. Options 1 and 2 are restrictive. Option 3 is demanding.

Test-Taking Strategy: Use the process of elimination. Remember that the depressed client requires a structured and stimulating program. Options 1 and 2 are too "restrictive" and offer little or no structure and stimulation. Option 3 is eliminated because of the high demands placed on the client. Review care to the client with depression if you had difficulty with this question.

Level of Cognitive Ability: Application
Client Needs: Safe, Effective Care Environment
Integrated Concept/Process: Nursing Process/Implementation
Content Area: Mental Health

Reference:
Varcarolis, E. (2002). *Foundations of psychiatric mental health nursing* (4th ed.). Philadelphia: W.B. Saunders, p. 461.

---

130. A nurse is in the process of giving the client a bed bath. During the procedure, the unit secretary calls the nurse on the intercom to ask the nurse to answer an emergency phone call. What would be the most appropriate nursing action?
1. Leave the door open so that the client can be monitored and answer the phone call

Answer: 4
Rationale: When an emergency phone call must be answered, one appropriate action is to ask another nurse to accept the call; however, this is not one of the options. If it is necessary for the nurse to answer the call and leave the room temporarily, the door should be closed or the room curtains pulled around the bathing area to provide privacy. To maintain safety, the call light should be placed within the client's reach.

2   Finish the bath before answering the phone call

3   Walk out of the room and answer the phone call

4   Put the call light within the client's reach and answer the phone call

Test-Taking Strategy: Use the process of elimination. Note the key words *emergency phone call.* This should assist in eliminating option 2. From the remaining options, the only option that addresses client safety and comfort is option 4. Review these safety measures if you had difficulty with this question.

Level of Cognitive Ability: Application
Client Needs: Safe, Effective Care Environment
Integrated Concept/Process: Nursing Process/Implementation
Content Area: Fundamental Skills

Reference:
Potter, P., & Perry, A. (2001). *Fundamentals of nursing* (5th ed.). St. Louis: Mosby, p. 1035.

---

131. A licensed practical nurse (LPN) has been instructed to move a client from the bed to a chair 1 day after a total knee replacement. The LPN reviews the physician's orders and would expect to note which of the following orders to protect the knee joint?

1   Apply a knee immobilizer before moving the client, and elevate the client's surgical leg while the client is seated

2   Apply a compression bandage around the dressing, and put ice on the knee while the client is seated

3   Lift the client to the bedside chair, leaving the continuous passive motion (CPM) machine in place

4   Obtain a walker to minimize weight bearing by the client on the affected leg

Answer: 1
Rationale: On the first postoperative day, the nurse assists the client in getting out of bed after stabilizing the affected joint with a knee immobilizer. The surgeon orders the weight-bearing limits on the affected leg. The leg is elevated while the client is sitting in the chair to minimize edema. A compression dressing should already be in place on the wound. The CPM machine is used only while the client is in bed. Ambulation is not started until the second postoperative day.

Test-Taking Strategy: Use the process of elimination. Focus on the issue to protect the knee joint. This will direct you to option 1 because a knee immobilizer will protect the joint. Review postoperative care after this procedure if you had difficulty with this question.

Level of Cognitive Ability: Comprehension
Client Needs: Safe, Effective Care Environment
Integrated Concept/Process: Nursing Process/Implementation
Content Area: Adult Health/Musculoskeletal

Reference:
Black, J., Hawks, J., & Keene, A. (2001). *Medical-surgical nursing: clinical management for positive outcomes* (6th ed.). Philadelphia: W.B. Saunders, p. 565.

---

132. A nurse in the physician's office receives a telephone call from a male client who states that he wants to kill himself and has a loaded gun on the table. The best nursing intervention is which of the following?

1   Insist that the client give you his name and address so that you can send the police immediately

2   Keep the client talking

3   Try to contact the physician

4   Keep the client talking and signal to another staff member to trace the call so that appropriate help can be sent

Answer: 4
Rationale: In a crisis, the nurse must take an authoritative, active role to promote the client's safety. When a client who has a loaded gun in his home verbalizes that he wants to kill himself, the client's safety is the primary concern. Keeping the client on the phone and getting help to the client is the best intervention. The word *insist* may anger the client and he might hang up. Keeping the client talking is only a part of the nursing intervention. Contacting the physician is not the most appropriate intervention at this time.

Test-Taking Strategy: Use the process of elimination, keeping the focus of safety in mind. Option 4 is the most global option and encompasses the necessary actions. Review emergency measures in a crisis related to suicide if you had difficulty with this question.

Level of Cognitive Ability: Application
Client Needs: Safe, Effective Care Environment
Integrated Concept/Process: Nursing Process/Implementation
Content Area: Mental Health

Reference:
Varcarolis, E. (2002). *Foundations of psychiatric mental health nursing* (4th ed.). Philadelphia: W.B. Saunders, p. 619.

---

133. A nurse in a long-term care facility determines the need to place a vest restraint on a client, but the client does not want a vest restraint applied. The best nursing action would be to:
1   Apply the restraint anyway
2   Contact the physician
3   Medicate the client with a sedative, then apply the restraint
4   Compromise with the client and use wrist restraints

Answer: 2
Rationale: The use of restraints should be avoided if possible. If the nurse determines that a restraint is necessary, the procedure should be discussed with the client's family and an order should be obtained from the physician. The physician's order protects the nurse from liability. The nurse should carefully explain to the client and the client's family the reasons that the restraint is necessary, the type of restraint selected, and the anticipated duration of restraint.

Test-Taking Strategy: Use the process of elimination. Eliminate option 1 first. If the nurse applied the restraint to a client who was refusing the procedure, the nurse could be charged with battery. Eliminate option 3 next because it is similar to option 1, and the nurse could be charged with battery. Option 4 could be an unsafe and ineffective procedure if the vest restraint was initially considered necessary. Review the issues surrounding the use of restraints if you had difficulty with this question.

Level of Cognitive Ability: Application
Client Needs: Safe, Effective Care Environment
Integrated Concept/Process: Nursing Process/Implementation
Content Area: Fundamental Skills

Reference:
Potter, P., & Perry, A. (2001). *Fundamentals of nursing* (5th ed.). St. Louis: Mosby, p. 1039.

---

134. A client is being discharged from the hospital and will receive oxygen therapy at home. The nurse is reinforcing instructions with the client and family about oxygen safety measures in the home. Which of the following statements indicates that the client needs further instruction?
1   "I realize that I should check the oxygen level of the portable tank on a consistent basis."
2   "I will keep my scented candles within 5 feet of my oxygen tank."

Answer: 2
Rationale: Oxygen is a highly combustible gas. Although it will not spontaneously burn or cause an explosion, oxygen can easily cause a fire to ignite in a client's room if it comes in contact with a spark from a cigarette, candle, or electrical equipment. Oxygen in high concentrations is highly combustible and causes fire to spread quickly. The client should contact the physician if shortness of breath occurs.

Test-Taking Strategy: Use the process of elimination and note the key words *needs further instruction*. Remembering that oxygen is a highly combustible gas will assist in directing you to option 2.

3 "I will not sit in front of my fire-place (wood burning) with my oxygen on."

4 "I will call the physician if I experience any shortness of breath."

If you had difficulty with this question, review teaching points related to home care and oxygen.

Level of Cognitive Ability: Comprehension
Client Needs: Safe, Effective Care Environment
Integrated Concept/Process: Teaching/Learning
Content Area: Fundamental Skills

Reference:
Potter, P., & Perry, A. (2001). *Fundamentals of nursing* (5th ed.). St. Louis: Mosby, p. 1181.

---

135. A nurse is preparing to administer a continuous tube feeding via a feeding pump. The nurse notes that the electrical cord for the pump has only two prongs. Which of the following is the most appropriate action?

1 Use the plug anyway
2 Contact the physician
3 Run the pump on the battery
4 Obtain a 3-prong grounded plug

Answer: 4
Rationale: Electrical equipment must be maintained in good working order and should be grounded. The third longer prong in an electrical plug is the ground. Theoretically, the ground prong carries any stray electrical current back to the ground. The other two prongs carry the power to the piece of electrical equipment. There is no reason to contact the physician. Running the pump on the battery is not the most appropriate nursing action because the battery will run out, especially because the feeding is continuous.

Test-Taking Strategy: Use the process of elimination. Note the key words *only two prongs*. Principles of basic electrical safety should assist in directing you to the correct option. Review these principles if you had difficulty with this question.

Level of Cognitive Ability: Application
Client Needs: Safe, Effective Care Environment
Integrated Concept/Process: Nursing Process/Implementation
Content Area: Fundamental Skills

Reference:
Potter, P., & Perry, A. (2001). *Fundamentals of nursing* (5th ed.). St. Louis: Mosby, p. 1046.

---

136. A nurse is questioning a client about potential hazards in the home environment. Which of the following items in the home if identified by the client is an indication that the client needs instruction about safety?

1 Skid-resistant, small area rugs in the living room
2 Clothes hamper at the end of the hallway
3 Area rugs on the stairs
4 Carpeted stairs secured with carpet tacks

Answer: 3
Rationale: Area rugs and runners should not be used on or near stairs. Any carpeting on the stairs should be secured with carpet tacks. Injuries in the home frequently result from small rugs on the stairs and floor, wet spots on the floor, and clutter on bedside tables, closet shelves, the top of the refrigerator, and bookshelves. Care should also be taken to ensure that end tables are secure and have stable straight legs. Nonessential items should be placed in drawers to eliminate clutter

Test-Taking Strategy: Use the process of elimination and note the key words *needs instruction*. Recalling the principles related to home safety will assist in directing you to the correct option. Review these principles if you had difficulty with this question.

Level of Cognitive Ability: Comprehension
Client Needs: Safe, Effective Care Environment

Integrated Concept/Process: Nursing Process/Evaluation
Content Area: Fundamental Skills

Reference:
Potter, P., & Perry, A. (2001). *Fundamentals of nursing* (5th ed.). St. Louis: Mosby, p. 1021.

---

137. A hospitalized client with a history of alcohol abuse tells the nurse, "I am leaving now. I have to go. I don't want anymore treatment. I have things that I have to do right away." The client has not been discharged. In fact, the client is scheduled for an important diagnostic test to be performed in 1 hour. After the nurse discusses the client's concerns with the client, the client dresses and begins to walk out of the hospital room. The most appropriate nursing action is which of the following?
1   Restrain the client until the physician can be reached
2   Call security to block all exit areas
3   Tell the client that he or she cannot return to this hospital again if he or she leaves now
4   Notify the registered nurse (RN)

Answer: 4
Rationale: A nurse can be charged with false imprisonment if a client is made to wrongfully believe that he or she cannot leave the hospital. Most health care facilities have documents that the client is asked to sign that relate to the client's responsibilities when the client leaves against medical advice (AMA). The LPN should notify the RN who will ask the client to sign this document before leaving. The RN should request that the client wait to speak to the physician before leaving, but if the client refuses to do so, the nurse cannot hold the client against his or her will. Restraining the client and calling security to block exits constitutes false imprisonment. Any client has a right to health care and cannot be told otherwise.

Test-Taking Strategy: Use the process of elimination. Keeping the concept of false imprisonment in mind, eliminate options 1 and 2 because they are similar. Eliminate option 3, knowing that any client has a right to health care. Review the points related to false imprisonment if you had difficulty with this question.

Level of Cognitive Ability: Application
Client Needs: Safe, Effective Care Environment
Integrated Concept/Process: Nursing Process/Implementation
Content Area: Fundamental Skills

Reference:
Brent, N. (2002) *Nurses and the law* (2nd ed.). Philadelphia: W.B. Saunders, p. 115.

---

138. Two nurses are in the cafeteria having lunch in a quiet secluded area. A physical therapist from the physical therapy department joins the nurses. During lunch, the nurses discuss a client who was physically abused. After lunch, the physical therapist provides therapy to the abused client and asks the client questions about the physical abuse. The client discovers that the nurses told the therapist about the abuse situation and is emotionally harmed. The consequences associated with the nurses' discussion about the client are most appropriately associated with which of the following?
1   None, because they were in a quiet secluded area
2   They can be charged with slander

Answer: 2
Rationale: Defamation occurs when information that causes damage to someone else's reputation is communicated to a third party either in writing (libel) or verbally (slander). The most common examples are giving out inaccurate or inappropriate information from the medical record; discussing clients, families, or visitors in public areas; or speaking negatively about co-workers. This situation can cause emotional harm to the client, and the nurses could be charged with slander. This situation also violates the client's right to confidentiality.

Test-Taking Strategy: Use the process of elimination and knowledge about the law and legal responsibilities of the nurse in protecting the client to answer the question. Eliminate options 1 and 4 first. From the remaining options, it is necessary to know that slander involves verbal discussion about a client. Review this legal responsibility if you had difficulty with this question.

3   They can be charged with libel
4   None, because the physical thera-
     pist is involved in the client's care

Level of Cognitive Ability: Comprehension
Client Needs: Safe, Effective Care Environment
Integrated Concept/Process: Nursing Process/Implementation
Content Area: Fundamental Skills

Reference:
Potter, P., & Perry, A. (2001). *Fundamentals of nursing* (5th ed.). St. Louis: Mosby, p. 426.

---

139. A nurse is assisting in planning care for a client diagnosed with deep vein thrombosis (DVT) of the left leg. Which of the following interventions would the nurse plan to avoid in the care of this client?
1   Application of moist heat to the left leg
2   Administration of acetaminophen (Tylenol) as prescribed
3   Elevation of the left leg
4   Ambulation in the hall once per shift

Answer: 4
Rationale: Standard management of the client with DVT includes bed rest for 5 to 7 days as prescribed, limb elevation, relief of discomfort with warm moist heat and analgesics as needed, anticoagulant therapy, and monitoring for signs of pulmonary embolism. Ambulation is contraindicated because it increases the likelihood of dislodgement of the thrombus, which would travel to the lungs as a pulmonary embolism.

Test Taking Strategy: Use the process of elimination. Note the key word *avoid*. Application of heat and limb elevation are indicated to reduce inflammation and edema, so these options are eliminated. Tylenol relieves discomfort and is also indicated. This leaves ambulation, which could lead to pulmonary embolism. Review care to the client with DVT if you had difficulty with this question.

Level of Cognitive Ability: Application
Client Needs: Safe, Effective Care Environment
Integrated Concept/Process: Nursing Process/Planning
Content Area: Adult Health/Cardiovascular

Reference:
Black, J., Hawks, J., & Keene, A. (2001). *Medical-surgical nursing: clinical management for positive outcomes* (6th ed.). Philadelphia: W.B. Saunders, p. 1422.

---

140. A nurse administers the morning dose of digoxin (Lanoxin) to a client. When charting the medication, the nurse discovers that a dose of 0.25 mg was administered rather than the prescribed dose of 0.125 mg. Which of the following actions will the nurse take?
1   Administer an additional 0.125 mg
2   Tell the client that the dose administered was not the total amount and administer the additional dose
3   Tell the client that too much medication was administered and an error was made
4   Complete an incident report

Answer: 4
Rationale: In accordance with the agency's policies, nurses are required to file incident reports when a situation arises that could or did cause client harm. If a dose of 0.125 mg was prescribed, and a dose of 0.25 mg was administered, then the client received too much medication. Additional medication is not required and in fact could be detrimental. The client should be informed when an error has occurred but in a professional manner so as not to cause fear and concern. In many situations, the physician will discuss this with the client.

Test-Taking Strategy: Use the process of elimination. Simple math calculation will assist in eliminating both options 1 and 2. From the remaining options, select option 4 because it is the nurse's responsibility to complete this form. Review nursing responsibilities related to medication errors if you had difficulty with this question.

Level of Cognitive Ability: Application
Client Needs: Safe, Effective Care Environment
Integrated Concept/Process: Nursing Process/Implementation
Content Area: Fundamental Skills

Reference:
Brent, N. (2002) *Nurses and the law* (2nd ed.). Philadelphia: W.B. Saunders, p. 105.

---

141. A client has an indwelling urinary catheter. The nurse would plan to ensure that the nursing assistant does not:
1 Use soap and water to cleanse the perineal area
2 Keep the drainage bag below the level of the bladder
3 Prevent kinks in the tubing
4 Let the drainage tubing rest under the client's leg

Answer: 4
Rationale: Proper care of an indwelling catheter is especially important to prevent infection. The nurse and all caregivers must use strict aseptic technique when emptying the drainage bag or obtaining urine specimens. The perineal area is cleansed thoroughly using mild soap and water at least twice a day and after a bowel movement. The drainage bag is kept below the level of the bladder to prevent urine from being trapped in the bladder, and for the same reason, the drainage tubing is not placed under the client's leg. The tubing must drain freely at all times.

Test-Taking Strategy: Use the process of elimination and note the key word *not*. Eliminate option 1 first, as this is a basic standard of care for the client with an indwelling catheter. Option 3 is consistent with principles of care and will assist in promoting drainage. From the remaining options, recall that option 2 promotes drainage, and option 4 could impede drainage. Thus the answer to the question is option 4. Review care to the client with an indwelling urinary catheter if you had difficulty with this question.

Level of Cognitive Ability: Application
Client Needs: Safe, Effective Care Environment
Integrated Concept/Process: Nursing Process/Implementation
Content Area: Fundamental Skills

Reference:
Potter, P., & Perry, A. (2001). *Fundamentals of nursing* (5th ed.). St. Louis: Mosby, p. 1412.

---

142. A client is scheduled for bronchoscopy. The nurse gives which of the following measures the highest priority?
1 Restricting the diet to clear liquids on the day of the test
2 Asking the client about allergies to shellfish
3 Obtaining an informed consent for an invasive procedure
4 Administering preprocedure antibiotics prophylactically

Answer: 3
Rationale: Bronchoscopy requires that an informed consent be obtained from the client before the procedure. The client is kept NPO for at least 6 hours before the procedure. It is unnecessary to inquire about allergies to shellfish before this procedure because no contrast dye is injected. There is also no need for prophylactic antibiotics.

Test-Taking Strategy: This question can be answered by recalling that bronchoscopy is an invasive procedure and requires an informed consent specific for this procedure. If this question was difficult, review this procedure.

Level of Cognitive Ability: Application
Client Needs: Safe, Effective Care Environment

Integrated Concept/Process: Nursing Process/Implementation
Content Area: Adult Health/Respiratory

Reference:
Black, J., Hawks, J., & Keene, A. (2001). *Medical-surgical nursing: clinical management for positive outcomes* (6th ed.). Philadelphia: W.B. Saunders, p. 200.

---

143. A client with urolithiasis is being evaluated to determine the type of stone that is being formed. The nurse would provide the client with which item to assist in this process?
1   A calorie count sheet
2   A strainer
3   An intake and output record
4   A vital signs graphic sheet

Answer: 2
Rationale: The urine is strained to catch small stones that can be sent to the laboratory for analysis. Once the type of stone is determined, an individualized plan of care and prevention is developed. Options 1, 3, and 4 will not assist in determining the stone type.

Test-Taking Strategy: Use the process of elimination. Note that the question asks for an item that will help to determine the type of stone. Therefore, even if several of the options may be appropriate for use with the client with urolithiasis, you must select the one that is specific for this purpose. Begin by eliminating options 3 and 4, as these items give information about vital signs and fluid balance, but do not provide data that will help determine the type of stone. From the remaining options, choose option 2, knowing that straining the urine would allow possible capture of small stones that could then be sent to the laboratory for analysis. Review care to the client with urolithiasis if you had difficulty with this question.

Level of Cognitive Ability: Application
Client Needs: Safe, Effective Care Environment
Integrated Concept/Process: Nursing Process/Implementation
Content Area: Adult Health/Renal

Reference:
Black, J., Hawks, J., & Keene, A. (2001). *Medical-surgical nursing: clinical management for positive outcomes* (6th ed.). Philadelphia: W.B. Saunders, pp. 882-883.

---

144. A child is hospitalized with an undiagnosed exanthema (rash) that covers the trunk profusely and is sparse on the extremities. The child was exposed to varicella 2 weeks ago. The most appropriate nursing intervention will be to:
1   Allow the child to play in the playroom until orders are received from the physician
2   Place the child in a private room on strict isolation
3   Immediately place the child in any available bed
4   Check the progression of the exanthema and report it to physician

Answer: 2
Rationale: The child with undiagnosed exanthema should be placed on strict isolation in a private room. Varicella causes a profuse rash on the trunk with a sparse rash on the extremities. It is important to prevent the spread of this communicable disease by placing the child in isolation until further diagnosis and treatment is made. Options 1, 3, and 4 are incorrect.

Test-Taking Strategy: Use the process of elimination. Option 2 prevents the child from exposing other children and keeps staff, visitors, and others at minimal risk. Option 1 exposes other children or the environment unnecessarily to varicella. Admitting the child to "any" room is inappropriate. Checking the progression of the exanthema is correct, but it is not the most appropriate immediate intervention. Review care to the child with exanthema if you had difficulty with this question.

Level of Cognitive Ability: Application
Client Needs: Safe, Effective Care Environment

Integrated Concept/Process: Nursing Process/Implementation
Content Area: Child Health

Reference:
Wong, D., & Hockenberry-Eaton, M. (2001). *Wong's essentials of pediatric nursing* (6th ed.). St. Louis: Mosby, p. 456.

---

145. Before administering an intermittent tube feeding, a nurse aspirates 40 mL of undigested formula from the client's nasogastric tube. Before administering the tube feeding, the nurse does which the following with the 40 mL of gastric aspirate?

1 Discards it properly and records it as output on the client's I&O record
2 Pours it into the nasogastric tube through a syringe with the plunger removed
3 Mixes it with the formula and pours it into the nasogastric tube through a syringe without a plunger
4 Dilutes it with water and injects it into the nasogastric tube by putting pressure on the plunger

Answer: 2
Rationale: After checking residual feeding contents, gastric contents are reinstilled into the stomach by removing the syringe bulb or plunger and pouring the gastric contents via the syringe into the nasogastric tube. Gastric contents should be reinstilled to maintain the client's electrolyte balance. The gastric aspirate need not be mixed with water or formula, nor should it be discarded or injected by putting pressure on the plunger.

Test-Taking Strategy: Use the process of elimination. Remembering that removal of the gastric contents could disturb the client's electrolyte balance will assist in eliminating option 1. Eliminate option 4 because of the word *pressure*. Recalling that aspirated gastric contents should be immediately replaced will assist in directing you to the correct option. Review this procedure if you had difficulty with this question.

Level of Cognitive Ability: Application
Client Needs: Safe, Effective Care Environment
Integrated Concept/Process: Nursing Process/Implementation
Content Area: Fundamental Skills

Reference:
Potter, P., & Perry, A. (2001). *Fundamentals of nursing* (5th ed.). St. Louis: Mosby, p. 1358.

---

146. A nurse has an order to obtain a urinalysis from a client with an indwelling urinary catheter. To prevent contamination of the specimen, the nurse would avoid which of the following?

1 Obtaining the specimen from the urinary drainage bag
2 Clamping the tubing of the drainage bag
3 Aspirating a sample from the port on the drainage system
4 Wiping the port with an alcohol swab before inserting the syringe

Answer: 1
Rationale: A urine specimen is not taken from the urinary drainage bag. Urine undergoes chemical changes while sitting in the bag; therefore it does not necessarily reflect current client status. In addition, it may become contaminated with bacteria from opening the system.

Test-Taking Strategy: Note the key word *avoid*. Use the process of elimination, bearing in mind the issue of preventing contamination. This thought process should assist in directing you to the correct option. If this question was difficult review this procedure.

Level of Cognitive Ability: Application
Client Needs: Safe, Effective Care Environment
Integrated Concept/Process: Nursing Process/Implementation
Content Area: Fundamental Skills

Reference:
Potter, P., & Perry, A. (2001). *Fundamentals of nursing* (5th ed.). St. Louis: Mosby, p. 1402.

147. A client requests pain medication from the nurse. After administration of the intramuscular (IM) injection, the nurse would do which of the following first?

1 Recap the needle
2 Assist the client to ambulate to aid in absorption
3 Massage the injection site with alcohol
4 Place the syringe on the overbed table

Answer: 3

Rationale: The nurse should first massage the injection site lightly after an IM injection to assist in medication absorption. The needle is not recapped or placed on the overbed table. The needle and syringe are placed in the appropriate puncture resistant receptacle. The client in pain should not be ambulated to aid in medication absorption.

Test-Taking Strategy: Use the process of elimination and note the key word *first*. Visualize this procedure and use knowledge of the principles related to the safe administration of IM medication to direct you to option 3. Review this procedure if you had difficulty with this question.

Level of Cognitive Ability: Application
Client Needs: Safe, Effective Care Environment
Integrated Concept/Process: Nursing Process/Implementation
Content Area: Fundamental Skills

Reference:
Potter, P., & Perry, A. (2001) *Fundamentals of nursing* (5th ed.). St. Louis: Mosby, p. 944.

---

148. A child is seen in the health care clinic and initial testing for human immunodeficiency virus (HIV) is performed because of the child's exposure to HIV infection. Which of the following home care instructions would the nurse provide to the parents of the child?

1 Avoid all immunizations until the diagnosis is established
2 Avoid sharing toothbrushes
3 Wipe up any blood spills with soap and water and allow to air dry
4 Wash hands with half strength bleach if they come in contact with the child's blood

Answer: 2

Rationale: Immunizations must be kept up to date. Blood spills are wiped up with a paper towel; the area is then washed with soap and water, rinsed with bleach and water, and allowed to air dry. Hands are washed with soap and water if they come in contact with blood. Parents are instructed that toothbrushes are not to be shared.

Test-Taking Strategy: Use the process of elimination. Eliminate option 1 first because of the word *all*. Eliminate option 3 next based on the knowledge that blood spills should be cleaned with a bleach solution. Eliminate option 4 because bleach would be very irritating and caustic to the skin. If you had difficulty with this question, review home care instructions for the child exposed to HIV infection.

Level of Cognitive Ability: Application
Client Needs: Safe, Effective Care Environment
Integrated Concept/Process: Teaching/Learning
Content Area: Child Health

Reference:
Wong, D., & Hockenberry-Eaton, M. (2001). *Wong's essentials of pediatric nursing* (6th ed.). St. Louis: Mosby, p. 359.

---

149. A nurse is preparing to leave the room of a client with a tracheostomy. The nurse ensures that the client has which of the following means of communication readily available before leaving the room?

Answer: 2

Rationale: Before leaving the room, the nurse ensures that the call bell is readily available. The client who cannot speak must have a means of contacting the nurse who is not in the room. The other options facilitate communication when the nurse is already present in the client's room.

1 Pen and paper
2 Call bell
3 Picture board
4 Letter board

Test-Taking Strategy: Use the process of elimination and knowledge of basic principles of communication to answer this question. The key words in the question are *tracheostomy* and *leaving the room*. Remember that options that are similar are often incorrect. With this in mind, eliminate options 1, 3, and 4. Review these methods of communication if you had difficulty with this question.

Level of Cognitive Ability: Application
Client Needs: Safe, Effective Care Environment
Integrated Concept/Process: Communication and Documentation
Content Area: Adult Health/Respiratory

Reference:
Lewis, S., Heitkemper, M., & Dirksen, S. (2000). *Medical-surgical nursing: assessment and management of clinical problems* (5th ed.). St. Louis: Mosby, p. 598.

---

150. A nurse is reinforcing instructions with a client being discharged from the hospital with home oxygen. Which statement by the client indicates a need for further instruction?
1 "I should place the oxygen concentrator tightly in a corner."
2 "I should keep open flames at least 10 feet away from the oxygen source."
3 "No one can smoke near the oxygen."
4 "I should keep the oxygen tank secured in a holder."

Answer: 1
Rationale: There should be no open flames or smoking within 10 feet of the oxygen source. The tank should remain secured in its holder, and the concentrator should be away from walls or other close quarters (to allow adequate air circulation around the unit). The oxygen source should also be removed from sources of heat and sunlight.

Test-Taking Strategy: Use the process of elimination. Note the key words *need for further instruction*. Remembering that similar options are not likely to be correct will assist you in eliminating options 2 and 3. Use basic nursing knowledge about oxygen in selecting option 1 instead of option 4. Review safety measures related to oxygen use if you had difficulty with this question.

Level of Cognitive Ability: Comprehension
Client Needs: Safe, Effective Care Environment
Integrated Concept/Process: Teaching/Learning
Content Area: Adult Health/Respiratory

Reference:
Potter, P., & Perry, A. (2001). *Fundamentals of nursing* (5th ed.). St. Louis: Mosby, p. 1181.

---

151. A nurse is collecting data regarding home safety from an older client who is at risk for falls. The nurse determines that which of the following items in the home poses a potential risk for the client?
1 Scatter rugs
2 Shower seat
3 Railings on staircase
4 Bathroom handrails

Answer: 1
Rationale: The incidence of falls by older clients can be reduced by the use of bathroom safety equipment such as a shower seat and handrails. In addition, the home should have railings on all staircases and ample lighting. Scatter rugs could potentially cause the older client to fall and should be removed or at least secured with a nonskid backing.

Test-Taking Strategy: Use the process of elimination. The issue stated in the question is a factor in the home that poses a risk to the client. Begin to answer by eliminating options 3 and 4, which provide physical support to the client and pose no risk. Using this same line of reasoning, eliminate option 2, the shower seat. Review measures to prevent falls if you had difficulty with this question.

Level of Cognitive Ability: Comprehension
Client Needs: Safe, Effective Care Environment
Integrated Concept/Process: Nursing Process/Data Collection
Content Area: Adult Health/Musculoskeletal

Reference:
Potter, P., & Perry, A. (2001). *Fundamentals of nursing* (5th ed.). St. Louis: Mosby, p. 1020.

---

152. A physician tells a nurse that a client admitted with a neurological problem will be scheduled for magnetic resonance imaging (MRI). The nurse questions the physician about this procedure based on a client history of which of the following?
1   Prosthetic valve replacement?
2   Cardiac dysrhythmias
3   Chronic airflow limitation
4   Heart failure

Answer: 1
Rationale: The client scheduled for MRI removes all metallic objects because of the magnetic field generated by the device. A careful history is done to determine if any metal objects have been implanted in the client, such as orthopedic hardware, pacemakers, artificial heart valves, aneurysm clips, or intrauterine devices. These may heat up, become dislodged, or malfunction during the procedure. The client may be ineligible if there is a significant risk. The remaining options pose no risk to the client scheduled for MRI.

Test-Taking Strategy: Use the process of elimination and focus on the issue: contraindications to MRI. Noting the word *magnetic* in the name of the test will direct you to option 1. Review this diagnostic test if you had difficulty with this question.

Level of Cognitive Ability: Application
Client Needs: Safe, Effective Care Environment
Integrated Concept/Process: Nursing Process/Data Collection
Content Area: Adult Health/Neurological

Reference:
Lewis, S., Heitkemper, M., & Dirksen, S. (2000). *Medical-surgical nursing: assessment and management of clinical problems* (5th ed.). St. Louis: Mosby, p. 1030.

---

153. A clinic nurse is providing instructions to a mother whose child was diagnosed with rubeola (red measles). To prevent the infection from spreading to her other children, the mother asks the nurse how the measles are transmitted. The nurse informs the mother that rubeola is transmitted by which the following?
1   Airborne particles
2   Fecal-oral route
3   Saliva
4   Contact with sweat

Answer: 1
Rationale: Rubeola is transmitted via airborne particles or by direct contact with infectious droplets. Options 2, 3, and 4 are incorrect.

Test-Taking Strategy: Knowledge regarding the route of transmission of rubeola is required to answer this question. Review the route of transmission of this infectious disease if you had difficulty with this question.

Level of Cognitive Ability: Application
Client Needs: Safe, Effective Care Environment
Integrated Concept/Process: Teaching/Learning
Content Area: Child Health

Reference:
Wong, D., & Hockenberry-Eaton, M. (2001). *Wong's essentials of pediatric nursing* (6th ed.). St. Louis: Mosby, p. 460.

---

154. A nurse is called to a client's room by another nurse. When the nurse arrives at the room, the nurse discovers that a fire has occurred in the client's waste basket. The first nurse has removed the client from the room. What is the second nurse's next action?

1 Evacuate the unit
2 Extinguish the fire
3 Confine the fire
4 Activate the fire alarm

Answer: 4
Rationale: Remember the acronym RACE to set priorities if a fire occurs. R stands for rescue. A stands or alarm. C stands for confine. E stands for extinguish. In this situation, the client has been rescued from the immediate vicinity of the fire. The next action is to activate the fire alarm.

Test-Taking Strategy: Use the RACE acronym to set priorities to answer the question. If you had difficulty with this question, review fire safety.

Level of Cognitive Ability: Application
Client Needs: Safe, Effective Care Environment
Integrated Concept/Process: Nursing Process/Implementation
Content Area: Fundamental Skills

Reference:
Potter, P., & Perry, A. (2001). *Fundamentals of nursing* (5th ed.). St. Louis: Mosby, p. 114.

---

155. A nurse is providing instructions to a mother of a child diagnosed with rubeola (red measles). Which of the following information does the nurse provide to the mother regarding the infectious period for this type of measles?

1 Ranges from 1 to 2 days before the onset of symptoms to 4 days after rash appearance
2 Ranges from 10 days before the onset of symptoms to 15 days after rash appearance
3 Unknown but is thought to extend from the prodromal period until the appearance of the rash
4 Usually ranges from 1 to 2 days

Answer: 1
Rationale: Rubeola has an infectious period that ranges from 1 to 2 days before the onset of symptoms to 4 days after rash appearance. Option 2 identifies the infectious period for rubella (German measles). Option 3 identifies erythema infectiosum (fifth disease). Option 4 identifies the infectious period for mumps, which is usually 1 to 2 days (7 days before swelling to 9 days after onset).

Test-Taking Strategy: Use the process of elimination. Knowledge regarding the infectious period for rubeola is required to answer this question. Review this infectious disease if you had difficulty with this question.

Level of Cognitive Ability: Application
Client Needs: Safe, Effective Care Environment
Integrated Concept/Process: Nursing Process/Implementation
Content Area: Child Health

Reference:
Wong, D., & Hockenberry-Eaton, M. (2001). *Wong's essentials of pediatric nursing* (6th ed.). St. Louis: Mosby, p. 460.

---

156. A licensed practical nurse (LPN) employed in a long-term care facility is making the assignments for the day. When delegating a task, the LPN gives authority and responsibility to a team member regarding the task by:

Answer: 2
Rationale: Authority for task completion is not given to the team member by directing or participating but by allowing the team member to be responsible for completing the task on his or her own. Options 1, 3, and 4 do not delegate authority and responsibility to the person performing the task.

1 Suggesting how to complete the task
2 Waiting for the team member to report the results of the completed task
3 Completing the task for the team member
4 Checking to be sure the task is complete

Test-Taking Strategy: Use the process of elimination. Note the similarity in options 1, 3, and 4. These options all have the LPN involved in task completion. Review the principles related to delegation if you had difficulty with this question.

Level of Cognitive Ability: Application
Client Needs: Safe, Effective Care Environment
Integrated Concept/Process: Nursing Process/Implementation
Content Area: Fundamental Skills

Reference:
Potter, P., & Perry, A. (2001). *Fundamentals of nursing* (5th ed.). St. Louis: Mosby, p. 359.

---

157. A licensed practical nurse (LPN) is watching a student nurse insert an indwelling bladder catheter. The LPN would intervene if the student were observed doing which of the following?
1 Lubricating the catheter tip with water-soluble jelly
2 Stopping catheter advancement just as urine appears in the catheter tubing
3 Inflating the balloon with more than the stated balloon capacity
4 Coiling the tubing of the collection bag

Answer: 2
Rationale: The catheter should be advanced 1 to 2 inches beyond the point where the flow of urine is first noted. This ensures that the balloon is fully in the bladder before it is inflated. Each of the other options represents correct procedure. The catheter tip is lubricated for easier insertion. Extra fluid is needed to fill the lumen that runs between the external port and the balloon at the tip of the catheter. The tubing should be coiled, not kinked, and the collection bag should be placed lower than the level of the bladder.

Test-Taking Strategy: Use the process of elimination and note the key word *intervene*. Recalling that the catheter is advanced 1 to 2 inches after urine is seen will direct you to option 2. Review this procedure if you had difficulty with this question.

Level of Cognitive Ability: Application
Client Needs: Safe, Effective Care Environment
Integrated Concept/Process: Nursing Process/Implementation
Content Area: Adult Health/Renal

Reference:
Perry, A., & Potter, A. (2002). *Clinical nursing skills & techniques* (5th ed.). St. Louis: Mosby, p. 411.

---

158. A nurse is reviewing the physician's orders for a client with acute pancreatitis. Which of the following, if noted in the client's record, would the nurse question?
1 Morphine sulfate for pain
2 Nothing by mouth (NPO) status
3 Intravenous fluids
4 Histamine H$_2$ antagonist

Answer: 1
Rationale: Medications such as meperidine (Demerol) are administered for pain. Morphine sulfate and other opioids are usually avoided because they cause spasms of Oddi's sphincter. The client is given nothing by mouth (NPO) during acute pancreatitis to rest the pancreas, and IV fluids are administered. Histamine H2 antagonists are usually prescribed to decrease hydrochloric acid, thus decreasing the production of pancreatic enzymes.

Test-Taking Strategy: Use the process of elimination and note the key words *would the nurse question*. Recalling the pathophysiology of acute pancreatitis will direct you to option 1. If you had difficulty with this question, review the therapeutic management of the client with acute pancreatitis.

Level of Cognitive Ability: Analysis
Client Needs: Safe, Effective Care Environment
Integrated Concept/Process: Nursing Process/Implementation
Content Area: Adult Health/Gastrointestinal

Reference:
Black, J., Hawks, J., & Keene, A. (2001). *Medical-surgical nursing: clinical management for positive outcomes* (6th ed.). Philadelphia: W.B. Saunders, p. 1196.

---

159. An emergency room nurse asks a licensed practical nurse (LPN) to assist in preparing a client who has sustained a gunshot wound for surgery. The LPN removes the client's clothing and places a hospital gown on the client to prepare the client for the surgical procedure. Which of the following indicates the most appropriate nursing action regarding the client's clothing, which is stained with blood?
1 Discard the clothing
2 Give the clothing to the family member or significant other
3 Place the clothing in a paper bag
4 Place the clothing in a plastic bag

Answer: 3
Rationale: Any evidence of crime discovered during an examination is saved and recorded. Documentation of evidence includes the bodily location from which the evidence was obtained and when or to whom it was delivered. Evidence should be maintained in its original condition. Clothing is stored in a paper bag instead of plastic to prevent decomposition. If clothing must be cut off the client, special attention is taken not to destroy evidence inadvertently.

Test-Taking Strategy: Use the process of elimination. Note the key word *shooting* and identify the issue of the question, which involves a legal consideration regarding evidence related to a crime. Therefore eliminate options 1 and 2. From the remaining options, recalling that articles can decompose in a plastic bag will direct you to option 3. Review emergency care to a client involved in a crime if you had difficulty with this question.

Level of Cognitive Ability: Application
Client Needs: Safe, Effective Care Environment
Integrated Concept/Process: Nursing Process/Implementation
Content Area: Fundamental Skills

Reference:
Potter, P., & Perry, A. (2001). *Fundamentals of nursing* (5th ed.). St. Louis: Mosby, p. 425.

---

160. A nurse has been caring for a client with cancer of the lung. The nurse arrives at 7 AM and begins to collect data about the client. The client reports severe pain to the nurse, even though pain medication was administered several times during the night. The nurse notes that the client has been complaining of this severe pain every morning during the last 3 days, although pain medication was received during the night. The same nurse has cared for this client for the last 3 nights. The nurse suspects that the night nurse is not administering the pain medication to the client as prescribed. According to the Nurse Practice Act, which of the following would the nurse who discovered the occurrence do?

Answer: 2
Rationale: The Nurse Practice Acts require reporting the suspicion of impaired nurses. The Board of Nursing has jurisdiction over the practice of nursing and may develop plans for treatment and supervision. The suspicion should be reported to the nursing supervisor, who then notifies the Board of Nursing. Option 1 can cause further injury to the client. Option 3 and 4 will not alert the health care agency of the problem.

Test-Taking Strategy: Use the process of elimination. Option 1 can be easily eliminated first because this action can cause further injury to this client. Use principles of prioritizing and focus on the issue of ethical and legal responsibilities to answer the question. The nurse should report the information and alert the health care agency of the potential problem, which will lead to further investigation and action. Review these ethical and legal issues if you had difficulty with this question.

1   Wait until the next morning and talk to the night nurse
2   Report the information to the nursing supervisor
3   Notify the impaired nurse organization
4   Call the police

Level of Cognitive Ability: Application
Client Needs: Safe, Effective Care Environment
Integrated Concept/Process: Nursing Process/Implementation
Content Area: Fundamental Skills

Reference:
Potter, P., & Perry, A. (2001). *Fundamentals of nursing* (5th ed.). St. Louis: Mosby, p. 424.

---

161. A nurse caring for a hospitalized client helps the family prepare a birthday party for the client. When the family arrives and the party starts, the nurse enters the room and takes photographs of the client and the family. Which violation has the nurse committed?
1   Breach of confidentiality
2   Invasion of privacy
3   Assault
4   Negligence

Answer: 2
Rationale: Invasion of privacy takes place when someone unreasonably intrudes into an individual's private affairs; this includes taking photographs of the client without the client's consent. Confidentiality is threatened when the nurse discusses the client's health care or other private issues with another without the client's consent. Assault occurs when a person causes another to fear harmful or offensive contact. Negligence involves actions that are below the standards of care.

Test-Taking Strategy: Use the process of elimination. Focusing on the key words *takes photographs* should direct you to option 2. Review situations that violate client rights if you had difficulty with this question.

Level of Cognitive Ability: Comprehension
Client Needs: Safe, Effective Care Environment
Integrated Concept/Process: Nursing Process/Implementation
Content Area: Fundamental Skills

Reference:
Potter, P., & Perry, A. (2001). *Fundamentals of nursing* (5th ed.). St. Louis: Mosby, p. 425.

---

162. A nurse administers digoxin (Lanoxin) 0.25 mg instead of the prescribed order of 0.125 mg. The nurse discovers the error while charting the medication. The nurse completes an incident report and notifies the physician of the incident. Which of the following would be the next appropriate nursing action?
1   Send the incident report to the risk-management department
2   Make a copy of the incident report and send it to the physician's office
3   Document the incident in the client's record
4   Place the incident report in the client's record

Answer: 3
Rationale: The incident report is confidential and privileged information. It should not be copied or placed in the client's record or have any reference made to it in the client's record. It is the physician's responsibility to sign the incident report before it is sent to the risk-management department. A copy should not be made or sent to the physician's office. The incident report is not a substitute for a complete entry in the client's record concerning the incident.

Test-Taking Strategy: Use the process of elimination and note the key word *next*. Recalling the purpose of an incident report and the nurse's responsibilities regarding the report and documentation will direct you to option 3. If you had difficulty with this question or are unfamiliar with incident reports, review the nurse's responsibilities regarding these documents.

Level of Cognitive Ability: Application
Client Needs: Safe, Effective Care Environment
Integrated Concept/Process: Nursing Process/Implementation
Content Area: Fundamental Skills

Reference:
Potter, P., & Perry, A. (2001). *Fundamentals of nursing* (5th ed.). St. Louis: Mosby, p. 440.

---

163. A client with an infection is receiving antibiotics by intramuscular (IM) injections. Because this client is also on anticoagulant therapy, the nurse knows that safety for this client would most appropriately include which of the following?
  1   Application of a pressure bandage to the site after each IM injection
  2   Prolonged pressure applied to the IM site after injections
  3   Decreasing the IM needle size
  4   Doubling the dose of anticoagulant

Answer: 2
Rationale: Anticoagulants place the client at risk for bleeding. Prolonged pressure over the site of an IM injection will assist in preventing bleeding into the tissues surrounding the injection site. A pressure bandage is not an appropriate measure and is also unnecessary. Decreasing the IM needle size may be helpful but is not the most appropriate action. Option 4 is incorrect.

Test-Taking Strategy: Use the process of elimination and note the key words *most appropriately*. Option 4 can be easily eliminated. From the remaining options, select option 2 because this is the most appropriate action and is necessary after every IM injection. Review safety measures for a client taking an anticoagulant if you had difficulty with this question.

Level of Cognitive Ability: Application
Client Needs: Safe, Effective Care Environment
Integrated Concept/Process: Nursing Process/Implementation
Content Area: Pharmacology

Reference:
Lehne, R. (2001). *Pharmacology for nursing care* (4th ed.). Philadelphia: W.B. Saunders, p. 1562.

---

164. A nurse brings a client the morning medications. The client states, "I don't want them. They don't help worth a hoot anyway." The nurse's most appropriate response is which of the following?
  1   "Well, you have a right to refuse them."
  2   "You don't seem to feel your pills are working?"
  3   "Just take the pills. I'm too busy for this nonsense."
  4   "I'll have the doctor order different pills."

Answer: 2
Rationale: Open-ended questions, such as reflection, are appropriate therapeutic communication strategies. Although option 1 is true, it is not the most appropriate response. Options 3 and 4 are inappropriate responses to the client.

Test-Taking Strategy: Use therapeutic communication techniques to answer the question. Remember to always address the client's feelings and concerns. This will direct you to option 2. Review therapeutic communication techniques if you had difficulty with this question.

Level of Cognitive Ability: Application
Client Needs: Safe, Effective Care Environment
Integrated Concept/Process: Communication and Documentation
Content Area: Fundamental Skills

Reference:
Potter, P., & Perry, A. (2001). *Fundamentals of nursing* (5th ed.). St. Louis: Mosby, p. 459.

---

165. When a medication is being administered, which of the following is the safest and most accurate way for the nurse to verify the identity of a client?

Answer: 4
Rationale: One of the five rights in medication administration is the *right client*, which can only be accurately verified by checking the identity band. The client may be also asked his or her name,

1 Ask the client to state his or her name
2 Ask another nurse to verify identity
3 Call out the client's name
4 Check the identity band

but this action may not be reliable, particularly if the client has periods of confusion. Options 2 and 3 can result in a medication error.

Test-Taking Strategy: Use the process of elimination and knowledge of the five rights in medication administration. If you had difficulty with this question, review these five rights.

Level of Cognitive Ability: Comprehension
Client Needs: Safe, Effective Care Environment
Integrated Concept/Process: Nursing Process/Implementation
Content Area: Fundamental Skills

Reference:
Potter, P., & Perry, A. (2001). *Fundamentals of nursing* (5th ed.). St. Louis: Mosby, p. 903.

---

166. A nurse has developed a plan of care for a client diagnosed with cerebrovascular accident (CVA). The nurse would be most concerned with which of the following aspects of care for this client when the client begins to ambulate?
1 Hydration
2 Hygiene
3 Elimination
4 Safety

Answer: 4
Rationale: Safety is the primary concern when the client is ambulating. Although hydration, hygiene, and elimination are also concerns in the plan of care, safety is the priority.

Test-Taking Strategy: Use the process of elimination. Noting the key words *begins to ambulate* will direct you to option 4. Review care to the client with a CVA who is beginning to ambulate if you had difficulty with this question.

Level of Cognitive Ability: Comprehension
Client Needs: Safe, Effective Care Environment
Integrated Concept/Process: Nursing Process/Planning
Content Area: Fundamental Skills

Reference:
Lewis, S., Heitkemper, M., & Dirksen, S. (2000). *Medical-surgical nursing: assessment and management of clinical problems* (5th ed.). St. Louis: Mosby, p. 1665.

---

167. A nurse demonstrates awareness of the single most important infection control technique when the nurse does which of the following?
1 Uses gloves when giving a bed bath
2 Washes hands before and after every client contact
3 Uses sterile gloves to provide perineal care
4 Uses sterile technique for an abdominal dressing change

Answer: 2
Rationale: The most important infection control measure is prevention of the spread of infection, which is accomplished by frequent hand washing. Options 1 and 4 are correct techniques, but are not the most important infection control technique. Using sterile gloves for perineal care is not necessary and is costly. Clean gloves are sufficient for this procedure.

Test-Taking Strategy: Use the process of elimination. Note the key words *single most important*. Recalling the basics of infection control will direct you to option 2. Review the importance of hand washing if you had difficulty with question.

Level of Cognitive Ability: Application
Client Needs: Safe, Effective Care Environment
Integrated Concept/Process: Nursing Process/Implementation
Content Area: Fundamental Skills

Reference:
Potter, P., & Perry, A. (2001). *Fundamentals of nursing* (5th ed.). St. Louis: Mosby, p. 852.

---

168. A client has been placed on contact precautions. The most appropriate nursing intervention to include in the plan of care to prevent the spread of infection is which of the following?

1 Perform meticulous hand washing frequently

2 Wear a mask and a gown with all client contacts

3 Restrict all visitors

4 Wear sterile gloves for all contacts with the client

Answer: 1

Rationale: When the client is on contact precautions, a mask is not necessary. A mask is necessary for respiratory precautions. Sterile gloves are not required for all client contacts, although clean gloves may be worn. All visitors need not be restricted from visiting if they are instructed in the measures to prevent infection. Meticulous and frequent hand washing is necessary.

Test-Taking Strategy: Focus on the key words *contact precautions*. Use the process of elimination, keeping this focus in mind. Eliminate options 2, 3, and 4 because of the absolute word *all*. Review the measures for contact precautions if you had difficulty with this question.

Level of Cognitive Ability: Application
Client Needs: Safe, Effective Care Environment
Integrated Concept/Process: Nursing Process/Planning
Content Area: Fundamental Skills

Reference:
Potter, P., & Perry, A. (2001). *Fundamentals of nursing* (5th ed.). St. Louis: Mosby, p. 838.

---

169. A nurse is assisting in the care of a client with hyperparathyroidism. The nurse does which of the following to help safely minimize effects of the disease process?

1 Assist the client to ambulate in the hall 3 times a day for 15 minutes

2 Explain the benefits of a diet high in milk products

3 Encourage the liberal use of calcium carbonate (Tums) antacids

4 Restrict fluids to 1000 mL per day

Answer: 1

Rationale: The client with hyperparathyroidism is predisposed to hypercalcemia and to renal calculi formation; therefore ambulation is important. A diet high in milk products would add to the client's calcium load. Calcium carbonate contains calcium and is therefore not the best choice as an antacid. Fluids should not be restricted because fluids aid in excreting calcium via the kidneys and prevent the formation of calcium-containing renal stones.

Test-Taking Strategy: Use the process of elimination. Knowledge that the client is predisposed to hypercalcemia is needed to answer the question. This would help you to eliminate options 2 and 3 first. Recalling that fluid would help reduce the likelihood of developing renal stones will direct you to option 1 from the remaining options. If you had difficulty with this question, review care to the client with hyperparathyroidism.

Level of Cognitive Ability: Application
Client Needs: Safe, Effective Care Environment
Integrated Concept/Process: Nursing Process/Implementation
Content Area: Adult Health/Endocrine

Reference:
Ignatavicius, D., & Workman, M. (2002). *Medical-surgical: critical thinking for collaborative care* (4th ed.). Philadelphia: W.B. Saunders, p. 1437.

170. A nurse is evaluating a client's readiness for discharge and is performing a home safety assessment to determine if there are any environmental hazards in the home. Which of the following statements, if made by the client, would the nurse further investigate?

1. "I use smoke detectors in my home."
2. "I have removed the scatter rugs from the house."
3. "I live in a house that is one-floor."
4. "I don't have any nightlights in the house."

Answer: 4

Rationale: If the client tells the nurse that there are no nightlights in the home, the nurse should further investigate the situation. Nightlights assist in preventing falls by clients who may need to get up during the night. Options 1, 2, and 3 do not pose an environmental hazard in the home.

Test-Taking Strategy: Use the process of elimination focusing on the key words *further investigate*. Look for the option that identifies an environmental hazard to the client. This will direct you to option 4. Review environmental hazards if you had difficulty with this question.

Level of Cognitive Ability: Comprehension
Client Needs: Safe, Effective Care Environment
Integrated Concept/Process: Nursing Process/Evaluation
Content Area: Fundamental Skills

Reference:
Potter, P., & Perry, A. (2001). *Fundamentals of nursing* (5th ed.). St. Louis: Mosby, p. 1021.

---

171. A nurse is caring for a client with a hiatal hernia. To prevent tracheal aspiration, the nurse would do which of the following?

1. Administer antacids prn
2. Instruct the client to not smoke
3. Instruct the client to lose weight
4. Elevate the head of bed on 4- to 6-inch blocks

Answer: 4

Rationale: Regurgitation with tracheal aspiration is a major complication of a hiatal hernia. Although antacids, avoidance of smoking, and losing weight will assist in alleviating the discomfort that can occur, these measures will not prevent aspiration.

Test-Taking Strategy: Use the process of elimination. Note the issue of the question: to prevent tracheal aspiration. Options 1, 2, and 3 are all interventions that may be used with the client with a hiatal hernia, but they do not prevent regurgitation and aspiration. Option 4 is the only option that will assist in preventing this from occurring. Review care to the client with a hiatal hernia if you had difficulty with this question.

Level of Cognitive Ability: Application
Client Needs: Safe, Effective Care Environment
Integrated Concept/Process: Nursing Process/Implementation
Content Area: Adult Health/Gastrointestinal

Reference:
Lewis, S., Heitkemper, M., & Dirksen, S. (2000). *Medical-surgical nursing: assessment and management of clinical problems* (5th ed.). St. Louis: Mosby, p. 1095.

---

172. A licensed practical nurse (LPN) is assigned to assist in caring for a client undergoing peritoneal dialysis. The client complains of shoulder pain while the nurse is providing care to the client. The nurse would do the following?

1. Administer a narcotic analgesic
2. Infuse the dialysate more slowly

Answer: 4

Rationale: The occurrence of shoulder pain during peritoneal dialysis is caused by irritation of the diaphragm by the dialysate. The appropriate nursing action is to elevate the head of the bed. This position uses gravity to move the dialysate away from the diaphragm. The nurse would not adjust the rate of the infusion, stop the infusion, or administer a narcotic analgesic. The LPN should notify the registered nurse of

3 Stop the dialysis and drain the abdomen
4 Elevate the head of the bed

the client's complaint after appropriately positioning the client.

Test-Taking Strategy: Use the process of elimination. Options 2 and 3 are similar and should be eliminated. To choose from the remaining options, it is necessary to know that the shoulder pain results from diaphragmatic irritation. Combining this knowledge with the principle of gravity will direct you to option 4. Review the complications associated with peritoneal dialysis and the appropriate nursing interventions if you had difficulty with this question.

Level of Cognitive Ability: Application
Client Needs: Safe, Effective Care Environment
Integrated Concept/Process: Nursing Process/Implementation
Content Area: Adult Health/Renal

Reference:
Lewis, S., Heitkemper, M., & Dirksen, S. (2000). *Medical-surgical nursing: assessment and management of clinical problems* (5th ed.). St. Louis: Mosby, p. 1324.

---

173. The nurse notes an 85-year-old client has become extremely agitated 2 days after surgery to repair a fractured hip. Which of the following nursing actions would be most appropriate?
1 Walk up behind the client and gently place the hand on the client's shoulder while speaking
2 Speak to the client at the entrance of the room to avoid any violent episodes
3 Speak and move slowly toward the client
4 Wait until the client's agitation has subsided before approaching the client

Answer: 3
Rationale: If the client is agitated, the nurse should speak and move slowly toward the client. Any sudden moves or speaking too quickly may cause the client to have a violent episode. Walking up behind the client may cause the client to become startled and react violently. Remaining at the entrance of the room may make the client feel alienated. If the client's agitation is not addressed, it will only increase.

Test-Taking Strategy: Use the process of elimination and the principles related to preventing violent episodes. One of the most basic is to avoid further agitation. Remember to be empathetic to the client but avoid actions that would startle the client. Review these measures if you had difficulty with this question.

Level of Cognitive Ability: Application
Client Needs: Safe, Effective Care Environment
Integrated Concept/Process: Nursing Process/Implementation
Content Area: Fundamental Skills

Reference:
Potter, P., & Perry, A. (2001). *Fundamentals of nursing* (5th ed.). St. Louis: Mosby, p. 230.

---

174. A 17-year-old female client is about to be discharged with her new baby. Which of the following statements if made by the client indicates the need for further teaching regarding care of her baby?
1 "I have locks on all my cabinets that have my cleaning supplies."

Answer: 2
Rationale: A baby car seat should never be placed in the front seat because of the potential for injury on impact. Any cabinets that contain dangerous items that the baby could swallow should be locked. Microwaves should never be used to heat bottle formula because it could burn and even scald the baby's mouth. Even though the bottle may feel warm, it could contain hot spots that could severely damage the baby's mouth. It is perfectly safe to

2   "I have a car seat that I will put in the front seat to keep my baby safe."

3   " I will not use the microwave to heat my baby's formula."

4   "I keep all my pots and pans in my lower cabinets."

leave pots and pans in the lower cabinets, as long as they are not made of glass, for the baby to investigate when he or she begins to explore the environment. Glass items if broken could harm the baby.

Test-Taking Strategy: Note the key words *need for further teaching.* Use the process of elimination to identify the option that would cause injury to the baby. Review these safety measures if you had difficulty with this question.

Level of Cognitive Ability: Comprehension
Client Needs: Safe, Effective Care Environment
Integrated Concept/Process: Nursing Process/Evaluation
Content Area: Maternity

Reference:
McKinney, E., Ashwill, J., Murray, S. et al. (2000). *Maternal-child nursing.* Philadelphia: W.B. Saunders, p. 96.

---

175. A nurse is discussing the home environment with a client preparing for discharge to determine if there are any fire hazards in the home. Which of the following statements by the client should the nurse further explore?

1   "I use smoke detectors and change the batteries faithfully every 2 years."

2   "I keep my matches on a very high shelf."

3   "My space heaters are located 3 feet from any items or furniture."

4   "I should plan and practice escape routes in case of a fire."

Answer: 1
Rationale: Smoke detectors should be used; however, the batteries should be changed yearly. Options 2, 3, and 4 identify correct actions regarding fire safety in the home.

Test-Taking Strategy: Note the key words *further explore.* Recalling that smoke detector batteries should be changed yearly will direct you to option 1. Review fire safety measures if you had difficulty with this question.

Level of Cognitive Ability: Comprehension
Client Needs: Safe, Effective Care Environment
Integrated Concept/Process: Nursing Process/Evaluation
Content Area: Fundamental Skills

Reference:
Potter, P., & Perry, A. (2001). *Fundamentals of nursing* (5th ed.). St. Louis: Mosby, p. 1022.

---

176. A nurse has administered an injection to a client. After the injection, the nurse accidentally drops the syringe on the floor. Which of the following actions by the nurse is appropriate?

1   Carefully pick up the syringe from the floor and gently recap the needle

2   Carefully pick up the syringe from the floor and dispose of it in a sharps container

3   Recap the needle and then use forceps to discard the syringe

4   Call the housekeeping department to pick up the syringe

Answer: 2
Rationale: Syringes should never be recapped in any circumstances to prevent being stuck by a contaminated needle. Syringes should always be placed in sharps container immediately after use to prevent injury from a needle stick. It is not appropriate to ask housekeeping to pick up the syringe.

Test-Taking Strategy: Use the process of elimination. Eliminate options 1 and 3 because they are similar. Use principles related to Standard Precautions to direct you to option 2. Review the procedure for discarding needles if you had difficulty with this question.

Level of Cognitive Ability: Application
Client Needs: Safe, Effective Care Environment
Integrated Concept/Process: Nursing Process/Implementation
Content Area: Fundamental Skills

Reference:
Potter, P., & Perry, A. (2001). *Fundamentals of nursing* (5th ed.). St. Louis: Mosby, p. 930.

---

177. After discussing the use of restraints with a client and family, a physician has written an order for wrist restraints to be applied to a client. The nurse instructs the nursing assistant to apply the restraints. When checking the client, which of the following observations would indicate that the nursing assistant performed unsafe care?

1   A hitch knot was used to secure the restraints
2   Restraints were released every 2 hours
3   Restraints were applied snugly and tightly
4   The call light was placed within reach of the client's hand

Answer: 3
Rationale: Restraints should never be applied tightly because they could impair circulation. A hitch knot should be used because it can easily be released in an emergency. Restraints must be released every 2 hours to inspect the skin, assess circulation, and provide range of motion. The call light must always be placed within the client's reach so the client can use it to call for assistance.

Test-Taking Strategy: Note the key words *performed unsafe care*. Use the process of elimination, noting the key word *tightly* in option 3. Review care to the client with restraints if you had difficulty with this question.

Level of Cognitive Ability: Comprehension
Client Needs: Safe, Effective Care Environment
Integrated Concept/Process: Nursing Process/Evaluation
Content Area: Fundamental Skills

Reference:
Potter, P., & Perry, A. (2001). *Fundamentals of nursing* (5th ed.). St. Louis: Mosby, p. 1039.

---

178. A nurse is preparing to perform morning care on a client. Which of the following describes the correct way for the nurse to wash his or her hands?

1   Turn on the water; allow the warm water to wet the hands; apply soap to the hands and rub them vigorously; keep hands pointed downward and rinse the hands; dry the hands using a paper towel; turn the water faucet off with the paper towel
2   Turn on the water; allow the warm water to wet the hands; apply soap to the hands and rub them vigorously; keep hands pointed upward and rinse the hands; dry the hands using a paper towel; turn the water faucet off with the paper towel
3   Turn on the water; allow the warm water to wet the hands; apply soap to the hands and rub them vigorously; keep hands pointed downward and rinse the hands using a paper towel to dry them; turn the water off with the clean hands
4   Turn on the water; allow the cold water to wet the hands; apply soap

Answer: 1
Rationale: Warm water should be used for hand washing because it increases the sudsing action of the soap. Hands should be pointed downward to enable the unsanitary material to fall off the skin. The faucet should be turned off by using towels to prevent the hands from becoming recontaminated.

Test-Taking Strategy: Use the process of elimination and visualize the procedure. Recalling that warm water must be used and care must be taken to avoid recontaminating the hands will direct you to option 1. Review the procedure for hand washing if you had difficulty with this question.

Level of Cognitive Ability: Comprehension
Client Needs: Safe, Effective Care Environment
Integrated Concept/Process: Nursing Process/Implementation
Content Area: Fundamental Skills

Reference:
Potter, P., & Perry, A. (2001). *Fundamentals of nursing* (5th ed.). St. Louis: Mosby, p. 854.

to the hands and rub them vigorously; keep hands pointed upward;
rinse the hands using a paper towel;
turn the water off with the clean
hands

---

179. Which of the following items would be appropriate for the nurse to wear if there is the potential for body fluid to splatter in the mouth or nose while caring for the client?

1 Gown
2 Goggles
3 Mask
4 Cap

Answer: 3
Rationale: A mask would offer full protection of the nose and mouth. Goggles would protect the eyes from getting injured. A gown would protect the nurse's uniform. A cap would protect the nurse's hair.

Test-Taking Strategy: Note the key words *mouth or nose*. The only item that would protect these areas is a mask. Review Standard Precautions if you had difficulty with this question.

Level of Cognitive Ability: Application
Client Needs: Safe, Effective Care Environment
Integrated Concept/Process: Nursing Process/Implementation
Content Area: Fundamental Skills

Reference:
Potter, P., & Perry, A. (2001). *Fundamentals of nursing* (5th ed.). St. Louis: Mosby, p. 858.

---

180. A nurse assigned to care for a client with a diagnosis of active tuberculosis will be wearing a particulate respirator mask. Which of the following indicates that the nurse understands how this mask operates?

1 Readjusts the nose piece if air is detected escaping around the nose
2 Obtains another particulate respirator if there is leakage at the respirator mask edge
3 Inhales forcefully while placing both hands on the respirator
4 A fit check is only necessary when the nurse is putting the mask on for the first time

Answer: 1
Rationale: It is important that no air escapes around the nose while wearing the respirator mask. The strap is adjusted if air is escaping around the respirator mask edge; obtaining another particulate respirator is not necessary. It is important to exhale forcefully while placing both hands over the apparatus. It is necessary to perform a fit check each time the nurse uses the mask.

Test-Taking Strategy: Knowledge regarding the principles related to using the particulate respirator mask is required to answer this question. Review these principles if you had difficulty with this question.

Level of Cognitive Ability: Comprehension
Client Needs: Safe, Effective Care Environment
Integrated Concept/Process: Nursing Process/Implementation
Content Area: Fundamental Skills

Reference:
Potter, P., & Perry, A. (2001). *Fundamentals of nursing* (5th ed.). St. Louis: Mosby, p. 858.

---

181. A nurse is assigned to care for four clients. The nurse implements which of the following to prevent the spread of infection from client to client?

1 Reads about performing treatments in the policy and procedure manual

Answer: 2
Rationale: Proper hand washing is the best way to prevent the spread of infection. Reading the policy and procedure manual does not guarantee that infection will not spread. All procedures do not require sterile technique. Clean technique alone is not always appropriate.

2 Uses proper hand washing techniques when necessary

3 Performs sterile technique with all procedures

4 Uses clean technique with all procedures

Test-Taking Strategy: Focus on the issue: preventing the spread of infection. Recalling the importance of hand washing will direct you to option 2. Review the importance of hand washing if you had difficulty with this question.

Level of Cognitive Ability: Application
Client Needs: Safe, Effective Care Environment
Integrated Concept/Process: Nursing Process/Implementation
Content Area: Fundamental Skills

Reference:
Potter, P., & Perry, A. (2001). *Fundamentals of nursing* (5th ed.). St. Louis: Mosby, p. 1022.

---

182. A nurse must collect a midstream urine specimen from a female client. Which of the following indicates that the nurse understands the principles of using proper technique to collect the specimen?

1 Cleanses the meatus with antiseptic pads using upward strokes

2 Lets go of the labia once it is cleansed and ask the client to urinate

3 Makes sure that the fingers avoid touching the inside of the collection container

4 Instructs the client to urinate in the container after the labia have been cleansed

Answer: 3
Rationale: The inside of the container is sterile and sterility must be maintained. Fingers touching the inside would contaminate the container. The meatus should be cleansed from front to back (towards the anus). Upward strokes would carry bacteria from the anal region. The labia should remain open during the procedure. The client should urinate a small amount into the toilet before urinating into the specimen container to allow some of the organisms near the meatus to leave the area.

Test-Taking Strategy: Use the process of elimination and identify the option that would prevent contamination. This will direct you to option 3. Review the procedure for collecting a midstream urine specimen if you had difficulty with this question.

Level of Cognitive Ability: Application
Client Needs: Safe, Effective Care Environment
Integrated Concept/Process: Nursing Process/Implementation
Content Area: Fundamental Skills

Reference:
Potter, P., & Perry, A. (2001). *Fundamentals of nursing* (5th ed.). St. Louis: Mosby, p. 863.

---

183. A nurse is giving a bed bath to a client and notes the need for another towel. Which nursing action will the nurse take first?

1 Go to the linen room and get the towel

2 Wash his or her hands before leaving the client's room

3 Borrow the roommate's towel

4 Use a bath blanket as a towel

Answer: 2
Rationale: To avoid spreading the client's germs, the nurse's hands must be washed before leaving the client's room. It is never appropriate to borrow other clients' supplies because this will spread germs. It is not appropriate to use a bath blanket as a towel.

Test-Taking Strategy: Note the key word *first*. Use knowledge regarding the basic principles related to bathing a client and visualize the situation to direct you to option 2. Review these basic principles if you had difficulty with this question.

Level of Cognitive Ability: Application
Client Needs: Safe, Effective Care Environment
Integrated Concept/Process: Nursing Process/Implementation
Content Area: Fundamental Skills

Reference:
Potter, P., & Perry, A. (2001). *Fundamentals of nursing* (5th ed.). St. Louis: Mosby, p. 1074.

---

184. A nurse is determining a family member's ability to use sterile gloves to perform a dressing change. Which statement would indicate to the nurse that the family member requires further teaching?

1 "I know that I can use the inner wrapper as a sterile field."

2 "If I touch the glove on the counter, I should open another pair."

3 "I don't have to worry about washing my hands because I have sterile gloves."

4 "Whichever glove I decide to put on first is up to me."

Answer: 3

Rationale: Hands must always be washed (even though sterile gloves are used) to keep germs from spreading. The inner wrapper makes an excellent area for usage because it is sterile. If the gloves touch anything unsterile, they must be considered contaminated and a new package of sterile gloves must be used. Which glove is put on first is up to the individual as long as sterile technique is not compromised.

Test-Taking Strategy: Use the process of elimination, recalling the principles of sterile technique. Noting the key words *requires further teaching* will direct you to option 3. Review these principles if you had difficulty with this question.

Level of Cognitive Ability: Comprehension
Client Needs: Safe, Effective Care Environment
Integrated Concept/Process: Nursing Process/Evaluation
Content Area: Fundamental Skills

Reference:
Potter, P., & Perry, A. (2001). *Fundamentals of nursing* (5th ed.). St. Louis: Mosby, p. 864.

---

185. A nurse is preparing to leave a client's room and must remove a gown, mask, and gloves before leaving the room. Which of the following interventions could lead to the spread of infection?

1 While removing the gown, avoids rolling it from inside out

2 Takes the gloves off first before removing the gown

3 Washes hands after the entire procedure has been completed

4 Using ungloved hands, removes the gown using the neckties

Answer: 1

Rationale: The gown must be rolled from inside out to prevent the organisms on the outside of the gown from contaminating other areas. Gloves are considered the most contaminated protective items the nurse wears and therefore must be removed first. Hands should be washed after removing the protective items to eliminate any germs still present. Ungloved hands should be used to remove the gown to prevent contaminating the back of the gown with germs from the gloves.

Test-Taking Strategy: Note the key words *lead to the spread of infection.* Visualize this procedure and use the process of elimination with this focus in mind. Review these measures to prevent infection if you had difficulty with this question.

Level of Cognitive Ability: Application
Client Needs: Safe, Effective Care Environment
Integrated Concept/Process: Nursing Process/Implementation
Content Area: Fundamental Skills

Reference:
Potter, P., & Perry, A. (2001). *Fundamentals of nursing* (5th ed.). St. Louis: Mosby, p. 866.

---

186. A nurse is caring for a hospitalized child with rubeola (red measles). Which of the following precautions would the

Answer: 3

Rationale: Rubeola is transmitted via airborne particles or direct contact with infectious droplets. The treatment of rubeola is

nurse institute when caring for the child?

1   Wearing gloves
2   Wearing a gown
3   Wearing a mask
4   Wearing a gown, gloves, and a mask

symptomatic, whether the child is hospitalized or remains at home. If hospitalized, however, the child will require respiratory isolation. During the febrile period, the child should be restricted to quiet activities and bed rest. Respiratory isolation for a child with rubeola requires masks for those in close contact with the child. Gowns and gloves are not specifically indicated. Strict hand washing is advised after touching the child or contaminated objects and before caring for another child. Articles that are contaminated should be bagged and labeled before reprocessing.

Test-Taking Strategy: Note the key word *hospitalized*. Recalling that rubeola is transmitted via airborne particles or direct contact with infectious droplets will direct you to option 3. Review this infectious disease if you had difficulty with this question.

Level of Cognitive Ability: Application
Client Needs: Safe, Effective Care Environment
Integrated Concept/Process: Nursing Process/Implementation
Content Area: Child Health

Reference:
Wong, D., & Hockenberry-Eaton, M. (2001). *Wong's essentials of pediatric nursing* (6th ed.). St. Louis: Mosby, p. 460.

---

187. A nurse has checked a client's vision and is addressing safety needs in relation to deficits experienced from normal age-related changes. Which statement by the client indicates a need for further discussion about safety?

1   "I should have bright orange strips of tape installed at the edge of stairs."
2   "I should avoid nighttime driving."
3   "I should have a high-gloss paint put on the walls to increase light reflection."
4   "I should keep the lights turned on in the stairways and hallways at night."

Answer: 3
Rationale: Age-related changes in the eye such as diminished or absent pupillary response and decreased retinal blood supply can cause night blindness, inability to see because of glare, and deficits with depth and color perception. Using high gloss paint on walls will increase glare and make it more difficult for the client to see. All of the other options are appropriate safety measures.

Test-Taking Strategy: Note the key words *need for further discussion*. Look for the option that would not enhance the client's safety. Recalling that high gloss will cause a glare will easily direct you to option 3. Review these safety measures if you had difficulty with this question.

Level of Cognitive Ability: Comprehension
Client Needs: Safe, Effective Care Environment
Integrated Concept/Process: Self-Care
Content Area: Fundamental Skills

Reference:
Potter, P., & Perry, A. (2001). *Fundamentals of nursing* (5th ed.). St. Louis: Mosby, p. 1653.

---

188. A nurse gives a client one nitroglycerin tablet sublingual as ordered for the client's chest pain. The nurse then informs the client that he or she will be back in 5 minutes to reassess the chest pain. Which of the following should the

Answer: 3
Rationale: Nitroglycerin causes vasodilation of the coronary vessels and can lead to a decrease in the client's blood pressure causing light-headedness and dizziness. Therefore the nurse evaluates the client's environment to be sure that the side rails are up. Next, the nurse would ensure that the client's call light is within reach.

nurse check first before leaving the room?
1   Phone is within reach
2   Call light is within reach
3   Side rails are up
4   TV is on

Options 1 and 4 are not a priority for this client because the phone and TV provide stimulus, which can cause stress and aggravate chest pain.

Test-Taking Strategy: Use the process of elimination and note the key word "first." Recalling the side effects of this medication will direct you to option 3. Review these side effects if you had difficulty with this question.

Level of Cognitive Ability: Application
Client Needs: Safe, Effective Care Environment
Integrated Concept/Process: Nursing Process/Implementation
Content Area: Adult Health/Cardiovascular

Reference:
Lewis, S., Heitkemper, M., & Dirksen, S. (2000). *Medical-surgical nursing: assessment and management of clinical problems* (5th ed.). St. Louis: Mosby, p. 858.

---

189. A nurse is caring for an 8-month old infant with a diagnosis of febrile seizures. In planning care, the nurse would anticipate the need for which of the following items?
1   A padded tongue blade taped to the head of the bed
2   Restraints
3   A code cart at the bedside
4   Padded sides on the crib

Answer: 4
Rationale: Padded crib sides will protect the child from injury during seizure activity. A padded tongue blade should never be used. During a seizure, nothing should be placed in a child's mouth and the child should be placed in a side-lying position but not be restrained. A code cart should be available but need not be placed at the bedside.

Test-Taking Strategy: Use the process of elimination, recalling that safety is an issue during seizure activity. If you are unfamiliar with the precautions to take when seizure activity is a risk, review these precautions.

Level of Cognitive Ability: Application
Client Needs: Safe, Effective Care Environment
Integrated Concept/Process: Nursing Process/Planning
Content Area: Child Health

Reference:
Wong, D., & Hockenberry-Eaton, M. (2001). *Wong's essentials of pediatric nursing* (6th ed.). St. Louis: Mosby, p. 1101.

---

190. A licensed practical nurse (LPN) has been asked to do a safety survey at a children's day care center. All of the children cared for at the center are ages 1 to 3 years. Of the following safety hazards, which presents the greatest hazard to the toddler at the center?
1   Toys with small, loose parts in the playroom
2   A swimming pool in the neighbor's gated yard
3   A hot water heater set above 120° F

Answer: 1
Rationale: Toys in the playroom should be the first concern because the toddler will play in this area. Options 2 and 4 identify safety hazards that are not in the toddlers' play area and would not be the first priority. Water temperature should be a priority in a toddler's home where scalding could occur during bathing; this would be a secondary consideration in a day care setting.

Test-Taking Strategy: Note the key words *greatest hazard* and focus on the setting, the day care center. This focus and the process of elimination will direct you to option 1. Review safety in a day care center if you had difficulty with this question.

4 Toxic plants located in the front yard of the center

Level of Cognitive Ability: Comprehension
Client Needs: Safe, Effective Care Environment
Integrated Concept/Process: Nursing Process/Data Collection
Content Area: Child Health

Reference:
Wong, D., & Hockenberry-Eaton, M. (2001). *Wong's essentials of pediatric nursing* (6th ed.). St. Louis: Mosby, p. 378.

---

191. A nurse is reinforcing instructions to the mother of a preschool child with hemophilia. The nurse instructs the mother to do which of the following to promote a safe but normal environment?
1 Insist that the child wear a helmet and elbow pads during all waking hours
2 Restrict the child from playing in an outdoor playground
3 Examine toys and the play area for sharp objects
4 Allow the child to use play equipment only when a parent or older sibling is present

Answer: 3
Rationale: Examining toys and equipment in the play area will prevent potential injuries. Protective equipment may be necessary when the child first becomes mobile, but by the preschool age, this equipment should only be needed during bike riding and other activities that present a risk of injury. Outdoor playgrounds can present hazards, and activities in these areas should be supervised rather than restricted. The child is overprotected if allowed to play only when directly supervised by a family member. Parents should reduce their anxiety and give the child some independence.

Test-Taking Strategy: Use the process of elimination. Eliminate options 1, 2, and 4 because of the words *all*, *restrict*, and *only*. Review these safety measures if you had difficulty with this question.

Level of Cognitive Ability: Application
Client Needs: Safe, Effective Care Environment
Integrated Concept/Process: Teaching/Learning
Content Area: Child Health

Reference:
Wong, D., & Hockenberry-Eaton, M. (2001). *Wong's essentials of pediatric nursing* (6th ed.). St. Louis: Mosby, p. 998.

---

192. A nurse is assisting in providing emergency treatment for a client in ventricular tachycardia. The registered nurse (RN) is preparing to defibrillate the client. The licensed practical nurse understands that which action by the RN provides for the safest environment during a defibrillation attempt?
1 Hand the charged paddles separately to the RN who is defibrillating
2 Place no lubricant on the paddles
3 Holding the client's upper torso stable while the defibrillation is performed
4 Perform a visual and verbal check of "all clear"

Answer: 4
Rationale: Safety during defibrillation is essential for preventing injury to the client and to the personnel assisting with the procedure. The person performing the defibrillation ensures that all personnel are standing clear of the bed by a verbal and visual check of "all clear." Charged paddles should never be handed to other personnel. For the shock to be effective, some type of conductive medium (lubricant, gel) must be placed between the paddles and the skin. The client is not touched during the defibrillation procedure.

Test-Taking Strategy: Use the process of elimination and focus on the issue: safe principles of defibrillation. Option 4 involves a verbal and visual check of "all clear," providing for the safety of all involved. Review the principles related to safety and defibrillation if you had difficulty with this question.

Level of Cognitive Ability: Application
Client Needs: Safe, Effective Care Environment

Integrated Concept/Process: Nursing Process/Implementation
Content Area: Adult Health/Cardiovascular

Reference:
Lewis, S., Heitkemper, M., & Dirksen, S. (2000). *Medical-surgical nursing: assessment and management of clinical problems* (5th ed.). St. Louis: Mosby, p. 934.

---

193. A nurse has oriented a new employee to basic procedures for continuous ECG monitoring. The nurse should intervene if the orientee did which of the following while initiating cardiac monitoring on a client?

1   Cleansed the skin with Betadine (povidone iodine) before applying electrodes
2   Clipped small areas of hair under the area planned for electrode placement
3   Stated the need to change the electrodes every 24 hours and inspect the skin
4   Stated the availability of hypoallergenic electrodes for clients who are sensitive

Answer: 1
Rationale: The skin is cleansed with soap and water (not Betadine), wiped with denatured alcohol, and allowed to air dry before electrodes are applied. The other three options are correct.

Test-Taking Strategy: Use the process of elimination. The word *intervene* makes you look for an incorrect item. Eliminate options 3 and 4 because they are reasonable actions and are correct. From the remaining options, remember that Betadine is used to cleanse the skin, usually before some type of invasive procedure that breaks the skin barrier. ECG monitoring does not break the skin. Review the procedure for applying ECG electrodes if you had difficulty with this question.

Level of Cognitive Ability: Application
Client Needs: Safe, Effective Care Environment
Integrated Concept/Process: Nursing Process/Implementation
Content Area: Adult Health/Cardiovascular

Reference:
Lewis, S., Heitkemper, M., & Dirksen, S. (2000). *Medical-surgical nursing: assessment and management of clinical problems* (5th ed.). St. Louis: Mosby, p. 811.

---

194. A nurse is assisting in planning care for a suicidal client admitted to a mental health unit. To provide a caring, therapeutic environment, which of the following is included in the nursing care plan?

1   Placing the client in a private room to ensure privacy
2   Establishing a therapeutic relationship and conveying unconditional positive regard
3   Placing the client in charge of a meaningful unit activity such as a morning chess tournament
4   Maintaining a distance of 12 inches at all times to assure the client that control will be provided

Answer: 2
Rationale: The establishment of a therapeutic relationship with the suicidal client increases feelings of acceptance. Whereas the suicidal behavior and thinking of the client are unacceptable, the use of unconditional positive regard acknowledges the client in a human-to-human context and increases the client's sense of self-worth. Placing the client in a private room is not necessary unless the client's condition is extremely acute because the isolation would intensify the client's feelings of worthlessness. Placing the client in charge of the morning chess game is a premature intervention that can overwhelm and cause the client to fail, which can reinforce the client's feelings of worthlessness. Distances of 18 inches or less between two individuals constitute intimate space. Invasion of this space may be misinterpreted by the client and increase his or her tension and feelings of helplessness.

Test-Taking Strategy: Use the process of elimination and focus on the issue of providing a caring, therapeutic environment. Eliminate option 1 because a private room is not a safe and therapeutic intervention. Option 3 may produce feelings of worthlessness. Eliminate option 4 because a distance of 12 inches is restrictive. Option 2 is the only option that addresses a therapeutic environment. Review care to the suicidal client if you had difficulty with this question.

Level of Cognitive Ability: Application
Client Needs: Safe, Effective Care Environment
Integrated Concept/Process: Nursing Process/Planning
Content Area: Mental Health

Reference:
Varcarolis, E. (2002). *Foundations of psychiatric mental health nursing* (4th ed.). Philadelphia: W.B. Saunders, p. 648.

---

195. Seizure precautions have been ordered for a client. The nurse would plan to avoid doing which of the following when planning care for the client?
1   Monitor the client closely while the client is showering
2   Maintain the bed in the lowest position
3   Turn on the lights in the room at night
4   Assist the client to ambulate in the hallway

Answer: 3
Rationale: A quiet, restful environment is provided as part of seizure precautions. This includes undisturbed times for sleep and a night light for safety. The client should be accompanied during activities such as bathing and walking, so that assistance is readily available and injury is minimized if a seizure begins. The bed is maintained in the low position for safety.

Test-Taking Strategy: Use the process of elimination and note the word *avoid*. This guides you to look for an option that represents incorrect planning on the part of the nurse. Eliminate options 1 and 4 because they indicate safe planning. Eliminate option 2 next, because it also represents an item that plans for client safety. Review care to the client with orders for seizure precautions if you had difficulty with this question.

Level of Cognitive Ability: Application
Client Needs: Safe, Effective Care Environment
Integrated Concept/Process: Nursing Process/Planning
Content Area: Adult Health/Neurological

Reference:
Black, J., Hawks, J., & Keene, A. (2001). *Medical-surgical nursing: clinical management for positive outcomes* (6th ed.). Philadelphia: W.B. Saunders, p. 1926.

---

196. A client with active tuberculosis is admitted to the medical-surgical unit. When planning a bed assignment, the nurse follows proper acid-fast bacteria isolation precautions when he or she does which of the following?
1   Transfers the client to the intensive care unit
2   Assigns the client to a double room because intravenous antibiotics will be administered
3   Assigns the client to a double room and places a "strict hand washing" sign outside the door
4   Places the client in a·private, well-ventilated room

Answer: 4
Rationale: According to category-specific (respiratory) isolation precautions, acid-fast bacteria isolation always requires a private room. The room is well ventilated and should have at least 6 exchanges of fresh air per hour and be ventilated to the outside if possible. Therefore option 4 is the only appropriate option.

Test-Taking Strategy: Use the process of elimination. Note that the question states "active tuberculosis." Eliminate options 2 and 3 because they are similar involving a double room. Next, eliminate option 1 by focusing on the client's diagnosis. Review care to the client with active TB if you had difficulty with this question.

Level of Cognitive Ability: Application
Client Needs: Safe, Effective Care Environment
Integrated Concept/Process: Nursing Process/Planning
Content Area: Adult Health/Respiratory

Reference:
Black, J., Hawks, J., & Keene, A. (2001). *Medical-surgical nursing: clinical management for positive outcomes* (6th ed.). Philadelphia: W.B. Saunders, p.628.

---

197. A nurse is caring for a client in pelvic traction. Which of the following physician's orders would the nurse determine requires clarification?

  1 Apply the girdle snugly over the client's pelvis and iliac crest
  2 Raise the head of the bed 30 degrees
  3 Observe for pressure points over the iliac crest
  4 Keep the client in good alignment

Answer: 2

Rationale: The foot of the bed is raised to prevent the client from being pulled down in bed by the traction. The head of the bed is usually kept flat, and good body alignment is maintained. The girdle should be applied snugly so that it does not slip off. The skin should be checked for pressure sores.

Test-Taking Strategy: Use the process of elimination and note the key words *requires clarification*. Options 3 and 4 are fundamental principles and are eliminated first. From the remaining options, visualizing the procedure will assist in directing you to the correct option. If you had difficulty with this question, review the procedure for pelvic traction.

Level of Cognitive Ability: Comprehension
Client Needs: Safe, Effective Care Environment
Integrated Concept/Process: Nursing Process/Evaluation
Content Area: Adult Health/Musculoskeletal

Reference:
Lewis, S., Heitkemper, M., & Dirksen, S. (2000). *Medical-surgical nursing: assessment and management of clinical problems* (5th ed.). St. Louis: Mosby, p. 1774.

---

198. A client is admitted to the long-term care facility with a diagnosis of Parkinson's disease. The nurse gives information regarding the client's condition to a visitor assumed to be a family member. The nurse has violated which legal concept of the nurse-client relationship?

  1 Invasion of privacy
  2 Incompetency
  3 Teaching and learning principles
  4 Communication techniques

Answer: 1

Rationale: Discussing a client's condition without the client's permission violates the client's rights and places the nurse in legal jeopardy. This action by the nurse invades privacy and affects the confidentiality issue with Client Rights. Incompetency could lead to negligence, but this legal concept is not related to the issue identified in the question. Teaching and learning principles are considered concepts of standards of practice. Communication techniques relate to a nurse-client relationship.

Test-Taking Strategy: Use the process of elimination. Focus on the issue of the question: sharing information, which constitutes an invasion of privacy. If you had difficulty with this question, review Client Rights.

Level of Cognitive Ability: Comprehension
Client Need: Safe, Effective Care Environment
Integrated Concept/Process: Nursing Process/Implementation
Content Area: Fundamental Skills

Reference:
Potter, P., & Perry, A. (2001). *Fundamentals of nursing* (5th ed.). St. Louis: Mosby, p. 905.

199. A nurse is collecting data regarding the client's risk for falls. The nurse would recognize that which of the following factors does not put the client at added risk?
1 Cataracts
2 Episodes of dizziness
3 Use of nitroglycerin
4 Use of orthopedic shoes

Answer: 4
Rationale: Several factors can increase the client's risk for falls: impaired vision, medications that cause dizziness or orthostatic hypotension, and problems with balance and coordination. Cataracts represent a vision impairment, which could increase the client's risk. Dizziness obviously increases the likelihood of a fall. Nitroglycerin could cause orthostatic hypotension, which is also a potential risk. Orthopedic shoes are specially fitted for the client and are generally sturdy and safe.

Test-Taking Strategy: Use the process of elimination and note the key word *not*. To select the correct option, evaluate each of the items in terms of the potential of that item to make the client fall. Orthopedic shoes are beneficial to the client and are therefore the answer to this question as stated. Review the risk factors for falls if you had difficulty with this question.

Level of Cognitive Ability: Comprehension
Client Needs: Safe, Effective Care Environment
Integrated Concept/Process: Nursing Process/Data Collection
Content Area: Fundamental Skills

Reference:
Potter, P., & Perry, A. (2001). *Fundamentals of nursing* (5th ed.). St. Louis: Mosby, p. 264.

200. A client has a synthetic cast on the right leg. The client asks if it would be possible to take a shower. Based on review of the data related to the injury and type of cast, the best response to the client would be which of the following?
1 "The cast padding will not dry."
2 "It is not safe for you to shower alone."
3 "Hot water may soften the synthetic cast."
4 "It may lead to a serious infection."

Answer: 2
Rationale: It may be unsafe for the client to shower alone because the client may slip and fall. Water does not damage the synthetic cast; however, the client should know that it may take awhile for the cast padding to dry. Water may soften a plaster cast but has no effect on a synthetic cast. A shower will not cause an infection.

Test-Taking Strategy: Use the process of elimination. Note the key words *synthetic* and *best response*. Use Maslow's Hierarchy of Needs theory. Option 2 addresses the issue of safety. Review care to the client with a synthetic cast if you had difficulty with this question.

Level of Cognitive Ability: Application
Client Needs: Safe, Effective Care Environment
Integrated Concept/Process: Nursing Process/Implementation
Content Area: Adult Health/Musculoskeletal

Reference:
Black, J., Hawks, J., & Keene, A. (2001). *Medical-surgical nursing: clinical management for positive outcomes* (6th ed.). Philadelphia: W.B. Saunders, p. 602.

201. A client is scheduled for elective cardioversion to treat chronic high-rate atrial fibrillation. The nurse determines that the client is not yet ready for the procedure if the:

Answer: 3
Rationale: Digoxin may be withheld for up to 48 hours before cardioversion because it increases ventricular irritability and may cause ventricular dysrhythmias after countershock. The client typically receives a dose of an IV sedative or antianxiety agent.

1   Client's digoxin (Lanoxin) has been withheld for the last 48 hours
2   Client has received a dose of midazolam (Versed) intravenously
3   Client is wearing a nasal cannula delivering oxygen at 2 L per minute
4   Defibrillator has the synchronizer turned on and is set at 50 joules

The defibrillator is switched to synchronizer mode to time the delivery of the electrical impulse to coincide with the QRS and to avoid the T wave, which could cause ventricular fibrillation. Energy level is typically set at 50 to 100 joules. During the procedure, any oxygen is removed temporarily because oxygen supports combustion, and a fire could result from electrical arcing.

Test-Taking Strategy: Note the key words *not yet ready*. Visualizing the procedure and recalling the concepts related to oxygen combustion will direct you to option 3. If you had difficulty with this question, review the descriptions and procedures related to cardioversion.

Level of Cognitive Ability: Analysis
Client Needs: Safe, Effective Care Environment
Integrated Concept/Process: Nursing Process/Evaluation
Content Area: Adult Health/Cardiovascular

Reference:
Black, J., Hawks, J., & Keene, A. (2001). *Medical-surgical nursing: clinical management for positive outcomes* (6th ed.). Philadelphia: W.B. Saunders, p. 1568.

---

202. A physician has written an order for the preoperative client to have "enemas until clear." The nurse has administered three enemas and the client is still passing brown liquid stool. Which of the following actions should the nurse take next?
1   Wait 30 minutes and then administer another enema
2   Continue to administer the enemas
3   Administer an oil retention enema
4   Notify the physician

Answer: 4
Rationale: Up to three enemas may be given when there is an order for enemas until clear. If more than three are necessary, the nurse should call the physician (or act based on agency policy). Excessive enemas could cause fluid and electrolyte depletion. Options 1 and 2 are incorrect for these reasons. An oil retention enema (option 3) is an enema that is used to soften dry, hard stool.

Test-Taking Strategy: Use the process of elimination and consider the physiological effects that can occur with enema administration. Eliminate options 1 and 2 because they are similar. Recalling that an oil retention enema is an enema that is used to soften dry, hard stool will assist in eliminating option 3. Review the various types of enemas if you had difficulty with this question.

Level of Cognitive Ability: Application
Client Needs: Safe, Effective Care Environment
Integrated Concept/Process: Nursing Process/Implementation
Content Area: Fundamental Skills

Reference:
Potter, P., & Perry, A. (2001). *Fundamentals of nursing* (5th ed.). St. Louis: Mosby, p. 1461.

---

203. A nurse enters the laundry room to empty a bag of dirty linens and discovers a fire in the laundry room. The nurse activates the alarm, closes the laundry room door, and obtains the fire extinguisher to extinguish the fire. To prepare to use the fire extinguisher the nurse first:

Answer: 2
Rationale: A fire can be extinguished by smothering it with a blanket or using a fire extinguisher. To use the extinguisher, the pin is pulled first. The extinguisher should then be aimed at the base of the fire. The handle of the extinguisher is then squeezed and the fire is extinguished by sweeping the extinguisher from side to side to coat the area evenly. Although the nurse should be cautious

1 Squeezes the handle on the extinguisher

2 Pulls the pin on the fire extinguisher

3 Puts on a pair of gloves before touching the extinguisher

4 Puts on a mask before using the extinguisher

when using an extinguisher, it is not necessary to don gloves or a mask. These actions also would delay the process of extinguishing the fire.

Test-Taking Strategy: Use the process of elimination. Eliminate options 3 and 4 first because these actions would delay the process of extinguishing the fire. Remember the mnemonic PASS to prioritize in the use of a fire extinguisher: P = Pull the pin; A = Aim at the base of the fire; S = Squeeze the handle; S = Sweep from side to side to coat the area evenly. If you had difficulty with this question, review the appropriate use of a fire extinguisher.

Level of Cognitive Ability: Application
Client Needs: Safe, Effective Care Environment
Integrated Concept/Process: Nursing Process/Implementation
Content Area: Fundamental Skills

Reference:
Potter, P., & Perry, A. (2001). *Fundamentals of nursing* (5th ed.). St. Louis: Mosby, p. 1044.

---

204. A nurse is caring for a client receiving chemotherapy. On review of the morning laboratory results, the nurse notes that the white blood cell count is extremely low and the client is immediately placed on neutropenic precautions. The client's breakfast tray arrives and the nurse inspects the meal and prepares to bring the tray into the client's room. Which of the following actions would the nurse take before bringing the meal to the client?

1 Remove the fresh orange from the breakfast tray

2 Remove the coffee from the breakfast tray

3 Call the dietary department and ask for disposable utensils

4 Ask the client if he or she feels like eating at this time

Answer: 1
Rationale: In the immunocompromised client, a low bacteria diet is implemented. This includes avoiding fresh fruits and vegetables and thorough cooking of all foods. It is not necessary to remove the coffee from the tray. Disposable utensils are used for clients who are infectious and present a risk of transmitting an infection to others. It is best to encourage the client to eat because nutrition is very important for a client receiving chemotherapy who is immunocompromised.

Test-Taking Strategy: Use the process of elimination. Focus on the issue of the question: neutropenic precautions. Eliminate option 4 because this is not the best measure for the client who requires nutrition. Eliminate option 2 because there is no reason for it. Knowing that fresh fruits and vegetables present a threat to this client, or knowing that disposable utensils are used for the client who is infectious will easily direct you to the correct option. Review interventions for the client with hematological toxicity if you had difficulty with this question.

Level of Cognitive Ability: Application
Client Needs: Safe, Effective Care Environment
Integrated Concept/Process: Nursing Process/Implementation
Content Area: Adult Health/Oncology

Reference:
Black, J., Hawks, J., & Keene, A. (2001). *Medical-surgical nursing: clinical management for positive outcomes* (6th ed.). Philadelphia: W.B. Saunders, p. 392.

---

205. A nurse is assigned to care for a client on contact precautions. When reviewing the client's record, the nurse notes that the

Answer: 1
Rationale: Goggles are worn to protect the mucous membranes of the eye during interventions that may produce splashes of blood,

client has a nosocomial infection caused by methicillin-resistant, *Staphylococcus aureus* (MRSA). The client has an abdominal wound that requires irrigation and has a tracheostomy attached to a mechanical ventilator that requires frequent suctioning. The nurse gathers supplies before entering the client's room. Which of the following protective items will the nurse need to care for this client?

1   Gloves, gown, and goggles
2   Gloves and goggles
3   Gloves, gown, and shoe protectors
4   Gloves and a gown

body fluids, secretions, and excretions. In addition, contact precautions require that gloves be used and a gown worn if direct client contact is anticipated. Shoe protectors are not necessary.

Test-Taking Strategy: Use the process of elimination. Note the key words *contact precautions, irrigation,* and *frequent suctioning.* Visualizing the nursing care required in performing these procedures will direct you to option 1. Review Transmission-Based Precautions if you had difficulty with this question.

Level of Cognitive Ability: Application
Client Needs: Safe, Effective Care Environment
Integrated Concept/Process: Nursing Process/Implementation
Content Area: Fundamental Skills

Reference:
Potter, P., & Perry, A. (2001). *Fundamentals of nursing* (5th ed.). St. Louis: Mosby, p. 859.

---

206. A nurse who is assigned to work with a hospitalized client would do which of the following to maintain standard precautions?

1   Dispose of sharps, needles, and syringes in a labeled plastic bag
2   Institute protective measures when the potential for exposure to body fluids or blood exists
3   Conduct hand washing only before donning gloves
4   Use protective equipment, such as masks and gloves, when collecting data from client

Answer: 2
Rationale: Protective measures are necessary when exposure is likely or anticipated but is not necessary for all client contact or for data collection. Sharps, needles, and syringes must be disposed of in puncture-resistant containers. Hand washing must be done before and after all procedures and client contact, regardless of the use of gloves.

Test-Taking Strategy: Use the process of elimination. Eliminate option 3 first because of the absolute word *only.* Next eliminate option 1 because of the words *plastic bag.* From the remaining options, recalling that protective measures are necessary when exposure is likely or anticipated will direct you to option 2. Review these measures if you had difficulty with this question.

Level of Cognitive Ability: Application
Client Needs: Safe, Effective Care Environment
Integrated Concept/Process: Nursing Process/Implementation
Content Area: Fundamental Skills

Reference:
Potter, P., & Perry, A. (2001). *Fundamentals of nursing* (5th ed.). St. Louis: Mosby, p. 858.

---

207. Spironolactone (Aldactone) is prescribed for a client with hypertension. The licensed practical nurse (LPN) would consult with the registered nurse (RN) before giving which medication already prescribed for the client?

1   Potassium chloride (Slow -K)
2   Docusate sodium (Colace)
3   Warfarin sodium (Coumadin)
4   Digoxin (Lanoxin)

Answer: 1
Rationale: Spironolactone is a potassium-sparing diuretic and places the client at risk for hyperkalemia. If a potassium supplement were prescribed, the nurse would question the order. Docusate sodium is a stool softener. Warfarin sodium is an anticoagulant.

Test-Taking Strategy: Use the process of elimination and knowledge of the medication classification of spironolactone. Recalling that this medication is a potassium-sparing diuretic will direct you to option 1. Review this medication if you had difficulty with this question.

Level of Cognitive Ability: Application
Client Needs: Safe, Effective Care Environment
Integrated Concept/Process: Nursing Process/Implementation
Content Area: Pharmacology

Reference:
Hodgson, B., & Kizior, R. (2003). *Saunders nursing drug handbook 2003.* Philadelphia: W.B. Saunders, p. 1028.

---

208. A clinic nurse is caring for a pregnant woman with acquired immunodeficiency syndrome (AIDS) who is exhibiting signs of fever, weight loss, and candidiasis. The nurse would place highest priority on which of the following interventions?
  1 Provide clear information about the consequences of AIDS on the unborn child
  2 Use disposable gloves when in contact with nonintact skin
  3 Provide emotional support to the mother
  4 Assess history for AIDS risk factors

Answer: 2
Rationale: Standard precautions should be used when caring for a pregnant client with AIDS. Options 1 and 3 are part of the plan of care, but according to Maslow's Hierarchy of Needs theory they have a lesser priority. Option 4 is not a timely intervention because the client has acquired the virus.

Test-Taking Strategy: Use the process of elimination and note the key words *highest priority*. Use Maslow's Hierarchy of Needs theory to eliminate options 1 and 3. From the remaining options, noting that the client has AIDS will eliminate option 4. Review care to the client with AIDS if you had difficulty with this question.

Level of Cognitive Ability: Application
Client Needs: Safe, Effective Care Environment
Integrated Concept/Process: Nursing Process/Implementation
Content Area: Maternity

Reference:
Burroughs, A., & Leifer, G. (2002). *Maternity nursing* (8th ed.). Philadelphia: W.B. Saunders, p. 377.

---

209. A nurse would put on gloves to perform which of the following nursing interventions when working with a neonate?
  1 Providing cord care
  2 Changing the infant's clothes
  3 Discharging the infant
  4 Feeding the infant

Answer: 1
Rationale: Standard precautions indicate that unsterile, clean gloves should be worn when touching nonintact skin. The nurse wears gloves when changing the baby's diaper and providing cord care. Gloves are not necessary for the activities in options 2, 3, and 4.

Test-Taking Strategy: Use the process of elimination. Recalling the principle that wearing gloves is necessary when in contact with nonintact skin will direct you to option 1. If you are unfamiliar with standard precautions, review these principles.

Level of Cognitive Ability: Application
Client Needs: Safe, Effective Care Environment
Integrated Concept/Process: Nursing Process/Implementation
Content Area: Maternity

Reference:
McKinney, E., Ashwill, J., Murray, S. et al. (2000). *Maternal-child nursing.* Philadelphia: W.B. Saunders, p. 574.

210. An adult client with heart failure has a change in diet order from NPO to clear liquids. An additional order is written to change digoxin (Lanoxin), 0.25 mg intravenously every morning to digoxin (Lanoxin) 0.25 mg orally TID. Which of the following actions by the nurse has the highest priority?
1   Give the client a bowl of chicken broth
2   Review the latest serum digoxin level
3   Check the results of the daily potassium level
4   Withhold the digoxin, and consult with the registered nurse (RN)

Answer: 4
Rationale: The usual maintenance dose of digoxin is 0.125 to 0.5 mg daily. The RN should be consulted because the order is written for three times daily, which would exceed the usual daily dose. The RN would then clarify the order with the physician. This action has the highest priority for client safety.

Test-Taking Strategy: Use the process of elimination and note the key words *highest priority*. Note the change in the physician's orders from *daily* to *TID*. This will assist in directing you to option 4. Review this medication if you had difficulty with this question.

Level of Cognitive Ability: Application
Client Needs: Safe, Effective Care Environment
Integrated Concept/Process: Nursing Process/Implementation
Content Area: Pharmacology

Reference:
Hodgson, B., & Kizior, R. (2003). *Saunders nursing drug handbook 2003.* Philadelphia: W.B. Saunders, p. 348.

---

211. A nurse is assigned to care for a hospitalized client. Which of the following interventions in the general plan of care specifically upholds an item listed in the Client Bill of Rights?
1   Maintain accurate and current client information
2   Consult with other health care team members about discharge planning
3   Incorporate available and appropriate teaching reference materials
4   Act in a manner that reinforces the client's dignity

Answer: 4
Rationale: Option 4 reflects the items identified in the Client Bill of Rights. The other nursing interventions reflect competent care but are not directly mentioned in this document.

Test-Taking Strategy: Use the process of elimination and focus on the issue: Client Bill of Rights. Recalling these rights will direct you to option 4. Review these rights if you had difficulty with this question.

Level of Cognitive Ability: Comprehension
Client Needs: Safe, Effective Care Environment
Integrated Concept/Process: Nursing Process/Implementation
Content Area: Fundamental Skills

Reference:
Potter, P., & Perry, A. (2001). *Fundamentals of nursing* (5th ed.). St. Louis: Mosby p. 905.

---

212. A nurse is assigned to care for a client with hypoparathyroidism. Which of the following interventions would the nurse focus on if the priority of care were to maintain a safe environment for this client?
1   Keeping the client comfortably cool
2   Keeping the bed in a modified Trendelenburg position
3   Applying chest and ankle restraints after raising the side rails
4   Implementing seizure precautions

Answer: 4
Rationale: Hypoparathyroidism causes deficiency of parathyroid hormone that leads to low serum calcium levels. Untreated hypocalcemia can cause tetany and seizure activity. The nurse should anticipate such a complication and institute seizure precautions to maintain a safe environment. The client's temperature does not elevate with this disorder. This disorder does not cause hypovolemia, which leads to hypotension and requires the modified Trendelenburg position. Option 3 could cause injury to the client if seizure activity occurred.

Test-Taking Strategy: Use the process of elimination and recall the pathophysiology associated with hypoparathyroidism. Focusing on the key words *safe environment* will direct you to option 4. Review this disorder if you had difficulty with this question.

Level of Cognitive Ability: Application
Client Needs: Safe, Effective Care Environment
Integrated Concept/Process: Nursing Process/Implementation
Content Area: Adult Health/Endocrine

Reference:
Lewis, S., Heitkemper, M., & Dirksen, S. (2000). *Medical-surgical nursing: assessment and management of clinical problems* (5th ed.). St. Louis: Mosby, p. 1416.

---

213. A nurse is beginning an intermittent enteral feeding. Which of the following nursing actions has the highest priority?
   1   Add blue food coloring to the formula
   2   Determine proper tube placement
   3   Measure intake and output each shift
   4   Weigh the client beforehand

Answer: 2
Rationale: The highest priority is determining tube placement. Initiating a tube feeding without checking placement places the client at risk for aspiration, which can lead to pneumonia. Blue food coloring would be added if the client were diagnosed as being at high risk for aspiration. Options 3 and 4 are routine care items for a client receiving enteral feedings but are not the highest priority.

Test-Taking Strategy: Use the process of elimination. Note the key words *highest priority*. Use the ABCs—airway, breathing, and circulation. This will assist in directing you to option 2. Remember, initiating a tube feeding without checking placement places the client at risk for aspiration. Review enteral feedings if you had difficulty with this question.

Level of Cognitive Ability: Application
Client Needs: Safe, Effective Care Environment
Integrated Concept/Process: Nursing Process/Implementation
Content Area: Fundamental Skills

Reference:
Lewis, S., Heitkemper, M., & Dirksen, S. (2000). *Medical-surgical nursing: assessment and management of clinical problems* (5th ed.). St. Louis: Mosby, p. 1057.

---

214. A client is being discharged to return home after a spinal fusion with insertion of a Harrington rod. The nurse would suggest a consultation with the continuing care nurse regarding the need for follow-up modification of the home environment if the client stated which of the following?
   1   The bedroom and bath are on the second floor of the home
   2   The bathroom has hand railings in the shower
   3   The family has rented a commode for use by the client
   4   There are three steps to get up to the front door

Answer: 1
Rationale: Stair climbing may be restricted or limited for several weeks after spinal fusion with instrumentation. Options 2 and 3 are useful to the client. Option 4 would not cause as many problems as option 1.

Test-Taking Strategy: Use the process of elimination. Options 2 and 3 are useful to the client and can be eliminated first. To discriminate between options 1 and 4 (both of which involve stairs), you should determine that option 4 is least problematic, whereas option 1 poses a significant problem to the client who is restricted from stair climbing. Review activity restrictions required after this procedure if you had difficulty with this question.

Level of Cognitive Ability: Comprehension
Client Needs: Safe, Effective Care Environment

Integrated Concept/Process: Nursing Process/Planning
Content Area: Adult Health/Musculoskeletal

Reference:
Black, J., Hawks, J., & Keene, A. (2001). *Medical-surgical nursing: clinical management for positive outcomes* (6th ed.). Philadelphia: W.B. Saunders, p. 1987.

---

215. A nurse caring for a client at home notes the presence of multiple straight and wavy threadlike lines beneath the client's skin. The nurse suspects the presence of scabies. Which of the following precautions will the nurse institute until the physician is contacted?
    1   Donning a mask and gloves
    2   Putting on a pair of gloves
    3   Putting on a gown and gloves
    4   Avoiding sitting on the client's furniture

Answer: 3
Rationale: The Centers for Disease Control and Prevention recommends the wearing of gowns and gloves for close contact with a person infested with scabies. Masks are not necessary. Transmission via clothing and other inanimate objects is uncommon. Scabies is usually transmitted from person to person by direct skin contact. All contacts that the client has had should be treated at the same time.

Test-Taking Strategy: Consider the mode of transmission of scabies and use the process of elimination in answering the question. Because scabies is transmitted by direct skin contact, eliminate options 1, 2, and 4. If you had difficulty with this question, review standard precautions and transmission mode of scabies.

Level of Cognitive Ability: Application
Client Needs: Safe, Effective Care Environment
Integrated Concept/Process: Nursing Process/Implementation
Content Area: Adult Health/Integumentary

Reference:
Potter, P., & Perry, A. (2001). *Fundamentals of nursing* (5th ed.). St. Louis: Mosby, p. 858.

---

216. A nurse in a well baby clinic is providing safety instructions to a mother of a 1-month-old infant. Which safety instruction is most appropriate at this age?
    1   Cover electrical outlets
    2   Remove hazardous objects from low places
    3   Lock all poisons
    4   Never shake the infant's head

Answer: 4
Rationale: The most important age-appropriate instruction is not to shake or vigorously jiggle the baby's head. Options 1, 2, and 3 become important instructions to provide to the mother as the child reaches the age of 6 months and begins to explore the environment.

Test-Taking Strategy: Use the process of elimination. Focus on the age of the infant to direct you to the correct option. A 1-month-old is not at a developmental level to explore the environment, which will assist in eliminating options 1, 2, and 3. Review age appropriate safety measures if you had difficulty with this question.

Level of Cognitive Ability: Comprehension
Client Needs: Safe, Effective Care Environment
Integrated Concept/Process: Teaching/Learning
Content Area: Child Health

Reference:
Wong, D., & Hockenberry-Eaton, M. (2001). *Wong's essentials of pediatric nursing* (6th ed.). St. Louis: Mosby, p. 370.

217. A nurse is caring for a 9-month-old child after cleft palate repair. The nurse has applied elbow restraints to the child. The mother visits the child and asks the nurse to remove the restraints. Which of the following is the most appropriate nursing action?
1   Remove both restraints
2   Tell the mother that the restraints cannot be removed
3   Remove a restraint from one extremity
4   Loosen the restraints but tell the mother that they cannot be removed

Answer: 3
Rationale: Elbow restraints are used after cleft palate repair to prevent the child from touching the repair site, which could cause accidental rupture and tearing of the sutures. The restraints can be removed one at a time only if a parent or nurse is in constant attendance. Options 1, 2, and 4 are inaccurate nursing actions.

Test-Taking Strategy: Use the process of elimination. Eliminate options 2 and 4 first because they are similar. From the remaining options recall the purpose of the restraints after this surgical procedure. This will assist in directing you to option 3, the safest nursing action. Review postoperative nursing interventions after cleft palate repair if you had difficulty with this question.

Level of Cognitive Ability: Application
Client Needs: Safe, Effective Care Environment
Integrated Concept/Process: Nursing Process/Implementation
Content Area: Child Health

Reference:
Schulte, E. Price, D., & Gwin, J. (2001). *Thompson's pediatric nursing* (8th ed.). Philadelphia: W.B. Saunders, p. 90.

---

218. A nurse is caring for a hospitalized child with rubella (German measles). Which of the following precautions would the nurse institute while caring for this child?
1   Contact isolation
2   Reverse isolation procedures
3   Enteric precautions
4   Protective isolation

Answer: 1
Rationale: Care of a child with rubella involves airborne precautions and contact isolation. Contact isolation requires masks, gowns, and gloves for contact with any infectious material. Contaminated articles must be bagged and labeled before reprocessing. Options 2, 3, and 4 are not specific to the care of a child with rubella.

Test-Taking Strategy: Use the process of elimination. Eliminate options 2 and 4 because they are similar. Knowledge that transmission of rubella is by direct contact with infectious droplets will direct you to option 1. Review the method of transmission of rubella if you had difficulty with this question.

Level of Cognitive Ability: Application
Client Needs: Safe, Effective Care Environment
Integrated Concept/Process: Nursing Process/Implementation
Content Area: Child Health

Reference:
Wong, D., & Hockenberry-Eaton, M. (2001). *Wong's essentials of pediatric nursing* (6th ed.). St. Louis: Mosby, p. 462.

---

219. A nurse is caring for a child who was diagnosed with erythema infectiosum (fifth disease). The mother asks the nurse how this disease is transmitted. The nurse informs the mother that fifth disease is transmitted by which of the following routes?
1   Airborne particles
2   Fecal-oral route

Answer: 1
Rationale: Fifth disease is transmitted via airborne particles, respiratory droplets, blood, blood products, or transplacental means. Options 2, 3, and 4 are incorrect regarding the mode of transmission of fifth disease.

Test-Taking Strategy: Knowledge regarding the mode of transmission of fifth disease is required to answer this question.

3 Saliva
4 Contact with sweat

Review this infectious disease if you had difficulty with this question.

Level of Cognitive Ability: Application
Client Needs: Safe, Effective Care Environment
Integrated Concept/Process: Teaching/Learning
Content Area: Child Health

Reference:
Wong, D., & Hockenberry-Eaton, M. (2001). *Wong's essentials of pediatric nursing* (6th ed.). St. Louis: Mosby, p. 458.

---

220. A nurse is caring for a child with bronchiolitis. The cause of the disorder is respiratory syncytial virus (RSV). Which of the following precautions will the nurse institute when caring for the child to decrease the spread of organisms?
1 Respiratory isolation
2 Contact isolation
3 Enteric precautions
4 Protective isolation

Answer: 2
Rationale: RSV can live on paper or skin for up to 1 hour and on cribs or other nonporous surfaces for up to 6 hours. Although RSV is not airborne it is highly communicable and it is usually transferred by the hands. Meticulous hand washing decreases the spread of organisms. Personnel who care for these children should maintain contact isolation, which includes wearing gloves and gowns and practicing good hand washing.

Test-Taking Strategy: Knowledge regarding the method of transmission of RSV is required to answer this question. Review this virus and its mode of transmission if you had difficulty with this question.

Level of Cognitive Ability: Application
Client Needs: Safe, Effective Care Environment
Integrated Concept/Process: Nursing Process/Implementation
Content Area: Child Health

Reference:
Wong, D., & Hockenberry-Eaton, M. (2001). *Wong's essentials of pediatric nursing* (6th ed.). St. Louis: Mosby, p. 841.

---

221. A nurse administers medications to the wrong client. During the investigation of the incident, it was determined that the nurse failed to check the client's identification bracelet before administering the medications. The nurse evaluates the situation and determines that negligence has occurred because negligence is:
1 Defined as the failure to meet established standards of care
2 Defined as a crime that results in the injury of a client
3 Strictly prohibited by the state's Nurse Practice Act
4 Strictly prohibited by the institution's own policies

Answer: 1
Rationale: The legal definition of negligence is the failure to meet accepted standards of care. Option 2 is an incorrect definition of negligence, although injury may have come to the client as a result of error. Both the institution and the Nurse Practice Act have provisions that identify and discourage acts of negligence.

Test-Taking Strategy: Use the process of elimination. Option 3 and 4 are true in that the purpose of the Nurse Practice Act and institutional policies and procedures is to protect the public from harm, but they identify and discourage acts of negligence rather than "strictly prohibit" negligence. From the remaining options, select option 1 because it is more global. Review the concepts related to negligence if you had difficulty with this question.

Level of Cognitive Ability: Comprehension
Client Needs: Safe, Effective Care Environment
Integrated Concept/Process: Nursing Process/Evaluation
Content Area: Fundamental Skills

Reference:
Potter, P., & Perry, A. (2001). *Fundamentals of nursing* (5th ed.). St. Louis: Mosby, p. 425.

---

222. Which activity by the family of an infant with respiratory syncytial virus (RSV) who is receiving ribavirin (Virazole) would indicate a knowledge deficit regarding the management of the disease process?
1 The infant's grandfather, who has asthma, is told he may not visit
2 The family wears a gown, gloves, mask, and hair covering when they visit the infant
3 Before leaving the infant's room, all family members wash their hands
4 The infant's pregnant aunt visits the infant

Answer: 4
Rationale: Whenever anyone is receiving ribavirin, there are precautions to prevent exposure to the medication. Everyone who enters the room while the client is receiving ribavirin should wear a gown, mask, gloves, and hair covering. Anyone who is pregnant or considering pregnancy and anyone with a history of respiratory problems or reactive airway disease should not care for or visit anyone who is receiving ribavirin. Good hand washing is necessary before leaving the room because hand washing prevents the spread of germs.

Test-Taking Strategy: Use the process of elimination. Noting the key words *indicate a knowledge deficit* will assist in directing you to option 4. Review this medication and these precautions if you had difficulty with this question.

Level of Cognitive Ability: Comprehension
Client Needs: Safe, Effective Care Environment
Integrated Concept/Process: Nursing Process/Evaluation
Content Area: Child Health

Reference:
Hodgson, B., & Kizior, R. (2003). *Saunders nursing drug handbook 2003.* Philadelphia: W.B. Saunders, p. 974.

---

223. A nurse receives a telephone call from the laboratory and is told that an initial report of a urine culture identifies the presence of several different organisms. The nurse evaluates that this most likely means which of the following?
1 Client has a bladder infection
2 Client has a kidney infection
3 Specimen was contaminated
4 Specimen was mishandled in the laboratory

Answer: 3
Rationale: The presence of multiple organisms in a urine culture usually indicates that contamination has occurred. The urinary tract is normally sterile, and infection, if it occurs, is usually with one organism. A repeat of the urine culture is indicated.

Test-Taking Strategy: Use the process of elimination. Note the key words *most likely*. There is no information in the question indicating that the laboratory personnel mishandled the specimen. A urine culture will not discriminate between bladder or kidney infection; the clinical picture would help to differentiate this. Remember that specimen contamination is the most frequent reason that multiple organisms are cultured; most urinary tract infections are caused by a single organism such as *Escherichia coli*. Review the causes of specimen contamination if you had difficulty with this question.

Level of Cognitive Ability: Comprehension
Client Needs: Safe, Effective Care Environment
Integrated Concept/Process: Nursing Process/Evaluation
Content Area: Fundamental Skills

Reference:
Potter, P., & Perry, A. (2001). *Fundamentals of nursing* (5th ed.). St. Louis: Mosby, p. 1402.

224. A nurse is evaluating the client's use of a cane for left-sided weakness. The nurse would intervene and correct the client if the nurse observed the client doing which of the following?

1. Holding the cane on the right side
2. Keeping the cane 6 inches out to the side of the right foot
3. Moving the cane when the right leg is moved
4. Leaning on the cane when the right leg swings through

Answer: 3

Rationale: The cane is held on the stronger side to minimize stress on the affected extremity and provide a wide base of support. The cane is held 6 inches lateral to the fifth toe. The cane is moved forward with the affected leg. The client leans on the cane for added support while the stronger side swings through.

Test-Taking Strategy: Focus on the key words *would intervene and correct the client*. Knowing that the cane is held on the stronger side helps you eliminate options 1 and 2 first. To discriminate between the remaining options, recall that the client moves the cane with the weaker leg and leans on it for support when the stronger leg swings through. Review the use of a cane if you had difficulty with this question.

Level of Cognitive Ability: Comprehension
Client Needs: Safe, Effective Care Environment
Integrated Concept/Process: Nursing Process/Evaluation
Content Area: Adult Health/Musculoskeletal

Reference:
Potter, P., & Perry, A. (2001). *Fundamentals of nursing* (5th ed.). St. Louis: Mosby, p. 1008.

---

225. A nurse instructs a mother caring for an infant with acute infectious diarrhea about measures to prevent the spread of pathogens. Which action by the mother indicates a need for further teaching?

1. Washes the infant's hands after changing the diaper
2. Applies a cloth diaper snugly after cleaning the perineum
3. Restrains the infant's hands when changing the diaper
4. Places the soiled diaper in a sealed, double plastic bag

Answer: 2

Rationale: Cloth diapers do not have elastic in the legs. This could allow for seepage of the infectious stool and cause the spread of pathogens. Also, the liquid stool makes the diaper wet, which also promotes the spread of disease. Disposable, plastic diapers have elastic in the legs, high absorbency, and plastic on the outside. These features decrease transmission of pathogens. Option 1 prevents the spread of pathogens through hand washing. Option 3 prevents the child from coming into contact with the infectious material. Option 4 identifies appropriate disposal of infectious waste.

Test-Taking Strategy: Note the key words *need for further teaching*. Use the principles of Standard (Universal) Precautions, which include hand washing, proper disposal of body fluids and waste, and avoiding contact with body fluid. The only option that does not accurately reflect these precautions is option 2. Review these precautions if you had difficulty with this question.

Level of Cognitive Ability: Comprehension
Client Needs: Safe, Effective Care Environment
Integrated Concept/Process: Teaching/Learning
Content Area: Child Health

Reference:
Murray, S., McKinney, E. & Gorrie, T. (2002). *Foundations of maternal-newborn nursing* (3rd ed.). Philadelphia: W.B. Saunders, p. 1099.

FILL-IN-THE-BLANK

A nurse is told that an assigned client has acquired multidrug-resistant *Staphylococcus aureus* (MRSA). In addition to standard precautions, the nurse places the client on which type of transmission-based precautions?
Answer: _____

Answer: Contact precautions
Rationale: Contact precautions are precautions that include standard precautions and the use of barrier precautions such as gloves and impermeable gowns. Contact precautions are used for clients with diarrhea or draining wounds not contained by a sterile dressing, or clients who have acquired antibiotic-resistant infections. The goal of these precautions is to eliminate disease transmission resulting either from direct contact with the client or indirect contact through an intermediary infected object or surface that has been in contact with the client, such as instruments, linens, or dressing materials.

Test-Taking Strategy: Focus on the client's diagnosis and think about the method of transmission of the infection to others. Recalling that MRSA can be transmitted by contact with the infecting organism will assist in answering the question. Review contact precautions if you had difficulty with this question.

Level of Cognitive Ability: Application
Client Needs: Safe, Effective Care Environment
Integrated Concept/Process: Nursing Process/Implementation
Content Area: Fundamental Skills

Reference:
Linton, A. & Maebius, N. (2003). *Introduction to medical-surgical nursing* (3rd ed.). Philadelphia: W.B. Saunders, p. 141.

MULTIPLE-RESPONSE – SELECT ALL THAT APPLY

A nurse is caring for a client with leukemia who is receiving chemotherapy. The nurse reviews the client's laboratory results and notes that the client's neutrophil count is less than 1000 cells/mm3. Select all nursing interventions that specifically apply to the care of the client.
___   Pad the side rails
___   Restrict visitors with colds or respiratory infections
___   Implement a low bacteria diet that excludes fresh fruits and vegetables and milk products
___   Avoid invasive procedures as much as possible
___   Monitor the temperature every 2 to 4 hours
___   Place a clean mask on the client if the client needs to leave the room for a diagnostic test
___   Encourage the client to shower daily

Answer:
___   Restrict visitors with colds or respiratory infections
___   Implement a low bacteria diet that excludes fresh fruits and vegetables and milk products
___   Avoid invasive procedures as much as possible
___   Monitor the temperature every 2 to 4 hours
___   Place a clean mask on the client if the client needs to leave the room for a diagnostic test
___   Encourage the client to shower daily

Rationale: A client who has a low neutrophil count is at risk for infection. Therefore interventions are aimed at preventing this occurrence. Individuals with a cold or respiratory infection should not be in contact with the client. Because clients with low white blood cell counts often become infected with their own microorganisms through their gastrointestinal tract, a low bacteria diet is prescribed. Invasive procedures are avoided as much as possible to prevent the entrance of microorganisms into the client's body and the client's temperature is monitored frequently to detect an early sign of infection. The client should wear a clean mask when outside the room, especially in heavily traveled public

_____ Remove all hazards and sharp objects from the environment
_____ Place the client in a semi-private room
_____ Keep the door to the client's room closed at all times
_____ Measure the abdominal girth daily

areas such as corridors, elevators, and waiting rooms. The client should be encouraged to shower daily to remove bacteria from the skin and perianal area. The client should be placed in a private room. The door to the room may be left open and a "Compromised Host Precaution" sign should be placed on the door. The incorrect interventions for this question would be implemented if the client had thrombocytopenia and was at risk for bleeding.

Test-Taking Strategy: Note that the client has a low neutrophil count. Recalling that this low count places a client at risk for infection will assist in identifying the appropriate interventions. Review the interventions for the client at risk for infection if you had difficulty with this question.

Level of Cognitive Ability: Application
Client Needs: Safe, Effective Care Environment
Integrated Concept/Process: Nursing Process/Implementation
Content Area: Adult Health/Oncology

References:
Linton, A. & Maebius, N. (2003). *Introduction to medical-surgical nursing* (3rd ed.). Philadelphia: W.B. Saunders, pp. 540; 546.

REFERENCES

Bauer, B., & Hill, S. (2000). *Mental health nursing.* Philadelphia: W.B. Saunders.

Black, J., Hawks, J., & Keene, A. (2001). *Medical-surgical nursing: clinical management for positive outcomes* (6th ed.). Philadelphia: W.B. Saunders.

Brent, N. (2002) *Nurses and the law* (2nd ed.). Philadelphia: W.B Saunders.

Burroughs, A., & Leifer, G. (2002). *Maternity nursing* (8th ed.). Philadelphia: W.B. Saunders.

deWit, S. (2001). *Fundamental concepts and skills for nursing.* Philadelphia: W.B. Saunders.

Hill, S., & Bauer, B. (2000). *Mental health nursing.* Philadelphia: W.B. Saunders.

Hodgson, B., & Kizior, R. (2003). *Saunders nursing drug handbook 2003.* Philadelphia: W.B. Saunders.

Ignatavicius, D., & Workman, M. (2002). *Medical-surgical nursing: critical thinking for collaborative care* (4th ed.). Philadelphia: W.B. Saunders.

Lehne, R. (2001). *Pharmacology for nursing care* (4th ed.). Philadelphia: W.B. Saunders.

Lewis, S., Heitkemper, M., & Dirksen, S. (2000). *Medical-surgical nursing: assessment and management of clinical problems* (5th ed.). St. Louis: Mosby.

Linton, A., & Maebius, N. (2003). *Introduction to medical-surgical nursing* (3rd ed.). Philadelphia: W.B. Saunders.

Lueckenotte, A. (2002). *Gerontologic nursing* (2nd ed.). St. Louis: Mosby.

McKinney, E., Ashwill, J., Murray, S. et al. (2000). *Maternal-child nursing.* Philadelphia: W.B. Saunders.

Murray, S., McKinney, E., & Gorrie, T. (2002). *Foundations of maternal-newborn nursing* (3rd ed.). Philadelphia: W.B. Saunders.

Perry, A., & Potter, A. (2002). *Clinical nursing skills & techniques* (5th ed.). St. Louis: Mosby.

Potter, P., & Perry, A. (2001). *Fundamentals of nursing* (5th ed.). St. Louis: Mosby.

Schulte, E. Price, D., & Gwin, J. (2001). *Thompson's pediatric nursing* (8th ed.). Philadelphia: W.B. Saunders.

Varcarolis, E. (2002). *Foundations of psychiatric mental health nursing* (4th ed.). Philadelphia: W.B. Saunders.

Williams, S. (2001). *Basic nutrition & diet therapy* (11th ed.). St. Louis: Mosby.

Wong, D., & Hockenberry-Eaton, M. (2001). *Wong's essentials of pediatric nursing* (6th ed.). St. Louis: Mosby.

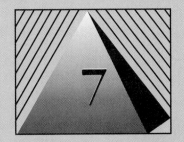

Health Promotion and Maintenance

1. A nurse is reinforcing instructions with the hypertensive client about dietary modifications to control the health problem. The nurse would use which of the following meal selections as the best sample menu for the client?

1 Hot dog in a bun, sauerkraut, baked beans
2 Turkey, baked potato, salad with oil and vinegar
3 Scallops, french fries, salad with bleu cheese dressing
4 Corned beef, fresh carrots, boiled potato

Answer: 2

Rationale: Foods from the meat group that are higher in sodium include bacon, luncheon meat, chipped or corned beef, kosher meat, smoked or salted meat or fish, peanut butter, and a variety of shellfish. Options 1, 3, and 4 are incorrect.

Test-Taking Strategy: Use the process of elimination. Eliminate the hot dog and corned beef first (options 1 and 4) because they are processed meats, which would be higher in sodium (the sauerkraut in option 1 is high in sodium also). The shellfish and the commercial dressing help you eliminate option 3 next. Review foods high in sodium if you had difficulty with this question.

Level of Cognitive Ability: Application
Client Needs: Health Promotion and Maintenance
Integrated Concept/Process: Teaching/Learning
Content Area: Adult Health/Cardiovascular

Reference:
Williams, S. (2001). *Basic nutrition & diet therapy* (11th ed.). St. Louis: Mosby, p. 366.

---

2. A nurse is reinforcing home care instructions to a client with chronic venous insufficiency secondary to deep vein thrombosis. The nurse would tell the client to avoid which of the following activities?

1 Wearing elastic hose for at least 6 to 8 weeks
2 Sitting in chairs that allow the feet to touch the floor
3 Sleeping with the foot of the bed elevated
4 Elevating the head of the bed 6 inches during sleep

Answer: 4

Rationale: Clients with chronic venous insufficiency are advised to avoid crossing the legs, sitting in chairs where the feet do not touch the floor, standing or sitting for prolonged periods of time, and wearing garters or sources of pressure above the legs (such as girdles). The client should wear elastic hose for 6 to 8 weeks and perhaps for life. The client should sleep with the foot of the bed (not the head of the bed) elevated to promote venous return during sleep.

Test-Taking Strategy: Use the process of elimination. Note the key word *avoid*. Use the concept of gravity when answering questions that relate to peripheral vascular problems. Venous problems are characterized by insufficient drainage of blood from the legs returning to the heart. Thus interventions should be directed toward promoting flow of blood from the legs and to the heart. Only option 4 does not promote venous drainage, making it the answer to the question as stated. Review teaching points for the client with venous insufficiency if you had difficulty with this question.

Level of Cognitive Ability: Application
Client Needs: Health Promotion and Maintenance
Integrated Concept/Process: Teaching/Learning
Content Area: Adult Health/Cardiovascular

Reference:
Black, J., Hawks, J., & Keene, A. (2001). *Medical-surgical nursing: clinical management for positive outcomes* (6th ed.). Philadelphia: W.B. Saunders, p. 1425.

---

3. A nurse has reinforced instructions to the hypertensive client about nonfood items that contain sodium. The nurse determines that the client understands the information presented if the client states that which of the following may be used?
1   Cold remedies
2   Toothpaste
3   Demineralized water
4   Mouthwash

Answer: 3
Rationale: Sodium intake can be increased by use of several types of products, including toothpaste and mouthwashes; over-the-counter (OTC) medications such as analgesics, antacids, cough remedies, laxatives, and sedatives; and softened water, as well as some mineral waters. Clients are advised to read labels for sodium content. Water that is bottled, distilled, deionized, or demineralized may be used for drinking and cooking.

Test-Taking Strategy: Use the process of elimination. The wording of the question directs you to seek the item that is low in sodium. Remember that several OTC medications and products contain significant levels of sodium. This will assist in eliminating options 1, 2, and 4. Finally, look at the word *demineralized*, which means having the minerals removed. An option such as this would be a good choice when selecting an item low in sodium. Review low sodium nonfood items if you had difficulty with this question.

Level of Cognitive Ability: Comprehension
Client Needs: Health Promotion and Maintenance
Integrated Concept/Process: Nursing Process/Evaluation
Content Area: Adult Health/Cardiovascular

Reference:
Williams, S. (2001) *Basic nutrition & diet therapy* (11th ed.). St. Louis: Mosby, p. 366.

---

4. A nurse is reinforcing instructions with a client about how to perform a three-point gait with crutches. Which of the following instructions would the nurse provide to the client?
1   Simultaneously move both crutches and the affected leg forward, then move the unaffected leg forward
2   Advance the right crutch and the left foot forward, then bring the right foot and left crutch forward

Answer: 1
Rationale: A three-point gait or orthopedic gait is used for amputees and orthopedic clients. It requires that the client have normal use of one leg and both arms. The client is instructed to simultaneously move both crutches and the affected leg forward, then the unaffected leg should move forward. Options 2 and 3 identify a four-point gait. Option 4 identifies a swing-through gait.

Test-Taking Strategy: Use the process of elimination. Note the key words *three-point gait*. This will assist in eliminating options 2, 3, and 4 because these gaits do not represent a three-point gait.

3 Move the right crutch, the left foot, the left crutch, and then the right foot forward

4 Move both crutches forward and then swing both feet forward to the crutches

Review client instructions regarding a three-point gait if you had difficulty with this question.

Level of Cognitive Ability: Application
Client Needs: Health Promotion and Maintenance
Integrated Concept/Process: Nursing Process/Implementation
Content Area: Adult Health/Musculoskeletal

Reference:
deWit, S. (2001). *Fundamental concepts and skills for nursing.* Philadelphia: W.B. Saunders, p. 829.

---

5. A nurse is reinforcing instructions with a client about the use of crutches and is teaching the client the method for ascending and descending stairs. When instructing the client about ascending the stairs, the nurse tells the client to do which of the following?

1 Move the unaffected leg up first, followed by the affected leg and crutches

2 Move the crutches and unaffected leg down, followed by the affected leg

3 Move both crutches up the stair, followed by the affected leg and then the unaffected leg

4 Move both crutches up the stair, followed by the unaffected leg and then the affected leg

Answer: 1
Rationale: To go up the stairs the client should move the unaffected leg up first. Then the client moves the affected leg and crutches up. When going down the stairs, the client should move the crutches and the affected leg, then move the unaffected leg.

Test-Taking Strategy: When answering this question, attempt to visualize the process of going up and down stairs with the use of crutches. If you can remember "good-up, and bad-down" you will easily answer this question. When going up the stairs, the good leg or unaffected leg moves first. When going down the stairs, the bad or affected leg moves first. Review crutch-walking techniques if you had difficulty with this question.

Level of Cognitive Ability: Application
Client Needs: Health Promotion and Maintenance
Integrated Concept/Process: Teaching/Learning
Content Area: Adult Health/Musculoskeletal

Reference:
deWit, S. (2001). *Fundamental concepts and skills for nursing.* Philadelphia: W.B. Saunders, p. 827.

---

6. A client being discharged to go home is prescribed enoxaparin (Lovenox) 30 mg subcutaneously twice a day for 7 days. The nurse is asked to reinforce teaching with the client about administration of the medication. The nurse plans to tell the client which of the following?

1 Aspirate the syringe before pushing down on the plunger

2 Massage the skin after giving the injection

3 Push the skin flat and taut before injecting the medication

4 A 25- to 27-gauge, 5/8-inch needle is attached to the syringe

Answer: 4
Rationale: With subcutaneous injection of enoxaparin, the administration technique is the same as for subcutaneous heparin. The nurse teaches the client that a 25- to 27-gauge needle is attached to the syringe to prevent hematoma formation at the injection site. The client should use a "bunching" technique to inject the medication deep into fatty abdominal tissue. The nurse teaches the client not to aspirate before injecting and not to massage the injection site.

Test-Taking Strategy: To select the correct option, recall that enoxaparin is a subcutaneously administered anticoagulant medication. With this in mind, you can select the statement that is standard subcutaneous injection procedure. Apply the principles related to administering heparin by subcutaneous injection to assist in answering the question. Review the procedure for administering enoxaparin if you had difficulty with this question.

Level of Cognitive Ability: Application
Client Needs: Health Promotion and Maintenance

Integrated Concept/Process: Nursing Process/Planning
Content Area: Adult Health/Cardiovascular

Reference:

Hodgson, B., & Kizior, R. (2003). *Saunders nursing drug handbook 2003.* Philadelphia: W.B. Saunders, p. 398.

---

7. A nurse has reinforced instructions with a client who has an arterial ischemic leg ulcer about wound care and self-management of the health problem. Which statement by the client indicates a need for further instructions?
  1. "I should elevate my legs above heart level at least 1 hour each day."
  2. "I should apply lanolin lotion to my feet but not between my toes."
  3. "I should not go barefoot."
  4. "I should cut my toenails straight across."

Answer: 1

Rationale: Foot care instructions for the client with peripheral arterial ischemia are the same instructions given to the client with diabetes mellitus (options 2, 3, and 4). The client with arterial disease, however, should avoid raising the legs above heart level unless instructed to do so as part of an exercise program (such as Buerger-Allen exercises), or unless venous stasis is also present. Even so, legs would be elevated for approximately 30 seconds to 2 minutes at a time, not for 1 hour.

Test-Taking Strategy: Note the key words *need for further instructions.* Use principles related to care of clients with peripheral arterial disease to answer this question. The words *arterial ischemic* cue you to enlist the aid of gravity to enhance blood flow. With this in mind, you can eliminate all of the incorrect options. Review teaching points related to the client with peripheral arterial ischemia if you had difficulty with this question.

Level of Cognitive Ability: Application
Client Needs: Health Promotion and Maintenance
Integrated Concept/Process: Teaching/Learning
Content Area: Adult Health/Cardiovascular

Reference:

Black, J., Hawks, J., & Keene, A. (2001). *Medical-surgical nursing: clinical management for positive outcomes* (6th ed.). Philadelphia: W.B. Saunders, p. 1416.

---

8. A young woman has just been diagnosed with rheumatic heart disease. The client's husband asks the nurse why the client must tell the dentist about this condition before dental cleaning or other work. The nurse tells the client's husband that the condition should be reported for which of the following reasons?
  1. So that the dentist will use a type of lidocaine that doesn't contain epinephrine
  2. So that the dentist will use a lower speed drill when doing dental work
  3. So that prophylactic antibiotic therapy will be prescribed
  4. To prevent the client from going into heart failure

Answer: 3

Rationale: The client with a history of rheumatic heart disease is at risk for developing infective endocarditis. The client should notify all physicians and dentists about this previous health problem. The physician or dentist will then initiate prophylactic antibiotic therapy before any procedure that is invasive or that could result in bleeding. The other options are not related to the question.

Test-Taking Strategy: To answer this question correctly, it is necessary to understand that the client with rheumatic heart disease must have prophylactic antibiotic therapy before undergoing invasive procedures. Recalling this concept will direct you to option 3. Review this disease if you had difficulty with this question.

Level of Cognitive Ability: Application
Client Needs: Health Promotion and Maintenance
Integrated Concept/Process: Nursing Process/Implementation
Content Area: Adult Health/Cardiovascular

Reference:
Black, J., Hawks, J., & Keene, A. (2001). *Medical-surgical nursing: clinical management for positive outcomes* (6th ed.). Philadelphia: W.B. Saunders, p. 1484.

---

9. A nurse is caring for a client who experiences frequent episodes of bronchial asthma. The nurse is reinforcing home care instructions about measures to reduce aggravation of the condition. The nurse tells the client that which of the following is least likely to help the client's condition?
- **1** Buying a humidifier
- **2** Damp dusting the furniture
- **3** Having the chimney cleaned
- **4** Having the furnace serviced

Answer: 1
Rationale: Environmental allergens and organisms that can cause infection are likely to aggravate asthma. These irritants can be reduced by having the chimney cleaned and by dusting with a damp cloth. Having the furnace serviced will eliminate dirt and soot from the system and detect if carbon monoxide is leaking or present. A humidifier will increase the moisture in the air but may also increase the growth of mold and mildew, which would not be helpful for this client.

Test-Taking Strategy: Use the process of elimination and note the key words *least likely*. Recalling the factors that contribute to asthma will direct you to option 1. Review these home care measures if you had difficulty with this question.

Level of Cognitive Ability: Application
Client Needs: Health Promotion and Maintenance
Integrated Concept/Process: Self-Care
Content Area: Adult Health/Respiratory

Reference:
Black, J., Hawks, J., & Keene, A. (2001). *Medical-surgical nursing: clinical management for positive outcomes* (6th ed.). Philadelphia: W.B. Saunders, p. 1639.

---

10. A client with respiratory disease is experiencing activity intolerance related to fatigue and dyspnea after physical exertion. The nurse suggests which of the following goals that will best improve the client's functioning?
- **1** Reduce caloric intake by half to allow more energy for breathing
- **2** Begin taking a light sedative medication each night to ensure a good night's sleep
- **3** Gradually increase ambulation and completion of small tasks daily
- **4** Stay in one room of the house to decrease episodes of fatigue and dyspnea

Answer: 3
Rationale: The client should try to gradually increase activity and mobility each day. The client should not reduce caloric intake by half because the client will not have sufficient energy for respiration. Rather, the client should take in adequate calories but eat small frequent meals each day. The client needs adequate rest, but relying on a sedative each night could foster dependence. Finally, the client should not stay in one room of the house because doing so will not increase endurance and will also foster feelings of seclusion and social isolation.

Test-Taking Strategy: Use the process of elimination and focus on the issue—the goal that will best improve the client's tolerance of activity. Option 3 is the only option that relates to activity. Review the goals for the client with activity intolerance if you had difficulty with this question.

Level of Cognitive Ability: Application
Client Needs: Health Promotion and Maintenance
Integrated Concept/Process: Self-Care
Content Area: Adult Health/Respiratory

Reference:
Johnson, M., Bulechek, G., Dochterman, J. et al. (2001). *Nursing diagnoses, outcomes, and interventions.* St. Louis: Mosby, p. 41.

11. Captopril (Capoten) has been prescribed for a hospitalized client with hypertension, and the nurse provides instructions to the client about the medication. The nurse evaluates that the client understands how to take this medication if the client states an intention to do which of the following?
1   Sit upright and stand slowly
2   Drink larger amounts of water
3   Eat foods that are high in potassium
4   Take in large amounts of high fiber foods

Answer: 1
Rationale: Captopril is an antihypertensive medication (angiotensin-converting enzyme inhibitor). Orthostatic hypotension is a concern for clients taking antihypertensive medications. Clients are advised to avoid standing in one position for long periods of time, change positions slowly, and avoid extreme warmth (showers, bath, weather). Clients are also taught to recognize the symptoms of orthostatic hypotension, including dizziness, light-headedness, weakness, and syncope. The other options are not necessary, and option 2 could aggravate the hypertension.

Test-Taking Strategy: Use the process of elimination. Recalling that captopril is an antihypertensive will direct you to option 1, because the risk of orthostatic hypotension is present with all types of antihypertensives. Review this medication if you had difficulty with this question.

Level of Cognitive Ability: Comprehension
Client Needs: Health Promotion and Maintenance
Integrated Concept/Process: Nursing Process/Evaluation
Content Area: Adult Health/Cardiovascular

Reference:
Hodgson, B., & Kizior, R. (2003). *Saunders nursing drug handbook 2003.* Philadelphia: W.B. Saunders, p. 166.

12. A client is 39 years old, has three children, and is a waitress. The nurse recognizes that this client is most at risk for developing which of the following peripheral vascular disorders?
1   Varicose veins
2   Thrombophlebitis
3   Acute arterial embolism
4   Arterial insufficiency

Answer: 1
Rationale: Varicose veins are more common after the age of 30 in clients who have occupations that require prolonged standing. The condition also occurs more frequently in pregnant women, obese individuals, and those with a positive family history of varicose veins or systemic problems, such as heart disease. Conservative treatment in these individuals focuses on promoting venous return to the heart. There is no information in the question to indicate prolonged immobility (option 2), risk of cardiac thrombus (option 3), or added risk of arterial insufficiency (option 4).

Test-Taking Strategy: Use the process of elimination and knowledge of the risk factors for development of varicose veins. Focusing on the key words *peripheral vascular* will direct you to option 1. Review these risk factors if you had difficulty with this question.

Level of Cognitive Ability: Comprehension
Client Needs: Health Promotion and Maintenance
Integrated Concept/Process: Nursing Process/Data Collection
Content Area: Adult Health/Cardiovascular

Reference:
Black, J., Hawks, J., & Keene, A. (2001). *Medical-surgical nursing: clinical management for positive outcomes* (6th ed.). Philadelphia: W.B. Saunders, p. 1426.

13. A nurse is giving a client general information about acceptable foods to include on a sodium-restricted diet. The nurse tells the client that which of the following is a good selection from the bread food group?

1 Instant rice
2 Commercial stuffing
3 Frozen bread dough
4 Corn meal

Answer: 4
Rationale: Clients on a sodium-restricted diet should avoid whenever possible the use of commercially prepared products, which often contain sodium as a preservative. Products made with natural grains that do not have added salt are the best food items.

Test-Taking Strategy: Use the process of elimination. Recalling that many commercially prepared products contain sodium will direct you to option 4. Review sodium-restricted diets if you had difficulty with this question.

Level of Cognitive Ability: Application
Client Needs: Health Promotion and Maintenance
Integrated Concept/Process: Teaching/Learning
Content Area: Adult Health/Cardiovascular

Reference:
Williams, S. (2001) *Basic nutrition & diet therapy* (11th ed.). St. Louis: Mosby, p. 366.

---

14. A client with hypercholesterolemia is beginning to limit the intake of dietary cholesterol. The nurse tells the client to choose which of the following meat choices because it is lowest in fat?

1 Skinless chicken
2 Prime grade beef
3 Liver
4 Bacon

Answer: 1
Rationale: The best meat choices to lower the intake of cholesterol include lean cuts of beef with the fat trimmed, lamb, pork (except spare ribs), veal (except ground), skinless poultry, fish, and shellfish. Meats that have larger amounts of cholesterol include prime grades of beef, pork spare ribs, goose, duck, organ meats (liver, brain, kidney), sausage, bacon, luncheon meats, frankfurters, and caviar.

Test-Taking Strategy: Use the process of elimination and focus on the issue, the meat choice lowest in fat. Noting the word *skinless* in option 1 will assist in directing you to this option. Review low-fat foods if you had difficulty with this question.

Level of Cognitive Ability: Application
Client Needs: Health Promotion and Maintenance
Integrated Concept/Process: Nursing Process/Implementation
Content Area: Adult Health/Cardiovascular

Reference:
Williams, S. (2001) *Basic nutrition & diet therapy* (11th ed.). St. Louis: Mosby, p. 237.

---

15. A nurse has provided instructions about body mechanics and low back care to the client with a herniated lumbar disk. Which statement by the client indicates a need for further instructions?

1 "I should swim or walk to strengthen my back muscles."
2 "I should bend at the knees to pick up objects."

Answer: 3
Rationale: Clients should get out of bed by sliding toward the mattress edge. The client should then roll onto one side and push up from the bed using one or both arms. The client should keep the back straight as the legs are swung over the side. Proper body mechanics includes bending at the knees, not the waist, to lift objects. The client should increase dietary fiber and fluids to prevent straining at stool, which would increase intraspinal pressure. Walking and swimming are excellent exercises for strengthening lower back muscles.

3 "I should get out of bed by sitting up straight and swinging my legs over the side."

4 "I should increase the amount of fluid and fiber in my diet."

Test-Taking Strategy: Use the process of elimination and note the key words *need for further instructions.* Eliminate options 1 and 2 first, as they are correct actions. Choose option 3 instead of option 4 by knowing either that sitting up straight causes strain on lower back muscles, or that straining at stool increases intraspinal pressure. Review teaching points for the client with a herniated lumbar disk if you had difficulty with this question.

Level of Cognitive Ability: Comprehension
Client Needs: Health Promotion and Maintenance
Integrated Concept/Process: Teaching/Learning
Content Area: Adult Health/Musculoskeletal

Reference:
Potter, P., & Perry, A. (2001). *Fundamentals of nursing* (5th ed.). St. Louis: Mosby, p. 1004.

---

16. A nurse has instructed a client with chronic airflow limitation (CAL) about energy conservation techniques. Which statement by the client indicates a need for further instructions?

1 "I should not hold my breath during activities requiring exertion."

2 "I should limit activities that involve much arm movement."

3 "I should sit when performing activities that do not require much movement."

4 "I should perform all activities early in the day when I am most rested."

Answer: 4
Rationale: The client should alternate activities with rest periods to conserve energy. The client should also sit when performing activities that do not require exertion, such as sewing or ironing. The client should limit activities involving arm movements because these will increase dyspnea. The client should not hold the breath for the same reason.

Test-Taking Strategy: Use the process of elimination and note the key words *indicates a need for further instruction.* Focusing on the issue, energy conservation techniques will direct you to option 4. Review these measures if you had difficulty with this question.

Level of Cognitive Ability: Comprehension
Client Needs: Health Promotion and Maintenance
Integrated Concept/Process: Teaching/Learning
Content Area: Adult Health/Respiratory

Reference:
Black, J., Hawks, J., & Keene, A. (2001). *Medical-surgical nursing: clinical management for positive outcomes* (6th ed.). Philadelphia: W.B. Saunders, p. 1702.

---

17. A nurse teaches a client with chronic airflow limitation (CAL) about positions that help breathing during dyspneic episodes. Which position if identified by the client indicates a need for further teaching?

1 Lying on the back in semi-Fowler's position

2 Sitting up and leaning on a table

3 Sitting up with elbows resting on knees

4 Standing and leaning against a wall

Answer: 1
Rationale: The client should use the positions identified in options 2, 3, and 4. These allow for maximal chest expansion and decreased use of the accessory muscles of respiration. The client should not lie on the back because it reduces movement of a large area of the client's chest wall. Sitting is better than standing whenever possible. If no chair is available, then leaning against a wall while standing allows accessory muscles to be used for breathing, and not posture control.

Test-Taking Strategy: Use the process of elimination and note the key words *need for further teaching.* Visualize each position identified in the options and note that options 2, 3, and 4 are similar and involve a position in which the client leans forward. Review the positions that assist in breathing if you had difficulty with this question.

Level of Cognitive Ability: Comprehension
Client Needs: Health Promotion and Maintenance
Integrated Concept/Process: Self-Care
Content Area: Adult Health/Respiratory

Reference:
Black, J., Hawks, J., & Keene, A. (2001). *Medical-surgical nursing: clinical management for positive outcomes* (6th ed.). Philadelphia: W.B. Saunders, p. 1702.

---

18. A nurse reinforces instructions with a client about monoamine oxidase (MAO) inhibitor toxicity. The nurse determines that the client is aware of the signs of toxicity when the client tells the nurse that he or she will report:

1   Insomnia
2   Low-grade fever
3   Excessive fatigue
4   Lethargy

Answer: 1
Rationale: Acute toxicity of MAO inhibitors is manifested by restlessness, anxiety, and insomnia. Dizziness and hypertension may also occur. Options 2, 3, and 4 are not signs of toxicity.

Test-Taking Strategy: Use the process of elimination. Options 3 and 4 can be eliminated first because they are similar. From the remaining options, it is necessary to know the signs of toxicity associated with these medications. Review these signs if you had difficulty with this question.

Level of Cognitive Ability: Comprehension
Client Needs: Health Promotion and Maintenance
Integrated Concept/Process: Teaching/Learning
Content Area: Mental Health

Reference:
Lehne, R. (2001). *Pharmacology for nursing care* (4th ed.). Philadelphia: W.B. Saunders, p. 322.

---

19. Methylphenidate hydrochloride (Ritalin) is prescribed for a 10-year-old male child diagnosed with attention deficit hyperactivity disorder. The nurse reinforces instructions to the mother about administration of the medication and determines that the mother understands when the mother responds by saying:

1   "I will give my child the medication at bedtime so that he will be rested and alert for school the next day."
2   "I will give my child the medication after meals to obtain the full effects of the medication."
3   "I will give my child the medication at breakfast and lunch to prevent insomnia."
4   "I will give my child the medication with water to prevent kidney damage."

Answer: 3
Rationale: Methylphenidate hydrochloride is a central nervous system (CNS) stimulant that can cause insomnia. This can be prevented by taking the medication orally 30 to 45 minutes before breakfast and lunch and avoiding taking the medication in the evening. Option 4 is unrelated to the administration of the medication.

Test-Taking Strategy: Use the process of elimination. Recalling that this medication is a CNS stimulant will direct you to option 3. Review this medication if you had difficulty with this question.

Level of Cognitive Ability: Comprehension
Client Needs: Health Promotion and Maintenance
Integrated Concept/Process: Teaching/Learning
Content Area: Mental Health

Reference:
Hodgson, B., & Kizior, R. (2003). *Saunders nursing drug handbook 2003.* Philadelphia: W.B. Saunders, p. 728.

20. Lithium carbonate (Eskalith) is prescribed for a client who is breastfeeding her healthy newborn delivered 2 weeks ago. The nurse provides information about the medication to the client and makes which statement?
1 "This medication is perfectly safe for new mothers and will help to stabilize your mood."
2 "You can safely breast-feed your baby because this medication is not excreted in breast milk."
3 "This medication is not safe for new mothers because of the extreme hormonal fluctuations you are currently experiencing."
4 "You are unable to breastfeed your baby because this medication is excreted in breast milk."

Answer: 4
Rationale: Lithium carbonate is contraindicated in pregnancy and in breastfeeding mothers. The client will be taught that breastfeeding is not possible while taking this medication and will be instructed to notify the physician immediately if pregnancy is even suspected or is being planned. Options 1 and 2 are incorrect and option 3 is inaccurate information.

Test-Taking Strategy: Use the process of elimination. Eliminate options 1 and 2 because they are similar. Eliminate option 3 next because hormonal changes are not directly related to the use of this medication. Review the contraindications associated with the use of lithium if you had difficulty with this question.

Level of Cognitive Ability: Application
Client Needs: Health Promotion and Maintenance
Integrated Concept/Process: Nursing Process/Implementation
Content Area: Mental Health

Reference:
Hodgson, B., & Kizior, R. (2003). *Saunders nursing drug handbook 2003.* Philadelphia: W.B. Saunders, p. 671.

---

21. A nurse is reinforcing instructions to a client who will be receiving clozapine (Clozaril). Which statement by the client indicates an understanding of the use of the medication?
1 "I can take over-the-counter medications as long as they do not contain alcohol."
2 "I can drink alcohol as long as it is limited amounts."
3 "It is all right to drive because the medication does not cause sedation."
4 "I should report to the clinic in a week for follow-up laboratory studies."

Answer: 4
Rationale: Clients should be taught the toxic and side effects of the medication and the need for a weekly white blood cell (WBC) count. The client should be instructed to avoid over-the-counter medications, alcohol, and central nervous system (CNS) medications because of the potential for severe medication interactions. The client should immediately report lethargy, weakness, fever, sore throat, malaise, mucous membrane ulceration, or other possible signs of infection. Because the medication causes sedation the client should refrain from operating machinery, driving, or other tasks that require alertness until the response to the medication is established.

Test-Taking Strategy: Knowledge regarding the client teaching points related to the use of clozapine is necessary to answer this question. If you had difficulty with this question or are unfamiliar with this medication review this content.

Level of Cognitive Ability: Comprehension
Client Needs: Health Promotion and Maintenance
Integrated Concept/Process: Teaching/Learning
Content Area: Mental Health

Reference:
Hodgson, B., & Kizior, R. (2003). *Saunders nursing drug handbook 2003.* Philadelphia: W.B. Saunders, p. 269.

---

22. A nurse is reinforcing instructions to the spouse of a client with Alzheimer's disease. Donepezil hydrochloride (Aricept) has been prescribed for the client. The

Answer: 4
Rationale: Donepezil hydrochloride is a cholinergic medication and is to be taken in the evening before bedtime. The medication should be taken with food; therefore a snack should be provided

nurse tells the spouse that it is best to administer the medication:

1   In the morning with the breakfast meal
2   On an empty stomach 1 hour before the noontime meal
3   At 5 PM with dinner and an antacid
4   In the evening before bedtime with a snack

to the client when the medication is administered. Options 1, 2, and 3 are incorrect.

Test-Taking Strategy: Knowledge regarding the administration of this medication is necessary to answer this question. If you are unfamiliar with the teaching points related to the administration of this medication, review this content.

Level of Cognitive Ability: Application
Client Needs: Health Promotion and Maintenance
Integrated Concept/Process: Nursing Process/Implementation
Content Area: Mental Health

Reference:
Hodgson, B. & Kizior, R. (2003). *Saunders nursing drug handbook 2003.* Philadelphia: W.B. Saunders, p. 375.

---

23. Imipramine hydrochloride (Tofranil) has been prescribed for a client with depression. After 6 weeks of therapy, the client has not demonstrated a noticeable change in behavior and the physician has decided to increase the dose of the medication. Which information would the nurse provide to the client regarding the addition of an increased dose to the medication regimen?

1   Take the additional dose in the morning with the present dose
2   Take the additional dose and the usual dose at bedtime
3   Take the usual dose in the morning and the additional dose at bedtime
4   Take the usual dose in the morning and the additional dose at noontime with lunch

Answer: 2
Rationale: Dosage increases should be made at bedtime because the medication causes sedation. Dose titration is a slow process that may take weeks to months. The medication may be given as a single dose at bedtime to minimize sedation that may occur during the day.

Test-Taking Strategy: Use the process of elimination. Recalling that the medication causes sedation will assist in directing you to the correct option. If you had difficulty with this question, review the appropriate administration schedule of this medication.

Level of Cognitive Ability: Application
Client Needs: Health Promotion and Maintenance
Integrated Concept/Process: Nursing Process/Implementation
Content Area: Mental Health

Reference:
Hodgson, B., & Kizior, R. (2003). *Saunders nursing drug handbook 2003.* Philadelphia: W.B. Saunders, p. 580.

---

24. Lithium carbonate (Eskalith) is prescribed for a client with bipolar disorder. The nurse reinforces instructions to the client regarding the administration of the medication and makes which statement to the client?

1   "Take the medication 1 hour before meals."
2   "Decrease sodium intake while taking this medication."
3   "Limit the intake of alcohol while on the medication."
4   "Drink at least 2 to 3 liters of fluid per day."

Answer: 4
Rationale: Lithium should be administered with meals. The client should be instructed to maintain a regular diet and an average salt intake to keep the serum lithium level in the therapeutic range. The client is instructed to avoid alcohol and to drink 2 to 3 liters of liquids per day during initial therapy and 1 to 1.5 liters per day during the remainder of therapy.

Test-Taking Strategy: Knowledge regarding client instructions related to the administration of lithium is necessary to answer this question. If you are unfamiliar with this medication or had difficulty with answering this question, review these client teaching points.

Level of Cognitive Ability: Application
Client Needs: Health Promotion and Maintenance

Integrated Concept/Process: Teaching/Learning
Content Area: Mental Health

Reference:
Hodgson, B., & Kizior, R. (2003). *Saunders nursing drug handbook 2003.* Philadelphia: W.B. Saunders, p. 672.

---

25. Lorazepam (Ativan) has been prescribed for a client for the management of anxiety, and the nurse reinforces instructions to the client regarding the administration of the medication. Which statement by the client indicates a need for further instructions?

1 "I should avoid driving or other activities requiring alertness until the response to the medication is known."

2 "I should not skip medication doses or double missed doses."

3 "I should double a dose if a dose was missed."

4 "I should avoid the use of alcohol while taking the medication."

Answer: 3

Rationale: The client should be instructed to take the medication exactly as directed and not to skip or double the doses. The client should also be instructed not to increase doses or to abruptly withdraw the medication. Abrupt withdrawal may cause tremors, nausea, vomiting, and abdominal or muscle cramps. The client is advised to avoid driving or other activities requiring alertness until response to the medication in known. Clients are also instructed to avoid alcohol or other central nervous system depressants while taking this medication.

Test-Taking Strategy: Use the process of elimination and note the key words *need for further instructions.* Recalling the general principles related to medication administration will direct you to option 3. Review this medication if you had difficulty with this question.

Level of Cognitive Ability: Comprehension
Client Needs: Health Promotion and Maintenance
Integrated Concept/Process: Teaching/Learning
Content Area: Mental Health

Reference:
Hodgson, B., & Kizior, R. (2003). *Saunders nursing drug handbook 2003.* Philadelphia: W.B. Saunders, p. 683.

---

26. Methylphenidate (Ritalin) is prescribed for a child with attention deficit hyperactivity disorder (ADHD) and the nurse reinforces instructions to the mother regarding the administration of the medication. Which statement by the mother would indicate a need for further instructions?

1 "I will administer the medication with the noon meal."

2 "I will keep the medication tightly capped and away from direct heat."

3 "I should inform the school nurse that my child is taking this medication."

4 "I should avoid giving the medications on Saturdays and Sundays to provide a drug holiday."

Answer: 4

Rationale: The nurse should suggest that the parents discuss medication holidays, which can help avoid the side effects of growth delays, with their primary health care provider. The nurse should tell the parents to administer the medication at noon because the stimulant effects may keep the child awake if administered after this time. The medication should be kept dry, tightly capped, and away from direct heat, and the parents should be encouraged to inform a school official about proper administration of this medication.

Test-Taking Strategy: Use the process of elimination. Note the key words *need for further instructions.* Reading each option carefully will direct you to option 4 because general principles related to medication administration indicate that parents should not be instructed to discontinue or hold medication on particular days unless specifically prescribed by the physician. If you had difficult with this question, review the teaching points related to the administration of this medication.

Level of Cognitive Ability: Comprehension
Client Needs: Health Promotion and Maintenance

Integrated Concept/Process: Teaching/Learning
Content Area: Mental Health

Reference:
Hodgson, B., & Kizior, R. (2003). *Saunders nursing drug handbook 2003.* Philadelphia: W.B. Saunders, p. 728.

---

27. A nurse is reinforcing discharge instructions to a client who is taking phenelzine sulfate (Nardil). Which of the following foods would the nurse instruct the client to avoid while taking this medication?
1   Red meat
2   Chicken
3   Bananas
4   Plums

Answer: 3
Rationale: Phenelzine sulfate is a monoamine oxidase inhibitor (MAOI) antidepressant. The client needs to be instructed to avoid foods that require bacteria or mold for their preparation or preservation, or those that contain tyramine. These food items include cheese, sour cream, beer, wine, pickles herring, liver, figs, raisins, bananas, avocados, soy sauce, yeast extracts, yogurt, papaya, broad beans, meat tenderizers, or foods or fluids containing excessive amounts of caffeine such as coffee, tea, or chocolate. The client is also instructed to avoid over-the-counter preparations used for hay fever, colds, or weight reduction. The client should also avoid alcohol.

Test-Taking Strategy: Use the process of elimination recalling that this medication is a MAOI. Knowledge regarding the food items that are necessary to be avoided while taking this medication will direct you to option 3. If you are unfamiliar with this medication and with the food items that would need to be avoided, review this content.

Level of Cognitive Ability: Application
Client Needs: Health Promotion and Maintenance
Integrated Concept/Process: Teaching/Learning
Content Area: Mental Health

Reference:
Hodgson, B., & Kizior, R. (2003). *Saunders nursing drug handbook 2003.* Philadelphia: W.B. Saunders, p. 881.

---

28. A nurse has taught a client with acute renal failure (ARF) to include high-quality proteins in the diet. The nurse determines that the client has not fully understood the instructions if the client selects which food that is a low-quality protein source?
1   Chicken
2   Fish
3   Eggs
4   Sweet potatoes

Answer: 4
Rationale: High quality proteins come from animal sources and include such foods as eggs, chicken, meat, and fish. Low quality proteins derive from plant sources and include vegetables and foods made from grains. Because the renal diet is limited in protein, it is important that the proteins ingested are of high quality.

Test-Taking Strategy: Use the process of elimination and note the key words *has not fully understood.* Remember that when options are similar, they are not likely to be correct. In this case, the chicken, eggs, and fish are similar because they are derived from animal sources; sweet potatoes are a vegetable. Review foods that are high-quality protein foods if you had difficulty with this question.

Level of Cognitive Ability: Comprehension
Client Needs: Health Promotion and Maintenance

Integrated Concept/Process: Teaching/Learning
Content Area: Adult Health/Renal

Reference:
Williams, S. (2001) *Basic nutrition & diet therapy* (11th ed.). St. Louis: Mosby, p. 48.

---

29. A nurse is teaching a client with chronic renal failure about diet and fluid restriction. The nurse tells the client that which of the following dessert items from the dietary menu represents the best choice?
1   Ice cream
2   Sherbet
3   Angel food cake
4   Jell-O

Answer: 3
Rationale: Dietary fluid includes anything that is liquid at room temperature. This includes items such as ice cream, sherbet, and Jell-O. With clients on a fluid-restricted diet, it is helpful to avoid "hidden" fluids to whatever extent is possible. This allows the client more fluid for drinking, which can help alleviate thirst.

Test-Taking Strategy: Use the process of elimination. Remember that options that are similar are not likely to be correct. Evaluation of each of the options shows that the incorrect options contain a greater amount of fluid. In addition, these items are fluid at room temperature, and therefore must be counted as fluid in the daily allotment. Review items to be avoided while on fluid restriction if you had difficulty with this question.

Level of Cognitive Ability: Application
Client Needs: Health Promotion and Maintenance
Integrated Concept/Process: Teaching/Learning
Content Area: Adult Health/Renal

Reference:
Williams, S. (2001) *Basic nutrition & diet therapy* (11th ed.). St. Louis: Mosby, p. 294.

---

30. A nurse is giving suggestions to the client with chronic renal failure (CRF) about ways to reduce pruritis from uremia. The nurse tells the client to avoid which of the following types of skin care products?
1   Lanolin-based lotion
2   Bath oil
3   Mild soap
4   Astringent facial cleansing pads

Answer: 4
Rationale: The client with CRF often has dry skin, accompanied by itching (pruritis) from uremia. The client should use mild soaps, lotions, and bath water oils to reduce dryness without increasing skin irritation. Products that contain perfumes or alcohol increase dryness and pruritis, and should be avoided.

Test-Taking Strategy: Use the process of elimination and note the key word *avoid*. Options 1 and 2 are similar because they enhance skin moisture and should therefore be eliminated. From the remaining options, select option 4 instead of option 3, knowing that the client should avoid irritating products on the skin. Review measures that reduce pruritis in the client with renal failure if you had difficulty with this question.

Level of Cognitive Ability: Application
Client Needs: Health Promotion and Maintenance
Integrated Concept/Process: Self-Care
Content Area: Adult Health/Renal

Reference:
Black, J., Hawks, J., & Keene, A. (2001). *Medical-surgical nursing: clinical management for positive outcomes* (6th ed.). Philadelphia: W.B. Saunders, p. 1286.

31. A nurse has reinforced instructions to a client with chronic renal failure (CRF) about medication therapy used in its treatment. The nurse determines that the client has a clear understanding of the medications if the client states that which of the following medications is not used to enhance red blood cell (RBC) production?
1   Calcium carbonate (Tums)
2   Epoetin (Epogen)
3   Ferrous sulfate (Feosol)
4   Folic acid (Folvite)

Answer: 1
Rationale: Calcium carbonate is a calcium salt that is used as a phosphate binder in the client with CRF. It has nothing to do with treatment of anemia. Folic acid is a vitamin that is needed for RBC production, and it is usually deficient in the client with CRF. Iron supplements (ferrous sulfate) are needed to produce adequate hemoglobin. Epoetin stimulates the production of RBCs because it is an external source of erythropoietin.

Test-Taking Strategy: Use the process of elimination. Note the key words *not used* and focus on the issue, enhance RBC production. Recall the pathophysiology and medication therapy used in the treatment of anemia in the CRF client. Knowledge regarding the actions and uses of the medications presented in the options will direct you to option 1. Review the medications identified in the options if you had difficulty with this question.

Level of Cognitive Ability: Comprehension
Client Needs: Health Promotion and Maintenance
Integrated Concept/Process: Teaching/Learning
Content Area: Adult Health/Renal

Reference:
Hodgson, B., & Kizior, R. (2003). *Saunders nursing drug handbook 2003.* Philadelphia: W.B. Saunders, p. 158.

32. A client has been given a prescription for levothyroxine sodium (Synthroid). The nurse is asked to reinforce instructions to the client about this medication and tells the client that an expected effect is:
1   Lowered body temperature
2   Decreased acid production
3   Increased energy level
4   Gain in weight

Answer: 3
Rationale: Levothyroxine sodium is a synthetically prepared thyroid hormone that increases body metabolism. The client feels this effect as an increase in energy level. Other effects are weight loss and increased body temperature. It does not affect acid production in the gastrointestinal tract.

Test-Taking Strategy: Begin to answer this question by recalling that this medication replaces thyroid hormone. Knowledge of the effects of this hormone will direct you to option 3. Review the effects of this medication if you had difficulty with this question.

Level of Cognitive Ability: Application
Client Needs: Health Promotion and Maintenance
Integrated Concept/Process: Teaching/Learning
Content Area: Adult Health/Endocrine

Reference:
Hodgson, B., & Kizior, R. (2003). *Saunders nursing drug handbook 2003.* Philadelphia: W.B. Saunders, p. 660.

33. A nurse has taught a client with hyperaldosteronism about dietary changes needed to manage the condition. The nurse determines that the client understands the information presented if the

Answer: 1
Rationale: Clients with hyperaldosteronism should follow a low-sodium diet as an adjunct to medical management to decrease serum sodium levels. For this reason, salty foods are to be avoided. Potassium intake (oranges) should be maintained

client states a need to decrease which of the following types of foods?

1   Salty snacks
2   Oranges
3   Whole grain breads
4   Red meats

because the client is at risk for hypokalemia. The diet should have adequate protein, carbohydrates, and fat to maintain a normal body weight (options 3 and 4).

Test-Taking Strategy: Use the process of elimination. Recalling that aldosterone is a mineralocorticoid that helps to regulate sodium and potassium levels will assist in eliminating options 3 and 4 first. To choose correctly from the remaining options, you must understand the physiological function of aldosterone. Review dietary measures for the client with hyperaldosteronism if you had difficulty with this question.

Level of Cognitive Ability: Comprehension
Client Needs: Health Promotion and Maintenance
Integrated Concept/Process: Teaching/Learning
Content Area: Adult Health/Endocrine

Reference:
Black, J., Hawks, J., & Keene, A. (2001). *Medical-surgical nursing: clinical management for positive outcomes* (6th ed.). Philadelphia: W.B. Saunders, p. 1135.

---

34. A client has undergone laser surgery to remove two nevi. The nurse includes which of the following statements when reinforcing discharge instructions to the client?

1   "Scrub the affected areas daily to prevent infection."
2   "Expect frequent episodes of discomfort after the procedure."
3   "Protect the areas from direct sunlight for at least 3 months."
4   "Report any swelling or redness to the physician immediately."

Answer: 3
Rationale: The area should be cleansed gently with half strength hydrogen peroxide twice a day as prescribed after the initial dressing is removed (24 hours postprocedure). There should be minimal or no discomfort after the procedure, and, if present, it should be easily relieved with acetaminophen (Tylenol). Redness and swelling are expected after this procedure. After laser surgery removal of any type of skin lesion, the skin should be protected from direct sunlight for at least 3 months.

Test-Taking Strategy: Use the process of elimination. To answer this question correctly, you must be familiar with laser surgery and elements of self after-care. Read each option carefully and use the process of elimination. The word *scrub* in option 1, *frequent* in option 2, and *immediately* in option 4 should assist in eliminating these options. Review client teaching points after laser therapy if you had difficulty with this question.

Level of Cognitive Ability: Application
Client Needs: Health Promotion and Maintenance
Integrated Concept/Process: Self-Care
Content Area: Adult Health/Integumentary

Reference:
Black, J., Hawks, J., & Keene, A. (2001). *Medical-surgical nursing: clinical management for positive outcomes* (6th ed.). Philadelphia: W.B. Saunders, p. 1326.

---

35. A nurse is reinforcing measures with the client with Addison's disease about ways to prevent addisonian crisis. The nurse tells the client to:

1   Eat a diet high in protein

Answer: 3
Rationale: Addisonian crisis is triggered by stressful events such as emotional crises, illness, injury, or surgery. The client should minimize the risk of infection and illness whenever possible. If the client becomes ill, doses of adrenocortical replacement

2 Eat a diet high in glucose

3 Avoid stressful situations whenever possible

4 Stop medication therapy if infection or illness occurs

medication are increased. There are no specific dietary alterations used to manage this disorder.

Test-Taking Strategy: Use the process of elimination. Recalling that medication therapy should not be interrupted will assist in eliminating option 4. From the remaining options, recall that stressful events will cause a crisis. Review the causes of addisonian crisis if you had difficulty with this question.

Level of Cognitive Ability: Application
Client Needs: Health Promotion and Maintenance
Integrated Concept/Process: Nursing Process/Implementation
Content Area: Adult Health/Endocrine

Reference:
Black, J., Hawks, J., & Keene, A. (2001). *Medical-surgical nursing: clinical management for positive outcomes* (6th ed.). Philadelphia: W.B. Saunders, p. 1122.

---

36. A client newly diagnosed with type 1 diabetes mellitus exercises daily. When reinforcing instructions about medication therapy, the nurse tells this client to inject the daily dose of insulin:

1 In any site, but do it after exercise

2 In a site that will not be exercised

3 Only in the abdomen before exercise

4 Only in the arm before exercise

Answer: 2
Rationale: Exercise of a body part increases the rate of absorption of the insulin from that site. For this reason, the client should inject insulin into an area that will not be exercised. This will help the client to avoid hypoglycemia from rapid insulin absorption. Insulin should be administered at the time prescribed by the physician.

Test-Taking Strategy: Use the process of elimination. Eliminate options 3 and 4 because of the absolute word *only*. Use general knowledge about principles of exercise and diabetes to choose option 2 instead of option 1. Review client teaching points related to diabetes and exercise if you had difficulty with this question.

Level of Cognitive Ability: Application
Client Needs: Health Promotion and Maintenance
Integrated Concept/Process: Nursing Process/Implementation
Content Area: Adult Health/Endocrine

Reference:
Black, J., Hawks, J., & Keene, A. (2001). *Medical-surgical nursing: clinical management for positive outcomes* (6th ed.). Philadelphia: W.B. Saunders, p. 1167.

---

37. A nurse is assisting in developing a teaching plan for a client with diabetes mellitus about proper foot care. The nurse suggests including which of the following in the plan?

1 Cut the toenails down to the nail plate

2 Place a heating pad on the feet if they become chilled

3 Apply lotion to dry skin areas except between the toes

Answer: 3
Rationale: The client should apply lotion to the feet to prevent dryness and cracking, but lotion should not be applied between the toes because of the risk of skin breakdown resulting from moisture. The client should cut the toenails straight across at the level of the contour of the toe. The client should wear shoes that are closed at the heel and toe to prevent injury to the feet, regardless of the season. The client should also avoid other potential sources of injury to the feet, such as the application of direct heat to the feet, which could result in burns. The client should avoid exposure of the feet to excessive heat or cold.

4 Wear open heel and toe shoes in warm weather

Test-Taking Strategy: Use the process of elimination. Recalling that the client with diabetes mellitus is at risk for infection if an injury occurs to the feet will direct you to option 3. Options 1, 2, and 4 place the client at risk for injury. If you had difficulty with this question, review diabetic foot care.

Level of Cognitive Ability: Application
Client Needs: Health Promotion and Maintenance
Integrated Concept/Process: Nursing Process/Planning
Content Area: Adult Health/Endocrine

Reference:
Black, J., Hawks, J., & Keene, A. (2001). *Medical-surgical nursing: clinical management for positive outcomes* (6th ed.). Philadelphia: W.B. Saunders, p. 1184.

---

38. A nurse is reinforcing instructions regarding skin care to a client receiving external radiation therapy to the chest area. The nurse tells the client to do which of the following?
  1 Avoid the use of lotions on the area being treated
  2 Use deodorants only once daily
  3 Limit sun exposure to three times a week
  4 Wear snug-fitting clothing to prevent irritation

Answer: 1
Rationale: The client is instructed to avoid the use of lotions on the area being treated. The client should be instructed to avoid exposure to the sun. Deodorant should not be used during treatment to the chest area. The client should wear loose-fitting clothing over the area.

Test-Taking Strategy: Use the process of elimination. Focus on the issue of avoiding any substance or materials that can irritate skin in the area receiving the radiation. This will direct you to option 1. Review skin care measures for the client receiving external radiation if you had difficulty with this question.

Level of Cognitive Ability: Application
Client Needs: Health Promotion and Maintenance
Integrated Concept/Process: Nursing Process/Implementation
Content Area: Adult Health/Oncology

Reference:
Black, J., Hawks, J., & Keene, A. (2001). *Medical-surgical nursing: clinical management for positive outcomes* (6th ed.). Philadelphia: W.B. Saunders, p. 380.

---

39. Hyperphosphatemia has been diagnosed in a client. The nurse plans to teach the client to eliminate which of the following beverages from the diet?
  1 Coffee
  2 Tea
  3 Carbonated beverages
  4 Grape juice

Answer: 3
Rationale: Foods that are naturally high in phosphates should be avoided by the client with hyperphosphatemia. These include fish, eggs, milk products, vegetables, whole grains, and carbonated beverages. Coffee, tea, and grape juice are not high in phosphates.

Test-Taking Strategy: Use the process of elimination and focus on the client's diagnosis. Eliminate options 1 and 2 first because they are similar. It is necessary to know which of the remaining items are high in phosphates. Review these items if you had difficulty with this question.

Level of Cognitive Ability: Application
Client Needs: Health Promotion and Maintenance
Integrated Concept/Process: Teaching/Learning
Content Area: Fundamental Skills

Reference:
Williams, S. (2001). *Basic nutrition & diet therapy* (11th ed.). St. Louis: Mosby, p. 408.

---

40. A nurse has conducted dietary teaching with a client diagnosed with iron deficiency anemia. The nurse evaluates that the client understood the information if the client states a need to increase intake of which of the following foods?
1   Refined white bread
2   Egg whites
3   Pineapple
4   Kidney beans

Answer: 4
Rationale: The client with iron deficiency anemia should increase intake of foods that are naturally high in iron. The best sources of dietary iron are red meat, liver and other organ meats, blackstrap molasses, and oysters. Other good sources of iron are kidney beans, whole wheat bread, egg yolk, spinach, kale, turnip tops, beet greens, carrots, raisins, and apricots.

Test-Taking Strategy: Use the process of elimination and focus on the client's diagnosis. Recalling foods high in iron will direct you to option 4. Review foods high in iron if you had difficulty with this question.

Level of Cognitive Ability: Comprehension
Client Needs: Health Promotion and Maintenance
Integrated Concept/Process: Nursing Process/Evaluation
Content Area: Fundamental Skills

Reference:
Williams, S. (2001). *Basic nutrition & diet therapy* (11th ed.). St. Louis: Mosby, p. 127.

---

41. A nurse is reinforcing home care instructions with a client who has sickle cell disease. The nurse instructs the client to avoid which of the following that could trigger a sickle cell crisis?
1   Mild exercise
2   Fluid overload
3   Warm weather
4   Infection

Answer: 4
Rationale: The client should avoid infections, which can increase metabolic demand and cause dehydration, triggering a sickle cell crisis. The client should also avoid dehydration from other causes. Warm weather and mild exercise need not be avoided, but the client should take measures to avoid dehydration during these occurrences. Fluid intake is important in preventing dehydration. Finally, the client should avoid high altitudes or flying in nonpressurized aircraft because of their lesser oxygen tension.

Test-Taking Strategy: Use the process of elimination and note the key word *avoid*. Recalling that infection increases metabolic demand and can cause dehydration will direct you to option 4. Review the causes of sickle cell crisis if you had difficulty with this question.

Level of Cognitive Ability: Application
Client Needs: Health Promotion and Maintenance
Integrated Concept/Process: Teaching/Learning
Content Area: Fundamental Skills

Reference:
Ignatavicius, D., & Workman, M. (2002). *Medical-surgical nursing: critical thinking for collaborative care* (4th ed.). Philadelphia: W.B. Saunders, p. 840.

42. A woman is seen in the prenatal clinic and complains of morning sickness. Which of the following self-care measures will the nurse suggest to the client?

  1 To eat toast for breakfast
  2 To eat fatty or spicy foods only at the noontime meal
  3 To eat three well-balanced meals every day
  4 To eat a dry cracker before getting out of bed in the morning

Answer: 4

Rationale: Morning sickness is common during the first trimester and is associated with increased levels of human chorionic gonadotropin and changes in carbohydrate metabolism. It most often occurs on arising, although a few women experience it throughout the day. Self-care measures include eating a dry cracker or toast before getting out of bed, eating small frequent meals, avoiding fatty or spicy foods, and rising slowly from a lying or sitting position to avoid orthostatic hypotension

Test-Taking Strategy: Use the process of elimination. Focusing on the issue of the question, morning sickness, will direct you to option 4. Review measures to assist with morning sickness if you had difficulty with this question.

Level of Cognitive Ability: Application
Client Needs: Health Promotion and Maintenance
Integrated Concept/Process: Self-Care
Content Area: Maternity

Reference:
Burroughs, A., & Leifer, G. (2002). *Maternity nursing* (8th ed.). Philadelphia: W.B. Saunders, p. 238.

---

43. A client in her third trimester of pregnancy is seen in the clinic and is complaining of urinary frequency. Which of the following self-care measures will the nurse suggest to the client?

  1 Avoid emptying the bladder frequently
  2 Drink at least 2000 mL of fluid per day
  3 Avoid large amounts of fluids during the day
  4 Restrict fluid intake in the evening

Answer: 2

Rationale: Urinary frequency is present in the first trimester and late in the third trimester because of the pressure placed on the bladder by the enlarged uterus. Self-care measures for urinary frequency include emptying the bladder frequently (every 2 hours) and drinking at least 2000 mL of fluid a day. Options 1, 3, and 4 are incorrect and could lead to urinary stasis (option 1) and fluid volume deficit (options 3 and 4).

Test-Taking Strategy: Use the process of elimination. Eliminate options 3 and 4 first because they are similar and inappropriate measures. Eliminate option 1 next because it does not make sense to avoid emptying the bladder frequently. This action could lead to urinary stasis and cause discomfort in the woman. Review measures that will assist with the discomfort of urinary frequency if you had difficulty with this question.

Level of Cognitive Ability: Application
Client Needs: Health Promotion and Maintenance
Integrated Concept/Process: Self-Care
Content Area: Maternity

Reference:
Burroughs, A., & Leifer, G. (2002). *Maternity nursing* (8th ed.). Philadelphia: W.B. Saunders, p. 56.

---

44. A maternity client is seen in the health care clinic and is complaining of ankle edema. After diagnostic evaluation it is determined that the blood pressure is within

Answer: 4

Rationale: Ankle edema is a common occurrence during pregnancy and is caused by decreased venous return from the feet because of gravity. It is a minor discomfort as long as hypertension normal limits and proteinuria is not present. The nurse reinforces self-care measures to the client. Which of the following self-care measures would not be a component of the instructions?

1   Elevating the feet at hip level during the day
2   Wearing supportive stockings or hose
3   Avoiding standing in one position or place for long periods
4   Avoiding frequent rest periods

and proteinuria are not present. Self-care measures for ankle edema include elevating the feet at hip level during the day, taking frequent rest periods, wearing supportive stockings or hose, and avoiding standing in one position or place for long periods.

Test-Taking Strategy: Use the process of elimination. Note the key word *not*. Read each option carefully and visualize its effect in relation to ankle edema. You should easily be directed to option 4. Review the measures to alleviate ankle edema if you had difficulty with this question.

Level of Cognitive Ability: Application
Client Needs: Health Promotion and Maintenance
Integrated Concept/Process: Self-Care
Content Area: Maternity

Reference:
Burroughs, A., & Leifer, G. (2002). *Maternity nursing* (8th ed.). Philadelphia: W.B. Saunders, p. 57.

---

45. A client is seen in the prenatal clinic and is complaining of heartburn. The nurse reinforces self-care measures to the client to prevent heartburn. What statement by the client indicates a need for further instructions?

1   "I should eat small frequent meals."
2   "I should avoid fatty or spicy foods."
3   "I should lie down after eating."
4   "I should drink approximately 2000 mL of fluid per day."

Answer: 3
Rationale: Heartburn is associated with regurgitation of gastric acid contents into the esophagus. Self-care for heartburn includes eating small frequent meals, avoiding fatty or spicy foods, remaining upright for 30 minutes after eating, drinking approximately 2000 mL of fluid per day, and taking antacids that contain aluminum hydroxide or a combination of magnesium hydroxide and aluminum hydroxide as prescribed by the physician.

Test-Taking Strategy: Use the process of elimination and note the key words *need for further instructions*. Recalling the cause of heartburn and careful reading of the options will direct you to option 3. Additionally, visualize each option in terms of its effect on the development of heartburn. Review measures to relieve or prevent heartburn if you had difficulty with this question.

Level of Cognitive Ability: Comprehension
Client Needs: Health Promotion and Maintenance
Integrated Concept/Process: Teaching/Learning
Content Area: Maternity

Reference:
Burroughs, A., & Leifer, G. (2002). *Maternity nursing* (8th ed.). Philadelphia: W.B. Saunders, p. 56.

---

46. A nurse working in a prenatal clinic is reviewing the records of a number of clients scheduled for prenatal visits today. The nurse recognizes that the client most at risk for abruptio placentae is the one with which characteristic?

1   Is 26 years old
2   A primipara

Answer: 3
Rationale: Research has shown that the highest incidence of this disorder occurs in women who smoke, or use alcohol, cocaine, and caffeine during pregnancy. Other risk factors include having more than five pregnancies, advanced age, and heavy physical labor.

Test-Taking Strategy: Use the process of elimination. Focusing on the issue, risk for abruptio placentae, will direct you to option 3.

3 Continues to use cocaine
4 Exercises moderately

Review the risk factors related to abruptio placentae if you had difficulty with this question.

Level of Cognitive Ability: Comprehension
Client Needs: Health Promotion and Maintenance
Integrated Concept/Process: Nursing Process/Data Collection
Content Area: Maternity

Reference:
Burroughs, A., & Leifer, G. (2002). *Maternity nursing* (8th ed.). Philadelphia: W.B. Saunders, p. 227.

---

47. A nurse has reinforced instructions to a postpartum client regarding postpartum exercises. Which statement by the client indicates an understanding of the exercises?
1 "Any exercises should be delayed for 4 weeks to allow healing time."
2 "Strenuous exercises will be started while in the hospital to evaluate tolerance."
3 "I should alternately contract and relax the muscles of the perineal area."
4 "The postpartum exercises can result in stress urinary incontinence."

Answer: 3
Rationale: Kegel's exercises are extremely important to strengthen the muscle tone of the perineal area. Postpartum exercises can begin soon after birth. The initial exercises should be simple with progression to increasingly strenuous exercises. Postpartum exercises will not result in stress urinary incontinence.

Test-Taking Strategy: Use the process of elimination and knowledge of the benefit of exercise to assist in answering the question. Eliminate options 1 and 2 because of the words *any* and *strenuous*. Careful reading of option 4 will assist in eliminating this option. Review the purpose and benefit of postpartum exercises if you had difficulty with this question.

Level of Cognitive Ability: Comprehension
Client Needs: Health Promotion and Maintenance
Integrated Concept/Process: Teaching/Learning
Content Area: Maternity

Reference:
Burroughs, A., & Leifer, G. (2002). *Maternity nursing* (8th ed.). Philadelphia: W.B. Saunders, p. 215.

---

48. A nurse employed in a well-baby clinic is evaluating the language and communication developmental milestones of a 2-month-old infant. The nurse understands that which of the following begins to occur in the infant at this developmental age?
1 Use of gestures
2 Babbling sounds
3 Cooing sounds
4 Increased interest in sounds

Answer: 3
Rationale: Between the ages of 1 and 3 months, the infant will produce cooing sounds. Babbling sounds are common between the ages of 3 and 4 months. An increased interest in sounds occurs between 6 and 8 months, and the use of gestures occurs between 9 and 12 months.

Test-Taking Strategy: Use the process of elimination. Noting the age of the infant will assist in eliminating options 1 and 4. From the remaining options, focus on the age to direct you to option 3. Review these developmental milestones if you had difficulty with this question.

Level of Cognitive Ability: Comprehension
Client Needs: Health Promotion and Maintenance
Integrated Concept/Process: Nursing Process/Data Collection
Content Area: Child Health

Reference:
Schulte, E. Price, D., & Gwin, J. (2001). *Thompson's pediatric nursing* (8th ed.). Philadelphia: W.B. Saunders, p. 164.

---

49. A nurse is assigned to care for a hospitalized preschooler who is in traction. The nurse determines that the most appropriate play activity for the child is which of the following?
1 Finger painting
2 Reading from a large picture book
3 Hand sewing a picture
4 Listening to music

Answer: 1

Rationale: In the preschooler, play is simple and imaginative. The preschooler likes to build and create things. For a bedridden child, the nurse should provide an activity that provides stimulation. Option 2 is most appropriate for an infant or young child, option 3 for a school-aged child, and option 4 is for an adolescent.

Test-Taking Strategy: Use the process of elimination and note the age-group of the child. Option 2 can be eliminated because this activity is most appropriate for an infant or young child. Next, eliminate option 4, knowing that this activity is most appropriate for an adolescent. From the remaining options, recalling that play is simple, imaginative, and creative for the preschooler will assist in directing you to option 1. Review age-related activities and toys if you had difficulty with this question.

Level of Cognitive Ability: Comprehension
Client Needs: Health Promotion and Maintenance
Integrated Concept/Process: Nursing Process/Implementation
Content Area: Child Health

Reference:
Schulte, E., Price, D., & Gwin, J. (2001). *Thompson's pediatric nursing* (8th ed.). Philadelphia: W.B. Saunders, p. 212.

---

50. A nurse is reinforcing instructions to parents of a 10-year-old child with hemophilia regarding appropriate activities. Which of the following activities would be safe to suggest for the child?
1 Jogging
2 Football
3 Archery
4 Skateboarding

Answer: 3

Rationale: Activity guidelines for children with hemophilia are categorized into those that are usually safe, those that are riskier and should be discouraged, and those in which the risks outweigh the benefits and are not recommended. Archery, badminton, fishing, golf, hiking, Ping-Pong, swimming, and walking are usually considered safe for those with hemophilia. Options 1, 2, and 4 are riskier and are not recommended for individuals with hemophilia.

Test-Taking Strategy: Focus on the complications associated with this disorder to assist in answering the question. Use the process of elimination, noting that options 1, 2, and 4 are activities that will most likely cause a risk of trauma and bleeding. If you had difficulty with this question, review the appropriate play activities for a child with hemophilia.

Level of Cognitive Ability: Application
Client Needs: Health Promotion and Maintenance
Integrated Concept/Process: Teaching/Learning
Content Area: Child Health

Reference:
Schulte, E., Price, D., & Gwin, J. (2001). *Thompson's pediatric nursing* (8th ed.). Philadelphia: W.B. Saunders, p. 235.

51. A nurse reinforces home care instructions to a client with multiple sclerosis (MS). Which of the following would the nurse include in the instructions?
1 To avoid pregnancy
2 To restrict fluid intake to 1000 mL daily
3 To maintain a low-fiber diet
4 To avoid taking hot baths or showers

Answer: 4
Rationale: Because fatigue can be precipitated by warm temperatures, the client is instructed to take cool baths and maintain a cool environmental temperature. A high-fiber diet and an adequate fluid intake of 2000 mL daily are encouraged to prevent alterations in elimination and bowel patterns. The client should not be told to avoid pregnancy, but the nurse should assist the client in making informed decisions regarding pregnancy.

Test-Taking Strategy: Use the process of elimination. Eliminate option 1 first because it is inappropriate to tell a client to avoid pregnancy. Eliminate options 2 and 3 next because these measures would be unhealthy and would promote alterations in elimination patterns for this client. Review teaching points related to the client with MS if you had difficulty with this question.

Level of Cognitive Ability: Application
Client Needs: Health Promotion and Maintenance
Integrated Concept/Process: Nursing Process/Implementation
Content Area: Adult Health/Musculoskeletal

Reference:
Black, J., Hawks, J., & Keene, A. (2001). *Medical-surgical nursing: clinical management for positive outcomes* (6th ed.). Philadelphia: W.B. Saunders, p. 2015.

52. A nurse has reinforced instructions to a mother about the use of safety seats in car travel for an infant. Which of the following statements if made by the mother indicates an understanding of the instructions?
1 "I will restrain my infant in a car seat in the front seat in a semireclined rear-facing position."
2 "I will restrain my infant in a car seat in the front seat in a semireclined in a face-forward position."
3 "I will restrain my infant in a car seat in the middle back seat in a semireclined rear-facing position."
4 "I will restrain my infant in a car seat in the middle back seat in a semireclined face-forward position."

Answer: 3
Rationale: Infants who weigh less than 20 pounds should be restrained in a car seat in a semireclined, rear-facing position to allow the seat and infant's spine to bear the forces of impact should a collision occur. The infant should never face forward or ride in the front seat.

Test-Taking Strategy: Use the process of elimination. Visualize each of the descriptions in the options, focusing on safety. This should direct you to option 3. If you had difficulty with this question, review safety measures for the infant.

Level of Cognitive Ability: Comprehension
Client Needs: Health Promotion and Maintenance
Integrated Concept/Process: Teaching/Learning
Content Area: Child Health

Reference:
Schulte, E. Price, D., & Gwin, J. (2001). *Thompson's pediatric nursing* (8th ed.). Philadelphia: W.B. Saunders, p. 216.

53. A child who was bitten in the arm by a neighborhood dog is brought to the emergency room. The nurse cleanses the wound as prescribed and continues to collect data on the child. Which of the following is the priority question

Answer: 2
Rationale: When a bite occurs, the injury site of the bite should be cleansed carefully and the child should be given tetanus prophylaxis as prescribed if immunizations are not up to date. Option 3 is not an important consideration. The mother may not have the answers to the questions listed in the incorrect options. Options

for the nurse to ask the mother of the child?

1 "Did the dog have rabies?"
2 "Are the child's immunizations up to date?"
3 "How old is the dog?"
4 "Did the dog have all of its recommended shots?"

1 and 4 identify information that may have to be obtained, but it is not the priority question.

Test-Taking Strategy: Use the process of elimination and note the key word *priority*. Note that the correct option is the only one that focuses on the needs of the child. If you are unfamiliar with the care of a child who receives a dog bite, review this content.

Level of Cognitive Ability: Application
Client Needs: Health Promotion and Maintenance
Integrated Concept/Process: Nursing Process/Data Collection
Content Area: Child Health

Reference:
Wong, D., & Hockenberry-Eaton, M. (2001). *Wong's essentials of pediatric nursing* (6th ed.). St. Louis: Mosby, p. 1175.

---

54. A nurse is reinforcing instructions to the mother of an infant who is seen in the clinic for recurrent episodes of otitis media. Which statement by the mother indicates an understanding of the methods to decrease the risk of recurrence?
1 "I will hold my infant in an upright position during feeding."
2 "I will allow the infant to have a bottle during nap time."
3 "I will maintain bottle feeding as long as possible."
4 "I will stop breastfeeding as soon as possible."

Answer: 1
Rationale: To decrease the risk of recurrent otitis media, the mother should be encouraged to breastfeed during infancy and to discontinue bottle feeding as soon as possible. The infant is also fed while he or she is in an upright position and should never be given a bottle while in bed. The mother is also instructed not to smoke in the child's presence because passive smoking increases the risk of otitis media.

Test-Taking Strategy: Use the process of elimination. Option 2 can be eliminated first. Recalling that breastfeeding offers some protection by providing maternal antibodies will assist in eliminating options 3 and 4. Review the measures related to preventing otitis media if you had difficulty with this question.

Level of Cognitive Ability: Comprehension
Client Needs: Health Promotion and Maintenance
Integrated Concept/Process: Teaching/Learning
Content Area: Child Health

Reference:
Wong, D., & Hockenberry-Eaton, M. (2001). *Wong's essentials of pediatric nursing* (6th ed.). St. Louis: Mosby, p. 837.

---

55. A nurse is reinforcing instructions to a mother of a 2-year-old child who will be receiving ear drops for a diagnosis of otitis media. Which statement by the mother indicates an understanding of the procedure for administering the ear drops?
1 "I will pull the child's ear up and back."
2 "I will wear gloves when I administer the ear drops."
3 "I will hold the child in a sitting position when I administer the ear drops."

Answer: 4
Rationale: The ear should be pulled down, back, and out when ear drops are being administered to a 2-year-old child. In an adult, the ear is pulled up and back. Gloves need not be worn by the parent but hand washing should be performed before and after the procedure. The child should be placed in a side-lying position, with the affected ear facing upward to allow gravity to assist the flow of medication down the ear canal.

Test-Taking Strategy: Use the process of elimination. Note that options 1 and 4 describe the ear position for administering medication. This similarity should provide you with the clue that one of these options may be correct. Recalling the anatomy of the

4 "I will pull the child's ear down, back and out."

2-year-old child's ear canal will assist in directing you to option 4. Review this procedure if you had difficulty with this question.

Level of Cognitive Ability: Comprehension
Client Needs: Health Promotion and Maintenance
Integrated Concept/Process: Teaching/Learning
Content Area: Child Health

Reference:
Wong, D., & Hockenberry-Eaton, M. (2001). *Wong's essentials of pediatric nursing* (6th ed.). St. Louis: Mosby, p. 795.

---

56. An adolescent client asks the nurse questions about the transmission of the Epstein-Barr virus (infectious mononucleosis). The nurse tells the adolescent that the disease is transmitted by which of the following?
1 Close intimate contact
2 Respiratory droplets
3 Fecal-oral route
4 Airborne particles

Answer: 1
Rationale: Epstein-Barr virus is transmitted by contact with infectious saliva, close intimate contact with an infectious individual, or contact with infected blood. The infectious period is unknown. The virus is commonly shed before clinical onset of the disease until 6 months or longer after recovery. Options 2, 3, and 4 are incorrect.

Test-Taking Strategy: Use the process of elimination. Eliminate options 2 and 4 first because they are similar. From the remaining options it is necessary to know the route of transmission of infectious mononucleosis. If you are unfamiliar with this infectious disease, review this content.

Level of Cognitive Ability: Application
Client Needs: Health Promotion and Maintenance
Integrated Concept/Process: Teaching/Learning
Content Area: Child Health

Reference:
Wong, D., & Hockenberry-Eaton, M. (2001). *Wong's essentials of pediatric nursing* (6th ed.). St. Louis: Mosby, p. 543.

---

57. A child with juvenile rheumatoid arthritis (JRA) is seen in the clinic for a routine visit. The child tells the nurse that he or she has a difficult time getting out of bed in the morning because of early morning stiffness. Which of the following responses to the child is most appropriate?
1 "This is a normal occurrence with your disorder."
2 "You should be sure you are taking medications as prescribed and on schedule."
3 "It might help to use a sleeping bag at night to stay warm."
4 "A warm bath at bedtime will prevent early morning stiffness."

Answer: 3
Rationale: Getting out of bed in the morning is often a difficult task for a child with JRA because of the early morning stiffness that occurs. A warm morning bath is helpful. An alternative is to have the child use a sleeping bag at night to stay warm, an electric blanket with a timer that turns on 1 hour before the child awakens, or a water bed to ease the stiffness.

Test-Taking Strategy: Use the process of elimination to answer the question and focus on the issue, morning stiffness. Option 3 is the only option that addresses this issue. If you have difficulty with this question, review the measures that will relieve morning stiffness for the child with JRA.

Level of Cognitive Ability: Application
Client Needs: Health Promotion and Maintenance
Integrated Concept/Process: Self-Care
Content Area: Child Health

Reference:
Wong, D., & Hockenberry-Eaton, M. (2001). *Wong's essentials of pediatric nursing* (6th ed.). St. Louis: Mosby, p. 1238.

---

58. A nurse is reinforcing instructions to the mother of a child with a diagnosis of exercise-induced asthma. The nurse instructs the mother and child that the best sport or activity is which of the following?

1 Track
2 Swimming indoors
3 Gymnastics
4 Weight lifting

Answer: 2

Rationale: Indoor swimming is frequently recommended for children with asthma because the air is humidified. With adequate treatment, however, a child with asthma can participate in most physical activities.

Test-Taking Strategy: Note the key word *best*. This may indicate that one or all of the options may be correct. Think about each activity in terms of its effect on the respiratory system and use the process of elimination. This should direct you to option 2. If you had difficulty with this question, review home care measures for the child with asthma.

Level of Cognitive Ability: Application
Client Needs: Health Promotion and Maintenance
Integrated Concept/Process: Teaching/Learning
Content Area: Child Health

Reference:
Wong, D., & Hockenberry-Eaton, M. (2001). *Wong's essentials of pediatric nursing* (6th ed.). St. Louis: Mosby, p. 856.

---

59. A nurse reinforces instructions to the mother of the child with acute nasal pharyngitis regarding the administration of nose drops. Which statement by the mother indicates an understanding of the use of the drops?

1 "I should administer the nose drops 15 minutes after I feed the child."
2 "If the nose drops don't help within 1 week, I should call the physician."
3 "I should administer the nose drops 15 minutes before feeding the child."
4 "I should administer a cough suppressant at the same time that I administer the nose drops."

Answer: 3

Rationale: Nose drops are most helpful when administered 15 minutes before feeding and at bedtime. Instilling two drops and waiting 5 minutes before instilling more drops if prescribed increases the effectiveness when administering nose drops. Parents should be cautioned against using vasoconstrictive decongestant nose drops for more than 3 days because of the risk of rebound congestion. Cough suppressants are not recommended because they impair removal of secretions, thus increasing the risk of secondary infection.

Test-Taking Strategy: Use the process of elimination. Eliminate option 4 because it is unrelated to the question and is inaccurate. From the remaining options, think about the effect that each action will have on the child. It is best to relieve congestion before feeding so the child is able to consume sufficient nutrients. Review the procedure for administering nose drops in a child if you had difficulty with this question.

Level of Cognitive Ability: Comprehension
Client Needs: Health Promotion and Maintenance
Integrated Concept/Process: Teaching/Learning
Content Area: Child Health

Reference:
Wong, D., & Hockenberry-Eaton, M. (2001). *Wong's essentials of pediatric nursing* (6th ed.). St. Louis: Mosby, p. 795.

60. A client asks the nurse about the measures that will prevent Lyme disease in her children. The nurse suggests which of the following measures to the client?
1 Insect repellant should be applied to the entire body except around the eyes and mouth
2 A tick should be removed by pulling it out of the skin using the fingernails
3 Children should wear long pants, long-sleeved shirts, and hats when in wooded or grassy areas
4 If a tick falls off a pet, it will die and not be a concern for the family members

Answer: 3
Rationale: Children should wear long pants, long-sleeved shirts, and hats when in wooded or grassy areas. Ticks should be removed with tweezers as close to the skin as possible. Repellants should be used with caution and should not be applied to the hands to avoid contact with the child's eyes and mouth. Commercially prepared products should be used on pets to keep them free of ticks. If a tick falls off a pet, it can travel, contact an individual, and attach to the skin.

Test-Taking Strategy: Use the process of elimination. Knowledge about the use of insect repellants will assist in eliminating option 1. Option 2 can be eliminated next by knowing that direct contact with the tick should be avoided. From the remaining options, select option 3 because this intervention will protect from contact with a tick. Review preventive measures related to avoiding insect bites if you had difficulty with this question.

Level of Cognitive Ability: Application
Client Needs: Health Promotion and Maintenance
Integrated Concept/Process: Self-Care
Content Area: Child Health

Reference:
Wong, D., & Hockenberry-Eaton, M. (2001). *Wong's essentials of pediatric nursing* (6th ed.). St. Louis: Mosby, p. 1173.

61. A clinic nurse provides dietary instructions to the mother of a 3-year-old child who was seen in the health care clinic for a complaint of mild diarrhea. Which statement by the mother would indicate a need for further instructions?
1 "I should avoid foods that are high in starch such as mashed potatoes and noodles."
2 "I should encourage my child to drink clear liquids."
3 "It is alright to give my child active-culture yogurt."
4 "I should avoid giving my child any raw fruits or vegetables."

Answer: 1
Rationale: When children older than 2 years of age have mild or moderate diarrhea, the mother should be instructed to give foods high in starch such as breads, crackers, rice, mashed potatoes, and noodles, because these are easily absorbed during diarrhea. Clear liquids are encouraged and milk and milk products should be eliminated except for active-culture yogurt, which is digested by lactobacillus organisms. Raw fruits and vegetables, beans, spices, and any other foods that cause loose stools should be avoided.

Test-Taking Strategy: Use the process of elimination and note the key words *indicates a need for further instructions*. Focusing on the child's diagnosis will direct you to option 1. Review these measures if you had difficulty with this question.

Level of Cognitive Ability: Comprehension
Client Needs: Health Promotion and Maintenance
Integrated Concept/Process: Teaching/Learning
Content Area: Child Health

Reference:
Wong, D., & Hockenberry-Eaton, M. (2001). *Wong's essentials of pediatric nursing* (6th ed.). St. Louis: Mosby, p. 890.

62. A school-aged child with type 1 diabetes mellitus is seen in the health care clinic. The nurse reinforces instructions to the

Answer: 3
Rationale: Because exercise lowers glucose levels, the child must be taught how to prevent hypoglycemia. The child should try to

child regarding food and exercise because the child has told to nurse that she will begin soccer practice. Which of the following instructions will the nurse provide to the child?

1   Avoid insulin on the day of soccer practice
2   Eat lunch 1 hour earlier on the day of soccer practice
3   Eat an extra snack of carbohydrates before the soccer starts
4   The soccer activity should be delayed for 1 more year

schedule activities to avoid exercising when an insulin dose is peaking and should be instructed to eat extra snacks of 15 to 30 grams of carbohydrates for each 45 to 60 minutes of exercise. The extra snack before practice will avert the hypoglycemia. Options 1 and 2 are inaccurate management measures for the child with diabetes mellitus. Option 4 is unnecessary.

Test-Taking Strategy: Use the process of elimination and knowledge regarding the effects of insulin to answer this question. Option 4 can be eliminated because it is inappropriate. From the remaining options, eliminate options 1 and 2 because they are inappropriate options for the management of diabetes. If you had difficulty with this question, review management of diabetes mellitus in a child.

Level of Cognitive Ability: Application
Client Needs: Health Promotion and Maintenance
Integrated Concept/Process: Self-Care
Content Area: Child Health

Reference:
Wong, D., & Hockenberry-Eaton, M. (2001). *Wong's essentials of pediatric nursing* (6th ed.). St. Louis: Mosby, p. 1135.

---

63. A nurse is reinforcing home care instructions to the mother of a child with human immunodeficiency virus (HIV) infection. Which of the following statements if made by the mother indicates a need for further instructions?

1   "I should not allow my child to share toothbrushes with the other children."
2   "I should call the physician if my child has a fever greater that 101° F."
3   "I should delay the polio virus vaccine."
4   "If any blood spills occur from a cut on my child, I should wash the spill with soap and water, rinse it with bleach and water, and allow it to air dry."

Answer: 3
Rationale: The mother should be instructed to keep immunizations up to date. Inactivated polio vaccine is administered. The other options are correct instructions regarding the care of the child with HIV infection.

Test-Taking Strategy: Use the process of elimination. Note the key words *indicates a need for further instructions*. Recalling that immunizations should always be kept up to date for any child will direct you to option 3. If you are unfamiliar with the home care measures for a child with HIV infection, review this content.

Level of Cognitive Ability: Comprehension
Client Needs: Health Promotion and Maintenance
Integrated Concept/Process: Teaching/Learning
Content Area: Child Health

Reference:
Wong, D., & Hockenberry-Eaton, M. (2001). *Wong's essentials of pediatric nursing* (6th ed.). St. Louis: Mosby, p. 1020.

---

64. A nurse is reinforcing instructions to the mother of a child who had a plaster cast applied to a lower arm after fracture of the radius. Which of the following statements if made by the mother indicates a need for further instructions?

1   "A fan directed toward the cast can help it dry."

Answer: 3
Rationale: Fans can be directed toward the cast to assist drying. Ice can be applied to the casted area, and the casted extremity should be elevated with pillows to prevent swelling. The fingers of the casted extremity should be the same color and temperature as the other extremity. When bathing or showering the child, the mother should be instructed to cover the cast to keep it dry.

2 "I should keep the cast from becoming wet and cover it with plastic when I bathe or shower my child."

3 "The fingers of the casted arm will probably be cooler than those on the other arm, which is normal for the first few days."

4 "I should elevate the arm on a pillow to help prevent swelling."

Test-Taking Strategy: Note the key words *indicates a need for further instructions.* Use the ABCs—airway, breathing, and circulation—to assist in answering the question. This will direct you to option 3. If you had difficulty with this question, review discharge instructions for the child with a cast.

Level of Cognitive Ability: Comprehension
Client Needs: Health Promotion and Maintenance
Integrated Concept/Process: Teaching/Learning
Content Area: Child Health

Reference:
Wong, D., & Hockenberry-Eaton, M. (2001). *Wong's essentials of pediatric nursing* (6th ed.). St. Louis: Mosby, p. 1213.

---

65. A clinic nurse is reinforcing instructions to the mother of a child with impetigo. The nurse tells the mother to notify the physician if which of the following occurs?
    1 Increased urinary output
    2 Swelling around the eyes
    3 Lesions located around the mouth
    4 Lesions that appear as honey-colored crusts

Answer: 2
Rationale: If impetigo is caused by beta-hemolytic streptococci, the child should be observed for periorbital edema or blood in the urine, which may signal the development of acute glomerulonephritis. Option 1 is unrelated to impetigo. Impetigo lesions are usually located around the mouth and nose but may also be located on the extremities. Secondary lesions of impetigo are thick honey-colored crusts that are lightly attached to the lesions.

Test-Taking Strategy: Use the process of elimination and knowledge of the complications that can occur with this disorder. Eliminate options 3 and 4 because they are characteristics of this skin infection. From the remaining options it is necessary to know that glomerulonephritis is a complication, and that periorbital edema is a sign of glomerulonephritis. Review the characteristics and complications of impetigo if you had difficulty with this question.

Level of Cognitive Ability: Application
Client Needs: Health Promotion and Maintenance
Integrated Concept/Process: Nursing Process/Implementation
Content Area: Child Health

Reference:
Wong, D., & Hockenberry-Eaton, M. (2001). *Wong's essentials of pediatric nursing* (6th ed.). St. Louis: Mosby, p. 1162.

---

66. A nurse has reinforced instructions to the mother of a child with tinea pedis (athlete's foot). Which of the following statements if made by the mother indicates a need for further instructions?
    1 "My child should wash the feet daily and keep them dry."
    2 "I should apply talcum powder or antifungal powder to my child's feet twice daily."
    3 "My child should wear socks until the infection is gone."

Answer: 4
Rationale: With a fungal infection of the foot, the client should be instructed to wash the feet daily and keep them dry. Nonventilated athletic shoes should be allowed to dry thoroughly between wearing. The child should wear heavy cotton socks and change the socks at least twice a day because the socks will absorb sweat and keep the feet dry. Talcum powder or antifungal powder applied twice daily may help keep the feet dry.

Test-Taking Strategy: Use the process of elimination. Note the key words *indicates a need for further instructions.* Noting the word *nylon* in option 4 will direct you to this option. If you are unfamiliar

4   "If my child wears socks, they should be lightweight and nylon."

with these measures or had difficulty with this question, review this content.

Level of Cognitive Ability: Comprehension
Client Needs: Health Promotion and Maintenance
Integrated Concept/Process: Teaching/Learning
Content Area: Child Health

Reference:
Wong, D., & Hockenberry-Eaton, M. (2001). *Wong's essentials of pediatric nursing* (6th ed.). St. Louis: Mosby, p. 1164.

---

67. A nurse is reinforcing instructions to the mother of a child diagnosed with pediculosis capitis. Which statement by the mother indicates a need for further instructions?
  1   "I should apply antilice sprays to my child before bedtime."
  2   "I should soak combs and brushes in antilice shampoo for 15 minutes."
  3   "I should wash the bedding and linens in hot water and dry on a hot setting."
  4   "I should perform thorough house cleaning to remove any remaining lice or nits."

Answer: 1
Rationale: Antilice sprays are unnecessary and should never be used on a child. Combs and brushes should be boiled or soaked in antilice shampoo or water hotter than 140° F for 15 minutes. Bedding and linens should be washed with hot water and dried on a hot setting, and items that cannot be washed should be dry-cleaned or sealed in plastic bags in a warm place for a period of three weeks. Thorough home cleaning is necessary to remove any remaining lice or nits. Parents should vacuum floors, play areas, and furniture to remove any hairs that may carry live nits.

Test-Taking Strategy: Use the process of elimination and note the key words *need for further instructions*. Recalling that antilice sprays are unnecessary and should never be used on a child will direct you to this option. If you had difficulty with this question, review home care measures for the child with pediculosis.

Level of Cognitive Ability: Application
Client Needs: Health Promotion and Maintenance
Integrated Concept/Process: Teaching/Learning
Content Area: Child Health

Reference:
Wong, D., & Hockenberry-Eaton, M. (2001). *Wong's essentials of pediatric nursing* (6th ed.). St. Louis: Mosby, p. 1169.

---

68. A nurse is caring for a paraplegic client with a spinal cord injury (SCI) who is preparing for discharge from the hospital. The nurse would reinforce home care instructions to the client's wife if the wife said that she plans to do which of the following to try to prevent episodes of autonomic dysreflexia?
  1   Ensure that there are no wrinkles on the sheets underneath the client
  2   Keep a chart for managing bowel elimination
  3   Keep the air conditioner set on high
  4   Make sure that bladder catheterizations are done on time

Answer: 3
Rationale: Causes of autonomic dysreflexia include bladder distention, bowel distention from constipation or fecal impaction, and stimulation of the skin from pain, pressure, or changes in temperature. The client and family should learn the triggering factors, methods of preventing them from occurring, and how to manage an episode. Options 1, 2, and 4 are actions that will help prevent occurrences, whereas option 3 could trigger one.

Test-Taking Strategy: Use the process of elimination. The easiest way to answer questions of this nature is to remember that autonomic dysreflexia is caused by noxious stimuli to the bowel, bladder, or skin. With this in mind, you can easily eliminate each of the incorrect options. Review this complication of an SCI if you had difficulty with this question.

Level of Cognitive Ability: Comprehension
Client Needs: Health Promotion and Maintenance
Integrated Concept/Process: Teaching/Learning
Content Area: Adult Health/Neurological

Reference:
Ignatavicius, D., & Workman, M. (2002). *Medical-surgical: critical thinking for collaborative care* (4th ed.). Philadelphia: W.B. Saunders, p. 931.

---

69. A nurse is reinforcing medication information to a client receiving phenytoin (Dilantin). The nurse tells the client which of the following?
    1 Good oral hygiene is needed, including brushing and flossing
    2 The daily medication dose should be taken before a serum drug level is drawn
    3 The medication dose may be self-adjusted depending on side effects
    4 Alcohol may be used in moderation while taking this medication

Answer: 1
Rationale: The client should perform good oral hygiene and have regular dental examinations because gingival hyperplasia is a side effect of this medication. Other instructions include having a serum drug level drawn before taking the daily dose, taking the dose at the same time each day to keep the blood level of the medication constant, and avoiding abruptly stopping the medication. The client may not self-adjust dosage levels. The client should avoid alcohol and should check with the physician before taking over-the-counter (OTC) medications.

Test-Taking Strategy: Use the process of elimination. Options 3 and 4 can be eliminated first using general principles related to medication therapy. From the remaining options, remember that medications are not generally taken just before drawing therapeutic serum levels because the results would be artificially high. This leaves oral hygiene as the correct answer because of the risk of gingival hyperplasia. Review teaching points for the client taking phenytoin if you had difficulty with this question.

Level of Cognitive Ability: Application
Client Needs: Health Promotion and Maintenance
Integrated Concept/Process: Teaching/Learning
Content Area: Adult Health/Neurological

Reference:
Hodgson, B., & Kizior, R. (2003). *Saunders nursing drug handbook 2003.* Philadelphia: W.B. Saunders, p. 892.

---

70. A nurse is caring for the client with hemiparesis of the left arm and leg who is preparing for discharge. To be most effective in helping the client's rehabilitation and self-care, the nurse tells the family to place personal care articles in which of the following locations?
    1 Just out of the client's reach, on the left side
    2 Just out of the client's reach, on the right side
    3 Within the client's reach, on the left side
    4 Within the client's reach, on the right side

Answer: 4
Rationale: Hemiparesis is a weakness of the face, arm, and leg on one side. The client with one-sided hemiparesis benefits from having objects placed on the unaffected side and within reach (option 4). Other helpful activities with hemiparesis include range of motion exercises to the affected side and muscle strengthening exercises to the unaffected side.

Test-Taking Strategy: Use the process of elimination. Begin to answer this question by eliminating options 1 and 2 as potentially hazardous to the client. Note the key words *most effective.* It is most effective to place objects on the side that the client can move. Review care to the client with hemiparesis if you had difficulty with this question.

Level of Cognitive Ability: Application
Client Needs: Health Promotion and Maintenance
Integrated Concept/Process: Self-Care
Content Area: Adult Health/Neurological

Reference:
Ignatavicius, D., & Workman, M. (2002). *Medical-surgical nursing: critical thinking for collaborative care* (4th ed.). Philadelphia: W.B. Saunders, p. 980.

---

71. A nurse assigned to a client with cerebrovascular accident who has left homonymous hemianopsia is planning measures to help the client overcome the deficit. The nurse would plan to do which of the following to assist the client with rehabilitation?
  1 Remind the client to turn the head to scan the left visual field
  2 Discourage the client from wearing his or her own eyeglasses
  3 Place objects in the client's left field of vision
  4 Approach the client from the left field of vision

Answer: 1
Rationale: Homonymous hemianopsia is loss of one half of the visual field. The client with homonymous hemianopsia should have objects placed in the intact field of vision, and the nurse should also approach the client from the intact side. The nurse instructs the client to scan the environment to overcome the visual deficit and does client teaching from within the intact field of vision. The nurse encourages the use of personal eyeglasses, if they are available.

Test-Taking Strategy: Use the process of elimination. To answer this question accurately, you must be able to distinguish between homonymous hemianopsia and unilateral neglect. Clients are approached differently with these two deficits. The similarity is that the client must be taught to scan the environment, which is also the answer to this question. Review care to the client with homonymous hemianopsia and review the differences between homonymous hemianopsia and unilateral neglect if you had difficulty with this question.

Level of Cognitive Ability: Application
Client Needs: Health Promotion and Maintenance
Integrated Concept/Process: Nursing Process/Planning
Content Area: Adult Health/Neurological

Reference:
Ignatavicius, D., & Workman, M. (2002). *Medical-surgical: critical thinking for collaborative care* (4th ed.). Philadelphia: W.B. Saunders, p. 981.

---

72. A nurse is reinforcing instructions with the client with myasthenia gravis and the client's family about prevention of myasthenic and cholinergic crises. The nurse evaluates that the client has best understood this information if the client states a need to do which of the following?
  1 Adhere to a schedule for muscle strengthening exercises
  2 Eat large, well-balanced meals every day
  3 Do all chores early in the day while less fatigued

Answer: 4
Rationale: Inadequate or inappropriate medication therapy can result in either myasthenic or cholinergic crisis. It is important for the client to take medications correctly to maintain blood levels that are within the therapeutic range. Clients with myasthenia gravis are taught to space out activities during the day to conserve energy and restore muscle strength. Muscle strengthening exercises are not helpful and can fatigue the client. Overeating can aggravate symptoms, as can exposure to heat, crowds, erratic sleep habits, and emotional stress.

Test-Taking Strategy: Use the process of elimination. If you know that common causes of myasthenic and cholinergic crises are

4 Take medications on time to maintain therapeutic blood levels

undermedication and overmedication, respectively, you should be able to eliminate each of the incorrect options. No other option would prevent both of those complications. Review the causes of myasthenic and cholinergic crisis if you had difficulty with this question.

Level of Cognitive Ability: Comprehension
Client Needs: Health Promotion and Maintenance
Integrated Concept/Process: Nursing Process/Evaluation
Content Area: Adult Health/Neurological

Reference:
Ignatavicius, D., & Workman, M. (2002). *Medical-surgical: critical thinking for collaborative care* (4th ed.). Philadelphia: W.B. Saunders, p. 962.

---

73. A nurse is reinforcing discharge instructions with a client with myasthenia gravis, and has discussed methods to minimize the risk of aspiration during meals. The nurse evaluates that the client needs reinforcement of the information given if the client states a need to do which of the following while eating?
1 Swallow when the chin is tipped slightly downward to the chest
2 Lift the head while swallowing liquids
3 Sit straight in the chair while eating
4 Cut food into very small pieces and chew thoroughly

Answer: 2
Rationale: The client avoids swallowing any type of food or drink with the head lifted upward, which could actually cause aspiration by opening the glottis. The client should also refrain from talking with food in the mouth (glottis is open). The client should sit upright while eating, cut food into very small pieces, chew thoroughly, and tip the chin downward to swallow.

Test-Taking Strategy: Use the process of elimination. Note the key words *client needs reinforcement*. Note that options 1 and 2 oppose each other. This makes it likely that one of the two is correct. Remember that lifting the head opens the airway. This will direct you to option 2. Review care to the client with myasthenia gravis if you had difficulty with this question.

Level of Cognitive Ability: Comprehension
Client Needs: Health Promotion and Maintenance
Integrated Concept/Process: Nursing Process/Evaluation
Content Area: Adult Health/Neurological

Reference:
Ignatavicius, D., & Workman, M. (2002). *Medical-surgical: critical thinking for collaborative care* (4th ed.). Philadelphia: W.B. Saunders, p. 965.

---

74. A nurse is reinforcing teaching with a client with Parkinson's disease about measures to maintain mobility. The nurse would include which of the following suggestions in discussions with the client?
1 Sit in soft, deep chairs that are wide and comfortable
2 Buy clothes with snaps and buttons to maintain finger dexterity
3 Exercise in the early evening to combat end-of-the-day fatigue
4 Rock back and forth to initiate movement if bradykinesia occurs

Answer: 4
Rationale: The client with Parkinson's disease experiences bradykinesia and can be taught to rock back and forth to initiate movement. The client should avoid sitting in soft, deep chairs, because they make returning to a standing position difficult. The client should buy clothes with Velcro fasteners and slide locking buckles to support independence in dressing. The client should exercise in the morning when energy levels are highest.

Test-Taking Strategy: Use the process of elimination and focus on the issue of the question. Eliminate option 3 as the least helpful measure. Choose correctly from the remaining options by recalling that a key feature of the disease is bradykinesia. The correct option will correct this problem, but the others will not. Review care to the client with Parkinson's disease if you had difficulty with this question.

Level of Cognitive Ability: Application
Client Needs: Health Promotion and Maintenance
Integrated Concept/Process: Self-Care
Content Area: Adult Health/Neurological

Reference:
Ignatavicius, D., & Workman, M. (2002). *Medical-surgical: critical thinking for collaborative care* (4th ed.). Philadelphia: W.B. Saunders, p. 911.

---

75. A nurse is telling a client with right-sided trigeminal neuralgia about strategies to minimize episodes of pain. The nurse tells the client to avoid which of the following activities that could trigger an episode?
1   Using mouthwash during times when tooth brushing is painful
2   Eating foods that are very hot or very cold
3   Washing the face with cotton balls
4   Chewing on the left side of the mouth

Answer: 2
Rationale: Pressure and temperature changes often trigger an episode of pain with trigeminal neuralgia. For this reason, the client should avoid eating or drinking foods or beverages that are very hot or very cold. The client should chew on the unaffected side of the mouth and eat a soft diet. If tooth brushing triggers pain, the client may choose instead to rinse the mouth after a meal. Facial pain can be minimized by using cotton pads and room-temperature water to wash the face.

Test-Taking Strategy: Use the process of elimination and note the key word *avoid*. Recalling that the pain of trigeminal neuralgia is triggered by mechanical or thermal stimuli will direct you to option 2. Very hot or cold foods are likely to trigger the pain, not relieve it. Review care measures for the client with trigeminal neuralgia if you had difficulty with this question.

Level of Cognitive Ability: Application
Client Needs: Health Promotion and Maintenance
Integrated Concept/Process: Nursing Process/Implementation
Content Area: Adult Health/Neurological

Reference:
Ignatavicius, D., & Workman, M. (2002). *Medical-surgical: critical thinking for collaborative care* (4th ed.). Philadelphia: W.B. Saunders, p. 969.

---

76. A nurse is giving a client with Bell's palsy instructions about how to preserve muscle tone in the face and prevent denervation. The nurse tells the client to avoid which of the following?
1   Exercises such as wrinkling the forehead and whistling
2   Use of an electrical stimulator device
3   Exposure of the face to cold and drafts
4   Gentle face massage

Answer: 3
Rationale: Prevention of muscle atrophy with Bell's palsy is accomplished with the use of facial massage, facial exercises, and electrical stimulation of the nerves. Local application of heat to the face may improve blood flow and provide comfort. Exposure to cold or drafts is avoided.

Test-Taking Strategy: Use the process of elimination. Note the key word *avoid*. The issue of the question is how to *preserve muscle tone*. Option 3 is the only option that does not focus on this issue. Review measures that will preserve muscle tone in the client with Bell's palsy if you had difficulty with this question.

Level of Cognitive Ability: Application
Client Needs: Health Promotion and Maintenance
Integrated Concept/Process: Teaching/Learning
Content Area: Adult Health/Neurological

Reference:
Ignatavicius, D., & Workman, M. (2002). *Medical-surgical: critical thinking for collaborative care* (4th ed.). Philadelphia: W.B. Saunders, p. 971.

---

77. An older client with osteoporosis is at risk for falls. The nurse instructs the client to avoid which of the following to maintain safety in the home?

1   Removing the mat from the bathtub
2   Obtaining a shower chair
3   Making sure railings are sturdy and secure
4   Placing a night light in the hall

Answer: 1
Rationale: Home modifications to reduce the risk for falls includes use of sturdy and secure railings on all staircases and ample lighting. Bathroom safety equipment includes using a shower chair, placing handrails in the shower and near the toilet, and keeping a mat in the tub to prevent slipping.

Test-Taking Strategy: Use the process of elimination. Note the key word *avoid*. Begin to answer this question by eliminating options 2 and 3. Both of these items provide physical support to the client and are needed. A night light will enhance vision for the client using the bathroom at night and is also warranted. The only remaining option, which is the correct answer, is removing the bath mat. Remember that mats prevent slips and falls. Review the basic measures related to the prevention of falls if you had difficulty with this question.

Level of Cognitive Ability: Application
Client Needs: Health Promotion and Maintenance
Integrated Concept/Process: Self-Care
Content Area: Adult Health/Musculoskeletal

Reference:
deWit, S. (2001). *Fundamental concepts and skills for nursing.* Philadelphia: W.B. Saunders, p. 839.

---

78. A client has had a bone scan done. The nurse instructs the client to do which of the following after the procedure?

1   Eat only small meals for the remainder of the day
2   Drink plenty of water for a day or two
3   Report any feelings of nausea or flushing
4   Ambulate at least three times before the end of the day

Answer: 2
Rationale: No activity or dietary restrictions are necessary after a bone scan. The client is encouraged to drink large amounts of water for 24 to 48 hours to flush the radioisotope from the system. There are no hazards to the client or staff from the minimal amount of radioactivity of the isotope. The client would not experience nausea or flushing because contrast dye is not used for this procedure. In addition, those sensations would likely be experienced at the time of dye injection, not after it.

Test-Taking Strategy: Use the process of elimination. There is no purpose for options 1 or 4 so eliminate these options first. Nausea and flushing could accompany dye injection during a procedure, but this procedure uses radioisotopes. Therefore eliminate option 3. The only option left is encouraging fluids, which will speed elimination of the isotope from the client's system. Review care to a client after a bone scan if you had difficulty with this question.

Level of Cognitive Ability: Application
Client Needs: Health Promotion and Maintenance
Integrated Concept/Process: Nursing Process/Implementation
Content Area: Adult Health/Musculoskeletal

Reference:
Ignatavicius, D., & Workman, M. (2002). *Medical-surgical: critical thinking for collaborative care* (4th ed.). Philadelphia: W.B. Saunders, p. 1113.

---

79. A nurse is planning to teach the client with a left arm cast about stiff or "frozen" shoulder as a complication of having the cast in place. The nurse tells the client that which of the following actions by the client would contribute to this occurrence?
1 Making a fist with the hand of the left arm
2 Using a sling on the left arm
3 Lifting the left arm over the head
4 Lifting the right arm over the head

Answer: 2
Rationale: Immobility and the weight of a casted arm may cause the shoulder above an arm fracture to become stiff. The use of slings further immobilizes the shoulder and may be contraindicated. The shoulder of a casted arm should be lifted over the head periodically as a preventive measure. Making fists with the left hand provides good isometric exercise to maintain muscle strength. Range of motion of the affected fingers is also a useful general measure. Lifting the right arm is irrelevant to the situation in the question.

Test-Taking Strategy: Use the process of elimination. Note the key words *contribute to this occurrence*. Visualize each of the movements and think about the muscle groups that are moved with each. Option 4 is unrelated to the client's problem and is eliminated first. Recalling that immobility can lead to a stiff or "frozen" shoulder will direct you to option 2. Review teaching points related to a client with an arm cast if you had difficulty with this question.

Level of Cognitive Ability: Application
Client Needs: Health Promotion and Maintenance
Integrated Concept/Process: Nursing Process/Implementation
Content Area: Adult Health/Musculoskeletal

Reference:
Ignatavicius, D., & Workman, M. (2002). *Medical-surgical: critical thinking for collaborative care* (4th ed.). Philadelphia: W.B. Saunders, p. 1135.

---

80. A nurse is reviewing a set of specific leg exercises with a client immobilized in right skeletal leg traction. The nurse tells the client that which of the following movements should be avoided as potentially harmful?
1 Performing active range of motion (ROM) to the right ankle and knee
2 Doing quadriceps-setting and gluteal-setting exercises
3 Pulling up on the trapeze
4 Flexing and extending the feet

Answer: 1
Rationale: Exercise is indicated within therapeutic limits for the client in skeletal traction to maintain muscle strength and range of motion. The client should not, however, do active ROM to the involved joints, because it would disrupt the pull of the traction force. The client may pull up on the trapeze, perform active ROM with uninvolved joints, and do isometric muscle-setting exercises (such as quadriceps- and gluteal-setting exercises). The client may also flex and extend the feet.

Test-Taking Strategy: Use the process of elimination. The wording of the question tells you that the correct option will be a type of exercise that is not indicated for this client. Use knowledge of the principles of traction and client mobility, and note the key word *active* in the correct option. Review these concepts if you had difficulty with this question.

Level of Cognitive Ability: Application
Client Needs: Health Promotion and Maintenance
Integrated Concept/Process: Nursing Process/Implementation
Content Area: Adult Health/Musculoskeletal

Reference:
Ignatavicius, D., & Workman, M. (2002). *Medical-surgical nursing: critical thinking for collaborative care* (4th ed.). Philadelphia: W.B. Saunders, p. 1136.

---

81. A client with thromboangiitis obliterans (Buerger's disease) asks the nurse what can be done to alleviate the symptoms. In reinforcing instructions about this disorder and symptom control, the nurse tells the client which of the following?
1   Analgesics are primarily used to control the symptom of pain
2   Warmth, exercise, and smoking cessation are most helpful
3   There is no current treatment
4   Surgery is the most successful therapy

Answer: 2
Rationale: The main goals of treatment for thromboangiitis obliterans are the same as for peripheral arterial insufficiency. Thus the client is taught measures to increase circulation, which include enhancing vasodilation through warmth, exercise, and smoking cessation.

Test-Taking Strategy: Use the process of elimination. Option 3 is unrealistic and is eliminated first. From the remaining options, recalling that the measures used to treat peripheral arterial insufficiency are also useful in treating this disorder will direct you to option 2. Review therapeutic management in Buerger's disease if you had difficulty with this question.

Level of Cognitive Ability: Application
Client Needs: Health Promotion and Maintenance
*Integrated Concept/Process:*Teaching/Learning
Content Area: Adult Health/Cardiovascular

Reference:
Ignatavicius, D., & Workman, M. (2002). *Medical-surgical: critical thinking for collaborative care* (4th ed.). Philadelphia: W.B. Saunders, p. 761.

---

82. A nurse is reviewing the teaching plan for a client who is receiving phenelzine sulfate (Nardil). The nurse plans to reinforce which of the following instructions noted on the plan?
1   Avoid aged cheeses
2   Avoid cherries and blueberries
3   Avoid digitalis preparations
4   Avoid vasodilators

Answer: 1
Rationale: Phenelzine sulfate is in the monoamine oxidase (MAO) inhibitor class of antidepressant medications. Clients taking MAO inhibitors must avoid aged cheeses, alcoholic beverages, avocados, bananas, caffeine, chocolate, meat tenderizers, pickled herring, raisins, sour cream, yogurt, and soy sauce. Medications to avoid include amphetamines, antiasthmatic agents, tricyclic antidepressants, and serotonin reuptake inhibitor (SRI) antidepressants. Clients should also avoid antihistamines, antihypertensive medications, levodopa, and meperidine hydrochloride (Demerol).

Test-Taking Strategy: Use the process of elimination and knowledge regarding this medication to answer this question. All the food and medication groups listed in options 2, 3, and 4 are allowed. If you had difficulty with this question review this medication.

Level of Cognitive Ability: Application
Client Needs: Health Promotion and Maintenance

Integrated Concept/Process: Teaching/Learning
Content Area: Pharmacology

Reference:
Hodgson, B., & Kizior, R. (2003). *Saunders nursing drug handbook 2003.* Philadelphia: W.B. Saunders, p. 881.

---

83. Which of the following strategies would be included when teaching parents how to prevent infection in their infant after surgical repair of an inguinal hernia?
1   Change the diapers as soon as they become damp
2   Report a fever immediately
3   Soak the infant in a tub bath twice a day for the next 5 days
4   Restrict the infant's physical activity

Answer: 1
Rationale: Changing diapers as soon as they become damp helps reduce the chance of irritation or infection of the incision. Parents are instructed to change diapers more frequently than usual during the day and once or twice during the night. A fever could indicate the presence of an infection. Parents are instructed to give the child sponge baths instead of tub baths for 2 to 5 days. No restrictions are placed on the infant's activity.

Test-Taking Strategy: Use the process of elimination. The question asks for strategies to prevent infection. Focusing on this issue and recalling the factors that cause infection will direct you to option 1. Review these measures to prevent infection if you had difficulty with this question.

Level of Cognitive Ability: Application
Client Needs: Health Promotion and Maintenance
Integrated Concept/Process: Teaching/Learning
Content Area: Child Health

Reference:
Schulte, E. Price, D., & Gwin, J. (2001). *Thompson's pediatric nursing* (8th ed.). Philadelphia: W.B. Saunders, p. 134.

---

84. A client is experiencing difficulty using an incentive spirometer. The nurse teaches the client that which of the following variables may interfere with effective use of the device?
1   Breathing through the nose
2   Forming a tight seal around the mouthpiece with the lips
3   Inhaling slowly
4   Removing the mouthpiece to exhale

Answer: 1
Rationale: Incentive spirometry is not effective if the client breathes through the nose. The client should exhale, form a tight seal around the mouthpiece, inhale slowly, hold for the count of 3, and remove the mouthpiece to exhale. The client should repeat the exercise approximately 10 times every hour for best results.

Test-Taking Strategy: Use the process of elimination and note the words *may interfere.* Visualize the use of the incentive spirometer to direct you to option 1. Review the use of this device if you had difficulty with this question.

Level of Cognitive Ability: Application
Client Needs: Health Promotion and Maintenance
Integrated Concept/Process: Teaching/Learning
Content Area: Adult Health/Respiratory

Reference:
deWit, S. (2001). *Fundamental concepts and skills for nursing.* Philadelphia: W.B. Saunders, p. 535.

85. A client with a respiratory disorder is unsure of the position to use to breathe more easily. The nurse teaches the client to do which of the following?
1 Lie on the side with the head of the bed at a 45-degree angle
2 Sit upright in bed with the arms crossed over the chest
3 Sit on the edge of the bed with the arms leaning on an overbed table
4 Sit in a reclining chair tilted slightly back and elevate the feet

Answer: 3
Rationale: Proper positioning can decrease episodes of dyspnea in a client. Such positions include sitting upright while leaning on an overbed table, sitting upright in a chair with the arms resting on the knees, and leaning against a wall while standing.

Test-Taking Strategy: Use the process of elimination. Option 1 restricts expansion of the lateral wall of a lung and is eliminated first. Option 2 restricts movement of the anterior and posterior walls and is also eliminated. Option 3 does not restrict expansion of any lung segment, whereas option 4 restricts posterior lung expansion. Review care to the client with a respiratory disorder if you had difficulty with this question.

Level of Cognitive Ability: Application
Client Needs: Health Promotion and Maintenance
Integrated Concept/Process: Teaching/Learning
Content Area: Adult Health/Respiratory

Reference:
Black, J., Hawks, J., & Keene, A. (2001). *Medical-surgical nursing: clinical management for positive outcomes* (6th ed.). Philadelphia: W.B. Saunders, p. 1702.

86. A client with acquired immunodeficiency syndrome (AIDS) is experiencing fatigue. The nurse teaches the client which of the following strategies to conserve energy after discharge?
1 Stand in the shower instead of taking a bath
2 Bathe before eating breakfast
3 Sit for as many activities as possible
4 Group all tasks to be performed early in the morning

Answer: 3
Rationale: The client is taught to conserve energy by sitting for as many activities as possible, including dressing, shaving, preparing food, and ironing. The client should also sit in a shower chair instead of standing while bathing. The client should prioritize activities (eating breakfast before bathing), and should intersperse each major activity with a period of rest. Frequent short rest periods are more effective than fewer longer ones.

Test-Taking Strategy: Use the process of elimination. Answer this question by considering the amount of exertion required by the client to perform each of the activities listed in the options. Options 1 and 4 are obviously taxing for the client and are eliminated first. From the remaining options, recall that bathing may take away energy that could be used for eating, and is not helpful. Review measures that conserve energy if you had difficulty with this question.

Level of Cognitive Ability: Application
Client Needs: Health Promotion and Maintenance
Integrated Concept/Process: Teaching/Learning
Content Area: Adult Health/Respiratory

Reference:
Black, J., Hawks, J., & Keene, A. (2001). *Medical-surgical nursing: clinical management for positive outcomes* (6th ed.). Philadelphia: W.B. Saunders, p. 2209.

87. A nurse has reinforced instructions with a client with pleurisy about strategies to promote comfort during recuperation. The nurse evaluates that the client has understood the instructions if the client states that he or she will do which of the following?
1 Try to take only small, shallow breaths
2 Splint the chest wall during coughing and deep breathing
3 Lie as much as possible on the unaffected side
4 Take as much pain medication as possible

Answer: 2

Rationale: The client with pleurisy should splint the chest wall during coughing and deep breathing, which is necessary to prevent atelectasis. The client should also lie on the affected side to minimize movement of the affected chest wall. The client should not take only small, shallow breaths because this promotes atelectasis. The client should take medication prudently to allow coughing, deep breathing, and adequate levels of comfort.

Test-Taking Strategy: Use the process of elimination. Option 4 is obviously incorrect and is eliminated first. Eliminate option 1 next because taking small, shallow breaths would promote atelectasis. Lying on the unaffected side would stretch the chest wall on the affected side, increasing discomfort. Therefore eliminate option 3. Option 2 promotes lung expansion while minimizing client discomfort. Review care to the client with pleurisy if you had difficulty with this question.

Level of Cognitive Ability: Comprehension
Client Needs: Health Promotion and Maintenance
Integrated Concept/Process: Nursing Process/Evaluation
Content Area: Adult Health/Respiratory

Reference:
Black, J., Hawks, J., & Keene, A. (2001). *Medical-surgical nursing: clinical management for positive outcomes* (6th ed.). Philadelphia: W.B. Saunders, p. 1450.

88. A client is to be discharged on warfarin (Coumadin) therapy and the nurse reinforces medication instructions with the client. Which statement by the client would indicate further teaching is needed?
1 "This medicine thins my blood and allows me to clot slower."
2 "I should have a prothrombin level checked in 2 weeks."
3 "If I notice any increased bleeding or bruising, I should call my doctor."
4 "I should increase foods high in vitamin K in my diet."

Answer: 4

Rationale: Warfarin sodium is an oral anticoagulant that is used mainly to prevent thromboembolic events such as thrombophlebitis, pulmonary embolism, and embolism formation caused by atrial fibrillation. Oral anticoagulants prolong the clotting time and are monitored by the prothrombin time (PT) and the International Normalized Ratio (INR). Client education should include signs and symptoms of toxic effects and dietary restrictions such as limiting foods high in vitamin K (leafy green vegetables, liver, cheese, and egg yolk), as these food items increase clotting times.

Test-Taking Strategy: Note the key words *further teaching is needed.* Recalling the purpose of warfarin therapy and the role vitamin K plays in the clotting mechanism will direct you to option 4. If you had difficulty with this question, review client education points related to this medication.

Level of Cognitive Ability: Comprehension
Client Needs: Health Promotion and Maintenance
Integrated Concept/Process: Teaching/Learning
Content Area: Pharmacology

Reference:
Hodgson, B., & Kizior, R. (2003). *Saunders nursing drug handbook 2003.* Philadelphia: W.B. Saunders, p. 1170.

89. A teenager returns to the gynecological (GYN) clinic for a follow-up visit for a sexually transmitted disease (STD). Which statement by the client indicates the need for teaching?
   1   "I always make sure my boyfriend uses a condom."
   2   "I know you won't tell my parents I'm sick."
   3   "My boyfriend doesn't have to come in for treatment."
   4   "I finished all the antibiotic, just like you said."

Answer: 3
Rationale: In treating STDs, all sexual contacts must be notified and treated with medication. Clients should always use a condom with any sexual contact. Any treatment at a GYN clinic for teenagers is confidential, and parents will not be contacted, even if the client is younger than 18 years of age. Clients should always finish a medication ordered by the health care provider.

Test-Taking Strategy: Use the process of elimination and note the key words *need for further teaching*. Knowledge of safe sex practices and the treatment of STDs will assist in answering this question. Review this content if you had difficulty with this question.

Level of Cognitive Ability: Comprehension
Client Needs: Health Promotion and Maintenance
Integrated Concept/Process: Nursing Process/Evaluation
Content Area: Child Health

Reference:
Wong, D., & Hockenberry-Eaton, M. (2001). *Wong's essentials of pediatric nursing* (6th ed.). St. Louis: Mosby, p. 552.

---

90. A nurse is reinforcing instructions with a client recently diagnosed with diabetes mellitus about blood glucose monitoring. The nurse tells the client to report glucose levels that exceed which of the following?
   1   150 mg/dL
   2   200 mg/dL
   3   250 mg/dL
   4   350 mg/dL

Answer: 3
Rationale: It is standard practice to teach the client to report blood glucose levels that exceed 250 mg/dL unless otherwise instructed by the physician. Options 1 and 2 do not warrant reporting, whereas option 4 is dangerously high and the level should have been reported before it became that high.

Test-Taking Strategy: Use the process of elimination and note the key word *exceed*. Recalling the principles related to blood glucose monitoring and the ramifications of the results will direct you to option 3. Review this area of teaching for diabetic clients if you had difficulty with this question.

Level of Cognitive Ability: Application
Client Needs: Health Promotion and Maintenance
Integrated Concept/Process: Teaching/Learning
Content Area: Adult Health/Endocrine

Reference:
Black, J., Hawks, J., & Keene, A. (2001). *Medical-surgical nursing: clinical management for positive outcomes* (6th ed.). Philadelphia: W.B. Saunders, p. 1158.

---

91. A client has a new prescription for timolol maleate (Betimol). The nurse determines that the client has not fully understood instructions given about the medication if the client stated which of the following?
   1   Take the pulse daily and hold the dose if it is less than 60 beats per minute

Answer: 3
Rationale: Common client teaching points about beta-adrenergic blocking agents include to take the pulse daily and hold for a rate under 60 beats per minute (and notify the physician), not to discontinue or change the medication dose, to keep enough medication on hand so as not to run out, to change positions slowly, not to take over-the-counter medications (especially decongestants, cough, and cold preparations) without consulting the physician, and to carry medical identification

2 Use caution with driving because drowsiness is a side effect

3 Taper or discontinue the medication once the client feels well

4 Have enough medication on hand to last through weekends and vacations

stating a beta-blocker is in use. Drowsiness is a side effect of the medication.

Test-Taking Strategy: Use the process of elimination. Note the key words *has not fully understood.* Option 1 is a correct action, and option 2 is a known effect of the medication, so these are eliminated first. A client should not run out of any prescribed medications, which eliminates option 4. This leaves option 3 as the correct answer, which is also an important point for many prescribed medications. Antihypertensive medications should never be discontinued by the client without physician approval. Review this medication if you had difficulty with this question.

Level of Cognitive Ability: Comprehension
Client Needs: Health Promotion and Maintenance
Integrated Concept/Process: Nursing Process/Evaluation
Content Area: Pharmacology

Reference:
Hodgson, B., & Kizior, R. (2003). *Saunders nursing drug handbook 2003.* Philadelphia: W.B. Saunders, p. 1088.

---

92. A nurse has reinforced medication instructions to a client receiving benazepril (Lotensin). The nurse would evaluate that the client needs further instruction if the client stated a need to do which of the following?

1 Change positions slowly

2 Report signs and symptoms of infection

3 Monitor blood pressure every week

4 Use salt substitutes and eat foods high in potassium

Answer: 4
Rationale: The client taking an angiotensin-converting enzyme inhibitor is instructed to take the medication exactly as prescribed, monitor blood pressure weekly, and continue with other lifestyle changes to control hypertension. The client should change positions slowly to avoid orthostatic hypotension; report fever, mouth sores, and sore throat (signs of neutropenia) to the physician; and avoid salt substitutes and foods high in potassium (which can cause hyperkalemia).

Test-Taking Strategy: Use the process of elimination. Note the key words *needs further instruction.* Knowing that options 1 and 3 are standard instructions with antihypertensive therapy, you would eliminate these first. To choose correctly between the remaining options, you should know that side effects of this medication include neutropenia and hyperkalemia. Review this medication if you had difficulty with this question.

Level of Cognitive Ability: Comprehension
Client Needs: Health Promotion and Maintenance
Integrated Concept/Process: Nursing Process/Evaluation
Content Area: Pharmacology

Reference:
Hodgson, B., & Kizior, R. (2003). *Saunders nursing drug handbook 2003.* Philadelphia: W.B. Saunders, p. 112.

---

93. The nurse has reinforced instructions about the use of sublingual nitroglycerin tablets. The client has an order for PRN use if chest pain occurs. The nurse would evaluate that the client understands the

Answer: 3
Rationale: Nitroglycerin may be self-administered sublingually 5 to 10 minutes before an activity that triggers chest pain. Tablets should be discarded 6 months after opening the bottle. Nitroglycerin is very unstable and is affected by heat and cold, so

instructions if the client stated a need to do which of the following?

1 Avoid using the medication until chest pain actually begins and intensifies

2 Take aspirin to treat headache that occurs with early use of nitroglycerin

3 Discard unused tablets 6 months after the bottle is opened

4 Keep the nitroglycerin in a pocket close to the body

it should not be kept close to the body (warmth); instead it should be kept in a jacket pocket or purse. Headache often occurs with early use and diminishes in time. Acetaminophen (Tylenol) may be used to treat headache.

Test-Taking Strategy: Use the process of elimination. Knowing that nitroglycerin is unstable helps you eliminate option 4. It is good practice to take nitroglycerin before activities or stressors that cause chest pain, because this prevents or reduces myocardial ischemia. Therefore eliminate option 1. Aspirin is not the best analgesic to take for headache because it is irritating to the stomach and could interfere with other medications a client may be taking. This leaves option 3 as the correct answer. Review the points to teach regarding this medication if you had difficulty with this question.

Level of Cognitive Ability: Comprehension
Client Needs: Health Promotion and Maintenance
Integrated Concept/Process: Nursing Process/Evaluation
Content Area: Pharmacology

Reference:
Hodgson, B., & Kizior, R. (2002). *Saunders nursing drug handbook 2002.* Philadelphia: W.B. Saunders, p. 802.

---

94. A nurse is reviewing teaching needs for an older client with diabetes mellitus who takes insulin daily and has a history of diabetic ketoacidosis (DKA). Which of the following statements, if made by the client's wife, indicates that further teaching is necessary?

1 "If the grandchildren are sick, they probably shouldn't come to visit."

2 "I should call the doctor if he has nausea or abdominal pain lasting for more than 1 or 2 days."

3 "If he is vomiting, I shouldn't give him any insulin."

4 "I should call the doctor if he develops a fever."

Answer: 3
Rationale: Infection and illness can trigger DKA; therefore options 1, 2, and 4 are accurate statements. Stopping insulin administration is another causal factor of DKA.

Test-Taking Strategy: Use the process of elimination. Note the key words *further teaching is necessary.* Eliminate options 1 and 4 first because they both relate to infection and are therefore similar. From the remaining options, recall the causes of DKA. This should assist in directing you to option 3. If you had difficulty with this question, review the precipitating factors associated with DKA.

Level of Cognitive Ability: Comprehension
Client Needs: Health Promotion and Maintenance
Integrated Concept/Process: Teaching/Learning
Content Area: Adult Health/Endocrine

Reference:
Black, J., Hawks, J., & Keene, A. (2001). *Medical-surgical nursing: clinical management for positive outcomes* (6th ed.). Philadelphia: W.B. Saunders, p. 1190.

---

95. A nurse is caring for a client with chronic venous insufficiency resulting from deep vein thrombosis and reinforces teaching about the disorder. Which statement by the client indicates a need for further instructions?

Answer: 1
Rationale: Clients with chronic venous insufficiency are advised to avoid crossing the legs, sitting in chairs where the feet don't touch the floor, and wearing garters or sources of pressure on the legs (such as girdles). The client should wear elastic hose for 6 to 8 weeks, and perhaps for life. The client should sleep

1　"I can cross my legs at the knee, but not the ankle."
2　"I should elevate the foot of my bed 6 inches during sleep."
3　"I should avoid prolonged standing or sitting."
4　"I should continue to wear elastic hose for at least 6 to 8 weeks."

with the foot of the bed elevated to promote venous return during sleep.

Test-Taking Strategy: Note the key words *need for further instructions*. Consider the concept of gravity when answering questions that relate to peripheral vascular problems. Venous problems are characterized by insufficient drainage of blood from the legs returning to the heart. Thus interventions should be aimed at promoting flow of blood from the legs and to the heart. Only option 1 does not promote venous drainage. Review care to the client with chronic venous insufficiency if you had difficulty with this question.

Level of Cognitive Ability: Comprehension
Client Needs: Health Promotion and Maintenance
Integrated Concept/Process: Teaching/Learning
Content Area: Adult Health/Cardiovascular

Reference:
Black, J., Hawks, J., & Keene, A. (2001). *Medical-surgical nursing: clinical management for positive outcomes* (6th ed.). Philadelphia: W.B. Saunders, p. 1425.

---

96. A nurse is reinforcing discharge instructions to the client with varicose vein stripping and ligation done as outpatient surgery. The nurse would give which of the following directions to the client?
1　Maintain bed rest for the first 3 days
2　Ambulate for 5 to 10 minutes twice a day beginning the day after surgery
3　Elevate the foot of the bed while in bed
4　Remove elastic hose after 24 hours

Answer: 3
Rationale: Standard postoperative care after vein ligation and stripping consists of bed rest for 24 hours, with ambulation for 5 to 10 minutes every 2 hours thereafter. Continuous elastic compression of the leg is maintained for 1 week after the procedure, followed by long-term use of elastic hose. The foot of the bed should be elevated to promote venous drainage.

Test-Taking Strategy: Use the process of elimination and knowledge of concepts related to blood flow and immobility to answer this question. Options 1 and 4 will promote venous stasis, so they are eliminated first. From the remaining options, recalling that the client should ambulate more frequently than twice daily will direct you to option 3. Review postoperative teaching points about care after varicose vein stripping and ligation if you had difficulty with this question.

Level of Cognitive Ability: Application
Client Needs: Health Promotion and Maintenance
Integrated Concept/Process: Teaching/Learning
Content Area: Adult Health/Cardiovascular

Reference:
Black, J., Hawks, J., & Keene, A. (2001). *Medical-surgical nursing: clinical management for positive outcomes* (6th ed.). Philadelphia: W.B. Saunders, p. 1427.

---

97. A perinatal client has been instructed on the prevention of genital tract infections. Which of the following statements made

Answer: 4
Rationale: Condoms should be used to minimize the spread of sexually transmitted infectious diseases. Wearing tight clothes

by the client would indicate understanding of the instructions?

1 "I should avoid the use of condoms."
2 "I can douche anytime I want."
3 "I can wear my tight-fitting jeans."
4 "I should choose underwear with a cotton panel liner."

irritates the genital area and does not allow for air circulation. Douching is to be avoided. Wearing items with a cotton panel liner allows for air movement in and around the genital area.

Test-Taking Strategy: Use the process of elimination. Note the key words *understanding of the instructions.* Options 1, 2, and 3 are all incorrect statements regarding client self-care. If you had difficulty with this question, review prevention measures associated with genital tract infections.

Level of Cognitive Ability: Comprehension
Client Needs: Health Promotion and Maintenance
Integrated Concept/Process: Self-Care
Content Area: Maternity

Reference:
Murray, S., McKinney, E., & Gorrie, T. (2002). *Foundations of maternal-newborn nursing* (3rd ed.). Philadelphia: W.B. Saunders, p. 959.

---

98. A client who sustained a major burn is resuming an oral diet. The nurse encourages the client to eat a variety of which of the following types of foods to best help in continued wound healing and tissue repair?

1 High carbohydrate and low protein
2 High fat and low carbohydrate
3 High protein and high fat
4 High protein and high carbohydrate

Answer: 4
Rationale: To promote adequate healing and meet continued high metabolic needs, the client with a major burn should eat a diet that is high in calories, protein, and carbohydrates. This type of diet also keeps the client in positive nitrogen balance. There is no need to increase the amount of fat in the diet.

Test-Taking Strategy: Use the process of elimination. Focus on the key words *wound healing and tissue repair.* Use principles of nutrition as they relate to healing tissues to answer this question. This will direct you to option 4. If you had difficulty with this question, review nutrition necessary for healing and tissue repair.

Level of Cognitive Ability: Application
Client Needs: Health Promotion and Maintenance
Integrated Concept/Process: Nursing Process/Implementation
Content Area: Adult Health/Integumentary

Reference:
Black, J., Hawks, J., & Keene, A. (2001). *Medical-surgical nursing: clinical management for positive outcomes* (6th ed.). Philadelphia: W.B. Saunders, p. 1352.

---

99. A nurse has taught the client with myxedema about dietary changes to help manage the disorder. The nurse evaluates that the client understood the information if the client states that it is permissible to continue eating which of the following foods?

1 Beef liver, carrots, and fried potatoes
2 Shrimp, green beans, and butter
3 Peanut butter, cheese, and red meat

Answer: 4
Rationale: Clients with myxedema or hypothyroidism have decreased metabolic demands from reduced metabolic rate. For this reason they often experience weight gain. The diet should be low in calories overall and yet be representative of all food groups. Option 4 is the only group that contains solely low-calorie foods.

Test-Taking Strategy: Use the process of elimination. Remember that when there is more than one part to an option, all of the parts of the option must be correct for the option to be correct. With this in mind, analyze each option in terms of dietary

4 Apples, whole-grain breads, and low-fat milk

content. The correct option is the one that promotes weight reduction by being low in fat and calories. Review care to the client with myxedema if you had difficulty with this question.

Level of Cognitive Ability: Comprehension
Client Needs: Health Promotion and Maintenance
Integrated Concept/Process: Nursing Process/Evaluation
Content Area: Adult Health/Endocrine

Reference:
Black, J., Hawks, J., & Keene, A. (2001). *Medical-surgical nursing: clinical management for positive outcomes* (6th ed.). Philadelphia: W.B. Saunders, p. 1093.

---

100. A nurse demonstrates to a mother how to correctly take an axillary temperature to determine if a child has a fever. Which action by the mother would indicate a need for further teaching?
1 She selects a mercury thermometer with a slender tip
2 She holds the thermometer in the axilla for 1 minute
3 She records the actual temperature reading and route
4 She places the thermometer in the center of the axilla

Answer: 2
Rationale: An axillary temperature should be taken for at least 5 minutes to be most accurate. Options 1, 3, and 4 are correct steps for taking an axillary temperature.

Test-Taking Strategy: Use the process of elimination. Note the key words *need for further teaching.* The words *1 minute* in option 2 will direct you to this option. If you had difficulty with this question, review the procedure for obtaining an axillary temperature.

Level of Cognitive Ability: Comprehension
Client Needs: Health Promotion and Maintenance
Integrated Concept/Process: Nursing Process/Evaluation
Content Area: Child Health

Reference:
Schulte, E. Price, D., & Gwin, J. (2001). *Thompson's pediatric nursing* (8th ed.). Philadelphia: W.B. Saunders, p. 32.

---

101. A nurse instructs a client about a low-fat diet. The client would indicate understanding of this diet by choosing which of the following foods?
1 Liver, potato salad, and sherbet
2 Shrimp and bacon salad
3 Turkey breast, boiled rice, and angel food cake
4 Lean hamburger steak, macaroni and cheese

Answer: 3
Rationale: Major sources of fats include organ meats and red meats, salad dressings, eggs, butter, and cheese. All options except the correct one contain high-fat foods.

Test-Taking Strategy: Use the process of elimination. Eliminate options 2 and 4 first because both a hamburger steak and bacon are high in fat. From the remaining options, look at the foods closely. Option 3 does not contain any high-fat foods. Potato salad will contain mayonnaise, which is high in fat. If you had difficulty with this question, review those foods that contain fat.

Level of Cognitive Ability: Comprehension
Client Needs: Health Promotion and Maintenance
Integrated Concept/Process: Teaching/Learning
Content Area: Fundamental Skills

Reference:
Williams, S. (2001). *Basic nutrition & diet therapy* (11th ed.). St. Louis: Mosby, p. 384.

102. A client has renal calculi composed of uric acid. The nurse is teaching the client dietary measures to prevent further development of uric acid calculi. Which of the following statements would indicate that the client understands these dietary measures?
1   "I would avoid milk and dairy products."
2   "I would avoid foods such as spinach, chocolate, and tea."
3   "I would avoid foods such as fish with fine bones and organ meats."
4   "I should drink cranberry juice."

Answer: 3
Rationale: With a uric acid stone, the client should limit intake of foods high in purines. Organ meats, sardines, herring, and other high-purine foods are eliminated from the diet. Foods with moderate levels of purines, such as red and white meats and some seafood are also limited. Options 1 and 2 are necessary dietary measures for calculi composed of calcium phosphate or calcium oxalate. Cranberry juice is commonly recommended to help lower the pH of urine, rendering it more acid to prevent the development of urinary tract infections. However, uric acid stones form most readily in acid urine and would therefore be contraindicated in this client with uric acid stone formation.

Test-Taking Strategy: Use the process of elimination and note the key words *uric acid*. Remembering simply that organ meats contain purines will assist in directing you to the correct option. If you had difficulty with this question, review foods to avoid with uric acid calculi.

Level of Cognitive Ability: Comprehension
Client Needs: Health Promotion and Maintenance
Integrated Concept/Process: Teaching/Learning
Content Area: Adult Health/Renal

Reference:
Williams, S. (2001). *Basic nutrition & diet therapy* (11th ed.). St. Louis: Mosby, p. 412.

103. A nurse is providing follow-up instructions to a client who received a Mantoux skin test in the physician's office on a Monday. The nurse tells the client to return to the physician's office to have the results read on which of the following days?
1   Tuesday or Wednesday
2   Wednesday or Thursday
3   Thursday or Friday
4   The next Monday

Answer: 2
Rationale: The Mantoux skin test for tuberculosis is read in 48 to 72 hours. The client should return to the clinic on Wednesday or Thursday.

Test-Taking Strategy: Use the process of elimination. Recalling that the Mantoux skin test results must be read within 48 to 72 hours will direct you to option 2. Review this test if you had difficulty with this question.

Level of Cognitive Ability: Application
Client Needs: Health Promotion and Maintenance
Integrated Concept/Process: Nursing Process/Implementation
Content Area: Adult Health/Respiratory

Reference:
deWit, S. (2001). *Fundamental concepts and skills for nursing.* Philadelphia: W.B. Saunders, p. 696.

104. A nurse is teaching the client with acquired immunodeficiency syndrome how to avoid food-borne illnesses. The nurse teaches the client to avoid which of the following items, to prevent infections?
1   Raw oysters
2   Bottled water

Answer: 1
Rationale: The client is taught to avoid raw or undercooked seafood, meat, poultry, and eggs. The client should also avoid unpasteurized milk and dairy products. Fruits that the client peels are safe, as are bottled beverages. The client may be taught to avoid sorbitol, but this is to diminish diarrhea and has nothing to do with food-borne infections.

3 Products with sorbitol
4 Bananas

Test-Taking Strategy: Use the process of elimination and focus on the issue of the question, to prevent infection. Sorbitol produces diarrhea but is unrelated to food-borne illness, so option 3 is eliminated first. Bottled water is safe, which eliminates option 2. Eliminate option 4 because the client is taught that fruits that are peeled are safe. Review items to avoid to prevent infection if you had difficulty with this question.

Level of Cognitive Ability: Application
Client Needs: Health Promotion and Maintenance
Integrated Concept/Process: Teaching/Learning
Content Area: Fundamental Skills

Reference:
Black, J., Hawks, J., & Keene, A. (2001). *Medical-surgical nursing: clinical management for positive outcomes* (6th ed.). Philadelphia: W.B. Saunders, p. 2200.

---

105. A client with histoplasmosis has an order for ketoconazole (Nizoral). The nurse tells the client to do which of the following while taking this medication?
1 Take the medication on an empty stomach
2 Take the medication with an antacid
3 Avoid exposure to sunlight
4 Limit alcohol to 2 oz per day

Answer: 3
Rationale: The client should be taught that ketoconazole is an antifungal medication. It should be taken with food or milk, and antacids should be avoided for 2 hours after it is taken. The client should avoid concurrent use of alcohol, because the medication is hepatotoxic. The client should also avoid exposure to sunlight because the medication increases photosensitivity.

Test-Taking Strategy: Use the process of elimination. Begin to answer this question by eliminating options 2 and 4. Many medications are not well absorbed if an antacid is given concurrently. There are also many medications with which alcohol use is contraindicated for the duration of the therapy. To discriminate between options 1 and 3, you should know that the medication causes photophobia and that it should be taken with food or milk. Review this medication if you had difficulty with this question.

Level of Cognitive Ability: Application
Client Needs: Health Promotion and Maintenance
Integrated Concept/Process: Nursing Process/Implementation
Content Area: Pharmacology

Reference:
Hodgson, B., & Kizior, R. (2003). *Saunders nursing drug handbook 2003.* Philadelphia: W.B. Saunders, p. 631.

---

106. A male client being discharged who initially denied that he drank alcohol before admission now admits that he has a drinking problem. The client states he will *get some help* so he will live a healthier lifestyle. The nurse plans a meeting between a representative of which of the following groups and the client before discharge?

Answer: 2
Rationale: Alcoholics Anonymous is a major self-help organization for the treatment of alcoholism. Option 1 is a group for families of alcoholics. Option 3 is for parents of children who abuse substances. Option 4 is for nicotine addicts.

Test-Taking Strategy: Use the process of elimination. If you are unfamiliar with these support groups, note the relationship between *drinking* in the question and *Alcoholics* in the correct

1 Al Anon	option. Familiarize yourself with the purpose of specific support groups if you had difficulty with this question.
2 Alcoholics Anonymous	
3 Families Anonymous	
4 Fresh Start	

Level of Cognitive Ability: Application
Client Needs: Health Promotion and Maintenance
Integrated Concept/Process: Nursing Process/Implementation
Content Area: Mental Health

Reference:
Varcarolis, E. (2002). *Foundations of psychiatric mental health nursing* (4th ed.). Philadelphia: W.B. Saunders, p. 772.

---

107. A nurse is planning to teach a teenage client about sexuality. The nurse would begin the instruction by doing which of the following?

1 Determining the client's knowledge about sexuality

2 Providing written information about sexually transmitted diseases

3 Informing the client about the dangers of pregnancy

4 Advising the teen to maintain sexual abstinence until marriage

Answer: 1

Rationale: The first step in the teaching and learning process is to determine the client's knowledge. The other options may be later steps, depending on the data obtained.

Test-Taking Strategy: Use the nursing process and select the option that gathers data. This will direct you to option 1. Remember, when teaching, determining motivation, interest, and level of knowledge comes before providing information. If you had difficulty with this question, review the principles of teaching and learning.

Level of Cognitive Ability: Application
Client Needs: Health Promotion and Maintenance
Integrated Concept/Process: Teaching/Learning
Content Area: Child Health

Reference:
Schulte, E. Price, D., & Gwin, J. (2001). *Thompson's pediatric nursing* (8th ed.). Philadelphia: W.B. Saunders, p. 304.

---

108. A nurse provides suggestions to parents about the appropriate actions to take when their toddler has a temper tantrum. Which statement by the parents indicates an understanding of the actions to take?

1 "I will send my child to a room alone for 10 minutes after every tantrum."

2 "I will reward my child with candy at the end of each day without a tantrum."

3 "I will give frequent reminders that only bad children have tantrums."

4 "I will ignore the tantrums as long as there is no physical danger."

Answer: 4

Rationale: Ignoring a negative attention-seeking behavior is considered the best way to discourage it, provided the child is safe from injury. Option 1 gives attention to the tantrum and also exceeds the recommended time of 1 minute per year of age for time-out. Providing candy for rewards is unhealthy and unlikely to be effective at the end of a day. Option 3 is untrue and negative.

Test-Taking Strategy: Use Maslow's Hierarchy of Needs theory. Recalling that safety is a primary concern will direct you to option 4. Review these measures if you had difficulty with this question.

Level of Cognitive Ability: Comprehension
Client Needs: Health Promotion and Maintenance
Integrated Concept/Process: Nursing Process/Evaluation
Content Area: Child Health

Reference:
Schulte, E. Price, D., & Gwin, J. (2001). *Thompson's pediatric nursing* (8th ed.). Philadelphia: W.B. Saunders, p. 161.

109. A nurse provides medication instructions to a male client who has been prescribed disulfiram (Antabuse). Which of the following statements, if made by the client, would indicate the need for further instructions about the medication?
1 "As long as I don't drink alcohol, I'll be fine."
2 "I must be careful taking cold medicines."
3 "I'll have to check my aftershave lotion."
4 "I'll have to be more careful with the ingredients I use for cooking."

Answer: 1
Rationale: Clients who are taking disulfiram must be taught that substances containing alcohol can trigger an adverse reaction. Sources of hidden alcohol include foods (soups, sauces, vinegars), medicine (cold medicine, mouthwashes), and skin preparations (alcohol rubs, aftershave lotions).

Test-Taking Strategy: Use the process of elimination and note the key words *need for further instructions*. Recalling that disulfiram is used with clients who have alcoholism and that any form of alcohol should be avoided with this medication will direct you to option 1. Review the client teaching points related to this medication if you had difficulty with this question.

Level of Cognitive Ability: Comprehension
Client Needs: Health Promotion and Maintenance
Integrated Concept/Process: Teaching/Learning
Content Area: Pharmacology

Reference:
Hodgson, B., & Kizior, R. (2003). *Saunders nursing drug handbook 2003.* Philadelphia: W.B. Saunders, p. 365.

---

110. Which client statement indicates that the client needs further teaching about testicular self-examination (TSE)?
1 "I feel the spermatic cord in back and going upward."
2 "I know to report any small lumps."
3 "I examine myself after I take a warm shower."
4 "I examine myself every 2 months."

Answer: 4
Rationale: TSE should be performed every month. Small lumps or abnormalities should be reported. The spermatic cord finding is normal. After a warm bath or shower, the scrotum is relaxed, making it easier to perform TSE.

Test-Taking Strategy: Use the process of elimination. Remembering that breast self-examination should be performed monthly may assist in recalling that TSE is also performed monthly. If you had difficulty with this question, review the procedure for TSE.

Level of Cognitive Ability: Comprehension
Client Needs: Health Promotion and Maintenance
Integrated Concept/Process: Teaching/Learning
Content Area: Adult Health/Oncology

Reference:
Black, J., Hawks, J., & Keene, A. (2001). *Medical-surgical nursing: clinical management for positive outcomes* (6th ed.). Philadelphia: W.B. Saunders, p. 41.

---

111. A nurse determines that a client with Cushing's syndrome understands the hospital discharge instructions if the client makes which of these statements?
1 "I should eat foods low in potassium."
2 "I should take aspirin rather than acetaminophen (Tylenol) for a headache."

Answer: 3
Rationale: Cortisol (secreted in Cushing's syndrome) stimulates the secretion of gastric acid, which can result in peptic ulcers and gastrointestinal (GI) bleeding. The client should check the stools for signs of GI bleeding. Option 1 is incorrect because potassium-rich foods should be encouraged to correct hypokalemia. Option 2 is incorrect because aspirin can increase the risk for gastric bleeding and skin bruising. Option 4 is incorrect because Cushing's syndrome does not affect temperature changes in lower extremities.

3 "I should check the color of my stools."

4 "I should check the temperature of my legs at least once a day."

Test-Taking Strategy: Knowledge regarding the pathophysiology related to Cushing's syndrome is necessary to answer this question. Review this disorder if you had difficulty with this question.

Level of Cognitive Ability: Comprehension
Client Needs: Health Promotion and Maintenance
Integrated Concept/Process: Nursing Process/Evaluation
Content Area: Adult Health/Endocrine

Reference:
Black, J., Hawks, J., & Keene, A. (2001). *Medical-surgical nursing: clinical management for positive outcomes* (6th ed.). Philadelphia: W.B. Saunders, p. 1126.

---

112. A client is on a diet designed to avoid concentrated sugars. The nurse determines that the client understands the diet plan if which of these diets is selected?

1 Strawberry yogurt, lettuce salad, coffee

2 Chicken salad, tomato, Jell-O, tea and honey

3 Peanut butter and jelly sandwich, sherbet, cola

4 Tuna sandwich, lettuce salad, watermelon, herbal tea

Answer: 4
Rationale: Concentrated sugars are found in fruit yogurt, gelatin desserts, prepared drink mixes, jelly, and sherbet.

Test-Taking Strategy: Use the process of elimination. Read each food item in each option, noting that options 1, 2, and 3 contain foods high in concentrated sugars. Review foods containing concentrated sugars if you had difficulty with this question.

Level of Cognitive Ability: Comprehension
Client Needs: Health Promotion and Maintenance
Integrated Concept/Process: Nursing Process/Evaluation
Content Area: Fundamental Skills

Reference:
Williams, S. (2001). *Basic nutrition & diet therapy* (11th ed.). St. Louis: Mosby, p. 26.

---

113. A nurse is assisting in planning home care instructions for a client with diabetes mellitus who takes insulin. The nurse is told that the blood work reveals a glycosylated hemoglobin (HbA_{1c}) of 10%. In planning home care instructions, the nurse interprets this laboratory finding as indicating which of the following?

1 Normal value and that the client is managing blood glucose control well

2 Low value and that the client is not managing blood glucose control well

3 High value and that the client is not managing blood glucose control well

4 Value that does not offer information about client management of the disease

Answer: 3
Rationale: Glycosylated hemoglobin is a measure to determine the degree of glucose control in diabetic clients over a period of time and is not influenced by dietary management a day or two before the test is done. A level higher than 70% indicates poor glucose control.

Test-Taking Strategy: Knowledge about the glycosylated hemoglobin test is necessary to answer this question. Review this test if you had difficulty with this question.

Level of Cognitive Ability: Analysis
Client Needs: Health Promotion and Maintenance
Integrated Concept/Process: Nursing Process/Planning
Content Area: Adult Health/Endocrine

Reference:
Black, J., Hawks, J., & Keene, A. (2001). *Medical-surgical nursing: clinical management for positive outcomes* (6th ed.). Philadelphia: W.B. Saunders, p. 1155.

114. A nurse is reinforcing instructions to a client with type 1 diabetes mellitus about management of hypoglycemic reactions. The nurse instructs the client that hypoglycemia most likely occurs during what time interval after insulin administration?
1 Onset
2 Peak
3 Duration
4 Anytime

Answer: 2
Rationale: Insulin reactions are most likely to occur during the peaking of the insulin, when the medication is at its maximum action. Peak action depends on type of insulin, amount, injection site, and other factors.

Test-Taking Strategy: Use the process of elimination and remember that insulin is a hypoglycemic agent. The work *peak* means the *highest point.* Remembering this should assist in directing you to the correct option. If you had difficulty with this question, review the occurrence of hypoglycemia when a client is taking insulin.

Level of Cognitive Ability: Application
Client Needs: Health Promotion and Maintenance
Integrated Concept/Process: Teaching/Learning
Content Area: Adult Health/Endocrine

Reference:
Black, J., Hawks, J., & Keene, A. (2001). *Medical-surgical nursing: clinical management for positive outcomes* (6th ed.). Philadelphia: W.B. Saunders, p. 1179.

115. A nurse has reinforced instructions to a client with chronic obstructive pulmonary disease (COPD) regarding home care measures. Which statement, if made by the client, would indicate a need for further teaching about nutrition?
1 "I will certainly try to drink 3 liters of fluid every day."
2 "It's best to eat three large meals a day so I will get all my nutrients."
3 "I will not eat as much cabbage as I once did."
4 "I will rest a few minutes before I eat."

Answer: 2
Rationale: Adequate fluid intake helps to liquefy pulmonary secretions. Large meals distend the abdomen and elevate the diaphragm, which may hinder breathing. Gas-forming foods may cause bloating, which interferes with normal diaphragmatic breathing. Resting before eating may decrease the fatigue that is often associated with COPD.

Test-Taking Strategy: Use the process of elimination. Note the key words *need for further teaching.* Recalling that an overdistended abdomen will have harmful effects on a client's respiratory system will direct you to option 2. Also, option 2 suggests that the only way to obtain all of the daily nutrients is by eating three large meals a day; this of course is false. If you had difficulty with this question, review nutrition and the client with a chronic respiratory disorder.

Level of Cognitive Ability: Comprehension
Client Needs: Health Promotion and Maintenance
Integrated Concept/Process: Teaching/Learning
Content Area: Adult Health/Respiratory

Reference:
Black, J., Hawks, J., & Keene, A. (2001). *Medical-surgical nursing: clinical management for positive outcomes* (6th ed.). Philadelphia: W.B. Saunders, p. 1702.

116. A nurse is reinforcing instructions to a hospitalized client with pneumonia about home care measures. Which statement, if made by the client, indicates that the client needs further discharge teaching?

Answer: 4
Rationale: Deep breathing and coughing exercises should be practiced for 6 to 8 weeks after the client is discharged from the hospital to keep the alveoli expanded and promote the removal of lung secretions. If the entire regimen of antibiotics is not taken,

1 "I will take all of my antibiotics even if I do feel 100% better."

2 "I understand that it may be weeks before my usual sense of well-being returns."

3 "It is a good idea for me to take a nap every afternoon for the next couple of weeks."

4 "You can toss out that incentive spirometry as soon as I leave for home."

the client may experience a relapse. Adequate rest is needed to maintain progress toward recovery. The period of convalescence with pneumonia is often lengthy, and it may be weeks before the client feels a sense of well-being.

Test-Taking Strategy: Use the process of elimination. Note the key words *needs further discharge teaching*. The issue of the question is *pneumonia*. Options 1, 2, and 3 are accurate, whereas option 4 is inaccurate. In addition, the use of an incentive spirometer has a direct relationship to the pneumonia, which is the issue of the question. If you had difficulty with this question, review teaching points for the client with pneumonia.

Level of Cognitive Ability: Comprehension
Client Needs: Health Promotion and Maintenance
Integrated Concept/Process: Teaching/Learning
Content Area: Adult Health/Respiratory

Reference:
Black, J., Hawks, J., & Keene, A. (2001). *Medical-surgical nursing: clinical management for positive outcomes* (6th ed.). Philadelphia: W.B. Saunders, p. 1715.

---

117. A nurse is planning to reinforce home care instructions with a client who is newly diagnosed with tuberculosis (TB) about how to prevent the spread of TB. Which of the following strategies would be least effective in preventing the spread of this infection?

1 Teach the client to cover the mouth when coughing

2 Teach the client to sterilize dishes at home

3 Teach the client to properly dispose of tissues

4 Teach the client that close contacts should be tested for TB

Answer: 2
Rationale: Options 1, 3, and 4 would assist in breaking the chain of infection. Not only would option 2 be impractical, but there is no evidence to suggest that sterilizing dishes would break the TB chain of infection.

Test-Taking Strategy: The issue of the question is to prevent the spread of TB. Use the process of elimination, noting the key words *least effective*. Recalling the mode of transmission of TB will easily direct you to the correct option. Review home care principles related to TB, if you had difficulty with this question.

Level of Cognitive Ability: Application
Client Needs: Health Promotion and Maintenance
Integrated Concept/Process: Teaching/Learning
Content Area: Adult Health/Respiratory

Reference:
Black, J., Hawks, J., & Keene, A. (2001). *Medical-surgical nursing: clinical management for positive outcomes* (6th ed.). Philadelphia: W.B. Saunders, p. 2199.

---

118. A nurse has completed reinforcing discharge instructions with the parents of a child with glomerulonephritis. Which of the following statements, if made by the parents, indicates that further teaching is necessary?

1 "We'll check the blood pressure every day."

Answer: 3
Rationale: After discharge, parents should allow the child to return to his or her normal routine and activities with adequate periods allowed for rest. Participating in karate 1 week after discharge would be unrealistic and too rapid an increase in activity level. Options 1, 2, and 4 are correct measures.

Test-Taking Strategy: Use the process of elimination and note the key words *further teaching is necessary*. If you are unfamiliar with

2 "We'll be eating a lot of vegetables and not add extra salt to food."

3 "It'll be so good to have my child back in karate next week."

4 "We'll test the urine for albumin every week."

this disorder, read the options carefully. It would make sense to select option 3 because karate is an aggressive exercise. If you had difficulty with this question, review client teaching points for glomerulonephritis.

Level of Cognitive Ability: Comprehension
Client Needs: Health Promotion and Maintenance
Integrated Concept/Process: Teaching/Learning
Content Area: Child Health

Reference:
Wong, D., & Hockenberry-Eaton, M. (2001). *Wong's essentials of pediatric nursing* (6th ed.). St. Louis: Mosby, p. 1046.

---

119. A nurse is reinforcing discharge instructions with the parents of a child who had sustained a head injury and is now on tapering doses of dexamethasone sodium phosphate (Decadron). The nurse would include which of the following statements in the parent teaching?
1 "This medication decreases chances of infections."
2 "This medication is tapered to minimize side effects."
3 "If your child's face becomes puffy, the medication dose should be increased."
4 "This medication is tapered to decrease chances of rebounding of cerebral edema."

Answer: 4
Rationale: Rebounding of cerebral edema is a side effect of abrupt dexamethasone withdrawal. Option 2 is incorrect because tapering, although necessary, is not done for the purpose of decreasing side effects. Option 1 is incorrect because this medication decreases inflammation, not infection. Option 3 is incorrect; facial "mooning" is a common side effect of this medication that disappears when the medication is discontinued.

Test-Taking Strategy: Use the process of elimination. It is also important to understand the principles and impact of tapering medication. Remembering that tapering is necessary to prevent rebounding will assist in directing you to the correct option. If you had difficulty with this question, review information about this medication.

Level of Cognitive Ability: Application
Client Needs: Health Promotion and Maintenance
Integrated Concept/Process: Teaching/Learning
Content Area: Pharmacology

Reference:
Hodgson, B., & Kizior, R. (2003). *Saunders nursing drug handbook 2003.* Philadelphia: W.B. Saunders, pp. 326-327.

---

120. An 18-year-old female is admitted to an inpatient unit with the diagnosis of anorexia nervosa. Health promotion should focus on which of the following?
1 Helping the client identify and examine dysfunctional thoughts and beliefs
2 Emphasizing social interaction with other clients
3 Providing a supportive environment
4 Examining intrapsychic conflicts and past issues

Answer: 1
Rationale: Health promotion focuses on helping clients recognize and analyze dysfunctional thoughts, as well as identify and examine values and beliefs that maintain these thoughts. Providing a supportive environment is important but is not as critical as option 1. Emphasizing social interaction is not appropriate at this time. Examining intrapsychic conflicts and past issues is not directly related to the client's problem.

Test-Taking Strategy: Use the process of elimination. Option 1 is the only option that is specifically client centered. This option also focuses on identifying client issues related to the diagnosis. Review care to the client with anorexia nervosa if you had difficulty with this question.

Level of Cognitive Ability: Application
Client Needs: Health Promotion and Maintenance
Integrated Concept/Process: Nursing Process/Planning
Content Area: Mental Health

Reference:
Varcarolis, E. (2002). *Foundations of psychiatric mental health nursing* (4th ed.). Philadelphia: W.B. Saunders, p. 420.

---

121. A nurse is assisting in planning care for a client with a C5 spinal cord injury. The nurse suggests which client outcome for the plan of care?
1 Regains bladder and bowel control
2 Performs activities of daily living independently
3 Maintains intact skin
4 Independently transfer to and from a wheelchair

Answer: 3
Rationale: C5 spinal cord injury results in quadriplegia with no sensation below the clavicle, including most of the arms and hands. The client maintains partial movement of the shoulders and elbows. Maintaining intact skin is a key outcome for the client with a spinal cord injury. The remaining options are inappropriate for the client with this type of injury.

Test-Taking Strategy: Use the process of elimination. Eliminate options 2 and 4 first because they are similar. Knowledge of the effects of a C5 spinal cord injury will assist in eliminating option 1. Review the effects of this type of injury if you had difficulty with this question.

Level of Cognitive Ability: Application
Client Needs: Health Promotion and Maintenance
Integrated Concept/Process: Nursing Process/Planning
Content Area: Adult Health/Neurological

Reference:
Black, J., Hawks, J., & Keene, A. (2001). *Medical-surgical nursing: clinical management for positive outcomes* (6th ed.). Philadelphia: W.B. Saunders, p. 2059.

---

122. A client who sustained a thoracic cord injury 1 year ago returns to the physician's office with a small reddened area on the coccyx. The client has no sensation in the area. After instructing the client to relieve pressure on the area using a turning schedule, which action by the nurse is most appropriate?
1 Ask a family member to check the skin daily
2 Schedule the client to return to the physician's office daily for a skin check
3 Teach the client to feel for broken areas
4 Teach the client to use a mirror for skin assessment

Answer: 4
Rationale: The client should be encouraged to be as independent as possible. The most effective method of skin self-assessment is to use a special mirror to view the skin. Options 1 and 2 involve others in performing a task that the client can perform independently. Option 3 is an inaccurate technique, because redness cannot be felt. Option 4 is the only option that addresses client self-assessment of the issue of the question, which is redness.

Test-Taking Strategy: Use the process of elimination. Independence is the key in rehabilitation of clients. Recalling this concept will direct you to option 4. Review home care measures for the client with a spinal cord injury if you had difficulty with this question.

Level of Cognitive Ability: Comprehension
Client Needs: Health Promotion and Maintenance
Integrated Concept/Process: Self-Care
Content Area: Adult Health/Neurological

Reference:
Black, J., Hawks, J., & Keene, A. (2001). *Medical-surgical nursing: clinical management for positive outcomes* (6th ed.). Philadelphia: W.B. Saunders, p. 2068.

---

123. A client with diabetes mellitus has received instructions about foot care. Which of the following statements would indicate that the client needs further instructions about foot care?

1 "The best time to cut my nails is after bathing."

2 "Cotton stockings should be worn to absorb excess moisture."

3 "The cuticles of my nails must be cut to prevent overgrowth."

4 "My feet should be inspected daily using a mirror."

Answer: 3
Rationale: Trimming or cutting the cuticles of the nails can lead to injury to the foot because the skin may be scratched. Even small injuries can be dangerous to the diabetic, who has decreased peripheral vascular circulation. A manicure stick can be used to gently clean the cuticle. Nails should be cut straight across, preferably after a bath because that is when the nails are the softest. Wearing white cotton stockings is best, and the client should inspect the feet daily.

Test-Taking Strategy: Use the process of elimination and note the key words *needs further instructions*. Select the option that could result in altered skin integrity. Using this principle, eliminate options 1, 2, and 4. Review diabetic foot care if you had difficulty with this question.

Level of Cognitive Ability: Comprehension
Client Needs: Health Promotion and Maintenance
Integrated Concept/Process: Self-Care
Content Area: Adult Health/Endocrine

Reference:
Black, J., Hawks, J., & Keene, A. (2001). *Medical-surgical nursing: clinical management for positive outcomes* (6th ed.). Philadelphia: W.B. Saunders, p. 2063.

---

124. A client is taking propranolol (Inderal) for the treatment of hypertension. The nurse tells the client that concurrent use of which of the following items may aggravate the hypertension?

1 Furosemide (Lasix)

2 Insulin

3 Nasal decongestants

4 Digoxin (Lanoxin)

Answer: 3
Rationale: Some nasal decongestants contain stimulants. Clients on beta–adrenergic-blocking agents such as propranolol should avoid concurrent use of nasal decongestants because doing so could cause rebound hypertension and bradycardia. Furosemide has an additive hypotensive effect. Digoxin has an additive bradycardic effect. The insulin effect may be altered by propranolol, which requires adjustment of insulin dosage.

Test-Taking Strategy: Use the process of elimination and note the key words *aggravate the hypertension*. Recalling the items that will increase blood pressure will direct you to option 3. Review the effects of the items in the options on the blood pressure if you had difficulty with this question.

Level of Cognitive Ability: Application
Client Needs: Health Promotion and Maintenance
Integrated Concept/Process: Nursing Process/Implementation
Content Area: Pharmacology

Reference:
Hodgson, B., & Kizior, R. (2003). *Saunders nursing drug handbook 2003.* Philadelphia: W.B. Saunders, pp. 941-943.

125. A client has received a prescription for lisinopril (Prinivil). The nurse reinforces medication instructions and tells the client that which of the following frequent side effects may occur?
1 Hypertension
2 Polyuria
3 Hypothermia
4 Cough

Answer: 4
Rationale: Cough is a frequent side effect of therapy with any of the angiotensin-converting enzyme inhibitors. Hypertension is not a side effect and is the reason to administer the medication. Fever is an occasional side effect. Proteinuria is another common side effect, but not polyuria.

Test-Taking Strategy: To answer this question accurately, it is necessary to be familiar with this medication and its side effects. Note the word *frequent*. If this question was difficult, review the side effects of this medication.

Level of Cognitive Ability: Application
Client Needs: Health Promotion and Maintenance
Integrated Concept/Process: Nursing Process/Implementation
Content Area: Pharmacology

Reference:
Lehne, R. (2001). *Pharmacology for nursing care* (4th ed.). Philadelphia: W.B. Saunders, p. 444.

---

126. Lithium carbonate (Eskalith) is prescribed for a client. Which of the following statements indicate that the client understands the prescribed lithium carbonate regimen?
1 "My last blood test showed that my salt level is normal."
2 "I keep my medication next to the milk in the refrigerator so that I can remember to take it every day."
3 "It is not difficult to restrict my water intake."
4 "I am careful to avoid eating foods high in potassium."

Answer: 1
Rationale: Lithium replaces sodium ions in the cells and induces excretion of sodium and potassium from the body. Client teaching includes maintenance of sodium in the daily diet and increased fluid intake (at least 1 to 1.5 L/day) during maintenance. Lithium is stored at room temperature and protected from light and moisture.

Test-Taking Strategy: Use the process of elimination. Remembering that lithium is a salt will assist in directing you to the correct option. If you had difficulty with this question, review this medication.

Level of Cognitive Ability: Comprehension
Client Need: Health Promotion and Maintenance
Integrated Concept/Process: Nursing Process/Evaluation
Content Area: Pharmacology

Reference:
Hodgson, B., & Kizior, R. (2003). *Saunders nursing drug handbook 2003.* Philadelphia: W.B. Saunders, p. 672.

---

127. An elderly client is given a prescription for haloperidol (Haldol). The nurse reinforces instructions with the client and family and tells the family to report any signs of pseudoparkinsonism. Which of the following symptoms would the nurse instruct the family to monitor for?
1 Stooped posture, shuffling gait
2 Muscle weakness, decreased salivation

Answer: 1
Rationale: Pseudoparkinsonism is a common extrapyramidal side effect of antipsychotic medications. This condition is characterized by a stooped posture, shuffling gait, masklike facial appearance, drooling, tremors, and pill-rolling motions of fingers. Hyperreflexia and aphasia are not characteristic of pseudoparkinsonism.

Test-Taking Strategy: Knowledge regarding the characteristics of pseudoparkinsonism is necessary to answer the question. Review

3 Tremors, hyperreflexia
4 Motor restlessness, aphasia

these characteristics and the effects of antipsychotic medications if you had difficulty with this question.

Level of Cognitive Ability: Application
Client Needs: Health Promotion and Maintenance
Integrated Concept/Process: Teaching/Learning
Content Area: Pharmacology

Reference:
Hodgson, B., & Kizior, R. (2003). *Saunders nursing drug handbook 2003.* Philadelphia: W.B. Saunders, p. 542.

---

128. A client on tranylcypromine (Parnate) requests information about foods that are contraindicated while on this medication. The nurse tells the client that which of the following foods can be safely included in the diet?
1 Raisins
2 Smoked fish
3 Yogurt
4 Oranges

Answer: 4
Rationale: Tranylcypromine is classified as a monoamine inhibitor, and as such tyramine-containing food should be avoided. Types of food to be avoided include, but are not limited to, those in options 1, 2, and 3. In addition, beer, wine, caffeine beverages, pickled meats, yeast preparations, avocados, bananas, and plums are to be avoided. Oranges are permissible.

Test-Taking Strategy: Use the process of elimination. Note the similarities in options 1, 2, and 3. Options 1, 2, and 3 are foods that are processed or contain some type of additive. If you had difficulty with this question, review foods high in tyramine.

Level of Cognitive Ability: Application
Client Needs: Health Promotion and Maintenance
Integrated Concept/Process: Nursing Process/Implementation
Content Area: Pharmacology

Reference:
Hodgson, B., & Kizior, R. (2003). *Saunders nursing drug handbook 2003.* Philadelphia: W.B. Saunders, p. 1115.

---

129. A nurse is giving instructions to a client with peptic ulcer disease about symptom management. The nurse tells the client to do which of the following?
1 Eat slowly and chew food thoroughly
2 Eat large meals to absorb gastric acid
3 Limit intake of water
4 Use aspirin to relieve gastric pain

Answer: 1
Rationale: The client with a peptic ulcer is taught to eat smaller, frequent meals to help keep the gastric secretions neutralized. The client should eat slowly and chew thoroughly to prevent excess gastric acid secretion. The client should drink at least 6 to 8 glasses of water per day to dilute gastric acid. The use of aspirin is avoided, because it is irritating to gastric mucosa.

Test-Taking Strategy: Use the process of elimination. Focus on the client's diagnosis and use knowledge of concepts related to digestion and knowledge of substances that are known gastric irritants to direct you to option 1. Review teaching points related to the client with peptic ulcer disease if you had difficulty with this question.

Level of Cognitive Ability: Application
Client Needs: Health Promotion and Maintenance
Integrated Concept/Process: Teaching/Learning
Content Area: Adult Health/Gastrointestinal

Reference:
Black, J., Hawks, J., & Keene, A. (2001). *Medical-surgical nursing: clinical management for positive outcomes* (6th ed.). Philadelphia: W.B. Saunders, p. 712.

---

130. A client with a hiatal hernia asks the nurse about the types of juices that will not aggravate the condition. The nurse instructs the client to drink which type of juice?
1 Tomato juice
2 Orange juice
3 Grapefruit juice
4 Apple juice

Answer: 4
Rationale: Substances that are irritating to the client with a hiatal hernia include tomato products and citrus fruits, which should be avoided. Because caffeine stimulates gastric acid secretion, beverages that contain caffeine, such as coffee, tea, cola, and cocoa, are also eliminated from the diet.

Test-Taking Strategy: Use the process of elimination. Eliminate options 1, 2, and 3 because they are similar and are irritating to the gastrointestinal system. Apple juice is the least irritating substance. Review the food items that are least irritating for the client with hiatal hernia if you had difficulty with this question.

Level of Cognitive Ability: Application
Client Needs: Health Promotion and Maintenance
Integrated Concept/Process: Teaching/Learning
Content Area: Adult Health/Gastrointestinal

Reference:
Black, J., Hawks, J., & Keene, A. (2001). *Medical-surgical nursing: clinical management for positive outcomes* (6th ed.). Philadelphia: W.B. Saunders, pp. 696; 698.

---

131. A nurse's teaching plan for the client with seizures includes reinforcing information about the safe use of phenytoin (Dilantin). The nurse instructs the client to do which of the following?
1 Take the anticonvulsant for life
2 Not skip a dose without expecting the occurrence of a serious effect
3 Realize that seizures cannot be completely controlled
4 Discontinue driving a car

Answer: 2
Rationale: In some well-controlled cases, the medication can eventually be discontinued. In some states, a client can drive a car if the client has had no seizures for a year. Option 2 alerts the client to the seriousness of the condition; that is, skipping a dose places the client at risk for status epilepticus.

Test-Taking Strategy: Use the process of elimination. General principles related to medication administration will direct you to option 2. Review care to the client taking phenytoin if you had difficulty with this question.

Level of Cognitive Ability: Application
Client Needs: Health Promotion and Maintenance
Integrated Concept/Process: Teaching/Learning
Content Area: Pharmacology

Reference:
Hodgson, B., & Kizior, R. (2003). *Saunders nursing drug handbook 2003.* Philadelphia: W.B. Saunders, p. 891.

---

132. A hospitalized client with a spinal cord injury (SCI) experiences bladder spasms and reflex incontinence. In preparing for discharge, the nurse reinforces instruc-

Answer: 4
Rationale: Caffeine in the diet can contribute to bladder spasms and reflex incontinence. Therefore it should be eliminated from the diet of the client with a SCI. Limiting fluid intake does not

tions and tells the client to do which of the following?
1   Limit fluid intake to 1000 mL in 24 hours
2   Take own temperature every day
3   Catheterize self every 2 hours PRN to prevent spasm
4   Avoid caffeine in the diet

prevent spasm and could place the client at further risk of urinary tract infection. Self-monitoring of temperature would be useful in detecting infection, but does nothing to alleviate bladder spasms. Self-catheterization every 2 hours is too frequent and serves no useful purpose.

Test-Taking Strategy: Use the process of elimination and focus on the issues: bladder spasms and reflex incontinence. Eliminate options 1 and 3 first because they increase the client's risk of urinary tract infection and are therefore not appropriate. Choose option 4 instead of option 2 because option 2 would be used to detect infection and does not deal with spasm and incontinence. Review care to the client with a SCI if you had difficulty with this question.

Level of Cognitive Ability: Application
Client Needs: Health Promotion and Maintenance
Integrated Concept/Process: Teaching/Learning
Content Area: Adult Health/Neurological

Reference:
Black, J., Hawks, J., & Keene, A. (2001). *Medical-surgical nursing: clinical management for positive outcomes* (6th ed.). Philadelphia: W.B. Saunders, p. 2059.

---

133. A client with atherosclerosis asks the nurse about dietary modifications to lower the risk of heart disease. The nurse encourages the client to eat which of the following foods that will lower the risk of heart disease?
1   Baked chicken with skin
2   Fresh cantaloupe
3   Broiled cheeseburger
4   Mashed potato with gravy

Answer: 2
Rationale: To lower the risk of heart disease, the diet should be low in saturated fat with the appropriate number of total calories. The diet should include fewer red meats and more white meat, with the skin removed. Dairy products used should be low in fat, and foods with high amounts of empty calories should be avoided.

Test-Taking Strategy: Use the process of elimination. Eliminate options 1 and 3 first, because of the fat content of the described meats. Choose option 2 instead of option 4 because fresh fruits and vegetables are naturally low in fat. Review foods low in fat if you had difficulty with this question.

Level of Cognitive Ability: Application
Client Needs: Health Promotion and Maintenance
Integrated Concept/Process: Nursing Process/Implementation
Content Area: Adult Health/Cardiovascular

Reference:
Williams, S. (2001) *Basic nutrition & diet therapy* (11th ed.). St Louis: Mosby, p. 356.

---

134. A client is being discharged and allowed to return home after angioplasty that used the right femoral area as the catheter insertion site. The nurse reinforces instructions to the client and explains that which of the following signs and

Answer: 4
Rationale: The client may feel some mild discomfort at the catheter insertion site after angioplasty. This is usually relieved by analgesics such as acetaminophen (Tylenol). The client is taught to report to the physician any neurovascular changes to the affected leg, bleeding or bruising at the insertion site, and signs

symptoms may be expected after the procedure?

1   Coolness or discoloration of the right foot
2   Temperature as high as 101° F
3   Large area of bruising in the right groin
4   Mild discomfort in the right groin

of local infection such as drainage at the site or increased temperature.

Test-Taking Strategy: Use the process of elimination. Knowing that bleeding and infection are complications of the procedure guides you to eliminate options 2 and 3. You would choose option 4 instead of option 1 by knowing that neurovascular status should not be impaired by the procedure, or by knowing that the area may be mildly uncomfortable. Review postprocedure expectations if you had difficulty with this question.

Level of Cognitive Ability: Application
Client Needs: Health Promotion and Maintenance
Integrated Concept/Process: Nursing Process/Implementation
Content Area: Adult Health/Cardiovascular

Reference:
Black, J., Hawks, J., & Keene, A. (2001). *Medical-surgical nursing: clinical management for positive outcomes* (6th ed.). Philadelphia: W.B. Saunders, p. 1406.

---

135. A nurse is teaching dietary modifications to a hypertensive client. The nurse encourages which of the following snack foods that will be acceptable for this client?

1   Cheese and crackers
2   Honeydew melon slices
3   Frozen pizza
4   Canned tomato soup

Answer: 2
Rationale: Sodium should be avoided by the client with hypertension. Fresh fruits and vegetables are naturally low in sodium. Hypertensive clients are also advised to keep fat intake to less than 30% of the total daily calories. Each of the incorrect options contains high amounts of sodium.

Test-Taking Strategy: Use the process of elimination. Recall that the client with hypertension should limit sodium intake. Eliminate options 1, 3, and 4 because they are similar. The correct option is not only a fruit but also the only unprocessed food in the choices given. Review the foods low in sodium if you had difficulty with this question.

Level of Cognitive Ability: Application
Client Needs: Health Promotion and Maintenance
Integrated Concept/Process: Nursing Process/Implementation
Content Area: Adult Health/Cardiovascular

Reference:
Williams, S. (2001) *Basic nutrition & diet therapy* (11th ed.). St Louis: Mosby, p. 366.

---

136. A nurse is reinforcing instructions to a client who will be discharged to return home with a halo vest. Which of the following instructions would the nurse include in the discussion?

1   Have the spouse use the metal frame to assist the client to sit upright
2   Perform pin care three times a week, using hydrogen peroxide or alcohol

Answer: 4
Rationale: The metal frame is never used or pulled on for turning or lifting. Pin care should be performed at least once a day using soap and water with cotton-tipped swabs or alcohol swabs. The bolts should never be loosened except in an emergency, and the physician should be notified if the bolts loosen. The client is instructed to carry the correct size wrench in case of an emergency requiring cardiopulmonary resuscitation (CRP). In such a situation, the anterior portion of the vest, including the anterior bolts, must be loosened, and the

3   Loosen the bolts once a day for bathing

4   Carry the correct size wrench to loosen the bolts in an emergency

posterior portion should remain in place to provide stability for the spine during CPR.

Test-Taking Strategy: Try to visualize the appearance of a halo vest. Eliminate option 2 first because pin care should be done at least once a day. Eliminate option 1 because pulling on the frame will disrupt the stabilization of the fracture and possibly lead to serious complications. Bolts should never be loosened except in an emergency situation. Review teaching points related to this device if you had difficulty with this question.

Level of Cognitive Ability: Application
Client Needs: Health Promotion and Maintenance
Integrated Concept/Process: Teaching/Learning
Content Area: Adult Health/Neurological

Reference:
Black, J., Hawks, J., & Keene, A. (2001). *Medical-surgical nursing: clinical management for positive outcomes* (6th ed.). Philadelphia: W.B. Saunders, p. 2054.

---

137. A client is taking iron supplements to treat iron-deficiency anemia. The nurse tells the client to do which of the following while on iron therapy?
1   Avoid taking the iron with milk or antacids
2   Limit intake of meat, fish, and poultry
3   Eat a low-fiber diet
4   Limit intake of fluids

Answer: 1
Rationale: The client should avoid taking iron with milk or antacids, which decreases the absorption of iron. The client should also avoid taking iron with food if possible. The client should increase natural sources of iron, such as meats, fish, and poultry. Finally, the client should take in sufficient fiber and fluids to prevent constipation, which is a side effect of therapy.

Test-Taking Strategy: Use the process of elimination. Begin to answer this question by eliminating options 3 and 4, knowing that constipation is a side effect of iron therapy. From the remaining options, recalling the nutritional contents of meat products will assist in eliminating option 2. Remember that milk products or antacids impair absorption of certain medications. Review this medication if you had difficulty with this question.

Level of Cognitive Ability: Application
Client Needs: Health Promotion and Maintenance
Integrated Concept/Process: Nursing Process/Implementation
Content Area: Pharmacology

Reference:
Black, J., Hawks, J., & Keene, A. (2001). *Medical-surgical nursing: clinical management for positive outcomes* (6th ed.). Philadelphia: W.B. Saunders, p. 2104.

---

138. A client with a colostomy complains to the nurse of appliance odor. The nurse recommends that the client consume which of the following deodorizing foods?
1   Yogurt
2   Mushrooms

Answer: 1
Rationale: Foods that help to eliminate odor from a colostomy include yogurt, buttermilk, spinach, beet greens, and parsley. Foods that cause odor include alcohol, beans, turnips, radishes, asparagus, onions, cucumbers, mushrooms, cabbage, eggs, and fish.

3 Cucumbers
4 Eggs

Test-Taking Strategy: Use the process of elimination. Remember foods that cause gas in the client with normal gastrointestinal function also cause gas in the gastrointestinal tract of the client with a colostomy. Review these gas-forming foods if you had difficulty with this question.

Level of Cognitive Ability: Application
Client Needs: Health Promotion and Maintenance
Integrated Concept/Process: Nursing Process/Implementation
Content Area: Adult Health/Gastrointestinal

Reference:
Black, J., Hawks, J., & Keene, A. (2001). *Medical-surgical nursing: clinical management for positive outcomes* (6th ed.). Philadelphia: W.B. Saunders, p. 786.

---

139. A nurse is reinforcing instructions about colostomy care to a client. The nurse demonstrates correct cutting of the appliance by making the circle how much larger than the client's stoma?
1 1/16 inch
2 1/8 inch
3 1/4 inch
4 1/2 inch

Answer: 2
Rationale: The size of the opening for the appliance is generally cut 1/8-inch larger than the size of the client's stoma. This minimizes the amount of exposed skin but does not cause pressure on the stoma itself. Options 1, 3, and 4 are incorrect.

Test-Taking Strategy: Use the process of elimination. Begin to answer this question by eliminating options 3 and 4 because they leave too much skin area exposed for possible irritation by gastrointestinal contents. From the remaining options, eliminate option 1 because 1/16 inch is extremely small and not realistic. Review care to the client with a colostomy if you had difficulty with this question.

Level of Cognitive Ability: Application
Client Needs: Health Promotion and Maintenance
Integrated Concept/Process: Nursing Process/Implementation
Content Area: Adult Health/Gastrointestinal

Reference:
Black, J., Hawks, J., & Keene, A. (2001). *Medical-surgical nursing: clinical management for positive outcomes* (6th ed.). Philadelphia: W.B. Saunders, p. 785.

---

140. A 10-year-old child is diagnosed with type I diabetes mellitus. The nurse prepares to reinforce diabetic teaching to the child and family and plans to teach:
1 The child's teacher to monitor insulin requirements and administer the child's insulin
2 The child to monitor insulin requirements and administer own insulin
3 The parents to always be available to monitor the child's insulin requirements
4 All the friends and family involved with the child's activities to monitor the child's insulin requirements

Answer: 2
Rationale: Most children 9 years old and older can understand the principles of monitoring their own insulin requirements. They are usually responsible enough to determine the appropriate intervention needed to maintain their health. Options 1, 3, and 4 do not support the growth and development level of this child.

Test-Taking Strategy: Use the process of elimination and growth and development concepts. The age of the child indicates that the child is able to control and be responsible for the health care situation. Eliminate option 4 first because of the absolute word *all* and because this option is unrealistic. Eliminate option 1 next because the teacher will not take responsibility for health care interventions. Eliminate option 3 because the parents cannot always be available. If you had difficulty with this question, review growth and development of a 10-year-old child.

Level of Cognitive Ability: Application
Client Needs: Health Promotion and Maintenance
Integrated Concept/Process: Nursing Process/Planning
Content Area: Child Health

Reference:
Schulte, E. Price, D., & Gwin, J. (2001). *Thompson's pediatric nursing* (8th ed.). Philadelphia: W.B. Saunders, p. 288.

---

141. A nurse is assisting in developing a plan of care for a client who attempted suicide. The nurse understands that the discharge plans for the client should focus on which of the following?
1 Weekly follow-up appointments
2 Contracts and immediately available crisis resources
3 Encouraging family and friends to always be with the client
4 Providing phone numbers for the hospital

Answer: 2
Rationale: Crisis times may occur between appointments. Contracts encourage the client to be responsible for keeping a promise. This gives the client control. Option 3 is unrealistic. Providing phone numbers will not ensure available and immediate crisis resources.

Test-Taking Strategy: Use the process of elimination. The issue of the question relates to the availability of immediate crisis resources for the client if needed. Eliminate option 3 first because it is unrealistic. Options 1 and 4 will not necessarily provide immediate resources. Review care to the client with suicide if you had difficulty with this question.

Level of Cognitive Ability: Application
Client Needs: Health Promotion and Maintenance
Integrated Concept/Process: Nursing Process/Planning
Content Area: Mental Health

Reference:
Varcarolis, E. (2002). *Foundations of psychiatric mental health nursing* (4th ed.). Philadelphia: W.B. Saunders, p. 641.

---

142. A nurse has instructed a client with hepatitis about measures to control fatigue. Which statement by the client indicates a need for further instructions?
1 "I should plan rest periods after meals."
2 "I should not engage in activity to the point of becoming overly tired."
3 "I can perform personal hygiene if I am not fatigued."
4 "I should complete all daily activities in the morning when I am most rested."

Answer: 4
Rationale: A client with hepatitis has tremendous metabolic demands that lead to fatigue and interfere with activities of daily living (ADLs.) The nurse encourages ADLs unless they cause excessive fatigue. The client is advised to plan rest periods after activities such as meals. Activities should be spaced throughout the day with frequent planned rest periods. Clients who engage in excessive activity too early in the recovery stage may experience a relapse.

Test-Taking Strategy: Note the key words *need for further instructions*. Use the process of elimination and the basic principles associated with a balance of rest and activities to answer the question. By the process of elimination, the only option that does not provide this balance is option 4. Review measures to alleviate fatigue in the client with hepatitis if you had difficulty with this question.

Level of Cognitive Ability: Comprehension
Client Needs: Health Promotion and Maintenance
Integrated Concept/Process: Teaching/Learning
Content Area: Adult Health/Gastrointestinal

Reference:
Black, J., Hawks, J., & Keene, A. (2001). *Medical-surgical nursing: clinical management for positive outcomes* (6th ed.). Philadelphia: W.B. Saunders, p. 1228.

---

143. A client who is on haloperidol (Haldol) 5 mg at bedtime also receives benztropine (Cogentin) 1 mg at the same time. The nurse reinforces instructions and tells the client that the benztropine is given to do which of the following?
  1   Decrease extrapyramidal side effects (EPS)
  2   Enhance sleep
  3   Enhance the effects of haloperidol
  4   Enhance the anticholinergic effects of the medications

Answer: 1
Rationale: Haloperidol is a neuroleptic medication that may cause the client to experience EPS. Antiparkinsonian medications such as benztropine are given to decrease the symptoms of EPS. Options 2, 3, and 4 are incorrect.

Test-Taking Strategy: Knowledge regarding the purpose of administering these medications in combination is necessary to answer the question. If you had difficulty with this question, review the purposes of these medications.

Level of Cognitive Ability: Application
Client Needs: Health Promotion and Maintenance
Integrated Concept/Process: Teaching/Learning
Content Area: Pharmacology

Reference:
Hodgson, B., & Kizior, R. (2003). *Saunders nursing drug handbook 2003.* Philadelphia: W.B. Saunders, p. 114.

---

144. A nurse provides instructions about measures to relieve the discomfort to a client with jaundice who is experiencing pruritus. Which statement by the client indicates a need for further instructions?
  1   "I should wear loose cotton clothing."
  2   "I should use tepid water for bathing."
  3   "I should maintain a warm house temperature."
  4   "I should avoid alkaline soaps."

Answer: 3
Rationale: Pruritus is caused by the accumulation of bile salts in the skin and results from obstructed biliary excretion. Antihistamines may relieve the itching, as will tepid water or emollient baths. The client should avoid alkaline soap and wear loose, soft cotton clothing. The client is instructed to keep the room cool.

Test-Taking Strategy: Use the process of elimination. Note the key words *need for further instructions.* Recalling that heat causes vasodilation will assist in answering this question. This principle should direct you to option 3 as the measure to avoid in the treatment of pruritus. If you had difficulty with this question, review the measures that assist in alleviating pruritus.

Level of Cognitive Ability: Comprehension
Client Needs: Health Promotion and Maintenance
Integrated Concept/Process: Teaching/Learning
Content Area: Adult Health/Gastrointestinal

Reference:
Black, J., Hawks, J., & Keene, A. (2001). *Medical-surgical nursing: clinical management for positive outcomes* (6th ed.). Philadelphia: W.B. Saunders, p. 1283.

145. A client is being discharged after a bronchoscopy that was performed the previous day. The nurse reinforces discharge instructions to the client. Which client statement indicates a need for further teaching?

1 "I can expect to cough up bright red blood."
2 "I will stop smoking my cigarettes."
3 "I will get help immediately if I start having trouble breathing."
4 "I will use the throat lozenges as directed by the physician until my sore throat goes away."

Answer: 1

Rationale: After the procedure, the client should be observed for signs of respiratory distress, including dyspnea, changes in respiratory rate, use of accessory muscles, and changes in or absent lung sounds. Expectorated secretions are inspected for hemoptysis. The client should avoid smoking. A sore throat is common and lozenges would be helpful as directed.

Test-Taking Strategy: Use the process of elimination. Note the key words *indicates a need for further teaching*. Option 2 and 3 can be easily eliminated first. From the remaining options, remember that bright red bleeding indicates active bleeding. Review bronchoscopy postprocedure care if you had difficulty with this question.

Level of Cognitive Ability: Comprehension
Client Needs: Health Promotion and Maintenance
Integrated Concept/Process: Teaching/Learning
Content Area: Adult Health/Respiratory

Reference:
Black, J., Hawks, J., & Keene, A. (2001). *Medical-surgical nursing: clinical management for positive outcomes* (6th ed.). Philadelphia: W.B. Saunders, p. 200.

---

146. A client who is on chlorpromazine (Thorazine) is preparing for discharge. The nurse is asked to reinforce instructions regarding the medication to the client. The nurse tells the client to do which of the following?

1 Adhere to a strict tyramine-restricted diet
2 Watch for signs and symptoms of relapse of depression
3 Avoid prolonged exposure to the sun
4 Have the therapeutic blood levels measured, because there is a narrow range between the therapeutic and toxic levels of the medication

Answer: 3

Rationale: Chlorpromazine is an antipsychotic medication often used in the treatment of psychosis. Photosensitivity is a side effect of the phenothiazine class of antipsychotic medications, to which chlorpromazine (Thorazine) belongs. Options 1, 2, and 4 are unrelated to the administration of this medication.

Test-Taking Strategy: Use the process of elimination. Because chlorpromazine is an antipsychotic, not an antidepressive medication, option 2 can be eliminated. Eliminate option 1 because this option relates to medications that are monoamine oxidase inhibitors. There is not a narrow range between therapeutic and toxic levels such as with lithium; therefore eliminate option 4. If you had difficulty with this question, review information about this medication.

Level of Cognitive Ability: Application
Client Needs: Health Promotion and Maintenance
Integrated Concept/Process: Teaching/Learning
Content Area: Pharmacology

Reference:
Hodgson, B., & Kizior, R. (2003). *Saunders nursing drug handbook 2003.* Philadelphia: W.B. Saunders, p. 233.

---

147. A nurse is evaluating a client's understanding about the signs and symptoms of hyperglycemia. Which statement by the client best reflects an accurate understanding?

Answer: 3

Rationale: Fatigue, dry skin, polyuria, and polydipsia are classic symptoms of hyperglycemia. Fatigue occurs because of lack of energy from inability of the body to use glucose. Dry skin occurs secondary to dehydration related to polyuria. Polydipsia

1 "I may become diaphoretic and faint."
2 "I should take an extra diabetic tablet if my blood sugar level is greater than 300."
3 "I may notice signs of fatigue, dry skin, polyuria, and polydipsia."
4 "I should restrict my fluid intake if my blood sugar level is greater than 250 mg."

occurs secondary to fluid loss. Diaphoresis is associated with hypoglycemia. Clients should not take extra oral hypoglycemic agents to reduce an elevated blood glucose level; to reduce hyperglycemia, regular insulin is used because of its rapid response. A client with hyperglycemia becomes dehydrated secondary to the osmotic effect of elevated glucose. Therefore the client must increase fluid intake.

Test-Taking Strategy: Use the process of elimination. Focusing on the issue, signs and symptoms, will assist in eliminating options 2 and 4. From the remaining options, discriminating between signs of hypoglycemia and hyperglycemia will direct you to option 3. Review these signs if you had difficulty with this question.

Level of Cognitive Ability: Comprehension
Client Needs: Health Promotion and Maintenance
Integrated Concept/Process: Nursing Process/Evaluation
Content Area: Adult Health/Endocrine

Reference:
Black, J., Hawks, J., & Keene, A. (2001). *Medical-surgical nursing: clinical management for positive outcomes* (6th ed.). Philadelphia: W.B. Saunders, p. 1155.

---

148. A client taking famotidine (Pepcid) asks the nurse what would be the best medication to take for a headache. Which of the following medications would the nurse advise the client to take?
1 Aspirin (acetylsalicylic acid, ASA)
2 Ibuprofen (Motrin)
3 Acetaminophen (Tylenol)
4 Naproxen (Naprosyn)

Answer: 3
Rationale: The client is taking famotidine, a histamine-receptor antagonist. This implies that the client has a disorder characterized by gastrointestinal (GI) irritation. The only listed medication that is not irritating to the GI tract is acetaminophen. The others could aggravate an already existing GI problem.

Test-Taking Strategy: To answer this question accurately, it is necessary to know the reason behind histamine receptor antagonist use. Recalling that this medication is used for GI irritation will direct you to option 3. Review these medications if you had difficulty with this question.

Level of Cognitive Ability: Application
Client Needs: Health Promotion and Maintenance
Integrated Concept/Process: Nursing Process/Implementation
Content Area: Pharmacology

Reference:
Hodgson, B., & Kizior, R. (2003). *Saunders nursing drug handbook 2003.* Philadelphia: W.B. Saunders, p. 442.

---

149. A nurse is teaching a client taking cyclosporine (Sandimmune) after renal transplant about the medication. The nurse tells the client to be especially alert for which of the following?
1 Signs of infection
2 Hypotension

Answer: 1
Rationale: Cyclosporine is an immunosuppressant medication used to prevent transplant rejection. The client should be especially alert for signs and symptoms of infection while taking this medication, and report them to the physician if experienced. The client is also taught about other side effects of the medication including hypertension, increased facial hair, tremors, gingival hyperplasia, and gastrointestinal complaints.

3 Weight loss
4 Hair loss

Test-Taking Strategy: Use the process of elimination. Recalling that this medication is an immunosuppressant and that the client is at risk for infection will direct you to option 1. Review this information because it involves a fundamental concept in transplant medication therapy.

Level of Cognitive Ability: Application
Client Needs: Health Promotion and Maintenance
Integrated Concept/Process: Teaching/Learning
Content Area: Pharmacology

Reference:
Hodgson, B., & Kizior, R. (2003). *Saunders nursing drug handbook 2003.* Philadelphia: W.B. Saunders, p. 293.

---

150. A client has undergone surgery for glaucoma. The nurse reinforces with the client which of the following discharge instructions?
   1 Wound healing usually takes 12 weeks
   2 Expect that vision will be permanently impaired to a small degree
   3 A shield or eye patch should be worn to protect the eye
   4 The sutures are removed after 1 week

Answer: 3
Rationale: After ocular surgery, the client should wear a shield or eye patch to protect the eye. Healing occurs in approximately 6 weeks. After the postoperative inflammation subsides, the client's vision should return to the preoperative level of acuity. Most sutures used are absorable.

Test-Taking Strategy: Use Maslow's Hierarchy of Needs theory to answer this question and note that the client has had eye surgery. Safety is the issue. This will direct you to option 3. If you had difficulty with this question, review postoperative teaching points following eye surgery.

Level of Cognitive Ability: Application
Client Needs: Health Promotion and Maintenance
Integrated Concept/Process: Self-Care
Content Area: Adult Health/Eye

Reference:
Black, J., Hawks, J., & Keene, A. (2001). *Medical-surgical nursing: clinical management for positive outcomes* (6th ed.). Philadelphia: W.B. Saunders, p. 1819.

---

151. A client has undergone surgery for cataract removal. The nurse instructs the client to call the physician for which of the following complaints?
   1 A sudden decrease in vision
   2 Eye pain relieved by acetaminophen (Tylenol)
   3 Small amounts of dried matter on eyelashes after sleep
   4 Gradual resolution of eye redness

Answer: 1
Rationale: The client should report a noticeable or sudden decrease in vision to the physician. The client is taught to take acetaminophen, which is usually effective in relieving discomfort. The eye may be slightly reddened postoperatively, but this should gradually resolve. Small amounts of dried material may be present on the lashes after sleep. This is expected, and the material should be removed with a warm, damp facecloth.

Test-Taking Strategy: Focus on the issue: the need to call the physician. Noting the key words *sudden decrease* in option 1 will direct you to this option. Review client instructions after this surgery if you had difficulty with this question.

Level of Cognitive Ability: Application
Client Needs: Health Promotion and Maintenance

Integrated Concept/Process: Teaching/Learning
Content Area: Adult Health/Eye

Reference:
Black, J., Hawks, J., & Keene, A. (2001). *Medical-surgical nursing: clinical management for positive outcomes* (6th ed.). Philadelphia: W.B. Saunders, p. 1814.

---

152. A nurse is assigned to care for a client diagnosed with cirrhosis and ascites. Which of the following dietary measures will the nurse expect to be prescribed for the client?
1   Decreased fat intake
2   Decreased carbohydrates
3   Calorie restriction of 1500 daily
4   Sodium restriction

Answer: 4
Rationale: If the client has ascites, sodium and possibly fluids should be restricted in the diet. Fat restriction is not necessary. Total daily calories should range between 2000 and 3000. The diet should supply sufficient carbohydrates to maintain weight and ample protein to rebuild tissue, but not enough protein to precipitate hepatic encephalopathy.

Test-Taking Strategy: Focus on the client's diagnosis. Recalling the definition of ascites will direct you to option 4. If you had difficulty with this question, review dietary measures for the client with cirrhosis and ascites.

Level of Cognitive Ability: Comprehension
Client Needs: Health Promotion and Maintenance
Integrated Concept/Process: Nursing Process/Planning
Content Area: Adult Health/Gastrointestinal

Reference:
Black, J., Hawks, J., & Keene, A. (2001). *Medical-surgical nursing: clinical management for positive outcomes* (6th ed.). Philadelphia: W.B. Saunders, p. 1253.

---

153. A nurse is preparing a client with a diagnosis of multiple myeloma for discharge. Which of the following instructions will the nurse reinforce?
1   Restrict fluid intake to 1500 mL daily
2   Maintain bed rest
3   Maintain a high-calorie, low-fiber diet
4   Notify the physician if anorexia and nausea persists

Answer: 4
Rationale: Clients with multiple myeloma should be taught to watch for signs of hypercalcemia and to report them immediately to the physician. Anorexia, nausea, vomiting, polyuria, weakness and fatigue, constipation, and dehydration are signs of moderate hypercalcemia. A fluid intake of about 3000 mL daily is necessary to dilute the calcium overload and prevent protein from precipitating in the renal tubules. Activity is encouraged. Although a high-calorie diet is encouraged, a diet low in fiber will lead to constipation.

Test-Taking Strategy: Use the process of elimination, recalling that hypercalcemia is a concern in multiple myeloma Eliminate option 2 first knowing that bed rest is not indicated. Next eliminate option 1 because this amount of fluid is rather low. Finally, eliminate option 3 because of the low-fiber diet stated in the option. Review the signs of hypercalcemia if you had difficulty in selecting the correct option.

Level of Cognitive Ability: Analysis
Client Needs: Health Promotion and Maintenance
Integrated Concept/Process: Teaching/Learning
Content Area: Adult Health/Oncology

Reference:
Black, J., Hawks, J., & Keene, A. (2001). *Medical-surgical nursing: clinical management for positive outcomes* (6th ed.). Philadelphia: W.B. Saunders, p. 2120.

---

154. A nurse reinforces home care instructions to a client hospitalized for a transurethral resection of the prostate (TURP). Which statement by the client indicates a need for further instructions?
1 "I should avoid strenuous activity for 4 to 6 weeks."
2 "I should maintain a daily intake of 6 to 8 glasses of water daily."
3 "I should avoid lifting items weighing more than 30 pounds."
4 "I should include prune juice in my diet."

Answer: 3

Rationale: The client should be advised to avoid strenuous activity for 4 to 6 weeks and to avoid lifting items weighing more than 20 pounds. The client should consume at least 6 to 8 glasses daily of nonalcoholic fluids to minimize clot formation. Straining during defecation for at least 6 weeks after surgery is avoided to prevent bleeding. Prune juice is a satisfactory bowel stimulant.

Test-Taking Strategy: Use the process of elimination. Focusing on the key words *need for further instructions* will assist in eliminating options 1 and 2. Considering the anatomical location of the surgical procedure, it would be reasonable to think that constipation should be avoided; therefore eliminate option 4. Lifting items weighing 30 pounds is excessive. Keeping this principle in mind will assist in directing you to option 3. Review TURP discharge teaching points if you had difficulty with this question.

Level of Cognitive Ability: Comprehension
Client Needs: Health Promotion and Maintenance
Integrated Concept/Process: Teaching/Learning
Content Area: Adult Health/Renal

Reference:
Black, J., Hawks, J., & Keene, A. (2001). *Medical-surgical nursing: clinical management for positive outcomes* (6th ed.). Philadelphia: W.B. Saunders, p. 958.

---

155. A nurse reinforces discharge instructions to a client after a mastectomy and axillary lymph node dissection. Which of the following would the nurse include in the instructions?
1 Avoid the use of insect repellent
2 Cut cuticles on nails using a clean cuticle scissor
3 Wear protective gloves when doing the dishes
4 Avoid the use of lanolin hand cream on the affected arm

Answer: 3

Rationale: After axillary node dissection, the affected arm may swell and if injured can cause complications such as infection. The client should use insect repellent to avoid bites and stings. Picking at or cutting cuticles should be avoided. Lanolin hand cream should be applied several times daily. Protective gloves should be worn while doing dishes and cleaning.

Test-Taking Strategy: Focus on the issue: preventing altered skin integrity and thus infection. Keeping this concept in mind will assist in eliminating options 1, 2, and 4, which could potentially lead to a skin alteration. Review the client teaching points related to mastectomy and lymph node dissection if you had difficulty with this question.

Level of Cognitive Ability: Application
Client Needs: Health Promotion and Maintenance
Integrated Concept/Process: Self-Care
Content Area: Adult Health/Oncology

Reference:
Ignatavicius, D., & Workman, M. (2002). *Medical-surgical: critical thinking for collaborative care* (4th ed.). Philadelphia: W.B. Saunders, p. 1746.

156. A camp nurse provides instruction about protecting the skin from the sun to parents who are preparing their children for a camping adventure. Which of the following would not be included in the instructions?

1   Sun screens with a sun protection factor (SPF) of 15 or more is recommended
2   Sun screen will not be necessary on cloudy days
3   Pack a hat, long-sleeved shirt, and long pants for the child
4   Select tightly woven materials for greater protection from sun rays

Answer: 2

Rationale: Sun rays are as damaging to the skin on cloudy or hazy days as they are on sunny days. Sun screens with a SPF of 15 or more are recommended and should be applied before exposure to the sun and reapplied frequently and liberally at least every 2 hours. A hat, long-sleeved shirt, and long pants should be worn when out in the sun. Tightly woven materials provide greater protection from the sun rays.

Test-Taking Strategy: Note the key word *not*. Recalling the concept that the ultraviolet rays can be damaging regardless of cloudiness or haziness will assist in directing you to option 2. Eliminate options 1, 3, and 4 because these measures provide the greatest protection from the sun. Review guidelines about how to protect the skin from the damaging rays of the sun if you had difficulty with this question.

Level of Cognitive Ability: Application
Client Needs: Health Promotion and Maintenance
Integrated Concept/Process: Nursing Process/Implementation
Content Area: Fundamental Skills

Reference:
Black, J., Hawks, J., & Keene, A. (2001). *Medical-surgical nursing: clinical management for positive outcomes* (6th ed.). Philadelphia: W.B. Saunders, p. 1305.

157. A client is receiving a course of chemotherapy for a diagnosis of lung cancer. The nurse reinforces which of the following home care instructions to the client?

1   A bathroom can be shared with any of the other members of the family
2   Urinary and bowel excreta is not considered contaminated
3   Disposable plates and plastic utensils must be used during the entire course of chemotherapy
4   Contaminated linens should be washed separately and then washed a second time

Answer: 4

Rationale: The client may excrete the chemotherapeutic agent for 48 hours or more after administration, depending on the medication administered. During this time, blood, emesis, and excreta may be considered contaminated, and the client should not share a bathroom with children or pregnant women. Any contaminated linens or clothing should be washed separately and then washed a second time. The second wash may be done with the rest of the household laundry if necessary. All contaminated disposable items should be sealed in plastic bags and disposed of as hazardous waste.

Test-Taking Strategy: Use the process of elimination. Eliminate options 1 and 2 first because the concepts in each are similar. Eliminate option 3 next because it would seem unreasonable to have to use disposable utensils for the *entire* course of therapy. Review client teaching points related to chemotherapy if you had difficulty with this question.

Level of Cognitive Ability: Application
Client Needs: Health Promotion and Maintenance
Integrated Concept/Process: Teaching/Learning
Content Area: Adult Health/Oncology

Reference:
Ignatavicius, D., & Workman, M. (2002). *Medical-surgical nursing: critical thinking for collaborative care* (4th ed.). Philadelphia: W.B. Saunders, p. 432.

158. A nurse is caring for a client with bowel cancer who recently received a course of chemotherapy and has developed stomatitis. The nurse reinforces instructions to the client regarding the stomatitis. Which statement by the client indicates a need for further instructions?
1 "I should drink foods and liquids that are cold."
2 "I should avoid foods with spices."
3 "I should eat soft foods."
4 "I should avoid citrus fruits and juices."

Answer: 1
Rationale: Stomatitis is a term used to describe inflammation and ulceration of the mucosal lining of the mouth. Dietary modifications for this condition include avoiding extremely hot or cold foods, spices, and citrus fruits and juices. The client should be instructed to eat soft foods and take nutritional supplements as prescribed.

Test-Taking Strategy: Note the key words *need for further instructions*. Knowledge that stomatitis is an inflammation of the mucosal lining of the mouth will assist in eliminating those options that include measures to reduce further irritation. Eliminate options 2, 3, and 4 because these measures will prevent further discomfort. Review client teaching points for stomatitis if you had difficulty with this question.

Level of Cognitive Ability: Application
Client Needs: Health Promotion and Maintenance
Integrated Concept/Process: Teaching/Learning
Content Area: Adult Health/Oncology

Reference:
Ignatavicius, D., & Workman, M. (2002). *Medical-surgical: critical thinking for collaborative care* (4th ed.). Philadelphia: W.B. Saunders, p. 434.

159. A nurse prepares to reinforce instructions to a postpartum client who has developed breast engorgement. Which of the following instructions would the nurse provide to the client?
1 Feed the infant less frequently, every 4 to 6 hours, using bottle-feeding in between
2 Apply cool packs to both breasts 20 minutes before a feeding
3 Avoid the use of a bra during engorgement
4 During feeding, gently massage the breast from the outer areas to the nipple

Answer: 4
Rationale: The client with breast engorgement should be advised to feed frequently, at least every 2 1/2 hours for 15 to 20 minutes per side. Moist heat should be applied to both breasts for about 20 minutes before a feeding. Between feedings, the mother should wear a supportive bra. During a feeding, it is helpful to gently massage the breast from the outer areas to the nipple to stimulate letdown and flow of milk.

Test-Taking Strategy: Consider the manifestations that occur with engorgement and eliminate those options that will not assist in increasing the flow of milk. With this concept in mind, you should be able to eliminate options 1 and 2. From the remaining options, select option 4 because massage would assist in the flow of milk. In addition, a supportive bra would reduce the discomfort that occurs with this condition. If you had difficulty with this question, review the measures for breast engorgement.

Level of Cognitive Ability: Application
Client Needs: Health Promotion and Maintenance
Integrated Concept/Process: Self-Care
Content Area: Maternity

Reference:
McKinney, E., Ashwill, J., Murray, S. et al. (2000). *Maternal-child nursing.* Philadelphia: W.B. Saunders, p. 595.

160. A client in the third trimester of pregnancy arrives at the physician's office and tells the nurse that she frequently has a backache. Which of the following instructions would the nurse provide to the client to ease the backache?
1. Sleep in a supine position on a firm mattress
2. Maintain correct posture
3. Eat small meals frequently
4. Elevate the legs when sitting

Answer: 2
Rationale: To provide relief from backache, the nurse would advise the client to use good posture and body mechanics, perform pelvic rock exercises, and wear flat supportive shoes. The client would also be instructed to avoid overexertion and sleep in the lateral position on a firm mattress. Back massage is also helpful. Eating small meals would more specifically help relieve dyspnea. Leg elevation assists the client with varicosities.

Test-Taking Strategy: Use the process of elimination, keeping in mind that the issue of the question is backache. This should assist in eliminating options 3 and 4 because they are unrelated to the relief of backache. From the remaining options, recalling that the lateral position is most appropriate will direct you to option 2. Review relief measures for backache if you had difficulty with this question.

Level of Cognitive Ability: Application
Client Needs: Health Promotion and Maintenance
Integrated Concept/Process: Nursing Process/Implementation
Content Area: Maternity

Reference:
McKinney, E., Ashwill, J., Murray, S. et al. (2000). *Maternal-child nursing.* Philadelphia: W.B. Saunders, p. 280.

---

161. A nurse reinforces dietary instructions with a client receiving spironolactone (Aldactone). Which of the following foods would the nurse instruct the client to avoid while taking this medication?
1. Crackers
2. Shrimp
3. Apricots
4. Popcorn

Answer: 3
Rationale: Spironolactone is a potassium-sparing diuretic, and the client should avoid foods high in potassium such as whole grain cereals, legumes, meat, bananas, apricots, orange juice, potatoes, and raisins. Option 3 provides the highest source of potassium and should be avoided.

Test-Taking Strategy: Use the process of elimination and note the key word *avoid*. Begin by eliminating options 1 and 4 because they are food items that are similar. Remembering that fruits, vegetables, and fresh meats are high in potassium will assist in directing you to option 3 as the food to avoid. Review the foods high in potassium if you had difficulty with this question.

Level of Cognitive Ability: Application
Client Needs: Health Promotion and Maintenance
Integrated Concept/Process: Teaching/Learning
Content Area: Pharmacology

Reference:
Hodgson, B., & Kizior, R. (2003). *Saunders nursing drug handbook 2003.* Philadelphia: W.B. Saunders, p. 1030.

162. Oral lactulose (Chronulac) is prescribed for a client with a hepatic disorder. The nurse reinforces instructions to the client about this medication. Which of the following instructions would not be part of the teaching plan?

1 The medication may be taken with milk
2 Increase fluid intake while taking the medication
3 Increase fiber in the diet
4 Notify the physician if nausea occurs

Answer: 4

Rationale: Lactulose retains ammonia in the colon and promotes increased peristalsis and bowel evacuation, expelling ammonia from the colon. The medication should be taken with water, juice, or milk to aid in softening the stool. An increased fluid intake and a high-fiber diet will promote defecation. If nausea occurs, the client should be instructed to drink cola or eat unsalted crackers or dry toast.

Test-Taking Strategy: Use the process of elimination and note the key word *not*. Eliminate options 2 and 3 first because they are similar in that they will both promote defecation. Remembering that the client can be provided measures to relieve nausea without having to notify the physician will direct you to option 4. Review this medication if you had difficulty with this question.

Level of Cognitive Ability: Application
Client Needs: Health Promotion and Maintenance
Integrated Concept/Process: Teaching/Learning
Content Area: Pharmacology

Reference:
Hodgson, B., & Kizior, R. (2003). *Saunders nursing drug handbook 2003.* Philadelphia: W.B. Saunders, p. 638.

---

163. A client with leukemia receives a course of chemotherapy. The nurse is told that the client's neutrophil count is 600/mm^3. The nurse reinforces which of the following instructions to the client for home care?

1 Avoid eating any raw fruits or vegetables
2 Avoid aspirin or medications containing aspirin
3 Avoid straining at bowel movements
4 Use an electric shaver for shaving

Answer: 1

Rationale: Neutrophil counts should range between 3000 and 5800/mm^3. A low neutrophil count places the client at risk for infection. A client at risk for infection should avoid exposure to individuals with colds or infections. All live plants, flowers, or objects that harbor bacteria, such as stuffed animals, should be removed from the client's environment. The client should be on a low-bacteria diet that excludes raw fruits and vegetables. Options 2, 3, and 4 are measures that would be implemented if the client was at risk for bleeding.

Test-Taking Strategy: Recall that a low neutrophil count places the client at risk for infection. Remembering that the issue of the question relates to infection will assist in eliminating options 2, 3, and 4 because these options identify measures that reduce the risk of bleeding. Review the measures that reduce the risk of infection if you had difficulty with this question.

Level of Cognitive Ability: Application
Client Needs: Health Promotion and Maintenance
Integrated Concept/Process: Nursing Process/Implementation
Content Area: Adult Health/Oncology

Reference:
Ignatavicius, D., & Workman, M. (2002). *Medical-surgical: critical thinking for collaborative care* (4th ed.). Philadelphia: W.B. Saunders, p. 435.

164. A child admitted to the hospital for sickle cell crisis is preparing for discharge. The nurse reinforces instructions to the parents about measures to prevent a crisis. Which of the following would not be included in the instructions?
1   Avoid high altitudes and air travel
2   Increase oral fluid intake
3   Notify the physician if vomiting or diarrhea occurs
4   Increase the dose of the analgesic as soon as the pain begins

Answer: 4
Rationale: The parents should be provided with information on how to prevent crises from occurring with the child, such as avoiding high altitudes and flying in nonpressurized planes because oxygen tension is lowered under these conditions. Dehydration should be avoided, and the parents should call the physician if vomiting, diarrhea, high fever, or any other cause of water loss develops in the child. Analgesics should not be increased.

Test-Taking Strategy: Note the key word "not." Knowledge regarding the causes of crises will assist in answering this question. However, using basic principles related to client instructions regarding medications will assist in directing you to option 4. Clients should not be instructed to increase medication unless specifically prescribed. If you had difficulty with this question, review the causes of sickle cell crisis.

Level of Cognitive Ability: Application
Client Needs: Health Promotion and Maintenance
Integrated Concept/Process: Teaching/Learning
Content Area: Child Health

Reference:
Wong, D., & Hockenberry-Eaton, M. (2001). *Wong's essentials of pediatric nursing* (6th ed.). St. Louis: Mosby, p. 989.

165. A nurse is reinforcing instructions to a client who received cryosurgery for a localized cervical tumor. The nurse tells the client which of the following?
1   To call the physician if a watery discharge occurs
2   To call the physician if the discharge remains odorous in 1 week
3   To avoid tub baths
4   That pain indicates a complication of procedure

Answer: 3
Rationale: Mild pain may occur and continue for several days after this procedure. A clear watery discharge is expected for several weeks. This is followed by discharge containing debris, which may be odorous. If the discharge continues longer than 8 weeks, an infection is suspected. Healing takes about 10 weeks. Showers or sponge baths should be taken during this time and tub baths and sitz baths should be avoided.

Test-Taking Strategy: Use the process of elimination. Consider the area of the body where this procedure is performed. It would seem likely that the client would be instructed to avoid tub baths after this procedure. Review teaching points related to this procedure if you had difficulty with this question.

Level of Cognitive Ability: Application
Client Needs: Health Promotion and Maintenance
Integrated Concept/Process: Nursing Process/Implementation
Content Area: Adult Health/Oncology

Reference:
Ignatavicius, D., & Workman, M. (2002). *Medical-surgical: critical thinking for collaborative care* (4th ed.). Philadelphia: W.B. Saunders, p. 1774.

166. A nurse reinforces instructions to a client taking digoxin (Lanoxin) 0.25 mg daily. Which of the following client

Answer: 1
Rationale: Digoxin is an antidysrhythmic. The most common early manifestations of toxicity are gastrointestinal (GI) disturbances,

statements would indicate a need for further instructions?
1 "I will take my prescribed antacid if I become nauseated."
2 "It is important to have my blood drawn when prescribed."
3 "I will check my pulse before I take my medication."
4 "I will carry a medication identification (ID) card with me."

such as anorexia, nausea, and vomiting. Digoxin blood levels should be obtained as prescribed to monitor for therapeutic plasma levels (0.5 to 2.0 ng/mL). The client is instructed to take the pulse, hold the medication if the pulse is below 60 beats per minute, and notify the physician. The client is instructed to wear or carry an ID bracelet or card.

Test-Taking Strategy: Note the key words *need for further instructions*. Remembering that GI disturbances are the earliest signs of digoxin toxicity will assist in directing you to option 1. Review this medication and signs of toxicity if you had difficulty with this question.

Level of Cognitive Ability: Comprehension
Client Needs: Health Promotion and Maintenance
Integrated Concept/Process: Teaching/Learning
Content Area: Pharmacology

Reference:
Hodgson, B., & Kizior, R. (2003). *Saunders nursing drug handbook 2003.* Philadelphia: W.B. Saunders, p. 350.

---

167. A nurse is caring for a client with possible cholelithiasis who is being prepared for a cholangiogram. Which client statement indicates that the client understands the purpose of a cholangiogram as described by the nurse?
1 "They are going to 'look at' my gallbladder and ducts."
2 "This procedure will drain my gallbladder."
3 "My gallbladder will be irrigated."
4 "They will put medication in my gallbladder."

Answer: 1
Rationale: A cholangiogram is for diagnostic purposes. It outlines both the gallbladder and the ducts, so gallstones that have moved into the ductal system can be detected. X-rays are used to visualize the biliary duct system after an intravenous injection of radiopaque dye.

Test-Taking Strategy: Use the process of elimination. Note that options 2, 3, and 4 are similar because they involve some form of treatment. Option 1 involves assessment of the gallbladder. If you had difficulty with this question, review the purpose of this procedure.

Level of Cognitive Ability: Comprehension
Client Needs: Health Promotion and Maintenance
Integrated Concept/Process: Nursing Process/Evaluation
Content Area: Adult Health/Gastrointestinal

Reference:
Ignatavicius, D., & Workman, M. (2002). *Medical-surgical: critical thinking for collaborative care* (4th ed.). Philadelphia: W.B. Saunders, p. 1327.

---

168. A nurse is providing immediate postprocedure care to a client who had a thoracentesis. The goal is that the client will exhibit normal respiratory functioning, and the nurse reinforces instructions to assist the client to achieve this goal. Which statement by the client would indicate that further instructions are needed?

Answer: 2
Rationale: After the procedure, the client is usually turned onto the unaffected side for 1 hour to facilitate lung expansion. Tachypnea, dyspnea, cyanosis, retractions, or diminished breath sounds, which may indicate pneumothorax, should be reported. A chest x-ray study may be performed to evaluate the effectiveness of the procedure. Subcutaneous emphysema may follow this procedure, because air in the pleural cavity leaks into subcutaneous tissues. The tissues feel like lumpy paper and crackle when

1   "I will let you know at once if I have trouble breathing."

2   "I will lie on my affected side for an hour."

3   "I can expect a chest x-ray to be done shortly."

4   "I will notify you if I feel a crackling sensation on my chest."

palpated (crepitus). Usually subcutaneous emphysema causes no problems unless it is increasing and constricting vital organs such as the trachea.

Test-Taking Strategy: Note the key words *further instructions are needed.* Note that option 2 states *the affected side for an hour.* Recalling that the client should be placed on the unaffected side for 1 hour to facilitate lung expansion will easily direct you to this option. Review postprocedure care after a thoracentesis if you had difficulty with this question.

Level of Cognitive Ability: Comprehension
Client Needs: Health Promotion and Maintenance
Integrated Concept/Process: Nursing Process/Evaluation
Content Area: Adult Health/Respiratory

Reference:
Ignatavicius, D., & Workman, M. (2002). *Medical-surgical: critical thinking for collaborative care* (4th ed.). Philadelphia: W.B. Saunders, p. 485.

---

169. A nurse is evaluating a client's adjustment to a new diagnosis of coronary heart disease before hospital discharge. Of the following questions, which one would the nurse ask to obtain the most useful information from the client?

1   "Do you have anyone at home to help with housework and shopping?"

2   "How do you feel about the lifestyle changes you are planning to make?"

3   "Do you understand the use of your new medications?"

4   "Are you going to book your follow-up physician visit?"

Answer: 2
Rationale: All questions relate to aspects of posthospital care, but only option 2 explores the client's feelings about the disease. Exploring feelings will assist in determining the clients adjustment to the diagnosis.

Test-Taking Strategy: Use therapeutic communication techniques. Focusing on the issue, determining the client's adjustment to a new diagnosis, will direct you to option 2. Also note that options 1, 3, and 4 are close-ended questions. Review therapeutic communication techniques if you had difficulty with this question.

Level of Cognitive Ability: Application
Client Needs: Health Promotion and Maintenance
Integrated Concept/Process: Nursing Process/Data Collection
Content Area: Fundamental Skills

Reference:
Potter, P., & Perry, A. (2001). *Fundamentals of nursing* (5th ed.). St. Louis: Mosby, p. 459.

---

170. A client recently diagnosed with angina pectoris asks the nurse how to prevent future angina attacks. The nurse includes which of the following instructions in a teaching session?

1   Eat fewer, larger meals for more efficient digestion

2   Plan all activities for early in the morning, when the client is most rested

3   Adjust medication doses freely until symptoms do not recur

Answer: 4
Rationale: Anginal episodes are triggered by events such as eating large or heavy meals, straining during bowel movements, smoking, overexertion, and experiencing emotional upset or temperature extremes. Medication therapy is monitored and regulated by the physician.

Test-Taking Strategy: Note the key words *prevent future angina attacks.* Basic knowledge of the causes of chest pain and the principles related to medication therapy helps to eliminate the incorrect options. If you had difficulty with this question, review teaching points for the client with angina.

4   Dress appropriately in very cold or very hot weather

Level of Cognitive Ability: Application
Client Needs: Health Promotion and Maintenance
Integrated Concept/Process: Self-Care
Content Area: Adult Health/Cardiovascular

Reference:
Ignatavicius, D., & Workman, M. (2002). *Medical-surgical nursing: critical thinking for collaborative care* (4th ed.). Philadelphia: W.B. Saunders, p. 631.

---

171. A nurse is caring for a client who has just returned to the nursing unit after an intravenous pyelogram (IVP). Which of the following would be a priority for the nurse in the postprocedure care of this client?
1   Encouraging increased intake of oral fluids
2   Ambulating the client in the hallway
3   Encouraging the client to try to void frequently
4   Maintaining the client on bed rest

Answer: 1
Rationale: After an IVP, the client should increase fluid intake to aid in the clearance of the dye used for the procedure. It is unnecessary to void frequently after the procedure. The client is usually allowed activity as tolerated, without any specific activity guidelines.

Test-Taking Strategy: Note the key word *priority*. Option 3 has no useful purpose and is eliminated first. You would choose correctly among the remaining options by knowing that there are no activity guidelines after this procedure. Alternatively, you could choose correctly if you know that fluids are necessary to promote clearance of the dye from the client's system. Review postprocedure care after an IVP if you had difficulty with this question.

Level of Cognitive Ability: Application
Client Needs: Health Promotion and Maintenance
Integrated Concept/Process: Nursing Process/Implementation
Content Area: Adult Health/Renal

Reference:
Ignatavicius, D., & Workman, M. (2002). *Medical-surgical: critical thinking for collaborative care* (4th ed.). Philadelphia: W.B. Saunders, p. 737.

---

172. A nurse has collected nutritional data from a client with a diagnosis of cystitis. The nurse determines that which of the following beverages should be encouraged to minimize recurrence of cystitis?
1   Coffee
2   Tea
3   Water
4   White wine

Answer: 3
Rationale: Caffeine and alcohol can irritate the bladder. Therefore beverages that contain alcohol and caffeine such as coffee, tea, and wine are avoided to reduce the risk of recurrence. Water helps flush bacteria out of the bladder, and an intake of 6 to 8 glasses per day is encouraged.

Test-Taking Strategy: Use the process of elimination. Option 4 should be eliminated first because alcohol intake is not encouraged for any disorder. Options 1 and 2 are similar because both contain caffeine, and they are eliminated because it is unlikely that either is the correct answer. Review the measures that reduce the recurrence of cystitis if you had difficulty with this question.

Level of Cognitive Ability: Comprehension
Client Needs: Health Promotion and Maintenance
Integrated Concept/Process: Nursing Process/Implementation
Content Area: Adult Health/Renal

Reference:
Ignatavicius, D., & Workman, M. (2002). *Medical-surgical: critical thinking for collaborative care* (4th ed.). Philadelphia: W.B. Saunders, p. 1617.

---

173. A nurse has reinforced instructions to a female client with cystitis about measures to prevent recurrence. The nurse evaluates that the client needs further instruction if the client verbalizes a need to do which of the following?
  1 Take bubble baths for more effective hygiene
  2 Wear underwear made of cotton or with cotton panels
  3 Drink a glass of water and void after intercourse
  4 Avoid wearing pantyhose while wearing slacks

Answer: 1
Rationale: Measures to prevent cystitis include increasing fluid intake to 3 liters per day; eating an acid-ash diet; wiping front to back after urination; taking showers instead of tub baths; drinking water and voiding after intercourse; avoiding bubble baths, feminine hygiene sprays, or perfumed toilet tissue or sanitary pads; and wearing clothes that "breathe" (cotton pants, no tight jeans, no pantyhose under slacks). Other measures include teaching pregnant women to void every 2 hours and instructing menopausal women to use estrogen vaginal creams to restore vaginal pH.

Test-Taking Strategy: Note the key words *needs further instruction.* Eliminate option 3 first, knowing that drinking water is a basic measure to prevent cystitis. Next, eliminate options 2 and 4 because they are similar. Review teaching measures to prevent cystitis if you had difficulty with this question.

Level of Cognitive Ability: Comprehension
Client Needs: Health Promotion and Maintenance
Integrated Concept/Process: Nursing Process/Evaluation
Content Area: Adult Health/Renal

Reference:
Ignatavicius, D., & Workman, M. (2002). *Medical-surgical: critical thinking for collaborative care* (4th ed.). Philadelphia: W.B. Saunders, p. 1618.

---

174. A client with pyelonephritis is being discharged from the hospital. The nurse reinforces instructions to prevent recurrence. The nurse determines that the client understands the information that was given if the client states an intention to do which of the following?
  1 Report signs and symptoms of urinary tract infection (UTI) if they persist for more than 1 week
  2 Take the prescribed antibiotics until all symptoms subside
  3 Return to the physician's office for scheduled follow-up urine cultures
  4 Modify fluid intake for the day based on the previous day's output

Answer: 3
Rationale: The client with pyelonephritis should take the full course of antibiotic therapy that has been prescribed and return to the physician's office for follow-up urine cultures if so instructed. The client should learn the signs and symptoms of UTI and report them immediately if they occur. The client should use all measures recommended to prevent cystitis, which includes forcing fluids to 3 liters per day.

Test-Taking Strategy: Use the process of elimination. Begin to answer this question by eliminating option 1 because urinary tract infection symptoms should never go unreported for a week. Option 2 is eliminated next because antibiotics should be taken for the full course of treatment to adequately eliminate the infection. From the remaining options, recalling that the client needs follow-up urine cultures helps you to choose option 3 instead of option 4, which is not an appropriate option. Review the measures that prevent this infection if you had difficulty with this question.

Level of Cognitive Ability: Comprehension
Client Needs: Health Promotion and Maintenance

Integrated Concept/Process: Nursing Process/Evaluation
Content Area: Adult Health/Renal

Reference:
Ignatavicius, D., & Workman, M. (2002). *Medical-surgical: critical thinking for collaborative care* (4th ed.). Philadelphia: W.B. Saunders, p. 1646.

---

175. A client with nephrotic syndrome needs dietary teaching about how diet can help counteract the effects of altered renal function. The nurse would include which of the following statements in the instructions to the client?

1　"Force fluids throughout the day."
2　"Add salt during cooking to replace sodium lost in the urine."
3　"Increase your intake of fish, meat, and eggs."
4　"Increase your intake of fatty foods to prevent protein loss."

Answer: 3
Rationale: Sodium is limited in the nephrotic syndrome diet to help control edema, which is part of the clinical picture. Fluids are not limited unless hyponatremia is present, but the client is not encouraged to force fluids. Protein is increased unless the glomerular filtration rate is impaired. This helps to replace protein lost in the urine and ultimately helps in controlling edema. Hyperlipidemia, which results from the liver's synthesis of lipoproteins in response to hypoalbuminemia, is also part of the clinical picture. Increasing fatty food intake would not be helpful in this circumstance.

Test-Taking Strategy: Begin to answer this question by recalling that nephrotic syndrome is characterized by fluid retention and hypoalbuminemia. This would help you eliminate options 1 and 2 first. To choose between the remaining options, knowing that hyperlipidemia accompanies nephrotic syndrome would help you to choose option 3 instead of option 4. You could also choose correctly recalling that hypoalbuminemia is part of the clinical picture, and that the foods in option 3 are good sources of protein. Review dietary measures for the client with nephrotic syndrome if you had difficulty with this question.

Level of Cognitive Ability: Application
Client Needs: Health Promotion and Maintenance
Integrated Concept/Process: Nursing Process/Implementation
Content Area: Adult Health/Renal

Reference:
Ignatavicius, D., & Workman, M. (2002). *Medical-surgical: critical thinking for collaborative care* (4th ed.). Philadelphia: W.B. Saunders, p. 1654.

---

176. A nurse is giving the client with polycystic kidney disease instructions in replacing elements lost in the urine because of impaired kidney function. The nurse instructs the client to increase intake of which of the following in the diet?

1　Sodium and potassium
2　Sodium and water
3　Water and phosphorus
4　Calcium and phosphorus

Answer: 2
Rationale: Clients with polycystic kidney disease waste sodium rather than retain it, and therefore need an increase in sodium and water in the diet. Potassium, calcium, and phosphorus require no special attention.

Test-Taking Strategy: In reviewing the possible answers to this question, notice that either sodium or phosphorus appears in each of the options. Remember also that when an option has two parts to it, both of the parts must be correct for the option to be correct. Knowing this, begin to answer this question by eliminating options 3 and 4 first, because the disorder causes sodium, not phosphorus, to be wasted. From the remaining options, recall that when the kidney excretes sodium, water is carried with it.

This will direct you to option 2. Review the manifestations associated with polycystic kidney disease if you had difficulty with this question.

Level of Cognitive Ability: Application
Client Needs: Health Promotion and Maintenance
Integrated Concept/Process: Nursing Process/Implementation
Content Area: Adult Health/Renal

Reference:
Ignatavicius, D., & Workman, M. (2002). *Medical-surgical: critical thinking for collaborative care* (4th ed.). Philadelphia: W.B. Saunders, p. 1643.

---

177. A client with acquired immunodeficiency syndrome is being treated for tuberculosis with isoniazid (INH). The nurse plans to do which of the following in administration of the medication?
1   Administer with an antacid to prevent gastrointestinal distress
2   Administer at least 1 hour before administering an aluminum antacid to prevent a medication interaction
3   Administer with food to prevent rapid absorption of isoniazid
4   Administer with a corticosteroid to maximize the effects of isoniazid

Answer: 2
Rationale: Aluminum hydroxide, a common ingredient in antacids, significantly decreases isoniazid absorption. Isoniazid should be administered at least 1 hour before aluminum antacids. Food does not affect the rate of absorption of isoniazid. Isoniazid administration with a corticosteroid decreases isoniazid effects and increases the corticosteroid effects.

Test-Taking Strategy: Use general principles related to medication administration. Remember, you would not usually administer a medication with an antacid because it would decrease absorption of the medication. Review this medication if you had difficulty with this question.

Level of Cognitive Ability: Application
Clients Needs: Health Promotion and Maintenance
Integrated Concept/Process: Nursing Process/Planning
Content Area: Pharmacology

Reference:
Hodgson, B., & Kizior, R. (2003). *Saunders nursing drug handbook 2003.* Philadelphia: W.B. Saunders, p. 616.

---

178. A client is treated in the physician's office for a sprained ankle after sustaining a fall. Before sending the client home, the nurse tells the client to avoid which of the following in the next 24 hours?
1   Applying a heating pad
2   Applying an elastic wrap
3   Resting the foot
4   Elevating the ankle on a pillow while sitting or lying down

Answer: 1
Rationale: Soft tissue injuries such as sprains are treated by RICE (rest, ice, compression, elevation) for the first 24 hours after the injury. Ice is applied intermittently for 20 to 30 minutes at a time. Heat is not used in the first 24 hours because it could increase venous congestion, which would increase edema and pain.

Test-Taking Strategy: Note the key word *avoid*. It is likely that sprains should be rested and elevated, so these options are eliminated. Use of an elastic wrap is also helpful in reducing the pain and swelling, so option 2 can also be eliminated. This leaves heat as the treatment to avoid in the first 24 hours. Review measures for a sprain if you had difficulty with this question.

Level of Cognitive Ability: Application
Client Needs: Health Promotion and Maintenance

Integrated Concept/Process: Nursing Process/Implementation
Content Area: Adult Health/Musculoskeletal

Reference:
Ignatavicius, D., & Workman, M. (2002). *Medical-surgical: critical thinking for collaborative care* (4th ed.). Philadelphia: W.B. Saunders, p. 1154.

---

179. A nurse has given dietary instructions to a client to minimize the risk of osteoporosis. The nurse determines that the client understands the instructions if the client verbalized to increase intake of which food item?
1   Rice
2   Yogurt
3   Sardines
4   Chicken

Answer: 2
Rationale: Calcium intake is important to minimize the risk of osteoporosis. The major dietary source of calcium is from dairy foods, including milk, yogurt, and a variety of cheeses. Calcium may also be added to certain products such as orange juice, which are then labeled as being "fortified" with calcium. Calcium supplements are available and recommended for those with typically low calcium intake.

Test-Taking Strategy: Use the process of elimination. Recall that calcium is needed to minimize the risk of osteoporosis. You should know that dairy products are rich in calcium, and that yogurt is a dairy product. Each of the incorrect options does not belong to this food group. Review foods high in calcium if you had difficulty with this question.

Level of Cognitive Ability: Analysis
Client Needs: Health Promotion and Maintenance
Integrated Concept/Process: Self-Care
Content Area: Adult Health/Musculoskeletal

Reference:
Ignatavicius, D., & Workman, M. (2002). *Medical-surgical: critical thinking for collaborative care* (4th ed.). Philadelphia: W.B. Saunders, p. 1098.

---

180. A nurse is assisting in conducting health screening for osteoporosis. The nurse would direct health promotion measures to which of the following clients, knowing he or she is at greatest risk of developing this disorder?
1   A 36-year-old male who has asthma
2   A 25-year-old female who jogs
3   A sedentary 65-year-old female who smokes cigarettes
4   A 70-year-old male who consumes excess alcohol

Answer: 3
Rationale: Risk factors for osteoporosis include being female, postmenopausal, of advanced age, or sedentary; consuming a low-calcium diet; using excessive alcohol; and smoking cigarettes. Long-term use of corticosteroids, anticonvulsants, and furosemide (Lasix) also increases the risk.

Test-Taking Strategy: Use the process of elimination. Option 2 is eliminated first. The 25-year-old female who jogs (exercise using the long bones) has negligible risk. The 36-year-old male with asthma is eliminated next because the only risk factor might be long-term corticosteroid use. From the remaining options, the 65-year-old female has greater risk (age, gender, postmenopausal, sedentary, smoking) than the 70-year-old male (age, alcohol consumption). Review the risk factors for osteoporosis if you had difficulty with this question.

Level of Cognitive Ability: Comprehension
Client Needs: Health Promotion and Maintenance
Integrated Concept/Process: Nursing Process/Data Collection
Content Area: Adult Health/Musculoskeletal

Reference:
Ignatavicius, D., & Workman, M. (2002). *Medical-surgical: critical thinking for collaborative care* (4th ed.). Philadelphia: W.B. Saunders, p. 1098.

181. A client with right-sided weakness must learn how to use a cane. Which of the following would the nurse plan to teach the client about the correct position of the cane?
1   Hold with the left hand, and place the cane in front of the left foot
2   Hold with the right hand, and place the cane in front of the right foot
3   Hold with the left hand, and place the cane 6 inches lateral to the left foot
4   Hold with the right hand, and place the cane 6 inches lateral to the right foot

Answer: 3
Rationale: The client is taught to hold the cane on the opposite side of the weakness because, with normal walking, the opposite arm and leg move together (called reciprocal motion). The cane is placed 6 inches lateral to the fifth toe.

Test-Taking Strategy: Use the process of elimination. Knowing that the cane is held at the client's side, not in front, helps you to eliminate options 1 and 2 first. Knowing that the preferred method is to have the cane positioned on the stronger side helps you to choose option 3 instead of option 4. Review client instructions for the use of a cane if you had difficulty with this question.

Level of Cognitive Ability: Application
Client Needs: Health Promotion and Maintenance
Integrated Concept/Process: Self-Care
Content Area: Adult Health/Musculoskeletal

Reference:
Potter, P., & Perry, A. (2001). *Fundamentals of nursing* (5th ed.). St. Louis: Mosby, p. 1008.

182. A nurse has reinforced instructions about prosthesis and stump care with a client who has a below-knee amputation. The nurse determines that the client has understood the instructions if the client states a need to do which the following?
1   Wear a clean nylon stump sock daily
2   Toughen the skin of the stump by rubbing it with alcohol
3   Prevent cracking of the skin of the stump by applying lotion daily
4   Use a mirror to inspect all areas of the stump each day

Answer: 4
Rationale: The client should wear a clean woolen stump sock each day. The stump is cleansed daily with a gentle soap and water, and is dried carefully. Alcohol is avoided because it could cause drying or cracking of the skin. Oils and creams are also avoided because they are too softening to the skin for safe prosthesis use. The client should inspect all surfaces of the stump daily for irritation, blisters, or breakdown.

Test-Taking Strategy: Use the process of elimination. Nylon is a synthetic material that does not allow the best air circulation and holds in moisture. For this reason, a stump sock is not made of nylon, and option 1 is incorrect. Either alcohol or lotion can interfere with the natural condition of the skin, increasing the likelihood of breakdown either from drying or from excess moisture. For these reasons, options 2 and 3 are also incorrect. By the process of elimination, the answer is option 4. It is very important that the client assess skin integrity of the stump at least daily. Review these home care measures if you had difficulty with this question.

Level of Cognitive Ability: Comprehension
Client Needs: Health Promotion and Maintenance
Integrated Concept/Process: Self-Care
Content Area: Adult Health/Musculoskeletal

Reference:
Ignatavicius, D., & Workman, M. (2002). *Medical-surgical: critical thinking for collaborative care* (4th ed.). Philadelphia: W.B. Saunders, p. 1149.

183. A nurse is ambulating a client with a right leg fracture who has an order for partial weight-bearing status. The nurse evaluates that the client demonstrates compliance with this restriction if the client does which the following?
1   Does not bear weight on the right leg
2   Allows the right leg only to touch the floor
3   Puts 30% to 50% of the weight on the right leg
4   Puts 60% to 80% of the weight on the right leg

Answer: 3

Rationale: The client who has partial weight-bearing status places 30% to 50% of the body weight on the affected limb. Full weight-bearing status is placing full weight on the limb. Non–weight-bearing status does not allow the client to let the limb touch the floor. Touch-down weight bearing allows the client to let the limb touch the floor but not bear weight. There is no classification for 60% to 80% weight bearing status.

Test-Taking Strategy: To answer this question, you should be familiar with the different categories of weight bearing. Begin by eliminating options 1 and 2 first, using general knowledge; the words *partial weight bearing* do not seem to fit either of these. Focusing on these words will also direct you to choose option 3 from the remaining options. Review the descriptions of weight bearing if you had difficulty with this question.

Level of Cognitive Ability: Comprehension
Client Needs: Health Promotion and Maintenance
Integrated Concept/Process: Nursing Process/Evaluation
Content Area: Adult Health/Musculoskeletal

Reference:
Black, J., Hawks, J., & Keene, A. (2001). *Medical-surgical nursing: clinical management for positive outcomes* (6th ed.). Philadelphia: W.B. Saunders, p. 614.

---

184. A nurse is planning measures to increase bed mobility for the client in skeletal leg traction. Which of the following items would the nurse consider to be most helpful for this client?
1   Television
2   Reading materials
3   Overhead trapeze
4   Fracture bedpan

Answer: 3

Rationale: The use of an overhead trapeze will help a client to move about in bed, and to get on and off the bedpan. This device has the greatest value in increasing overall bed mobility. A fracture bedpan is useful in reducing discomfort with elimination. Television and reading materials are helpful in reducing boredom and providing distraction.

Test-Taking Strategy: Note the words *most helpful* and focus on the issue: to increase bed mobility. Although all options are useful to the client in skeletal traction, the only one that helps with overall bed mobility is the trapeze. Review care to the client in skeletal traction if you had difficulty with this question.

Level of Cognitive Ability: Application
Client Needs: Physiological Integrity
Integrated Concept/Process: Nursing Process/Implementation
Content Area: Adult Health/Musculoskeletal

Reference:
Black, J., Hawks, J., & Keene, A. (2001). *Medical-surgical nursing: clinical management for positive outcomes* (6th ed.). Philadelphia: W.B. Saunders, p. 607.

185. A nurse has reinforced medication instructions to a client beginning anticonvulsant therapy with carbamazepine (Tegretol). The nurse determines that the client understands the use of the medication if the client states which of the following?
1 Drive as long as it is not at night
2 Use sunscreen when outdoors
3 Keep tissues handy because of excess salivation
4 Discontinue the medication if a fever or sore throat occurs

Answer: 2
Rationale: Carbamazepine acts by depressing synaptic transmission in the central nervous system (CNS). Because of this, the client should avoid driving or doing other activities that require mental alertness until the effect of the medication on the client is known. The client should use protective clothing and sunscreen to avoid photosensitivity reactions. The medication may cause dry mouth, and the client should be instructed to provide good oral hygiene and use sugarless candy or gum as needed. The medication should not be abruptly discontinued because this could cause return of seizures or status epilepticus. Fever and sore throat should be reported to the physician (leukopenia).

Test-Taking Strategy: Begin to answer this question by recalling that this is an anticonvulsant medication with CNS depressant properties. This would lead you to eliminate option 1 first, because driving in general could be hazardous. Option 4 is eliminated next because an anticonvulsant is not automatically discontinued if side effects or infection occurs; the physician should be called to determine an appropriate course of action. To choose between the remaining options, remembering that carbamazepine causes dry mouth may help you to eliminate option 3. Review this medication if you had difficulty with this question.

Level of Cognitive Ability: Analysis
Client Needs: Health Promotion and Maintenance
Integrated Concept/Process: Nursing Process/Evaluation
Content Area: Pharmacology

Reference:
Hodgson, B., & Kizior, R. (2003). *Saunders nursing drug handbook 2003.* Philadelphia: W.B. Saunders, p. 169.

186. A client with myasthenia gravis has difficulty chewing and has received a prescription for pyridostigmine (Mestinon). The nurse tells the client to take the medication:
1 Two hours after a meal
2 One hour before a meal
3 At bedtime
4 With food

Answer: 4
Rationale: Pyridostigmine is a cholinergic medication used to increase muscle strength for the client with myasthenia gravis. The medication is administered with food or milk.

Test-Taking Strategy: Use the process of elimination. Eliminate options 1, 2, and 3 because they are similar and indicate taking the medication without food. Review this medication if you had difficulty with this question.

Level of Cognitive Ability: Application
Client Needs: Health Promotion and Maintenance
Integrated Concept/Process: Nursing Process/Implementation
Content Area: Pharmacology

Reference:
Hodgson, B., & Kizior, R. (2003). *Saunders nursing drug handbook 2003.* Philadelphia: W.B. Saunders, p. 949.

187. A nurse reinforces discharge instructions with a client who has rheumatoid arthritis (RA). The instructions focus on measures to lessen discomfort and provide joint protection. Which of the following would be included in the instructions?
1   Change positions every hour
2   Lift items rather than sliding them
3   Perform prescribed exercises even if the joints are inflamed
4   Avoid stooping, bending, or overreaching

Answer: 4
Rationale: The client with RA should avoid remaining in one position and should change position or stretch every 20 minutes. To reduce efforts by joints, the client should slide objects rather than lift them. When the joints are inflamed, the client should avoid exercises and activities other than gentle range of motion. The client is instructed to avoid stooping, bending, or overreaching.

Test-Taking Strategy: Use the process of elimination. Eliminate option 1 because remaining in one position for 1 hour is excessive for a client with RA. Eliminate option 3 because joints should be rested if inflamed. Basic principles of body mechanics will assist in eliminating option 2 and directing you to option 4. Review principles for joint protection in RA if you had difficulty with this question.

Level of Cognitive Ability: Application
Client Needs: Health Promotion and Maintenance
Integrated Concept/Process: Self-Care
Content Area: Adult Health/Musculoskeletal

Reference:
Black, J., Hawks, J., & Keene, A. (2001). *Medical-surgical nursing: clinical management for positive outcomes* (6th ed.). Philadelphia: W.B. Saunders, p. 2147.

---

188. A nurse is caring for a client with arthritis. The client complains of difficulty instilling glaucoma eye drops because the arthritis causes the hands to shake. Which of the following instructions would the nurse provide to the client to alleviate this problem?
1   Keep the drops in the refrigerator so they will thicken and be easier to instill
2   Lie down on a bed or sofa to instill the eye drops
3   Tilt the head back to instill the eye drops
4   Ask a family member to instill the eye drops

Answer: 2
Rationale: Clients with arthritis or shaking hands have difficulty instilling their own eye drops. The client should be instructed to lie down on a bed or sofa. Tilting the head back can lead to loss of balance. Placing eye drops in a refrigerator should not be done unless specifically prescribed. Eye drop regimen for glaucoma requires accurate timing, and it is unreasonable to expect a family member to instill the drops. In addition, this discourages client independence.

Test-Taking Strategy: Use the process of elimination. Eliminate option 1 first because eye medication should not be refrigerated unless specifically prescribed. Option 4 does not promote and maintain client independence; in addition, no mention of family is made in the question. From the remaining options, select option 2 because it provides greater safety for the client. Review the methods of instilling eye drops if you had difficulty with this question.

Level of Cognitive Ability: Application
Client Needs: Health Promotion and Maintenance
Integrated Concept/Process: Self-Care
Content Area: Adult Health/Eye

Reference:
Perry, A., & Potter, P. (2002). *Clinical nursing skills & techniques* (5th ed.). St. Louis: Mosby, p. 471.

189. A nurse is providing dietary instructions to a client with pancreatitis. Which of the following foods would the nurse instruct the client to avoid?
1   Lentil soup
2   Bagel
3   Chili
4   Watermelon

Answer: 3
Rationale: The client should avoid alcohol, coffee and tea, spicy foods, and heavy meals, which stimulate pancreatic secretions and produce attacks of pancreatitis. The client is instructed in the benefit of eating small frequent meals that are high in protein, low in fat, and moderate to high in carbohydrates.

Test-Taking Strategy: Note the key word *avoid.* Use the process of elimination, noting that options 1, 2, and 4 are foods that are moderately bland. Option 3, chili, is a spicy food. Review foods that should be avoided in the client with pancreatitis if you had difficulty with this question.

Level of Cognitive Ability: Application
Client Needs: Health Promotion and Maintenance
Integrated Concept/Process: Nursing Process/Implementation
Content Area: Adult Health/Gastrointestinal

Reference:
Black, J., Hawks, J., & Keene, A. (2001). *Medical-surgical nursing: clinical management for positive outcomes* (6th ed.). Philadelphia: W.B. Saunders, p. 1196.

---

190. A scleral buckling procedure is performed on the client with retinal detachment, and the nurse reinforces home care instructions. Which statement by the client indicates a need for further instructions?
1   "I should clean my eye daily with sterile tap water and a clean white washcloth."
2   "I should wear an eye shield during naps and at night."
3   "I should avoid vigorous activity and heavy lifting."
4   "I should avoid air travel."

Answer: 1
Rationale: In a scleral buckling procedure, the sclera is compressed from the outside by Silastic sponges or silicone bands that are sutured in place permanently. In addition, an intraocular injection of an air or gas bubble, or both, may be used to apply pressure on the retina from the inside of the eye to hold the retina in place. If an air or gas bubble has been injected, it may take several weeks to be absorbed. Air travel is avoided because gas and air expand at high actitudes Vigorous activities and heavy lifting are avoided. An eye shield should be worn during naps and at night. The client is instructed to clean the eye with warm tap water using a clean washcloth.

Test-Taking Strategy: Note the key words *need for further instructions.* Reading carefully will assist in directing you to the correct option. It is not necessary to use sterile water to clean the eye, especially if a clean washcloth is used. Review client-teaching points after scleral buckling if you had difficulty with this question.

Level of Cognitive Ability: Application
Client Needs: Health Promotion and Maintenance
Integrated Concept/Process: Teaching/Learning
Content Area: Adult Health/Eye

Reference:
Black, J., Hawks, J., & Keene, A. (2001). *Medical-surgical nursing: clinical management for positive outcomes* (6th ed.). Philadelphia: W.B. Saunders, p. 1820.

---

191. A newborn receives the first dose of hepatitis B vaccine within 12 hours of birth. The nurse instructs the mother regarding

Answer: 1
Rationale: The vaccination schedule for an infant whose mother tests negative consists of a series of three immunizations given at

the immunization schedule for this vaccine and tells the mother that the second vaccine is administered at which of the following times?
1   1 to 2 months of age and then 4 months after the initial dose
2   6 months of age and then 8 months after the initial dose
3   8 months of age and then 1 year after the initial dose
4   3 years of age and then during the adolescent years

birth, 1 to 2 months of age, and then 4 months after the initial dose. An infant whose mother tests positive receives human B immune globulin along with the first dose of the hepatitis B vaccine within 12 hours of birth.

Test-Taking Strategy: Knowledge regarding the immunization schedule for hepatitis B vaccine is necessary to answer this question. Review this schedule if you are unfamiliar with it.

Level of Cognitive Ability: Application
Client Needs: Health Promotion and Maintenance
Integrated Concept/Process: Nursing Process/Implementation
Content Area: Child Health

Reference:
Wong, D., & Hockenberry-Eaton, M. (2001). *Wong's essentials of pediatric nursing* (6th ed.). St. Louis: Mosby, p. 361.

192. A nurse assists in performing health screening for scoliosis on children ages 9 through 15 years. Which of the following is the appropriate technique for this screening procedure?
1   Have the child stand with the arms extended over the head
2   Have the child stand with weight bearing on the right leg followed by the left leg
3   Have the child unclothed or wearing underpants only so the chest, back, and hips can be clearly seen
4   Take shoulder to foot measurements on the right and left side and compare measurements

Answer: 3
Rationale: The child should be unclothed or wearing underpants only so the chest, back, and hips can be clearly seen. The child is asked to stand with the weight equally on both feet, legs straight, and arms hanging loosely at both sides. Shoulder heights are observed for unequal alignment. Equal leg length is also checked.

Test-Taking Strategy: With knowledge regarding the anatomical location of this disorder, attempt to visualize the screening procedure identified in each option. This should assist in eliminating options 1, 2, and 4. If you had difficulty with this question, review this screening procedure.

Level of Cognitive Ability: Comprehension
Client Needs: Health Promotion and Maintenance
Integrated Concept/Process: Nursing Process/Data Collection
Content Area: Child Health

Reference:
Wong, D., & Hockenberry-Eaton, M. (2001). *Wong's essentials of pediatric nursing* (6th ed.). St. Louis: Mosby, p. 1230.

193. A nurse reinforces dietary instruction with the parents of a child with a diagnosis of cystic fibrosis. Which of the following would be a component of dietary management?
1   Low protein
2   Low fat
3   High calorie
4   Low sodium

Answer: 3
Rationale: Children with cystic fibrosis are managed with a high-calorie, high-protein diet, pancreatic enzyme replacement therapy, fat-soluble vitamin supplements, and if nutritional problems are severe, nighttime gastrostomy feedings or total parental nutrition. Fats are not restricted unless steatorrhea cannot be controlled by increased pancreatic enzymes. Sodium intake is unrelated to this disorder.

Test-Taking Strategy: Knowledge regarding the digestive problems and the dietary management in children with cystic fibrosis is necessary to answer this question. If you are unfamiliar with this content select option 3 because children require calories for growth and development and because this is the option that is different from the others. Review this content if you had difficulty with this question.

Level of Cognitive Ability: Application
Client Needs: Health Promotion and Maintenance
Integrated Concept/Process: Nursing Process/Implementation
Content Area: Child Health

Reference:
Wong, D., & Hockenberry-Eaton, M. (2001). *Wong's essentials of pediatric nursing* (6th ed.). St. Louis: Mosby, p. 863.

---

194. A nurse instructs an adolescent with iron deficiency anemia about the administration of oral iron preparations. The nurse tells the adolescent to take the iron with which of the following?
1 Water
2 Milk
3 Tomato juice
4 Apple juice

Answer: 3
Rationale: Iron should be administered with vitamin C rich fluids. Tomato juice contains a high content of ascorbic acid. Vitamin C enhances the absorption of the iron preparation.

Test-Taking Strategy: Recalling that vitamin C increases the absorption of iron will assist in answering this question. With this concept in mind, you can easily eliminate options 1 and 2. From the remaining options, select option 3 because this fluid contains the highest content of ascorbic acid. Review the procedure related to the administration of iron if you had difficulty with this question.

Level of Cognitive Ability: Application
Client Needs: Health Promotion and Maintenance
Integrated Concept/Process: Teaching/Learning
Content Area: Child Health

Reference:
Wong, D., & Hockenberry-Eaton, M. (2001). *Wong's essentials of pediatric nursing* (6th ed.). St. Louis: Mosby, p. 988.

---

195. A nurse is reinforcing instructions to a client who started taking a sustained-release preparation of procainamide (Pronestyl-SR). The nurse plans to teach the client which of the following about this medication?
1 Do not crush, chew, or break the sustained release tablets
2 The presence of tablet wax matrix in the stool indicates poor medication absorption
3 Take a double dose if a dose is missed
4 Monitoring of pulse rate and rhythm is unnecessary once this medication is begun

Answer: 1
Rationale: Procainamide is an antidysrhythmic that is available in sustained release form. The sustained release preparations should not be broken, chewed, or crushed. The SR form has a wax matrix that may be noted in the stool, which is not significant. If a dose is missed, a sustained-release tablet may be taken if remembered within 4 hours (2 hours for regular acting form); otherwise the dose should be omitted. Double dosing should not be done. The client or family member should be taught to monitor the client's pulse and report any change in rate or rhythm.

Test-Taking Strategy: Use the process of elimination. Recalling that procainamide is an antidysrhythmic, you may eliminate options 3 and 4 first. Basic knowledge of administration of sustained release medications will help you to choose option 1 instead of option 2. Review this medication if you had difficulty with this question.

Level of Cognitive Ability: Application
Client Needs: Health Promotion and Maintenance

Integrated Concept/Process: Nursing Process/Planning
Content Area: Pharmacology

Reference:
Clark, J., Queener, S., & Karb, V. (2002). *Pharmacologic basis of nursing practice* (6th ed). St. Louis: Mosby, p. 240.

---

196. A nurse has reinforced instructions with a client with a urinary catheter about home care after hospital discharge. The nurse evaluates that the client understands the instructions if the client states a need to drink at least how many glasses of water per day?
1   2 to 4
2   6 to 8
3   10 to 12
4   14 to 16

Answer: 2
Rationale: The client with a urinary catheter should have adequate fluid intake to dilute urinary particles and prevent infection. The nurse encourages the client to take in at least 2000 mL fluid per day, which is roughly equivalent to 6 to 8 glasses of water.

Test-Taking Strategy: Use the process of elimination. Eliminate options 3 and 4 first because these higher amounts can place undo distention on the bladder. From the remaining options, recalling general principles related to daily fluid intake will direct you to option 2. Review care to the client with a urinary catheter if you had difficulty with this question.

Level of Cognitive Ability: Comprehension
Client Needs: Health Promotion and Maintenance
Integrated Concept/Process: Nursing Process/Evaluation
Content Area: Adult Health/Renal

Reference:
Black, J., Hawks, J., & Keene, A. (2001). *Medical-surgical nursing: clinical management for positive outcomes* (6th ed.). Philadelphia: W.B. Saunders, p. 844.

---

197. A nurse is reinforcing home care instructions with a female client who has been diagnosed with recurrent trichomoniasis. Which statement by the client indicates a need for further instructions?
1   "I should perform good perineal hygiene."
2   "I should avoid sexual intercourse."
3   "I should discontinue treatment if my menstrual period begins."
4   "I should take metronidazole (Flagyl) for 7 days."

Answer: 3
Rationale: Treatment for a recurrent infection should be continued through the menstrual period because the vagina is more alkaline during this time and an exacerbation is likely to occur. Options 1, 2, and 4 are correct client statements. The client should refrain from sexual intercourse while the infection remains active. If this is not possible, a condom is recommended.

Test-Taking Strategy: Note the key words *need for further instructions* and use the process of elimination. Option 1 and option 2 can be easily eliminated. From the remaining options, select option 3 instead of option 4 because it is unlikely that treatment would be discontinued. If you had difficulty with this question review treatment for this protozoal infection.

Level of Cognitive Ability: Application
Client Needs: Health Promotion and Maintenance
Integrated Concept/Process: Teaching/Learning
Content Area: Fundamental Skills

Reference:
Potter, P., & Perry, A. (2001). *Fundamentals of nursing* (5th ed.). St. Louis: Mosby, p. 836.

198. A nurse is reinforcing home care instructions to a client recovering from a radical vulvectomy. Which statement by the client indicates a need for further instructions?
   1   "I should take showers rather than tub baths."
   2   "I should wipe from front to back after a bowel movement."
   3   "I should monitor for foul smelling perineal discharge."
   4   "Swelling of the groin or genital area is expected."

Answer: 4
Rationale: The physician should be notified if any swelling of the groin or genital area occurs. Options 1, 2, and 3 are accurate statements. Additionally the client should monitor for pain, redness, or tenderness in the calves, and for any signs of infection.

Test-Taking Strategy: Note the key words *need for further instructions*. Basic hygiene principles will assist in eliminating options 1 and 2. From the remaining options, select option 4 because swelling is not expected. Review client teaching points related to a radical vulvectomy if you had difficulty with this question.

Level of Cognitive Ability: Application
Client Needs: Health Promotion and Maintenance
Integrated Concept/Process: Teaching/Learning
Content Area: Adult Health/Oncology

Reference:
Black, J., Hawks, J., & Keene, A. (2001). *Medical-surgical nursing: clinical management for positive outcomes* (6th ed.). Philadelphia. W.B. Saunders, p. 1007.

---

199. A client with major depression is considering cognitive therapy. The client says to the nurse, "How does this treatment work?" The nurse makes which response to the client?
   1   "This type of therapy helps you examine how your thoughts and feelings contribute to your difficulties."
   2   "This type of therapy helps you examine how your past life has contributed to your problems."
   3   "This type of therapy helps you confront your fears by gradually exposing you to them."
   4   "This type of therapy will help you relax and develop new coping skills."

Answer: 1
Rationale: Cognitive therapy is frequently used with clients who have depression. This type of therapy is based on exploring the client's subjective experience. It includes examining the client's thoughts and feelings about situations as well as how these thoughts and feelings contribute and perpetuate the client's difficulties and mood. Options 2, 3, and 4 are incorrect descriptions.

Test-Taking Strategy: Focusing on the word *cognitive* will assist you in choosing the correct option. Look for a similar word or phrase used in the question and repeated in one of the options. Option 1 uses the word *thoughts* in describing the therapy. Review this type of therapy if you had difficulty with this question.

Level of Cognitive Ability: Application
Client Needs: Health Promotion and Maintenance
Integrated Concept/Process: Nursing Process/Implementation
Content Area: Mental Health

Reference:
Varcarolis, E. (1998). *Foundations of psychiatric mental health nursing* (3rd ed.). Philadelphia: W.B. Saunders. p. 469.

---

200. A nurse has reinforced dietary instructions to the client with acquired immunodeficiency syndrome about methods to maintain and increase weight. The nurse evaluates that the client would benefit from further instruction if the

Answer: 1
Rationale: The client should eat small, frequent meals throughout the day. The client also should take in nutrient-dense and high-calorie meals and snacks. The client is encouraged to eat favorite foods to maintain intake and plan meals that are easy to prepare. The client should also avoid taking fluids with

client stated a need to do which of the following?

1 Eat low calorie snacks between meals
2 Eat small, frequent meals throughout the day
3 Consume nutrient dense foods and beverages
4 Keep easy to prepare foods available in the home

meals to increase food intake before the client becomes satiated.

Test-Taking Strategy: Note the key words *would benefit from further instruction.* Because options 2, 3, and 4 are all measures that will maintain and increase weight, eliminate these options. The client should choose snacks that are high in calories, not low in calories. Review dietary measures that will maintain and increase weight if you had difficulty with this question.

Level of Cognitive Ability: Comprehension
Client Needs: Health Promotion and Maintenance
Integrated Concept/Process: Nursing Process/Evaluation
Content Area: Fundamental Skills

Reference:
Black, J., Hawks, J., & Keene, A. (2001). *Medical-surgical nursing: clinical management for positive outcomes* (6th ed.). Philadelphia: W.B. Saunders, p. 2210.

---

201. A nurse is caring for the client who had chest tube placement for drainage of empyema. The nurse has reinforced instructions about breathing exercises that will best promote respiratory function. The nurse evaluates that the client understands the instructions if the client properly demonstrates which of the following techniques?

1 Diaphragmatic and pursed-lip breathing
2 Incentive spirometry only
3 Deep breathing only
4 Diaphragmatic breathing

Answer: 1
Rationale: Respiratory exercises that promote normal respiratory function for the client with empyema include diaphragmatic and pursed-lip breathing. These exercises strengthen respiratory muscles and promote gas exchange.

Test-Taking Strategy: Use the process of elimination. Eliminate options 2, 3, and 4 because of the word *only*. Review breathing exercises that will best promote respiratory function if you had difficulty with this question.

Level of Cognitive Ability: Comprehension
Client Needs: Health Promotion and Maintenance
Integrated Concept/Process: Nursing Process/Evaluation
Content Area: Adult Health/Respiratory

Reference:
Black, J., Hawks, J., & Keene, A. (2001). *Medical-surgical nursing: clinical management for positive outcomes* (6th ed.). Philadelphia: W.B. Saunders, p. 1731.

---

202. A nurse has reinforced instructions with a postoperative thoracotomy client about how to perform arm and shoulder exercises after discharge. The nurse evaluates that the client has not learned the proper techniques if the client is observed doing which of the following movements on the affected side?

1 Moving the arm upward over the head and back down
2 Holding the hands crossed in front of the waist and raising them over the head

Answer: 4
Rationale: A variety of exercises that involve moving the shoulder and elbow joints are indicated after thoracotomy. These include shrugging the shoulders and moving them back and forth; moving the arms up and down, forward, and backward; holding the hands crossed in front of the waist and then raising them over the head; and holding the upper arm straight out while moving the lower arm up and down. Exercises that move only the wrist joint are of no use after this surgery.

Test-Taking Strategy: Note the key words *has not learned the proper techniques.* Note that options 1 and 2 move the shoulder joint. Option 3 moves the shoulder and elbow joint. Option 4 moves

3   Holding the upper arm straight out while moving the forearm up and down
4   Making circles with the wrist

only the wrist joint. Because the client should exercise the shoulder joint after thoracotomy, option 4 is the answer to the question. Review these postoperative exercises if you had difficulty with this question.

Level of Cognitive Ability: Comprehension
Client Needs: Health Promotion and Maintenance
Integrated Concept/Process: Nursing Process/Evaluation
Content Area: Adult Health/Respiratory

Reference:
Black, J., Hawks, J., & Keene, A. (2001). *Medical-surgical nursing: clinical management for positive outcomes* (6th ed.). Philadelphia: W.B. Saunders, p. 1647.

---

203. A nurse is reinforcing instructions with a client who has a histoplasmosis infection about prevention of future exposure to infectious sources. The nurse evaluates that the client needs further instruction if the client states that potential sources include which of the following?
    1   Grape arbors
    2   Mushroom cellars
    3   Floors of chicken houses
    4   Bird droppings

Answer: 1
Rationale: The client with histoplasmosis is taught to avoid exposure to potential sources of the fungus, which includes soil, bird droppings (especially starlings and blackbirds), floors of chicken houses and bat caves, and mushroom cellars.

Test-Taking Strategy: Note the key words *needs further instruction*. Eliminate options 3 and 4 first because they are similar. Because histoplasmosis is a fungus, there is increased exposure in areas where the fungus thrives. By the process of elimination, the least likely choice is the grape arbor, which is above ground and is not in a dark and damp area. Review the causes of this fungal infection if you had difficulty with this question.

Level of Cognitive Ability: Comprehension
Client Needs: Health Promotion and Maintenance
Integrated Concept/Process: Nursing Process/Evaluation
Content Area: Adult Health/Respiratory

Reference:
Black, J., Hawks, J., & Keene, A. (2001). *Medical-surgical nursing: clinical management for positive outcomes* (6th ed.). Philadelphia: W.B. Saunders, p. 1724.

---

204. A nurse is reinforcing instructions with a client with pulmonary sarcoidosis about long-term ongoing management. The nurse includes which of the following in the instructions?
    1   Need for daily corticosteroids
    2   Usefulness of home oxygen
    3   Need for follow-up chest films every 6 months
    4   Importance of using incentive spirometer daily

Answer: 3
Rationale: The client with pulmonary sarcoidosis should have follow-up chest films every 6 months to monitor disease progression. If an exacerbation occurs, treatment is given with systemic corticosteroids. These tend to give rapid improvement in symptoms. Home oxygen and ongoing use of incentive spirometer are not indicated.

Test-Taking Strategy: Use the process of elimination. Eliminate option 2 first because there is no specific information in the question to indicate a need for its use. Knowing that corticosteroids are used for exacerbation helps you to eliminate option 1. From the remaining options, it is necessary to know that serial monitoring with x-ray is needed to monitor progression of the disease. Review care to the client with pulmonary sarcoidosis if you had difficulty with this question.

Level of Cognitive Ability: Application
Client Needs: Health Promotion and Maintenance

Integrated Concept/Process: Nursing Process/Implementation
Content Area: Adult Health/Respiratory

Reference:
Black, J., Hawks, J., & Keene, A. (2001). *Medical-surgical nursing: clinical management for positive outcomes* (6th ed.). Philadelphia: W.B. Saunders, p. 1726.

---

205. A nurse has reinforced instructions with a client who has silicosis about prevention of self-exposure to silica dust. The nurse evaluates that the client understands the instructions if the client states a need to wear a mask for which of the following hobbies?
1   Pottery making
2   Woodworking
3   Painting
4   Gardening

Answer: 1
Rationale: Exposure to silica dust occurs with activities such as pottery making and stone masonry. Exposure to the finely ground silica, such as is used with soaps, polishes, and filters, is also dangerous. Options 2, 3, and 4 are safe activities.

Test-Taking Strategy: To answer this question, it is necessary to have an understanding of the materials that could emit silica dust. Eliminate gardening first, because silica is not a pesticide and is not found in the average soil. Recalling that silica is not inhaled in fumes, you may then eliminate woodworking or painting. By the process of elimination, you would choose pottery making as the correct option. Review this disorder if you had difficult with this question.

Level of Cognitive Ability: Comprehension
Client Needs: Health Promotion and Maintenance
Integrated Concept/Process: Nursing Process/Evaluation
Content Area: Adult Health/Respiratory

Reference:
Black, J., Hawks, J., & Keene, A. (2001). *Medical-surgical nursing: clinical management for positive outcomes* (6th ed.). Philadelphia: W.B. Saunders, p. 1726.

---

206. A nurse is conducting dietary teaching with a client who is hypocalcemic. The nurse encourages the client to increase intake of which of the following foods?
1   Apples
2   Chicken breast
3   Cheese
4   Cooked pasta

Answer: 3
Rationale: Products that are naturally high in calcium are dairy products, including milk, cheese, ice cream, and yogurt. High-calcium foods generally have greater than 100 mg of calcium per serving. The other options are foods that are low in calcium, which means that they have less than 25 mg of calcium per serving.

Test-Taking Strategy: Use the process of elimination and knowledge of the calcium content of foods. As a general rule, recall that dairy products are naturally high in calcium. If this question was difficult, review the foods high in calcium.

Level of Cognitive Ability: Application
Client Needs: Health Promotion and Maintenance
Integrated Concept/Process: Nursing Process/Implementation
Content Area: Fundamental Skills

Reference:
Black, J., Hawks, J., & Keene, A. (2001). *Medical-surgical nursing: clinical management for positive outcomes* (6th ed.). Philadelphia: W.B. Saunders, p. 249.

207. A client is diagnosed with hyperphosphatemia. The nurse encourages the client to limit intake of which of the following items that is aggravating the condition?

1   Bananas
2   Grapes
3   Coffee
4   Eggs

Answer: 4

Rationale: Foods that are naturally high in phosphates should be avoided by the client with hyperphosphatemia. These include fish, eggs, milk products, vegetables, whole grains, and carbonated beverages.

Test-Taking Strategy: Note the key words *limit intake*. Use knowledge related to the phosphate content of foods to answer this question. Review these foods and fluids if you had difficulty with this question.

Level of Cognitive Ability: Application
Client Needs: Health Promotion and Maintenance
Integrated Concept/Process: Nursing Process/Implementation
Content Area: Fundamental Skills

Reference:
Black, J., Hawks, J., & Keene, A. (2001). *Medical-surgical nursing: clinical management for positive outcomes* (6th ed.). Philadelphia: W.B. Saunders, p. 254.

---

208. A nurse assists in providing an educational session on the risk factors of cervical cancer to the women in a local community. The nurse understands that which of the following is not a risk factor for this type of cancer?

1   Caucasian race
2   Early age of first intercourse
3   Multiparity
4   Low socioeconomic class

Answer: 1

Rationale: Risk factors for cervical cancer include Black and Native American race, prostitution, early first pregnancy, untreated chronic cervicitis, sexually transmitted diseases, postpartum lacerations, partner with a history of penile or prostate cancer, and infection with human papillomavirus. Options 2, 3, and 4 identify risk factors.

Test-Taking Strategy: Note the key word *not*. Knowledge regarding the risk factors for cervical cancer is necessary to answer this question. Review these risk factors if you had difficulty with this question.

Level of Cognitive Ability: Comprehension
Client Needs: Health Promotion and Maintenance
Integrated Concept/Process: Nursing Process/Data Collection
Content Area: Adult Health/Oncology

Reference:
Black, J., Hawks, J., & Keene, A. (2001). *Medical-surgical nursing: clinical management for positive outcomes* (6th ed.). Philadelphia: W.B. Saunders, p. 370.

---

209. A nurse assists in teaching female clients how to prevent pelvic inflammatory disease (PID). Which of the following would be a component of the instructions?

1   Single sexual partners should be avoided
2   Consult with a gynecologist regarding placement of an intrauterine device (IUD)
3   Douche monthly
4   Avoid unprotected intercourse

Answer: 4

Rationale: Primary prevention for PID includes avoiding each of the following: unprotected intercourse, multiple sexual partners, the use of an IUD, and douching.

Test-Taking Strategy: Use the principle of exposure of the pelvic area as a cause of infection. With this concept in mind, you should be able to eliminate options 1, 2, and 3. Review preventive measures for PID if you had difficulty with this question.

Level of Cognitive Ability: Application

Client Needs: Health Promotion and Maintenance
Integrated Concept/Process: Teaching/Learning
Content Area: Fundamental Skills

Reference:
Black, J., Hawks, J., & Keene, A. (2001). *Medical-surgical nursing: clinical management for positive outcomes* (6th ed.). Philadelphia: W.B. Saunders, p. 988.

---

210. A nurse reinforces discharge teaching to a client after a vasectomy. Which statement by the client would indicate a need for further education?
  1   "If I have pain or swelling I can use an ice bag and take Tylenol."
  2   "I can use a scrotal support if I need to."
  3   "I can resume sexual intercourse whenever I want."
  4   "I don't need to practice birth control any longer."

Answer: 4
Rationale: After vasectomy, the client must continue to practice birth control until the follow-up semen analysis shows azoospermia, because live sperm are left in the ampulla of vas deferens. Options 1, 2, and 3 are appropriate statements.

Test-Taking Strategy: Note the key words *need for further education.* Considering the purpose of a vasectomy should assist in directing you to option 4. Options 1 and 2 can be eliminated because these measures assist in alleviating discomfort or swelling after the procedure. Option 3 can be eliminated because there would be no reason to avoid sexual intercourse unless the client was experiencing discomfort. Review these instructions if you had difficulty with this question.

Level of Cognitive Ability: Comprehension
Client Needs: Health Promotion and Maintenance
Integrated Concept/Process: Nursing Process/Evaluation
Content Area: Fundamental Skills

Reference:
Black, J., Hawks, J., & Keene, A. (2001). *Medical-surgical nursing: clinical management for positive outcomes* (6th ed.). Philadelphia: W.B. Saunders, p. 967.

---

211. A physician in a community clinic diagnoses prostatitis in a client. The nurse reinforces home care instructions to the client. Which statement by the client would indicate a need for further education?
  1   "I should take the antiinflammatory medications as prescribed."
  2   "The sitz baths will help my condition."
  3   "I should avoid sexual activity for 1 week."
  4   "There are no restrictions in my diet."

Answer: 3
Rationale: Interventions include antiinflammatory agents or short-term antimicrobial medication. Sitz baths and normal sexual activity are recommended. Dietary restrictions are not recommended unless the person finds them to be associated with manifestations.

Test-Taking Strategy: Note the key words *need for further education.* Eliminate option 1 first, using the general principles associated with medication prescriptions. Option 4 can be eliminated next because there is no specific relationship between diet and this disorder. From the remaining options, eliminate option 2 because it would seem reasonable that sitz baths would provide comfort. Review instructions for the client with prostatitis if you had difficulty with this question.

Level of Cognitive Ability: Comprehension
Client Needs: Health Promotion and Maintenance
Integrated Concept/Process: Nursing Process/Evaluation
Content Area: Fundamental Skills

Reference:
Black, J., Hawks, J., & Keene, A. (2001). *Medical-surgical nursing: clinical management for positive outcomes* (6th ed.). Philadelphia: W.B. Saunders, p. 962.

---

212. A nursing instructor asks a nursing student to identify the risk factors and methods of prevention of prostate cancer. Which of the following if stated by the student would indicate a need to review this information?
1 Men 50 years of age or older should be monitored with a yearly digital rectal examination
2 Men 50 years of age or older should be monitored with a prostate-specific antigen (PSA assay)
3 A high-fat diet will assist in preventing this type of cancer
4 Employment in fertilizer, textile, and rubber industries increases the risk of prostate cancer

Answer: 3
Rationale: A high intake of dietary fat is a risk factor for prostate cancer. Options 1, 2, and 4 are accurate statements regarding the risks and prevention measures related to this type of cancer.

Test-Taking Strategy: Note the key words *need to review*. Use the process of elimination and general risk factors related to cancer prevention to answer the question. By the wording of this question, you are looking for the option that is an incorrect statement. This should assist in directing you to option 3. Review the risk factors for prostate cancer if you had difficult with this question.

Level of Cognitive Ability: Comprehension
Client Needs: Health Promotion and Maintenance
Integrated Concept/Process: Teaching/Learning
Content Area: Fundamental Skills

Reference:
Black, J., Hawks, J., & Keene, A. (2001). *Medical-surgical nursing: clinical management for positive outcomes* (6th ed.). Philadelphia: W.B. Saunders, p. 958.

---

213. A nurse reinforces information to a married couple regarding measures to prevent infertility. Which of the following measures would not be a component of the discussion?
1 Avoid excessive intake of alcohol
2 Decrease exposure to environmental hazards
3 Eat a nutritious diet
4 Maintain warmth to the scrotum

Answer: 4
Rationale: Keeping the testes cool by avoiding hot baths and tight clothing appears to improve the sperm count. Avoiding factors that depress spermatogenesis, such as the use of drugs, alcohol, and marijuana, exposure to occupational and environmental hazards, and maintaining good nutrition, are key components to prevent infertility.

Test-Taking Strategy: Note the key word *not*. Eliminate option 3 first because maintenance of a nutritious diet is important in all situations. Eliminate options 1 and 2 next because these factors will affect spermatogenesis. Remembering that heat decreases motility of sperm will assist in directing you to the correct option. Review the measures that prevent infertility if you have difficulty with this question.

Level of Cognitive Ability: Application
Client Needs: Health Promotion and Maintenance
Integrated Concept/Process: Nursing Process/Implementation
Content Area: Fundamental Skills

Reference:
Black, J., Hawks, J., & Keene, A. (2001). *Medical-surgical nursing: clinical management for positive outcomes* (6th ed.). Philadelphia: W.B. Saunders, p. 1047.

214. A nurse reinforces home care instructions with a client preparing for discharge after a total hip replacement. Which statement by the client would indicate a need for further education?

1 "I should place a pillow between my knees when I lie down."
2 "I should wear a support stocking on my unaffected leg."
3 "I should not sit in one position for longer than 2 hours."
4 "I cannot drive a car for 6 weeks."

Answer: 3

Rationale: The client should be instructed not to sit continuously for longer than 1 hour and to stand, stretch, and take a few steps periodically. The client cannot drive a car for 6 weeks after surgery unless authorized by a physician. A support stocking should be worn on the unaffected leg and an Ace bandage on the affected leg until there is no swelling in the legs and feet, and full activities are resumed. The legs are abducted by placing a pillow between them when the client lies down.

Test-Taking Strategy: Note the key words *need for further education.* Recalling standard measures related to the postoperative period will assist in eliminating option 4. Knowing that leg abduction is maintained postoperatively during hospitalization may assist in eliminating option 1. From the remaining options, choose option 3, noting the time frame of 2 hours; this is a rather lengthy time period for this client to remain in one position. Review teaching points following total hip replacement if you had difficulty with this question.

Level of Cognitive Ability: Comprehension
Client Needs: Health Promotion and Maintenance
Integrated Concept/Process: Nursing Process/Evaluation
Content Area: Adult Health/Musculoskeletal

Reference:
Black, J., Hawks, J., & Keene, A. (2001). *Medical-surgical nursing: clinical management for positive outcomes* (6th ed.). Philadelphia: W.B. Saunders, p.619.

215. A nurse is caring for a pregnant woman who has had ruptured membranes for longer than 20 hours. The client is receiving intravenous antibiotics. The client asks the nurse why the medication is being given. The best response by the nurse is to tell the client that it will prevent which of the following?

1 Early-onset neonatal Group B streptococcus (GBS) disease
2 Transmission of a sexually transmitted disease to her partner
3 The development of chorioamnionitis
4 Maternal rheumatic fever

Answer: 1

Rationale: One of the Centers for Disease Control (CDC) prevention and treatment guidelines for early-onset neonatal GBS disease and maternal illness includes providing intrapartum antibiotics to women who develop risk conditions at the time of labor or rupture of membranes. A major risk factor for GBS includes prolonged rupture of membranes for more than 12 to 18 hours. Other risk factors include prolonged labor, high number of vaginal examinations during labor, low–birth-weight infants, premature onset of labor, and premature rupture of membranes.

Test-Taking Strategy: Use the process of elimination. Noting the word *antibiotics* in the question will direct you to option 1. If you had difficulty with this question, review GBS disease.

Level of Cognitive Ability: Application
Client Needs: Health Promotion and Maintenance
Integrated Concept/Process: Nursing Process/Implementation
Content Area: Maternity

Reference:
McKinney, E., Ashwill, J., Murray, S. et al. (2000). *Maternal-child nursing.* Philadelphia: W.B. Saunders, p. 681.

216. A client is diagnosed with hypothyroidism and is to begin thyroid supplements. The nurse reinforces instructions to the client about the medication. Which statement by the client would indicate the need for further education?
1 "I should take my daily dose every night at bedtime."
2 "I should call my physician if I develop any chest pain."
3 "I should speak to my physician when I begin to plan for parenthood."
4 "My appetite may increase because of the medication."

Answer: 1
Rationale: The client is instructed to take the medication in the morning to prevent insomnia. If the client experiences any chest pain, it may indicate overdose and the physician should be notified. The dose should be adjusted if the client is pregnant or plans to get pregnant. Gastrointestinal side effects from thyroid supplements include increased appetite, nausea, and diarrhea.

Test-Taking Strategy: Note the key words *need for further education.* You can easily eliminate options 2 and 3 based on basic principles related to medication therapy. Chest pain warrants follow-up evaluation, and pregnancy would require a review of the medication dosage. Because the disorder is hypothyroidism, you would expect a thyroid hormone to increase body metabolism. This should assist you in selecting option 1. Review the medications used in the treatment of hypothyroidism if you had difficulty with this question.

Level of Cognitive Ability: Comprehension
Client Needs: Health Promotion and Maintenance
Integrated Concept/Process: Nursing Process/Evaluation
Content Area: Adult Health/Endocrine

Reference:
Black, J., Hawks, J., & Keene, A. (2001). *Medical-surgical nursing: clinical management for positive outcomes* (6th ed.). Philadelphia: W.B. Saunders, p. 1090.

---

217. A nurse reinforces instructions to the client with diabetes mellitus about how to prevent diabetic ketoacidosis (DKA) on days when the client is feeling ill. Which statement by the client indicates a need for further education?
1 "I should stop my insulin if I am vomiting."
2 "I should call my physician if I am ill for more than 24 hours."
3 "I should monitor my blood glucose frequently."
4 "I should drink small quantities of fluid every 15 to 30 minutes."

Answer: 1
Rationale: The client should be instructed to take insulin even if he or she is vomiting and unable to eat. It is important to self-monitor blood glucose more frequently during illness—as often as every 2 to 4 hours. If the premeal blood glucose is greater than 250 mg/dL, the client should test for urine ketones and contact the physician. Options 2, 3, and 4 are accurate interventions.

Test-Taking Strategy: Note the key words *need for further education.* You should be able to eliminate options 2, 3, and 4. Recalling that insulin should be taken every day will assist in directing you to option 1. Review sick day rules for the diabetic client if you had difficulty with this question.

Level of Cognitive Ability: Comprehension
Client Needs: Health Promotion and Maintenance
Integrated Concept/Process: Self-Care
Content Area: Adult Health/Endocrine

Reference:
Black, J., Hawks, J., & Keene, A. (2001). *Medical-surgical nursing: clinical management for positive outcomes* (6th ed.). Philadelphia: W.B. Saunders, p. 1176.

---

218. A nurse is reinforcing instructions with a client with diabetes mellitus regarding hypoglycemia. Which statement by the

Answer: 2
Rationale: If a hypoglycemia reaction occurs, the client will need to consume 10 to 15 grams of carbohydrate. Six to eight ounces of

client would indicate a need for further education?

1. "Hypoglycemia can occur at any-time of the day or night."
2. "If hypoglycemia occurs, I should take my regular insulin as prescribed."
3. "If I feel sweaty or shaky I may be experiencing hypoglycemia."
4. "I can drink 8 ounces of 2% milk if hypoglycemia occurs."

2% milk contain this amount of carbohydrate. Tremors and diaphoresis are signs of mild hypoglycemia. Insulin is not taken as a treatment for hypoglycemia because the insulin will lower the blood glucose. Hypoglycemic reactions can occur at any time of the day or night.

Test-Taking Strategy: Note the key words *need for further education.* Think about the concept that in hypoglycemia the blood glucose is lowered. Insulin also lowers blood glucose; therefore insulin is not a treatment for this condition. Review the signs of hypoglycemia and the appropriate interventions if you had difficulty with this question.

Level of Cognitive Ability: Comprehension
Client Needs: Health Promotion and Maintenance
Integrated Concept/Process: Nursing Process/Evaluation
Content Area: Adult Health/Endocrine

Reference:
Black, J., Hawks, J., & Keene, A. (2001). *Medical-surgical nursing: clinical management for positive outcomes* (6th ed.). Philadelphia: W.B. Saunders, p. 1177.

---

219. A client with nephrolithiasis arrives at the clinic for a follow-up visit. The laboratory analysis of the stone that the client passed 1 week ago indicates that the stone is composed of calcium oxalate. Which of the following foods would the nurse instruct the client to avoid?

1. Lentils
2. Spinach
3. Lettuce
4. Pasta

Answer: 2
Rationale: Some food sources of oxalate include spinach, rhubarb, strawberries, chocolate, wheat bran, nuts, beets, and tea. Options 1, 3, and 4 are appropriate items to consume.

Test-Taking Strategy: Note the key word *avoid.* Knowledge regarding the foods that contain oxalate is necessary to answer this question. If you had difficulty identifying this food, review this content.

Level of Cognitive Ability: Application
Client Needs: Health Promotion and Maintenance
Integrated Concept/Process: Nursing Process/Implementation
Content Area: Adult Health/Renal

Reference:
Williams, S. (2001) *Basic nutrition & diet therapy* (11th ed.). St. Louis: Mosby, p. 413.

---

220. A nurse reinforces instructions to a new mother who is about to breastfeed her newborn infant. Which of the following instructions would not be part of the teaching?

1. Turn the newborn infant on its side facing the mother
2. When the newborn opens the mouth, draw the newborn the rest of the way onto the breast

Answer: 3
Rationale: The mother is instructed to avoid tilting the nipple upward or squeezing the areola and pushing it into the baby's mouth. Options 1, 2 and 4 are correct procedures for breast feeding.

Test-Taking Strategy: Note the key word *not.* Attempt to visualize the descriptions in each of the options. This will help you eliminate options 1, 2, and 4. Careful reading of option 3, noting the word *pushing* suggests force or resistance and should assist in directing you to this option. Review breastfeeding instructions if you had difficulty with this question.

3 Tilt the nipple upward or squeeze the areola, pushing it into the newborn infant's mouth

4 Place a clean finger in the side of the newborn infant's mouth to break the suction before removing the baby from the breast

Level of Cognitive Ability: Application
Client Needs: Health Promotion and Maintenance
Integrated Concept/Process: Nursing Process/Implementation
Content Area: Maternity

Reference:
McKinney, E., Ashwill, J., Murray, S. et al. (2000). *Maternal-child nursing.* Philadelphia: W.B. Saunders, p. 592.

---

221. A nurse reinforces instructions to a mother regarding the care of her child who is diagnosed with croup. Which statement by the mother indicates a need for further education?

1 "I will place a cool mist humidifier next to my child's bed."

2 "Sips of warm fluids during a croup attack will help."

3 "I will give Tylenol for the fever."

4 "I will give cough syrup every night at bedtime."

Answer: 4
Rationale: The mother should be instructed that cough syrup and cold medicines should not be administered because they may dry and thicken secretions. Sips of warm fluid will relax the vocal cords and thin mucus. A cool mist humidifier rather than a steam vaporizer is recommended because the child could accidentally tip the machine and be burned. Acetaminophen (Tylenol) will reduce the fever.

Test-Taking Strategy: Note the key words *need for further education.* Option 3 can be easily eliminated. Remembering that warm fluids dilute secretions will assist in eliminating option 2. From the remaining options, recalling that cough syrup dries secretions will assist in directing you to option 4. Review home care instructions for the child with croup if you had difficulty with this question.

Level of Cognitive Ability: Comprehension
Client Needs: Health Promotion and Maintenance
Integrated Concept/Process: Nursing Process/Evaluation
Content Area: Child Health

Reference:
Wong, D., & Hockenberry-Eaton, M. (2001). *Wong's essentials of pediatric nursing* (6th ed.). St. Louis: Mosby, pp. 840; 842.

---

222. A client with anxiety disorder is taking buspirone (BuSpar). The client tells the nurse that it is difficult to swallow the tablets. Which of the following would be the best instruction to provide to the client?

1 Purchase the liquid preparation with the next refill

2 Crush the tablets before taking them

3 Call the physician for a change in medication

4 Mix the tablet uncrushed in applesauce

Answer: 2
Rationale: Buspirone may be administered without regard to meals, and the tablets may be crushed. This medication is not available in liquid form. It is premature to advise the client to call the physician for a change in medication without first trying alternative interventions. Mixing the tablet uncrushed in applesauce will not ensure ease in swallowing.

Test-Taking Strategy: Use the process of elimination. You can easily eliminate option 3 first because in most situations there is a nursing intervention that can be instituted first. Next eliminate option 4 because this instruction will not ensure ease in swallowing. From the remaining options, it is necessary to know that this medication is not available in liquid form. In addition, many tablets can be crushed. Review this medication if you had difficulty with this question.

Level of Cognitive Ability: Application
Client Needs: Health Promotion and Maintenance

Integrated Concept/Process: Nursing Process/Implementation
Content Area: Pharmacology

Reference:
Hodgson, B., & Kizior, R. (2003). *Saunders nursing drug handbook 2003.* Philadelphia: W.B. Saunders, p. 148.

---

223. A nurse caring for a child with congestive heart failure reinforces instructions to the parents regarding the administration of digoxin (Lanoxin). Which statement by the mother indicates the need for further education?
  1 "If my child vomits after I give the medication, I will not repeat the dose."
  2 "I will check my child's pulse before giving the medication."
  3 "I will check the dose of the medication with my husband before I give the medication."
  4 "I will mix the medication with food."

Answer: 4
Rationale: The medication should not be mixed with food or formula because this method would not ensure that the child is receiving the entire dose of medication. Options 1, 2, and 3 are correct. In addition, if a dose is missed and is not identified until 4 or more hours later, that dose is not administered. If more than one consecutive dose is missed, the physician should be notified.

Test-Taking Strategy: Note the key words *need for further education.* General principles regarding medication administration to children should assist in directing you to the correct option. Mixing medications with formula or food may alter the effectiveness of the medication. Also, if the child does not consume the entire serving of formula or food, the total dose would not be administered. Review the administration of this medication if you had difficulty with this question.

Level of Cognitive Ability: Comprehension
Client Needs: Health Promotion and Maintenance
Integrated Concept/Process: Nursing Process/Evaluation
Content Area: Pharmacology

Reference:
Hodgson, B., & Kizior, R. (2003). *Saunders nursing drug handbook 2003.* Philadelphia: W.B. Saunders, p. 350.

---

224. A nurse reinforces home care instructions to the mother of a child who was hospitalized for heart surgery. Which of the following would be included in the teaching plan?
  1 The child may return to school 1 week after hospital discharge
  2 After bathing, rub lotion and sprinkle powder on the incision
  3 Allow the child to play outside for short periods
  4 Notify the physician if the child develops a fever greater than 100.5° F

Answer: 4
Rationale: After heart surgery, the child should not return to school until 3 weeks after hospital discharge; at that time the child should go to school half days for the first few days. No creams, lotions, or powders should be placed on the incision until it is completely healed and without scabs. The mother is instructed to omit play outside for several weeks. The physician needs to be notified if the child develops a fever greater than 100.5° F.

Test-Taking Strategy: Use the process of elimination, bearing in mind the potential for infection. Eliminate option 1 because of the time frame of 1 week. Eliminate option 3 because outside play can expose the child to infection and the risk of injury. Basic principles related to incision care should assist in eliminating option 2. Review these instructions if you had difficulty with this question.

Level of Cognitive Ability: Application
Client Needs: Health Promotion and Maintenance
Integrated Concept/Process: Teaching/Learning
Content Area: Child Health

Reference:
Wong, D., & Hockenberry-Eaton, M. (2001). *Wong's essentials of pediatric nursing* (6th ed.). St. Louis: Mosby, p. 962.

225. A nurse reinforces instructions to a client who will begin taking oral contraceptives. Which statement by the client would indicate the need for further education?

    1   "I will take one pill daily at the same time every day."

    2   "I will not need to use an additional birth control method once I start these pills."

    3   "If I miss a pill I should take it as soon as I remember."

    4   "If I miss two pills I will take them both as soon as I remember, and I will take two pills the next day also."

Answer: 2

Rationale: The client should be instructed to use a second birth control method during the first pill cycle. Options 1, 3, and 4 are correct. In addition, the client should be instructed that if she misses three pills, she should discontinue use for that cycle and use another birth control method.

Test-Taking Strategy: Note the key words *need for further education*. Knowledge regarding guidelines for oral contraceptive use is necessary to answer this question. It would seem reasonable, however, that during the first pill cycle, a second birth control method should be used to prevent conception. Review these guidelines if you had difficulty with this question.

Level of Cognitive Ability: Comprehension
Client Needs: Health Promotion and Maintenance
Integrated Concept/Process: Self-Care
Content Area: Pharmacology

Reference:
Murray, S., McKinney, E., & Gorrie, T. (2002). *Foundations of maternal-newborn nursing* (3rd ed.). Philadelphia: W.B. Saunders, p. 877.

FILL-IN-THE-BLANK

A client with myasthenia gravis reports the occurrence of difficulty chewing. The physician prescribes pyridostigmine bromide (Mestinon) to increase muscle strength for this activity. The nurse instructs the client to take the medication at what time, in relation to meals?
Answer: _____

Answer: Before meals

Rationale: Pyridostigmine is a cholinergic medication used to increase muscle strength for the client with myasthenia gravis. For the client who has difficulty chewing, the medication should be administered 30 minutes before meals to enhance the client's ability to eat.

Test-Taking Strategy: Focus on the issue: difficulty chewing. Knowing that the medication increases muscle strength will assist in determining that administering the medication 30 minutes before meals will provide the client the ability to chew the food. Review client teaching points related to this medication if you had difficulty with this question.

Level of Cognitive Ability: Application
Client Needs: Health Promotion and Maintenance
Integrated Concept/Process: Self Care
Content Area: Pharmacology

Reference:
Hodgson, B. & Kizior, R. (2003). *Saunders nursing drug handbook 2003.* Philadelphia: W.B. Saunders, p. 949.

MULTIPLE-RESPONSE – SELECT ALL THAT APPLY

A nurse is assisting in developing a teaching plan for a client who had ostomy surgery who will be caring for the ostomy at home. Select all instructions that should be included in the teaching plan.

____ Bathing and showering can be done with the appliance in place

____ Wear a snug article of clothing over the stoma to hold the appliance in place

____ Limit fluid intake to 1000 mL daily

____ Contact the physician if the stoma appears to bulge out

____ Avoid foods that cause excess gas

____ Traveling needs to be limited because of the differences in drinking water and food preparation that the client is used to

____ The United Ostomy Association can be contacted about information regarding living with an ostomy

____ Heavy lifting and strenuous activities are avoided for eight to twelve weeks following creation of the ostomy

Answer:

____ Bathing and showering can be done with the appliance in place

____ Contact the physician if the stoma appears to bulge out

____ Avoid foods that cause excess gas

____ The United Ostomy Association can be contacted about information regarding living with an ostomy

____ Heavy lifting and strenuous activities are avoided for 8 to 12 weeks after creation of the ostomy

Rationale: In the client with an ostomy, bathing and showering can be done with the appliance in place because the pouch and seal are waterproof. The client can wear regular clothing but should avoid snug clothing and direct pressure over the stoma. A fluid intake of at least 2000 mL a day should be maintained. The client is instructed to contact the physician if skin breakdown, prolapse (bulging out) of the stoma, or obstruction (output absent or markedly decreased) occurs. The client is taught about the foods to avoid, particularly those that cause excess gas and odor. Traveling does not need to be limited or restricted. If the client is planning to visit a country where drinking the water is not advised, the client is instructed not to irrigate the ostomy with the water. The United Ostomy Association, American Cancer Society, and the Crohn's and Colitis Foundations of America can be contacted about information regarding living with an ostomy. Heavy lifting and strenuous activities are avoided at first, and there are usually no restrictions after approximately 3 months after surgery.

Test-Taking Strategy: Focus on the issue: care to an ostomy. Focusing on this issue and recalling the specific client teaching points is needed to answer this question. Review client teaching points related to care to an ostomy if you had difficulty with this question.

Level of Cognitive Ability: Application
Client Needs: Health Promotion and Maintenance
Integrated Concept/Process: Self Care
Content Area: Adult Health/Gastrointestinal

Reference:
Linton, A. & Maebius, N. (2003). *Introduction to medical-surgical nursing* (3rd ed.). Philadelphia: W.B. Saunders, pp. 351-352.

REFERENCES

Black, J., Hawks, J., & Keene, A. (2001). *Medical-surgical nursing: clinical management for positive outcomes* (6th ed.). Philadelphia: W.B. Saunders.

Burroughs, A., & Leifer, G. (2002). *Maternity nursing* (8th ed.). Philadelphia: W.B. Saunders.

Clark, J., Queener, S., & Karb, V. (2002). *Pharmacologic basis of nursing practice* (6th ed.). St. Louis: Mosby.

deWit, S. (2001). *Fundamental concepts and skills for nursing.* Philadelphia: W.B. Saunders.

Ignatavicius, D., & Workman, M. (2002). *Medical-surgical nursing: critical thinking for collaborative care* (4th ed.). Philadelphia: W.B. Saunders.

Johnson, M., Bulechek, G., Dochterman, J. et al. (2001). *Nursing diagnoses, outcomes, and interventions.* St. Louis: Mosby.

Lehne, R. (2001). *Pharmacology for nursing care* (4th ed.). Philadelphia: W.B. Saunders.

Linton, A., & Maebius, N. (2003). *Introduction to medical-surgical nursing* (3rd ed.). Philadelphia: W.B. Saunders.

McKinney, E., Ashwill, J., Murray, S. et al. (2000). *Maternal-child nursing.* Philadelphia: W.B Saunders.

Murray, S., McKinney, E., & Gorrie, T. (2002). *Foundations of maternal-newborn nursing* (3rd ed.). Philadelphia: W.B. Saunders.

Perry, A., & Potter, P. (2002). *Clinical nursing skills & techniques* (5th ed.). St. Louis: Mosby.

Potter, P., & Perry, A. (2001). *Fundamentals of nursing* (5th ed.). St. Louis: Mosby.

Schulte, E., Price, D., & Gwin, J. (2001). *Thompson's pediatric nursing* (8th ed.). Philadelphia: W.B. Saunders.

Wong, D., & Hockenberry-Eaton, M. (2001). *Wong's essentials of pediatric nursing* (6th ed.). St. Louis: Mosby

Williams, S. (2001) *Basic nutrition & diet therapy* (11th ed.). St. Louis: Mosby.

Varcarolis, E. (2002). *Foundations of psychiatric mental health nursing* (4th ed.). Philadelphia: W.B. Saunders.

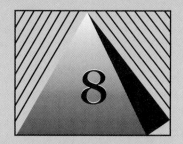

Psychosocial Integrity

1. A nurse is gathering data from a male client who has just been admitted to the hospital with a diagnosis of coronary artery disease. During the interviewing process the client tells the nurse that he has been quite stressed. The most therapeutic first action would be to:

1 Tell the client everybody is stressed these days
2 Encourage the client to verbalize the sources of stress in his life
3 Have the client write down the sources of stress in his life
4 Set up a psychiatric consult for the client

Answer: 2

Rationale: The nurse encourages the client to verbalize the stressors so that client strategies for coping with unavoidable stress can be explored. Option 1 does not address the client's concerns. Option 3 may be appropriate but is not the first action. Option 4 is not within the nurse's scope of practice.

Test-Taking Strategy: Use the process of elimination. Noting the key words *first action* will assist in directing you to option 2. Remember to focus on the client's feelings first. Review therapeutic communication techniques if you had difficulty with this question.

Level of Cognitive Ability: Application
Client Needs: Psychosocial Integrity
Integrated Concept/Process: Nursing Process/Implementation
Content Area: Adult Health/Cardiovascular

Reference:
Black, J., Hawks, J., & Keene, A. (2001). *Medical-surgical nursing: clinical management for positive outcomes* (6th ed.). Philadelphia: W.B. Saunders, p. 1454.

2. A nurse is caring for a female client admitted to the hospital with a diagnosis of angina pectoris. The nurse is gathering data from the client and during the interviewing process the client confidentially tells the nurse that she does recreational drugs, such as cocaine. Knowing the effect that this medication has on the heart, the nurse would:

1 Tell the client about the need to stop the drug
2 Explain to the client what the drug is doing to the heart

Answer: 3

Rationale: Option 3 is the best option. In this option, the nurse teaches the client about the effects of the drug, addresses the problem, and gets the client the needed help. Option 1 is incorrect because the client has an addiction and the client has to want to stop the drug. Option 2 does not address the fact that the client has a problem that she needs further help with. Option 4 is incorrect because what the client is telling the nurse is confidential; at this time, the nurse would violate the client's rights.

Test-Taking Strategy: Use the process of elimination and select the option that provides information to the client and at the same time assists the client with the problem. This will direct you to

3   Teach the client about the effects that cocaine has on the heart and plan to get the client further help
4   Report the client to the police for illegal drug use

option 3. If you had difficulty with this question, review care to the client with a drug addiction.

Level of Cognitive Ability: Application
Client Needs: Psychosocial Integrity
Integrated Concept/Process: Nursing Process/Implementation
Content Area: Mental Health

Reference:
Black, J., Hawks, J., & Keene, A. (2001). *Medical-surgical nursing: clinical management for positive outcomes* (6th ed.). Philadelphia: W.B. Saunders, p. 520.

---

3. A male client is admitted to the hospital with a diagnosis of myocardial infarction (MI). During the interviewing process, the client tells the nurse that the pain is probably related to the greasy cheeseburger he had for lunch. The nurse knows that this response from the client is common for people experiencing an MI and will be better able to help the client because:

1   A high fatty diet causes a MI
2   Denial is a major factor in not seeking immediate treatment
3   The client wants to blame something else for his problem

4   The client doesn't understand the factors that cause the disease process

Answer: 2
Rationale: An individual's first response to the pain that he or she is experiencing is denial because the individual can't believe that he or she is really having an MI. This in turn keeps the individual from seeking immediate medical treatment. Knowing that this is a common response, the nurse will be better able to help the client face the reality of the situation. Options 1 and 4 are not accurate. Although option 3 may be partially correct, option 2 is the most accurate option.

Test-Taking Strategy: Use the process of elimination and knowledge of the psychological effects that an individual experiences if they have a MI. Noting the key word *common* will assist in directing you to option 2. Review the psychosocial effects of a MI if you had difficulty with this question.

Level of Cognitive Ability: Comprehension
Client Needs: Psychosocial Integrity
Integrated Concept/Process: Nursing Process/Planning
Content Area: Adult Health/Cardiovascular

Reference:
Black, J., Hawks, J., & Keene, A. (2001). *Medical-surgical nursing: clinical management for positive outcomes* (6th ed.). Philadelphia: W.B. Saunders, p. 408.

---

4. A nurse is caring for a client with schizophrenia and documents in the client's record that the client has a flat affect. Which of the following most appropriately describes this behavior observed by the nurse?
1   A minimal emotional response
2   An immobile facial expression or blank look
3   An emotional response that is not congruent with the tone of the situation
4   Grimacing, giggling, or mumbling to oneself

Answer: 2
Rationale: A flat affect is an immobile facial expression or blank look. A blunted affect is indicated by a minimal emotional response. An inappropriate affect refers to an emotional response to a situation that is not congruent with the tone of the situation. A bizarre affect is especially prominent in the disorganized form of schizophrenia and is characterized by grimacing, giggling, or mumbling to oneself.

Test-Taking Strategy: Use the process of elimination. Note the words *flat* in the question and *blank* in the correct option. This relationship may assist you in identifying the correct option. Review these client behaviors if you had difficulty with this question.

Level of Cognitive Ability: Comprehension
Client Needs: Psychosocial Integrity

Integrated Concept/Process: Nursing Process/Data Collection
Content Area: Mental Health

Reference:
Bauer, B. & Hill, S. (2000). *Mental health nursing.* Philadelphia: W.B. Saunders, p.133.

---

5. A nurse assigned to care for a postpartum client will promote maternal-infant bonding when the nurse instructs the parents to:

1 Avoid using a high-pitched voice to speak to the infant

2 Allow the nursing staff to assume the infant care while in the hospital so they may rest

3 Hold and cuddle the infant closely each time the infant cries

4 Allow the infant to sleep in the parental bed between the parents

Answer: 3
Rationale: Holding and cuddling the infant closely initiates a positive experience for the mother. It is self-quieting and consoles the infant. The use of a high-pitched voice and participating in infant care are other methods of promoting paternal-infant attachment. An infant should not be allowed to sleep in the parental bed between parents not only because of the danger of suffocation, but also because the couple will require meaningful rest and time to be alone as a couple.

Test-Taking Strategy: Note the key word *promote* and use the process of elimination. Option 3 is the only option that addresses the issue of bonding. Review measures that will promote paternal-infant bonding if you had difficulty with this question.

Level of Cognitive Ability: Application
Client Needs: Psychosocial Integrity
Integrated Concept/Process: Nursing Process/Implementation
Content Area: Maternity

Reference:
McKinney, E., Ashwill, J., Murray, S. et al. (2000). *Maternal-child nursing.* Philadelphia: W.B Saunders, p. 498.

---

6. A nurse is assigned to care for a postpartum client. When collecting data regarding the new mother's parental anxieties, which client statement would indicate a potential problem with maternal-infant attachment?

1 "Why did this baby have to inherit my family's ugly toes?"

2 "I am too tired to fed him right now; let the nursery nurse do it this once."

3 "He has his daddy's deep blue eyes."

4 "I just feel weepy all the time."

Answer: 1
Rationale: Negativity about the baby's features may interfere with the mother's ability to bond with and care for the infant. Positive statements and identification with family members help the mother to identify with the infant, promoting attachment. Fatigue and mild postpartum depression are expected responses and may cause the mother to feel weepy and to request the staff to assume care of the infant temporarily; however, after a period of rest, she should begin to assume care for the infant.

Test-Taking Strategy: Focus on the issue of the question and the key words *potential problem with maternal attachment.* Use the process of elimination to direct you to option 1. Review factors that affect maternal-infant attachment if you had difficulty with this question.

Level of Cognitive Ability: Comprehension
Client Needs: Psychosocial Integrity
Integrated Concept/Process: Nursing Process/Data Collection
Content Area: Maternity

Reference:
McKinney, E., Ashwill, J., Murray, S. et al. (2000). *Maternal-child nursing.* Philadelphia: W.B Saunders, p. 498.

7. A nurse plans to counsel a postpartum client on caloric intake after discharge. Before the nurse can adequately advise the client, which of the following data is collected first?

  1 Method of infant feeding that the mother has chosen
  2 Concerns about weight gain
  3 Presence of fluoride in drinking water
  4 Cultural preferences

Answer: 1

Rationale: Nonlactating women require a balanced diet of approximately 300 calories a day less than that consumed during pregnancy. The lactating woman will require an increase of 500 calories a day above that consumed during pregnancy. Good nutrition, not weight loss or gain, is the focus of the postpartum diet. Cultural preferences are important but do not influence the amount of caloric intake required.

Test-Taking Strategy: Focus on the issue of the question and knowledge of the differences in nutritional requirements between the lactating and nonlactating mother. Noting the key word *first* will assist in directing you to option 1. Review dietary requirements in the postpartum period if you had difficulty with this question.

Level of Cognitive Ability: Comprehension
Client Needs: Psychosocial Integrity
Integrated Concept/Process: Nursing Process/Data Collection
Content Area: Maternity

Reference:
McKinney, E., Ashwill, J., Murray, S. et al. (2000). *Maternal-child nursing.* Philadelphia: W.B Saunders, p. 74.

8. A young adult male client with spinal cord injury (SCI) tells the nurse, "It's so depressing that I'll never get to have sex again." The nurse replies in a realistic way by making which of the following statements to the client?

  1 "You're young, so you'll adapt to this more easily than if you were older."
  2 "It must feel horrible to know you can never have sex again."
  3 "It is still possible to have a sexual relationship, but it is different."
  4 "Because of body reflexes, sexual functioning will be no different than before."

Answer: 3

Rationale: It is possible to have a sexual relationship after SCI, but it is different than what the client experienced before the injury. Males may experience reflex erections, although they may not ejaculate. Females can have adductor spasm. Sexual counseling may help the client to adapt to changes in sexuality after SCI. Options 1 and 4 are incorrect statements. Option 2 does not promote continued discussion of the client's concerns.

Test-Taking Strategy: Knowledge regarding the altered physiology after SCI and therapeutic communication techniques will assist in answering the question. Eliminate options 1 and 4 first because they are incorrect statements. Eliminate option 2 next because it is a communication block. Review the effects of a SCI and therapeutic communication techniques if you had difficulty with this question.

Level of Cognitive Ability: Application
Client Needs: Psychosocial Integrity
Integrated Concept/Process: Communication and Documentation
Content Area: Adult Health/Neurological

Reference:
Black, J., Hawks, J., & Keene, A. (2001). *Medical-surgical nursing: clinical management for positive outcomes* (6th ed.). Philadelphia: W.B. Saunders, p. 2060.

9. A family member of a client who was just diagnosed with a brain tumor is distraught and feeling guilty for not encouraging the client to seek medical evaluation

Answer: 2

Rationale: Signs and symptoms of brain tumor vary, depending on location, and may easily be attributed to another cause. Symptoms include headache, vomiting, visual disturbances, and

earlier. The nurse plans to incorporate which of the following items in formulating a response to the client's verbal concern?

1 It is true that brain tumors are easily recognizable

2 The symptoms of brain tumor may be easily attributed to another cause

3 Brain tumors are never detected until very late in their course

4 There are no symptoms of brain tumor

change in intellectual abilities or personality. Seizures occur in some clients. The family requires support to assist them in the normal grieving process. Options 1, 3, and 4 are incorrect.

Test-Taking Strategy: Use the process of elimination. Eliminate options 3 and 4 first because they contain the absolute words *never* and *no*, respectively. From the remaining options, it is necessary to know that the symptoms of brain tumor can be vague and may be easily attributed to another cause. Review this content area if you had difficulty with this question.

Level of Cognitive Ability: Application
Client Needs: Psychosocial Integrity
Integrated Concept/Process: Nursing Process/Planning
Content Area: Adult Health/Neurological

Reference:
Black, J., Hawks, J., & Keene, A. (2001). *Medical-surgical nursing: clinical management for positive outcomes* (6th ed.). Philadelphia: W.B. Saunders, p. 1932.

---

10. A male client is in a hip spica cast as a result of a hip fracture. On the day after the cast has been applied, the nurse finds the client surrounded by papers from his briefcase and planning a phone meeting. The nurse's interaction with the client should be based on the knowledge that:

1 Setting limits on a client's behavior is an essential aspect of the nursing role

2 Not keeping up with his job will increase his stress level

3 Immediate involvement in his job will keep him from becoming bored while on bed rest

4 Rest is an essential component in bone healing

Answer: 4
Rationale: Rest is an essential component of bone healing. The nurse can help the client understand the importance of rest and find ways to balance work demands with rest to promote healing. A nurse cannot demand that the client make changes but should encourage the client to make them. Doing work may relieve stress; however, in the immediate postcast period it may not be therapeutic. Stress should be kept at a minimum to promote bone healing.

Test-Taking Strategy: Use the process of elimination and focus on the issue, *rest.* Option 4 is the most global option and addresses the issue of the question. Review psychosocial and physical needs of the client after a hip fracture if you had difficulty with this question.

Level of Cognitive Ability: Comprehension
Client Needs: Psychosocial Integrity
Integrated Concept/Process: Nursing Process/Planning
Content Area: Adult Health/Musculoskeletal

Reference:
Black, J., Hawks, J., & Keene, A. (2001). *Medical-surgical nursing: clinical management for positive outcomes* (6th ed.). Philadelphia: W.B. Saunders, p. 588.

---

11. A licensed practical nurse (LPN) observes a nursing assistant talking in an unusually loud voice to a client with delirium. Which of these actions should the LPN take?

1 Speak to the nursing assistant immediately while in the client's room to solve the problem

2 Inform the client that everything is all right

Answer: 3
Rationale: The nurse must determine that the client is safe and then discuss the matter with the nursing assistant in an area where the conversation cannot be heard by the client. If the client hears the conversation, the client may become more confused or agitated. Options 1 and 4 could add to the client's confusion. Additionally, option 1 can embarrass the nursing assistant. Option 2 is a communication block.

3   Determine the client's safety, calmly ask the nursing assistant to join you outside the room, and inform the nursing assistant of the observation

4   Explain to the nursing assistant that yelling in the client's room is tolerated only if the client is talking loudly

Test-Taking Strategy: Use Maslow's Hierarchy of Needs theory and therapeutic communication techniques. Option 2 is eliminated first because it is a communication block. Next recall that safety needs are a priority. This will direct you to option 3. Review therapeutic communication techniques if you had difficulty with this question.

Level of Cognitive Ability: Application
Client Needs: Psychosocial Integrity
Integrated Concept/Process: Nursing Process/Implementation
Content Area: Mental Health

Reference:
Varcarolis, E. (2002). *Foundations of psychiatric mental health nursing* (4th ed.). Philadelphia: W.B. Saunders, p. 258.

---

12. A teenager who has celiac disease presents with profuse, watery, diarrhea after a pizza party the previous night. The client states, "I don't want to be different from my friends." The nurse determines that the client is at most risk for which psychosocial problem?

1   Lack of understanding about the disease process
2   Dehydration
3   Altered self-esteem
4   Celiac crisis

Answer: 3
Rationale: The client expresses concern over being *different*. Data provided in the question do not support a lack of understanding about the disease process. Dehydration and celiac crisis are physiological problems.

Test-Taking Strategy: Note the key words *psychosocial problem*. Focus on the data in the question and on the client's feelings of being "different." Option 3 is the only option that addresses this issue. Review the psychosocial issues of an adolescent with a chronic disorder if you had difficulty with this question.

Level of Cognitive Ability: Analysis
Client Needs: Psychosocial Integrity
Integrated Concept/Process: Nursing Process/Data Collection
Content Area: Child Health

Reference:
Wong, D., & Hockenberry-Eaton, M. (2001). *Wong's essentials of pediatric nursing* (6th ed.). St. Louis: Mosby, p. 927.

---

13. A nurse is assisting in developing a plan of care for a 1-month-old infant hospitalized for intussusception. Which measure would be most effective to provide psychosocial support for the parent-child relationship?

1   Encourage the parents to go home and get some sleep
2   Encourage the parents to room-in with their infant
3   Provide educational materials
4   Initiate home nutritional support as early as possible

Answer: 2
Rationale: Rooming-in is effective in reducing separation anxiety and preserving the parent-child relationship. It is stressful for the parents when a child is ill and hospitalized. Telling a parent to go home and sleep will not relieve this stress. Educational materials, although beneficial, will not provide psychosocial support for the parent-child relationship. Home nutritional support is not usually necessary to treat intussusception.

Test-Taking Strategy: Use the process of elimination and focus on the key words *provide psychosocial support*. Note that option 2 is the only option that provides an interaction between the child and parents. Review measures that provide psychosocial support for parents if you had difficulty with this question.

Level of Cognitive Ability: Application
Client Needs: Psychosocial Integrity

Integrated Concept/Process: Nursing Process/Planning
Content Area: Child Health

Reference:
Wong, D., & Hockenberry-Eaton, M. (2001). *Wong's essentials of pediatric nursing* (6th ed.). St. Louis: Mosby, p. 666.

---

14. The parents of a male infant who will have an inguinal hernia repair make the following comments. Which one of these comments would require follow-up evaluation by a nurse?
   1   "I understand surgery will repair the hernia."
   2   "We were told to give him sponge baths for a few days after surgery."
   3   "I'll need to buy extra diapers because we need to change them more frequently now."
   4   "I don't know if he will be able to father a child."

Answer: 4
Rationale: The anatomical location of hernias frequently causes more psychological concern to the parents than does the actual condition or treatment. Options 1, 2, and 3 all indicate the parents' accurate understanding.

Test-Taking Strategy: Focus on the key words *would require follow-up evaluation.* Option 4 reflects parental fear and identifies a need for further assistance. Review these parental concerns and care to the infant requiring inguinal hernia repair if you had difficulty with this question.

Level of Cognitive Ability: Analysis
Client Needs: Psychosocial Integrity
Integrated Concept/Process: Nursing Process/Data Collection
Content Area: Child Health

Reference:
Wong, D., & Hockenberry-Eaton, M. (2001). *Wong's essentials of pediatric nursing* (6th ed.). St. Louis: Mosby, p. 919.

---

15. A licensed practical nurse is assisting a school nurse to conduct a crisis intervention group. The clients are high school students whose classmate recently committed suicide at the school. The students are experiencing disbelief and reviewing details about finding the student dead in a bathroom. Based on this information, the nurse would first:
   1   Inquire how the students coped with death events in the past
   2   Reinforce the students' sense of growth through this death
   3   Reinforce the students' ability to work through this death event
   4   Inquire about the students' perception of their classmate's suicide

Answer: 4
Rationale: It is essential to first determine the students' view. Inquiring about the students' perception of the death will specifically identify the appraisal of the suicide and the meaning of the perception. Options 2 and 3 are similar in terms of attempts to foster clients' self-esteem. Such an approach is premature at this point. Although option 1 is exploratory, it does not address the "here and now" appraisal in terms of their classmate's suicide. Although the nurse is interested in how clients have coped in the past, this inquiry is not the most immediate.

Test-Taking Strategy: Use the process of elimination. Consider the issue of the question and select the option that deals with the "here and now." The nurse must first determine the client's perception or appraisal of the stressful event. Review the phases of crisis if you had difficulty with this question.

Level of Cognitive Ability: Application
Client Needs: Psychosocial Integrity
Integrated Concept/Process: Nursing Process/Data Collection
Content Area: Mental Health

Reference:
Varcarolis, E. (2002). *Foundations of psychiatric mental health nursing* (4th ed.). Philadelphia: W.B. Saunders, p. 627.

16. A hospitalized client has participated in substance abuse therapy group sessions and the nurse is monitoring the client's response to the sessions. Upon discharge, the client has consented to participate in Alcoholics Anonymous community groups. Which statement by the client would best indicate to the nurse that the client has well assimilated session topics and has processed information realistically for self-use?

1   "I know I'm ready to be discharged; I feel like I can say "no" and leave a group of friends if they are drinking. No problem."

2   "This group has really helped a lot. I know it will be different when I go home. But I'm sure that my family and friends will all help me like the people in this group have. They'll all help me...I know they will...they won't let me go back to old ways."

3   "I'm looking forward to leaving here; I know that I will miss all of you. So, I'm happy and I'm sad. I'm excited and I'm scared. I know it will be different out there. I know I have to make new friends and not hang around the local pubs. I know that I have to work hard to be strong and that everyone isn't going to be as helpful as you people. I know it isn't going to be easy. But, I'm going to try as hard as I can."

4   "I'll keep all my appointments; go to all my AA groups. I'll do everything I'm supposed to do. Nothing will go wrong that way."

Answer: 3

Rationale: In option 3 the client is expressing concern and ambivalence about discharge from the hospital. The client verbalizes reality in the appraisal about the changes that the client will have to initiate in lifestyle, as well as the fact that the client has to work hard and develop new friends and meeting places. Option 1 indicates client denial. In option 2, the client is relying heavily on others; the client's locus of control is external. In option 4, the client is concrete and procedure-oriented, but the client is unrealistic and states that "nothing will go wrong that way" if the client follows all the directions.

Test-Taking Strategy: Use the process of elimination. Select the option that identifies the most realistic client verbalization. This will direct you to option 3. Review the therapeutic effects of support groups if you had difficulty with this question.

Level of Cognitive Ability: Analysis
Client Needs: Psychosocial Integrity
Integrated Concept/Process: Nursing Process/Evaluation
Content Area: Mental Health

Reference:
Varcarolis, E. (2002). *Foundations of psychiatric mental health nursing* (4th ed.). Philadelphia: W.B. Saunders, p. 288.

---

17. A client recovering from a head injury becomes agitated at times. Which action will most likely calm this client?

1   Turn on the television to a musical program

2   Give the client a soft object to hold

3   Assign the client a new task to master

4   Make the client aware that the behavior is undesirable

Answer: 2

Rationale: Decreasing environmental stimuli aids in reducing agitation for the head-injured client. Option 1 increases stimuli. Option 3 does not simplify the environment; a new task may be frustrating. Option 4 identifies a nontherapeutic approach. The correct option helps to distract the client with a motor activity—holding a soft object.

Test-Taking Strategy: Use the process of elimination to identify options that may increase stimuli, agitation, and frustration. This should assist in directing you to the correct option. Review measures that will decrease agitation if you had difficulty with this question.

Level of Cognitive Ability: Application
Client Needs: Psychosocial Integrity

Integrated Concept/Process: Nursing Process/Implementation
Content Area: Adult Health/Neurological

Reference:
Black, J., Hawks, J., & Keene, A. (2001). *Medical-surgical nursing: clinical management for positive outcomes* (6th ed.). Philadelphia: W.B. Saunders, p. 2046.

---

18. A recovering postcerebrovascular accident (CVA) client has become irritable and angry about limitations. What is the best approach by the nurse to help the client regain motivation to succeed?
1   Allow longer and more frequent visitation by the spouse
2   Use supportive statements to correct behavior
3   State that with your experience you know how he or she feels
4   Ignore the behavior, knowing that the client is grieving

Answer: 2
Rationale: Post-CVA clients have many and varied needs. The client may need behavior pointed out so that correction can take place, as well as support and praise for accomplishments. Spouses of post-CVA clients are often grieving; therefore more visitations may not be helpful. Short visits are often encouraged. Stating that you know how someone feels is inappropriate. The client may be grieving or may have damage to cerebral inhibitory centers; however, the behavior should not be ignored.

Test-Taking Strategy: Use therapeutic communication techniques. Option 2 is the only option that addresses client feelings and supportive care. Review care to the client after a CVA if you had difficulty with this question.

Level of Cognitive Ability: Application
Client Needs: Psychosocial Integrity
Integrated Concept/Process: Nursing Process/Implementation
Content Area: Adult Health/Neurological

Reference:
Black, J., Hawks, J., & Keene, A. (2001). *Medical-surgical nursing: clinical management for positive outcomes* (6th ed.). Philadelphia: W.B. Saunders, p. 1965.

---

19. A client is admitted to the hospital with a broken hip and is experiencing periods of confusion. The nurse assists in developing a plan of care related to altered thought processes. The nurse understands that the psychosocial outcome that has the highest priority is:
1   Improved sleep patterns
2   Increased ability to concentrate and make decisions
3   Independently meeting self-care needs
4   Reducing family fears and anxiety

Answer: 2
Rationale: The client should be able to concentrate and make decisions. Once the client is able to do that, the nurse can work with the client to achieve the other outcomes. Options 1, 3, and 4 are goals secondary to option 2.

Test-Taking Strategy: Use the process of elimination. Look for the option that will have the greatest impact on the client's ability to function. Option 4 can be easily eliminated because it does not address the client of the question. Option 1 is unrelated to the primary issue. Option 3 is unrealistic at this time, considering the word *independently*. Option 2 will make the greatest difference in the client's ability to achieve options 1, 3, and 4. Review goals of care for the client with altered thought processes if you had difficulty with this question.

Level of Cognitive Ability: Analysis
Client Needs: Psychosocial Integrity
Integrated Concept/Process: Nursing Process/Planning
Content Area: Adult Health/Musculoskeletal

Reference:
Black, J., Hawks, J., & Keene, A. (2001). *Medical-surgical nursing: clinical management for positive outcomes* (6th ed.). Philadelphia: W.B. Saunders, p. 1918.

20. The client is a young woman dying from breast cancer. A defining characteristic of anticipatory grief is present when the client:

1 Verbalizes unrealistic goals and plans for the future

2 Discusses thoughts and feelings related to loss

3 Has prolonged emotional reactions and outbursts

4 Ignores untreated medical conditions that require treatment

Answer: 2

Rationale: The nurse can determine the client's stage of grief by observing behavior. This is extremely important so that an appropriate plan of care can be developed. Option 2 identifies anticipatory grief. Options 1, 3, and 4 are examples of dysfunctional grieving.

Test-Taking Strategy: Note the similarity in options 1, 3, and 4 and the words *unrealistic, prolonged,* and *ignores* in these options. These are examples of dysfunctional grieving. Review the stages of grief and anticipatory grief if you had difficulty with this question.

Level of Cognitive Ability: Analysis
Client Needs: Psychosocial Integrity
Integrated Concept/Process: Nursing Process/Data Collection
Content Area: Adult Health/Neurological

Reference:
Black, J., Hawks, J., & Keene, A. (2001). *Medical-surgical nursing: clinical management for positive outcomes* (6th ed.). Philadelphia: W.B. Saunders, p. 459.

---

21. A licensed practical nurse (LPN) notes that a client in labor is beginning to experience signs of shock from hemorrhage secondary to a partial inversion of the uterus. The LPN immediately notifies the registered nurse. The client asks in an apprehensive voice, "What is happening to me? I feel so funny and I know I am bleeding. Am I dying?" The nurse bases the response on the fact that the client is feeling:

1 Panic secondary to shock

2 Fear and anxiety related to the unexpected and ambiguous sensations

3 Anticipatory grieving related to the fear of dying

4 Depression related to postpartum hormonal changes

Answer: 2

Rationale: Feelings of loss of control because of the unknown are common causes of anxiety. Apprehension and feelings of impending doom are also associated with shock, but the case situation does not suggest panic at this point. Anticipatory grieving occurs when there is knowledge of the impending loss, but is not operative in a sudden situational crisis such as this one. It is far too early for the onset of postpartum depression.

Test-Taking Strategy: Use the process of elimination noting the words *apprehensive voice* in the question. Note the relationship between the words *I feel so funny* in the question and *unexpected and ambiguous sensations* in the correct option. Review the causes of anxiety if you had difficulty with this question.

Level of Cognitive Ability: Application
Client Needs: Psychosocial Integrity
Integrated Concept/Process: Nursing Process/Implementation
Content Area: Maternity

Reference:
McKinney, E., Ashwill, J., Murray, S. et al. (2000). *Maternal-child nursing.* Philadelphia: W.B Saunders, p. 31.

---

22. A nurse has just assessed the fetal status of a client with a diagnosis of partial placental abruption of 20 weeks' gestation. The client is experiencing new bleeding and reports less fetal movement. The nurse informs the client that the physician has been notified. The client begins to cry quietly while holding her abdomen with

Answer: 3

Rationale: Anticipatory grieving occurs when a client has knowledge of an impending loss. The first stages of anticipatory grieving may be characterized by shock, emotional numbness, disbelief, and strong emotions such as tears, screaming, or anger. Anticipatory grieving is appropriate when any signs of fetal distress accelerate. There is no indication of pain or confusion or that the death of the fetus has occurred.

her hands. She murmurs, "No, no, you can't go my little man." The nurse recognizes the client's behavior as an indication of:

1 Pain related to abdominal pain
2 Confusion secondary to shock
3 Grieving, anticipatory related to perceived potential loss
4 Situational crisis related to the death of fetus and to fear and loss

Test-Taking Strategy: Focus on the data in the question and use the process of elimination. Options 1 and 2 can be eliminated because there is no indication of pain or confusion. Note that in this situation, there is a situational crisis with feelings of grief, but no loss has occurred at this point; therefore eliminate option 4. Review the characteristics of anticipatory grieving if you had difficulty with this question.

Level of Cognitive Ability: Analysis
Client Needs: Psychosocial Integrity
Integrated Concept/Process: Nursing Process/Data Collection
Content Area: Maternity

Reference:
McKinney, E., Ashwill, J., Murray, S. et al. (2000). *Maternal-child nursing.* Philadelphia: W.B Saunders, p. 925.

---

23. A postoperative client has been vomiting and ileus has been diagnosed. The physician orders insertion of a nasogastric tube. The nurse explains the purpose and insertion procedure to the client. The client says to the nurse, "I'm not sure I can take any more of this treatment." The most appropriate response by the nurse is:

1 "It is your right to refuse any procedure. I'll notify the physician."
2 "You are feeling tired and frustrated with your recovery from surgery?"
3 "If you don't have this tube put down, you will just continue to vomit."
4 "Let the doctor put the tube down so you can get well."

Answer: 2
Rationale: Option 2 assists the client in expressing and exploring feelings, which can lead to problem solving. The other options are examples of barriers to effective communication in that the nurse does not address the client's concerns.

Test-Taking Strategy: Use therapeutic communication techniques. Option 2 is an open-ended question and is a communication tool. It also focuses on the client's feelings. Review these techniques if you had difficulty with this question.

Level of Cognitive Ability: Application
Client Needs: Psychosocial Integrity
Integrated Concept/Process: Communication and Documentation
Content Area: Adult Health/Gastrointestinal

Reference:
Potter, P., & Perry, A. (2001). *Fundamentals of nursing* (5th ed.). St. Louis: Mosby, p. 459.

---

24. A client is admitted to the hospital with a bowel obstruction secondary to a recurrent malignancy. The physician inserts a Miller-Abbott tube. After the procedure the client asks the nurse, "Do you think this is worth all this trouble?" The most appropriate action or response by the nurse is:

1 Stay with the client and be silent
2 "Are you wondering whether you are going to get better? "
3 "Let's give this tube a chance."
4 "I remember a case similar to yours and the tube relieved the obstruction."

Answer: 2
Rationale: The nurse uses therapeutic communication tools when assisting a client with a chronic terminal illness to express feelings. The nurse listens attentively to the client and uses clarifying and focusing to assist the client in expressing their feelings. Responding with inappropriate silence (option 1), changing the subject (option 3), and offering false reassurance (option 4) are examples of barriers to communication.

Test-Taking Strategy: Use therapeutic communication techniques. Option 2 encourages the client to verbalize. Options 1, 3, and 4 are blocks to communication. Review these techniques if you had difficulty with this question.

Level of Cognitive Ability: Application
Client Needs: Psychosocial Integrity

Integrated Concept/Process: Communication and Documentation
Content Area: Adult Health/Oncology

Reference:
Potter, P., & Perry, A. (2001). *Fundamentals of nursing* (5th ed.). St. Louis: Mosby, p. 460.

---

25. A client receiving total parenteral nutrition and intralipids says to the nurse, "I was always overweight until I had this illness. I'm not sure I want to get that fat. The other IVs are probably enough." What is the best initial response by the nurse?

1 "Fatty acids are essential for life. You'll develop deficiencies without the fats."

2 "I think you need to discuss this decision with the physician."

3 "Tell me how being ill has affected the way you think of yourself."

4 "I understand what you mean. I've dieted most of my life."

Answer: 3
Rationale: Clients receiving long-term parenteral nutrition are at risk for development of essential fatty acid deficiency. However, the client's response requires more than an informational response initially. The nurse uses tools of therapeutic communication to assist the client to express feelings and deal with the aspects of illness and treatment. Blocks to communication, such as giving information too soon (option 1), placing the client's feelings on hold (option 2), and giving opinions (option 4) will not assist the client in coping effectively.

Test-Taking Strategy: Use therapeutic communication techniques. Option 3 is the only option that encourages the client to express feelings. Review these techniques if you had difficulty with this question.

Level of Cognitive Ability: Application
Client Needs: Psychosocial Integrity
Integrated Concept/Process: Communication and Documentation
Content Area: Fundamental Skills

Reference:
Potter, P., & Perry, A. (2001). *Fundamentals of nursing* (5th ed.). St. Louis: Mosby, p. 1374.

---

26. A client has terminal cancer and is using narcotic analgesics for pain relief. The client is concerned about becoming addicted to the pain medication. The nurse allays this anxiety by:

1 Explaining to the client that his or her fears are justified but should be of no concern in the final stages of illness

2 Encouraging the client to hold off as long as possible between doses of pain medication

3 Telling the client to take lower doses of medications even though the pain is not well controlled

4 Explaining to the client that addiction rarely occurs in people who are taking medication to relieve pain

Answer: 4
Rationale: Clients who are on narcotics often have well-founded fears about addiction, even in the face of pain. The nurse has a responsibility to give correct information about the likelihood of addiction while still maintaining adequate pain control. Addiction is rare for individuals who are taking medication to relieve pain. Allowing the client to be in pain, as in options 2 and 3, is not acceptable nursing practice. Option 1 is correct only in that it acknowledges the client's fear, but addressing the final stages of illness is inappropriate at this time.

Test-Taking Strategy: Use the process of elimination. Eliminate options 2 and 3 because these are not acceptable nursing practices. Eliminate option 1 because it is only partially correct. Review pain management if you had difficulty with this question.

Level of Cognitive Ability: Application
Client Needs: Psychosocial Integrity
Integrated Concept/Process: Caring
Content Area: Adult Health/Oncology

Reference:
deWit, S. (2001). *Fundamental concepts and skills for nursing.* Philadelphia: W.B. Saunders, p. 191.

27. A client is highly anxious about receiving chest physical therapy (CPT) for the first time. In planning for the client's care, the nurse proceeds in reassuring the client that:
1 There are no risks associated with this procedure
2 CPT will resolve all of the client's respiratory symptoms
3 CPT will assist in mobilizing secretions to enhance more effective breathing
4 CPT will assist the client to cough more effectively

Answer: 3
Rationale: There are risks associated with this procedure and they include cardiac, gastrointestinal, neurological, and pulmonary complications. CPT is an intervention to assist in clearing secretions and will not resolve all respiratory symptoms. CPT will assist the client to cough indirectly if the secretions have been mobilized and the cough stimulus is present.

Test-Taking Strategy: Use the process of elimination. Eliminate options 1 and 2 because they contain the absolute terms *no* and *all*. The issue of the question is the purpose of CPT. Focusing on the issue will assist in directing you to select option 3 over option 4. Review the purpose of CPT if you had difficulty with this question.

Level of Cognitive Ability: Application
Client Needs: Psychosocial Integrity
Integrated Concept/Process: Nursing Process/Planning
Content Area: Adult Health/Respiratory

Reference:
Potter, P., & Perry, A. (2001). *Fundamentals of nursing* (5th ed.). St. Louis: Mosby, p. 1163.

---

28. A client with cardiomyopathy stops eating, takes long naps, and turns away from the nurse when the nurse talks to the client. The nurse identifies that the client may be experiencing which of the following?
1 Activity intolerance
2 Intractable pain
3 Mild discomfort
4 Depression

Answer: 4
Rationale: Depression is a common problem related to clients who have long-term and debilitating illness. Options 1, 2, and 3 are not associated with the data present in the question.

Test-Taking Strategy: Focus on the data provided in the question and use the process of elimination. Noting the words *stops eating, takes long naps, and turns away from the nurse* will direct you to option 4. Review the signs of depression if you had difficulty with this question.

Level of Cognitive Ability: Analysis
Client Needs: Psychosocial Integrity
Integrated Concept/Process: Nursing Process/Data Collection
Content Area: Adult Health/Cardiovascular

Reference:
Black, J., Hawks, J., & Keene, A. (2001). *Medical-surgical nursing: clinical management for positive outcomes* (6th ed.). Philadelphia: W.B. Saunders, p. 423.

---

29. Which short-term psychosocial intervention is important for a pregnant client hospitalized for stabilization of diabetes mellitus?
1 Teach the client and family about diabetes mellitus and its implications
2 Provide emotional support and education about altered family processes related to the pregnant client's hospitalization

Answer: 2
Rationale: The short-term psychosocial well-being of the family is at risk because of the hospitalization of a diabetic mother. Teaching about diabetes is a long-term intervention related to diabetes and is more physiological in nature. Options 3 and 4 are unrelated to diabetes, are physiological, and are more related to pregnancy-induced hypertension.

Test-Taking Strategy: Use the process of elimination and note the key word *psychosocial*. Eliminate options 3 and 4 because they are unrelated to diabetes and are physiological. From the remaining

3 Protect from risk of injury secondary to convulsions

4 Be alert to the risks of early labor and birth

options, note the words *short-term psychosocial intervention*. This should direct you to option 2. Review the psychosocial aspects of care for a pregnant client with diabetes mellitus if you had difficulty with this question.

Level of Cognitive Ability: Comprehension
Client Needs: Psychosocial Integrity
Integrated Concept/Process: Nursing Process/Planning
Content Area: Maternity

Reference:
McKinney, E., Ashwill, J., Murray, S. et al. (2000). *Maternal-child nursing.* Philadelphia: W.B Saunders, p. 1462.

---

30. A new parent is trying to make the decision whether or not to have her baby boy circumcised. Which of the following is the best response to assist the mother in making a decision?

1 "I had my son circumcised, and I am so glad!"

2 "Circumcision is a difficult decision, but your physician is the best, and you know it's better to get it done now than later!"

3 "Circumcision is a difficult decision. There are various controversies surrounding circumcision. Here, read this pamphlet that discusses the pros and cons and we will talk after you read to answer any questions that you have."

4 "You know, they say it prevents cancer and sexually transmitted diseases, so I would definitely have my son circumcised!"

Answer: 3
Rationale: Various controversies have surrounded circumcision. Providing written information to the client will give the mother the information she needs to make an educated and informed decision. Options 1, 2, and 4 identify nontherapeutic communication techniques In that they offer personal opinion and advice to the client. The nurse's personal thoughts and feelings should not be part of the educational process.

Test-Taking Strategy: Use the process of elimination. Eliminate options 1 and 4 because they are similar. In addition, options 1, 2, and 4 are communication blocks because the nurse is providing a personal opinion to the client. Informed decision making is the key point when selecting the correct option in this question. Review therapeutic communication techniques and teaching/learning principles if you had difficulty with this question.

Level of Cognitive Ability: Application
Client Needs: Psychosocial Integrity
Integrated Concept/Process: Communication and Documentation
Content Area: Maternity

Reference:
McKinney, E., Ashwill, J., Murray, S. et al. (2000). *Maternal-child nursing.* Philadelphia: W.B Saunders, p. 577.

---

31. A nurse is assisting in planning care for a client who is experiencing anxiety after a myocardial infarction. Which nursing intervention should be included in the plan of care?

1 Provide detailed explanations of all procedures

2 Administer cyclobenzaprine (Flexeril) to promote relaxation

3 Limit family involvement during the acute phase

4 Answer questions with factual information

Answer: 4
Rationale: Accurate information reduces fear, strengthens the nurse-client relationship, and assists the client to deal realistically with the situation. Providing detailed information may increase the client's anxiety. Information should be provided simply and clearly. Cyclobenzaprine is a skeletal muscle relaxant and is used in the short-term treatment of muscle spasms. Limiting family involvement may or may not be helpful; the client's family may be a source of support for the client.

Test-Taking Strategy: Use the process of elimination. Avoid selecting options with strong adjectives, such as *detailed* as in option 1. Eliminate option 2 because medication should not be the first intervention to alleviate anxiety. In addition, this medication is used to relieve muscle spasms. From the remaining options, eliminate option 3 because limiting family involvement does not reduce anxiety in all situations. Review measures to relieve anxiety if you had difficulty with this question.

Level of Cognitive Ability: Application
Client Needs: Psychosocial Integrity
Integrated Concept/Process: Nursing Process/Planning
Content Area: Adult Health/Cardiovascular

Reference:
Black, J., Hawks, J., & Keene, A. (2001). *Medical-surgical nursing: clinical management for positive outcomes* (6th ed.). Philadelphia: W.B. Saunders, p. 1600.

---

32. A client recovering from an acute myocardial infarction will be discharged from the hospital the next day. Which client action on the evening before discharge suggests that the client is in the denial phase of grieving?
  1 Requests a sedative for sleep at 10:00 PM
  2 Expresses hesitancy to leave the hospital
  3 Walks up and down three flights of stairs unsupervised
  4 Consumes 25% of foods and fluids for supper

Answer: 3
Rationale: Ignoring activity limitations and avoidance of lifestyle changes are signs of denial in the stages of grieving. Walking three flights of stairs should be a supervised activity during the rehabilitation process. Option 1 is an appropriate client action on the evening before discharge. Option 2, expressing hesitancy to leave, may be a manifestation of anxiety or fear, not of denial. Option 4, anorexia, is a manifestation of depression, not denial.

Test-Taking Strategy: Focus on the issue, the denial phase. Use the process of elimination. Option 1 is an appropriate client action. Option 2 identifies anxiety or fear. Option 4 identifies depression. Option 3 is the only option that suggests denial in the client. Review the signs of denial if you had difficulty with this question.

Level of Cognitive Ability: Analysis
Client Needs: Psychosocial Integrity
Integrated Concept/Process: Nursing Process/Data Collection
Content Area: Adult Health/Cardiovascular

Reference:
Black, J., Hawks, J., & Keene, A. (2001). *Medical-surgical nursing: clinical management for positive outcomes* (6th ed.). Philadelphia: W.B. Saunders, p. 408.

---

33. Which of the following statements if made by a client indicates a positive coping mechanism to be used during treatment for Hodgkin's disease?
  1 "I have selected a wig even though I will miss my own hair."
  2 "I know losing my hair won't bother me."
  3 "I will not leave the house bald."
  4 "I will be one of the few who don't lose their hair."

Answer: 1
Rationale: A combination of radiation and chemotherapy often causes alopecia in clients with Hodgkin's disease. To use positive coping mechanisms, the client must identify personal feelings and use problem-solving positive interventions to deal with the side effects of treatment.

Test-Taking Strategy: Use the process of elimination and note the key words *positive coping mechanism*. Options 2 and 3 involve avoidance. Option 4 indicates denial. Option 1 is the only option that addresses a positive coping mechanism. Review positive coping mechanisms if you had difficulty with this question.

Level of Cognitive Ability: Analysis
Client Needs: Psychosocial Integrity
Integrated Concept/Process: Nursing Process/Evaluation
Content Area: Adult Health/Oncology

Reference:
Black, J., Hawks, J., & Keene, A. (2001). *Medical-surgical nursing: clinical management for positive outcomes* (6th ed.). Philadelphia: W.B. Saunders, p. 408.

---

34. A client is admitted to the hospital with diabetic ketoacidosis (DKA). The client's daughter says to the nurse, "My mother died last month, and now this. I've been trying to follow all of the instructions from the doctor. What have I done wrong?" The nurse's best response would be:

1   "Maybe we can keep your father in the hospital for a while longer to give you a rest."
2   "An emotional stress, such as your mother's death, can trigger DKA even though you are following the prescribed regimen to the letter."
3   "You should talk to the social worker about getting you someone at home who is more capable in managing a diabetic's care."
4   "Tell me what you think you did wrong."

Answer: 2
Rationale: Environment, infection, or an emotional stressor can initiate the pathophysiological mechanism of DKA. Option 1 is inappropriate and is not cost effective. Options 3 and 4 substantiate the daughters' feelings of guilt.

Test-Taking Strategy: Use the process of elimination. Note that the daughter, not the client, is the client of the question. This will assist in eliminating option 1, in addition to the fact that this option is inappropriate and is not cost effective. Options 3 and 4 devalue the client (the daughter) and block therapeutic communication. Review therapeutic communication techniques if you had difficulty with this question.

Level of Cognitive Ability: Application
Client Needs: Psychosocial Integrity
Integrated Concept/Process: Communication and Documentation
Content Area: Adult Health/Endocrine

Reference:
Potter, P., & Perry, A. (2001). *Fundamentals of nursing* (5th ed.). St. Louis: Mosby, p. 459.

---

35. A nurse is assisting with planning goals for a victim of rape. Which short-term initial goal is inappropriate?

1   The client will resolve feelings of fear and anxiety related to the rape trauma
2   The client will experience physical healing of the wounds that were incurred at the time of the rape
3   The client will verbalize feelings about the rape event
4   The client will participate in the treatment plan by keeping appointments and following through with treatment options

Answer: 1
Rationale: Short-term goals will include the beginning stages of dealing with the rape trauma. Clients will be expected initially to keep appointments, participate in care, begin to explore feelings, and begin to heal the physical wounds that were inflicted at the time of the rape. The resolution of feelings is a long-term goal.

Test-Taking Strategy: Note the key words *inappropriate* and *short-term initial goal*. Noting the word *resolved* in option 1 should provide you with the clue that this option is a long-term goal. Review care to the client who is a victim of rape if you had difficulty with this question.

Level of Cognitive Ability: Application
Client Needs: Psychosocial Integrity
Integrated Concept/Process: Nursing Process/Planning
Content Area: Mental Health

Reference:
Varcarolis, E. (2002). *Foundations of psychiatric mental health nursing* (4th ed.). Philadelphia: W.B. Saunders, p. 723.

36. A client is admitted to a surgical unit with a diagnosis of cancer. The client is scheduled for surgery in the morning. When the nurse enters the room and begins the surgical preparation, the client states, "I'm not having surgery, you must have the wrong person! My test results were negative. I'll be going home tomorrow." The nurse recognizes that the defense mechanism that the client is exhibiting is:

1 Psychosis
2 Denial
3 Delusions
4 Displacement

Answer: 2

Rationale: Defense mechanisms protect against anxiety. Denial is the defense mechanism that "blocks out" painful or anxiety-inducing events or feelings. In this case, the client cannot deal with the upcoming surgery for cancer and therefore denies that he or she is ill. Displacement is acting out in anger or frustration with people who did not arouse those feelings. Options 1 and 3 are not defense mechanisms.

Test-Taking Strategy: Use the process of elimination and focus on the issue, defense mechanisms. Options 1 and 3 are eliminated first because these are not defense mechanisms. From the remaining options, focusing on the data in the question will direct you to option 2. Review defense mechanisms if you had difficulty with this question.

Level of Cognitive Ability: Comprehension
Client Needs: Psychosocial Integrity
Integrated Concept/Process: Nursing Process/Data Collection
Content Area: Adult Health/Oncology

Reference:
Varcarolis, E. (2002). *Foundations of psychiatric mental health nursing* (4th ed.). Philadelphia: W.B. Saunders, p. 288.

37. A nurse who works in an industrial setting is given a memo that indicates that a large number of employees will be laid off in the next 2 weeks. A review of previous layoffs suggested that workers experienced role crises, indecision, and depression. Using this data, the nurse assists in planning for the layoff by suggesting to:

1 Help the workers acquire unemployment benefits to avoid a gap in income
2 Reduce the staff in the occupational health department of the industrial setting
3 Notify the insurance carriers of the upcoming event to assist with potential health alterations
4 Identify referral, counseling, and vocational rehabilitative services for the employees being laid off

Answer: 4

Rationale: A review of data should lead to a comprehensive conclusion based directly on the data. In this case, option 4 is the only conclusion. The other options may or may not need to occur. The nurse would need to know more about the industry to determine whether option 1, 2, or 3 would be necessary or possible.

Test-Taking Strategy: Use the process of elimination and focus on the data in the question. Options 1, 2, and 3 are more industry-specific, and one would need to know more about the industrial setting than is presented in the question. In addition, option 4 is a global option. Review the purpose of referral, counseling, and rehabilitative services if you had difficulty with this question.

Level of Cognitive Ability: Application
Client Needs: Psychosocial Integrity
Integrated Concept/Process: Nursing Process/Planning
Content Area: Mental Health

Reference:
Varcarolis, E. (2002). *Foundations of psychiatric mental health nursing* (4th ed.). Philadelphia: W.B. Saunders, p. 798.

38. A primigravida client is seen by the physician and a urinary tract infection is diagnosed. The client has repeatedly verbalized concern regarding safety of the

Answer: 4

Rationale: The primary concern for this client is safety of her fetus, not herself. There is no information in the question to support options 1, 2, and 3.

fetus. The nurse determines that which of the following is the priority concern at this time?
1 Pain
2 Embarrassment
3 Nutritional requirements
4 Fear

Test-Taking Strategy: Focus on the issue of the question and the data provided in the question. There is no information in the question to support options 1, 2, and 3. Review the defining characteristics of fear if you had difficulty with this question.

Level of Cognitive Ability: Comprehension
Client Needs: Psychosocial Integrity
Integrated Concept/Process: Nursing Process/Data Collection
Content Area: Maternity

Reference:
Burroughs, A., & Leifer, G. (2002). *Maternity nursing* (8th ed.). Philadelphia: W.B. Saunders, p. 243.

---

39. When planning interventions for the pregnant client with newly diagnosed sickle cell anemia, the most important psychosocial intervention at this time would be which of the following?
    1 Provide all information regarding the disease
    2 Allow the client to be alone if she is crying
    3 Provide emotional support
    4 Avoid the topic of the disease

Answer: 3
Rationale: The most important psychosocial intervention is providing emotional support to the client and family. Option 1 overwhelms the client with information while the client is trying to cope with the news of the disease. Option 2 is only appropriate if the client requests to be alone. Option 4 is similar to option 1 and is nontherapeutic. Supportive therapy allows the client to express feelings, explore alternatives, and make decisions in a safe, caring environment.

Test-Taking Strategy: Use the process of elimination. Eliminate option 1 and option 4 because of the words *all* and *avoid*. In addition, these actions are nontherapeutic. From the remaining options, remember that the client's feelings are the priority and that an important role of the nurse is to provide emotional support. Review psychosocial issues related to sickle cell anemia if you had difficulty with this question.

Level of Cognitive Ability: Application
Client Needs: Psychosocial Integrity
Integrated Concept/Process: Nursing Process/Implementation
Content Area: Maternity

Reference:
Burroughs, A., & Leifer, G. (2002). *Maternity nursing* (8th ed.). Philadelphia: W.B. Saunders, p. 238.

---

40. A nurse is assisting in caring for a newborn with suspected erythroblastosis fetalis immediately after delivery. The nurse makes which therapeutic statement to the parents at this time?
    1 "You must have many concerns. Please ask me any questions."
    2 "This is a common neonatal problem; you shouldn't be concerned."
    3 "There is no need to worry. We have the most updated equipment in this hospital."

Answer: 1
Rationale: Parental concern and anxiety are expected and are related to the care of the newborn with erythroblastosis fetalis. This anxiety results from a lack of knowledge about disease process, treatment, and expected outcomes. Parents need to be encouraged to verbalize concerns and participate in care as appropriate.

Test-Taking Strategy: Use the process of elimination. Eliminate options 2 and 3 because they are similar and saying basically the same thing. In addition, they are blocks to communication. The wording in option 4 would frighten the parents. Remember to address clients' feelings and concerns. Review therapeutic communication techniques if you had difficulty with this question.

4   "Your newborn is very sick. The next 24 hours are most crucial."

Level of Cognitive Ability: Application
Clients Needs: Psychosocial Integrity
Integrated Concept/Process: Communication and Documentation
Content Area: Maternity

Reference:
Potter, P., & Perry, A. (2001). *Fundamentals of nursing* (5th ed.). St. Louis: Mosby, p. 460.

---

41. A licensed practical nurse (LPN) is assisting a school nurse in weighing all the high school students. One of the teenagers, who has type 1 diabetes mellitus, has gained 15 pounds since last year with no gain in height. The LPN is told that the student eats alone in the cafeteria at lunch time. Based on this data, the LPN is most concerned that the student may have:
1   Bulimia nervosa
2   Depression
3   An alcohol abuse problem
4   An insulin deficiency

Answer: 2
Rationale: Diabetic teenagers are at risk for depression and suicide, which is frequently manifested by changing insulin and eating patterns. Social isolation is another clue. Remember weight loss is a symptom of type 1 diabetes, and an insulin deficiency would have the same effect. Bulimic clients may be of normal weight but control weight gain by purging. Alcohol abuse is more likely to be related to weight loss.

Test-Taking Strategy: Use the process of elimination and focus on the data presented in the question. Eliminate options 1, 3, and 4 because weight gain would not occur in these conditions. Review the signs associated with depression if you had difficulty with this question.

Level of Cognitive Ability: Analysis
Client Needs: Psychosocial Integrity
Integrated Concept/Process: Nursing Process/Data Collection
Content Area: Child Health

Reference:
Schulte, E. Price, D., & Gwin, J. (2001). *Thompson's pediatric nursing* (8th ed.). Philadelphia: W.B. Saunders, p. 342.

---

42. A nurse is conducting a session with a class of high school students about the risk of sexually transmitted diseases (STD). What opening statement will best encourage participation within the group?
1   "At the end of the class, condoms will be distributed to everyone in the class."
2   "The topic today is very personal. For this reason, anything shared with the group will remain confidential."
3   "Please feel free to share your personal experiences with the group."
4   "Our goal today is to describe ways to prevent acquiring a sexually transmitted disease."

Answer: 2
Rationale: The correct option states the rules for confidentiality, which will help develop a trust in sharing sensitive issues with the group. Option 1 may be an incentive for those attending to stay, but infers that participation is not required to get the reward. Option 3 offers the opportunity to share personal experiences but no protection of confidentiality. Option 4 is a good introduction to the topic but doesn't foster trust, especially with those who may already have a STD.

Test-Taking Strategy: Use the process of elimination and focus on the issue: confidentiality, trust building, and sharing. Eliminate option 4, which focuses on content, and option 1, which addresses format. Option 2 is more global than option 3 and addresses the issue of confidentiality. Review teaching/learning principles if you had difficulty with this question.

Level of Cognitive Ability: Application
Client Needs: Psychosocial Integrity
Integrated Concept/Process: Nursing Process/Implementation
Content Area: Child Health

Reference:
Schulte, E. Price, D., & Gwin, J. (2001). *Thompson's pediatric nursing* (8th ed.). Philadelphia: W.B. Saunders, p. 337.

---

43. A nurse is assisting in planning care for a client with an intrauterine fetal demise. Which of the following is not an appropriate goal for this client?
1   The woman and her family will express their grief about the loss of their desired infant
2   The woman and her family will discuss plans for going home without the infant
3   The woman and her family will contact their pastor or grief counselor for support after discharge
4   The woman will recognize that thoughts of worthlessness and suicide are normal after a loss

Answer: 4

Rationale: It is important for the nurse to determine whether the couple is undergoing the normal grieving process. Signs that are a cause for concern and not part of the normal grieving process include thoughts of worthlessness and suicide. The woman should be referred to a mental heath provider if she exhibits any of these symptoms. Options 1, 2, and 3 are appropriate goals.

Test-Taking Strategy: Use the process of elimination and note the key word *not*. You should easily be directed to option 4 because thoughts of suicide and worthlessness are cause for concern. These feelings are not normal but instead are indicative of a serious problem. Review psychosocial reactions after loss if you had difficulty with this question.

Level of Cognitive Ability: Application
Client Needs: Psychosocial Integrity
Integrated Concept/Process: Nursing Process/Planning
Content Area: Maternity

Reference:
McKinney, E., Ashwill, J., Murray, S. et al. (2000). *Maternal-child nursing.* Philadelphia: W.B Saunders, p. 925.

---

44. A client with severe preeclampsia is admitted to the hospital. She is a student at a local college and insists on continuing her studies while in the hospital despite being instructed to rest. The nurse notes that the client studies several hours a day between numerous visits from fellow students, family, and friends. Which nursing approach should initially be included in the plan of care?
1   Instructing the client that the health of the baby is more important than her studies at this time
2   Asking her why she is not complying with the order of rest
3   Including a significant other in helping the client understand the need for rest
4   Developing a routine with the client to balance studies and rest needs

Answer: 4

Rationale: Option 4 involves the client in the decision making. In options 1 and 2, the nurse is judging the client's opinion and asking probing questions. This will cause a breakdown in communication. Option 3 persuades the client's significant others to disagree with the client's action. This could cause problems with the client's self-esteem and also affect the nurse-client relationship.

Test-Taking Strategy: Use therapeutic communication techniques and the process of elimination. Eliminate options 1, 2, and 3 because these are blocks to communication. Option 4 is therapeutic and the most thorough nursing action because it addresses rest and studies and involves the client in the decision-making process. Review therapeutic communication techniques if you had difficulty with this question.

Level of Cognitive Ability: Application
Client Needs: Psychosocial Integrity
Integrated Concept/Process: Nursing Process/Implementation
Content Area: Maternity

Reference:
McKinney, E., Ashwill, J., Murray, S. et al. (2000). *Maternal-child nursing.* Philadelphia: W.B Saunders, p. 814.

45. A pregnant client is newly diagnosed as having gestational diabetes. She is crying and keeps repeating. "What have I done to cause this? If I could only live my life over." The nurse identifies that the client is experiencing which problem?

1   A disturbance in self-concept related to a complication of pregnancy
2   A lack of understanding regarding diabetic self-care during pregnancy
3   A disturbance in body image related to complications of pregnancy
4   A risk for injury to the fetus related to maternal distress

Answer: 1

Rationale: The client is putting the blame for the diabetes on herself, lowering her self-concept or image. She is expressing fear and grief. There is no information in the question to support options 2, 3, and 4.

Test-Taking Strategy: Use the data presented in the question to assist you in selecting the correct option. The words *what have I done* should assist in eliminating options 2 and 4. From the remaining options, focusing on the data in the question should direct you to option 1. Review the defining characteristics of a disturbance in self-concept if you had difficulty with this question.

Level of Cognitive Ability: Comprehension
Client Needs: Psychosocial Integrity
Integrated Concept/Process: Nursing Process/Data Collection
Content Area: Maternity

Reference:
McKinney, E., Ashwill, J., Murray, S. et al. (2000). *Maternal-child nursing.* Philadelphia: W.B Saunders, p. 923.

---

46. A client says to the nurse, "I'm going to die and I wish my family would stop hoping for a 'cure'! I get so angry when they carry on like this! After all, I'm the one who's dying." The most therapeutic response by the nurse is:

1   "You're feeling angry that your family continues to hope for you to be 'cured'?"
2   "I think we should talk more about your anger with your family."
3   "Well, it sounds like you're being pretty pessimistic."
4   "Have you shared your feelings with your family?"

Answer: 1

Rationale: Reflection is the therapeutic communication technique that redirects the client's feelings back to validate what the client is saying. In option 2, the nurse attempts to use focusing, but the attempt addresses a premature statement. In option 3, the nurse makes a judgment and is nontherapeutic. In option 4, the nurse is attempting to assess the client's ability to openly discuss feelings with family members.

Test-Taking Strategy: Use therapeutic communication techniques to eliminate options 2, 3, and 4. Review these techniques if you had difficulty with this question.

Level of Cognitive Ability: Application
Client Needs: Psychosocial Integrity
Integrated Concept/Process: Communication and Documentation
Content Area: Mental Health

Reference:
Varcarolis, E. (2002). *Foundations of psychiatric mental health nursing* (4th ed.). Philadelphia: W.B. Saunders, p. 255.

---

47. A nurse is caring for an older adult client who says, "I don't want to talk with you. You're only a nurse, I'll wait for my doctor." Which of the following nursing responses would be the most therapeutic?

1   "I'll leave you now and call your physician."
2   "I'm assigned to work with you. Your doctor placed you in my hands."

Answer: 3

Rationale: The nurse uses the therapeutic communication of reflection to redirect the client's feelings back for validation. Note that the nurse does not reflect a negative in option 3 but focuses on the client's desire to talk with the physician. Options 1, 2, and 4 are nontherapeutic. Remember that the nurse places the client's well-being first and foremost while engaged in nursing care.

Test-Taking Strategy: This question tests your knowledge of the appropriate therapeutic communication for clients who are using

3 "So you're saying that you want to talk to your physician?"
4 "I'm angry with the way you've dismissed me. I am your nurse not your servant."

a defensive statement that is aimed to drive others away. You can easily eliminate options 2 and 4 because these are nontherapeutic responses. Option 1 is a social response and intervention that reinforces the client's continuation of this behavior. Review therapeutic communication techniques if you had difficulty with this question.

Level of Cognitive Ability: Application
Client Needs: Psychosocial Integrity
Integrated Concept/Process: Communication and Documentation
Content Area: Fundamental Skills

Reference:
Varcarolis, E. (2002). *Foundations of psychiatric mental health nursing* (4th ed.). Philadelphia: W.B. Saunders, p. 255.

---

48. A female client and her newborn infant have undergone human immunodeficiency virus (HIV) testing, and the test results for both clients have turned out positive. The news is devastating and the mother is crying. The most appropriate nursing action at this time is to:
1 Call an HIV counselor and make an appointment for them
2 Describe the progressive stages and treatments for HIV
3 Examine with the mother how she got HIV
4 Listen quietly while the mother talks and cries

Answer: 4
Rationale: This client has just received devastating news and needs to have someone present with her as she begins to cope with this issue. The nurse needs to sit and actively listen while the mother talks and cries. Calling an HIV counselor may be helpful, but it is not what the client needs at this time. The other options are not appropriate for this stage of coping with the news that both she and the infant are HIV-positive.

Test-Taking Strategy: Use the process of elimination. Noting the key words *at this time* will assist in eliminating options 2 and 3. From the remaining options, remember to address the client's feelings and to support the client. Review therapeutic communication techniques if you had difficulty with this question.

Level of Cognitive Ability: Application
Client Needs: Psychosocial Integrity
Integrated Concept/Process: Nursing Process/Implementation
Content Area: Maternity

Reference:
McKinney, E., Ashwill, J., Murray, S. et al. (2000). *Maternal-child nursing.* Philadelphia: W.B Saunders, p. 680.

---

49. A nurse employed in a home care agency is assigned to provide care to a recently widowed, retired military man who is estranged from his only child because he was discharged from the service for being homosexual. When the nurse arrives at the client's home, the ordinarily immaculate house is in chaos, and the client is disheveled, with alcohol on his breath. Which of the following statements by the nurse would be most therapeutic?
1 "You seem to be having a very troubling time."

Answer: 1
Rationale: The most therapeutic statement is the one that helps the client to explore his situation and to express his feelings. Option 1 identifies the use of reflection and will assist the client to begin to ventilate feelings. As the client begins to do so, the nurse can assist the client to discuss the reasons behind alienation from his only child. In option 2, the nurse uses humor to avoid therapeutic intimacy and effective problem solving. In option 3, the nurse uses social communication. In option 4, the nurse uses admonishment and tries to shame the client, which is not therapeutic. This belittles the client, causes anger, and may evoke "acting out" by the client.

Test-Taking Strategy: Use therapeutic communication techniques. Option 1 is the only option that addresses the client's feelings.

2 "I can see this isn't a good time to visit."

3 "What are you doing? How much are you drinking and for how long?"

4 "Do you think your wife would want you to behave like this?"

Review therapeutic communication techniques if you had difficulty with this question.

Level of Cognitive Ability: Application
Client Needs: Psychosocial Integrity
Integrated Concept/Process: Communication and Documentation
Content Area: Mental Health

Reference:
Varcarolis, E. (2002). *Foundations of psychiatric mental health nursing* (4th ed.). Philadelphia: W.B. Saunders, p. 253.

---

50. A client says to the nurse, "I don't do anything right. I'm such a loser." The most appropriate response is:

1 "You do things right all the time."

2 "Everything will get better."

3 "You don't do anything right?"

4 "You are not a loser, you are sick."

Answer: 3
Rationale: Option 3 allows the client to verbalize feelings. With this statement, the nurse can learn more about what the client really means. This option repeats the client's statement and allows the communication to stay open. Options 1, 2, and 4 are closed statements and do not encourage the client to explore further.

Test-Taking Strategy: Use therapeutic communication techniques. Remember to address the client's feelings. Option 3 is the only option that identifies a therapeutic response. Review these techniques if you had difficulty with this question.

Level of Cognitive Ability: Application
Client Needs: Psychosocial Integrity
Integrated Concept/Process: Communication and Documentation
Content Area: Mental Health

Reference:
Varcarolis, E. (2002). *Foundations of psychiatric mental health nursing* (4th ed.). Philadelphia: W.B. Saunders, p. 254.

---

51. A client who is experiencing suicidal thoughts says to the nurse, "It just doesn't seem worth it anymore. Why not just end it all." The nurse would gather data from the client by using which of the following responses?

1 "I'm sure your family is worried about you."

2 "I know you have had a stressful night."

3 "Did you sleep at all last night?"

4 "Tell me what you mean by that?"

Answer: 4
Rationale: Option 4 allows the client to tell the nurse more about what the current thoughts are. Option 1 is false reassurance and may block communication. Options 2 and 3 change the subject and also block communication.

Test-Taking Strategy: Use therapeutic communication techniques. Note the key words *gather data*. Options 1 and 2 can be eliminated because they do not reflect data collection. Both options 3 and 4 relate to further data collection, but option 4 is directly related to the issue of the question and provides the opportunity for the client to express thoughts. Review therapeutic communication techniques if you had difficulty with this question.

Level of Cognitive Ability: Application
Client Needs: Psychosocial Integrity
Integrated Concept/Process: Communication and Documentation
Content Area: Mental Health

Reference:
Varcarolis, E. (2002). *Foundations of psychiatric mental health nursing* (4th ed.). Philadelphia: W.B. Saunders, p. 253.

52. A mother says to the nurse, "I am afraid that my child might have another febrile seizure." Which response by the nurse is most therapeutic?

1 "Why worry about something that you cannot control?"
2 "Most children will never experience a second seizure."
3 "Tell me what frightens you the most about seizures."
4 "Acetaminophen (Tylenol) can prevent another seizure from occurring."

Answer: 3

Rationale: Option 3 is the only response that is an open-ended statement and provides the mother with an opportunity to express feelings. Option 1 is incorrect because it blocks communication by giving a flippant response to an expressed fear. Options 2 and 4 are incorrect because the nurse is giving false assurance that a seizure will not reoccur or can be prevented in this child.

Test-Taking Strategy: Note the key words *most therapeutic*. Use the process of elimination, seeking the option that encourages the client to express feelings. Options 1, 2, and 4 are nontherapeutic and block communication. Review therapeutic communication techniques if you had difficulty with this question.

Level of Cognitive Ability: Application
Client Needs: Psychosocial Integrity
Integrated Concept/Process: Communication and Documentation
Content Area: Child Health

Reference:
Wong, D., & Hockenberry-Eaton, M. (2001). *Wong's essentials of pediatric nursing* (6th ed.). St. Louis: Mosby, p. 126.

53. A mother has just given birth to a baby who has a cleft lip and palate. When planning to talk to this mother, the nurse should recognize that this client needs be allowed to work through which of these emotions before maternal-bonding can occur?

1 Anger
2 Grief
3 Guilt
4 Depression

Answer: 2

Rationale: The mother must first be assisted to grieve for the anticipated child that she did not have. Once this is accomplished, the mother can begin to focus on bonding with the infant she gave birth to. Options 1, 3, and 4 are incorrect because they are only one component of the grief process.

Test-Taking Strategy: Use the process of elimination. The key words are *to work through. . . before maternal-bonding can occur*. Options 1, 3, and 4 are incorrect because each is only one component of the grief process. Option 2 is the most global option. Review the grief process if you had difficulty with this question.

Level of Cognitive Ability: Comprehension
Client Needs: Psychosocial Integrity
Integrated Concept/Process: Nursing Process/Planning
Content Area: Maternity

Reference:
Wong, D., & Hockenberry-Eaton, M. (2001). *Wong's essentials of pediatric nursing* (6th ed.). St. Louis: Mosby, p. 923.

54. A client scheduled for cardiac stress testing expresses a fear of the heart "giving out" during the procedure. The nurse attempts to discuss these fears with the client. Which client behavior indicates a barrier to communication?

1 Client asks numerous questions about the stress test

Answer: 4

Rationale: Expressions of fear, anxiety, and frustration are examples of effective client communication. These expressions are identified in options 1, 2, and 3. Refusal to speak is a physical barrier to effective communication.

Test-Taking Strategy: Use the process of elimination. Note the key words *barrier to communication*. Options 1, 2, and 3 contain

2 Client verbally expresses fears regarding own mortality

3 Client is frustrated because the test needs to be performed

4 Client does not talk about procedure

evidence of effective communication. Not talking indicates a barrier. Review the barriers to communication if you had difficulty with this question.

Level of Cognitive Ability: Comprehension
Client Needs: Psychosocial Integrity
Integrated Concept/Process: Nursing Process/Data Collection
Content Area: Adult Health/Cardiovascular

Reference:
Potter, P., & Perry, A. (2001). *Fundamentals of nursing* (5th ed.). St. Louis: Mosby, p. 459.

---

55. After vaginal delivery of a large for gestational age (LGA) male infant, the nurse wraps the infant in a warm blanket and hands him to his mother. The mother demonstrates reluctance to touch the baby and verbalizes concern over the infant's facial bruising. To enhance maternal-infant attachment, the nurse responds:

1 "Because the bruising is painful, it is advisable that you not touch the baby's face."

2 "The bruising is caused by polycythemia, which usually leads to jaundice."

3 "It is a normal finding in large babies and nothing to be concerned about."

4 "The bruising is temporary, and it is important to interact with your infant."

Answer: 4
Rationale: The mother of an LGA infant with facial bruising may be reluctant to interact with the infant because of concern about causing additional pain to the infant. The bruising is temporary. Option 1 advises the mother not to touch the baby's face because the bruising is painful; however, touch is an important component of the attachment process. Touching the infant gently with fingertips should be encouraged. The LGA infant may have polycythemia, which can contribute to bruising, but the bruising is not caused by the polycythemia. Option 3 appears to be an appropriate response, but it does not address the issue of the question.

Test-Taking Strategy: Use the process of elimination. Note the relationship of the word *attachment* in the question and the word *interact* in the correct option. Review the concepts related to maternal-infant attachment if you had difficulty with this question.

Level of Cognitive Ability: Application
Client Needs: Psychosocial Integrity
Integrated Concept/Process: Nursing Process/Implementation
Content Area: Maternity

Reference:
McKinney, E., Ashwill, J., Murray, S. et al. (2000). *Maternal-child nursing.* Philadelphia: W.B Saunders, p. 755.

---

56. A client with myasthenia gravis is ready to return home. The client confides that she is concerned that her husband will no longer find her physically attractive. The nurse plans to:

1 Encourage the client to start a support group

2 Insist that the client reach out and face this fear

3 Tell the client not to dwell on the negative

4 Encourage the client to share her feelings with her husband

Answer: 4
Rationale: Sharing feelings with her husband directly address the issue of the question. Encouraging the client to start a support group will not address the client's immediate and individual concerns. Options 2 and 3 are blocks to communication and avoid the client's concern.

Test-Taking Strategy: Focus on the issue and use the process of elimination. Option 4 is the only option that addresses the client's immediate concern. Remember, address the client's feelings first. Review therapeutic communication techniques if you had difficulty with this question.

Level of Cognitive Ability: Application
Client Needs: Psychosocial Integrity
Integrated Concept/Process: Nursing Process/Planning
Content Area: Adult Health/Neurological

Reference:
Potter, P., & Perry, A. (2001). *Fundamentals of nursing* (5th ed.). St. Louis: Mosby, p. 459.

---

57. A 9-year-old child is hospitalized for 2 months after a car accident. The best way to promote psychosocial development of this child is to plan for:
  1 Tutoring to keep the child up-to-date with schoolwork
  2 A phone to call family and friends
  3 Computer games, TV, and videos at the bedside
  4 A portable radio and tape player with headphones

Answer: 1
Rationale: The developmental task of the school-aged child is industry versus inferiority. The child achieves success by mastering skills and knowledge. Maintaining school work provides for accomplishment and prevents feelings of inferiority from lagging behind the class. The other options provide diversion and are of lesser importance for a child of this age.

Test-Taking Strategy: Note the age of the child and determine the developmental task for this child. Options 2, 3, and 4 address social and diversional issues, whereas option 1 specifically addresses psychosocial development. Review growth and development related to the school-aged child if you had difficulty with this question.

Level of Cognitive Ability: Application
Client Needs: Psychosocial Integrity
Integrated Concept/Process: Nursing Process/Planning
Content Area: Child Health

Reference:
Wong, D., & Hockenberry-Eaton, M. (2001). *Wong's essentials of pediatric nursing* (6th ed.). St. Louis: Mosby, p. 710.

---

58. A client who is in halo traction, says to the nurse, "I can't get used to this contraption. I can't see properly on the side and I keep misjudging where everything is." The most therapeutic response by the nurse is:
  1 "Halo traction involves many difficult adjustments. Practice scanning with your eyes after standing up, before you move."
  2 "No one ever gets used to that thing! It's horrible. Many of our sports people who are in it complain vigorously."
  3 "Why do you feel like this when you could have died from a broken neck? This is the way it is for several months. You need to accept it more, don't you think?"
  4 "If I were you, I would have had the surgery rather than suffer like this."

Answer: 1
Rationale: The therapeutic communication technique that the nurse uses in option 1 is reflection. The nurse then offers a problem-solving strategy that helps increase peripheral vision for the client. In option 2, the nurse provides a social response that contains emotionally charged language and could increase the client's anxiety. In option 3, the nurse uses excessive questioning and gives advice, which is nontherapeutic. In option 4, the nurse undermines the client's faith in the medical treatment being used by giving advice that is insensitive and unprofessional.

Test-Taking Strategy: Use the process of elimination, seeking the option that represents a therapeutic communication technique. This will direct you to option 1. Review therapeutic communication techniques if you had difficulty with this question.

Level of Cognitive Ability: Application
Client Needs: Psychosocial Integrity
Integrated Concept/Process: Communication and Documentation
Content Area: Adult Health/Neurological

Reference:
Varcarolis, E. (2002). *Foundations of psychiatric mental health nursing* (4th ed.). Philadelphia: W.B. Saunders, p. 255.

59. An older client has been admitted to the hospital with a hip fracture. The nurse assists in preparing a plan for the client and identifies desired outcomes. Which client statement most appropriately supports a positive adjustment to the alterations experienced in mobility?

1 "I wish you nurses would leave me alone! You are always telling me what to do!"
2 "What took you so long? I called for you 30 minutes ago."
3 "Hurry up and go away. I want to be alone."
4 "I find it difficult to concentrate since the doctor talked with me about the surgery tomorrow."

Answer: 4

Rationale: Option 1 demonstrates acting out by the client. Opt[...] is a demanding response. Option 3 demonstrates withdrawal beha[...]ior. Demanding, acting-out, and withdrawn clients have not coped or adjusted with injury or disease. Option 4 is reflective of a person with moderate anxiety. This client statement most appropriately supports a positive adjustment.

Test-Taking Strategy: Focus on the issue *positive adjustment*. Also, remember that age and limited mobility, combined with medications, often contribute to anxiety and confusion. This should assist in directing you to option 4. Review the characteristics that indicate a positive adjustment if you had difficulty with this question.

Level of Cognitive Ability: Comprehension
Client Needs: Psychosocial Integrity
Integrated Concept/Process: Nursing Process/Evaluation
Content Area: Adult Health/Musculoskeletal

Reference:
Black, J., Hawks, J., & Keene, A. (2001). *Medical-surgical nursing: clinical management for positive outcomes* (6th ed.). Philadelphia: W.B. Saunders, p. 284.

---

60. The best way to help parents of a premature infant develop attachment behaviors is to:

1 Encourage parents to touch and speak to their infant
2 Place family pictures in the infant's view
3 Report only positive qualities and progress to parents
4 Provide information on infant development and stimulation

Answer: 1

Rationale: Parents' involvement through touch and voice establishes and initiates the attachment process in the relationship. Their active participation builds confidence and supports the parenting role. Providing information and emphasizing only positives do not relate to the attachment process. Family pictures are ineffective for an infant.

Test-Taking Strategy: Use the process of elimination. The clients of the question are the parents and the issue is attachment. The only option that addresses attachment behaviors is option 1. Review infant-parent bonding concepts if you had difficulty with this question.

Level of Cognitive Ability: Application
Client Needs: Psychosocial Integrity
Integrated Concept/Process: Nursing Process/Implementation
Content Area: Maternity

Reference:
Murray, S., McKinney, E., & Gorrie, T. (2002). *Foundations of maternal-newborn nursing* (3rd ed.). Philadelphia: W.B. Saunders, p. 825.

---

61. A client angrily tells the nurse that the doctor purposefully provided wrong information. Which of the following nursing responses would hinder therapeutic communication?

1 "I'm certain the doctor would not lie to you."

Answer: 1

Rationale: Option 1 hinders communication by disagreeing with the client. This technique could make the client defensive and block further communication. Options 2 and 3 attempt to clarify what the client is referring to. Option 4 attempts to explore if the client is comfortable talking to the doctor about this issue and encourages direct confrontation.

describe the information
re referring to?"
ure what information you
g to."
comfortable talking to
about this."

Test-Taking Strategy: Use the process of elimination noting the key word *hinder.* Disagreeing with or challenging a client's response will hinder or block therapeutic communication. Therapeutic communication addresses client concerns, seeks clarification, acknowledges feelings, or encourages open and direct communication. Review therapeutic communication techniques if you had difficulty with this question.

Level of Cognitive Ability: Application
Client Needs: Psychosocial Integrity
Integrated Concept/Process: Communication and Documentation
Content Area: Fundamental skills

Reference:
Potter, P., & Perry, A. (2001). *Fundamentals of nursing* (5th ed.). St. Louis: Mosby, p. 459.

---

62. A client with major depression says to the nurse, "I should have died. I've always been a failure." The most therapeutic response by the nurse is:
1   "I see a lot of positive things in you."
2   "Feeling like a failure is part of your illness."
3   "You've been feeling like a failure for some time now?"
4   "You still have a great deal to live for."

Answer: 3
Rationale: Responding to the feelings expressed by a client is an effective therapeutic communication technique. The correct option is an example of the use of restating. Options 1, 2, and 4 block communication because they minimize the client's experience and do not facilitate exploration of the client's expressed feelings.

Test-Taking Strategy: Use therapeutic communication techniques. Select the option that directly addresses client feelings and concerns. Option 3 is the only option that is stated in the form of a question and is open-ended and thus will encourage the verbalization of feelings. Review therapeutic communication techniques if you had difficulty with this question.

Level of Cognitive Ability: Application
Client Needs: Psychosocial Integrity
Integrated Concept/Process: Communication and Documentation
Content Area: Mental Health

Reference:
Varcarolis, E. (2002). *Foundations of psychiatric mental health nursing* (4th ed.). Philadelphia: W.B. Saunders, p. 253.

---

63. Two months after a right mastectomy for breast cancer, the client comes to the physician's office for a follow-up appointment. The client was told that the risk for cancer in the left breast existed. When asked about the breast self-examination (BSE) practices since the surgery, the client replies, "I don't need to do that any more." This response may indicate:
1   Change in body image
2   Change in family role
3   Denial
4   Grief and mourning

Answer: 3
Rationale: The coping strategy of denying or minimizing a health problem is manifested in anxiety-producing health situations, especially those that may be life-threatening. Denial can lead to avoidance of self-care measures such as performing BSE. Options 1, 2, and 4 are not associated with the data in the question.

Test-Taking Strategy: Use the data presented in the question to select the correct option. Note the client statement "I don't need to do that any more." Eliminate option 1 and 2 because they are not directly related to the client's statement. From the remaining options, select option 3 based of the client's statement, which reflects denial. Review the indicators of denial if you had difficulty with this question.

Level of Cognitive Ability: Comprehension
Client Needs: Psychosocial Integrity
Integrated Concept/Process: Nursing Process/Evaluation
Content Area: Adult Health/Oncology

Reference:
Varcarolis, E. (2002). *Foundations of psychiatric mental health nursing* (4th ed.). Philadelphia: W.B. Saunders, p. 270.

---

64. In planning the care of a client dying of cancer, one of the nurse's goals is to have the client verbalize acceptance of impending death. Which of the following statements indicates to the nurse that this goal has been met?
1 "I'll be ready to die when my children finish school."
2 "I just want to live until my 100th birthday."
3 "I want to go to my daughter's wedding. Then I'll be ready to die."
4 "I'd like to have my family here when I die."

Answer: 4
Rationale: Acceptance is often characterized by plans for death. Often the client wants loved ones near. Options 1, 2, and 3 all reflect the bargaining stage of coping in which the client tries to negotiate with his or her God or with fate.

Test-Taking Strategy: Use the process of elimination. Note the similarity in options 1, 2, and 3. These options all demonstrate negotiating for something else to happen before death occurs. Option 4 is the option that reflects acceptance. Review the stages of death and dying if you had difficulty with this question.

Level of Cognitive Ability: Comprehension
Client Needs: Psychosocial Integrity
Integrated Concept/Process: Nursing Process/Evaluation
Content Area: Adult Health/Oncology

Reference:
Varcarolis, E. (2002). *Foundations of psychiatric mental health nursing* (4th ed.). Philadelphia: W.B. Saunders, p. 270.

---

65. Which of the following nursing interventions would the nurse implement for the oncology client who has a body image disturbance related to alopecia?
1 Teach the client proper dental hygiene with the use of a foam toothbrush
2 Teach the client the importance of rinsing the mouth after eating
3 Tell the client about the use of wigs that are often paid for by health insurance
4 Tell the client to use cosmetics to hide medication-induced rashes

Answer: 3
Rationale: The temporary or permanent thinning or loss of hair, known as alopecia, is common in oncology clients receiving chemotherapy. This often causes a body image disturbance that can be addressed by the use of wigs, hats, or scarves.

Test-Taking Strategy: Use the process of elimination. Eliminate option 1 and 2 because they are addressing a similar issue, other than alopecia. Select option 3 over option 4 because cosmetics are not always prescribed for use when a client has a rash. Also, knowledge of the definition of alopecia will direct you to option 3. Review the effects of alopecia if you had difficulty with this question.

Level of Cognitive ability: Application
Client Needs: Psychosocial Integrity
Integrated Concept/Process: Nursing Process/Implementation
Content Area: Adult Health/Oncology

Reference:
Black, J., Hawks, J., & Keene, A. (2001). *Medical-surgical nursing: clinical management for positive outcomes* (6th ed.). Philadelphia: W.B. Saunders, p. 1271.

66. In reviewing the record of a client with schizophrenia, the nurse notes that the physician has documented that the client has a bizarre affect. Which of the following would the nurse expect to note in the client based on this documentation?

1 An immobile facial expression or blank look
2 Minimal emotional response
3 An emotional response that is not congruent with the tone of the situation
4 Grimacing, giggling, or mumbling to oneself

Answer: 4

Rationale: A bizarre affect is especially prominent in the disorganized form of schizophrenia. Grimacing, giggling, and mumbling to oneself are included under this heading. Bizarre affect is marked when the client is unable to relate logically to the environment. A flat affect is an immobile facial expression or blank look. A blunted affect is a minimal emotional response, commonly seen in schizophrenia. In schizophrenia, the client's outward affect may not coincide with inner emotions. An inappropriate affect refers to an emotional response to a situation that is not congruent with the tone of the situation.

Test-Taking Strategy: Use the process of elimination. Note the word *bizarre* in the question and the client behaviors identified in option 4. This relationship may assist you in answering the question. Review these client behaviors if you had difficulty with this question.

Level of Cognitive Ability: Comprehension
Client Needs: Psychosocial Integrity
Integrated Concept/Process: Nursing Process/Data Collection
Content Area: Mental Health

Reference:
Bauer, B., & Hill, S. (2000). *Mental health nursing.* Philadelphia: W.B. Saunders, p.124.

67. A nurse is caring for a client who recently had a bilateral adrenalectomy. Which of the following interventions is essential for the nurse to include in the client's plan of care?

1 Prevent social isolation
2 Discuss changes in body image
3 Consider occupational therapy
4 Avoid stressful situations

Answer: 4

Rationale: Adrenalectomy can lead to adrenal insufficiency. Adrenal hormones are essential in maintaining homeostasis in response to stressors. Options 1, 2, and 3 are not directly related to the client's diagnosis.

Test-Taking Strategy: Focus on the client's diagnosis. Recalling that an adrenalectomy can lead to adrenal insufficiency and recalling the relationship of an adrenalectomy to the stress response will direct you to option 4. Review the effects of an adrenalectomy if you had difficulty with this question.

Level of Cognitive Ability: Application
Client Needs: Psychosocial Integrity
Integrated Concept/Process: Nursing Process/Planning
Content Area: Adult Health/Endocrine

Reference:
Black, J., Hawks, J., & Keene, A. (2001). *Medical-surgical nursing: clinical management for positive outcomes* (6th ed.). Philadelphia: W.B. Saunders, p. 1132.

68. Which statement made by a client with anorexia nervosa would indicate to the nurse that treatment has been effective?

1 "I no longer have a weight problem."
2 "I don't want to starve myself anymore."

Answer: 4

Rationale: Anorexia nervosa is usually seen in adolescent girls who try to establish identity and control by self-imposed starvation. Options 1, 2, and 3 are verbalizations of the client's intentions. Option 4 is a measurable action that can be verified.

3   "I'll eat until I don't feel hungry."
4   "My friends and I went out to lunch today."

Test-Taking Strategy: Use the process of elimination. Note the key words *treatment has been effective.* Select the option that is measurable and can be verified. Option 4 is the only measurable action. Review goals of care for the client with anorexia nervosa if you had difficulty with this question.

Level of Cognitive Ability: Analysis
Client Needs: Psychosocial Integrity
Integrated Concept/Process: Nursing Process/Evaluation
Content Area: Mental Health

Reference:
Varcarolis, E. (2002). *Foundations of psychiatric mental health nursing* (4th ed.). Philadelphia: W.B. Saunders, p. 420.

---

69. A nurse is admitting a client with a diagnosis of anorexia nervosa to the mental health unit. The nurse assists in planning care knowing that which of the following is not a characteristic of this disorder?
1   Personal relationships tend to become more superficial and distant
2   Social contacts are avoided because of the fear of being invited to eat and being discovered
3   The client is preoccupied with food and meal planning, especially for others
4   The client with anorexia will usually keep the weight near normal

Answer: 4
Rationale: As anorexia nervosa develops, personal relationships tend to become more superficial and distant. Social contacts are avoided because of the fear of being invited to eat and being discovered. The client is preoccupied with food and meal planning (especially for others), their own caloric intake throughout the day, and methods to avoid eating. Anorexic persons are likely to become very emaciated and will not maintain their near normal body weight.

Test-Taking Strategy: Use the process of elimination. Note the key word *not* in the stem of the question. Recalling that the client with anorexia nervosa becomes very emaciated and will not maintain their near normal body weight will direct you to option 4. Review the characteristics associated with this disorder if you had difficulty with this question.

Level of Cognitive Ability: Application
Client Needs: Psychosocial Integrity
Integrated Concept/Process: Nursing Process/Planning
Content Area: Mental Health

Reference:
Varcarolis, E. (2002). *Foundations of psychiatric mental health nursing* (4th ed.). Philadelphia: W.B. Saunders, p. 420.

---

70. A client who is to be discharged with a temporary colostomy says to the nurse, "I know I've changed this thing once, but I just don't know how I'll do it by myself when I'm home alone. Can't I stay here until the doctor puts it back?" Which of the following is the most therapeutic response by the nurse?
1   "So you're saying that you don't feel comfortable on your own yet even though you've practiced changing your colostomy bag once."
2   "Well, your insurance will not pay for a longer stay just to practice

Answer: 3
Rationale: The client is expressing feelings of helplessness and abandonment. Option 3 assists in meeting this need. Option 1 restates but focuses on the issue of helplessness. Option 2 provides what is probably accurate information but the words *just to practice* can be interpreted by the client as belittling. Option 4 provides information that the client already knows and then problem-solves by using a client-centered action that would probably overwhelm the client.

Test-Taking Strategy: Use the process of elimination. Focus on the issue of the question, fear and dependency. Eliminate options 2 and 4 first. From the remaining options, remember the issue of the question and address the client's feelings and concerns.

changing your colostomy, so you'll have to fight it out with them."

3 "Going home to care for yourself still feels pretty overwhelming? I will ask the registered nurse to schedule you for home visits until you're feeling more comfortable."

4 "This is only temporary, but you need to hire a nurse companion until your surgery."

Option 1 is restating, but focuses on the issue of helplessness. Option 3 addresses both fear and dependency needs. Review the psychosocial issues related to a colostomy if you had difficulty with this question.

Level of Cognitive Ability: Application
Client Needs: Psychosocial Integrity
Integrated Concept/Process: Communication and Documentation
Content Area: Adult Health/Gastrointestinal

Reference:
Potter, P., & Perry, A. (2001). *Fundamentals of nursing* (5th ed.). St. Louis: Mosby, p. 459.

---

71. A client is diagnosed as having schizophrenia and is unable to speak, although nothing is wrong with the organs of communication. The nurse understands that this condition is referred to as:
1 Pressured speech
2 Verbigeration
3 Poverty of speech
4 Mutism

Answer: 4
Rationale: Mutism is absence of verbal speech. The client does not communicate verbally despite intact physical structural ability to speak. Pressured speech refers to rapidity of speech, reflecting the client's racing thoughts. Verbigeration is the purposeless repetition of words or phrases. Poverty of speech means diminished amounts of speech or monotonic replies.

Test-Taking Strategy: Use the process of elimination. Focus on the issue: unable to speak. This should assist in eliminating options 1 and 2. Knowledge that poverty of speech indicates a diminished amount of speech will assist in eliminating option 3. If you had difficulty with this question, review these altered thought and speech patterns.

Level of Cognitive Ability: Comprehension
Client Needs: Psychosocial Integrity
Integrated Concept/Process: Nursing Process/Data Collection
Content Area: Mental Health

Reference:
Varcarolis, E. (2002). *Foundations of psychiatric mental health nursing* (4th ed.). Philadelphia: W.B. Saunders, p. 532.

---

72. A client tells the nurse, "I am a spy for the FBI. I am an eye, an eye in the sky." The nurse recognizes that this is an example of:
1 Loosened associations
2 Tangential speech
3 Clang associations
4 Echolalia

Answer: 3
Rationale: Repetition of words or phrases that are similar in sound and in no other way (rhyming) is one of the patterns of altered thought and language noted in schizophrenia. Loosened associations are a sign of disordered thought processes in which the person speaks with frequent changes of subject, and the content is only obliquely related, if at all, to the subject matter. Echolalia is an involuntary parrot-like repetition of words spoken by others. Tangential speech is characterized by a tendency to digress from an original topic of discussion, in which a common word connects two unrelated thoughts. Clang associations often take the form of rhyming.

Test-Taking Strategy: Use the process of elimination. Recalling that rhyming occurs in clang associations will direct you to option 3. Review altered thought and language patterns in schizophrenia if you had difficulty with this question.

Level of Cognitive Ability: Comprehension
Client Needs: Psychosocial Integrity
Integrated Concept/Process: Nursing Process/Data Collection
Content Area: Mental Health

Reference:
Varcarolis, E. (2002). *Foundations of psychiatric mental health nursing* (4th ed.). Philadelphia: W.B. Saunders, p. 532.

---

73. A nurse is assisting in planning the hospital discharge of a young male client newly diagnosed with type 1 diabetes mellitus. The client tells the nurse that he is concerned about self-administering insulin while in school with other students around. Which statement by the nurse best supports the client's need at this time?
  1 "You could contact the school nurse, who could provide a private area for you to take your insulin."
  2 "You could leave school early and take your insulin at home."
  3 "You shouldn't be embarrassed by your diabetes. Lots of people have this disease."
  4 "Oh, don't worry about that! You'll do fine!"

Answer: 1
Rationale: In the therapeutic caring relationship, the nurse offers information that will promote or assist the client to reach a decision that optimizes a sense of well-being. Option 2 requires a change in lifestyle. Options 3 and 4 are inappropriate statements and are similar in that they are both blocks to communication.

Test-Taking Strategy: Use the process of elimination. The issue of the question relates to a concern of self-administering insulin while in school. Eliminate options 3 and 4 because they are nontherapeutic responses and are not supporting to the client. Select option 1 because it promotes the client's ability to continue the present lifestyle, whereas option 2 changes the lifestyle. Review psychosocial issues related to diabetes mellitus if you had difficulty with this question.

Level of Cognitive Ability: Application
Client Needs: Psychosocial Integrity
Integrated Concept/Process: Communication and Documentation
Content Area: Child Health

Reference:
Potter, P., & Perry, A. (2001). *Fundamentals of nursing* (5th ed.). St. Louis: Mosby, p. 459.

---

74. A client who was admitted to the hospital for recurrent thyroid storm is preparing for discharge. The client is anxious about the illness and at times emotionally labile. Which of the following approaches would be most appropriate for the nurse to suggest including in the care plan for this client?
  1 Avoid teaching the client anything about the disease until he or she is emotionally stable
  2 Assist the client in identifying coping skills, support systems, and potential stressors
  3 Reassure the client that everything will be fine once they are in their home environment
  4 Confront the client and explain that the client must control the anxiety if the client wants to go home

Answer: 2
Rationale: It is normal for clients who experience thyroid storm to continue to be anxious and emotionally labile at the time of discharge. Confrontation in option 4 will only heighten the anxiety. Option 1 avoids the issue and option 3 provides false reassurance. The best intervention is to help the client cope with these changes in behavior and perhaps anticipate potential stressors so that symptoms will not be as severe.

Test-Taking Strategy: Use therapeutic communication techniques and focus on the issue, anxiety. This will direct you to option 2. Review care to the client with anxiety if you had difficulty with this question.

Level of Cognitive Ability: Application
Client Needs: Psychosocial Integrity
Integrated Concept/Process: Nursing Process/Planning
Content Area: Adult Health/Endocrine

Reference:
Black, J., Hawks, J., & Keene, A. (2001). *Medical-surgical nursing: clinical management for positive outcomes* (6th ed.). Philadelphia: W.B. Saunders, p. 409.

75. A client newly diagnosed with tuberculosis (TB) will be on respiratory isolation in the hospital for at least 2 weeks. Which of the following would be vital to prevent social isolation?
1   Remove the calendar and clock in the room so that the client will not obsess about time
2   Note whether the client has visitors
3   Give the client a roommate with TB who persistently tries to talk
4   Instruct all staff not to touch the client

Answer: 2
Rationale: The nurse should note whether the client has adequate visitation and social contact because the presence of others can offer positive stimulation. The calendar and clock are needed to promote orientation to time. A roommate who insists on talking could create sensory overload. Also, the client with TB should be in a private room. Touch may be important to help the client feel socially acceptable.

Test-Taking Strategy: Use the process of elimination. Note the key words *prevent social isolation.* Considering the basic principles related to sensory deprivation will direct you to option 2. Review the psychosocial issues related to the hospitalized client with TB if you had difficulty with this question.

Level of Cognitive Ability: Application
Client Needs: Psychosocial Integrity
Integrated Concept/Process: Nursing Process/Implementation
Content Area: Adult Health/Respiratory

Reference:
Black, J., Hawks, J., & Keene, A. (2001). *Medical-surgical nursing: clinical management for positive outcomes* (6th ed.). Philadelphia: W.B. Saunders, p. 1720.

---

76. A client was injured after drinking alcohol and falling into the coals of a fire. A circumferential burn wound to the left leg resulted from this accident. In report, the nurse is told that the client has just signed consent for amputation of the limb, and the procedure is scheduled for the next day. While caring for the client, the nurse notes that the client is upset and withdrawn. What is the most appropriate nursing action at this time?
1   Let the client have some time alone to grieve over the future loss of the limb
2   Remind the client that the injury was a result of alcohol abuse and refer him or her for counseling
3   Inform the physician of the client's depression and request medication to assist the client in coping with the diagnosis
4   Reflect back to the client that he or she appears upset

Answer: 4
Rationale: Reflection statements tend to elicit deeper awareness of feelings. In addition, option 4 validates the perception that the client is upset. Option 2 is inappropriate and a block to communication. Options 1 and 3 initiate interventions prematurely.

Test-Taking Strategy: Use therapeutic communication techniques. Select the option that encourages the client to express feelings. This will direct you to option 4. Review therapeutic communication techniques if you had difficulty with this question.

Level of Cognitive Ability: Application
Client Needs: Psychosocial Integrity
Integrated Concept/Process: Nursing Process/Implementation
Content Area: Mental Health

Reference:
Varcarolis, E. (2002). *Foundations of psychiatric mental health nursing* (4th ed.). Philadelphia: W.B. Saunders, p. 255.

---

77. Which of the following statements, if made by a client with left-sided Bell's palsy, requires further exploration by the nurse?

Answer: 4
Rationale: Bell's palsy is an inflammatory condition involving the facial nerve (cranial nerve VII). Bell's palsy is usually temporary in most of the clients affected. Symptoms resolve in several weeks to

1   "My left eye is tearing a lot."
2   "I have trouble closing my left eye lid."
3   "I can't taste anything on the left side."
4   "I don't know how I'll live with the effects of this stroke for the rest of my life."

months. Many clients fear that they have had a stroke when the symptoms of Bell's palsy appear, and they commonly believe that the paralysis is permanent. It is important for the nurse to identify these fears and formulate a plan for helping these clients deal with them. Options 1, 2, and 3 are expected findings in Bell's palsy.

Test-Taking Strategy: Use the process of elimination. Note the key words *requires further exploration.* Options 1, 2, and 3 identify expected findings in clients with Bell's palsy. Option 4 identifies an inaccurate understanding of the disorder and requires further exploration. Review this disorder if you had difficulty with this question.

Level of Cognitive Ability: Comprehension
Client Needs: Psychosocial Integrity
Integrated Concept/Process: Nursing Process/Evaluation
Content Area: Adult Health/Neurological

Reference:
Black, J., Hawks, J., & Keene, A. (2001). *Medical-surgical nursing: clinical management for positive outcomes* (6th ed.). Philadelphia: W.B. Saunders, p. 1997.

---

78. A nurse is assigned to assist in caring for a client newly diagnosed with diabetes mellitus who is anxious about the self-administration of insulin. Initially, the nurse would:
1   Teach a family member to give the client the insulin
2   Use an orange for the client to inject into until the client is less anxious
3   Insert the needle and have the client push in the plunger and remove the needle
4   Give the injection until the client feels confident enough to do so by himself or herself

Answer: 3
Rationale: Some clients find it difficult to insert a needle into their own skin. For these clients, the nurse might assist by selecting the site and inserting the needle. Then, as a first step in self-injection, the client can push in the plunger and remove the needle. Options 1 and 4 place the client into a dependent role. Option 2 is not realistic, in view of the issue of the question.

Test-Taking Strategy: Use the process of elimination and note the key word *initially.* Focusing on the issue, the self-administration of insulin, will direct you to option 3. Review the psychosocial issues related to the self-administration of insulin if you had difficulty with this question.

Level of Cognitive Ability: Application
Client Needs: Psychosocial Integrity
Integrated Concept/Process: Nursing Process/Implementation
Content Area: Adult Health/Endocrine

Reference:
Black, J., Hawks, J., & Keene, A. (2001). *Medical-surgical nursing: clinical management for positive outcomes* (6th ed.). Philadelphia: W.B. Saunders, p. 1162.

---

79. A client in labor has human immunodeficiency virus (HIV) and says to the nurse, "I know I will have a sick looking baby." Which of the following is the most appropriate response by the nurse?
1   "There is no reason to worry. Our neonatal unit offers the latest treatments available."

Answer: 2
Rationale: Option 2 is the most therapeutic response and the response that will elicit the best information from the client. It addresses the therapeutic communication technique of paraphrasing. Parents should know that their baby will not look sick from HIV at birth and that there will be a period of uncertainty before it is known whether the baby has acquired the infection.

2   "You have concerns about how HIV will affect your baby?"

3   "You are very sick, but your baby may not be."

4   "All babies are beautiful. I am sure your baby will be, too."

Test-Taking Strategy: Use therapeutic communication techniques. Eliminate option 1 because you would not tell the client *there is no reason to worry.* Options 3 and 4 provide false reassurances. Option 2 is an open-ended question that will provide an opportunity to the client to verbalize concerns. Review therapeutic communication techniques if you had difficulty with this question.

Level of Cognitive Ability: Application
Client Needs: Psychosocial Integrity
Integrated Concept/Process: Communication and Documentation
Content Area: Maternity

Reference:
McKinney, E., Ashwill, J., Murray, S. et al. (2000). *Maternal-child nursing.* Philadelphia: W.B Saunders, p. 814.

---

80. A client who is scheduled for an abdominal peritoneoscopy says to the nurse, "The doctor told me to restrict food and liquids for at least 8 hours before this procedure and to use a Fleet's enema 4 hours before coming to the hospital. Do people ever get into trouble with this procedure?" Which of the following is the most therapeutic response by the nurse?
   1   "Any invasive procedure brings risk with it. You need to report any shoulder pain immediately."
   2   "There are relatively few problems, especially if you are having local anesthesia, but vaginal bleeding should be reported immediately."
   3   "Trouble? There is never any trouble with this procedure. That's why the surgeon will use local anesthesia."
   4   "You seem to understand the preparation very well. Are you having concerns about the procedure?"

Answer: 4
Rationale: Abdominal peritoneoscopy is performed to directly visualize the liver, gallbladder, spleen, and stomach after the insufflation of carbon dioxide. During the procedure, a rigid laparoscope is inserted through a small incision in the abdomen. A microscope allows visualization of the organs and provides a way to collect a specimen for biopsy or to remove small tumors. The most therapeutic response is one that facilitates the client's expression of feelings and directly addresses the client's concerns. Options 1 and 2 will cause anxiety about the procedure. Option 3 is an inaccurate statement.

Test-Taking Strategy: Use therapeutic communication techniques. Option 4 is the most therapeutic response because it supports the data provided in the question and provides an opportunity for the client to verbalize concerns. Review these techniques if you had difficulty with this question.

Level of Cognitive Ability: Application
Client Needs: Psychosocial Integrity
Integrated Concept/Process: Communication and Documentation
Content Area: Adult Health/Gastrointestinal

Reference:
Black, J., Hawks, J., & Keene, A. (2001). *Medical-surgical nursing: clinical management for positive outcomes* (6th ed.). Philadelphia: W.B. Saunders, p. 276.

---

81. In assessing the client's emotional needs during a precipitate labor, the nurse can anticipate the client having:
   1   Less pain and anxiety than with a normal labor
   2   A need for support in maintaining a sense of control
   3   Fewer fears regarding the effect on the infant
   4   A sense of satisfaction regarding the quick labor

Answer: 2
Rationale: The client experiencing a precipitate labor may have more difficulty maintaining control because of the abrupt onset of labor and quick progression. This may be very different from previous labor experiences; therefore the client needs support from the nurse to understand and adapt to the rapid progression. The contractions often increase in intensity quickly, adding to the pain, anxiety, and lack of control. The client may also have an increased amount of concern about the effect of the labor on the baby. Lack of control over the situation, combined with increased pain and anxiety, can result in a decreased level of satisfaction

with the labor and delivery experience. Options 1, 3, and 4 imply a positive effect of the experience of precipitate labor.

Test-Taking Strategy: Use the process of elimination and recall that a precipitate labor has an abrupt onset and a quick progression. Note the key words *need for support* in option 2. Psychosocial questions often address the client's needs for support. Review the psychosocial issues related to this type of labor if you had difficulty with this question.

Level of Cognitive Ability: Comprehension
Client Needs: Psychosocial Integrity
Integrated Concept/Process: Nursing Process/Planning
Content Area: Maternity

Reference:
McKinney, E., Ashwill, J., Murray, S. et al. (2000). *Maternal-child nursing.* Philadelphia: W.B Saunders, p. 694.

---

82. A nurse is assisting in planning care for a client who presents in active labor with a history of a previous cesarean delivery. She complains of a "tearing" sensation in the lower abdomen. The client is upset and expresses concern for the safety of her baby. The most appropriate response from the nurse is:
1 "Don't worry, you are in good hands."
2 "I can understand that you are fearful. We are doing everything possible for your baby."
3 "You'll have to talk to your doctor about the tearing sensation."
4 "I don't have time to answer questions now. We'll talk later."

Answer: 2
Rationale: Clients have a concern for the safety of their baby during labor and delivery, especially when a problem arises. A calm attitude with realistic reassurances is an important aspect of client care. Dismissing or ignoring the client's concerns can lead to increased fear and lack of cooperation.

Test-Taking Strategy: Use therapeutic communication techniques. Avoid options that block therapeutic communication. Option 1 uses a cliché and false reassurance. Options 3 and 4 place the client's feelings "on hold." Choose the option that reflects acceptance of the client's feelings and provides realistic reassurances. This will direct you to option 2. Review therapeutic communication techniques if you had difficulty with this question.

Level of Cognitive Ability: Application
Client Needs: Psychosocial Integrity
Integrated Concept/Process: Communication and Documentation
Content Area: Maternity

Reference:
McKinney, E., Ashwill, J., Murray, S. et al. (2000). *Maternal-child nursing.* Philadelphia: W.B Saunders, p. 352.

---

83. During an initial physical examination of a newborn male, undescended testes (cryptorchidism) is discovered and these findings are shared with the parents. The nurse understands that if this condition is not corrected, which of the following could have a psychosocial impact?
1 Infertility
2 Malignancy
3 Feminization
4 Atrophy

Answer: 1
Rationale: Infertility could occur in this disorder because sperm production is decreased in the undescended testes. The psychological effects of an "empty scrotum" could affect the client's perception of self and the ability to reproduce. Options 2 and 4 are physiological concerns. Option 3 is not associated with this condition.

Test-Taking Strategy: Note the key words *psychosocial impact.* Options 2 and 4 are possible physical consequences of failure to treat cryptorchidism, not psychosocial consequences; therefore eliminate these options. Because all hormones responsible for secondary sex characteristics continue to be secreted directly into the bloodstream, option 3 is not correct. Review the psychosocial effects of this disorder if you had difficulty with this question.

Level of Cognitive Ability: Comprehension
Client Needs: Psychosocial Integrity
Integrated Concept/Process: Nursing Process/Planning
Content Area: Child Health

Reference:
Shulte, E., Price, D., Gwin, J. (2001). *Thompson's pediatric nursing* (8th ed.). Philadelphia: W.B. Saunders, p. 149.

---

84. Cranial surgery is performed on an adolescent who sustained a head injury. Which psychosocial complication would be of the most concern in the adolescent?
  1 Short-term memory loss
  2 Head area shaved for the surgical procedure
  3 Administration of phenobarbital (Luminal) medication
  4 Residual headaches

Answer: 2
Rationale: Body image is a main focus for the adolescent. Appearance is very important and is linked with peer acceptance. Loss of hair in the area of the head alters the adolescent's appearance. Option 1 could be a problem if memory loss interferes with remembering friends' names, directions, or school performance, but these are not as obvious as hair loss. Phenobarbital administration does not have psychosocial implications unless the adolescent refuses to take the medication. Residual headaches can be controlled by medication and stress reduction techniques.

Test-Taking Strategy: Use the process of elimination. Remember that adolescents' focus at this stage of growth and development is body image and how peers perceive them. Based on this issue, you can easily eliminate options 3 and 4. From the remaining options, select option 2 because this is the most obvious alteration in body image. Review psychosocial issues related to the adolescent if you had difficulty with this question.

Level of Cognitive Ability: Comprehension
Client Needs: Psychosocial Integrity
Integrated Concept/Process: Nursing Process/Planning
Content Area: Child Health

Reference:
McKinney, E., Ashwill, J., Murray, S. et al. (2000). *Maternal-child nursing*. Philadelphia: W.B Saunders, p. 152.

---

85. A mother with an infant with hydrocephalus is concerned about the complication of mental retardation. The mother states, "I'm not sure if I can care for my baby at home." The most appropriate response by the nurse is which of the following?
  1 "There is no reason to worry. You have a good pediatrician."
  2 "Mothers instinctively know what is best for their babies."

Answer: 3
Rationale: Paraphrasing is restating the mother's message in the nurse's own words. Option 3 addresses the therapeutic technique of paraphrasing. In options 1 and 2, the nurse is offering false reassurance, and these types of responses will block communication. In option 4, the nurse is minimizing the social needs involved with the baby's diagnosis, which is harmful for the nurse-parent relationship.

Test-Taking Strategy: Use therapeutic communication techniques and the process of elimination. Option 3 is the only

3   "You have concerns about your baby's condition and care?"

4   "All babies have individual needs."

therapeutic technique and addresses paraphrasing. This is the only option that will provide the client an opportunity to verbalize concerns. Review these techniques if you had difficulty with this question.

Level of Cognitive Ability: Application
Client Needs: Psychosocial Integrity
Integrated Concept/Process: Communication and Documentation
Content Area: Maternity

Reference:
Potter, P., & Perry, A. (2001). *Fundamentals of nursing* (5th ed.). St. Louis: Mosby, p. 459.

---

86. A preschooler is just diagnosed with impetigo. The child's mother tells the nurse, "But my children take baths every day." The most appropriate response by the nurse is which of the following?

1   "You are concerned about how your child got impetigo?"

2   "There is no need to worry, we will not tell daycare why your child is absent."

3   "Not only do you have to do a better job in keeping the children clean, you must also wash your hands more frequently."

4   "You should have seen the doctor before the wound became infected; then you would not have had to worry about the child having impetigo."

Answer: 1
Rationale: By paraphrasing what the parent tells the nurse, the nurse is addressing the parent's thoughts. Option 1 is the therapeutic technique of paraphrasing. All the other options are blocks to communication because they make the parent feel guilty for the child's illness.

Test-Taking Strategy: Use therapeutic communication techniques and the process of elimination. Option 1 is the only therapeutic technique and addresses paraphrasing. This is the only option that will provide the client an opportunity to verbalize concerns. Options 2, 3, and 4 are blocks to communication. Review these techniques if you had difficulty with this question.

Level of Cognitive Ability: Application
Client Needs: Psychosocial Integrity
Integrated Concept/Process: Communication and Documentation
Content Area: Child Health

Reference:
Potter, P., & Perry, A. (2001). *Fundamentals of nursing* (5th ed.). St. Louis: Mosby, p. 459.

---

87. Which is the best way to address the cultural needs of a child and family when the child is admitted to a health care facility?

1   Ask questions about cultural needs and explain to the family why the questions are being asked

2   Explain to the family that while the child is being treated, they need to discontinue cultural practices because they may be harmful to the child

3   Ignore cultural needs because they are not important to health care professionals

4   Address only those issues that directly affect the nurse's care of the child

Answer: 1
Rationale: When caring for individuals from different cultures, it is important to ask questions about specific cultural needs and means of treatment. An understanding of the family's beliefs and health practices is essential to successful interventions for that particular family. Options 2, 3, and 4 ignore the cultural beliefs and values of the client.

Test-Taking Strategy: Use the process of elimination and focus on the issue: cultural needs. Options 2, 3, and 4 are all similar in that they ignore the cultural practices and values of the client. Option 1 addresses the cultural needs of the family and the child. Review the concepts related to cultural needs if you had difficulty with this question.

Level of Cognitive Ability: Comprehension
Client Needs: Psychosocial Integrity

Integrated Concept/Process: Cultural Awareness
Content Area: Child Health

Reference:
Potter, P., & Perry, A. (2001). *Fundamentals of nursing* (5th ed.). St. Louis: Mosby, p. 457.

---

88. A client with a T1 spinal cord injury has just learned that the cord was completely severed. The client says, "I'm no good to anyone. I might as well be dead." The most appropriate response by the nurse is:
    1 "It makes me uncomfortable when you talk this way."
    2 "I'll ask the psychologist to see you about this."
    3 "You're not a useless person at all."
    4 "You are feeling pretty bad about things right now."

Answer: 4
Rationale: Restating and reflecting keeps the communication open and shows interest that will encourage the client to expand on the current feelings of unworthiness and loss that require exploration. The nurse blocks communication by showing discomfort or disapproval, or by postponing discussion of issues. Options 1, 2, and 3 block communication.

Test-Taking Strategy: Use therapeutic communication techniques and the process of elimination. Review these nursing statements considering the effect that they may produce on the client. Options 1, 2, and 3 clearly block communication. Option 4 identifies the therapeutic communication technique of restating and reflecting. Review these techniques if you had difficulty with this question.

Level of Cognitive Ability: Application
Client Needs: Psychosocial Integrity
Integrated Concept/Process: Communication and Documentation
Content Area: Adult Health/Neurological

Reference:
Potter, P., & Perry, A. (2001). *Fundamentals of nursing* (5th ed.). St. Louis: Mosby, p. 459.

---

89. A nurse enters the room of a client with myocardial infarction (MI) and finds the client quietly crying. After determining that there is no physiological reason for the client's distress, the nurse replies:
    1 "Do you want me to call your daughter?"
    2 "Can you tell me a little about what has you so upset?"
    3 "I understand how you feel. I'd cry too if I had a major heart attack."
    4 "Try not to be so upset. Psychological stress is bad for your heart."

Answer: 2
Rationale: Clients with MI often experience anxiety or fear. The nurse encourages the client to express concerns by showing genuine interest and concern, and by facilitating communication using therapeutic communication techniques. Options 1, 3, and 4 do not address the client's feelings or promote client verbalization.

Test-Taking Strategy: Use therapeutic communication techniques. Select the option that has an exploratory approach, because the question does not identify why the client is upset. Review these techniques if you had difficulty with this question.

Level of Cognitive Ability: Application
Client Needs: Psychosocial Integrity
Integrated Concept/Process: Communication and Documentation
Content Area: Adult Health/Cardiovascular

Reference:
Potter, P., & Perry, A. (2001). *Fundamentals of nursing* (5th ed.). St. Louis: Mosby, p. 459.

90. A male client with a recent complete T 4 spinal cord transection tells the nurse that he will walk as soon as spinal shock abates. Which of the following will provide the most accurate basis for planning a response?

1 To speed acceptance, the client needs reinforcement that he will not walk again

2 The client should move through the grieving process rapidly to benefit from rehabilitation

3 The client is projecting by insisting that walking is the rehabilitation goal

4 Denial can be protective while the client deals with the anxiety created by the new disability

Answer: 4

Rationale: During the adjustment period in the first few weeks after spinal cord injury, clients may use denial as a defense mechanism. Denial may decrease anxiety temporarily and is a normal part of grieving. After spinal shock abates, denial may impair rehabilitation if its use is prolonged or excessive. However, rehabilitation programs include psychological counseling to deal with grief. Options 1, 2, and 3 are inaccurate.

Test-Taking Strategy: Use the process of elimination. The words *speed acceptance, move through the grieving process rapidly*, and *walking is the rehabilitation goal* should be indicators that these are incorrect options. Focus on the client's statement, which is an indication of denial. Review the characteristics of denial if you had difficulty with this question.

Level of Cognitive Ability: Comprehension
Client Needs: Psychosocial Integrity
Integrated Concept/Process: Nursing Process/Planning
Content Area: Adult Health/Musculoskeletal

Reference:
Black, J., Hawks, J., & Keene, A. (2001). *Medical-surgical nursing: clinical management for positive outcomes* (6th ed.). Philadelphia: W.B. Saunders, p. 2065.

---

91. Maladaptive coping behavior can occur in response to a loss or change in the body associated with surgery. In this situation, the nurse would include which action in the nursing care plan?

1 Explain to the client that open grieving is abnormal

2 Discourage sharing feelings with others that have had similar experiences

3 Encourage the client to express feelings about body changes

4 Advise the client to seek psychological treatment immediately

Answer: 3

Rationale: Surgery can alter a client's body image. The onset of problems with coping with these changes may occur in the immediate or extended postoperative stage. Nursing interventions primarily involves providing psychological support, and the nurse should encourage the client to express feelings. Options 1, 2, and 4 are inaccurate interventions.

Test-Taking Strategy: Use therapeutic communication techniques. Remember options that block communication such as giving advice in option 4 and showing disapproval in options 1 and 2 are incorrect. Always focus on the client's feelings first. Review these therapeutic techniques if you had difficulty with this question.

Level of Cognitive Ability: Application
Client Needs: Psychosocial Integrity
Integrated Concept/Process: Nursing Process/Planning
Content Area: Fundamental Skills

Reference:
Black, J., Hawks, J., & Keene, A. (2001). *Medical-surgical nursing: clinical management for positive outcomes* (6th ed.). Philadelphia: W.B. Saunders, p. 311.

---

92. A client with pulmonary edema exhibits severe anxiety. The nurse is preparing to carry out the medically prescribed orders. Which approach should the nurse plan to best meet the needs of the client in a holistic manner?

Answer: 4

Rationale: Pulmonary edema is accompanied by extreme fear and anxiety. Because the client typically experiences a sense of impending doom, the nurse should remain with the client as much as possible. Options 1 and 2 do not provide for the psychological needs of the client in distress. Family members

1 Leave the client alone while gathering required equipment and medications

2 Give the client the call bell and encourage its use if the client feels worse

3 Ask a family member to stay with the client

4 Stay with the client and ask another nurse to gather equipment and supplies not already in the room

(option 3) can emotionally support the client but are not able to respond to physiological needs and symptoms. In fact, they are typically in psychological distress themselves.

Test-Taking Strategy: Use the process of elimination. The word *holistic* in the stem guides you to consider both physical and emotional needs of the client. This will direct you to option 4. Review care to the client with pulmonary edema if you had difficulty with this question.

Level of Cognitive Ability: Application
Client Needs: Psychosocial Integrity
Integrated Concept/Process: Nursing Process/Planning
Content Area: Adult Health/Respiratory

Reference:
Black, J., Hawks, J., & Keene, A. (2001). *Medical-surgical nursing: clinical management for positive outcomes* (6th ed.). Philadelphia: W.B. Saunders, p. 1748.

---

93. A family of a client with myocardial infarction is visibly anxious and upset about the client's condition. The nurse would plan to do which of the following to give the best support to the family?

1 Insist they go home to sleep at night, to keep up their own strength

2 Provide flexibility with visiting times according to the client's condition and family needs

3 Offer them coffee and other beverages on a regular basis

4 Ask the hospital chaplain to sit with them until the client's condition stabilizes

Answer: 2
Rationale: The use of flexible visiting hours meets the needs of the client and family in reducing the anxiety levels of both. Insisting that the family go home is nontherapeutic. Offering the family beverages does not provide support. Although the chaplain may provide support, it is unrealistic for the chaplain to stay until the client stabilizes; in addition, the religious preference of the family may not be compatible with this option.

Test-Taking Strategy: Use the process of elimination. The question asks for the *best* method of support. Options 1 and 4 may or may not be helpful, depending on the client and family situation. Coffee and beverages, while probably helpful to many visitors, do not provide the best support and can also be obtained in the hospital cafeteria. This leaves option 2 as the choice with most value. Review measures that provide support to the client and family if you had difficulty with this question.

Level of Cognitive Ability: Application
Client Needs: Psychosocial Integrity
Integrated Concept/Process: Nursing Process/Planning
Content Area: Adult Health/Cardiovascular

Reference:
Black, J., Hawks, J., & Keene, A. (2001). *Medical-surgical nursing: clinical management for positive outcomes* (6th ed.). Philadelphia: W.B. Saunders, p. 1602.

---

94. A client with unstable angina says to the nurse, "I'm so afraid something bad will happen." Which of the following actions by the nurse would be of most immediate help to the client?

1 Giving reassurance that nothing will happen to the client

2 Telephoning the client's family

Answer: 3
Rationale: When a client experiences fear, the nurse can provide a calm, safe environment by offering appropriate reassurance by the therapeutic use of touch, and by remaining with the client as much as possible.

Test-Taking Strategy: Use the process of elimination. Options 1 and 4 can be eliminated first. From the remaining options, focus

3 Staying with the client
4 Using television to distract the client

on the key words *of most immediate help*. This will direct you to option 3. Remember to provide support to the client. Review measures to provide support to the client if you had difficulty with this question.

Level of Cognitive Ability: Application
Client Needs: Psychosocial Integrity
Integrated Concept/Process: Nursing Process/Implementation
Content Area: Adult Health/Cardiovascular

Reference:
Black, J., Hawks, J., & Keene, A. (2001). *Medical-surgical nursing: clinical management for positive outcomes* (6th ed.). Philadelphia: W.B. Saunders, p. 1585.

---

95. A male client with Raynaud's disease tells the nurse that he has a stressful job and does not handle stressful situations well. The nurse should encourage the client to:
1 Change jobs
2 Consider a stress-management program
3 Seek help from a psychologist
4 Use ear plugs to minimize environmental noise

Answer: 2
Rationale: Stress can trigger the vasospasm that occurs with Raynaud's disease, so referral to a stress-management program or use of biofeedback training may be helpful. These measures teach clients a variety of techniques to reduce or minimize stress. Option 1 is unrealistic. Option 3 is not necessarily required at this time. Option 4 does not specifically address the issue.

Test-Taking Strategy: Use the process of elimination and focus on the issue: managing stress. Note the word *consider* in the correct option. This option provides the client with both assistance and the opportunity to make an independent decision. Review care to the client with Raynaud's disease if you had difficulty with this question.

Level of Cognitive Ability: Application
Client Needs: Psychosocial Integrity
Integrated Concept/Process: Nursing Process/Implementation
Content Area: Adult Health/Cardiovascular

Reference:
Black, J., Hawks, J., & Keene, A. (2001). *Medical-surgical nursing: clinical management for positive outcomes* (6th ed.). Philadelphia: W.B. Saunders, p. 1421.

---

96. A client has an oral endotracheal tube attached to a mechanical ventilator and is about to begin the weaning process. The nurse who is assisting in caring for the client determines that which of the following items, previously useful in minimizing the client's anxiety, should be limited?
1 Television
2 Radio
3 Family visitors
4 Antianxiety medications

Answer: 4
Rationale: Antianxiety medications and narcotic analgesics are used cautiously in the client being weaned from a mechanical ventilator. These medications may interfere with the weaning process by suppressing the respiratory drive. The client may exhibit anxiety during the weaning process for a variety of reasons; therefore distractions such as radio, television, and visitors are still very useful.

Test-Taking Strategy: To answer this question accurately, you should identify the items that could interfere with the client's strength, endurance, and respiratory drive in maintaining independent ventilation. Using this as the guideline will direct you to option 4. Side effects of these medications could include sedation, which could interfere with optimal respiratory function. Review the psychosocial effects of weaning from a mechanical ventilator if you had difficulty with this question.

Level of Cognitive Ability: Comprehension
Client Needs: Psychosocial Integrity
Integrated Concept/Process: Nursing Process/Implementation
Content Area: Adult Health/Respiratory

Reference:
Black, J., Hawks, J., & Keene, A. (2001). *Medical-surgical nursing: clinical management for positive outcomes* (6th ed.). Philadelphia: W.B. Saunders, p. 1655.

---

97. A client scheduled for pulmonary angiography is fearful about the procedure and asks the nurse if the procedure involves significant pain and radiation exposure. The nurse gives a response to the client that provides reassurance, understanding that:
1 The procedure is somewhat painful, but there is minimal exposure to radiation
2 Discomfort may occur with needle insertion, and there is minimal exposure to radiation
3 There is absolutely no pain, although a moderate amount of radiation must be used to get accurate results
4 There is very mild pain throughout the procedure, and the exposure to radiation is negligible

Answer: 2
Rationale: Pulmonary angiography involves minimal exposure to radiation. The procedure is painless, although the client may feel discomfort with insertion of the needle for the catheter that is used for dye injection. Options 1, 3, and 4 are incorrect.

Test-Taking Strategy: Use the process of elimination. Knowing that radiation exposure is minimal helps you to eliminate option 3 first. It is also helpful to know that the only discomfort occurs with needle insertion. This will direct you to option 2. Review this procedure if you had difficulty with this question.

Level of Cognitive Ability: Comprehension
Client Needs: Psychosocial Integrity
Integrated Concept/Process: Nursing Process/Implementation
Content Area: Adult Health/Respiratory

Reference:
Black, J., Hawks, J., & Keene, A. (2001). *Medical-surgical nursing: clinical management for positive outcomes* (6th ed.). Philadelphia: W.B. Saunders, p. 1376.

---

98. The client has an initial positive result of an enzyme-linked immunosorbent assay (ELISA) test for human immunodeficiency virus (HIV). The client begins to cry and asks the nurse what this means. The nurse is able to provide support to the client, using knowledge that:
1 The client is HIV-positive but the disease has been detected early
2 The client is HIV-positive but the client's CD4 cell count is high
3 There is a high rate of false-positive results with this test and more testing is needed before diagnosing the client's status as HIV positive
4 There are occasional false-positive readings with this test, which can be cleared up by repeating it one more time

Answer: 3
Rationale: If the ELISA test results are positive, the test is repeated. If it is positive a second time, the Western blot (a more specific test) is done to confirm the finding. The client is not considered HIV-positive unless the Western blot is positive. The ELISA is a fast and relatively inexpensive test, but it carries a high false-positive rate.

Test-Taking Strategy: Use the process of elimination. Recall that HIV infection is not diagnosed with a single laboratory test. With this in mind, eliminate options 1 and 2 first. To choose correctly between options 3 and 4, it is necessary to understand that the ELISA would be repeated, and a Western blot would be done to confirm these results. Review this content if you had difficulty with this question.

Level of Cognitive Ability: Comprehension
Client Needs: Psychosocial Integrity
Integrated Concept/Process: Nursing Process/Implementation
Content Area: Adult Health/Respiratory

Reference:
Black, J., Hawks, J., & Keene, A. (2001). *Medical-surgical nursing: clinical management for positive outcomes* (6th ed.). Philadelphia: W.B. Saunders, p. 2193.

99. A client diagnosed with cancer of the bladder has been experiencing fear related to the uncertain outcome of the upcoming cystectomy and urinary diversion. The nurse determines that the client is still fearful if the client makes which of the following statements?

1 "I'm so afraid I won't live through all this."
2 "What if I have no help at home after going through this awful surgery?"
3 "I'll never feel like myself once I can't go to the bathroom normally."
4 "I wish I'd never gone to the doctor at all."

Answer: 1

Rationale: In option 1, the client is expressing a fear of death related to cancer. The statement in option 2 reflects a risk for impaired home maintenance management. Option 3 reflects a body image disturbance. Option 4 is vague and nonspecific; further exploration would be required to associate this statement with fear.

Test-Taking Strategy: Use the process of elimination. Note the relationship between the word *fear* in the question and *afraid* in the correct option. This option clearly identifies the fear that the client is experiencing. Review the characteristics of fear if you had difficulty with this question.

Level of Cognitive Ability: Comprehension
Client Needs: Psychosocial Integrity
Integrated Concept/Process: Nursing Process/Data Collection
Content Area: Adult Health/Renal

Reference:
Black, J., Hawks, J., & Keene, A. (2001). *Medical-surgical nursing: clinical management for positive outcomes* (6th ed.). Philadelphia: W.B. Saunders, p. 399.

---

100. A client with renal cell carcinoma of the left kidney is scheduled for nephrectomy. The right kidney appears normal at this time. The client is anxious about whether dialysis will ultimately be a necessity. The nurse would plan to use which of the following information in discussions with the client?

1 There is absolutely no chance of needing dialysis because of the nature of the surgery
2 Dialysis could become likely, but it depends on how well the client complies with fluid restriction after surgery
3 One kidney is adequate to meet the needs of the body as long as it has normal function
4 There is a strong likelihood that the client will need dialysis within 5 to 10 years

Answer: 3

Rationale: Fears about having only one functioning kidney are common in clients who must undergo nephrectomy for renal cancer. These clients need emotional support and reassurance that the remaining kidney should be able to fully meet the body's metabolic needs, as long as it has normal function.

Test-Taking Strategy: Use the process of elimination. Eliminate option 1 first. An option that contains the words *absolutely no chance* is not likely to be correct. Knowing that there is no need for fluid restriction with a functioning kidney guides you to eliminate option 2 next. From the remaining options, remember that an individual can donate a kidney without adverse consequences or the need for dialysis. Applying that knowledge to this question would guide you to choose option 3 over option 4. Review the psychosocial effects of a nephrectomy if you had difficulty with this question.

Level of Cognitive Ability: Application
Client Needs: Psychosocial Integrity
Integrated Concept/Process: Nursing Process/Planning
Content Area: Adult Health/Oncology

Reference:
Black, J., Hawks, J., & Keene, A. (2001). *Medical-surgical nursing: clinical management for positive outcomes* (6th ed.). Philadelphia: W.B. Saunders, p. 861.

---

101. A plan of care for a client with a diagnosis of acute pulmonary edema should include strategies for:

1 Decreasing cardiac output
2 Increasing fluid volume

Answer: 4

Rationale: When cardiac output falls as a result of acute pulmonary edema, the sympathetic nervous system is stimulated. Stimulation of the sympathetic nervous system results in the flight-or-fight reaction that further impairs cardiac function.

3 Promoting a positive body image
4 Reducing anxiety

The goal of treatment is to increase cardiac output. Fluid volume should be decreased. Altered body image is not a common problem experienced by clients with acute pulmonary edema.

Test-Taking Strategy: Use the process of elimination. Considering the physiological manifestations of this condition will assist in eliminating options 1 and 2. From the remaining options, recalling that severe dyspnea occurs will assist in directing you to option 4. Review the psychosocial manifestations associated with this disorder if you had difficulty with this question.

Level of Cognitive Ability: Application
Client Needs: Psychosocial Integrity
Integrated Concept/Process: Nursing Process/Planning
Content Area: Adult Health/Cardiovascular

Reference:
Black, J., Hawks, J., & Keene, A. (2001). *Medical-surgical nursing: clinical management for positive outcomes* (6th ed.). Philadelphia: W.B. Saunders, p. 1746.

---

102. A client with acute renal failure (ARF) is having trouble remembering information and instructions because of an elevated blood urea nitrogen (BUN) level. The nurse would avoid doing which of the following when communicating with this client?
1 Give simple, clear directions
2 Explain treatments, using understandable language
3 Include the family in discussions related to care
4 Give thorough, complete explanations of treatment options

Answer: 4
Rationale: The client with ARF may have difficulty remembering information and instructions because of an increased BUN level and anxiety. Communication should be clear, simple, and understandable. The family is included whenever possible. It is the physician's responsibility to explain treatment options.

Test-Taking Strategy: Use the process of elimination and note the key word *avoid.* Recalling the basic principles of effective communication would allow you to recognize that options 1, 2, and 3 are helpful in maintaining effective communication. Review effective communication techniques if you had difficulty with this question.

Level of Cognitive Ability: Application
Client Needs: Psychosocial Integrity
Integrated Concept/Process: Communication and Documentation
Content Area: Adult Health/Renal

Reference:
Black, J., Hawks, J., & Keene, A. (2001). *Medical-surgical nursing: clinical management for positive outcomes* (6th ed.). Philadelphia: W.B. Saunders, p. 887.

---

103. A nurse working in a rehabilitation center witnesses a postoperative coronary artery bypass graft client and spouse arguing after a rehabilitation session. The most appropriate statement by the nurse to identify the feelings of the client is:
1 "You seem upset..."
2 "You shouldn't get upset. It will affect your heart."
3 "Oh, don't let this get you down."
4 "It will seem better tomorrow. Smile."

Answer: 1
Rationale: Therapeutic communication techniques assist the flow of communication and always focus on the client. Open-ended statements allow the client to verbalize, giving the nurse a direction or clarification of the true feelings. Additionally, acknowledging the client's feelings without inserting personal values or judgments is a method of therapeutic communication. Options 2, 3, and 4 do not encourage verbalization by the client.

Test-Taking Strategy: Use therapeutic communication techniques. Remembering to always focus on the client's feelings will direct you to option 1. Review these techniques if you had difficulty with this question.

Level of Cognitive Ability: Application
Client Needs: Psychosocial Integrity
Integrated Concept/Process: Communication and Documentation
Content Area: Adult Health/Cardiovascular

Reference:
Potter, P., & Perry, A. (2001). *Fundamentals of nursing* (5th ed.). St. Louis: Mosby, p. 459.

---

104. An acutely psychotic client displays increased motor activity. Which of the following medications, if prescribed, would the nurse administer?
1   Sertraline hydrochloride (Zoloft)
2   Haloperidol (Haldol)
3   Chloral Hydrate (Noctec)
4   Isocarboxazid (Marplan)

Answer: 2
Rationale: Antipsychotics are used to treat acute and chronic psychosis, especially when the client has increased psychomotor activity. A fast-acting, injectable agent would be the medication of choice in this situation. Antidepressants (options 1 and 4) and hypnotics (option 3) are not indicated in this situation.

Test-Taking Strategy: Use the process of elimination. Eliminate options 1 and 4 first because they are similar and are antidepressants. From the remaining options, focus on the data in the question and recall the classifications of the medications. This will direct you to option 2. Review these medications if you had difficulty with this question.

Level of Cognitive Ability: Application
Client Needs: Psychosocial Integrity
Integrated Concept/Process: Nursing Process/Implementation
Content Area: Pharmacology

Reference:
Hodgson, B., & Kizior, R. (2003). *Saunders nursing drug handbook 2003.* Philadelphia: W.B. Saunders, p. 540.

---

105. A client is admitted to the mental health unit with a diagnosis of panic disorder. The nurse would anticipate that the physician's order for a benzodiazepine would indicate:
1   Imipramine (Tofranil)
2   Alprazolam (Xanax)
3   Buproprion (Wellbutrin)
4   Doxepin (Sinequan)

Answer: 2
Rationale: Options 1, 3, and 4 are classified as antidepressants and act by stimulating the central nervous system (CNS) to elevate mood. Alprazolam, a benzodiazepine antianxiety agent, depresses the CNS and induces relaxation in panic disorders.

Test-Taking Strategy: Use the process of elimination. Eliminate options 1, 3, and 4 because they are similar and are antidepressants. Review these medications if you had difficulty with this question.

Level of Cognitive Ability: Comprehension
Client Needs: Psychosocial Integrity
Integrated Concept/Process: Nursing Process/Planning
Content Area: Pharmacology

Reference:
Hodgson, B., & Kizior, R. (2003). *Saunders nursing drug handbook 2003.* Philadelphia: W.B. Saunders, p. 31.

106. A client who has never been hospitalized before is having trouble initiating the stream of urine. Knowing that there is no pathological reason for this difficulty, the nurse avoids which of the following because it is the least helpful method of assisting the client?

1   Encouraging fluid intake
2   Providing privacy during voiding
3   Assisting the client to a commode behind a closed curtain
4   Closing the bathroom door during voiding

Answer: 3

Rationale: Lack of privacy may inhibit the ability of the client to void. Using a commode behind a curtain may inhibit voiding in some people. Use of a bathroom is preferable, and encouraging fluid intake will aid in urinary elimination.

Test-Taking Strategy: Use the process of elimination. Note the key words *avoids* and *least helpful*. Option 4 is most helpful and therefore is eliminated first. Knowing that options 1 and 2 are general nursing measures will direct you to option 3 as the least helpful method of assisting the client with elimination. Review these measures if you had difficulty with this question.

Level of Cognitive Ability: Application
Client Needs: Psychosocial Integrity
Integrated Concept/Process: Nursing Process/Implementation
Content Area: Adult Health/Renal

Reference:
Black, J., Hawks, J., & Keene, A. (2001). *Medical-surgical nursing: clinical management for positive outcomes* (6th ed.). Philadelphia: W.B. Saunders, p. 831.

107. A client tells the nurse, "My doctor says I can have the surgery and go home the same day, but I'm afraid. My husband's dead and my son is 3000 miles away. I'm alone, and what happens if something goes wrong? I'm not supposed to be up walking unless absolutely necessary." Which of the following nursing responses is most therapeutic?

1   "I know, I know. They say, 'Managed Care is no care'! Have you got an alarm system so that if you fall, it will alert someone to come? If worse comes to worse, call me and I'll come immediately."
2   "Don't worry. This procedure is done all the time without any problems. You'll be fine!"
3   "Your concern is well voiced. I advise you to call your son and insist he come home immediately! You can't be too careful."
4   "You seem very concerned about going home without help. Have you discussed your concerns with your doctor?"

Answer: 4

Rationale: In option 4, the nurse uses reflection to direct the client's feelings and concerns. In option 1, the nurse is ventilating the nurse's own anger, frustration, and powerlessness. In addition, the nurse is trying to solve problems for the client but is overly controlling and takes the decision-making out of the client's hands. In option 2, the nurse provides false reassurance and then minimizes the client's concerns. In option 3, the nurse is projecting the client's own fears and the problem-solving suggested by the nurse is histrionic and provokes fear and anxiety.

Test-Taking Strategy: Use therapeutic communication techniques. By the process of elimination, you should easily be able to eliminate options 1, 2, and 3. Remember that the priority is to address the client's feelings. Review therapeutic communication techniques if you had difficulty with this question.

Level of Cognitive Ability: Application
Client Needs: Psychosocial Integrity
Integrated Concept/Process: Communication and Documentation
Content Area: Fundamental Skills

Reference:
Potter, P., & Perry, A. (2001). *Fundamentals of nursing* (5th ed.). St. Louis: Mosby, p. 459.

108. While providing care, the client says, "My doctor just told me that my cancer has spread and that I have less than 6 months to live." Which of the following responses

Answer: 4

Rationale: The client has just received very distressing news. In the correct option, the nurse encourages the client to ventilate. Option 1 provides a social communication and false hope.

would be the most therapeutic for this client?

1 "I know it seems desperate but there have been a lot of break-throughs. Something might come along in a month or so to change your status drastically."

2 "I hope you'll focus on the fact that your doctor says you have 6 months to live and that you'll think of how you'd like to live it."

3 "I am sorry. There are no easy answers in times like this, are there?"

4 "I am sorry. Would you like to dis-cuss this with me some more?"

Option 2 is patronizing and stereotypical. Option 3 expresses the nurse's feelings rather than facilitating the client's feelings.

Test-Taking Strategy: Use therapeutic communication techniques. You can easily eliminate options 1 and 2. From the remaining options, note that option 4 is providing the opportunity for the client to express feelings. Review these techniques if you had dif-ficulty with this question.

Level of Cognitive Ability: Application
Client Needs: Psychosocial Integrity
Integrated Concept/Process: Communication and Documentation
Content Area: Adult Health/Oncology

Reference:
Potter, P., & Perry, A. (2001). *Fundamentals of nursing* (5th ed.). St. Louis: Mosby, p. 459.

---

109. A client with an endotracheal tube gets easily frustrated when trying to commu-nicate personal needs to the nurse. The nurse determines that which of the fol-lowing methods for communication may be the easiest for the client?

1 Have the family interpret needs
2 Use a picture or word board
3 Use a pad and paper
4 Devise a system of hand signals

Answer: 2
Rationale: The client with an endotracheal tube in place cannot speak and the nurse needs to devise an alternative communica-tion system with the client. Use of a picture or word board is the simplest method of communication because it requires only pointing at the word or object. A pad and pencil is an acceptable alternative, but it requires more client effort and more time. The use of hand signals may not be a reliable method because it may not meet all needs and is subject to misinterpretation. The family does not need to bear the burden of communicating the client's needs, and they may not understand them either.

Test-Taking Strategy: Use the process of elimination. Focus on the key words *easily frustrated* and *easiest*. Options 3 and 4 are obviously not the *easiest* and are therefore eliminated first. Because the family may not necessarily know what the client is trying to communicate, this option could add to the client's frustration. By elimination, the picture or word board is the eas-iest and the least frustrating for the client. Review these alter-native methods of communication if you had difficulty with this question.

Level of Cognitive Ability: Comprehension
Client Needs: Psychosocial Integrity
Integrated Concept/Process: Communication and Documentation
Content Area: Adult Health/Respiratory

Reference:
Black, J., Hawks, J., & Keene, A. (2001). *Medical-surgical nursing: clinical manage-ment for positive outcomes* (6th ed.). Philadelphia: W.B. Saunders, p. 1760.

---

110. A client has been receiving maprotiline hydrochloride (Ludiomil). The nurse notifies the health care provider if which of the following client responses to the medication is noted?

Answer: 3
Rationale: Maprotiline is an antidepressant used to treat various forms of depression and anxiety. The client is also often in psy-chotherapy while on this medication. Expected effects of the med-ication include improved sense of well-being, appetite, and sleep,

1 Increased sense of well-being
2 Reported decrease in anxiety
3 Increased drowsiness
4 Increased appetite

as well as a reduced level of anxiety. Common side effects to report to the health care provider include drowsiness, lethargy, and fatigue.

Test-Taking Strategy: Note the key words *notifies the health care provider.* Recall that the medication is an antidepressant. With this in mind, note that option 1, 2, and 4 are positive client responses. Review this medication if you had difficulty with this question.

Level of Cognitive Ability: Application
Client Needs: Psychosocial Integrity
Integrated Concept/Process: Nursing Process/Implementation
Content Area: Pharmacology

Reference:
Hodgson, B., & Kizior, R. (2003). *Saunders nursing drug handbook 2003.* Philadelphia: W.B. Saunders, p. 694.

---

111. A client who is to undergo thoracentesis is afraid of not being able to tolerate the procedure. The nurse provides support and reassurance by which of the following statements?
  1 "The procedure takes only 1 to 2 minutes, so you might try to get through it by mentally counting up to 120."
  2 "The needle is a little uncomfortable going in, but this is controlled by rhythmically breathing in and out. I'll be with you to coach your breathing."
  3 "The needle may be painful when it goes in, but you must remain still. I'll stay with you throughout the entire procedure and help you hold your position."
  4 "I'll be right by your side, but the procedure will be totally painless as long as you don't move."

Answer: 3
Rationale: The needle insertion for thoracentesis is painful for the client. The nurse tells the client how important it is to remain still during the procedure so that the needle does not injure visceral pleura or lung tissue. The nurse reassures the client during the procedure and helps the client hold the proper position.

Test-Taking Strategy: Use the process of elimination. Knowing that the client must remain still during the procedure helps you to eliminate option 2 first. Knowing that the procedure may be painful for the client and takes longer than 1 to 2 minutes helps you to eliminate options 1 and 4. Review this procedure if you had difficulty with this question.

Level of Cognitive Ability: Application
Client Needs: Psychosocial Integrity
Integrated Concept/Process: Communication and Documentation
Content Area: Adult Health/Respiratory

Reference:
Black, J., Hawks, J., & Keene, A. (2001). *Medical-surgical nursing: clinical management for positive outcomes* (6th ed.). Philadelphia: W.B. Saunders, p. 1648.

---

112. A client with chronic respiratory failure is dyspneic. The client responds to the dyspnea with anxiety, which worsens the feelings of dyspnea on the part of the client. The nurse would teach the client which of the following methods to best interrupt the dyspnea-anxiety-dyspnea cycle?
  1 Relaxation and breathing techniques
  2 Biofeedback and coughing techniques

Answer: 1
Rationale: The anxious client with dyspnea should be taught interventions to decrease anxiety, which include relaxation, biofeedback, guided imagery, and distraction. This will stop the escalation of feelings of dyspnea. The dyspnea can be further controlled by teaching the client respiratory techniques, which include pursed-lip and diaphragmatic breathing. Coughing techniques are useful, but breathing techniques are more effective. Limiting fluids will thicken secretions and is contraindicated. Increased dietary carbohydrates will increase production of carbon dioxide by the body and is also contraindicated.

3   Guided imagery and limiting fluids
4   Distraction and increased dietary carbohydrates

Test-Taking Strategy: Use the process of elimination and note the key word *best*. Because the first part of every option is helpful for anxiety reduction, focus on the second part of each option to select the correct choice. Limiting fluids and increasing carbohydrates are contraindicated; therefore eliminate options 3 and 4. Breathing techniques are more effective than coughing techniques, which help you to choose option 1 over option 2. Review care to the client with chronic respiratory failure if you had difficulty with this question.

Level of Cognitive Ability: Application
Client Needs: Psychosocial Integrity
Integrated Concept/Process: Teaching/Learning
Content Area: Adult Health/Respiratory

Reference:
Black, J., Hawks, J., & Keene, A. (2001). *Medical-surgical nursing: clinical management for positive outcomes* (6th ed.). Philadelphia: W.B. Saunders, p. 452.

---

113. A client who has had drainage of a pleural effusion is in pain. The nurse avoids which intervention in providing support to this client?
1   Offering verbal support and reassurance
2   Assisting the client to find positions of comfort
3   Leaving the client alone for an extended rest period
4   Providing pain medication for the client

Answer: 3
Rationale: The pain associated with drainage of pleural effusion is minimized by positioning the client for comfort and administering analgesics for relief of pain. The nurse also offers verbal support and understanding. All of these measures help the client to cope with the pain and discomfort associated with this problem. It is least helpful to leave the client alone for extended periods because the pain may be augmented by isolation.

Test-Taking Strategy: Use the process of elimination. Note the key word *avoids*. Basic knowledge of pain management techniques and the principles of nursing care will assist in directing you to option 3. Review effective pain management techniques if you had difficulty with this question.

Level of Cognitive Ability: Application
Client Needs: Psychosocial Integrity
Integrated Concept/Process: Caring
Content Area: Fundamental Skills

Reference:
Black, J., Hawks, J., & Keene, A. (2001). *Medical-surgical nursing: clinical management for positive outcomes* (6th ed.). Philadelphia: W.B. Saunders, p. 1742.

---

114. A nurse is caring for a client who has just experienced a pulmonary embolism. The client is restless and very anxious. The nurse plans to use which approach in communicating with this client?
1   Explaining each treatment in great detail
2   Having the family reinforce the nurse's directions
3   Giving simple, clear directions and explanations

Answer: 3
Rationale: The client who has suffered pulmonary embolism is fearful and apprehensive. The nurse effectively communicates with this client by staying with the client; providing simple, clear, and accurate information; and acting in a calm, efficient manner. Options 1, 2, and 4 will produce more anxiety for the client and family.

Test-Taking Strategy: Use the process of elimination. Options 1 and 4 represent the least effective communications strategies and may be eliminated first. Having the family reinforce the directions

4   Speaking very little to the client until the crisis is over

may place stress on the family. The nurse gives simple, clear information to the client who is in distress. Review care to the anxious client if you had difficulty with this question.

Level of Cognitive Ability: Application
Client Needs: Psychosocial Integrity
Integrated Concept/Process: Nursing Process/Planning
Content Area: Adult Health/Respiratory

Reference:
Black, J., Hawks, J., & Keene, A. (2001). *Medical-surgical nursing: clinical management for positive outcomes* (6th ed.). Philadelphia: W.B. Saunders, p. 1425.

---

115. A nurse is collecting data from a confused elderly client admitted to the hospital with a hip fracture. Which of the following data obtained by the nurse would not place the client at more risk for altered thought processes?
1   Stress induced by the fracture
2   Hearing aid available and in working order
3   Unfamiliar hospital setting
4   Eyeglasses left at home

Answer: 2
Rationale: Confusion in the older client with a hip fracture could result from the unfamiliar hospital setting, stress caused by the fracture, concurrent systemic diseases, cerebral ischemia, or side effects of medications. Use of eyeglasses and hearing aids enhances the client's interaction with the environment and can reduce disorientation and confusion.

Test-Taking Strategy: Use the process of elimination and note the key word *not*. The wording of the question asks you to look for an option that will keep the client at the highest possible level of functioning from a cognitive perspective. Stress from the fracture (option 1) and unfamiliar setting (option 3) are not likely to help the client's functional level and are eliminated first. Both eyeglasses and hearing aids are useful adjuncts in communicating with a client. Because the eyeglasses were left at home, they are of no use at the current time. Review the causes of confusion and disorientation in the hospitalized client if you had difficulty with this question.

Level of Cognitive Ability: Comprehension
Client Needs: Psychosocial Integrity
Integrated Concept/Process: Nursing Process/Data Collection
Content Area: Fundamental Skills

Reference:
Potter, P., & Perry, A. (2001). *Fundamentals of nursing* (5th ed.). St. Louis: Mosby, p. 459.

---

116. A client is admitted to the nursing unit following a below-the-knee amputation after sustaining a crush injury to the left foot and lower leg. The client tells the nurse, "I think I'm going crazy. I can feel my left foot itching." The nurse responds understanding that the client's statement is:
1   A normal response and indicates the presence of phantom limb sensation
2   A normal response and indicates the presence of phantom limb pain

Answer: 1
Rationale: Phantom limb sensations are felt in the area of the amputated limb. These can include itching, warmth, and cold. The sensations are due to intact peripheral nerves in the area amputated. Whenever possible, clients should be prepared for these sensations. The client may also feel painful sensations in the amputated limb, called phantom limb pain. The origin of the pain is less understood, but whenever possible the client should also be prepared for this occurrence.

Test-Taking Strategy: Use the process of elimination. Knowing that sensation and pain may be felt in the amputated limb helps

3 An abnormal response and indicates that the client needs more psychological support

4 An abnormal response and indicates that the client is in denial about the limb loss

you to eliminate options 3 and 4 first because the sensations are not abnormal responses. Select option 1 instead of option 2 because the client has described an itching sensation but has not complained of pain. Review care to the client after amputation if you had difficulty with this question.

Level of Cognitive Ability: Comprehension
Client Needs: Psychosocial Integrity
Integrated Concept/Process: Nursing Process/Implementation
Content Area: Adult Health/Neurological

Reference:
Ignatavicius, D., Workman, M. (2002). *Medical-surgical: critical thinking for collaborative care* (4th ed.). Philadelphia: W.B. Saunders, p. 1149.

---

117. A client who has had a spinal fusion and insertion of hardware is extremely concerned with the perceived lengthy rehabilitation period. The client expresses concerns about finances and the ability to return to prior employment. The nurse understands that the client's needs could best be addressed by referral to the:
1 Surgeon
2 Clinical nurse specialist
3 Social worker
4 Physical therapist

Answer: 3
Rationale: After spinal surgery, concerns about finances and employment are best handled by referral to a social worker. This health care member is aware of the best information about resources available to the client. The physical therapist has knowledge of techniques for increasing mobility and endurance. An occupational therapist would have knowledge of techniques for activities for daily living and items related to occupation, but this is not one of the options. The clinical nurse specialist and surgeon are not the best resources for providing specific information related to financial resources.

Test-Taking Strategy: An understanding of the roles of the various members of the health care team helps you to answer this question. Focusing on the issue, concern about finances, will direct you to the social worker as the optimal resource in this instance. Review the role of the social worker if you had difficulty with this question.

Level of Cognitive Ability: Comprehension
Client Needs: Psychosocial Integrity
Integrated Concept/Process: Nursing Process/Planning
Content Area: Fundamental Skills

Reference:
Potter, P., & Perry, A. (2001). *Fundamentals of nursing* (5th ed.). St. Louis: Mosby, p. 393.

---

118. A client is fearful about having an arm cast removed. Which of the following actions by the nurse would be the most helpful?
1 Telling the client that the saw makes a frightening noise
2 Reassuring the client that no one has had an arm lacerated yet
3 Stating that the hot cutting blades cause burns only very rarely
4 Showing the client the cast cutter and explaining how it works

Answer: 4
Rationale: Because of misconceptions about the cast cutting blade, clients may be fearful of having a cast removed. The nurse should show the cast cutter to the client before it is used and explain that the client may feel heat, vibration, and pressure. The cast cutter resembles a small electric saw with a circular blade. The nurse should reassure the client that the blade does not cut like a saw but instead cuts the cast by vibrating side to side.

Test-Taking Strategy: Use the process of elimination. Note the key words *most helpful*. Option 2 provides no information and may increase fear. Options 1 and 3 give accurate information but are not reassuring. Option 4 gives the client the most reassurance because it best prepares the client for what will occur when the cast is removed. Review care to the client preparing for cast removal if you had difficulty with this question.

Level of Cognitive Ability: Application
Client Needs: Psychosocial Integrity
Integrated Concept/Process: Nursing Process/Implementation
Content Area: Adult Health/Musculoskeletal

Reference:
Black, J., Hawks, J., & Keene, A. (2001). *Medical-surgical nursing: clinical management for positive outcomes* (6th ed.). Philadelphia: W.B. Saunders, p. 1141.

---

119. A client has just been told by the physician that an exercise stress test will be done to evaluate the client's status after recent episodes of more severe chest pain. As the nurse enters the examining room, the client states, "Maybe I shouldn't bother with this test. I wonder if I should just take more medication instead." The nurse's best response would be:
1   "Can you tell me more about how you're feeling?"
2   "Don't worry. Emergency equipment is available if it should be needed."
3   "Most people tolerate the procedure well without any complications."
4   "Don't you really want to control your heart disease?"

Answer: 1
Rationale: Anxiety and fear are often present before stress testing. The nurse uses questioning as a communication method to explore a client's feelings and concerns. The correct option is open-ended and is the only option that is phrased to engender trust and sharing of concerns by the client.

Test-Taking Strategy: Use the process of elimination and therapeutic communication techniques. Remembering to focus on the client's feelings will direct you to option 1. Review these techniques if you had difficulty with this question.

Level of Cognitive Ability: Application
Client Needs: Psychosocial Integrity
Integrated Concept/Process: Communication and Documentation
Content Area: Adult Health/Cardiovascular

Reference:
Potter, P. & Perry, A. (2001). *Fundamentals of nursing* (5th ed.). St. Louis: Mosby, p. 459.

---

120. A nurse is reinforcing home care instructions to the client with left-sided heart failure. The client interrupts saying, "What's the use? I'll never remember all of this, and I'll probably die anyway!" The nurse responds understanding that the client's response is most likely a result of:
1   The teaching strategies used by the nurse
2   Anger about the new medical regimen
3   Insufficient financial resources to pay for the medications
4   Anxiety about the ability to manage the disease process at home

Answer: 4
Rationale: Anxiety often develops after heart failure. The fear of death can persist, and there is often a long, difficult period of adjustment. Anxiety and fear further tax the failing heart. The nurse should take time to explore the concerns and fears of the client.

Test-Taking Strategy: Use the process of elimination and note that the client's statement comes suddenly in the middle of receiving home-care instructions. There is no evidence in the question to support options 1 or 3. Note the key words "I'll never remember all of this" in the question. This should direct you to option 4. Review the causes of anxiety if you had difficulty with this question.

Level of Cognitive Ability: Comprehension
Client Needs: Psychosocial Integrity
Integrated Concept/Process: Nursing Process/Implementation
Content Area: Adult Health/Cardiovascular

Reference:
Ignatavicius, D., Workman, M. (2002). *Medical-surgical nursing: critical thinking for collaborative care* (4th ed.). Philadelphia: W.B. Saunders, p. 710.

121. A client scheduled for an implanted port for intermittent chemotherapy treatments says, "I'm not sure if I can handle having a tube coming out of me all the time. What will my friends think?" The most appropriate nursing action is to:
1 Show the client various central line tubes and catheters
2 Explain that an implanted port is not visible under the skin
3 Notify the physician of the client's concerns
4 Explain that the client's friends probably will not see the tube under the clothing

Answer: 2
Rationale: What the client says in this situation indicates that the client should be educated about the implanted port. An implanted port is placed under the skin and is not visible. There is no visible tubing. Tubing is used only when the port is accessed intermittently and the IV line is connected. Showing the client various other tubes will not be beneficial because the client will not be using them. It is premature to notify the physician. Option 4 does not correct the client's confusion regarding the implanted port.

Test-Taking Strategy: Use the process of elimination and focus on the issue, an implanted port. Recalling that a port is placed under the skin will direct you to option 2. Review the concepts related to implanted ports and the teaching/learning process if you had difficulty with this question.

Level of Cognitive Ability: Application
Client Needs: Psychosocial Integrity
Integrated Concept/Process: Nursing Process/Implementation
Content Area: Fundamental Skills

Reference:
Ignatavicius, D., Workman, M. (2002). *Medical-surgical nursing: critical thinking for collaborative care* (4th ed.). Philadelphia: W.B. Saunders, p. 432.

122. A client displays signs of anxiety because of pain at an intravenous (IV) site. When explaining to the client that the IV line will need to be discontinued because of an infiltration, the nurse should say which of the following?
1 "This will be a totally painless experience. It is nothing to worry about."
2 "I'm sure it will be a real relief for you just as soon as I discontinue this IV for good."
3 "Just relax and take a deep breath. This procedure will not take long and will be over soon."
4 "I can see that you're anxious. Removal of the IV shouldn't be painful; however, the IV will need to be restarted in another location by the registered nurse."

Answer: 4
Rationale: Although discontinuing an IV line is a painless experience, it is not therapeutic to tell a client not to worry. Option 2 does not acknowledge the client's feelings and does not tell the client that an infiltrated IV line will need to be restarted. Option 3 does not address the client's feelings. The correct option addresses the client's anxiety and honestly informs the client that the IV line will need to be restarted. This option uses the therapeutic technique of giving information as well as acknowledging the client's feelings.

Test-Taking Strategy: When answering communication questions, remember to use therapeutic techniques. Option 4 is the only option that addresses the client's feelings. Remember always focus on the client's feelings. Review therapeutic communication techniques if you had difficulty with this question.

Level of Cognitive Ability: Application
Client Needs: Psychosocial Integrity
Integrated Concept/Process: Communication and Documentation
Content Area: Fundamental Skills

Reference:
Potter, P., & Perry, A. (2001). *Fundamentals of nursing* (5th ed.). St. Louis: Mosby, p. 459.

123. A toddler with suspected conjunctivitis is crying and refuses to sit still during the eye examination. Which of the following is the most appropriate statement to the child?

Answer: 2
Rationale: Fears in this age group can be decreased by getting the child actively involved in the examination. Option 1 gives advice and ignores the child's feelings. Although option 3

1 "If you will sit still, the exam will be over soon."

2 "Would you like to see the flashlight?"

3 "I know you are upset. We can do this exam later."

4 "Don't be scared, the light won't hurt you."

acknowledges feelings, it puts off the inevitable. Option 4 tells the child how to feel.

Test-Taking Strategy: Use knowledge regarding the stages of growth and development to answer the question. Note that the child is a toddler. Using the child's developmental level and the techniques of therapeutic communication will direct you to option 2. Review growth and development in relation to the toddler if you had difficulty with this question.

Level of Cognitive Ability: Application
Client Needs: Psychosocial Integrity
Integrated Concept/Process: Communication and Documentation
Content Area: Child Health

Reference:
Wong, D., & Hockenberry-Eaton, M. (2001). *Wong's essentials of pediatric nursing* (6th ed.). St. Louis: Mosby, p. 128.

---

124. A client with acute pyelonephritis is scheduled for a voiding cystourethrogram. The client has had other diagnostic tests, and the nurse observed that the client is timid and shy. The nurse interprets that this client would most likely benefit from increased support and teaching about the procedure because:

1 Radiopaque contrast is injected into the bloodstream

2 Radioactive contrast is injected into the bladder

3 The client must lie on an x-ray table in a cold, barren room

4 The client must void while the micturition process is filmed

Answer: 4
Rationale: Having to void in the presence of others can be very embarrassing for clients and may actually interfere with the client's ability to void. The nurse teaches the client about the procedure to try to minimize stress from lack of preparation and gives the client encouragement and emotional support. Screens may be used in the radiology department to provide privacy during this procedure.

Test-Taking Strategy: Use the process of elimination. Begin to answer this question by eliminating options 1 and 2 because the contrast material is inserted into the bladder by means of a catheter. From the remaining options it is necessary to know that the client has to void to allow filming of the movement of urine through the lower urinary tract. Review this procedure if you had difficulty with this question.

Level of Cognitive Ability: Comprehension
Client Needs: Psychosocial Integrity
Integrated Concept/Process: Nursing Process/Planning
Content Area: Adult Health/Renal

Reference:
Ignatavicius, D., & Workman, M. (2002). *Medical-surgical nursing: critical thinking for collaborative care* (4th ed.). Philadelphia: W.B. Saunders, p. 1607.

---

125. A female client in a manic state emerges from her room. She is topless and is making sexual remarks and gestures toward staff and peers. The best initial nursing action is to:

1 Quietly approach the client, escort her to her room, and assist her in getting dressed

Answer: 1
Rationale: A person who is experiencing mania lacks insight and judgment, has poor impulse control, and is highly excitable. The nurse must take control without creating increased stress or anxiety to the client. A quiet, firm approach while distracting the client (walking her to her room and assisting her with dressing) achieves the goal of having her dressed appropriately and preserving her psychosocial integrity. Options 2, 3, and 4 are inappropriate actions.

2 Approach the client in the hallway and insist that she go to her room

3 Confront the client on the inappropriateness of her behavior and offer her a time-out

4 Ask the other clients to ignore her behavior; eventually she will return to her room

Test-Taking Strategy: Use the process of elimination. The goal of the interaction is to have the client dress appropriately. Therefore option 4 is eliminated. Insisting that the client go to her room may meet with a great deal of resistance. Confronting the client and offering her a consequence of "time-out" may be meaningless to her. Review care to the client with mania if you had difficulty with this question.

Level of Cognitive Ability: Application
Client Needs: Psychosocial Integrity
Integrated Concept/Process: Nursing Process/Implementation
Content Area: Mental Health

Reference:
Varcarolis, E. (2002). *Foundations of psychiatric mental health nursing* (4th ed.). Philadelphia: W.B. Saunders, p. 500.

---

126. Both the client, who had cardiac surgery, and the family express anxiety about how to cope with the recuperative process after the client is discharged and they are home alone. The nurse would plan to tell the client and family about which available resource?
1 Local library
2 United Way
3 American Heart Association Mended Heart's Club
4 American Cancer Society Reach for Recovery

Answer: 3
Rationale: Most clients and families benefit from knowing that there are available resources to help them cope with the stress of self-care management at home. These can include telephone contact with the surgeon, cardiologist, and nurse; cardiac rehabilitation programs; and community support groups such as the American Heart Association Mended Heart's Club (a nationwide program with local chapters).

Test-Taking Strategy: Use the process of elimination. Of the four options, three list organizations and one is a library. Eliminate the library first because the client and family need resources to cope, implying the need for interactive processes. Focusing on the type of surgery addressed in the question will easily direct you to option 3. Review the purpose of this support group if you had difficulty with this question.

Level of Cognitive Ability: Application
Client Needs: Psychosocial Integrity
Integrated Concept/Process: Nursing Process/Planning
Content Area: Adult Health/Cardiovascular

Reference:
Black, J., Hawks, J., & Keene, A. (2001). *Medical-surgical nursing: clinical management for positive outcomes* (6th ed.). Philadelphia: W.B. Saunders, p. 1733.

---

127. An older client who has never been hospitalized before is ordered to have a 12-lead electrocardiogram (ECG). The nurse would best plan to alleviate the client's anxiety by providing which of the following explanations?
1 "The ECG can give the doctor information about what might be wrong with your heart."
2 "It's important to lie still during the procedure."

Answer: 4
Rationale: The ECG involves the use of painless electrodes, which are applied to the chest and limbs. It takes less than 5 minutes to complete and requires that the client lie still. The ECG measures the heart's electrical activity to determine rate, rhythm, and a variety of abnormalities.

Test-Taking Strategy: Use the process of elimination. Option 3 is an incorrect statement and is eliminated first. Of those remaining, options 1 and 2 are factual statements, but they are not stated to reduce anxiety. Option 4 is the only statement that is reassuring

3 "It should only take about 20 minutes to complete the ECG tracings."
4 "The ECG electrodes are painless and will record the electrical activity of the heart."

to the client. Review this exam and the measures to relieve anxiety if you had difficulty with this question.

Level of Cognitive Ability: Application
Client Needs: Psychosocial Integrity
Integrated Concept/Process: Communication and Documentation
Content Area: Adult Health/Cardiovascular

Reference:
deWit, S. (2001). *Fundamental concepts and skills for nursing.* Philadelphia: W.B. Saunders, p. 427.

---

128. A client with superficial varicose veins says to the nurse, "I hate these things. They're so ugly; I wish I could get them to go away." The nurse's best response would be:
1 "You should try sclerotherapy. It's great."
2 "What have you been told about varicose veins and their management?"
3 "There's not much you can do once you get them."
4 "I understand how you feel, but you know, they really don't look too bad."

Answer: 2
Rationale: The client is expressing distress about the physical appearance and has a risk for body image disturbance. The nurse collects data regarding what the client has been told. Options 1, 3, and 4 are nontherapeutic responses.

Test-Taking Strategy: Use the nursing process and therapeutic communication techniques to answer the question. This will direct you to option 2. Remember data collection is the first step of the nursing process. Review therapeutic communication techniques if you had difficulty with this question.

Level of Cognitive Ability: Application
Client Needs: Psychosocial Integrity
Integrated Concept/Process: Communication and Documentation
Content Area: Adult Health/Cardiovascular

Reference:
Potter, P., & Perry, A. (2001). *Fundamentals of nursing* (5th ed.). St. Louis: Mosby, p. 459.

---

129. A client who has been diagnosed with chronic renal failure has been told that hemodialysis will be required. The client becomes angry and states, "I'll never be the same now." The nurse determines that the client is experiencing which problem?
1 Depression
2 Disturbance in body image
3 Anxiety
4 Fear

Answer: 2
Rationale: The client with renal failure may become angry because of the need for dialysis and the permanence of the alteration. Because of the physical change and the change in lifestyle that may be required to manage a severe renal condition, the client may experience body image disturbance. Although options 1, 3, and 4 may occur, these problems are not associated with the data in the question.

Test-Taking Strategy: Use the process of elimination. Focus on the key words "I'll never be the same now." Note that the client's statement focuses on self, which is consistent with a disturbance in body image. This will direct you to option 2. Review the characteristics associated with a body image disturbance if you had difficulty with this question.

Level of Cognitive Ability: Comprehension
Client Needs: Psychosocial Integrity
Integrated Concept/Process: Nursing Process/Data Collection
Content Area: Adult Health/Renal

Reference:
Black, J., Hawks, J., & Keene, A. (2001). *Medical-surgical nursing: clinical management for positive outcomes* (6th ed.). Philadelphia: W.B. Saunders, p. 875.

---

130. A nurse observes that a client who is recovering from a myocardial infarction is crying silently. What action by the nurse would best explore the client's feelings?

  1 Enter the room and stand quietly at the bedside

  2 Sit by the client and discuss the news of the day

  3 Sit quietly by the client

  4 Assure the client that the condition will improve

Answer: 3

Rationale: Sitting quietly by the client conveys caring and acceptance. Option 1 may not encourage the client to express feelings because the nurse does not take an active part in identifying the client's feelings. Options 2 and 4 do not address the client's feelings and ignore the client's behavior.

Test-Taking Strategy: Use therapeutic communication techniques. Options 2 and 4 can be easily eliminated because they ignore the client's feelings. From the remaining options, option 3 is the option that conveys caring and acceptance. Review therapeutic communication techniques if you had difficulty with this question.

Level of Cognitive Ability: Application
Client Needs: Psychosocial Integrity
Integrated Concept/Process: Caring
Content Area: Adult Health/Cardiovascular

Reference:
Potter, P., & Perry, A. (2001). *Fundamentals of nursing* (5th ed.). St. Louis: Mosby, p. 459.

---

131. A client with the diagnosis of hyperparathyroidism says to the nurse, "I can't stay on this diet. It is too difficult for me." When intervening in this situation, the nurse should respond:

  1 "It is very important that you stay on this diet to avoid forming renal calculi."

  2 "It really isn't difficult to stick to this diet. Just avoid milk products."

  3 "Why do you think you find this diet plan difficult to adhere to?"

  4 "You are having a difficult time staying on this plan. Let's discuss this."

Answer: 4

Rationale: By paraphrasing this client's statement, the nurse can encourage the client to express feelings. The nurse also sends feedback to the client that the message was understood. An open-ended statement or question such as this prompts an information response. Option 1 is giving advice, which blocks communication. Option 2 devalues the client's feelings. Option 3 is requesting information that the client may not be able to express.

Test-Taking Strategy: Use therapeutic communication techniques. Option 4 is the only option that addresses the client's feelings. Review these techniques if you had difficulty with this question.

Level of Cognitive Ability: Application
Client Needs: Psychosocial Integrity
Integrated Concept/Process: Communication and Documentation
Content Area: Adult Health/Endocrine

Reference:
Potter, P., & Perry, A. (2001). *Fundamentals of nursing* (5th ed.). St. Louis: Mosby, p. 459.

---

132. A nurse caring for a client with newly diagnosed diabetes mellitus is assisting in developing a teaching plan. The nurse suggests checking which of the following first?

Answer: 2

Rationale: When diabetes mellitus is diagnosed, the client will usually go through the phases of grief including denial, fear, anger, bargaining, depression, and acceptance. Denial is the phase

1 The client's knowledge of the diabetic diet
2 The presence of denial regarding having diabetes
3 Fear of performing insulin administration
4 Feeling depressed about lifestyle changes

that is the most detrimental to the teaching and learning process. If the client is denying the fact that he or she has diabetes mellitus, the client probably will not listen to discussions about the disease or how to manage it. Denial must be identified before the nurse can develop a teaching plan.

Test-Taking Strategy: Use the process of elimination. All of the options may be appropriate; however, note that options 1, 3, and 4 are related to very specific components of the teaching. Option 2 is the most global, and considering the principles of teaching and learning, this aspect needs to be determined before teaching. Review the teaching and learning principles if you had difficulty with this question.

Level of Cognitive Ability: Comprehension
Client Needs: Psychosocial Integrity
Integrated Concept/Process: Nursing Process/Data Collection
Content Area: Adult Health/Endocrine

Reference:
Potter, P., & Perry, A. (2001). *Fundamentals of nursing* (5th ed.). St. Louis: Mosby, p. 491.

---

133. A nurse is reinforcing teaching with a client taking conjugated estrogen (Premarin). The nurse plans to address which psychosocial issue related to the medication?
1 The client should notify the physician if migraine headaches occur
2 Estrogen may cause mood and affect changes, and the medication may need to be discontinued if depression occurs
3 Estrogen should be used with caution by individuals with a family history of breast or reproductive cancer
4 Premarin may cause hyperglycemia and the client should be informed about signs and symptoms to report to the physician

Answer: 2
Rationale: Conjugated estrogen can cause changes in client affect, mood, and behavior. Aggression, depression, or both can also occur. Options 1, 3, and 4 are correct but address physiological needs. Option 2 is the only psychosocial need noted.

Test-Taking Strategy: Use the process of elimination and note the key word *psychosocial*. Eliminate options 1, 3, and 4 because the options address physiological issues. Review the psychosocial effects of this medication if you had difficulty with this question.

Level of Cognitive Ability: Application
Client Needs: Psychosocial Integrity
Integrated Concept/Process: Nursing Process/Planning
Content Area: Pharmacology

Reference:
Hodgson, B., & Kizior, R. (2003). *Saunders nursing drug handbook 2003.* Philadelphia: W.B. Saunders, p. 278.

---

134. A client with newly diagnosed diabetes mellitus has been seen in the clinic for 3 consecutive days because of hyperglycemia. The client says to the nurse, "I'm sorry to keep bothering you every day, but I just can't give myself those awful shots." The nurse's best response is:
1 "You must learn to give yourself the shots."
2 "I couldn't give myself a shot either."

Answer: 3
Rationale: It is important to determine and deal with a client's underlying fear of self-injection. The nurse should determine whether a client needs additional instructions. Scare tactics (option 1) should not be used. Positive reinforcement is necessary instead of focusing on negative behaviors (option 2). The nurse should not offer a change in regimen that can't be accomplished (option 4).

Test-Taking Strategy: Use therapeutic communication techniques and focus on the issue of the question. Options 1 and 2 are not

3 "I'm sorry you are having trouble with your injections. Has someone given you instructions on them?"

4 "Let me see if the doctor can change your medication."

therapeutic, and option 4 may give false reassurance about a change in medications. Option 3 focuses on the issue and is the therapeutic response. Review therapeutic communication techniques if you had difficulty with this question.

Level of Cognitive Ability: Application
Client Needs: Psychosocial Integrity
Integrated Concept/Process: Communication and Documentation
Content Area: Adult Health/Endocrine

Reference:
Potter, P., & Perry, A. (2001). *Fundamentals of nursing* (5th ed.). St. Louis: Mosby, p. 459.

---

135. A nurse asks a client with diabetes mellitus to ask his/her significant other(s) to attend an educational conference on self-administration of insulin. The client questions why a significant other needs to be included. The nurse's best response would be:

1 "Clients and families often work together to develop strategies for the management of diabetes."

2 "Family members can take you to the doctor."

3 "Family members are at risk of developing diabetes."

4 "Nurses need someone to call and check on a client's progress."

Answer: 1
Rationale: Families or significant others may be included in diabetes education to assist with adjustment to the diabetic regimen. Although options 2 and 3 may be accurate, they are not the most appropriate response in relation to the issue of the question. Option 4 devalues the client, disregards the issue of independence, and promotes powerlessness.

Test-Taking Strategy: Use the process of elimination, knowledge about diabetes mellitus, and therapeutic communication techniques. Option 1 addresses a collaborative response and addresses the client. Review psychosocial issues related to teaching if you had difficulty with this question.

Level of Cognitive Ability: Application
Client Needs: Psychosocial Integrity
Integrated Concept/Process: Nursing Process/Implementation
Content Area: Adult Health/Endocrine

Reference:
Potter, P., & Perry, A. (2001). *Fundamentals of nursing* (5th ed.). St. Louis: Mosby, p. 460.

---

136. A 22-year-old female client has recently been diagnosed with polycystic kidney disease. The nurse plans a series of discussions with the client that are intended to help her adjust to the disorder. The nurse would include which of the following items as part of one of these discussions?

1 Ongoing fluid restriction

2 Depression about massive edema

3 Risk of hypotensive episodes

4 Need for genetic counseling

Answer: 4
Rationale: Adult polycystic kidney disease is a hereditary disorder that is inherited as an autosomal dominant trait. Because of this, the client should have genetic counseling, as should the extended family. The client is likely to have hypertension, not hypotension. Massive edema is not part of the clinical picture for this disorder. Ongoing fluid restriction is unnecessary.

Test-Taking Strategy: Use the process of elimination. Because massive edema and the need for fluid restriction are not part of the clinical picture for the client with polycystic kidney disease, options 1 and 2 are eliminated first. From the remaining options you would need to know either that this disorder is hereditary in nature or that the client would exhibit hypertension, not hypotension. Review this disorder if you had difficulty with this question.

Level of Cognitive Ability: Application
Client Needs: Psychosocial Integrity
Integrated Concept/Process: Nursing Process/Planning
Content Area: Adult Health/Renal

Reference:
Black, J., Hawks, J., & Keene, A. (2001). *Medical-surgical nursing: clinical management for positive outcomes* (6th ed.). Philadelphia: W.B. Saunders, p. 871.

---

137. A nurse is caring for a client who is to undergo ureterolithotomy for urinary calculi removal. The nurse would not include which of the following during data collection in determining the client's readiness for surgery?

1 Understanding of the surgical procedure

2 Knowledge of the postoperative activities

3 Feelings or anxieties about the surgical procedure

4 Need for a visit from a member of a support group

Answer: 4

Rationale: Ureterolithotomy is removal of a calculus from the ureter using either a flank or abdominal incision. Since there is no urinary diversion created during this procedure, the client has no need for a visit from a member of a support group. The client should have an understanding of the same items as for any surgery, which includes knowledge of the procedure, expected outcome, and postoperative routines and discomfort. Concerns or anxieties before surgery should also be addressed.

Test-Taking Strategy: Use the process of elimination and note the key word *not*. Eliminate options 1 and 3 first because this data should be determined in the preoperative period. Knowing that this procedure does not involve urinary diversion helps you to choose option 4 over option 2 as the correct option. The client does need to know about postoperative activities but does not need a visit from a support group. Review the psychosocial issues related to this procedure if you had difficulty with this question.

Level of Cognitive Ability: Application
Client Needs: Psychosocial Integrity
Integrated Concept/Process: Nursing Process/Data Collection
Content Area: Adult Health/Renal

Reference:
Black, J., Hawks, J., & Keene, A. (2001). *Medical-surgical nursing: clinical management for positive outcomes* (6th ed.). Philadelphia: W.B. Saunders, p. 828.

---

138. A dying client's spouse says to the nurse, "I don't think I can come anymore and watch her die. It's 'chewing me up' too much!" The most therapeutic response is:

1 "I wish you'd focus on your wife's pain rather than yours. I know it's hard but this isn't about what's happening to you, you know."

2 "I know it's hard for you, but she would know if you're not there, and you'd feel guilty all the rest of your days."

3 "It's hard to watch someone you love die. You've been here with your wife every day. Are you taking any time for yourself?"

Answer: 3

Rationale: The husband is the client of this question. The most therapeutic response is the one that reflects the nurse's understanding of the client's stress and emotional pain. Option 1 is an example of a nontherapeutic, judgmental attitude. Option 2 makes a statement that the nurse cannot know is true (the wife may, in fact, not know whether the husband visits) and predicting guilt feelings is not appropriate. Option 4 is inappropriate because it fosters dependency and gives advice, which is nontherapeutic.

Test-Taking Strategy: Use the process of elimination and therapeutic communication techniques. Option 3 is the only option that addresses the client's feelings. Review these techniques if you had difficulty with this question.

Level of Cognitive Ability: Application
Client Needs: Psychosocial Integrity

4 "I think you're making the right decision. Your wife knows you love her. You don't have to come. I'll take care of her."

Integrated Concept/Process: Caring
Content Area: Fundamental Skills

Reference:
Potter, P., & Perry, A. (2001). *Fundamentals of nursing* (5th ed.). St. Louis: Mosby, p. 459.

---

139. An older client at a retirement center spits her food out and throws it on the floor during a Thanksgiving dinner in the community dining room. The client yells, "This turkey is dry and cold! I can't stand the food here!" Which of the following is the most therapeutic response by the nurse?

1 "Let me get you another serving that is more to your liking. Would you like to come visit the chef and select your own serving?"

2 "I think you had better return to your apartment, where a new meal will be served to you there."

3 "Now look what you've done! You're ruining this meal for the whole community. Aren't you ashamed of yourself?"

4 "One of the things that the residents of this group agreed on was that anyone who did not use appropriate behavior would be asked to leave the dining room. Please leave now."

Answer: 1
Rationale: The most therapeutic response identifies that the client's behavior stems from some troubled feelings the client is struggling with. Option 2 could provoke a regressive struggle between the nurse and client and cause more explosive behavior on the client's part. Option 3 is an angry, aggressive, nontherapeutic response, and is humiliating to the client. In option 4, the nurse is authoritative, but trying to expel the client would not be appropriate, and it might set up an aggressive struggle between the nurse and the client. Asking the client to accompany the nurse to the kitchen respects the client's need for control, removes the angry client from the dining room, and may offer the nurse an opportunity to identify what is happening to the client.

Test-Taking Strategy: Use therapeutic communication technique. Option 1 is the only option that focuses on the client's feelings. Review these techniques if you had difficulty with this question.

Level of Cognitive Ability: Application
Client Needs: Psychosocial Integrity
Integrated Concept/Process: Communication and Documentation
Content Area: Fundamental Skills

Reference:
Potter, P., & Perry, A. (2001). *Fundamentals of nursing* (5th ed.). St. Louis: Mosby, p. 459.

---

140. An older adult client with emphysema is at a physician's office for a follow-up visit. When it is time for the client to see the physician, the nurse finds the client at the front door of the office complex and the client is smoking. Which of the following statements if made by the nurse would be most therapeutic?

1 "Well, I can see you never got to the Stop Smoking clinic!"

2 "I notice that you are smoking. Did you explore the Stop Smoking Program at the Senior Citizens' Center?"

3 "I wonder if you realize that you are slowly killing yourself? Why prolong the agony? You can just jump off the bridge!"

Answer: 2
Rationale: Option 2 places the decision making in the client's hands and provides an avenue for the client to share what may be expressions of frustration at an inability to stop what is essentially a physiological addiction. Option 1 is an intrusive use of sarcastic humor that demeans the client. Option 3 is preachy and judgmental, and is an example of a countertransference issue for the nurse. Option 4 is a disciplinary remark and places a barrier between the nurse and client within the therapeutic relationship.

Test-Taking Strategy: This question tests your knowledge of the therapeutic communication technique for the nurse to use for a client who is failing to make adaptive decisions about health. Use the process of elimination and therapeutic communication techniques to direct you to option 2. Review these techniques if you had difficulty with this question.

Level of Cognitive Ability: Application

4 "I'm glad I caught you smoking! Now that your secret is out, let's decide what you are going to do?"

Client Needs: Psychosocial Integrity
Integrated Concept/Process: Communication and Documentation
Content Area: Adult Health/Respiratory

Reference:
Potter, P., & Perry, A. (2001). *Fundamentals of nursing* (5th ed.). St. Louis: Mosby, p. 460.

---

141. A client is to have arterial blood gases drawn by the respiratory therapist. While the respiratory therapist is performing the Allen test, the client says to the nurse, "What is he doing? No one else has done that!" On the basis of the understanding of this test, the nurse's most therapeutic response is:

1 "This is a routine precautionary step that simply makes certain your circulation is intact before obtaining a blood sample."

2 "Oh? You have questions about this? You should insist that everyone does this procedure before drawing up your blood."

3 "I assure you that this is the correct procedure. I cannot account for what others do."

4 "This step is crucial to safe blood withdrawal. I would not let anyone take my blood until they did this."

Answer: 1
Rationale: The Allen test is performed to assess collateral circulation in the hand before drawing blood from an artery. The nurse's most therapeutic response gives information. Option 2 is aggressive and controlling as well as nontherapeutic in its disapproving stance. Option 3 is defensive and nontherapeutic in offering false reassurance. Option 4 demonstrates client advocacy that is overly controlling and quite aggressive and undermining of treatment.

Test-Taking Strategy: Use the process of elimination and therapeutic communication techniques. Option 1 is the only therapeutic response and provides information to the client. Review therapeutic communication techniques if you had difficulty with this question.

Level of Cognitive Ability: Application
Client Needs: Psychosocial Integrity
Integrated Concept/Process: Communication and Documentation
Content Area: Adult Health/Cardiovascular

Reference:
Potter, P., & Perry, A. (2001). *Fundamentals of nursing* (5th ed.). St. Louis: Mosby, p. 460.

---

142. A male client reports difficulty concentrating, outbursts of anger, constant "keyed up" feelings, and poor peer relations. The nurse obtaining data from the client discovers that the symptoms started approximately 6 months previously. The client reveals that his best friend was killed in a drive-by shooting while they were sitting on the porch talking. The nurse suspects the client is experiencing:

1 Obsessive-compulsive disorder
2 Panic disorder
3 Posttraumatic stress disorder
4 Social phobia

Answer: 3
Rationale: Posttraumatic stress disorder is a response to an event that would be markedly distressing to almost anyone. Characteristic symptoms include sustained level of anxiety, difficulty sleeping, irritability, difficulty concentrating, or outbursts of anger. Obsessive-compulsive disorder refers to some repetitive thought or behavior. Panic disorder and social phobia are characterized by specific fear of an object or situation.

Test-Taking Strategy: Use the process of elimination and knowledge about the disorders identified in the options. Options 2 and 4 have similar symptoms and are eliminated first. The information described in the question is not characteristic of an obsessive-compulsive disorder. Therefore eliminate option 1. Review these disorders if you had difficulty with this question.

Level of Cognitive Ability: Comprehension
Client Needs: Psychosocial Integrity
Integrated Concept/Process: Nursing Process/Data Collection
Content Area: Mental Health

Reference:
Varcarolis, E. (2002). *Foundations of psychiatric mental health nursing* (4th ed.). Philadelphia: W.B. Saunders, p. 317.

143. A client who is reported by the staff to be very demanding says to the nurse, "I can't get any help with my care! I call and call but the nurses never answer my light. Last night one of them told me she had 'other patients besides me'! I'm very sick, but the nurses don't care!" Which of the following would be the most therapeutic response by the nurse?

1   "I think you are being very impatient. The nurses work very hard and come as quickly as they can."

2   "I can hear your anger. That nurse had no right to speak to you that way. I will report her to the Director. It won't happen again."

3   "It's hard to be in bed and have to ask for help. You call for a nurse who never seems to come."

4   "You poor thing! I'm so sorry this happened to you. That nurse should be reported!"

Answer: 3

Rationale: In option 3, the nurse displays empathy as she shares perceptions. Sharing perceptions asks the client to validate the nurse's understanding of what the client is feeling and thinking. It opens the door for the client to share concerns, fears, and anxieties. In option 1, the nurse is assertive and certainly defends the nursing staff. In option 2, the nurse expresses the client's frustration by labeling the client's feelings as "angry" and disapproving of the nursing staff. Option 4 is sympathetic and inappropriate regarding the negative comment about another nurse.

Test-Taking Strategy: Use therapeutic communication techniques and the process of elimination. Option 3 is the only option that encourages the client to express feelings. Review these therapeutic communication techniques if you had difficulty with this question.

Level of Cognitive Ability: Application
Client Needs: Psychosocial Integrity
Integrated Concept/Process: Communication and Documentation
Content Area: Fundamental Skills

Reference:
Potter, P., & Perry, A. (2001). *Fundamentals of nursing* (5th ed.). St. Louis: Mosby, p. 460.

---

144. A nurse is caring for a hospitalized client with an alcohol abuse disorder. In reviewing the client's discharge outcomes, the most positive outcome is that the client states that he or she will:

1   Continue to attend Alcoholics Anonymous (AA) meetings

2   Take a biofeedback class

3   Start an exercise program

4   Learn to play golf

Answer: 1

Rationale: All of the outcomes deserve support by the nurse, but option 1 will help the client abstain from alcohol and provide the client with a support group. Option 1 is the most positive outcome.

Test-Taking Strategy: Use the process of elimination and focus on the issue of the question, the most positive outcome. From the options presented, option 1 addresses the client's disorder. AA has the greatest potential to provide impulse control. Review care to the client with an alcohol abuse disorder if you had difficulty with this question.

Level of Cognitive Ability: Analysis
Client Needs: Psychosocial Integrity
Integrated Concept/Process: Nursing Process/Evaluation
Content Area: Mental Health

Reference:
Varcarolis, E. (2002). *Foundations of psychiatric mental health nursing* (4th ed.). Philadelphia: W.B. Saunders, p. 772.

---

145. An English-speaking Hispanic male has a long leg cast applied because of a right proximal fractured tibia. During rounds that night, the nurse finds the client restless, withdrawn, and quiet. Which of the following initial nurse statements would be most appropriate?

Answer: 2

Rationale: Option 2 is an open-ended statement and makes no assumptions about the client's physiological or emotional state. Option 1 is incorrect because the Hispanic male may deny feeling any pain when asked. Data collection is necessary before intervention so option 3 would be incorrect. False reassurance is never therapeutic, which makes option 4 incorrect.

1   "Are you uncomfortable?"
2   "Tell me what you are feeling?"
3   "I'll get your pain medication right away."
4   "You'll feel better in the morning."

Test-Taking Strategy: Use the process of elimination. The word *initial* in the stem of the question tells you that data collection and prioritization with a therapeutic communication technique is needed. Remember to focus on the client's feelings. Review these techniques if you had difficulty with this question.

Level of Cognitive Ability: Application
Client Needs: Psychosocial Integrity
Integrated Concept/Process: Communication and Documentation
Content Area: Adult Health/Musculoskeletal

Reference:
Potter, P., & Perry, A. (2001). *Fundamentals of nursing* (5th ed.). St. Louis: Mosby, pp. 127; 459.

---

146. A client was started on oral anticoagulant therapy while hospitalized. The client is now being discharged and going home and is intermittently confused. The nurse would evaluate that the client has the best support system for successful anticoagulant therapy monitoring if the client:
1   Has a good friend living next door who would take the client to the doctor
2   Has a home health aide coming to the house for 9 weeks
3   Lives with a daughter and son-in-law
4   Would have blood work drawn in the home by a local laboratory

Answer: 3
Rationale: Successful anticoagulant therapy has three components: taking the medication properly, having proper follow-up medical care, and doing serial follow-up blood work. Option 1 facilitates only medical care, option 2 facilitates only reminding the client to take the medication, and option 4 facilitates only blood work. The client who is intermittently confused may need support systems in place to enhance compliance with therapy. Option 3 addresses the best support system.

Test-Taking Strategy: Use the process of elimination and note that the client is intermittently confused. Focusing on the issue, the best support system, will direct you to option 3. Review appropriate support systems if you had difficulty with this question.

Level of Cognitive Ability: Analysis
Client Needs: Psychosocial Integrity
Integrated Concept/Process: Nursing Process/Evaluation
Content Area: Adult Health/Cardiovascular

Reference:
Potter, P., & Perry, A. (2001). *Fundamentals of nursing* (5th ed.). St. Louis: Mosby, p. 905.

---

147. A client who has undergone successful femoral-popliteal bypass grafting to the leg says to the nurse, "I hope everything goes well after this, and I don't lose my leg. I'm so afraid that I'll have gone through this for nothing." The nurse's best response is:
1   "I can understand what you mean. I'd be nervous too, if I were in your shoes."
2   "Stress isn't helpful for you. You should probably just relax and try

Answer: 3
Rationale: Clients frequently fear that they will ultimately lose a limb or become debilitated in some other way. The nurse reassures the client that participation in exercise, diet, and medication therapy, along with smoking cessation, can limit further plaque development. Option 1 feeds into the client's anxiety and is not therapeutic. Option 4 gives false reassurance, which is incorrect. Option 2 is meant to be reassuring, but offers no suggestions to empower the client.

Test-Taking Strategy: Use the process of elimination and therapeutic communication techniques. Option 3 acknowledges the

not to worry unless something actually happens."

3 "Complications are possible, but you have a good deal of control if you make the lifestyle adjustments we talked about."

4 "This surgery is so successful, that I wouldn't be concerned at all if I were you."

client's concerns and empowers the client to improve health, which will ultimately reduce concern about the risk of complications. Review therapeutic communication techniques if you had difficulty with this question.

Level of Cognitive Ability: Application
Client Needs: Psychosocial Integrity
Integrated Concept/Process: Communication and Documentation
Content Area: Adult Health/Cardiovascular

Reference:
Potter, P., & Perry, A. (2001). *Fundamentals of nursing* (5th ed.). St. Louis: Mosby, p. 460.

---

148. A client is scheduled to undergo pericardiocentesis for pericardial effusion. The nurse would best plan to alleviate the client's apprehension by:

1 Staying beside the client and giving information and encouragement during the procedure

2 Talking to the client from the foot of the bed to be available to get added supplies

3 Telling the client that the nurse will take care of another assigned client during the procedure so as to be available once the procedure is complete

4 Telling the client to watch television during the procedure as a distraction

Answer: 1
Rationale: Staying with the client and giving information and encouragement is most supportive to the client. Options 3 and 4 distance the nurse from a client in the psychosocial as well as a physical sense. The nurse should ask another caregiver to be available to get extra supplies if needed.

Test-Taking Strategy: Use the process of elimination and therapeutic techniques. Remember to provide support to the client and to always address the client's feelings and concerns. This will direct you to option 1. Review measures to provide client support if you had difficulty with this question.

Level of Cognitive Ability: Application
Client Needs: Psychosocial Integrity
Integrated Concept/Process: Nursing Process/Implementation
Content Area: Adult Health/Cardiovascular

Reference:
Potter, P., & Perry, A. (2001). *Fundamentals of nursing* (5th ed.). St. Louis: Mosby, p. 460.

---

149. A nurse reviews the nursing care plan for a male client taking spironolactone (Aldactone). The nurse notes that a nursing diagnosis of Body Image Disturbance is documented on the plan of care. The nurse understands that this has been documented based on which of the following side effects of the medication?

1 Edema and hirsutism
2 Weight gain and hair loss
3 Alopecia and muscle atrophy
4 Decreased libido and gynecomastia

Answer: 4
Rationale: The nurse should be alert to the fact that the client taking spironolactone may experience body image changes as a result of threatened sexual identity. These are related to decreased libido, gynecomastia in males, and hirsutism in females.

Test-Taking Strategy: Knowledge regarding the side effects associated with this medication will direct you to option 4. Review the side effects of this medication if you had difficulty with this question.

Level of Cognitive Ability: Comprehension
Client Needs: Psychosocial Integrity
Integrated Concept/Process: Nursing Process/Planning
Content Area: Pharmacology

Reference:
Hodgson, B., & Kizior, R. (2003). *Saunders nursing drug handbook 2003.* Philadelphia: W.B. Saunders, p. 1028.

150. Which of the following statements would be most appropriate for the nurse to make when talking with a hospitalized client who is recovering from the signs and symptoms of autonomic dysreflexia?
1 "I'm sure you now understand the importance of preventing this from occurring."
2 "Now that this problem is taken care of, I'm sure you'll be fine."
3 "How could your home care nurse let this happen?"
4 "I have some time if you would like to talk about what happened to you."

Answer: 4
Rationale: Offering time to the client encourages the client to discuss feelings. Options 1, 2, and 3 are blocks to communication. Options 1 and 3 show disapproval, and option 2 gives false reassurance.

Test-Taking Strategy: Use the process of elimination and select the option that is therapeutic. Always address the client's concerns and feelings first. Review therapeutic communication techniques if you had difficulty with this question.

Level of Cognitive Ability: Application
Client Needs: Psychosocial Integrity
Integrated Concept/Process: Communication and Documentation
Content Area: Adult Health/Neurological

Reference:
Potter, P., & Perry, A. (2001). *Fundamentals of nursing* (5th ed.). St. Louis: Mosby, p. 459.

---

151. A nurse is assisting a client with a spinal cord injury with activities of daily living. The client states, "I can't do this; I wish I were dead." The nurse's best response would be which of the following?
1 "Let's wash your back now."
2 "You wish you were dead?"
3 "I'm sure you are frustrated, but things will work out just fine for you."
4 "Why do you say that?"

Answer: 2
Rationale: Clarifying is a therapeutic technique involving restating what was said to obtain additional information. Option 1 changes the subject. Option 3 provides false reassurance. By asking why, in option 4, the nurse puts the client on the defensive. Options 1, 3, and 4 are nontherapeutic and block communication.

Test-Taking Strategy: Use therapeutic communication techniques. Option 2 identifies clarifying and restating and is the only option that will encourage the client to verbalize feelings and concerns. Review these techniques if you had difficulty with this question.

Level of Cognitive Ability: Application
Client Needs: Psychosocial Integrity
Integrated Concept/Process: Communication and Documentation
Content Area: Adult Health/Neurological

Reference:
Potter, P., & Perry, A. (2001). *Fundamentals of nursing* (5th ed.). St. Louis: Mosby, p. 460.

---

152. A 30-year-old client says to the nurse, "I want to die; I think about it sometimes, but I don't know how in the world to do it. My mother gave me this ring; I love it so; I think I'll give it to my grandchildren." Based on the client's statement, the nurse determines that:
1 There is no suicide risk noted
2 There is minimal suicide risk
3 Suicide has been attempted unsuccessfully

Answer: 4
Rationale: The words *I want to die* indicate a suicide risk. Any self-harm language must be viewed as serious. This situation gives no data related to self-harm history. Options 1, 2, and 3 are inaccurate interpretations.

Test-Taking Strategy: Use the process of elimination. Focusing on the statement made by the client will direct you to option 4. Review suicide assessment if you had difficulty with this question.

Level of Cognitive Ability: Analysis

4 The risk for suicide exists; continued data collection is needed

Client Needs: Psychosocial Integrity
Integrated Concept/Process: Nursing Process/Data Collection
Content Area: Mental Health

Reference:
Varcarolis, E. (2002). *Foundations of psychiatric mental health nursing* (4th ed.). Philadelphia: W.B. Saunders, p. 641.

---

153. Family members awaiting the outcome of a suicide attempt are tearful. Which response by the nurse would be most therapeutic to the family at this time?
1 "Don't worry, you have nothing to feel guilty about."
2 "Everything possible is being done."
3 "Let me check to see how long it will be before you can see your loved one."
4 "I can see you are worried."

Answer: 4
Rationale: Options 1, 2, and 3 are communication blocks. Option 1 labels the family's behavior without their validation. Option 2 uses clichés and false reassurance. Option 3 focuses on an important issue at an inappropriate time (family members are tearful). Option 4 uses the therapeutic technique of clarifying.

Test-Taking Strategy: Use therapeutic communication techniques. Option 4 identifies clarifying and is the only option that will encourage the family to verbalize feelings and concerns. Review these techniques if you had difficulty with this question.

Level of Cognitive Ability: Application
Client Needs: Psychosocial Integrity
Integrated Concept/Process: Communication and Documentation
Content Area: Mental Health

Reference:
Varcarolis, E. (2002). *Foundations of psychiatric mental health nursing* (4th ed.). Philadelphia: W.B. Saunders, p. 255.

---

154. Which of the following is important to include in caring for an 11-year-old child who has been abused?
1 Encourage the child to fear the abuser
2 Provide a care environment that allows for the development of trust
3 Teach the child to make wise choices when confronted with an abusive situation
4 Have the child point out the abuser if that person should visit while the child is hospitalized

Answer: 2
Rationale: The abused child usually requires long-term therapeutic support. The environment during the child's healing must include one in which trust and caring is provided for the child. Options 3 and 4 ask the child to behave with a maturity beyond that which would be expected for an 11-year-old. Option 1 reinforces fear.

Test-Taking Strategy: Use the process of elimination and the components of a therapeutic nurse-client relationship. Option 2 is the option that is most appropriate because it provides the child with a nurturing and supportive environment in which to begin the healing process. Review the psychosocial issues related to an abused child if you had difficulty with this question.

Level of Cognitive Ability: Application
Client Needs: Psychosocial Integrity
Integrated Concept/Process: Caring
Content Area: Child Health

Reference:
Varcarolis, E. (2002). *Foundations of psychiatric mental health nursing* (4th ed.). Philadelphia: W.B. Saunders, p. 692.

155. A nurse collects data from an older client and monitors for signs of potential abuse. The nurse understands that which of the following psychosocial factors place the client at risk for abuse?
1   The client is completely dependent upon family members for receiving food and medicine
2   The client shows signs and symptoms of depression
3   The client resides in a low-income neighborhood
4   The client has a chronic illness

Answer: 1
Rationale: Elder abuse is sometimes the result of frustration of adult children who find themselves caring for dependent parents. Increasing demands by parents for care and financial support can cause resentment and may be burdensome. Signs and symptoms of depression do not specifically indicate abuse. Issues of abuse are not bound to socioeconomic status. Option 4 is a physiological condition.

Test-Taking Strategy: Use the process of elimination and focus on the words *psychosocial factors*. Noting the key word *dependent* in option 1 will direct you to this option. If you had difficulty with this question, review the risk factors associated with elder abuse.

Level of Cognitive Ability: Comprehension
Client Needs: Psychosocial Integrity
Integrated Concept/Process: Nursing Process/Data Collection
Content Area: Mental Health

Reference:
Varcarolis, E. (2002). *Foundations of psychiatric mental health nursing* (4th ed.). Philadelphia: W.B. Saunders, p. 709.

---

156. The nurse is caring for a dying client who says, "What would you say if I asked you to be the executor for my will?" Which of the following nursing responses would be the most therapeutic?
1   "Why, I'd be honored to be the executor of your will."
2   "Is there any money in it? I adore money, but I am honest."
3   "Your confidence in me is an honor, but I would like to understand more about your thinking."
4   "I'd say, 'Great!' Don't worry. I'll carry out your will just as you want me to."

Answer: 3
Rationale: In option 3, the nurse uses the therapeutic communication of seeking clarification. In option 1, the nurse responds with a social communication with no assessment of the consequences, which demonstrates a lack of critical thinking and exploration of motivation or client needs. In option 2, the nurse uses histrionic language and crass ideation. In option 4, the nurse provides false reassurance, which is nontherapeutic.

Test-Taking Strategy: Use therapeutic communication techniques. Option 3 is the only option that is therapeutic and seeks to clarify the client's request. Review these techniques if you had difficulty with this question.

Level of Cognitive Ability: Application
Client Needs: Psychosocial Integrity
Integrated Concept/Process: Communication and Documentation
Content Area: Fundamental Skills

Reference:
Potter, P., & Perry, A. (2001). *Fundamentals of nursing* (5th ed.). St. Louis: Mosby, p. 459.

---

157. A client who is suffering from urticaria (hives) and pruritus, says to the nurse, "What am I going to do? I'm getting married next week and I'll probably be covered in this rash and itching like crazy." Which of the following is the most therapeutic response by the nurse?
1   "You're very troubled that this will extend into your wedding?"

Answer: 1
Rationale: The therapeutic communication technique that the nurse uses is reflection. In option 2, the nurse minimizes the client's anxiety and fears. In option 3, the nurse talks about antihistamines and asks the client to "wait and see." This is nontherapeutic because the nurse is making promises that may not be kept and because the response is close-ended and shuts of the client's expression of feelings. In option 4, the nurse uses humor inappropriately and with insensitivity.

2   "It's probably just due to prewedding jitters."

3   "The antihistamine will help a great deal, just you wait and see. "

4   "I hope your husband-to-be has a sense of humor."

Test-Taking Strategy: Use therapeutic communication techniques. Option 1 is the only option that encourages the client to express feelings. Review these techniques if you had difficulty with this question.

Level of Cognitive Ability: Application
Client Needs: Psychosocial Integrity
Integrated Concept/Process: Communication and Documentation
Content Area: Adult Health/Integumentary

Reference:
Potter, P., & Perry, A. (2001). *Fundamentals of nursing* (5th ed.). St. Louis: Mosby, p. 460.

---

158. A client with a spinal cord injury makes the following comments. Which comment warrants additional intervention by the nurse?

1   "I'm so angry this happened to me."

2   "I know I will have to make major adjustments in my life."

3   "I would like my family members to be here for my teaching sessions."

4   "I'm really looking forward to going home."

Answer: 1
Rationale: It is important to allow a spinal cord injury client to verbalize feelings. If the client indicates a desire to discuss feelings, the nurse should respond therapeutically. Options 2 and 3 indicate that the client understands changes will be occurring and that family involvement is best. Option 4 does not require further intervention.

Test-Taking Strategy: Use the process of elimination and note the key words *warrants additional intervention*. Options 2, 3, and 4 are similar in that the client expresses positive acceptance of the injury. In option 1, the client expresses a feeling warranting a need. Review psychosocial concerns related to a spinal cord injury if you had difficulty with this question.

Level of Cognitive Ability: Analysis
Client Needs: Psychosocial Integrity
Integrated Concept/Process: Nursing Process/Evaluation
Content Area: Adult Health/Neurological

Reference:
Black, J., Hawks, J., & Keene, A. (2001). *Medical-surgical nursing: clinical management for positive outcomes* (6th ed.). Philadelphia: W.B. Saunders, p. 2060.

---

159. A nurse is caring for a client with a grade II cerebral aneurysm rupture. The client becomes restless and anxious before visiting hours. The nurse determines that the client's behavior is likely related to:

1   The severity of the aneurysm rupture

2   Ineffective family coping

3   Body image disturbance

4   Spiritual distress

Answer: 3
Rationale: A grade II cerebral aneurysm rupture is a mild hemorrhage in which the client remains alert but has nuchal rigidity with possible neurological deficits, depending on the area of the hemorrhage. Because these clients remain alert, they are acutely aware of the neurological deficits and frequently have some degree of body image disturbance. Options 1, 2, and 4 do not relate to the data in the question.

Test-Taking Strategy: Use the process of elimination and knowledge of the effects of a grade II cerebral aneurysm rupture. Noting the key words *before visiting hours* will direct you to option 3. Review the effects of this disorder if you had difficulty with this question.

Level of Cognitive Ability: Analysis
Client Needs: Psychosocial Integrity
Integrated Concept/Process: Nursing Process/Data Collection
Content Area: Adult Health/Neurological

Reference:
Black, J., Hawks, J., & Keene, A. (2001). *Medical-surgical nursing: clinical management for positive outcomes* (6th ed.). Philadelphia: W.B. Saunders, p. 1942.

160. In planning care for a client with thromboangiitis obliterans (Buerger's disease), the nurse would incorporate measures to help the client cope with lifestyle changes needed to control the disease process. The nurse can best accomplish this by recommending a:

1 Smoking cessation program
2 Pain management clinic
3 Consult with a dietitian
4 Referral to a medical social worker

Answer: 1

Rationale: Smoking is highly detrimental to the client with Buerger's disease, and clients are recommended to stop completely. Because smoking is a form of chemical dependency, referral to a smoking cessation program may be helpful for many clients. For many clients, symptoms are relieved or alleviated once smoking stops. Options 2, 3, and 4 are not specifically related to this disorder.

Test-Taking Strategy: Use the process of elimination. Recalling that treatment goals for this disorder are the same as for peripheral vascular disease will direct you to option 1. Review this disorder if you had difficulty with this question.

Level of Cognitive Ability: Comprehension
Client Needs: Psychosocial Integrity
Integrated Concept/Process: Nursing Process/Implementation
Content Area: Adult Health/Cardiovascular

Reference:
Black, J., Hawks, J., & Keene, A. (2001). *Medical-surgical nursing: clinical management for positive outcomes* (6th ed.). Philadelphia: W.B. Saunders, p. 1422.

161. An examination of a 14-year-old child reveals bruises and bleeding in the genital area, cigarette burns on the chest, rope burns on the buttocks, and multiple old fractures. The child says, "I'm afraid to go home! My stepfather will be angry with me for telling on him!" The nurse's most therapeutic response is:

1 "I am sorry that this has happened to you but you will be safe here. Your physician has admitted you until further plans can be made."
2 "You can't go back there with that man. How do you think your mother will react?"
3 "You must know that your presence in the house will only tease your stepfather more."
4 "Let's keep this between you, me, and the physician until we can formulate further plans to assist you."

Answer: 1

Rationale: A child who is found to be physically and sexually assaulted should be admitted to the hospital. This will provide time for a more comprehensive evaluation while simultaneously protecting the child from further abuse. In option 2, the nurse does not respond with a calm and reassuring communication style, nor does the nurse maintain a professional attitude. Option 3 accuses the victim of 'teasing' the step-father and is incorrect. It is also judgmental, controlling, and demeaning. The nurse's suggestion in option 4 is not only inappropriate, but the statement is also collusive and passive in its stance.

Test-Taking Strategy: Use the process of elimination. Recalling that the priority issue is to protect the victim from the abuser will direct you to option 1. Review care to the abused child if you had difficulty with this question.

Level of Cognitive Ability: Application
Client Needs: Psychosocial Integrity
Integrated Concept/Process: Communication and Documentation
Content Area: Child Health

Reference:
Varcarolis, E. (2002). *Foundations of psychiatric mental health nursing* (4th ed.). Philadelphia: W.B. Saunders, p. 703.

162. A nurse is caring for a 15-year-old female client admitted to the hospital with a diagnosis of physical and sexual abuse by her father. That evening, the father angrily approaches the nurse and says, "I'm taking my daughter home. She's told me what you people are up to, and 'we're out of here'!" Which of the following would be the most therapeutic response by the nurse?

1 "Over my dead body you will! She's here and here she stays until the doctor says different, so get off my floor or I'll call hospital security and the police!"

2 "Listen to me. If you attempt to take your daughter from this unit, the police will only bring her back."

3 "Your daughter is ill and needs to be here. I know you want to help her to recover and that you will work to help everyone straighten out the circumstances that caused this. Go to the chapel and pray for your daughter and for your soul."

4 "You seem very upset. Let's talk at the nurse's station. I want to help you. I know you're very concerned and want to help your daughter. It will be best if you agree to let your daughter stay here for now."

Answer: 4

Rationale: When a child suspected of being abused is admitted to the hospital for further evaluation and protection, the physician usually attempts to get the parents to agree to the admission. If the parents refuse to agree to the admission, the hospital can request an immediate court order to retain the child for a specific length of time. In option 1, the nurse is angry and verbally abusive. It is clear that the nurse has decided that the father is guilty of child abuse. In addition, the nurse is so aggressive and challenging that she may antagonize the father and become a victim of violence as well. In option 2, the command to listen is somewhat demanding. Option 3 is pompous and lecturing.

Test-Taking Strategy: Use therapeutic communication techniques and focus on the client of the question, the father. Option 4 is the only option that addresses the father's behavior. Review these techniques if you had difficulty with this question.

Level of Cognitive Ability: Application
Client Needs: Psychosocial Integrity
Integrated Concept/Process: Communication and Documentation
Content Area: Child Health

Reference:
Varcarolis, E. (2002). *Foundations of psychiatric mental health nursing* (4th ed.). Philadelphia: W.B. Saunders, p. 709.

---

163. A client with peripheral arterial disease is being discharged from the hospital and going home. The client is occasionally forgetful about medication, exercise, and diet instructions; needs daily dressing changes to a small open area on the leg; has limited endurance for activities of daily living (ADLs); and lives alone in a one-story house. To best assist the client to adapt to self-care and disease management, the nurse suggests which follow-up service to be provided in the home?

1 Nursing, home health aide, physical therapy

2 Nursing, home health aide, speech therapy

3 Home health aide, physical therapy, and occupational therapy

4 Nursing, physical therapy, and occupational therapy

Answer: 1

Rationale: Home health care agencies provide a variety of services to clients, depending on individual need. The multidisciplinary team includes nurse, home health aides, social workers, and physical, occupational, and speech therapists. Nurses provide skilled nursing services. Home health aides can assist clients with ADLs, and physical therapists assist in rehabilitation and increasing musculoskeletal endurance. The occupational therapist would train clients to adapt to physical handicaps through new vocational skills and adaptive techniques for ADLs.

Test-Taking Strategy: Use the process of elimination. The question tells you that the client needs daily dressing changes (with which a nurse can help), is forgetful about the exercise program and has limited endurance (with which a physical therapist can help), and needs assistance with ADLs (which can be provided by a home health aide). Review the roles of each of these health care workers if you had difficulty with this question.

Level of Cognitive Ability: Application
Client Needs: Psychosocial Integrity

Integrated Concept/Process: Nursing Process/Implementation
Content Area: Fundamental Skills

Reference:
Potter, P., & Perry, A. (2001). *Fundamentals of nursing* (5th ed.). St. Louis: Mosby, p. 389.

---

164. A client with chronic arterial leg ulcers over the course of a year complains of pain and tells the nurse, "I'm so discouraged. The pain never seems to go away. I can't do anything, and I feel as though I'll never get better." The nurse determines that the client is experiencing which of the following problems?
1   Acute pain
2   Chronic pain
3   Fatigue
4   Ineffective coping

Answer: 2
Rationale: The major focus of the client's complaint is the experience of pain. Pain that has a duration of longer than 6 months is defined as chronic pain, not acute pain. Fatigue is a sense of exhaustion and decreased capacity for physical and mental work. Ineffective coping is impairment of adaptive behaviors and abilities of a person in meeting life's demands and roles.

Test-Taking Strategy: The focus of the question is on the client's pain. Expressions of discouragement by the client do not automatically indicate poor coping skills, which eliminates option 4. The question makes no mention of fatigue as the primary problem, so eliminate option 3. The question states that the ulcer has been an ongoing problem over the course of a year, which is the critical piece of data needed to discriminate chronic pain, not acute pain as the answer. Review the characteristics of chronic pain if you had difficulty with this question.

Level of Cognitive Ability: Comprehension
Client Needs: Psychosocial Integrity
Integrated Concept/Process: Nursing Process/Data Collection
Content Area: Adult Health/Cardiovascular

Reference:
Black, J., Hawks, J., & Keene, A. (2001). *Medical-surgical nursing: clinical management for positive outcomes* (6th ed.). Philadelphia: W.B. Saunders, p. 465.

---

165. A client with valvular heart disease is being considered for mechanical valve replacement. Which of the following items does the nurse know is essential to determine before the surgery is done?
1   The likelihood of the client experiencing body image problems
2   The ability to participate in a cardiac rehabilitation program
3   The physical demands of the client's lifestyle
4   The ability to comply with anticoagulant therapy for life

Answer: 4
Rationale: Mechanical valves carry the associated risk of thromboemboli, which necessitates long-term anticoagulation with warfarin (Coumadin). Option 1 is important but not essential. Not all clients who undergo valve replacement need cardiac rehabilitation, so option 2 can be eliminated. Knowing that mechanical valves are thrombogenic, select the option related to anticoagulant therapy.

Test-Taking Strategy: Use the process of elimination. The word *essential* guides you to look for a critical item. Focusing on the procedure being considered will direct you to option 4. Review care to the client after valve replacement if you had difficulty with this question.

Level of Cognitive Ability: Analysis
Client Needs: Psychosocial Integrity
Integrated Concept/Process: Nursing Process/Planning
Content Area: Adult Health/Cardiovascular

Reference:
Black, J., Hawks, J., & Keene, A. (2001). *Medical-surgical nursing: clinical management for positive outcomes* (6th ed.). Philadelphia: W.B. Saunders, p. 1502.

166. A client who has a history of depression has been prescribed nadolol (Corgard) in the management of angina pectoris. Which of the following items is a priority when the nurse plans to reinforce teaching with the client about the effects of nadolol?

1 High incidence of hyperglycemia
2 Possible exacerbation of depression
3 Risk of tachycardia
4 Probability of fatigue

Answer: 2
Rationale: Clients with depression or a history of depression have experienced an exacerbation of depression after beginning therapy with beta-adrenergic blocking agents. These clients should be monitored carefully if these agents are prescribed. Option 3 is incorrect because the medication would cause bradycardia, not tachycardia. Fatigue is a possible side effect, but is not a "priority" item. Beta-blockers can mask tachycardia, an early sign of hypoglycemia.

Test-Taking Strategy: Use the process of elimination. This question guides your response because it tells you the client has a history of depression. This will direct you to option 2. Review this medication if you had difficulty with this question.

Level of Cognitive Ability: Comprehension
Client Needs: Psychosocial Integrity
Integrated Concept/Process: Nursing Process/Planning
Content Area: Pharmacology

Reference:
Lehne, R. (2001). *Pharmacology for nursing care* (4th ed.). Philadelphia: W.B. Saunders, pp. 167-168.

---

167. A nurse is caring for a client with terminal cancer of the throat. The family approaches the nurse and tells that nurse that they have spoken to the physician regarding taking their loved one home. Which of the following services would be most supportive to the client and family at home?

1 American Cancer Society
2 American Lung Association
3 Hospice care
4 Local religious and social organizations

Answer: 3
Rationale: Hospice provides an environment that emphasizes caring rather than curing. The emphasis is on palliative care. One of the major goals of hospice care is for the client be free of pain and other symptoms that do not allow the client to maintain quality of life. An interdisciplinary approach is used. Options 1, 2, and 4 may provide services to the client but hospice care is most supportive.

Test-Taking Strategy: Use the process of elimination. Think about what each support service presented in the options will provide in meeting this client's needs. This will assist in directing you to option 3. Review these support services if you had difficulty with this question.

Level of Cognitive Ability: Comprehension
Client Needs: Psychosocial Integrity
Integrated Concept/Process: Nursing Process/Planning
Content Area: Adult Health/Oncology

Reference:
deWit, S. (2001). *Fundamental concepts and skills for nursing.* Philadelphia: W.B. Saunders, p. 189.

---

168. A licensed practical nurse (LPN) is planning to accompany a community health nurse who is visiting a shelter for the homeless to provide health services and education. The LPN assists in planning the visit knowing that which of the following health problems is least

Answer: 4
Rationale: Mental disorders, respiratory and cardiovascular diseases, and parasitic infestations are some of the most common health problems experienced by the homeless population.

Test-Taking Strategy: Use the process of elimination and note the key words *least likely.* Try to think about the environmental

likely experienced by the homeless population?
1   Mental disorders
2   Tuberculosis
3   Parasitic infestations
4   Renal calculi

conditions that the homeless individual is exposed to in answering this question. Options 2 and 3 can be eliminated in view of the crowded living conditions that exists and the close physical contact and sharing that occurs with the homeless in shelters. From the remaining options, select option 4 instead of option 1 because of the multiple social problems that occur in the homeless. Review the most common health problems associated with the homeless population if you had difficulty with this question.

Level of Cognitive Ability: Comprehension
Client Needs: Psychosocial Integrity
Integrated Concept/Process: Nursing Process/Planning
Content Area: Fundamental Skills

Reference:
Stone, S., McGuire, S., & Eigsti, D. (2002). *Comprehensive Community Health nursing* (6th ed.). St. Louis: Mosby, p. 411.

---

169. A client is hospitalized during an acute period of mania. The client is restless and pacing in the hallway, and slaps another client who is walking down the hall en route to a group meeting. Which statement by the nurse regarding the client's behavior would be least therapeutic?
1   "You're lucky that you didn't get hit right back!"
2   "You cannot hit other people. Come with me to your room now."
3   "If you are having difficulty controlling yourself right now, I will help you."
4   "I understand that you are not feeling well, but you cannot hurt others."

Answer: 1
Rationale: The client with mania may exhibit aggression. The nurse should respond using therapeutic communication techniques, and should set limits on the client's behavior. Option 1 is least therapeutic because it could aggravate the client and escalate the client's aggressive behavior. The statements in options 3 and 4 convey understanding and set limits on the client's behavior. The statement in option 2 sets limits on the client's behavior.

Test-Taking Strategy: Use the process of elimination. Note the key words *least therapeutic*. Option 1 could aggravate the client and escalate the client's behavior. Review therapeutic communication techniques if you had difficulty with this question.

Level of Cognitive Ability: Application
Client Needs: Psychosocial Integrity
Integrated Concept/Process: Communication and Documentation
Content Area: Mental Health

Reference:
Varcarolis, E. (2002). *Foundations of psychiatric mental health nursing* (4th ed.). Philadelphia: W.B. Saunders, p. 500.

---

170. A client has undergone two electroconvulsive therapy treatments (ECTs) during the past week and states to the nurse, "I'm starting to feel a little better, but it's scary too because I'm having trouble remembering things now." Which of the following responses by the nurse is most therapeutic?
1   "It must be disturbing to not be able to remember things. ECT causes a temporary memory loss,

Answer: 1
Rationale: Memory loss is an expected temporary effect of ECT. The client should be told that this may occur and that memory usually returns within a few weeks. Occasionally clients have memory loss that lasts up to 6 months. The nurse uses communication techniques that focus on the client's concerns and do not block further communication.

Test-Taking Strategy: Use the process of elimination. Eliminate options 3 and 4 first because they do not acknowledge the client's feelings and block further communication. Choose option 1 over

which many people recover from within a few weeks."

2 "That's too bad. Maybe you should keep a diary so you will have a reference of events as they happen to you."

3 "That does happen with ECT. It's just the price you pay for getting better, I suppose."

4 "Let's just hope you're forgetting bad things instead of good things!"

option 2 because it gives the client an explanation of the events, rather than focusing on a partial solution. Review the effects of ECT if you had difficulty with this question.

Level of Cognitive Ability: Application
Client Needs: Psychosocial Integrity
Integrated Concept/Process: Communication and Documentation
Content Area: Mental Health

Reference:
Varcarolis, E. (2002). *Foundations of psychiatric mental health nursing* (4th ed.). Philadelphia: W.B. Saunders, p. 479.

---

171. A client with a history of personality disorder has an appointment for counseling at the mental health clinic. Upon entering the facility, the client begins to fuss loudly about what the wind has done to her hair and asks the nurse if she likes the client's new lipstick. The nurse interprets that the client most likely has which of the following types of personality disorders?
1 Borderline
2 Histrionic
3 Narcissistic
4 Avoidant

Answer: 2
Rationale: The client with a histrionic personality disorder is overly concerned with impressing others, and they are often preoccupied with their appearance. Their emotional responses are often shallow and changeable, although they are also intense. The client with a borderline personality disorder tends to have intense needs that they seek to fulfill in relationships. The client with a narcissistic personality disorder has a great need for admiration, exploits others to meet own needs and desires, and has a lack of empathy for others. The client with an avoidant personality disorder is often preoccupied with a fear of rejection and criticism.

Test-Taking Strategy: Use the process of elimination and focus on the data in the question. Recalling the types of personality disorders and the characteristics that are common to each will direct you to option 2. Review the characteristics of these disorders if you had difficulty with this question.

Level of Cognitive Ability: Comprehension
Client Needs: Psychosocial Integrity
Integrated Concept/Process: Nursing Process/Data Collection
Content Area: Mental Health

Reference:
Varcarolis, E. (2002). *Foundations of psychiatric mental health nursing* (4th ed.). Philadelphia: W.B. Saunders, pp. 379; 387.

---

172. A client is being admitted to the inpatient unit with an admitting diagnosis of cluster A personality disorder. The nurse monitors this client for behavior that is:
1 Suspicious and eccentric
2 Manipulative and dramatic
3 Characterized by anger
4 Anxious and fearful

Answer: 1
Rationale: Clients with cluster A personality disorders often behave in a manner that is odd or eccentric. Suspicion of others is particularly typical in paranoid personality disorder, a cluster A disorder. Manipulative and dramatic behaviors are typical of some of the cluster B disorders. Anger, anxiety, and fearfulness are typical of clients with cluster C disorders.

Test-Taking Strategy: Knowledge regarding the characteristics of the various personality disorders is needed to answer this question. If you are unfamiliar with the characteristics of these various disorders, review this content.

Level of Cognitive Ability: Application
Client Needs: Psychosocial Integrity
Integrated Concept/Process: Nursing Process/Data Collection
Content Area: Mental Health

Reference:
Varcarolis, E. (2002). *Foundations of psychiatric mental health nursing* (4th ed.). Philadelphia: W.B. Saunders, p. 381.

---

173. A client on the psychiatric unit is displaying manipulative behavior. The nurse should avoid which of the following in working with this client?
1 Identify manipulative behaviors exhibited by the client
2 Communicate to the client the behaviors that are expected
3 Describe clearly the consequences of not staying within identified limits
4 Be prepared to argue with the client to ensure that views of a situation are shared

Answer: 4
Rationale: The nurse should avoid getting into arguments with the manipulative client. The other options listed are helpful interventions that will eventually assist the client to set limits on his or her own behavior.

Test-Taking Strategy: Use the process of elimination and note the key word *avoid*. This tells you that the correct option is an incorrect action on the part of the nurse. Use knowledge of the characteristics of this personality type to direct you to option 4. Review these interventions if you had difficulty with this question.

Level of Cognitive Ability: Application
Client Needs: Psychosocial Integrity
Integrated Concept/Process: Nursing Process/Implementation
Content Area: Mental Health

Reference:
Varcarolis, E. (2002). *Foundations of psychiatric mental health nursing* (4th ed.). Philadelphia: W.B. Saunders, p. 394.

---

174. A male client diagnosed with obsessive-compulsive disorder is upset and agitated, and is walking repeatedly around the unit following the same route each time. The client asks the nurse working the 3 to 11 shift to walk with him. Which of the following responses by the nurse would be most appropriate?
1 "I'm sorry but I'm too busy right now. Let me find someone else to do that with you."
2 "I can see that you're upset. I will walk with you and talk for awhile."
3 "No, it is bedtime. Let me walk you back to your room."
4 "Go to sleep now, but we can talk tomorrow afternoon."

Answer: 2
Rationale: This response in option 2 acknowledges the client's feelings and provides an avenue for release of the client's anxieties. Each of the incorrect options represents a block to communication. The wording of these responses does not indicate that the client is valued and does not acknowledge the client's feelings.

Test-Taking Strategy: Use therapeutic communication techniques. Eliminate each of the incorrect options because they do not deal with the client's concerns or promote further communication. Remember that the client's feelings need to be addressed first. Review these techniques if you had difficulty with this question.

Level of Cognitive Ability: Application
Client Needs: Psychosocial Integrity
Integrated Concept/Process: Communication and Documentation
Content Area: Mental Health

Reference:
Varcarolis, E. (2002). *Foundations of psychiatric mental health nursing* (4th ed.). Philadelphia: W.B. Saunders, p. 255.

175. An adolescent client who is serving a life sentence without parole has been transferred from maximum security and is being monitored by the nurse. In assisting in preparing a treatment plan for this client, the nurse will include which priority?
1 Assessment for suicidal risk
2 Rehabilitation
3 Assessment for homicidal risk
4 Vocational training

Answer: 1
Rationale: The nurse who is assisting in preparing a treatment plan for a client must employ a framework that integrates the built-in realities and limitations of the correctional setting and the compulsory regimen that has been created for the offender. The nurse's ability to assess for self-violence and suicide is critical. Option 2 is incorrect because while rehabilitation will be part of the care plan, it is not the priority for a client who has no hope of being freed. Option 3 is part of the lethality assessment, but first the assessment must deal with self-directed violence. Option 4 is incorrect because although vocational training will be included in a treatment plan, it is not the highest priority.

Test-Taking Strategy: Use the process of elimination and focus on the data in the question. Noting the key word *priority* will direct you to option 1. Review care to the forensic client if you had difficulty with this question.

Level of Cognitive Ability: Application
Client Needs: Psychosocial Integrity
Integrated Concept/Process: Nursing Process/Planning
Content Area: Mental Health

Reference:
Varcarolis, E. (2002). *Foundations of psychiatric mental health nursing* (4th ed.). Philadelphia: W.B. Saunders, p. 641.

176. A female forensic client, who killed her abusive husband by shooting him six times, is eligible for parole and asks the nurse, "Do you think I have a chance of being paroled?" Which of the following would be the most therapeutic response by the nurse?
1 "You have a promise of employment and regaining your children already lined up. I believe that the Parole Board will view your problem solving as a positive criterion."
2 "Let me tell you that most parole applications are denied the first time. Nevertheless, your good conduct record will be seriously considered."
3 "If I were you, I would not build up too much hope. Simply having a firm plan in place will not help your case. "
4 "Do you think you do?"

Answer: 1
Rationale: One item that the Parole Board will investigate is the client's ability to engage in strategic planning. The fact that the forensic client has plans for employment and regaining custody of children will be viewed in a positive way as an example of changed behavior. In option 2, the nurse is giving inaccurate information. In option 3, the nurse is giving an opinion, which is not therapeutic and is unprofessional. In option 4, the nurse is using a confrontational question, which is not therapeutic.

Test-Taking Strategy: Use the process of elimination and therapeutic communication techniques. Eliminate option 4 because the nurse is confrontational. Next, eliminate option 2 because it is inaccurate and option 3 because it is nontherapeutic. Review therapeutic communication techniques if you had difficulty with this question.

Level of Cognitive Ability: Application
Client Needs: Psychosocial Integrity
Integrated Concept/Process: Communication and Documentation
Content Area: Mental Health

Reference:
Varcarolis, E. (2002). *Foundations of psychiatric mental health nursing* (4th ed.). Philadelphia: W.B. Saunders, p. 253.

177. A nurse is caring for an older adult client with mild depression who says, "What do you think I should do about my home? My son thinks I should sell it and move into something smaller now that I'm alone." Which of the following is the most therapeutic response by the nurse?

1   "Oh no, I'm not getting into the middle of this. This is something only you can decide."

2   "What would you like to do? Do you feel you'd be happier in a smaller place? As your depression lifts, you'll be more able to decide what's best for you."

3   "Why not wait until you're feeling less depressed to make such an important decision? You've only been on your medication for four months."

4   "I agree with your son. As you age, you will find that smaller, one floor living is best."

Answer: 2

Rationale: The most therapeutic response is the one that encourages the client to make his or her own decisions. This approach provides the client with a sense of personal empowerment that will relieve the client's powerlessness. If the client is moderately or severely depressed, decision making is difficult. Option 1 is incorrect because the nurse provides a social not a therapeutic response, which may undermine the client's confidence, sense of support, and mutuality. Option 3 is incorrect because the nurse provides procrastination and avoidance as models for problem solving. Option 4 is incorrect because the nurse agrees with the client's son and makes a judgment that is unprofessional and not therapeutic.

Test-Taking Strategy: Use the process of elimination and therapeutic communication techniques focusing on the client feelings and concerns. Option 2 addresses the client's concerns directly. Review therapeutic communication techniques if you had difficulty with this question.

Level of Cognitive Ability: Application
Client Needs: Psychosocial Integrity
Integrated Concept/Process: Communication and Documentation
Content Area: Mental Health

Reference:
Varcarolis, E. (2002). *Foundations of psychiatric mental health nursing* (4th ed.). Philadelphia: W.B. Saunders, p. 253.

---

178. An adolescent is hospitalized for the evaluation and treatment of Tourette's disorder. The nurse reviews the client's record and notes that the client is exhibiting motor tics. Which of the following would the nurse most likely expect to note in the client?

1   Tongue protrusion
2   Grunting sounds
3   Consistent yelping sounds
4   Uttering of obscenities

Answer: 1

Rationale: Tourette's disorder involves motor and verbal tics that cause marked distress and significant impairment in social and occupational functioning. Motor tics usually involve the head but can also involve the torso and limbs. The most frequent first symptom is a single tic, such as eye blinking. Other motor tics include tongue protrusion, touching, squatting, hopping, skipping, retracing steps, and twirling when walking. Vocal tics include words and sounds as barks, grunts, yelps, clicks, snorts, sniffs, and coughs. Coprolalia, the uttering of obscenities, is present in a small number of cases.

Test-Taking Strategy: Note the key words *motor tics* in the question. Use the process of elimination noting that options 2, 3, and 4 all address verbal behaviors. Review the manifestations associated with this disorder if you had difficulty with this question.

Level of Cognitive Ability: Comprehension
Client Needs: Psychosocial Integrity
Integrated Concept/Process: Nursing Process/Data Collection
Content Area: Mental Health

Reference:
Varcarolis, E. (2002). *Foundations of psychiatric mental health nursing* (4th ed.). Philadelphia: W.B. Saunders, p. 874.

CHAPTER 8 Psychosocial Integrity 327

179. A nurse is preparing to collect data on a client suspected of having Alzheimer's disease. The nurse enters the client's room and asks the client, "How was your weekend?" The client responds by saying "It was great. I discussed politics with the President and he took me out to dinner." The nurse interprets that the client has exhibited which of the following defensive maneuvers?

1 Hiding
2 Confabulation
3 Perseveration
4 Apraxia

Answer: 2
Rationale: Confabulation is a defensive maneuver and is an unconscious attempt to maintain self-esteem. Hiding is a form of denial and an unconscious protective defense against the terrifying reality of losing one's place in the world. Perseveration is the repetition of phrases or behaviors and is often intensified under stress. Apraxia is not a defensive maneuver and is characterized by the loss of purposeful movement in the absence of motor or sensory impairment.

Test-Taking Strategy: Use the process of elimination and focus on the key words *defensive maneuvers*. Eliminate option 4 first because this is not a defensive maneuver. From the remaining options, focusing on the statement of the client should direct you to option 2. If you had difficulty with this question, review these defensive maneuvers.

Level of Cognitive Ability: Comprehension
Client Needs: Psychosocial Integrity
Integrated Concept/Process: Nursing Process/Data Collection
Content Area: Mental Health

Reference:
Varcarolis, E. (2002). *Foundations of psychiatric mental health nursing* (4th ed.). Philadelphia: W.B. Saunders, p. 587.

---

180. A female client who was attacked outside a mall is experiencing posttraumatic stress disorder. The client is visibly anxious about shopping in general and specifically avoids crowds and parking lots. The client expresses concern about these events and tells the nurse how upset she is about feeling this way. Which of the following is the most appropriate response by the nurse?

1 "Why don't you just go back there and get it 'out of your system'?"
2 "I can see that you are upset about this. Can we talk some more about it?"
3 "It's difficult now but try not to worry so much."
4 "Everything is going to be all right if you just give it more time."

Answer: 2
Rationale: Option 2 is the most therapeutic because it does not contain a communication block. The correct option indicates that the nurse is aware of the client's feelings and promotes continued communication. Each of the incorrect options fail to acknowledge the client's concerns and do not encourage further communication.

Test-Taking Strategy: Use therapeutic communication techniques. Option 2 is the only option that addresses the client's feelings. Review these techniques if you had difficulty with this question.

Level of Cognitive Ability: Application
Client Needs: Psychosocial Integrity
Integrated Concept/Process: Communication and Documentation
Content Area: Mental Health

Reference:
Varcarolis, E. (2002). *Foundations of psychiatric mental health nursing* (4th ed.). Philadelphia: W.B. Saunders, p. 253.

---

181. An agoraphobic client has been hospitalized for a relatively prolonged time. The client has become cooperative and communicative with peers. The client has also begun to make appropriate suggestions

Answer: 4
Rationale: The behavior demonstrated by the client is appropriate during hospitalization. There is no evidence in the question that the client is seeking attention, acting out (which is an attention-seeking behavior), or being manipulative.

during group discussions. The nurse concludes that the client's behavior is representative of:

1. Attention seeking
2. Acting out
3. Manipulation
4. Improvement

Test-Taking Strategy: Use the process of elimination. Focus on the data in the question. This should direct you to option 4. Review the indications of improvement in a client with a phobia if you had difficulty with this question.

Level of Cognitive Ability: Comprehension
Client Needs: Psychosocial Integrity
Integrated Concept/Process: Nursing Process/Evaluation
Content Area: Mental Health

Reference:
Varcarolis, E. (2002). *Foundations of psychiatric mental health nursing* (4th ed.). Philadelphia: W.B. Saunders, p. 313.

---

182. A client is not able to leave the home without checking several times to be sure the iron is turned off. The client then rechecks the lock each time after checking the iron. The client arrives late to many appointments and other functions because of this repetitive ritual and misses other engagements completely. The nurse interprets that the symptoms exhibited by this client are consistent with:

1. Posttraumatic stress disorder
2. Obsessive-compulsive disorder
3. Generalized anxiety disorder
4. Phobia

Answer: 2
Rationale: Obsessive-compulsive disorder is characterized by repetitive behavior that interferes with activities of daily living and functioning. Posttraumatic stress disorder occurs when a client continues to relive a traumatic event frequently, or avoids people and places associated with the event. Generalized anxiety disorder occurs when a client has excessive uncontrolled anxiety for more than 6 months. A phobia is an irrational fear of a situation or an object.

Test-Taking Strategy: Use the process of elimination. Focusing on the client's behavior identified in the question will direct you to option 2. Review the characteristics of the disorders presented in the options if you had difficulty with this question.

Level of Cognitive Ability: Comprehension
Client Needs: Psychosocial Integrity
Integrated Concept/Process: Nursing Process/Evaluation
Content Area: Mental Health

Reference:
Varcarolis, E. (2002). *Foundations of psychiatric mental health nursing* (4th ed.). Philadelphia: W.B. Saunders, p. 313.

---

183. A nurse is counseling a female alcoholic client and her husband. The husband tells the nurse that he worries about his wife "all the time," has helped "cover-up" her drinking, and would continue to "be there" for her, even though all of their children no longer speak to her because of her drinking. The nurse plans to refer the husband to a support group for:

1. Alcoholics
2. Substance abusers
3. Caregivers
4. Codependents

Answer: 4
Rationale: The description of the husband's behavior in the question is that of a codependent person. Codependence involves overresponsible behavior, which is doing for another person what that person could be doing for himself or herself. Option 1 identifies a support group for the client with the alcohol problem. Option 2 identifies a support group for a client with a drug problem. Option 3 identifies a support group for a caregiver that is involved with caring for a significant other on a daily basis.

Test-Taking Strategy: Focus on the data in the question. Noting that the client of the question is the husband will direct you to option 4. Review support groups if you had difficulty with this question.

Level of Cognitive Ability: Application
Client Needs: Psychosocial Integrity

Integrated Concept/Process: Nursing Process/Planning
Content Area: Mental Health

Reference:
Varcarolis, E. (2002). *Foundations of psychiatric mental health nursing* (4th ed.). Philadelphia: W.B. Saunders, p. 751.

---

184. A nurse has become friends with a second nurse working on the same clinical nursing unit. Over time, the nurse becomes aware that the friend is abusing narcotics. The nurse should encourage the friend to use which of the following resources initially to obtain help for this problem?
1 Primary care physician
2 Alcoholics Anonymous
3 Employee assistance program
4 State Board of Registration in Nursing

Answer: 3
Rationale: In larger organizations such as hospitals, there are often employee assistance programs that offer services such as information, counseling, and referral for employees experiencing a wide variety of problems, including substance abuse. This service may also provide an alternative to termination if the employee's job performance is affected because of the problem.

Test-Taking Strategy: Use the process of elimination. Note that the question contains the key word *initially*. This tells you that more than one option may be partially or totally correct. Eliminate option 2 first because it is designed for alcohol abuse, not narcotic abuse. Select option 3 instead of the other remaining options because of the wide range of services available. Review available resources for the client with a substance abuse problem if you had difficulty with this question.

Level of Cognitive Ability: Application
Client Needs: Psychosocial Integrity
Integrated Concept/Process: Nursing Process/Implementation
Content Area: Mental Health

Reference:
Varcarolis, E. (2002). *Foundations of psychiatric mental health nursing* (4th ed.). Philadelphia: W.B. Saunders, p. 773.

---

185. A client is hospitalized with a diagnosis of severe depression. The client is withdrawn, and exhibits poor motivation and concentration. The nurse should plan to involve the client in which of the following activities at this time?
1 Small group discussions
2 Simple two-person card games
3 Art therapy
4 Dance therapy

Answer: 2
Rationale: When the client is more severely depressed, the client should be involved in one-to-one activities that require little concentration, and that have no elements of being "right" or "wrong." As the client's condition improves, the client can become involved in activities with small groups (options 1, 3, and 4).

Test-Taking Strategy: Use the process of elimination. Remember that options that are similar are not likely to be correct. With this in mind, eliminate each of the incorrect options because they involve group activities. Review care to the client with severe depression if you had difficulty with this question.

Level of Cognitive Ability: Application
Client Needs: Psychosocial Integrity
Integrated Concept/Process: Nursing Process/Planning
Content Area: Mental Health

Reference:
Varcarolis, E. (2002). *Foundations of psychiatric mental health nursing* (4th ed.). Philadelphia: W.B. Saunders, p. 460.

186. A nurse is developing a plan of care for the client who is depressed. Which of the following is the most therapeutic nursing intervention to be included in the plan?

1 Be very cheerful and do not talk of anything that may be negative for the client
2 Avoid talking of serious issues that can depress the client
3 Promote superficial social discussions only for the first week
4 Be matter-of-fact, displaying a hopeful but not overly cheerful attitude

Answer: 4

Rationale: Employing a hopeful attitude that is not excessively cheery will combat the negative and gloomy affect, which is intrinsic to depression. Using a cheerful approach with the client can be interpreted by the client as belittling. A matter-of-fact approach will be more reassuring to the client and avoid any regressive struggles that might emerge. In option 1, the nurse is using a social, not therapeutic, approach. In option 2, the nurse is using a nontherapeutic approach. Remember, the client is working through a depression. Negative issues for the client will need to be discussed so that the client can explore effective coping skills. In option 3, the nurse uses a very nontherapeutic, social response.

Test-Taking Strategy: Use the process of elimination and knowledge regarding care for the client with depression to assist in answering the question. Note that option 4 is the most global option. Review these interventions if you had difficulty with this question.

Level of Cognitive Ability: Application
Client Needs: Psychosocial Integrity
Integrated Concept/Process: Nursing Process/Planning
Content Area: Mental Health

Reference:
Varcarolis, E. (2002). *Foundations of psychiatric mental health nursing* (4th ed.). Philadelphia: W.B. Saunders, p. 465.

187. A nurse is planning care for a client with an obsessive-compulsive disorder. The nurse would assign the highest priority to which of the following nursing interventions?

1 Educate the client about self-control techniques
2 Establish a trusting nurse-patient relationship
3 Monitor the client for abnormal behavior
4 Encourage participation in daily self-care and unit activities

Answer: 2

Rationale: Establishment of a trusting nurse-client relationship is the foundation for providing effective nursing care to the client with a mental health disorder. The nursing interventions identified in each of the other options may be appropriate, but are not of the highest priority.

Test-Taking Strategy: Use the process of elimination. Note that the stem of the question contains the key words *highest priority*. This tells you that there may be more than one correct option and that you must determine which one is most important. Recalling that a trusting relationship is the foundation for effective nursing care will direct you to option 2. Review the importance of a trusting relationship if you had difficulty with this question.

Level of Cognitive Ability: Application
Client Needs: Psychosocial Integrity
Integrated Concept/Process: Nursing Process/Implementation
Content Area: Mental Health

Reference:
Varcarolis, E. (2002). *Foundations of psychiatric mental health nursing* (4th ed.). Philadelphia: W.B. Saunders, p. 379.

188. The staff working in a mental health in-patient unit is reviewing the cases of selected clients with anxiety disorders. The nurse interprets that a client with which of the following problems is least likely to be treated with behavior therapy?
1 Obsessive-compulsive disorder
2 Posttraumatic stress disorder
3 Agoraphobia
4 Panic disorder

Answer: 2
Rationale: The client with posttraumatic stress disorder is not treated with behavior therapy. It may be treated with psychotherapy, family or group therapy, relaxation techniques, and vocational rehabilitation as needed. Each of the other disorders listed may be treated by use of behavior therapy.

Test-Taking Strategy: Specific knowledge about the management of each of the disorders listed in the options is needed to answer this question accurately. Review the various therapeutic modalities used in each of these disorders if you had difficulty with this question.

Level of Cognitive Ability: Analysis
Client Needs: Psychosocial Integrity
Integrated Concept/Process: Nursing Process/Planning
Content Area: Mental Health

Reference:
Varcarolis, E. (2002). *Foundations of psychiatric mental health nursing* (4th ed.). Philadelphia: W.B. Saunders, p. 331.

189. A nurse is assigned to care for a client with schizophrenia who has a nursing diagnosis of Disturbed Thought Processes documented in the care plan. The client exhibits defensive behaviors and relates suspicious thoughts. The nurse plans to use which approach when working with this client for the first time?
1 Frequently touch the client's arm when speaking
2 Avoid sitting too close to the client
3 Spend a long period of time with the client
4 Use a warm and close manner

Answer: 2
Rationale: The nurse should avoid sitting too close to the client. If the client perceives that personal space is invaded, the client's anxiety may increase. For the same reason, the nurse should limit the amount of time interacting with the client and should avoid touching the client. If it becomes necessary to touch the client, the nurse should ask permission first. The nurse's manner should be nonjudgmental and respectful. A warm and close manner could be threatening to the client who needs emotional distance.

Test-Taking Strategy: Use the process of elimination and focus on the data in the question. Noting the words *defensive behaviors and relates suspicious thoughts* will direct you to option 2. Review the techniques for caring for the schizophrenic client if you had difficulty with this question.

Level of Cognitive Ability: Application
Client Needs: Psychosocial Integrity
Integrated Concept/Process: Nursing Process/Planning
Content Area: Mental Health

Reference:
Varcarolis, E. (2002). *Foundations of psychiatric mental health nursing* (4th ed.). Philadelphia: W.B. Saunders, p. 537.

190. A client who has a long history of anti-social, acting-out behavior including polydrug abuse, numerous suicidal self-mutilation attempts, and prostitution says, "I'm ready to go straight now." Which of the following responses by the nurse would be the most therapeutic?

Answer: 2
Rationale: Clients who have a long history of antisocial behavior need to demonstrate motivation to change behaviors, not just verbalization. The nurse would be most therapeutic to assist the client to look at the behaviors that indicate the motivation to change. Option 2 is the only option that will accomplish this goal.

1   "Yeah, right. I've heard this from you before."

2   "Tell me what you believe will be different this time?"

3   "I disagree. I have seen absolutely no changes in your life to support your claims."

4   "That's so wonderful to hear!"

Test-Taking Strategy: Use the process of elimination. Option 1 is not therapeutic because it is insensitive and sarcastic. Option 3 is not therapeutic because it uses disagreeing rather than assisting the client to articulate how things will be different. Option 4 jumps to a conclusion with no data gathering and provides a social response; not a therapeutic one. Review therapeutic communication techniques if you had difficulty with this question.

Level of Cognitive Ability: Application
Client Needs: Psychosocial Integrity
Integrated Concept/Process: Communication and Documentation
Content Area: Mental Health

Reference:
Varcarolis, E. (2002). *Foundations of psychiatric mental health nursing* (4th ed.). Philadelphia: W.B. Saunders, p. 254.

---

191. A nurse is caring for a middle-aged female homeless client who is divorced and has just been evicted from her apartment because she is unemployed and cannot pay her rent. She says to the nurse, "I can't tell my son. He lives 80 miles away and barely gets by himself. I'm not his problem." Which of the following responses by the nurse would be the most therapeutic?

1   "O.K., let's call your ex-husband to see if he'll help you until you get on your feet."

2   "Yet if your son needed help, wouldn't you want to know about it and try to help as much as you could?"

3   "I could commit you for a few days to get you a safe place to sleep and some food."

4   "You can come home with me. I have an extra bedroom you can use until you get back on your feet."

Answer: 2
Rationale: The most therapeutic communication technique is clarification, which attempts to put vague ideas into words. It helps the client to view their own feelings and actions. In option 1, the nurse implements an insensitive and intrusive action. In option 3, the nurse is again insensitive and offers a solution, which may provide safety but strips the client of decision making. In option 4, the nurse is sympathetic, but the actions offered are social rather than professional.

Test-Taking Strategy: Use therapeutic communication techniques. Options 1, 3, and 4 are inappropriate. Option 2 focuses on the client's concern. Review therapeutic communication techniques if you had difficulty with this question.

Level of Cognitive Ability: Application
Client Needs: Psychosocial Integrity
Integrated Concept/Process: Communication and Documentation
Content Area: Mental Health

Reference:
Varcarolis, E. (2002). *Foundations of psychiatric mental health nursing* (4th ed.). Philadelphia: W.B. Saunders, p. 253.

---

192. A nurse is caring for a client in a mental health unit. The client says to the nurse, "You have beautiful eyes and you smell nice, Nurse." Which of the following responses would be the most therapeutic by the nurse?

1   "I'm not here to discuss my eyes or how I smell."

2   "Do you think you are being appropriate?"

3   "Thank you for noticing."

4   Say nothing in order to extinguish the client's inappropriate behavior

Answer: 1
Rationale: If a client makes a personal comment to the nurse, the nurse should respond directly regarding the purpose of the therapeutic relationship. The client's behavior should be confronted directly and then documented in the client's chart. Option 2 is confrontational but also judgmental and provides an opening for a regressive struggle. Option 3 is a social response, which can be misinterpreted by the client. Option 4 can be misinterpreted as the nurse wanting or liking the client's comments.

Test-Taking Strategy: Use the process of elimination and therapeutic communication techniques. Recalling that the nurse should maintain a therapeutic relationship will direct you to option 1. Review the components of a therapeutic relationship if you had difficulty with this question.

Level of Cognitive Ability: Application
Client Needs: Psychosocial Integrity
Integrated Concept/Process: Communication and Documentation
Content Area: Mental Health

Reference:
Varcarolis, E. (2002). *Foundations of psychiatric mental health nursing* (4th ed.). Philadelphia: W.B. Saunders, p. 222.

---

193. A nurse is working with a client during crisis intervention. Which statement by the client would indicate a successful outcome related to resolution of the crisis?
  1   "I still cannot return to work, but my concentration is better."
  2   "I have learned that my old ways of coping did not work. I have learned new ways of dealing with things."
  3   "I am sleeping better now."
  4   "I am going to have to work on repairing my relationship with my family."

Answer: 2
Rationale: A successful resolution of crisis indicates the acquisition of new knowledge and an opportunity for growth. Although options 1, 3, and 4 may be appropriate goals for the client, they do not specifically indicate a successful outcome.

Test-Taking Strategy: Use the process of elimination. Read each option carefully focusing on the key words *successful outcome*. Option 2 is the only option that indicates the acquisition of new behaviors in the client. Options 1, 3, and 4 do not indicate successful resolution of the crisis. Review the goals of crisis intervention if you had difficulty with this question.

Level of Cognitive Ability: Analysis
Client Needs: Psychosocial Integrity
Integrated Concept/Process: Nursing Process/Evaluation
Content Area: Mental Health

Reference:
Varcarolis, E. (2002). *Foundations of psychiatric mental health nursing* (4th ed.). Philadelphia: W.B. Saunders, p. 626.

---

194. A nurse working in a chronic mental health environment can be most successful in dealing with client crisis by:
  1   Recognizing that rehospitalization is necessary in the event of crisis
  2   Involving the family to support the client whenever crisis occurs
  3   Eliminating direct nursing interventions to allow the client to exercise problem-solving skills
  4   Identifying strengths and the healthy aspects of functioning that may compensate for weakness

Answer: 4
Rationale: The nurse working with chronically mentally ill clients in crisis should focus on client's strengths, modifying and setting realistic goals with the client, encouraging the client to take a more active role in the problem-solving process, and providing direct interventions as needed.

Test-Taking Strategy: Read the options carefully and use the process of elimination. Option 3 can be eliminated first because it is inappropriate to eliminate direct nursing interventions. Eliminate options 1 and 2 because they are not client focused. Note the key words *strengths* and *healthy* in option 4. These words will direct you to this option. Review the nurse's role in dealing with crisis if you had difficulty with this question.

Level of Cognitive Ability: Application
Client Needs: Psychosocial Integrity
Integrated Concept/Process: Nursing Process/Implementation
Content Area: Mental Health

Reference:
Varcarolis, E. (2002). *Foundations of psychiatric mental health nursing* (4th ed.). Philadelphia: W.B. Saunders, p. 627.

195. A nurse is assigned to care for a hospitalized client with a diagnosis of depression. When communicating with the client, which of the following would be the most appropriate statement by the nurse?
1   "You look nice this morning."
2   "I like the way you did your hair."
3   "You are wearing a new dress this morning."
4   "Don't worry, things will look up for you."

Answer: 3
Rationale: When depressed, a client sees the negative side of everything. The statement in option 1 can be interpreted by the client as "I didn't look nice yesterday morning." The statement in option 2 may be thought of by the client as something to be done to please the nurse. For example, the client may think, "If I did my hair another way maybe he or she will not like it." Neutral comments such as that identified in option 3 will avoid negative interpretations. The client should not be told "not to worry and that things will look up." This statement tends to minimize the client's feelings of guilt and worthlessness because the client cannot "look up or snap out of it" at this time.

Test-Taking Strategy: Note the diagnosis of the client and read each option carefully using the process of elimination to answer the question. Select the option that avoids negative interpretations. Neutral comments such as that identified in option 3 will avoid negative interpretations. Review therapeutic communication techniques for the depressed client if you had difficulty with this question.

Level of Cognitive Ability: Application
Client Needs: Psychosocial Integrity
Integrated Concept/Process: Communication and Documentation
Content Area: Mental Health

Reference:
Varcarolis, E. (2002). *Foundations of psychiatric mental health nursing* (4th ed.). Philadelphia: W.B. Saunders, p. 467.

196. A nurse is caring for a client who is experiencing psychomotor agitation. Which of the following activities would be most appropriate for the nurse to plan for the client?
1   Playing Ping-Pong
2   Playing chess
3   Playing simple card games
4   Reading magazines

Answer: 1
Rationale: In psychomotor agitation, it is best to provide activities that involve the use of hands and gross motor movements. These activities include Ping-Pong, volleyball, finger-painting, drawing, and working with clay. These activities give the client a more appropriate way of discharging motor tension. Options 3 and 4 are sedentary activities. Option 2 requires concentration and more intensive use of thought processes.

Test-Taking Strategy: Use the process of elimination. Note the diagnosis of the client and recall that activities that involve the use of hands and gross motor movements are best for this client. Eliminate option 2 because this activity will require concentration, which this client may not be able to do. Next eliminate options 3 and 4 because they will not provide a method of discharging motor tension. Review care to a client with psychomotor agitation if you had difficulty with this question.

Level of Cognitive Ability: Application
Client Needs: Psychosocial Integrity

Integrated Concept/Process: Nursing Process/Planning
Content Area: Mental Health

Reference:
Varcarolis, E. (2002). *Foundations of psychiatric mental health nursing* (4th ed.). Philadelphia: W.B. Saunders, p. 461.

---

197. When caring for a client with schizophrenia, the nurse documents that the client has an inappropriate affect. Which of the following best describes this type of behavioral response observed by the nurse?
  1 The client's emotional response to a situation is not congruent with the tone of the situation
  2 The client has an immobile facial expression or blank look
  3 The client displays minimal emotional responses
  4 The client is mumbling to himself or herself

Answer: 1
Rationale: An inappropriate affect refers to an emotional response to a situation that is not congruent with the tone of the situation. A flat affect is an immobile facial expression or blank look. A blunted affect is a minimal emotional response and expresses the client's outward affect. It may not coincide with the client's inner emotions. A bizarre affect such as grimacing, giggling, and mumbling to oneself is marked when the client is unable to relate logically to the environment.

Test-Taking Strategy: Knowledge regarding the behavioral responses in a client with schizophrenia is helpful to answer this question. Note the relationship between the words *inappropriate* in the question and *not congruent* in the correct option. If you are unfamiliar with the behaviors exhibited in a client with schizophrenia, review this content.

Level of Cognitive Ability: Comprehension
Client Needs: Psychosocial Integrity
Integrated Concept/Process: Nursing Process/Planning
Content Area: Mental Health

Reference:
Varcarolis, E. (2002). *Foundations of psychiatric mental health nursing* (4th ed.). Philadelphia: W.B. Saunders, p. 537.

---

198. A nurse is providing care to a paranoid client and notes that a nursing diagnosis of Disturbed Thought Processes is documented in the care plan. The nurse plans to avoid which of the following when caring for the client?
  1 Sitting with the client and holding the client's hand
  2 Using a nondefensive and nonjudgmental attitude
  3 Using simple and clear language when speaking to the client
  4 Diffusing angry and hostile verbal attacks with a nondefensive stand

Answer: 1
Rationale: When caring for a paranoid client, the nurse avoids any physical contact and does not touch the client. The nurse should ask the client's permission if touch is necessary because touch may be interpreted as a physical or sexual assault. The nurse should use simple and clear language when speaking to the client to prevent misinterpretation and to clarify the nurse's intent and actions. A nondefensive and nonjudgmental attitude provides an attitude in which feelings can be explored more easily. Angry and hostile verbal attacks should be diffused with a nondefensive stand. The anger a paranoid client expresses is often displaced, and when the staff becomes defensive, anger of both the client and staff escalates.

Test-Taking Strategy: Use the process of elimination. Note the key word *avoid* in the stem of the question. If you can recall that touch may be interpreted as a physical or sexual assault by the paranoid client, you will easily be directed to option 1. Review care to the client with paranoia if you had difficulty with this question.

Level of Cognitive Ability: Application
Client Needs: Psychosocial Integrity

Integrated Concept/Process: Nursing Process/Planning
Content Area: Mental Health

Reference:
Varcarolis, E. (2002). *Foundations of psychiatric mental health nursing* (4th ed.). Philadelphia: W.B. Saunders, p. 535.

---

199. A nurse is caring for a client with delirium who has become physically abusive. Which of the following initial nursing responses should be made to the client?

1 "You are not to hit me or anyone else. Tell me how you feel."
2 "If you hit me, I am putting you into restraints."
3 "The seclusion room is empty and that's where you will need to be if you threaten to hit me or anyone else."
4 "I will call the physician and order a shot for you if you continue to threaten to hit me or anyone else."

Answer: 1
Rationale: If the client's behavior becomes physically abusive, the nurse first sets limits on the behavior by saying, "You are not to hit me or anyone else. Tell me how you feel." Options 2, 3, and 4 threaten the client and are a violation of the client's rights.

Test-Taking Strategy: Use the process of elimination and knowledge of ethical and legal responsibilities to answer the question. Note that options 2, 3, and 4 all violate the client's rights. If you had difficulty with this question, review appropriate care to the client who is physically abusive.

Level of Cognitive Ability: Application
Client Needs: Psychosocial Integrity
Integrated Concept/Process: Nursing Process/Implementation
Content Area: Mental Health

Reference:
Varcarolis, E. (2002). *Foundations of psychiatric mental health nursing* (4th ed.). Philadelphia: W.B. Saunders, p. 579.

---

200. A male client with a diagnosis of schizophrenia tells the nurse that there are voices outside of the window telling him what do all the time. The client asks the nurse, "Can you hear them and what do you think I should tell them?" The most appropriate initial response by the nurse to the client is:

1 "What are the voices telling you?"
2 "Yes, I can hear them too."
3 "Maybe they will go away if you ignore them."
4 "You hear voices because you are ill."

Answer: 1
Rationale: When a client is experiencing an auditory hallucination, it is important initially to understand what the voices are saying or telling the client to do. Suicidal or homicidal messages, if heard by the client, necessitate initiating safety measures for all clients and members of the health care team. Options 2 and 3 are inappropriate and do not reinforce reality. Option 4 is inappropriate because it is telling the client that he is "ill."

Test-Taking Strategy: Use the process of elimination and the steps of the nursing process. Note the key word *initial* in the stem of the question. Use prioritization skills and therapeutic communication skills to assist in answering the question. Options 2, 3, and 4 are inappropriate communication techniques and should be eliminated. Option 1 is the only option that will provide the nurse with important additional data. If you had difficulty with this question, review the nursing interventions related to the client experiencing auditory hallucinations.

Level of Cognitive Ability: Application
Client Needs: Psychosocial Integrity
Integrated Concept/Process: Nursing Process/Implementation
Content Area: Mental Health

Reference:
Varcarolis, E. (2002). *Foundations of psychiatric mental health nursing* (4th ed.). Philadelphia: W.B. Saunders, p. 541.

201. A nurse is caring for a 7-year-old child with glomerulonephritis. When discussing the plan of care with the parents, the nurse notes that the parents are upset about the diagnosis. The nurse understands that a common initial reaction of parents to the diagnosis of glomerulonephritis is:

1   Fear of the complicated treatment regimen
2   Anger at the child for requiring hospitalization
3   Guilt that they did not seek treatment more quickly
4   Depression that the child may not be able to play sports

Answer: 3

Rationale: Guilt is a common reaction of the parents of a child diagnosed with glomerulonephritis. They blame themselves for not responding more quickly to the child's initial symptoms and may believe they could have prevented the development of glomerular damage. Options 1, 2, and 4 may also be reactions but are unlikely to occur initially.

Test-Taking Strategy: Use the process of elimination focusing on the key word *initial*. Noting that the clients of the question are the parents will assist in directing you to option 3. Review psychosocial parental reactions to a diagnosis of glomerulonephritis if you had difficulty with this question.

Level of Cognitive Ability: Comprehension
Client Needs: Psychosocial Integrity
Integrated Concept/Process: Nursing Process/Data Collection
Content Area: Child Health

Reference:
Schulte, E. Price, D., & Gwin, J. (2001). *Thompson's pediatric nursing* (8th ed.). Philadelphia: W.B. Saunders, p. 236.

---

202. A nurse is caring for a client with schizophrenia and documents that the client is experiencing poverty of speech. The nurse documents this finding based on which of the following observations?

1   Speech is adequate in amount but conveys little information because of vagueness, empty repetitions, or use of stereotypes or obscure phrases
2   Speech is restricted in amount and ranges from brief to monosyllabic one-word answers
3   The client stops talking in the middle of a sentence
4   The client remains silent

Answer: 2

Rationale: Poverty of speech is speech that is restricted in amount and ranges from brief to monosyllabic one-word answers. Poverty of content of speech is speech that is adequate in amount but conveys little information because of vagueness, empty repetitions, or use of stereotypes or obscure phrases. Blocking is when the client stops talking in the middle of a sentence and remains quiet.

Test-Taking Strategy: Use the process of elimination. Note the relationship between the words *poverty of speech* in the question and *speech is restricted in amount* in the correct option. If you are unfamiliar with the behaviors exhibited in a client with schizophrenia, review this content.

Level of Cognitive Ability: Comprehension
Client Needs: Psychosocial Integrity
Integrated Concept/Process: Communication and Documentation
Content Area: Mental Health

Reference:
Bauer, B., & Hill, S. (2000). *Mental health nursing*. Philadelphia: W.B. Saunders, p. 123.

---

203. An emergency room nurse is assisting in caring for a client with rape-trauma syndrome. Which of the following goals is most appropriate for the client?

1   Client will accept the trauma that has happened
2   Client will begin the healthy grief process

Answer: 2

Rationale: The client who has been raped is in the beginning stages of the grieving process. The acceptance phase does not occur immediately after the rape. The goal that states that the client will not experience psychological trauma is unrealistic. Clients use defense mechanisms to help with the anxiety and some defense mechanisms, such as denial, have been described to be helpful to the individual, especially in the immediate posttraumatic period.

3 Client will not experience psychological trauma
4 Client will not use defense mechanisms

Test-Taking Strategy: Use the process of elimination. Eliminate options 3 and 4 first because the client is experiencing psychological trauma and because the use of defense mechanisms is helpful to clients in traumatic situations. Eliminate option 1 because the immediate posttraumatic period is too early to accept the trauma. Review nursing care to the client with rape-trauma syndrome if you had difficulty with this question.

Level of Cognitive Ability: Application
Client Needs: Psychosocial Integrity
Integrated Concept/Process: Nursing Process/Planning
Content Area: Mental Health

Reference:
Bauer, B., & Hill, S. (2000). *Mental health nursing.* Philadelphia: W.B. Saunders, p. 192.

---

204. A male client comes to the clinic after losing all of his personal belongings in a flood. After identifying one of the client's problems as ineffective individual coping, the nurse and client plan goals. Which of the following is the least realistic goal?
1 The client will identify a realistic perception of stressors
2 The client will develop adaptive coping patterns
3 The client will express and share feelings regarding the present crisis
4 The client will stop blaming himself for the lack of flood insurance

Answer: 4
Rationale: Options 1, 2, and 3 identify a positive and realistic movement toward increased self-esteem and problem solving. Option 4 is unrealistic and there are no data in the question that indicate that the client lacked flood insurance.

Test-Taking Strategy: Use the process of elimination. Note the key words *least realistic.* The words *realistic* and *adaptive*, and the words *express and share feelings* in options 1, 2, and 3 respectively, identify positive and realistic goals. This should assist in directing you to option 4. In addition, there is nothing in the question that indicates that the client lacked flood insurance, as option 4 reflects. Review goals for the client with ineffective individual coping if you had difficulty with this question.

Level of Cognitive Ability: Application
Client Needs: Psychosocial Integrity
Integrated Concept/Process: Nursing Process/Planning
Content Area: Mental Health

Reference:
Johnson, M., Bulechek, G., Dochterman, J. et al. (2001). *Nursing diagnoses, outcomes, and interventions.* St. Louis: Mosby, p. 174.

---

205. A mental health nurse reviews the activity schedule for the day and determines that the best activity that a manic client could participate in is:
1 A book review
2 Badminton
3 Paint-by-number activity
4 Deep breathing or progressive relaxation group

Answer: 2
Rationale: A person who is experiencing mania is overactive and full of energy, lacks concentration, and has poor impulse control. The client needs an activity that will allow utilization of excess energy that will not endanger others during the process. Badminton is an exercise that uses the large muscle groups of the body and is a great way to expend the increased energy that this client is experiencing.

Test-Taking Strategy: Use the process of elimination. Options 1, 3, and 4 are similar and describe relatively sedate activities that require concentration, a quality that is lacking in the manic state. Such activities may lead to increased frustration and anxiety for the client. Review care to the client with mania if you had difficulty with this question.

Level of Cognitive Ability: Application
Client Needs: Psychosocial Integrity
Integrated Concept/Process: Nursing Process/Planning
Content Area: Mental Health

Reference:
Bauer, B., & Hill, S. (2000). *Mental health nursing.* Philadelphia: W.B. Saunders, p. 276.

---

206. A client is brought to the emergency room by the police after having seriously lacerated both wrists. The initial action that the nurse will undertake is to:
1 Examine and treat the wound sites
2 Secure and record a detailed history
3 Encourage and assist the client to ventilate feelings
4 Administer an antianxiety agent

Answer: 1
Rationale: The client is in physiological distress. It is likely that the serious lacerations have led to severe bleeding. Although options 2, 3, and 4 may be appropriate at some point, the initial action would need to be to treat the wounds.

Test-Taking Strategy: Use Maslow's Hierarchy of Needs theory to prioritize and note the key word *initial.* Physiological needs come first. Option 1 is the only option that addresses a physiological need. Review emergency care to the suicidal client if you had difficulty with this question.

Level of Cognitive Ability: Application
Client Needs: Psychosocial Integrity
Integrated Concept/Process: Nursing Process/Implementation
Content Area: Mental Health

Reference:
Varcarolis, E. (2002). *Foundations of psychiatric mental health nursing* (4th ed.). Philadelphia: W.B. Saunders, p. 643.

---

207. A home care nurse visits a client who is being cared for by her daughter. The nurse observes the client's daugher verbalizing threats to the client to place the client in a nursing home if she continues to refuse taking her medications. The nurse is concerned that the client is a victim of which form of victimization?
1 Emotional abuse
2 Neglect
3 Economic maltreatment
4 Sexual abuse

Answer: 1
Rationale: Emotional abuse is the infliction of mental anguish and includes threatening an individual with abandonment or institutionalization, such as a nursing home. Neglect is failure to provide care and can be in the form of physical, developmental, or educational. Economic maltreatment is illegal or improper exploitation of an individual's funds. Sexual abuse is any form of sexual contact or exposure without the individual's consent.

Test-Taking Strategy: Use the process of elimination. Note the relationship between the word "threats" in the question and option 1. Review the signs of emotional abuse if you had difficulty with this question.

Level of Cognitive Ability: Comprehension
Client Needs: Psychosocial Integrity
Integrated Concept/Process: Nursing Process/Data Collection
Content Area: Mental Health

Reference:
Varcarolis, E. (2002). *Foundations of psychiatric mental health nursing* (4th ed.). Philadelphia: W.B. Saunders, p. 694.

208. A woman is admitted to the in-client mental health unit. When asked her name, she responds, "I am Elizabeth, the Queen of England." The nurse recognizes this response as:
1 A visual illusion
2 An auditory hallucination
3 A grandiose delusion
4 A loose association

Answer: 3
Rationale: Delusion is an important personal belief that is almost certainly not true and resists modification. An illusion is a misperception or misinterpretation of externally real stimuli. A hallucination is a false perception. Loose association is thinking characterized by speech in which unrelated ideas shift from one subject to another.

Test-Taking Strategy: Use the process of elimination. Eliminate options 1 and 2 because the client is not having any visual or auditory disturbances. Eliminate option 4 because there is no indication of shifting from one subject to another. Making a reference to being a "queen" is a grandiose assumption. Review the characteristics of delusions if you had difficulty with this question.

Level of Cognitive Ability: Comprehension
Client Needs: Psychosocial Integrity
Integrated Concept/Process: Nursing Process/Data Collection
Content Area: Mental Health

Reference:
Varcarolis, E. (2002). *Foundations of psychiatric mental health nursing* (4th ed.). Philadelphia: W.B. Saunders, p. 531.

---

209. A nurse is assigned to care for a client with anorexia nervosa. The nurse reviews the client's health record and notes documentation of a nursing diagnosis: Ineffective Individual Coping related to dysfunctional cognition and maladaptive behaviors. Based on this documentation, the nurse would collect data regarding which of the following?
1 Client's eating patterns and food preferences and concerns about eating
2 Client's feelings about self and body weight
3 Previous and current coping skills
4 Client's sense of lack of control about the treatment plan

Answer: 3
Rationale: The nurse would most appropriately collect data regarding the client's previous and current coping skills. Assessing the client's eating patterns and food preferences and concerns about eating most appropriately relate to nutrition. Assessing the client's feelings about self and body weight most appropriately relates to body image disturbance. Assessing the client's sense of lack of control about the treatment plan most appropriately relates to powerlessness.

Test-Taking Strategy: Focus on the nursing diagnosis stated in the question to assist in directing you to the correct option. Note that option 3 is the only option that addresses the client's coping skills. This relationship should direct you to option 3. Review care to the client with anorexia nervosa if you had difficulty with this question.

Level of Cognitive Ability: Analysis
Client Needs: Psychosocial Integrity
Integrated Concept/Process: Nursing Process/Data Collection
Content Area: Mental Health

Reference:
Varcarolis, E. (2002). *Foundations of psychiatric mental health nursing* (4th ed.). Philadelphia: W.B. Saunders, p. 420.

---

210. A licensed practical nurse (LPN) is assisting a forensic psychiatric nurse in conducting a group session for female offender clients. Which of the following

Answer: 1
Rationale: The most useful survival skills for female offender clients in a group session would include effective problem-solving and coping skills to enhance the ability to manage stress.

would the LPN identify as a priority and plan to suggest to include in the group session with these clients?

1 Coping skills and stress management
2 Medication education
3 Self-defense skills
4 Psychodrama

Option 2 is incorrect because these clients do not normally receive medication. Option 3 is incorrect, although self-defense skills used to channel aggressive drive appropriately may be useful. Option 4 may be used to assist clients to express their feelings more appropriately but would not be a priority.

Test-Taking Strategy: Use the process of elimination. Focus on the issue, female offender clients, to direct you to option 1. If you had difficulty with this question, review the types of therapy described in the options and their uses.

Level of Cognitive Ability: Analysis
Client Needs: Psychosocial Integrity
Integrated Concept/Process: Nursing Process/Planning
Content Area: Mental Health

Reference:
Varcarolis, E. (2002). *Foundations of psychiatric mental health nursing* (4th ed.). Philadelphia: W.B. Saunders, p. 946.

---

211. A 67-year-old white male arrives at the emergency room complaining of increased anxiety and a sense of being "directionless" and "of no use to anyone." The client has recently retired from his job as a longshoreman. In planning for his care, the nurse knows that the client is suffering from a:

1 Situational crisis
2 Maturational crisis
3 Adventitious crisis
4 Nonspecific crisis

Answer: 2
Rationale: Maturational crises involve developmental crises at any transition point in life, such as marriage, pregnancy, or retirement. Situational crises are adverse happenings that disturb a person's functioning, such as death of a loved one, divorce, or illness. Adventitious crises involve unexpected accidents, such as floods or earthquakes. A nonspecific crisis is unrelated to this situation.

Test-Taking Strategy: Use the process of elimination. Note the key words in the question, *67-year-old* and *recently retired*. This should assist in directing you to option 2, maturational crisis. Review the types of crises if you had difficulty with this question.

Cognitive Level of Ability: Comprehension
Client Needs: Psychosocial Integrity
Integrated Concept/Process: Nursing Process/Planning
Content Area: Mental Health

Reference:
Varcarolis, E. (2002). *Foundations of psychiatric mental health nursing* (4th ed.). Philadelphia: W.B. Saunders, p. 617.

---

212. A client has been admitted to the hospital with a diagnosis of social phobia disorder. Which of the following behaviors would the nurse expect the client to exhibit?

1 Panic attack when leaving the house
2 Shortness of breath and palpitations when riding the elevator
3 Persistent hand washing before eating dinner

Answer: 4
Rationale: A social phobia is characterized by a fear of appearing stupid or inept in the presence of others and of doing something embarrassing. Thus the client becomes anxious when the attention is on him or her. Option 1 identifies agoraphobia, option 2 identifies claustrophobia, and option 3 identifies obsessive-compulsive behavior.

Test-Taking Strategy: Use the process of elimination and knowledge about the various types of phobias to answer this question. Focus on the key words *social phobia*. This should help

4   Fear of being humiliated in public, fear of speaking in public, and, specifically, fear of embarrassing self in front of others

direct you to the correct option. Review the characteristics of the various phobias if you had difficulty with this question.

Level of Cognitive Ability: Comprehension
Client Needs: Psychosocial Integrity
Integrated Concept/Process: Nursing Process/Data Collection
Content Area: Mental Health

Reference:
Varcarolis, E. (2002). *Foundations of psychiatric mental health nursing* (4th ed.). Philadelphia: W.B. Saunders, p. 311.

---

213. A client with aldosteronism has developed renal failure and says to the nurse, "This means that I will die very soon." The most appropriate response by the nurse is:
1   " Why do you feel this way?"
2   "You will do just fine."
3   "You sound discouraged today."
4   "I read that death is a beautiful experience"

Answer: 3
Rationale: Option 3 uses the therapeutic communication technique of reflection, and it clarifies and encourages further expression of the client's feelings. Option 1 may cause defensiveness and block communication. Options 2 and 4 avoid the client's concerns and provide false reassurance.

Test-Taking Strategy: Use the process of elimination. Remember to identify the use of communication blocks, such as the use of cliché, false reassurance, and requesting an explanation. Also, avoid the use of the word *why* when communicating with the client. Option 3 facilitates the client's expression of feelings. Review therapeutic communication techniques if you had difficulty with this question.

Level of Cognitive Ability: Application
Client Needs: Psychosocial Integrity
Integrated Concept/Process: Communication and Documentation
Content Area: Adult Health/Endocrine

Reference:
Potter, P., & Perry, A. (2001). *Fundamentals of nursing* (5th ed.). St. Louis: Mosby, p. 459.

---

214. A nurse is planning activities for a client who is severely depressed. Which of the following activities would be most appropriate to plan for this client?
1   Playing cards with the nurse
2   Role-playing during a group activity
3   Dance therapy
4   Ping-Pong with another client

Answer: 1
Rationale: When the client is severely depressed, the client should be involved in quiet one-to-one activities. Because concentration is impaired when the client is severely depressed, this strategy maximizes the potential for interacting and may minimize anxiety levels.

Test-Taking Strategy: Use the process of elimination. Note the key words *severely depressed*. Also note the words *with the nurse* in the correct option. The activities identified in options 2, 3, and 4 indicate interaction with individuals other than the nurse. If you had difficulty with this question, review care of the client who is severely depressed.

Level of Cognitive Ability: Comprehension
Client Needs: Psychosocial Integrity
Integrated Concept/Process: Nursing Process/Planning
Content Area: Mental Health

Reference:
Bauer, B., & Hill, S. (2000). *Mental health nursing.* Philadelphia: W.B. Saunders, p. 276.

---

215. A nurse is developing a plan of care for a client with depression and a problem with consuming adequate nutrition. Which of the following initial nursing interventions would the nurse include in the plan of care?

1 Offer low-calorie, high-protein snacks frequently throughout the day and evening

2 Offer high-protein, low-calorie fluids frequently throughout the day and evening

3 Allow the client to eat alone if the client prefers to do so

4 Ask the client to identify preferred foods and drinks

Answer: 4

Rationale: It is important to ask the client to identify preferred foods and drinks and to offer choices when possible. The client is more likely to eat the foods provided if choices are offered. The client should be offered high-calorie, high-protein fluids and snacks frequently throughout the day and evening. When possible, the nurse should remain with the client during meals. This strategy reinforces the idea that someone cares, can raise the client's self-esteem, and can serve as an incentive to eat.

Test-Taking Strategy: Use the process of elimination and note the key word *initial*. Eliminate options 1 and 2 first because they are similar. From the remaining options, recalling the basic principles related to nutrition and the importance of offering the client choices will direct you to option 4. Review effective measures related to the client with a problem with nutrition if you had difficulty with this question.

Level of Cognitive Ability: Application
Client Needs: Psychosocial Integrity
Integrated Concept/Process: Nursing Process/Implementation
Content Area: Mental Health

Reference:
Bauer, B., & Hill, S. (2000). *Mental health nursing.* Philadelphia: W.B. Saunders, p. 277.

---

216. A nurse is assigned to care for a client with depression. The nurse reviews the client's health record and notes documentation of a sleep pattern disturbance related to insomnia. Which of the following nursing interventions should be included in the plan of care?

1 Avoid rest periods after activities

2 Allow the client alone and quiet time before bedtime

3 Encourage the client to exercise before bedtime

4 Encourage the client to get up and dress and stay out of bed during the day

Answer: 4

Rationale: The client should be provided rest periods after activities during the day because fatigue can intensify feelings of depression. The nurse should spend more time with the client before bedtime because this intervention helps allay anxiety and increases feelings of security. Reduced environmental and physical stimuli should be provided in the evening, such as soft lights, soft music, and quiet activities. Exercise should be avoided before bedtime. The client should be encouraged to get up and dress and stay out of bed during the day because this routine minimizes sleep during the day and increases the likelihood of sleep at night.

Test-Taking Strategy: Use the process of elimination. Eliminate option 1 first because rest after activities is an important measure to avoid fatigue. Eliminate option 3 next because exercise before bedtime will cause additional stimulation. From the remaining options, focus on the issue of the question, insomnia. This will direct you to option 4. Review measures to promote rest and sleep in the client with depression if you had difficulty with this question.

Level of Cognitive Ability: Application
Client Needs: Psychosocial Integrity

Integrated Concept/Process: Nursing Process/Planning
Content Area: Mental Health

Reference:
Varcarolis, E. (2002). *Foundations of psychiatric mental health nursing* (4th ed.). Philadelphia: W.B. Saunders, p. 468.

---

217. A nurse is assigned to care for a client with mania. The nurse reviews the client's health record and notes documentation of a self-care deficit related to excessive hyperactivity. Which of the following would the nurse avoid when caring for the client?
1   Allow the client to select the clothes to wear
2   Give simple step-by-step reminders for hygiene and dress
3   Put the toothpaste on the brush for the client to brush the teeth
4   Hand the client the washcloth and instruct the client to wash the face

Answer: 1
Rationale: The nurse should supervise the choice of clothes, minimizing flamboyant and bizarre dress. The nurse should give simple step-by-step reminders for hygiene and dress and assist the client with specific directions regarding hygiene care. Distractibility and poor concentration in the manic client are countered by simple concrete instructions. Supervising the choice of clothing lessens the potential for ridicule when inappropriate dress is selected by the manic client. Ridicule lowers self-esteem and increases the need for manic defense.

Test-Taking Strategy: Use the process of elimination. Note the key word *avoid*. Note that options 2, 3, and 4 are similar in that they identify specific interventions in which the nurse assists the client. Review care related to self-care deficit in the manic client if you had difficulty with this question.

Level of Cognitive Ability: Application
Client Needs: Psychosocial Integrity
Integrated Concept/Process: Nursing Process/Implementation
Content Area: Mental Health

Reference:
Bauer, B., & Hill, S. (2000). *Mental health nursing.* Philadelphia: W.B. Saunders, p. 255.

---

218. The multidisciplinary health care team is developing a plan of care for a manic client. Which of the following medications would the nurse anticipate to be prescribed for the client?
1   Lithium carbonate (Eskalith)
2   Amitriptyline (Elavil)
3   Imipramine (Tofranil)
4   Trimipramine (Surmontil)

Answer: 1
Rationale: Lithium carbonate is the medication of choice for treating the manic phase of a bipolar disorder. It is a mood stabilizer and is the prototypical antimanic medication. It can calm manic clients, prevent or modify future manic episodes, and prevent future depressive episodes. The medications identified in options 2, 3, and 4 are tricyclic antidepressants used in the treatment of depression.

Test-Taking Strategy: Knowledge regarding the pharmacological treatment of manic disorders is required to answer this question. If you had difficulty with this question, review this medication and this disorder.

Level of Cognitive Ability: Comprehension
Client Needs: Psychosocial Integrity
Integrated Concept/Process: Nursing Process/Planning
Content Area: Pharmacology

Reference:
Hodgson, B., & Kizior, R. (2003). *Saunders nursing drug handbook 2003.* Philadelphia: W.B. Saunders, p. 670.

219. A nurse has reinforced discharge instructions with a client taking lithium carbonate (Eskalith). Which of the following client statements would indicate a need for further instructions?
1 "I should take the medication with my meals."
2 "I should avoid taking over-the-counter medications unless I check with my doctor first."
3 "I should lower my salt intake while taking the medication."
4 "I should have my blood levels checked frequently."

Answer: 3
Rationale: A normal diet and normal salt and fluid intake should be maintained while the client is on lithium. This agent decreases sodium reabsorption by the renal tubules, which could cause sodium depletion. A low-sodium intake causes a relative increase in lithium retention, which could lead to toxicity. The client should avoid taking any over-the-counter medications without checking first with the physician. Lithium is irritating to the gastric mucosa; therefore, the client should take the medication with meals. Because therapeutic and toxic dosage ranges are so close, lithium blood levels must be monitored very closely, more frequently at first, then once every several months thereafter.

Test-Taking Strategy: Use the process of elimination. Note the key words *need for further instructions*. Option 2 can be easily eliminated using basic principles related to medication administration. Knowledge that periodic blood levels need to be obtained will easily eliminate option 4. From the remaining options, recalling the relationship between a low-salt intake and lithium toxicity will easily direct you to option 3. Review teaching points related to lithium carbonate if you had difficulty with this question.

Level of Cognitive Ability: Comprehension
Client Needs: Psychosocial Integrity
Integrated Concept/Process: Teaching/Learning
Content Area: Pharmacology

Reference:
Hodgson, B., & Kizior, R. (2003). *Saunders nursing drug handbook 2003.* Philadelphia: W.B. Saunders, pp. 671-672.

220. A nurse is reviewing the record of a client with a diagnosis of schizophrenia and notes that the health care provider has documented that the client is thought-blocking. The nurse plans care for the client knowing that which of the following best describes this characteristic?
1 The client stops talking in the middle of a sentence
2 Speech is restricted in amount, consisting of brief, often monosyllabic or one-word answers
3 Speech is adequate in amount but conveys little information because of vagueness, empty repetitions, or the use of stereotypes or obscure phrases
4 Speech is adequate in amount but is unclear

Answer: 1
Rationale: Thought-blocking occurs when a client stops talking in the middle of a sentence and remains quiet. Poverty of speech occurs when there is a restriction in the amount of speech and answers consist of brief, often monosyllabic or one-word answers. Speech that is adequate in amount but conveys little information because of vagueness, empty repetitions, or the use of stereotypes or obscure phrases is described as poverty of content of speech.

Test-Taking Strategy: Use the process of elimination. Eliminate options 3 and 4 first because they are similar. From the remaining options, use the words *thought-blocking* to help direct you to option 1. Review client behaviors in schizophrenia if you had difficulty with this question.

Level of Cognitive Ability: Comprehension
Client Needs: Psychosocial Integrity
Integrated Concept/Process: Nursing Process/Planning
Content Area: Mental Health

Reference:
Bauer, B., & Hill, S. (2000). *Mental health nursing.* Philadelphia: W.B. Saunders, p. 271.

221. A nurse is giving a male client who recently suffered a myocardial infarction (MI) discharge instructions. The client tells the nurse that he is afraid that he can't go back to a normal life. The nurse would most effectively lessen the client's fear by:
1 Telling the client that his fears are not rational
2 Telling the client that his life has not changed
3 Acknowledging the client's fears and providing the client with information about a support group
4 Telling the client to talk it out with his significant other

Answer: 3

Rationale: A heart attack is a frightening experience. With this in mind, remember that the client and the family will need much help and support as they make the necessary adjustments. Option 3 lets the client know that the nurse has heard what the client said, acknowledges the client's feelings, and provides assistance. Options 1 and 2 are incorrect because the nurse does not acknowledge the client's concern. Similarly, option 4 avoids the client's concern.

Test-Taking Strategy: Use the process of elimination and therapeutic communication techniques to answer the question. Option 3 is the only option that addresses the client's concerns. Review therapeutic communication techniques if you had difficulty with this question.

Level of Cognitive Ability: Application
Client Needs: Psychosocial Integrity
Integrated Concept/Process: Nursing Process/Implementation
Content Area: Adult Health/Cardiovascular

Reference:
Potter, P., & Perry, A. (2001). *Fundamentals of nursing* (5th ed.). St. Louis: Mosby, p. 459.

222. A paranoid client says to the nurse, "The FBI is trying to harm me." Which of the following responses by the nurse would be most appropriate?
1 "The FBI is not going to harm you."
2 "You are in the hospital so you are safe from the FBI."
3 "I don't know about the FBI trying to harm you, but thinking that must be frightening."
4 "You're having auditory hallucinations at this time; the FBI will not hurt you."

Answer: 3

Rationale: When caring for the client with disturbed thought processes, the nurse needs to look for feelings behind the delusions and hallucinations. The client cannot logically discuss illogical material but perhaps can discuss feelings. The best response is option 3 because it addresses the client's feeling and reinforces reality.

Test-Taking Strategy: Use therapeutic communication techniques to answer the question. Options 1, 2, and 4 reinforce the client's belief that harm will occur. Option 3 is the only option that reinforces reality therapeutically. Review therapeutic communication techniques for the client experiencing altered thought processes if you had difficulty with this question.

Level of Cognitive Ability: Application
Client Needs: Psychosocial Integrity
Integrated Concept/Process: Communication and Documentation
Content Area: Mental Health

Reference:
Bauer, B., & Hill, S. (2000). *Mental health nursing.* Philadelphia: W.B. Saunders, p. 59.

223. A nurse is caring for a client with a diagnosis of anorexia nervosa. The nurse collects data from the client knowing that which of the following is not a characteristic of this disorder?

Answer: 3

Rationale: Anorexia nervosa is an eating disorder characterized by a determination to lose weight mainly by restricting food intake, even when emaciated. It generally occurs in young adults who have distorted views of the body's shape and weight and the self.

1 The client believes that control and autonomy will be experienced through dieting

2 The client has a distorted view of the body

3 The disorder is characterized by eating binges followed by maladaptive or inappropriate reparative behavior

4 The client is determined to lose weight mainly by restricting food intake, even when emaciated

Through dieting and weight loss, these persons believe they will experience control, autonomy, and competence. Bulimia nervosa is characterized by eating binges followed by maladaptive or inappropriate reparative behaviors, such as dieting and purging occurring at least two times each week for 3 or more months.

Test-Taking Strategy: Use the process of elimination. Note the key word *not* in the question. Recalling that eating binges occur in the client with bulimia nervosa will direct you to option 3 as the answer to this question. If you had difficulty with this question, review the characteristics of anorexia nervosa and bulimia nervosa.

Level of Cognitive Ability: Comprehension
Client Needs: Psychosocial Integrity
Integrated Concept/Process: Nursing Process/Data Collection
Content Area: Mental Health

Reference:
Bauer, B., & Hill, S. (2000). *Mental health nursing.* Philadelphia: W.B. Saunders, p. 174.

---

224. A nurse is assisting in developing a plan of care for a client with anorexia nervosa. Which of the following would be the most desirable goal for the client?
1 A daily weight gain of ¼ to ½ pound
2 A daily weight gain of 1 pound
3 A weekly weight gain of 5 pounds
4 A weekly weight gain of 7 pounds

Answer: 1
Rationale: A desirable target weight should be discussed with the client. Daily weight gains of ¼ to ½ pound are generally acceptable for the emaciated client. In the client with bulimia, weight stabilization without binge-purge behavior is expected.

Test-Taking Strategy: Use the process of elimination and knowledge regarding the basics related to nutrition and weight gain to direct you to option 1. Options 2, 3, and 4 can be easily eliminated because the amounts of weight gain are excessive. Also note that options 2 and 4 are similar. If you had difficulty with this question, review nutrition related to the client with anorexia nervosa.

Level of Cognitive Ability: Application
Client Needs: Psychosocial Integrity
Integrated Concept/Process: Nursing Process/Planning
Content Area: Mental Health

Reference:
Bauer, B., & Hill, S. (2000). *Mental health nursing.* Philadelphia: W.B. Saunders, p. 175.

---

225. A licensed practical nurse (LPN) is assisting in developing a plan of care for the client with anorexia nervosa. The registered nurse has formulated a nursing diagnosis of powerlessness. Which of the following goals would the LPN suggest for this client?
1 Client establishes healthy eating habits to achieve normal body weight

Answer: 3
Rationale: With a diagnosis of powerlessness, the most appropriate client goal would be that the client verbalizes an increased sense of control over self. The client should practice beginning assertive behavior skills, and should view the weight maintenance diet as evidence of self-control. Options 1, 2, and 4 are not directly related to powerlessness.

Test-Taking Strategy: Use the process of elimination. Note the relationship between *powerlessness* in the question and *sense of*

2 Client begins to implement a problem-solving approach to increase coping ability

3 Client verbalizes an increased sense of control over self

4 Client and family demonstrate increased efforts to clarify and resolve issues

control in the correct option. If you had difficulty with this question, review goals for the client with anorexia nervosa and powerlessness.

Level of Cognitive Ability: Analysis
Client Needs: Psychosocial Integrity
Integrated Concept/Process: Nursing Process/Planning
Content Area: Mental Health

Reference:
Bauer, B., & Hill, S. (2000). *Mental health nursing.* Philadelphia: W.B. Saunders, p. 175.

FILL-IN-THE-BLANK

A nurse is assisting in performing a physical assessment of an a 8-year-old child and notes the presence of swelling and lacerations in the genital area. The child is hesitant to answers questions that the nurse is asking and consistently looks at the mother in a fearful manner. The nurse suspects that the child is a victim of which type of abuse?
Answer: _____

Answer: Sexual abuse
Rationale: The most likely assessment findings in sexual abuse include difficulty walking or sitting; torn, stained or bloody underclothing; pain, swelling or itching of the genitals; and bruises, bleeding, or lacerations in the genital or anal area.

Test-Taking Strategy: Focus on the assessment findings noted in the question and on the issue, the type of abuse suspected. Noting the key words "swelling and lacerations in the genital area" will assist in answering the question. If you had difficulty with this question, review the assessment findings in a child suspected of sexual abuse.

Level of Cognitive Ability: Analysis
Client Needs: Psychosocial Integrity
Integrated Concept/Process: Nursing Process/Data Collection
Content Area: Mental Health

Reference:
Stuart, G. & Laraia, M. (2001). *Principles and practice of psychiatric nursing* (7th ed.). St. Louis: Mosby, p. 833.

MULTIPLE RESPONSE – SELECT ALL THAT APPLY

A nurse is caring for a client who is at risk for violent behavior. Select all interventions that will assist in preventing violent behavior if the client becomes agitated.
____ Speak in a calm low voice
____ Use short simple sentences
____ Maintain direct eye contact
____ Avoid laughing and smiling inappropriately
____ Avoid acknowledging the client's feelings

Answer:
____ Speak in a calm low voice
____ Use short simple sentences
____ Avoid laughing and smiling inappropriately
____ Assume a supportive stance that is at least 3 feet from the client

Rationale: Speaking to the client in a calm, low voice can help to decrease the client's agitation. Agitated clients often speak loudly and use profanity. It is important that nurses not respond by raising their voices because doing so will probably be perceived as

____ Face the client with the arms across the chest so that the client will be assured that the nurse is in control of the situation

____ Assume a supportive stance that is at least 3 feet from the client

competition and will further escalate a volatile situation. The nurse should use short, simple sentences and avoid laughing and smiling inappropriately. The nurse can help reduce agitation by acknowledging the client's feelings and reassuring the client that the staff is there to help. A posture that avoids intimidation should be assumed by the nurse. Placing the hands on the hips and crossing the arms across the chest are intimidating and communicate emotional distance and an unwillingness to help. The nurse should avoid intense direct eye contact. However, altering position so that the nurse's eyes are at the same level as those of the client's allows the client to communicate from an equal rather than an inferior position. In addition, the nurse should assume a supportive stance that is at least 3 feet from the client because intrusion into a client's personal space can be perceived as a threat and provoke aggression and violence.

Test-Taking Strategy: Focus on the issue: preventing violent behavior. Recalling that interventions are aimed at strengthening the therapeutic alliance with the client will assist in identifying the correct interventions. Review these interventions if you had difficulty with this question.

Level of Cognitive Ability: Application
Client Needs: Psychosocial Integrity
Integrated Concept/Process: Nursing Process/Implementation
Content Area: Mental Health

Reference:
Stuart, G. & Laraia, M. (2001). *Principles and practice of psychiatric nursing* (7th ed.). St. Louis: Mosby, pp. 645-646.

REFERENCES

Bauer, B., & Hill, S. (2000). *Mental health nursing.* Philadelphia: W.B. Saunders.

Black, J., Hawks, J., & Keene, A. (2001). *Medical-surgical nursing: clinical management for positive outcomes* (6th ed.). Philadelphia: W.B. Saunders.

Burroughs, A., & Leifer, G. (2002). *Maternity nursing* (8th ed.). Philadelphia: W.B. Saunders.

deWit, S. (2001). *Fundamental concepts and skills for nursing.* Philadelphia: W.B. Saunders.

Hodgson, B. & Kizior, R. (2003). *Saunders nursing drug handbook 2003.* Philadelphia: W.B. Saunders.

Ignatavicius, D., & Workman, M. (2002). *Medical-surgical nursing: critical thinking for collaborative care* (4th ed.). Philadelphia: W.B. Saunders.

Johnson, M., Bulechek, G., Dochterman, J. et al. (2001). *Nursing diagnoses, outcomes, and interventions.* St. Louis: Mosby.

Lehne, R., (2001). *Pharmacology for nursing care* (4th ed.). Philadelphia: W.B. Saunders.

McKinney, E., Ashwill, J., Murray, S. et al. (2000). *Maternal-child nursing.* Philadelphia: W.B Saunders.

Murray, S., McKinney, E., & Gorrie, T. (2002). *Foundations of maternal-newborn nursing* (3rd ed.). Philadelphia: W.B. Saunders.

Potter, P., & Perry, A. (2001). *Fundamentals of nursing* (5th ed.). St. Louis: Mosby.

Schulte, E. Price, D., & Gwin, J. (2001). *Thompson's pediatric nursing* (8th ed.). Philadelphia: W.B. Saunders.

Stone, S., McGuire, S., & Eigsti, D. (2002). *Comprehensive Community health nursing* (6th ed.). St. Louis: Mosby.

Stuart, G., & Laraia, M. (2001). *Principles and practice of psychiatric nursing* (7th ed.). St. Louis: Mosby.

Varcarolis, E. (2002). *Foundations of psychiatric mental health nursing* (4th ed.). Philadelphia: W.B. Saunders.

Wong, D., & Hockenberry-Eaton, M. (2001). *Wong's essentials of pediatric nursing* (6th ed.). St. Louis: Mosby.

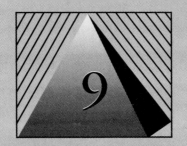

Physiological Integrity

---

1. A client with multiple sclerosis is being treated with diazepam (Valium) for painful muscle spasms. The nurse monitors the client knowing that a common side effect of diazepam is:

1 Urinary frequency
2 Headache
3 Increased salivation
4 Incoordination

Answer: 4
Rationale: Diazepam is a centrally acting skeletal muscle relaxant. Incoordination and drowsiness are common side effects resulting from the large doses of the medication that must be used to achieve desired effects. Options 1, 2, and 3 are not side effects.

Test-Taking Strategy: Use the process of elimination. Recalling that diazepam is used for muscle spasms directs you to think that this medication relaxes muscles. The only option that directly relates to this medication action is option 4. Review the action and side effects of this medication if you had difficulty with this question.

Level of Cognitive Ability: Comprehension
Client Needs: Physiological Integrity
Integrated Concept/Process: Nursing Process/Data Collection
Content Area: Pharmacology

Reference:
Hodgson, B., & Kizior, R. (2003). *Saunders nursing drug handbook 2003.* Philadelphia: W.B. Saunders, p. 336.

---

2. A client with epilepsy is taking the prescribed dose of phenytoin (Dilantin) to control seizures. A dilantin blood level is drawn and the nurse is told that the results reveal a level of 35 μg/mL. The nurse expects to note which of the following as a result of this laboratory result?

1 No effect. This is a normal therapeutic level
2 Lethargy
3 Tachycardia
4 Nystagmus

Answer: 2
Rationale: The therapeutic dilantin level is 10 to 20 μg/mL. Blood levels of phenytoin above 30 μg/mL produce lethargy.

Test-Taking Strategy: Knowledge regarding the normal dilantin level and the signs that occur in the client when the level rises is necessary to answer this question. Review this content if you had difficulty with this question.

Level of Cognitive Ability: Analysis
Client Needs: Physiological Integrity
Integrated Concept/Process: Nursing Process/Data Collection
Content Area: Pharmacology

Reference:
Hodgson, B., & Kizior, R. (2003). *Saunders nursing drug handbook 2003.* Philadelphia: W.B. Saunders, p. 891.

---

3. To reduce the risk of aspiration, the best position in which to place the child with cleft palate repair after feeding is which of the following?
1 On the right side
2 On the left side
3 Supine
4 Prone

Answer: 1
Rationale: The child with cleft palate repair is placed on the right side after feeding to reduce the chance of aspirating regurgitated formula. Options 2, 3, and 4 are incorrect positions.

Test-Taking Strategy: Use the process of elimination. Visualize the anatomical location of the stomach in answering this question. This assists in eliminating options 3 and 4. From the remaining options, remember that positioning on the right side aids in absorption and reduces the risk of aspiration. Review care of the child after this surgical procedure if you had difficulty with this question.

Level of Cognitive Ability: Application
Client Needs: Physiological Integrity
Integrated Concept/Process: Nursing Process/Implementation
Content Area: Child Health

Reference:
Wong, D., & Hockenberry-Eaton, M. (2001). *Wong's essentials of pediatric nursing* (6th ed.). St. Louis: Mosby, p. 915.

---

4. A nurse is assigned to care for a child with a diagnosis of hemophilia. The nurse reviews the child's health record and expects that which laboratory result will most likely be abnormal?
1 Bleeding time
2 Sedimentation rate
3 Clot retraction time
4 Partial thromboplastin time (PTT)

Answer: 4
Rationale: PTT measures the activity of thromboplastin, which is dependent on intrinsic factors. The intrinsic clotting factor VIII (antihemophilic factor) is deficient in hemophilia, resulting in a prolonged PTT. Options 1, 2, and 3 are not necessarily abnormal.

Test-Taking Strategy: Knowledge regarding the laboratory tests used to monitor hemophilia is necessary to answer this question. Review these laboratory tests if you had difficulty with this question.

Level of Cognitive Ability: Comprehension
Client Needs: Physiological Integrity
Integrated Concept/Process: Nursing Process/Data Collection
Content Area: Child Health

Reference:
Schulte, E., Price, D., & Gwin, J. (2001). *Thompson's pediatric nursing* (8th ed.). Philadelphia: W.B. Saunders, p. 235.

---

5. A nurse assigned to assist in caring for a client after a gastric resection is monitoring the drainage from a nasogastric (NG) tube. No drainage has been noted during the past 4 hours, and the client complains of severe nausea. The most appropriate nursing action would be which of the following?

Answer: 3
Rationale: Nausea and vomiting should not occur if the NG tube is patent. The NG tube should not be repositioned after gastric surgery because it is placed directly over the suture line. Only with a physician's order may the RN gently irrigate the NG tube with saline. In this situation, the RN should be notified.

1 Reposition the tube
2 Irrigate the tube
3 Notify the RN
4 Medicate for nausea

Test-Taking Strategy: Use the process of elimination. Note that this client had a surgical procedure that involved the gastric area. Additionally, recall that a nasogastric tube is placed near the surgical site. Note the key words *severe nausea*. This should alert you that the RN needs to be notified. Review postoperative nursing care after gastric surgery if you had difficulty with this question.

Level of Cognitive Ability: Application
Client Needs: Physiological Integrity
Integrated Concept/Process: Nursing Process/Implementation
Content Area: Adult Health/Gastrointestinal

Reference:
Ignatavicius, D., & Workman, M. (2002). *Medical-surgical nursing: critical thinking for collaborative care* (4th ed.). Philadelphia: W.B. Saunders, p. 1210.

---

6. A client with diabetes mellitus who takes insulin is receiving prenatal care. The nurse teaches the client about the early signs of hyperglycemia. The nurse evaluates that the teaching is effective when the client states that an early sign of hyperglycemia is which of the following?
1 Polyuria
2 Nervousness
3 Shakiness
4 Hunger

Answer: 1
Rationale: Polyuria is an early sign of hyperglycemia. Other signs can include polydipsia, polyphagia, dry mouth, increased appetite, fatigue, nausea, hot flushed skin, rapid deep breathing, abdominal cramps, acetone breath, headache, drowsiness, depressed reflexes, oliguria or anuria, stupor, and coma. Options 2, 3, and 4 are signs of hypoglycemia.

Test-Taking Strategy: Use the process of elimination. Options 2 and 3 are signs of hypoglycemia; they are similar and should be eliminated first. Recalling that hunger also is a sign of hypoglycemia assists in eliminating option 4. Review the signs of both hypoglycemia and hyperglycemia if you had difficulty with this question.

Level of Cognitive Ability: Comprehension
Client Needs: Physiological Integrity
Integrated Concept/Process: Nursing Process/Evaluation
Content Area: Maternity

Reference:
McKinney, E., Ashwill, J., Murray, S., James, S., Gorrie, T., & Droske, S. (2000). *Maternal-child nursing.* Philadelphia: W.B. Saunders, p. 1450.

---

7. An older female client is brought to the emergency room by a family member with whom she lives. The nurse notes that the client has poor hygiene, contractures, and decubitus ulcers on the sacrum, scapula, and heels. The nurse suspects that the client is a victim of which of the following?
1 Emotional abuse
2 Physical abuse
3 Psychological abuse
4 Sexual abuse

Answer: 2
Rationale: Victimization in the family takes many forms. When collecting data regarding a specific client situation, it is important to understand which form of abuse is being considered. Physical abuse can take the form of battering (hitting, slapping, striking), or can be more subtle, such as neglect (failure to meet basic needs). The data in the question do not indicate emotional, psychological, or sexual abuse.

Test-Taking Strategy: Use the process of elimination and focus on the data provided in the question. Option 2 in the only option that addresses the data in the question. Review signs of physical abuse if you had difficulty with this question.

Level of Cognitive Ability: Comprehension
Client Needs: Physiological Integrity
Integrated Concept/Process: Nursing Process/Data Collection
Content Area: Mental Health

Reference:
Bauer, B., & Hill, S. (2000). *Mental health nursing.* Philadelphia: W.B. Saunders,
  p. 206.

---

8. A client recovering from a craniotomy complains of a "runny nose." The most important nursing action in this situation is which of the following?
   1   Provide the client with tissues
   2   Tell the client to pat the drainage with the tissue
   3   Monitor the client for signs of a cold
   4   Notify the RN

Answer: 4
Rationale: If the client has sustained a craniocerebral injury or is recovering from a craniotomy, careful observation of any drainage from the eyes, ears, nose, or traumatic area is critical. Cerebrospinal fluid is colorless and generally nonpurulent, and its presence indicates a serious breach of cranial integrity. Any suspicious drainage should be reported immediately. Options 1, 2, and 3 are inappropriate nursing actions.

Test-Taking Strategy: Use the process of elimination and note the key words *most important*. This should provide you with the clue that there is a serious nature to the situation presented. Eliminate options 1 and 2 because they are similar. From the remaining options, recalling the signs of complications associated with craniotomy should assist in directing you to option 4. Review postoperative nursing care after craniotomy if you had difficulty with this question.

Level of Cognitive Ability: Application
Client Needs: Physiological Integrity
Integrated Concept/Process: Nursing Process/Implementation
Content Area: Adult Health/Neurological

Reference:
Ignatavicius, D., & Workman, M. (2002). *Medical-surgical nursing: critical thinking for collaborative care* (4th ed.). Philadelphia: W.B. Saunders, p. 1004.

---

9. A nurse is assigned to assist in caring for a client who has returned from the postanesthesia care unit after prostatectomy. The client has a three-way catheter with infusion of continuous bladder irrigation. The nurse determines that the flow rate is adequate if the color of the urinary drainage is which of the following?
   1   Dark cherry
   2   Concentrated yellow with small clots
   3   Clear as water
   4   Pale yellow or slightly pink

Answer: 4
Rationale: The infusion of bladder irrigant is not at a preset rate, but rather is increased or decreased to maintain urine that is a clear, pale, yellow color or that has just a slight pink tinge. The infusion rate should be increased if the drainage is cherry colored or if clots are seen. Correspondingly, the rate can be slowed down slightly if the returns are as clear as water.

Test-Taking Strategy: Use the process of elimination and eliminate option 2 as the least realistic of the described urine characteristics. Next, eliminate options 1 and 3 as reflecting inadequate and excessive flow, respectively. The urine should be pale yellow or pale pink with the proper flow rate of bladder irrigant. Review postoperative expectations after prostatectomy if you had difficulty with this question.

Level of Cognitive Ability: Comprehension
Client Needs: Physiological Integrity

Integrated Concept/Process: Nursing Process/Evaluation
Content Area: Adult Health/Renal

Reference:
Ignatavicius, D., & Workman, M. (2002). *Medical-surgical: critical thinking for collaborative care* (4th ed.). Philadelphia: W.B. Saunders, p. 1792.

---

10. A nurse is teaching a client with asthma how to use a peak flow meter. The nurse should tell the client which of the following?

1   Inhale an average-size breath
2   Form a loose seal with the mouth around the mouthpiece
3   Blow out as slowly as possible
4   Record the final position of the indicator

Answer: 4
Rationale: A peak flow meter is used to give an objective measure of the client's peak expiratory flow. The client is instructed to take the deepest possible breath, form a tight seal around the mouthpiece with the lips, and exhale forcefully and rapidly. The final position of the indicator on the meter is recorded.

Test-Taking Strategy: To answer this question correctly, it is necessary to be familiar with this piece of equipment and its use. Visualize the use of this piece of equipment to direct you to option 4. Review this commonly used device, which may be used to determine when medication adjustments are needed, if you had difficulty with this question.

Level of Cognitive Ability: Application
Client Needs: Physiological Integrity
Integrated Concept/Process: Teaching/Learning
Content Area: Adult Health/Respiratory

Reference:
Black, J., Hawks, J., & Keene, A. (2001). *Medical-surgical nursing: clinical management for positive outcomes* (6th ed.). Philadelphia: W.B. Saunders, p. 1639.

---

11. A mother of a child with celiac disease asks how long a special diet is necessary for the child. The nurse would most appropriately tell the mother which of the following?

1   A gluten-free diet must be followed for life
2   Adequate nutritional status helps to prevent celiac crisis
3   Supplemental vitamins, iron, and folate prevent complications
4   A lactose-free diet must be followed temporarily

Answer: 1
Rationale: The main nursing consideration with celiac disease is helping the child adhere to dietary management. Treatment of celiac disease consists primarily of dietary management with a gluten-free diet. Options 2, 3, and 4 are all true statements, but do not answer the mother's question. Children with untreated celiac disease may have lactose intolerance that usually improves with gluten withdrawal. Nutritional deficiencies resulting from malabsorption are treated with appropriate supplements.

Test-Taking Strategy: Use the process of elimination. Focus on the issue of the question about "the length of time a special diet is necessary." This focus directs you to the correct option. If you had difficulty with this question, review dietary requirements for celiac disease.

Level of Cognitive Ability: Application
Client Needs: Physiological Integrity
Integrated Concept/Process: Nursing Process/Implementation
Content Area: Child Health

Reference:
Wong, D., & Hockenberry-Eaton, M. (2001). *Wong's essentials of pediatric nursing* (6th ed.). St. Louis: Mosby, p. 927.

12. When providing the health history, the parents report that their 6-month-old male baby has been screaming and drawing the knees up to the chest. The parents state that the infant is passing jellylike stools mixed with blood and mucus. The nurse recognizes these signs and symptoms as indicating which of the following?
1 Hirschsprung's disease
2 Peritonitis
3 Intussusception
4 Appendicitis

Answer: 3
Rationale: The classic signs and symptoms of intussusception are acute, colicky abdominal pain with currant jellylike stools. Clinical manifestations of Hirschsprung's disease include constipation, abdominal distention, and ribbon-like, foul-smelling stools. Peritonitis is a serious complication that may follow intestinal obstruction and perforation. The most common symptom of appendicitis is colicky periumbilical or lower abdominal pain in the right quadrant.

Test-Taking Strategy: Use the process of elimination and knowledge regarding this disorder to answer the question. Focusing on the data in the question assists in directing you to option 3. If you had difficulty with this question, review the clinical manifestations of intussusception.

Level of Cognitive Ability: Comprehension
Client Needs: Physiological Integrity
Integrated Concept/Process: Nursing Process/Data Collection
Content Area: Child Health

Reference:
Wong, D., & Hockenberry-Eaton, M. (2001). *Wong's essentials of pediatric nursing* (6th ed.). St. Louis: Mosby, p. 923.

13. A nurse is caring for a burn client who has sustained thoracic burns and smoke inhalation and is at risk for impaired gas exchange. The nurse avoids which of the following actions as the least helpful in caring for this client?
1 Reposition the client from side to side every 2 hours
2 Position the client on the back only with the head of the bed at a 45-degree angle
3 Suction the airway on an as-needed basis
4 Provide humidified oxygen and incentive spirometry as prescribed

Answer: 2
Rationale: Aggressive pulmonary measures are used to prevent respiratory complications in the client who has impaired gas exchange as a result of a burn injury. These include turning and repositioning, positioning for comfort, using humidified oxygen, providing incentive spirometry, and suctioning the client on an as-needed basis. The least helpful measure is to keep the client in one single position. This ultimately leads to atelectasis and possible pneumonia.

Test-Taking Strategy: Note the key word *avoids*. This tells you that the answer to the question is an incorrect nursing action. Use basic nursing knowledge of respiratory support measures to eliminate each of the incorrect options. Also, note the word *only* in the correct option. Review these measures if you had difficulty with this question.

Level of Cognitive Ability: Application
Client Needs: Physiological Integrity
Integrated Concept/Process: Nursing Process/Implementation
Content Area: Adult Health/Integumentary

Reference:
Black, J., Hawks, J., & Keene, A. (2001). *Medical-surgical nursing: clinical management for positive outcomes* (6th ed.). Philadelphia: W.B. Saunders, p. 1344.

14. After the delivery of a newborn infant, a nurse assists in performing an initial assessment. The nurse obtains and docu-

Answer: 3
Rationale: One of the earliest indicators of successful adaptation of the newborn is the Apgar score. Scores range from 0 to 10.

ments an Apgar score of 4. This score indicates which of the following?

1 The infant is adjusting well to extrauterine life
2 The infant requires some resuscitative intervention
3 The infant is having difficulty adjusting to extrauterine life
4 This is an inaccurate score that should be immediately repeated

A score of 8 to 10 indicates that the infant is adjusting well to extrauterine life. A score of 4 to 7 often indicates that the infant requires some resuscitative intervention, such as oxygen. A score of less than 4 indicates that the infant is having difficulty adjusting to extrauterine life and requires vigorous resuscitation.

Test-Taking Strategy: Knowledge that Apgar scores range from 0 to 10 assists you in answering this question. Option 4 can be eliminated first. Noting that the score is 4 assists in directing you to option 3 from the remaining options. If you had difficulty with this question, review the Apgar score.

Level of Cognitive Ability: Comprehension
Client Needs: Physiological Integrity
Integrated Concept/Process: Nursing Process/Evaluation
Content Area: Maternity

Reference:
McKinney, E., Ashwill, J., Murray, S., James, S., Gorrie, T., & Droske, S. (2000). *Maternal-child nursing.* Philadelphia: W.B. Saunders, p. 399.

---

15. A client with a history of rheumatic heart disease asks the nurse why the client must tell the dentist about this condition before dental cleaning or other work. The nurse's response is based on the knowledge that:

1 The client is susceptible to reinfection unless prophylactic antibiotic therapy is given before treatment
2 The client is at risk for episodes of heart failure triggered by stressful events
3 The dentist should use a lidocaine solution that does not contain epinephrine
4 The dentist should be aware that the vibration of the drill could cause dysrhythmias

Answer: 1
Rationale: The client with a history of rheumatic heart disease is at risk for developing infective endocarditis. The client notifies all physicians and dentists about the history so prophylactic antibiotic therapy can be given before any invasive procedure, or if there is risk of bleeding.

Test-Taking Strategy: Use the process of elimination. Remember that prophylactic antibiotic treatment before any type of invasive procedure is indicated to prevent an episode of endocarditis. Knowledge of this concept should help you eliminate the incorrect options. Review this content if you had difficulty with this question.

Level of Cognitive Ability: Comprehension
Client Needs: Physiological Integrity
Integrated Concept/Process: Nursing Process/Implementation
Content Area: Adult Health/Cardiovascular

Reference:
Lewis, S., Heitkemper, M., & Dirksen, S. (2000). *Medical-surgical nursing: assessment and management of clinical problems* (5th ed.). St. Louis: Mosby, p. 962.

---

16. A nurse interprets a Mantoux tuberculin skin test as a significant finding. To most accurately diagnose tuberculosis (TB), the nurse should plan to consult with the physician to follow up the skin test with which procedure?

1 Chest radiograph
2 A computerized tomography (CT) scan of the chest
3 Sputum culture
4 Complete blood cell count

Answer: 3
Rationale: Although the findings on chest x-ray examination are important, it is not possible to make a diagnosis of TB solely on the basis of this examination because other diseases can mimic the appearance of TB. The demonstration of tubercle bacilli bacteriologically is essential for establishing a diagnosis. Microscopic examination of stained sputum smears for acid-fast bacilli is usually the first bacteriologic evidence of the presence of tubercle bacilli.

Test-Taking Strategy: Use the process of elimination. The important words in this question are *to most accurately diagnose tuberculosis.*

Analyze the probability of each option being the most accurate method of diagnosing tuberculosis as a follow-up to the Mantoux skin test. Review the tests used in diagnosing TB if you had difficulty with this question.

Level of Cognitive Ability: Application
Client Needs: Physiological Integrity
Integrated Concept/Process: Nursing Process/Planning
Content Area: Adult Health/Respiratory

Reference:
Lewis, S., Heitkemper, M., & Dirksen, S. (2000). *Medical-surgical nursing: assessment and management of clinical problems* (5th ed.). St. Louis: Mosby, p. 624.

---

17. A nurse has an order to suction the airway of an adult client and is using a wall suction unit. The nurse begins the procedure by setting the suction control dial at which of the following levels?
1 150 to 180 mmHg
2 100 to 120 mmHg
3 80 to 100 mmHg
4 50 to 60 mmHg

Answer: 2
Rationale: The correct pressure during suctioning of an adult using a wall suction unit is 120 to 180 mmHg. Correct suction pressure for infants and children is 60 to 110 mmHg.

Test-Taking Strategy: Use the process of elimination and focus on the issue, an adult client. To answer this question accurately, you must know fundamental principles associated with suctioning a client's airway. If this question was difficult, review the essentials of this fundamental nursing procedure.

Level of Cognitive Ability: Application
Client Needs: Physiological Integrity
Integrated Concept/Process: Nursing Process/Implementation
Content Area: Adult Health/Respiratory

Reference:
Perry, A., & Potter, P., (2002). *Clinical nursing skills & techniques* (5th ed.). St. Louis: Mosby, p. 371.

---

18. A nurse is obtaining Apgar scores for an infant immediately after birth. The nurse notes that the heart rate is less than 100 beats per minute (BPM), the respiratory effort is good, muscle tone indicates some extremity flexion, the newborn sneezes when suctioned by the bulb syringe, and the extremities are cyanotic. The nurse would most appropriately document which of the following Apgar scores for the newborn?
1 3
2 5
3 7
4 10

Answer: 3
Rationale: One of the earliest indicators of successful adaptation of the newborn is the Apgar score. Scores range from 0 to 10. The test assesses five areas to measure the infant's adaptation: heart rate (absent = 0; less than 100 BPM = 1; greater than 100 BPM = 2); respiratory effort (absent = 0; slow or irregular weak cry = 1; good, crying lustily = 2); muscle tone (limp or hypotonic = 0; some extremity flexion = 1; active, moving, and well flexed = 2); irritability or reflexes as measured by bulb suctioning (no response = 0; grimace = 1; cough, sneeze, or vigorous cry = 2); color (cyanotic or pale = 0; acrocyanotic, cyanosis of extremities = 1; pink = 2).

Test-Taking Strategy: Knowledge that Apgar scores range from 0 to 10 and of the measurements used in determining the score assists in answering this question. Focusing on the data in the question helps direct you to the correct option. If you had difficulty with this question, review Apgar scoring.

Level of Cognitive Ability: Comprehension
Client Needs: Physiological Integrity
Integrated Concept/Process: Communication and Documentation
Content Area: Maternity

Reference:
Murray, S., McKinney, E., & Gorrie, T. (2002). *Foundations of maternal-newborn nursing* (3rd ed.). Philadelphia: W.B. Saunders, p. 324.

---

19. A nurse in the newborn nursery is performing admission vital signs on a newborn. Which of the following findings indicates a normal axillary temperature?
  1   35.5° C
  2   37.5° C
  3   38.5° C
  4   39.5° C

Answer: 2
Rationale: The normal axillary temperature for a newborn ranges from 36.5° C to 37.5° C. The normal rectal temperature ranges from 36.5° C to 37.6° C.

Test-Taking Strategy: Knowledge regarding the normal axillary temperature of a newborn is necessary to answer this question. If you are unfamiliar with the normal ranges for newborn vital signs, review this content.

Level of Cognitive Ability: Comprehension
Client Needs: Physiological Integrity
Integrated Concept/Process: Nursing Process/Data Collection
Content Area: Maternity

Reference:
Murray, S., McKinney, E., & Gorrie, T. (2002). *Foundations of maternal-newborn nursing* (3rd ed.). Philadelphia: W.B. Saunders, p. 505.

---

20. A nursing instructor is observing a nursing student collecting data on a newborn admitted to the nursery after birth. The instructor asks the student about the anterior fontanel. Which of the following responses indicates inaccurate information regarding the fontanel?
  1   "It is diamond shaped."
  2   "It should be flat and soft."
  3   "It normally closes by 2 to 3 months of age."
  4   "It normally closes by 12 to 18 months of age."

Answer: 3
Rationale: The anterior fontanel is diamond shaped and located on the top of the head. It should be flat and soft and may range in size from almost nonexistent to 4 to 5 cm across. It normally closes by 12 to 18 months of age. The posterior fontanel closes by 2 to 3 months of age.

Test-Taking Strategy: Note the key word *inaccurate* in the question. Use the process of elimination, noting that options 3 and 4 both address a time frame regarding closure of the fontanel. Therefore, it is likely that one of these options is correct. Knowledge that the anterior fontanel normally closes by 12 to 18 months of age is necessary to answer the question correctly. Review normal newborn findings if you had difficulty with this question.

Level of Cognitive Ability: Comprehension
Client Needs: Physiological Integrity
Integrated Concept/Process: Teaching/Learning
Content Area: Maternity

Reference:
Murray, S., McKinney, E., & Gorrie, T. (2002). *Foundations of maternal-newborn nursing* (3rd ed.). Philadelphia: W.B. Saunders, p. 504.

21. A client is admitted to the hospital with a diagnosis of Cushing's syndrome. The nurse interprets that which of the following laboratory results is consistent with this health problem?

1 White blood cell (WBC) count 3200/mm^3
2 Blood urea nitrogen (BUN) 16 mg/dL
3 Potassium 3.6 mEq/L
4 Blood glucose 205 mg/dL

Answer: 4

Rationale: Cushing's syndrome is characterized by an excess of adrenocorticosteroid hormones. Abnormal laboratory findings that occur with this disorder are hyperkalemia, hyperglycemia, elevated WBC count, and elevated plasma cortisol and adrenocorticotropic hormone levels. These effects are the result of excess glucocorticoids and mineralocorticoids in the body. The WBC and potassium levels identified are low, whereas the BUN is normal and is an unrelated finding. Only the blood glucose is elevated.

Test-Taking Strategy: To answer this question accurately, you must understand this disorder and its effects on the body. If this question was difficult, review the clinical manifestations associated with Cushing's syndrome.

Level of Cognitive Ability: Analysis
Client Needs: Physiological Integrity
Integrated Concept/Process: Nursing Process/Data Collection
Content Area: Adult Health/Endocrine

Reference:
Lewis, S., Heitkemper, M., & Dirksen, S. (2000). *Medical-surgical nursing: assessment and management of clinical problems* (5th ed.). St. Louis: Mosby, p. 1435.

---

22. A client has just undergone transsphenoidal resection of a pituitary adenoma. The nurse includes which of the following in the plan of care?

1 Administer aspirin for a severe headache
2 Observe the client for frequent swallowing
3 Remove the nasal packing in 12 hours
4 Remind the client to cough and breathe deeply

Answer: 2

Rationale: The client should be observed for frequent swallowing, which could indicate postnasal drip after transsphenoidal surgery. This drainage could be cerebrospinal fluid. The nurse should report severe headache to the physician because it could indicate increased intracranial pressure. The surgeon removes the nasal packing after 24 hours in most cases. The client should be allowed to breathe deeply, but not cough. Coughing is contraindicated because it could increase intracranial pressure.

Test-Taking Strategy: Use the process of elimination. Recalling the anatomical location of this procedure assists you in eliminating options 1 and 4. From the remaining options, recall that packing is removed by the physician. Also, noting the time frame in option 3 helps you to eliminate this option. Review care of the client after this surgery if you had difficulty with this question.

Level of Cognitive Ability: Application
Client Needs: Physiological Integrity
Integrated Concept/Process: Nursing Process/Planning
Content Area: Adult Health/Endocrine

Reference:
Ignatavicius, D., & Workman, M. (2002). *Medical-surgical nursing: critical thinking for collaborative care* (4th ed.). Philadelphia: W.B. Saunders, p. 1407.

---

23. A client with Cushing's disease is admitted to the hospital after a motor vehicle accident that resulted in multiple lacerations. The nurse identifies which of the

Answer: 4

Rationale: The client with lacerations has a break in the body's first line of defense against infection. The client with Cushing's disease is at heightened risk for infection because of excess

following problems as the highest-priority concern based on the history of Cushing's disease?

1   Sensory-perceptual alterations
2   Altered health maintenance
3   Fluid volume deficit
4   Risk for infection

cortisol secretion, impaired antibody function, and decreased proliferation of lymphocytes. The client is at risk for fluid volume excess, not fluid volume deficit, with Cushing's disease. The client may have altered health maintenance, but there is insufficient information in the question to determine this. Sensory-perceptual alterations are an unrelated concern.

Test-Taking Strategy: Use the process of elimination. The key words in the question are *highest priority.* Recalling the pathophysiology related to this disorder and noting the key words *multiple lacerations* direct you to option 4. Review this disorder if you had difficulty with this question.

Level of Cognitive Ability: Analysis
Client Needs: Physiological Integrity
Integrated Concept/Process: Nursing Process/Data Collection
Content Area: Adult Health/Endocrine

Reference:
Lewis, S., Heitkemper, M., & Dirksen, S. (2000). *Medical-surgical nursing: assessment and management of clinical problems* (5th ed.). St. Louis: Mosby, p. 1438.

---

24. A client arrives at the nursing unit after abdominal surgery. A nasogastric (NG) tube is in place, and the physician has instructed that the NG tube be attached to intermittent suction. The nurse monitors the client knowing that the client is at risk for which of the following acid-base disorders?

1   Respiratory acidosis
2   Respiratory alkalosis
3   Metabolic acidosis
4   Metabolic alkalosis

Answer: 4
Rationale: Metabolic alkalosis can occur from vomiting or gastric suction because of the loss of acid through the suctioning. Options 1, 2, and 3 are incorrect because they are not likely to occur as a result of gastrointestinal (GI) suction.

Test-Taking Strategy: Use the process of elimination. Recalling that the loss of acid occurs through GI suctioning assists you in determining that an alkalosis can occur. Noting that the situation described in the question is not respiratory in nature directs you to option 4. Review the complications associated with GI suctioning if you had difficulty with this question.

Level of Cognitive Ability: Analysis
Client Needs: Physiological Integrity
Integrated Concept/Process: Nursing Process/Data Collection
Content Area: Adult Health/Gastrointestinal

Reference:
Lewis, S., Heitkemper, M., & Dirksen, S. (2000). *Medical-surgical nursing: assessment and management of clinical problems* (5th ed.). St. Louis: Mosby, p. 344.

---

25. A client has returned to the nursing unit after having computerized tomography (CT) scanning with a contrast medium. The nurse instructs the client to do which of the following after the procedure?

1   Do not take any medications for at least 8 hours
2   Eat lightly for the remainder of the day
3   Drink extra fluids during the day

Answer: 3
Rationale: After CT scanning, the client may resume all usual activities and diet. The contrast dye will cause diuresis, so the client should consume extra fluids to replace those that will be lost. Options 1, 2, and 4 are unnecessary.

Test-Taking Strategy: Use the process of elimination. Noting the words *contrast medium* in the question directs you to option 3. Review postprocedural care needed after CT scanning if you had difficulty with this question.

4   Rest quietly for the remainder of the day

Level of Cognitive Ability: Application
Client Needs: Physiological Integrity
Integrated Concept/Process: Nursing Process/Implementation
Content Area: Adult Health/Neurological

Reference:
Ignatavicius, D., & Workman, M. (2002). *Medical-surgical nursing: critical thinking for collaborative care* (4th ed.). Philadelphia: W.B. Saunders, p. 892.

---

26. A nurse is caring for a client who is recovering from a myelogram in which an oil-based contrast agent was used. The nurse maintains which of the following activity restrictions for the client?
   1   Bed rest for 6 to 8 hours, with the head of the bed flat
   2   Bed rest for 2 to 4 hours, with the head of the bed flat
   3   Bed rest for 6 to 8 hours, with the head of the bed elevated 15 to 30 degrees
   4   Bed rest for 2 to 4 hours, with the head of the bed elevated 15 to 30 degrees

Answer: 1
Rationale: After a myelogram, the client is placed on bed rest for 6 to 8 hours after the procedure. When a water-based contrast medium is used, the client is positioned with the head of the bed elevated 15 to 30 degrees. When an oil-based medium is used, the head of the bed is positioned flat, even though the contrast is aspirated out after the procedure.

Test-Taking Strategy: Use the process of elimination. This question is asking for knowledge of length of bed rest and head position. If you reason that the longer the bed rest, the less the likelihood of complications, you can narrow your choices to options 1 and 3. If you can remember that "oil rises, so keep the head low," you will be able to choose correctly between the remaining two options. Review care of the client after a myelogram if you had difficulty with this question.

Level of Cognitive Ability: Application
Client Needs: Physiological Integrity
Integrated Concept/Process: Nursing Process/Implementation
Content Area: Adult Health/Neurological

Reference:
Ignatavicius, D., & Workman, M. (2002). *Medical-surgical nursing: critical thinking for collaborative care* (4th ed.). Philadelphia: W.B. Saunders, p. 893.

---

27. A client is scheduled to have a serum glycosylated hemoglobin level drawn. The nurse determines that the client understands the nature of the test if the client makes which of the following statements about preparation?
   1   "I shouldn't eat red meat for 3 days before the test."
   2   "I shouldn't eat very fatty foods the day before the test."
   3   "I shouldn't eat anything after midnight."
   4   "I can eat and drink as usual before the test."

Answer: 4
Rationale: No special dietary preparation is necessary for this diagnostic test, which measures the amount of diabetic control during the previous 3 months. When circulating glucose levels are elevated, glucose molecules permanently attach themselves to red blood cells (RBCs). They remain on the RBCs for the rest of the life span (up to 120 days), thus giving some estimate of long-term diabetic control.

Test-Taking Strategy: Use the process of elimination. Recalling that the purpose of the test is to measure long-term glucose control helps you eliminate options 1, 2, and 3. Review this test if you had difficulty with this question.

Level of Cognitive Ability: Comprehension
Client Needs: Physiological Integrity
Integrated Concept/Process: Nursing Process/Evaluation
Content Area: Adult Health/Endocrine

Reference:
Chernecky, C., & Berger, B. (2001). *Laboratory tests and diagnostic procedures* (3rd ed.). Philadelphia: W.B. Saunders, p. 573.

28. A client with diabetes mellitus is brought to the urgent care center by the family. The client is lethargic and complains of dry mouth and thirst. The skin is warm and dry, and skin turgor is poor. The client has deep respirations and a fruity odor to the breath. The nurse concludes that the client is experiencing which of the following complications of diabetes mellitus?

1 Hypoglycemia
2 Stress-induced hypoglycemia
3 Diabetic ketoacidosis
4 Hyperglycemic hyperosmolar non-ketotic coma

Answer: 3
Rationale: Diabetic ketoacidosis is characterized by signs of dehydration, such as dry mouth, thirst, and poor skin turgor. The client's neurological status declines as the serum glucose level rises. The pulse becomes rapid and weak, whereas the respirations become deep. The breath has a fruity or acetone odor to it. The client also may complain of abdominal pain, nausea, and vomiting.

Test-Taking Strategy: Use the process of elimination. Remember that similar options are not likely to be correct; therefore, eliminate options 1 and 2 first. (Also, option 2 is not a clinical condition.) From the remaining options, recalling that a fruity odor to the breath characterizes ketoacidosis directs you to option 3. Review signs of diabetic ketoacidosis if you had difficulty with this question.

Level of Cognitive Ability: Analysis
Client Needs: Physiological Integrity
Integrated Concept/Process: Nursing Process/Data Collection
Content Area: Adult Health/Endocrine

Reference:
Lewis, S., Heitkemper, M., & Dirksen, S. (2000). *Medical-surgical nursing: assessment and management of clinical problems* (5th ed.). St. Louis: Mosby, p. 1394.

29. A nurse is collecting data from a client with hypoparathyroidism. The nurse would do which of the following to check for Chvostek's sign?

1 Inflate a BP cuff on the arm for 3 minutes
2 Tap the cheek below the area of the temple
3 Dorsiflex the foot briskly
4 Stroke upward on the soles of the feet

Answer: 2
Rationale: Hypoparathyroidism results in serum calcium levels that can cause tetany. This can be assessed by testing for Chvostek's sign (option 2) and Trousseau's sign (option 1). Option 3 describes a method of checking for Homan's sign. Option 4 describes assessment of the Babinski reflex.

Test-Taking Strategy: To answer this question accurately, you must be familiar with data collection techniques and the manifestations of hypoparathyroidism. Review these various techniques if you had difficulty with this question.

Level of Cognitive Ability: Application
Client Needs: Physiological Integrity
Integrated Concept/Process: Nursing Process/Data Collection
Content Area: Adult Health/Endocrine

Reference:
Lewis, S., Heitkemper, M., & Dirksen, S. (2000). *Medical-surgical nursing: assessment and management of clinical problems* (5th ed.). St. Louis: Mosby, p. 340.

30. A client with right-sided weakness has been taught how to use a cane. The nurse determines that the client has learned the

Answer: 1
Rationale: The client is taught to hold the cane on the opposite side of the weakness because the opposite arm and leg move

information correctly if the client positions the cane by holding it:

1 In the left hand and 6 inches lateral to the left foot
2 In the right hand and 6 inches lateral to the right foot
3 In the left hand and in front of the left foot
4 In the right hand and in front of the right foot

together (reciprocal motion) with normal walking. The cane is placed 6 inches lateral to the fifth toe.

Test-Taking Strategy: Use the process of elimination. Knowing that the cane is held at the client's side, not in front, helps you eliminate options 3 and 4 first. Recalling that the cane is positioned on the stronger side helps you eliminate option 2. Review client instructions for the use of a cane if you had difficulty with this question.

Level of Cognitive Ability: Comprehension
Client Needs: Physiological Integrity
Integrated Concept/Process: Self-Care
Content Area: Adult Health/Musculoskeletal

Reference:
Potter, P., & Perry, A. (2001). *Fundamentals of nursing* (5th ed.). St. Louis: Mosby, p. 1008.

---

31. A client has a long arm cast applied after a severe fracture of the left radius. The nurse assesses for which of the following signs and symptoms of compartment syndrome?

1 Absence of pain with passive movement of the left arm
2 Paralysis of the left hand not preceded by paresthesias
3 Pain that is relieved by narcotic analgesics
4 Aggravation of pain with elevation of the left arm

Answer: 4
Rationale: The pain of compartment syndrome is aggravated by limb elevation, which further impairs blood supply. This pain is not relieved by narcotic analgesics. The compartment is painful when moved. Paresthesias occur early in the syndrome, which progress to paralysis unless pressure in the compartment is relieved.

Test-Taking Strategy: Use the process of elimination. Recall that compartment syndrome impairs arterial circulation. Knowing that this pain would be aggravated by antigravity measures, such as elevating the limb, directs you to option 4. Review the signs of compartment syndrome if you had difficulty with this question.

Level of Cognitive Ability: Application
Client Needs: Physiological Integrity
Integrated Concept/Process: Nursing Process/Data Collection
Content Area: Adult Health/Musculoskeletal

Reference:
Lewis, S., Heitkemper, M., & Dirksen, S. (2000). *Medical-surgical nursing: assessment and management of clinical problems* (5th ed.). St. Louis: Mosby, p. 1786.

---

32. A client is learning to use a walker to aid in mobility after internal fixation of a hip fracture. The nurse corrects the client if the nurse notes that the client does which of the following?

1 Advances the walker with reciprocal motion
2 Supports body weight on the hands while moving the weaker leg
3 Holds the walker using the hand grips

Answer: 1
Rationale: The client should place the hands on the hand grips for stability. The client should lift the walker to advance it and lean forward slightly while moving it. The client walks into the walker, supporting the body weight on the hands while moving the weaker leg. A disadvantage of the walker is that it does not allow for reciprocal walking motion. If the client were to try to use this type of motion with a walker, it would advance forward one side at a time as the client was walking. This is incorrect because the client would not be supporting the weaker leg with the walker during ambulation.

4 Leans forward slightly when moving the walker

Test-Taking Strategy: Use the process of elimination. Note the key words *corrects the client,* which guides you to look for an incorrect movement. Holding the hand grips of the walker is obviously correct, so option 3 is eliminated first. Because the client must lean forward slightly to move the walker forward, option 4 is eliminated next. From the remaining options, recalling that the purpose of a walker is to provide support directs you to option 1. Review client instructions regarding the use of a walker if you had difficulty with this question.

Level of Cognitive Ability: Application
Client Needs: Physiological Integrity
Integrated Concept/Process: Nursing Process/Implementation
Content Area: Adult Health/Musculoskeletal

Reference:
Potter, P., & Perry, A. (2001). *Fundamentals of nursing* (5th ed.). St. Louis: Mosby, p. 1007.

---

33. A nurse is caring for a client with a left leg cast. The nurse suspects that the client has an infection under the cast if which of the following signs is noted?
1 Weakened left pedal pulse
2 Dependent left foot edema
3 Coolness and pallor of the left foot
4 Presence of a "hot spot" on the cast

Answer: 4
Rationale: Signs and symptoms of infection under a casted area include odor or purulent drainage from the cast and the presence of "hot spots," which are areas of the cast that are warmer than others. The physician should be notified if any of these occur. Signs of impaired circulation in the distal limb include coolness and pallor of the skin, diminished pulse, and edema.

Test-Taking Strategy: Use the process of elimination. Recall that the typical signs of infection include redness, swelling, heat, and purulent drainage. With these signs in mind, you can eliminate options 1 and 3. From the remaining options, recall that dependent edema does not necessarily indicate infection. Swelling would be continuous. The "hot spot" on the cast could signify infection underneath that area and is the correct answer to the question. Review these signs of infection if you had difficulty with this question.

Level of Cognitive Ability: Comprehension
Client Needs: Physiological Integrity
Integrated Concept/Process: Nursing Process/Data Collection
Content Area: Adult Health/Musculoskeletal

Reference:
Ignatavicius, D., & Workman, M. (2002). *Medical-surgical nursing: critical thinking for collaborative care* (4th ed.). Philadelphia: W.B. Saunders, p. 1136.

---

34. Treatment for a client with asthma has been changed from oral to inhalation therapy with beclomethasone (Vanceril). The client reports to the clinic and complains of weakness and anorexia. The client's blood glucose is 58 mg/dL, and blood pressure (BP) drops to 102/70 mmHg from 118/78 mmHg. The nurse interprets

Answer: 3
Rationale: Signs of adrenal insufficiency include anorexia and nausea, weakness and fatigue, hypotension, and hypoglycemia. The nurse should monitor for these signs of adverse medication effects whenever a client is switched from oral to inhalation glucocorticoid therapy, such as beclomethasone. Options 1, 2, and 4 are not associated with the use of this medication.

that the client may be experiencing which of the following adverse medication effects?
1   Circulatory collapse
2   Exacerbation of gastritis
3   Adrenal insufficiency
4   Diabetes mellitus

Test-Taking Strategy: To answer this question accurately, you must know the signs and symptoms of adrenal insufficiency and the adverse effects of beclomethasone. Recalling that this medication is a corticosteroid directs you to option 3. If this question was difficult, review this medication.

Level of Cognitive Ability: Analysis
Client Needs: Physiological Integrity
Integrated Concept/Process: Nursing Process/Data Collection
Content Area: Pharmacology

Reference:
Clark, J., Queener, S., & Karb, V. (2002). *Pharmacologic basis of nursing practice* (6th ed.). St Louis: Mosby, p. 337.

---

35. A female client has been given a prescription for erythromycin stearate (Erythrocin Stearate) to treat a respiratory infection. The nurse evaluates that the client does not understand instructions for medication use if the client states that it is necessary to report which of the following?
1   Furry overgrowth on the tongue
2   Loss of appetite
3   Vaginal itching or discharge
4   Foul-smelling diarrhea

Answer: 2
Rationale: The client is taught to report signs of superinfection while taking an antibiotic such as erythrocin stearate. These signs include furry overgrowth on the tongue, vaginal itching or discharge, and loose or foul-smelling stools. Loss of appetite is an unrelated sign.

Test-Taking Strategy: To answer this question accurately, you must know the common signs of superinfection and recall that they occur with antibiotic therapy. Review the adverse effects of this medication if you had difficulty with this question.

Level of Cognitive Ability: Analysis
Client Needs: Physiological Integrity
Integrated Concept/Process: Nursing Process/Evaluation
Content Area: Pharmacology

Reference:
Hodgson, B., & Kizior, R. (2003). *Saunders nursing drug handbook 2003.* Philadelphia: W.B. Saunders, p. 417.

---

36. A client has just returned to the nursing unit after having a bone scan. The nurse tells the client to do which of the following after this procedure?
1   Eat small frequent meals
2   Increase fluid intake
3   Call the nurse if nausea or flushing is felt
4   Walk in the hallway as much as possible

Answer: 2
Rationale: There are no special restrictions for diet or activity after a bone scan. The client is encouraged to drink large amounts of water for 24 to 48 hours to flush the radioisotope from the system. Options 1 and 4 are unnecessary. Option 3 is unrelated to this procedure.

Test-Taking Strategy: Use the process of elimination. There is no purpose for options 1 and 4, so these are eliminated first. Eliminate option 3 next for two reasons. First, the question relates to postprocedural concerns. Nausea and flushing accompany dye injection during a procedure. Second, this procedure uses radioisotopes rather than dye. The only option left is increasing fluids, which speeds elimination of the isotope from the client's system. Review postprocedural instructions after a bone scan if you had difficulty with this question.

Level of Cognitive Ability: Application
Client Needs: Physiological Integrity

Integrated Concept/Process: Nursing Process/Implementation
Content Area: Adult Health/Musculoskeletal

Reference:
Chernecky, C., & Berger, B. (2001). *Laboratory tests and diagnostic procedures* (3rd ed.). Philadelphia: W.B. Saunders, p. 261.

---

37. A nurse is collecting data from a client with a left arm fracture and is checking for impaired venous return distal to the fracture. Which of the following signs indicate that this is occurring?
1   Weakened left radial pulse
2   Continued pain despite medication
3   Pallor with blotchy cyanosis
4   Edema of the left hand

Answer: 4
Rationale: Impaired venous return is often marked by edema and can occur distal to the site of a fracture. Signs of arterial damage can result if an artery becomes contused, thrombosed, lacerated, or spastic. The other options are signs of arterial damage, which include pallor or blotchy cyanosis; variable, weakened, or absent distal pulse; pain; poor capillary refill; and distal paralysis or loss of sensation.

Test-Taking Strategy: Use the process of elimination and focus on the key words *impaired venous return*. Recalling the signs that accompany impairments of arterial and venous circulation directs you to option 4. If this question was difficult, review data collection techniques of circulatory status after fracture.

Level of Cognitive Ability: Analysis
Client Needs: Physiological Integrity
Integrated Concept/Process: Nursing Process/Data Collection
Content Area: Adult Health/Musculoskeletal

Reference:
Lewis, S., Heitkemper, M., & Dirksen, S. (2000). *Medical-surgical nursing: assessment and management of clinical problems* (5th ed.). St. Louis: Mosby, p. 1780.

---

38. An emergency medical services team arrives at the emergency room with a client who was in a severe automobile accident. The client is lethargic, the blood pressure is 98/50 mmHg, and the heart rate is 100 beats per minute. The client is bleeding profusely from a wound in the head, and it is suspected that the client has an internal injury. The physician orders intravenous fluids for the client to treat the suspected hypovolemia. Which of the following intravenous fluids would the nurse anticipate to be prescribed for the client?
1   5% dextrose
2   ½ normal saline
3   Lactated Ringer's solution
4   ¼ normal saline

Answer: 3
Rationale: Isotonic fluids are used clinically to treat hemorrhage, hypovolemia, and extracellular fluid deficit, and as an initial treatment for clinical dehydration. Examples of isotonic fluids are normal saline (0.9% NaCl), lactated Ringer's solution; replacement electrolyte solutions such as Normosol-R. 5% dextrose, ½ normal saline, and ¼ normal saline are examples of hypotonic solutions.

Test-Taking Strategy: Use the process of elimination. Note the key word *hypovolemia*. This key word, the understanding that isotonic solutions are used to treat hypovolemia, and the knowledge of isotonic solutions direct you to option 3. Review isotonic solutions if you had difficulty with this question.

Level of Cognitive Ability: Analysis
Client Needs: Physiological Integrity
Integrated Concept/Process: Nursing Process/Planning
Content Area: Fundamental Skills

Reference:
Ignatavicius, D., & Workman, M. (2002). *Medical-surgical nursing: critical thinking for collaborative care* (4th ed.). Philadelphia: W.B. Saunders, p. 1226.

39. A nurse is checking an IV site of a client, and an infiltration is suspected. Which of the following would the nurse note if an infiltration has occurred?
1   Coolness at the site
2   Warmth at the site
3   Redness at the site
4   Inflammation at the site

Answer: 1
Rationale: Signs of infiltration include edema and coolness at the site of insertion. The nurse should compare the site with the opposite extremity to note any swelling. Warmth and redness are noted in phlebitis, inflammation at the site, and infection.

Test-Taking Strategy: Use the process of elimination. Note the similarities in options 2, 3, and 4 in that they all indicate phlebitis or inflammation. Recalling that coolness at the IV insertion site indicates infiltration directs you to option 1. Review the signs of infiltration if you had difficulty with this question.

Level of Cognitive Ability: Comprehension
Client Needs: Physiological Integrity
Integrated Concept/Process: Nursing Process/Data Collection
Content Area: Fundamental Skills

Reference:
Potter, P., & Perry, A. (2001). *Fundamentals of nursing* (5th ed.). St. Louis: Mosby, p. 1235.

40. A nurse is monitoring the IV site of a client receiving an IV solution that contains potassium chloride. The nurse notes heat, redness, and tenderness at the site and suspects phlebitis. The nurse understands that which of the following is the most likely cause of the phlebitis?
1   The infusion of solution into the subcutaneous tissue
2   The inflammation of the vein
3   A local growth of microorganisms that gain entry through the venipuncture site
4   The collection of blood into the tissues

Answer: 2
Rationale: Phlebitis is caused by the inflammation of a vein from chemical irritants in the intravenous solution or medication, by mechanical irritation from the needle or cannula, or by accompanying local infection. Infiltration is the infusion of solution into the subcutaneous tissue. Infection is the local or systemic growth of microorganisms that gain entry into the body through the venipuncture site, and a hematoma is the collection of blood into the tissues that occurs during unsuccessful venipuncture or after the venipuncture site is discontinued.

Test-Taking Strategy: Use the process of elimination and note the key words *most likely*. Focus on the issue: phlebitis. The definition of this term should easily direct you to option 2. Review the causes of phlebitis if you had difficulty with this question.

Level of Cognitive Ability: Comprehension
Client Needs: Physiological Integrity
Integrated Concept/Process: Nursing Process/Data Collection
Content Area: Fundamental Skills

Reference:
Potter, P., & Perry, A. (2001). *Fundamentals of nursing* (5th ed.). St. Louis: Mosby, p. 1235.

41. A nurse is monitoring an IV site of a client receiving an IV solution and suspects thrombophlebitis. Which of the following signs would the nurse note if thrombophlebitis has occurred?
1   Coolness around the IV site
2   A hard or cordlike feeling along the vein

Answer: 2
Rationale: If phlebitis is present, the nurse notes heat, redness, tenderness, and swelling along the course of the vein. The vein may feel hard or cordlike with thrombophlebitis. Edema and coolness occur with infiltration. Inflammation at the site occurs with a local infection.

3 Inflammation at the IV site
4 Edema and coolness at the IV site

Test-Taking Strategy: Use the process of elimination. Focus on the key word *thrombophlebitis.* Eliminate options 1 and 4 first because they are similar. Recalling that inflammation is a sign of infection assists you in eliminating option 3 and directs you to option 2. Review the signs of thrombophlebitis if you had difficulty with this question.

Level of Cognitive Ability: Comprehension
Client Needs: Physiological Integrity
Integrated Concept/Process: Nursing Process/Data Collection
Content Area: Fundamental Skills

Reference:
Potter, P., & Perry, A. (2001). *Fundamentals of nursing* (5th ed.). St. Louis: Mosby, p. 1235.

---

42. A nurse is assisting in caring for a client with a central line who is receiving IV solutions. While caring for the client, the client suddenly develops tachycardia and dyspnea. Cyanosis is noted, and the nurse suspects an air embolism. Which of the following initial nursing actions is most appropriate?
1 Slow the IV rate
2 Provide emotional support for the client
3 Turn the client on the left side and lower the head of the bed
4 Elevate the head of the bed and monitor the vital signs

Answer: 3
Rationale: If an air embolism is suspected, the initial nursing action is to turn the client on the left side and to lower the head of the bed to trap the air in the right atrium. The tubing should be clamped, vital signs should be monitored, and the physician should be notified. Oxygen should be administered as prescribed, and emotional support should be given to the client. However, the initial nursing action is to position the client.

Test-Taking Strategy: Use the process of elimination. Eliminate option 2 first, recalling that physiological needs are the priority. Next eliminate option 1 because the IV is stopped, not slowed. Use the concepts of gravity to assist in selecting option 3 from the remaining options. If you had difficulty with this question, review the initial nursing actions that must be taken if an air embolism is suspected.

Level of Cognitive Ability: Application
Client Needs: Physiological Integrity
Integrated Concept/Process: Nursing Process/Implementation
Content Area: Fundamental Skills

Reference:
Potter, P., & Perry, A. (2001). *Fundamentals of nursing* (5th ed.). St. Louis: Mosby, p. 1375.

---

43. A client's serum digoxin level is 1.2 ng/mL. The nurse interprets that this level is which of the following?
1 Incorrectly reported
2 Above the therapeutic range
3 Below the therapeutic range
4 Within the therapeutic range

Answer: 4
Rationale: The normal therapeutic range for digoxin is 0.8 to 2.0 ng/mL. A level of 1.2 ng/mL is within the therapeutic range.

Test-Taking Strategy: To answer this question correctly, you must know the therapeutic range for digoxin. Because this is a commonly administered medication, it is helpful to memorize this value. Review this therapeutic range if you had difficulty with this question.

Level of Cognitive Ability: Comprehension
Client Needs: Physiological Integrity

Integrated Concept/Process: Nursing Process/Data Collection
Content Area: Pharmacology

Reference:
Hodgson, B., & Kizior, R. (2003). *Saunders nursing drug handbook 2003.* Philadelphia: W.B. Saunders, p. 350.

---

44. A client has been diagnosed with hyperthyroidism. The nurse assesses the client for which of the following complaints associated with this disorder?
1   Weight gain
2   Lethargy
3   Constipation
4   Heat intolerance

Answer: 4
Rationale: The client with hyperthyroidism has the metabolic manifestations of heat intolerance as well as increased metabolic rate and a low-grade fever. Some of the other symptoms include weight loss, restlessness, and diarrhea, which are the opposite of the symptoms presented in options 1, 2, and 3.

Test-Taking Strategy: Use the process of elimination. Noting the prefix to the name of the disorder *hyper-*, and recalling the function of the thyroid gland assist in directing you to the correct option. Review these symptoms if you had difficulty with this question.

Level of Cognitive Ability: Application
Client Needs: Physiological Integrity
Integrated Concept/Process: Nursing Process/Data Collection
Content Area: Adult Health/Endocrine

Reference:
Lewis, S., Heitkemper, M., & Dirksen, S. (2000). *Medical-surgical nursing: assessment and management of clinical problems* (5th ed.). St. Louis: Mosby, p. 1417.

---

45. A client has a history of hypothyroidism. The nurse assesses this client for which symptom of this disorder?
1   Weight loss
2   Diarrhea
3   Heat intolerance
4   Increased sleep

Answer: 4
Rationale: The client with hypothyroidism has decreased function of the thyroid gland. This often results in symptoms of weight gain, constipation, cold intolerance, and an increased need for sleep. The nurse questions the client for any of these manifestations.

Test-Taking Strategy: Use the process of elimination. Noting the prefix to the name of the disorder *hypo-*, and recalling the function of the thyroid gland assists in directing you to the correct option. Review these symptoms if you had difficulty with this question.

Level of Cognitive Ability: Application
Client Needs: Physiological Integrity
Integrated Concept/Process: Nursing Process/Data Collection
Content Area: Adult Health/Endocrine

Reference:
Lewis, S., Heitkemper, M., & Dirksen, S. (2000). *Medical-surgical nursing: assessment and management of clinical problems* (5th ed.). St. Louis: Mosby, p. 1416.

---

46. A client is being treated for diabetic ketoacidosis (DKA). The nurse monitors for which of the following as the most

Answer: 2
Rationale: The client being treated for DKA may experience hypokalemia. Potassium attaches to the insulin–glucose complex

serious electrolyte disturbance that can accompany this treatment?
1 Hyponatremia
2 Hypokalemia
3 Hypocalcemia
4 Hypomagnesemia

and is carried into the cell with it. As the client's serum glucose falls during treatment, hypokalemia also can ensue. The nurse monitors the serum potassium results during this treatment. Hypokalemia can lead to cardiac dysrhythmias.

Test-Taking Strategy: Use the process of elimination and recall the pathophysiology of DKA and its treatment. Recalling the process of glucose transport into the cells assists in directing you to option 2. Review the treatment of DKA if you had difficulty with this question.

Level of Cognitive Ability: Application
Client Needs: Physiological Integrity
Integrated Concept/Process: Nursing Process/Data Collection
Content Area: Adult Health/Endocrine

Reference:
Lewis, S., Heitkemper, M., & Dirksen, S. (2000). *Medical-surgical nursing: assessment and management of clinical problems* (5th ed.). St. Louis: Mosby, p. 1396.

---

47. A client has an order to receive glyburide (Micronase) once each day. The nurse schedules this medication so that it is administered at which of the following times?
1 ½ hour before breakfast
2 2 hours after breakfast
3 With the noon meal
4 At bedtime

Answer: 1
Rationale: Glyburide is an oral hypoglycemic agent that is administered once a day. It should be given ½ hour before breakfast to have the best effect in preventing postprandial hyperglycemia. The other options are incorrect.

Test-Taking Strategy: Use the process of elimination. Recalling that this medication is an oral hypoglycemic agent and that it should be given before the first meal of the day directs you to option 1. If this question was difficult, review oral hypoglycemic therapy and this medication.

Level of Cognitive Ability: Application
Client Needs: Physiological Integrity
Integrated Concept/Process: Nursing Process/Implementation
Content Area: Adult Health/Endocrine

Reference:
Hodgson, B., & Kizior, R. (2003). *Saunders nursing drug handbook 2003.* Philadelphia: W.B. Saunders, p. 530.

---

48. A client with abdominal pain has a history of duodenal ulcer. To assist in determining whether the etiology of the pain is recurrence of the ulcer, the nurse asks the client which of the following about the pain?
1 If it is accompanied by nausea and vomiting
2 If it is experienced just after a meal
3 If it is relieved with eating
4 If it radiates down the right arm

Answer: 3
Rationale: The most frequent manifestation of a duodenal ulcer is pain that is relieved by food intake. Clients with this condition generally describe the pain as a burning, heavy, sharp, or "hungry" pain that often localizes in the midepigastric area. Pain that occurs after a meal characterizes gastric ulcer. Nausea and vomiting are also more typical in the client with a gastric ulcer. Option 4 is unrelated to duodenal ulcer.

Test-Taking Strategy: Use the process of elimination. Begin to answer this question by eliminating option 4, which is unrelated to a duodenal ulcer. From the remaining options, recalling the differences between the symptoms of duodenal and gastric ulcer directs you to option 3. Review these differences if you had difficulty with this question.

Level of Cognitive Ability: Application
Client Needs: Physiological Integrity
Integrated Concept/Process: Nursing Process/Data Collection
Content Area: Adult Health/Gastrointestinal

Reference:
Phipps, W., Monahan., J., Sands, J. et al. (2003) *Medical surgical nursing: health and illness perspectives* (7th ed.). St. Louis: Mosby, p. 1030.

---

49. A client has undergone esophagogastroduodenoscopy (EGD). The nurse assesses which of the following items immediately upon the client's return to the clinical nursing unit?
1 Temperature
2 Complaints of heartburn
3 Return of the gag reflex
4 Sore throat

Answer: 3
Rationale: The nurse immediately assesses the return of the gag reflex, which protects the client's airway. The client's vital signs are monitored also. A sudden sharp increase in temperature could indicate perforation of the gastrointestinal tract, which would be accompanied by other signs, such as pain. Monitoring for sore throat and heartburn are also important; however, the client's airway is still the priority.

Test-Taking Strategy: Use the process of elimination and the ABCs (airway, breathing, and circulation). Note that the question contains the key word *immediately*. This tells you that more than one or all of the options may be partially or totally correct. Review care to the client after EGD if you had difficulty with this question.

Level of Cognitive Ability: Application
Client Needs: Physiological Integrity
Integrated Concept/Process: Nursing Process/Data Collection
Content Area: Adult Health/Gastrointestinal

Reference:
Black, J., Hawks, J., & Keene A. (2001). *Medical-surgical nursing: clinical management for positive outcomes* (6th ed.). Philadelphia. W. B. Saunders, p. 658.

---

50. A nurse is assessing for stoma retraction in a client who has recently undergone colostomy. The nurse would observe to see if the stoma is:
1 Narrowed and flattened
2 Protruding and swollen
3 Sunken and hidden
4 Dark and bluish in color

Answer: 3
Rationale: Stoma retraction is characterized by sinking of the stoma, which makes it harder to see. A stoma with a narrowed opening at the level of either the skin or the fascia is said to be stenosed. A prolapsed stoma is one in which bowel protrudes through the stoma, causing an elongated and swollen appearance. Ischemia of the stoma would be associated with a dusky or bluish color.

Test-Taking Strategy: Use the process of elimination. Noting the key word *retraction* assists in directing you to the correct option. If this question was difficult, review the complications of a stoma.

Level of Cognitive Ability: Application
Client Needs: Physiological Integrity
Integrated Concept/Process: Nursing Process/Data Collection
Content Area: Adult Health/Gastrointestinal

Reference:

Black, J., Hawks, J., & Keene A. (2001). *Medical-surgical nursing: clinical management for positive outcomes* (6th ed.). Philadelphia. W. B. Saunders, p. 784.

51. A client with acute pancreatitis is experiencing severe pain from the disorder. The nurse would avoid placing the client in which of the following positions?
1 Upright and leaning forward
2 Side-lying with legs flexed
3 Semi-Fowler's
4 Recumbent

Answer: 4

Rationale: The pain of pancreatitis is aggravated by either lying supine or walking because the pancreas is located retroperitoneally, and the edema and the inflammation intensify the irritation of the posterior peritoneal wall with these positions. Positions such as semi-Fowler's, being upright, leaning forward, and with the legs flexed (especially the left leg) may reduce some of the pain associated with pancreatitis.

Test-Taking Strategy: Use the process of elimination and note the key word *avoid*. Remember that options that are similar are not likely to be correct, which helps you eliminate options 1 and 3. From the remaining options, visualize the pancreas and the potential effects from stretching associated with the various positions listed. This directs you to option 4. Review this disorder if you had difficulty with this question.

Level of Cognitive Ability: Application
Client Needs: Physiological Integrity
Integrated Concept/Process: Nursing Process/Implementation
Content Area: Adult Health/Gastrointestinal

Reference:

Ignatavicius, D., & Workman, M. (2002). *Medical-surgical nursing: critical thinking for collaborative care* (4th ed.). Philadelphia: W.B. Saunders, p. 1224.

52. A nurse is completing the preprocedural checklist before a client is sent for bronchoscopy. The nurse determines that the client is not adequately prepared for the procedure if which of the following is noted?
1 There is no signed informed consent
2 The client has had nothing by mouth since midnight
3 Sedation has been administered
4 Dentures have been removed

Answer: 1

Rationale: The client must sign an informed consent because the procedure is invasive. The client is not allowed to eat or drink for 6 hours before the procedure. If the client wears contact lenses, dentures, or another prosthesis, it is removed before the client is given preprocedural sedation.

Test-Taking Strategy: Use the process of elimination. Note the key words *not adequately prepared*. Recalling that this procedure is invasive and that invasive procedures require an informed consent directs you to the correct option. Review preprocedural care regarding this procedure if you had difficulty with this question.

Level of Cognitive Ability: Comprehension
Client Needs: Physiological Integrity
Integrated Concept/Process: Nursing Process/Evaluation
Content Area: Adult Health/Respiratory

Reference:

Ignatavicius, D., & Workman, M. (2002). *Medical-surgical nursing: critical thinking for collaborative care* (4th ed.). Philadelphia: W.B. Saunders, p. 486.

53. A client is told that a tuberculin skin test has positive results and asks the nurse what this means. The nurse tells the client that the test result means which of the following?
1 Active tuberculosis (TB)
2 Exposure to TB
3 A history of TB
4 No TB

Answer: 2
Rationale: A test in a client who is not immunosuppressed is considered positive for TB if there is an area of induration that measures 10 mm or more. The reading is generally done 48 to 72 hours after the testing solution is planted in the forearm. A positive result indicates that the client has been exposed to TB and requires further diagnostic work-up. It does not indicate the presence of active disease.

Test-Taking Strategy: To answer this question accurately, you must know the significance of positive results for TB skin testing. Review the procedure for interpreting these results if you had difficulty with this question.

Level of Cognitive Ability: Application
Client Needs: Physiological Integrity
Integrated Concept/Process: Nursing Process/Implementation
Content Area: Adult Health/Respiratory

Reference:
Black, J., Hawks, J., & Keene, A. (2001). *Medical-surgical nursing: clinical management for positive outcomes* (6th ed.). Philadelphia: W.B. Saunders, p. 1719.

54. A client is wearing an oxygen cannula that delivers a flow rate of 2 liters per minute. The nurse is told that a set of arterial blood gases (ABGs) on room air will be obtained. The nurse interprets this to mean a need to do which of the following with the oxygen?
1 Change to a Venturi face mask before the ABGs are drawn
2 Remove the oxygen at least 15 min. before the ABGs are drawn
3 Remove before the ABGs are drawn
4 Leave unchanged and the ABGs should be drawn

Answer: 3
Rationale: The client should have the oxygen removed before the ABGs are drawn. When the physician is deciding whether to discontinue oxygen therapy, ABGs will be obtained on room air and evaluated to see how the client tolerates oxygen removal.

Test-Taking Strategy: Use the process of elimination. Noting the key words *room air* directs you to option 3. Review the procedures for obtaining ABCs if you had difficulty with this question.

Level of Cognitive Ability: Comprehension
Client Needs: Physiological Integrity
Integrated Concept/Process: Nursing Process/Implementation
Content Area: Adult Health/Respiratory

Reference:
Black, J., Hawks, J., & Keene, A. (2001). *Medical-surgical nursing: clinical management for positive outcomes* (6th ed.). Philadelphia: W.B. Saunders, pp. 1641-1642.

55. A client who has emphysema has an arterial blood gas (ABG) drawn. The results indicate a pH of 7.31. Based on the pH result, the nurse interprets that which of the following conditions is present?
1 Acidosis
2 Alkalosis
3 Compensation
4 Decompensation

Answer: 1
Rationale: Acidosis is defined as a pH of less than 7.35, whereas alkalosis is defined as a pH of greater than 7.45. There are not adequate data in the question to determine compensation or decompensation.

Test-Taking Strategy: Use the process of elimination. Recalling the physiology related to the body pH directs you to option 1. Review the interpretation of ABGs if you had difficulty with this question.

Level of Cognitive Ability: Comprehension
Client Needs: Physiological Integrity

Integrated Concept/Process: Nursing Process/Data Collection
Content Area: Adult Health/Respiratory

Reference:
Black, J., Hawks, J., & Keene, A. (2001). *Medical-surgical nursing: clinical management for positive outcomes* (6th ed.). Philadelphia: W.B. Saunders, p. 264.

---

56. A nurse is caring for a child with erythema infectiosum (Fifth disease). Which of the following clinical manifestations does the nurse expect to note in the child?
1 Small bluish-white spots with a red base found on the buccal mucosa
2 Pinkish rose maculopapular rash on the face, neck, and scalp
3 Reddish and pinpoint petechiae spots found on the soft palate
4 An intense fiery red edematous rash on the cheeks

Answer: 4
Rationale: Option 1 describes Koplik spots, which are found in rubeola (red measles). Options 2 and 3 are clinical manifestations related to rubella (German measles). Fifth disease is characterized by the presence of an intense fiery red edematous rash on the cheeks, which gives an appearance that the child has been slapped.

Test-Taking Strategy: Use the process of elimination. Recalling the "slapped cheek" appearance associated with Fifth disease directs you to the correct option. Review the clinical manifestations associated with this disease if you had difficulty with this question.

Level of Cognitive Ability: Comprehension
Client Needs: Physiological Integrity
Integrated Concept/Process: Nursing Process/Data Collection
Content Area: Child Health

Reference:
Schulte, E., Price, D., & Gwin, J. (2001). *Thompson's pediatric nursing* (8th ed.). Philadelphia: W.B. Saunders, p. 242.

---

57. A nurse is caring for a child admitted to the hospital with nonspecific symptoms of headache, fever, anorexia, and restlessness. A rash is noted on the palms and soles of the feet and on the remainder of the body. The child is diagnosed with Rocky Mountain spotted fever (RMSF). Which of the following medications does the nurse anticipate will be prescribed for the child?
1 Tetracycline hydrochloride (Achromycin)
2 Thioguanine
3 Thiotepa (Thioplex)
4 Ticlopidine hydrochloride (Ticlid)

Answer: 1
Rationale: With early detection, tetracycline hydrochloride and chloramphenicol (Chloromycetin) have been found to be effective in treating RMSF. These medications inhibit the growth of the organism. However, if vascular damage has already occurred, the medications may not alter the course of the disease. Antibiotic therapy is continued until the child has had no fever for at least 2 to 3 days. The usual duration of therapy is 6 to 10 days. Thioguanine and thiotepa are antineoplastic medications. Ticlopidine hydrochloride is a platelet aggregation inhibitor.

Test-Taking Strategy: Use the process of elimination. Knowledge regarding the treatment for RMSF is necessary to answer this question. If you were familiar with the classifications of the medications identified in the options, you would easily be directed to option 1. Tetracycline hydrochloride is the only antibiotic. Review the treatment for RMSF if you had difficulty with this question.

Level of Cognitive Ability: Analysis
Client Needs: Physiological Integrity
Integrated Concept/Process: Nursing Process/Planning
Content Area: Pharmacology

Reference:
Hodgson, B., & Kizior, R. (2003). *Saunders nursing drug handbook 2003.* Philadelphia: W.B. Saunders, p. 1070.

58. A nurse is caring for a child with a diagnosis of human immunodeficiency virus (HIV). The nurse plans care based on which of the following accurate descriptions of this disorder?

1 It is an acquired cell-mediated immunodeficiency disorder
2 It is an inflammatory autoimmune disease that affects the connective tissue of the heart, joints, and subcutaneous tissues
3 It is a chronic multisystem autoimmune disease characterized by the inflammation of connective tissue
4 It is a febrile generalized vasculitis of unknown etiology

Answer: 1
Rationale: HIV infection is an acquired cell-mediated immunodeficiency disorder causing a wide spectrum of illnesses in children ranging from no symptoms to mild and moderate symptoms to severe symptoms. Acquired immunodeficiency syndrome represents the most severe illness. Option 2 identifies rheumatic fever. Option 3 identifies systemic lupus erythematosus, and option 4 identifies Kawasaki disease.

Test-Taking Strategy: Use the process of elimination. Note the relationship between immunodeficiency in the question and the correct option. If you had difficulty with this question, review information about this disease.

Level of Cognitive Ability: Comprehension
Client Needs: Physiological Integrity
Integrated Concept/Process: Nursing Process/Planning
Content Area: Child Health

Reference:
Schulte, E., Price, D., & Gwin, J. (2001). *Thompson's pediatric nursing* (8th ed.). Philadelphia: W.B. Saunders, p. 101.

---

59. A nurse is collecting data on a child suspected of having rheumatic fever (RF). The nurse plans to obtain specific data about the child's recent illnesses and asks the parent which question?

1 "Has the child had a recent streptococcal infection of the throat?"
2 "Has the child had a recent ear infection?"
3 "Has the child had a recent case of otitis media?"
4 "Has the child had a recent case of pneumonia?"

Answer: 1
Rationale: Rheumatic fever characteristically presents 1 to 3 weeks after an untreated or partially treated group A β-hemolytic streptococcal infection of the upper respiratory tract. The questions asked in options 2, 3, and 4 are not specifically related to RF, although they may be part of the data-collection process.

Test-Taking Strategy: Use the process of elimination. Options 2 and 3 can be eliminated first because they are similar. From the remaining options, you must know that RF can follow a streptococcal infection of the upper respiratory tract. Review the etiology associated with RF if you had difficulty with this question.

Level of Cognitive Ability: Comprehension
Client Needs: Physiological Integrity
Integrated Concept/Process: Nursing Process/Data Collection
Content Area: Child Health

Reference:
Schulte, E., Price, D., & Gwin, J. (2001). *Thompson's pediatric nursing* (8th ed.). Philadelphia: W.B. Saunders, p. 276.

---

60. A nurse is preparing to care for a hospitalized child with rheumatic fever (RF) and is told that the child has erythema marginatum. Which of the following does the nurse expect to see documented in the child's record?

1 Tender painful joints, especially the elbows, knees, ankles, and wrists
2 Inflammation of all parts of the heart, primarily the mitral valve

Answer: 4
Rationale: Erythema marginatum is characterized by red skin lesions that start as flat or slightly raised macules, usually over the trunk and spread peripherally. Option 1 identifies polyarthritis. Option 2 identifies carditis. Option 3 identifies chorea.

Test-Taking Strategy: Use the process of elimination. Noting the relationship between the words *erythema* in the question and *red* in option 4 assists you in answering this question. Review the manifestations of this disorder if you had difficulty with this question.

3 Involuntary movements affecting the legs, arms, and face

4 Red skin lesions that started as flat or slightly raised macules over the trunk, and spread peripherally

Level of Cognitive Ability: Comprehension
Client Needs: Physiological Integrity
Integrated Concept/Process: Nursing Process/Data Collection
Content Area: Child Health

Reference:
Schulte, E., Price, D., & Gwin, J. (2001). *Thompson's pediatric nursing* (8th ed.). Philadelphia: W.B. Saunders, p. 277.

---

61. A nurse is monitoring a child with a nasogastric tube. The nurse reviews the child's health care record and notes that the laboratory values indicate a potassium level of 3.2 mEq/L. Which of the following clinical manifestations does the nurse expect to note in the child?

1 Muscle weakness
2 Increased bowel sounds
3 Elevated blood pressure
4 Nausea

Answer: 1
Rationale: Hypokalemia is indicated by a potassium level of less that 3.5 mEq/L. Clinical manifestations include muscle weakness, paralysis, leg cramps, decreased bowel sounds, weak and irregular pulse, and cardiac dysrhythmias (tachycardia or bradycardia). Clinical manifestations may also include hypotension, ileus, irritability, and fatigue. Nausea may or may not occur.

Test-Taking Strategy: Knowledge regarding the normal potassium level assists you in determining that the child is experiencing hypokalemia. From this point, knowledge of the clinical manifestations associated with hypokalemia directs you to option 1. Review these manifestations if you had difficulty with this question.

Level of Cognitive Ability: Analysis
Client Needs: Physiological Integrity
Integrated Concept/Process: Nursing Process/Data Collection
Content Area: Child Health

Reference:
Wong, D., & Hockenberry-Eaton, M. (2001). *Wong's essentials of pediatric nursing* (6th ed.). St. Louis: Mosby, p. 393.

---

62. A nurse is preparing to administer an immunization to an 11-year-old child. Which of the following sites does the nurse select as the best area to administer the intramuscular (IM) injection?

1 Posterior lateral aspect of the thigh
2 Anterolateral aspect of the thigh
3 Deltoid muscle
4 Ventral gluteal muscle

Answer: 4
Rationale: The ventral gluteal site may be used for IM injections in older children. In children who have not yet developed the gluteal muscle (those younger than 2 years of age), the preferred site for IM injections is the anterolateral aspect of the thigh. The deltoid muscle can be used in children 18 months or older; however, in an 11-year-old child, the ventral gluteal muscle is the preferred site. Option 1 is an inappropriate site for an injection.

Test-Taking Strategy: Use the process of elimination. Option 1 can be easily eliminated first. Note the age of the child in the question and the key word *best*. Visualize each of these body areas to help you choose the correct option. If you had difficulty with this question, review sites for IM injections.

Level of Cognitive Ability: Application
Client Needs: Physiological Integrity
Integrated Concept/Process: Nursing Process/Implementation
Content Area: Child Health

Reference:
Schulte, E., Price, D., & Gwin, J. (2001). *Thompson's pediatric nursing* (8th ed.). Philadelphia: W.B. Saunders, p. 363.

63. A nurse employed in a physician's office is administering immunizations to a child. The nurse ensures that which of the following is available as the priority item during the administration of a vaccine?
1 Diphenhydramine hydrochloride (Benadryl)
2 ⅞-inch needle
3 Pediatric syringes
4 Epinephrine (Adrenalin)

Answer: 4
Rationale: Any immunization may cause an anaphylactic reaction. All physicians offices and clinics administering immunizations must have epinephrine 1:1000 available. Pediatric syringes are needed to administer the immunization. Generally, a needle that is ⅞-inch or longer is adequate to administer immunizations for a normal 4-month-old infant. Diphenhydramine hydrochloride is not normally needed unless specifically prescribed by the physician. The priority item, however, is the epinephrine.

Test-Taking Strategy: Use the process of elimination. Noting the key word *priority* and recalling the risk associated with the potential for anaphylactic reaction directs you to option 4. Review the risks associated with the administration of immunizations if you had difficulty with this question.

Level of Cognitive Ability: Application
Client Needs: Physiological Integrity
Integrated Concept/Process: Nursing Process/Planning
Content Area: Child Health

Reference:
Schulte, E., Price, D., & Gwin, J. (2001). *Thompson's pediatric nursing* (8th ed.). Philadelphia: W.B. Saunders, p. 119.

64. A client who experienced a single rib fracture 3 days earlier is breathing shallowly and splinting the injured area by leaning against the bed mattress, chair, and other supports. The nurse plans care knowing that the client is at risk for developing which of the following complications?
1 Atelectasis and pneumonia
2 Hemoptysis and fever
3 Pneumothorax and infection
4 Deep vein thrombosis and atelectasis

Answer: 1
Rationale: The client with fractured ribs is predisposed to atelectasis and pneumonia because of the effects of shallow breathing, which leads to decreased coughing, accumulation of secretions, and subsequent pneumonia. The client could have hemoptysis or pneumothorax at the time of injury if the rib pierced lung tissue or the pleural cavity, but these complications are not likely to occur after the first 24 to 48 hours following the injury. Fever is a symptom, not a complication. Deep vein thrombosis is often a result of immobility, which is not indicated in the question.

Test-Taking Strategy: The key words in the question are *shallowly* and *splinting*. This tells you that the client is not fully expanding the lungs, which should lead you to conclude that the client is at risk for atelectasis and pneumonia. If this question was difficult, review these fundamental principles.

Level of Cognitive Ability: Comprehension
Client Needs: Physiological Integrity
Integrated Concept/Process: Nursing Process/Planning
Content Area: Adult Health/Respiratory

Reference:
Black, J., Hawks, J., & Keene, A. (2001). *Medical-surgical nursing: clinical management for positive outcomes* (6th ed.). Philadelphia: W.B. Saunders, p. 1769.

65. A client is recovering from flail chest. The nurse evaluates that the client status is most favorable if which of the following respiratory data are noted?
1   Respiratory rate 24 breaths per minute, oxygen saturation 99%
2   Respiratory rate 22 breaths per minute, oxygen saturation 93%
3   Respiratory rate 18 breaths per minute, oxygen saturation 98%
4   Respiratory rate 16 breaths per minute, oxygen saturation 90%

Answer: 3
Rationale: The normal respiratory rate is 12 to 22 breaths per minute, whereas the normal oxygen saturation range is 95% to 100%. Options 1, 2, and 4 do not represent normal values. Option 3 is the only option that identifies values that fall within normal parameters.

Test-Taking Strategy: Use the process of elimination. Note the key words *most favorable* in the question. Recalling the normal respiratory rate and the normal oxygen saturation directs you to option 3. Review these normal values if you had difficulty with this question.

Level of Cognitive Ability: Analysis
Client Needs: Physiological Integrity
Integrated Concept/Process: Nursing Process/Evaluation
Content Area: Adult Health/Respiratory

Reference:
Black, J., Hawks, J., & Keene, A. (2001). *Medical-surgical nursing: clinical management for positive outcomes* (6th ed.). Philadelphia: W.B. Saunders, pp. 1629; 1639.

---

66. A nurse is assisting in planning care for a client with respiratory failure. The highest priority of the nurse is to plan care that focuses on which of the following?
1   Optimizing nutrition
2   Maintaining fluid balance
3   Conserving energy
4   Preventing Valsalva maneuver

Answer: 3
Rationale: The care of the client in respiratory failure is focused on maintaining effective respirations and conserving energy. Fluid balance and nutrition are important, but energy conservation takes priority. Energy conservation conserves oxygen. Option 4 is unrelated to the question.

Test-Taking Strategy: Use the process of elimination and note the key words *respiratory failure* and *highest priority*. Focusing on the disorder and recalling that energy conservation conserves oxygen assists in directing you to option 3. Review care to the client with respiratory failure if you had difficulty with this question.

Level of Cognitive Ability: Application
Client Needs: Physiological Integrity
Integrated Concept/Process: Nursing Process/Planning
Content Area: Adult Health/Respiratory

Reference:
Ignatavicius, D., & Workman, M. (2002). *Medical-surgical nursing: critical thinking for collaborative care* (4th ed.). Philadelphia: W.B. Saunders, p. 599.

---

67. A nurse is collecting urine for a culture and sensitivity on a 1-year-old child. The nurse attaches a urine specimen bag to the perineum of the child after cleansing the perineum meticulously. After 30 minutes, the nurse checks the child to see whether the specimen has been obtained and notes that the child has not voided. Which of the following actions is most appropriate?

Answer: 1
Rationale: In infants and non–toilet-trained children, a urine specimen may be collected by attaching a bag to the perineum. The perineal area must be meticulously cleansed and the specimen collected within 30 minutes. If the child or infant does not void within 30 minutes, the bag is changed. Urine can be collected by urethral catheterization, but this is not the best method because it introduces bacteria into the bladder. The physician need not be notified.

1 Change the urine collection bag
2 Check in another 30 minutes to see whether the child has voided
3 Notify the physician that the specimen cannot be obtained
4 Catheterize the child

Test-Taking Strategy: Use the process of elimination and note the key words *culture and sensitivity*. Eliminate option 3 first because there is no indication that the physician should be notified. Eliminate option 4 next because of the invasive nature of this procedure. Noting the key words assists in directing you to choose option 1 from the remaining options. Review the procedure for obtaining a urine specimen for culture from an infant or a child if you had difficulty with this question.

Level of Cognitive Ability: Application
Client Needs: Physiological Integrity
Integrated Concept/Process: Nursing Process/Implementation
Content Area: Child Health

Reference:
Wong, D., & Hockenberry-Eaton, M. (2001). *Wong's essentials of pediatric nursing* (6th ed.). St. Louis: Mosby, p. 775.

---

68. A child is diagnosed with glomerulonephritis. The mother asks the nurse what the diagnosis means. The nurse bases the response on which of the following?
1 It is the backflow or reflux of urine from the bladder into the ureters and possibly the kidneys
2 It is a condition in which the child is unable to control bladder functions
3 It occurs when one or both testes fail to descend through the inguinal canal and to the scrotal sac
4 It is characterized by inflammation of the capillaries contained in the glomerulus

Answer: 4
Rationale: Glomerulonephritis is characterized by inflammation of the capillaries contained in the glomerulus. It can result from different causes, such as an infection, systemic disease process, or primary defect in the glomerulus itself. Option 1 describes vesicoureteral reflux. Option 2 describes enuresis. Option 3 describes cryptorchidism.

Test-Taking Strategy: Use the process of elimination. Note the relationship between the words *glomerulonephritis* in the question and *glomerulus* in the correct option. If you are unfamiliar with this disorder, this strategy may assist in directing you to the correct option. Review the physiology associated with this disorder if you had difficulty with this question.

Level of Cognitive Ability: Comprehension
Client Needs: Physiological Integrity
Integrated Concept/Process: Nursing Process/Implementation
Content Area: Child Health

Reference:
Wong, D., & Hockenberry-Eaton, M. (2001). *Wong's essentials of pediatric nursing* (6th ed.). St. Louis: Mosby, p. 1046.

---

69. A client with rheumatoid arthritis has been prescribed aspirin (acetylsalicylic acid) 1000 mg daily in divided doses. The nurse has reinforced instructions with the client regarding the medication. Which statement by the client indicates the need for further instructions?
1 "I will take the aspirin 1 hour before meals."
2 "I will watch for signs of bleeding."
3 "I will avoid activities that may cause bruising."

Answer: 1
Rationale: The client with rheumatoid arthritis may be prescribed a dose of aspirin of 1000 to 1600 mg a day. At these high doses, aspirin is frequently toxic. In addition, aspirin must be taken four times per day to sustain therapeutic blood levels, and such frequent doses often lead to problems with compliance with the medication regimen. Clients should be instructed to take aspirin with food and watch for clinical manifestations of gastrointestinal (GI) bleeding, easy bruising, and tinnitus (ringing in the ears).

Test-Taking Strategy: Use the process of elimination and note the key words *need for further instructions*. Eliminate options 2 and 3

4 "I will call my doctor if ringing in my ears occurs."

first because they are similar and both relate to the potential for bleeding. With this concept in mind, select option 1 instead of option 4 as the answer to this question because aspirin taken on an empty stomach can produce GI irritation and possible bleeding. Review teaching points related to the administration of aspirin if you had difficulty with this question.

Level of Cognitive Ability: Comprehension
Client Needs: Physiological Integrity
Integrated Concept/Process: Teaching/Learning
Content Area: Pharmacology

Reference:
Hodgson, B., & Kizior, R. (2003). *Saunders nursing drug handbook 2003.* Philadelphia: W.B. Saunders, p. 85.

---

70. Hypospadias is diagnosed in a newborn infant. The mother asks the nurse about the disorder. The nurse bases the response to the mother on which of the following?
1 It is a congenital anomaly in which the actual opening of the urethral meatus is below the normal placement on the glans penis
2 It occurs when one or both testes fail to descend through the inguinal canal into the scrotal sac
3 It is a congenital anomaly in which the actual opening of the urethral meatus is dorsal to the urethral opening
4 It is a congenital anomaly characterized by the extrusion of the urinary bladder to the outside of the body

Answer: 1
Rationale: Hypospadias is a congenital anomaly in which the actual opening of the urethral meatus is below the normal placement on the glans penis. Option 2 describes cryptorchidism. Option 3 describes epispadias. Option 4 describes bladder exstrophy.

Test-Taking Strategy: Use the process of elimination. Note the relationship between the prefix in the name of the disorder, *hypo-,* and the word *below* in the correct option. This strategy may assist in directing you to the correct option if you are unfamiliar with this disorder. Review this disorder if you had difficulty with the question.

Level of Cognitive Ability: Comprehension
Client Needs: Physiological Integrity
Integrated Concept/Process: Nursing Process/Implementation
Content Area: Child Health

Reference:
Wong, D., & Hockenberry-Eaton, M. (2001). *Wong's essentials of pediatric nursing* (6th ed.). St. Louis: Mosby, p. 220.

---

71. A nurse is reviewing the record of an infant admitted to the newborn nursery. The nurse notes that the physician has documented bladder exstrophy. Which of the following does the nurse expect to note in the infant?
1 Undescended or hidden testes
2 The opening of the urethral meatus below the normal placement on the glans penis
3 The opening of the urethral meatus on the ventral side of the glans penis
4 The urinary bladder on the outside of the body

Answer: 4
Rationale: Bladder exstrophy is a congenital anomaly characterized by the extrusion of the urinary bladder to the outside of the body through a defect in the lower abdominal wall. Option 1 describes cryptorchidism. Option 2 describes hypospadias. Option 3 describes epispadias.

Test-Taking Strategy: Use the process of elimination. Note the relationship between the prefix in the name of the disorder, *ex-,* and the word *outside* in the correct option. This strategy may assist in directing you to the correct option if you are unfamiliar with this disorder. Review information about this disorder if you had difficulty with this question.

Level of Cognitive Ability: Comprehension

Client Needs: Physiological Integrity
Integrated Concept/Process: Nursing Process/Data Collection
Content Area: Child Health

Reference:
Wong, D., & Hockenberry-Eaton, M. (2001). *Wong's essentials of pediatric nursing* (6th ed.). St. Louis: Mosby, p. 1042.

---

72. A nurse is reinforcing discharge instructions to the parents of a child who underwent a myringotomy with insertion of tympanostomy tubes. Which of the following does the nurse include in the instructions?
1   If any reddish drainage occurs, call the physician immediately
2   Encourage the child to blow the nose gently
3   Allow the child to swim as long as it is in a chlorinated swimming pool
4   Notify the physician if the child complains of any pain or has a fever

Answer: 4
Rationale: Postoperatively, a small amount of reddish drainage is normal for the first few days after surgery; however, the parents should report any heavier bleeding or bleeding that occurs after 3 days. The parents also should be instructed to report any fever or increased pain. The child should not blow the nose for 7 to 10 days. Baths and lake water are potential sources of bacterial contamination, and chlorinated swimming pools can be irritative to the tympanic membranes. The child should place earplugs or cotton balls covered with petroleum jelly in the ears during baths and shampoos. Swimming is allowed only with earplugs and with the physician's approval. Diving and swimming deeply underwater are prohibited.

Test-Taking Strategy: Use the process of elimination. Noting both the anatomical location of this surgical procedure and the key words *insertion of tympanostomy tubes* assists in directing you to option 4. Additionally, a general teaching guideline to remember is that the physician should be notified if a fever occurs. Review teaching points related to this procedure if you had difficulty with this question.

Level of Cognitive Ability: Application
Client Needs: Physiological Integrity
Integrated Concept/Process: Teaching/Learning
Content Area: Child Health

Reference:
Wong, D., & Hockenberry-Eaton, M. (2001). *Wong's essentials of pediatric nursing* (6th ed.). St. Louis: Mosby, p. 836.

---

73. A nurse has reinforced instructions to a mother regarding the care of her 10-year-old child with pharyngitis. Which statement by the mother indicates a need for further instructions?
1   "Antibiotics should be taken for the entire prescribed course."
2   "I should encourage my child to gargle with saline."
3   "I should apply warm compresses to my child's throat."
4   "I should bring my child to the clinic in 3 days for a repeat throat culture."

Answer: 4
Rationale: Antibiotics should be taken for the entire prescribed course, even if the child is feeling better and is free of symptoms. The older child may gargle with saline. Warm or cool compresses may be applied to the throat. A follow-up with repeat throat culture should be done 3 to 5 days after completing the course of the antibiotics.

Test-Taking Strategy: Note the key words *need for further instructions*. Use the process of elimination and general principles related to the effects of antibiotic therapy to answer the question. Careful reading of option 4 indicates that a throat culture after 3 days will not provide useful information regarding resolution of the infection. Review teaching guidelines related to pharyngitis if you had difficulty with this question.

Level of Cognitive Ability: Comprehension
Client Needs: Physiological Integrity
Integrated Concept/Process: Teaching/Learning
Content Area: Child Health

Reference:
Wong, D., & Hockenberry-Eaton, M. (2001). *Wong's essentials of pediatric nursing* (6th ed.). St. Louis: Mosby, p. 833.

---

74. A nurse is caring for a child after a tonsillectomy. Fluids are prescribed for the child. Which of the following would be most appropriate for the nurse to offer to the child?
1 Carbonated beverage
2 Orange juice
3 Ice cream
4 Apple juice

Answer: 4
Rationale: Clear, cool liquids are offered to the child when the child is fully awake. Citrus, carbonated, and extremely hot or cold liquids are avoided because they irritate the throat. Milk and milk products, including puddings and ice cream, are avoided initially until the child has tolerated clear liquids well. This is done because milk products can coat the throat and cause the child to clear it, thus increasing the risk of bleeding.

Test-Taking Strategy: Note the key words *most appropriate*. Focus on the surgical procedure and use the process of elimination. Eliminate option 1 first because of the word *carbonated*. Eliminate option 2 next because orange is a citrus product. Eliminate option 3 because milk can coat the throat and cause the child to attempt to clear it. Review nursing care after tonsillectomy if you had difficulty with this question.

Level of Cognitive Ability: Application
Client Needs: Physiological Integrity
Integrated Concept/Process: Nursing Process/Implementation
Content Area: Child Health

Reference:
Wong, D., & Hockenberry-Eaton, M. (2001). *Wong's essentials of pediatric nursing* (6th ed.). St. Louis: Mosby, p. 834.

---

75. The mother of a 6-year-old child arrives at the emergency room stating that the child has been complaining of a sore throat. The child has a high fever, and acute epiglottitis is diagnosed. The emergency room nurse plans care knowing that which of the following is not a clinical manifestation associated with this disorder?
1 It is usually viral in nature
2 It has an abrupt onset
3 It may rapidly progress to complete airway obstruction and death
4 It causes swelling and inflammation of the epiglottis

Answer: 1
Rationale: Acute epiglottitis is caused by bacteria, usually haemophilus influenzae, type B. Viral epiglottitis is rare. The other options are accurate descriptions of this respiratory disorder.

Test-Taking Strategy: Use the process of elimination and note the key word *not* in the question. Options 3 and 4 are similar and can be eliminated first. Knowledge regarding the clinical manifestations associated with epiglottitis is needed to select correctly from the remaining options. Review this life-threatening disorder if you had difficulty with this question.

Level of Cognitive Ability: Application
Client Needs: Physiological Integrity
Integrated Concept/Process: Nursing Process/Planning
Content Area: Child Health

Reference:
Wong, D., & Hockenberry-Eaton, M. (2001). *Wong's essentials of pediatric nursing* (6th ed.). St. Louis: Mosby, p. 837.

76. Ribavirin (Virazole) is prescribed for a child with respiratory syncytial virus. The nurse prepares to administer this medication by which of the following routes?
1 Subcutaneous
2 Oral
3 Intravenous
4 Via face mask

Answer: 4
Rationale: Ribavirin is an antiviral respiratory medication that is used to inhibit viral replication. Administration is via hood, face mask, or oxygen tent.

Test-Taking Strategy: Knowledge regarding the route of administration of this medication is necessary to answer this question. Review this medication if you had difficulty with this question.

Level of Cognitive Ability: Application
Client Needs: Physiological Integrity
Integrated Concept/Process: Nursing Process/Implementation
Content Area: Child Health

Reference:
Wong, D., & Hockenberry-Eaton, M. (2001). *Wong's essentials of pediatric nursing* (6th ed.). St. Louis: Mosby, p. 842.

---

77. A client seen in the health care clinic is scheduled for several diagnostic procedures. An abdominal aorta sonogram, a barium enema, an upper gastrointestinal (GI) series, and a small bowel series are prescribed. Which of the following should the nurse schedule first?
1 Barium enema
2 Upper GI series
3 Small bowel series
4 Abdominal aorta sonogram

Answer: 4
Rationale: The abdominal aorta sonogram should be performed before intestinal barium tests, or after the barium is cleared from the system. The barium obstructs the view when the abdominal aorta sonogram is obtained. The tests identified in options 1, 2, and 3 use barium for the visualization of these organs during diagnostic study.

Test-Taking Strategy: Use the process of elimination. Note the similarities among options 1, 2, and 3. All of these diagnostic tests use barium for the visualization of these organs during diagnostic study. Bearing this in mind, consider the effect of the barium in relation to visualizing the structures when the sonogram is performed. Review the diagnostic tests presented in the options if you are unfamiliar with them.

Level of Cognitive Ability: Application
Client Needs: Physiological Integrity
Integrated Concept/Process: Nursing Process/Implementation
Content Area: Adult Health/Gastrointestinal

Reference:
Chernecky, C., & Berger, B. (2001). *Laboratory tests and diagnostic procedures* (3rd ed.). Philadelphia: W.B. Saunders, p. 111.

---

78. A nurse is assigned to care for a child with a diagnosis of atrial septal defect. The nurse plans care knowing that which of the following is characteristic of this type of defect?
1 It is an opening between the two atria and allows oxygenated and unoxygenated blood to mix
2 It is an opening between the two ventricles and allows oxygenated and unoxygenated blood to mix

Answer: 1
Rationale: Atrial septal defect is an opening between the two atria that allows oxygenated blood and unoxygenated blood to mix. Left-to-right shunting of blood occurs because of the higher pressure on the left side of the heart. Ventricular septal defect is an opening between the two ventricles allowing oxygenated and unoxygenated blood to mix. Patent ductus arteriosus involves an artery that connects the aorta and pulmonary artery during fetal life. Atrioventricular canal defect occurs as a result of inappropriate fetal development of endocardial cushions.

3 It involves an artery that connects the aorta and the pulmonary artery during fetal life

4 It occurs as a result of inappropriate fetal development of endocardial cushions

Test-Taking Strategy: Use the process of elimination. Noting the words *atrial* in the question and *atria* in the correct option assists in directing you to option 1. Review the characteristics of this disorder if you had difficulty with this question.

Level of Cognitive Ability: Comprehension
Client Needs: Physiological Integrity
Integrated Concept/Process: Nursing Process/Planning
Content Area: Child Health

Reference:
Wong, D., & Hockenberry-Eaton, M. (2001). *Wong's essentials of pediatric nursing* (6th ed.). St. Louis: Mosby, p. 939.

---

79. A client has been prescribed isoniazid (INH) in the treatment of tuberculosis (TB). While the client is receiving this medication, the nurse plans to monitor the results of periodic measurements of which of the following?

1 Hemoglobin and hematocrit
2 Blood urea nitrogen (BUN) and creatinine
3 Hepatic enzymes
4 Vision testing

Answer: 3
Rationale: The client taking isoniazid is at risk for hepatotoxicity. For this reason, the client's hepatic enzymes are measured before and periodically during medication therapy. BUN and creatinine are measured during therapy with streptomycin, which is a nephrotoxic medication. Vision testing is done during treatment with ethambutol (Myambutol). Hemoglobin and hematocrit values are unrelated to the medication addressed in the question.

Test-Taking Strategy: Use the process of elimination. To answer this question accurately, you must be familiar with the various medications that are used to treat TB and their associated adverse or toxic effects. Review these medications if you had difficulty with this question.

Level of Cognitive Ability: Analysis
Client Needs: Physiological Integrity
Integrated Concept/Process: Nursing Process/Data Collection
Content Area: Pharmacology

Reference:
Hodgson, B., & Kizior, R. (2003). *Saunders nursing drug handbook 2003.* Philadelphia: W.B. Saunders, p. 616.

---

80. A client is at risk for pulmonary embolism (PE) because of a postoperative state and immobility. The nurse monitors the client for which most common symptom of PE?

1 Dry cough
2 Diaphoresis
3 Apprehension
4 Sudden onset of chest pain

Answer: 4
Rationale: The most common symptom of PE is a sudden onset of chest pain. The next most frequent symptoms are dyspnea and tachypnea. Other manifestations include tachycardia, diaphoresis, cough, fever, hemoptysis, and syncope.

Test-Taking Strategy: Use the process of elimination and note the key words *most common*. Recalling the manifestations associated with PE directs you to option 4. Review these manifestations if you had difficulty with this question.

Level of Cognitive Ability: Application
Client Needs: Physiological Integrity
Integrated Concept/Process: Nursing Process/Data Collection
Content Area: Adult Health/Respiratory

Reference:
Black, J., Hawks, J., & Keene, A. (2001). *Medical-surgical nursing: clinical management for positive outcomes* (6th ed.). Philadelphia: W.B. Saunders, p. 606.

---

81. A nurse is preparing to administer quinapril hydrochloride (Accupril) to a client with hypertension. The nurse understands that this medication belongs to which of the following medication classifications?

1 Angiotensin-converting enzyme (ACE) inhibitor
2 Thiazide diuretic
3 Loop diuretic
4 Calcium-channel blocker

Answer: 1
Rationale: Quinapril hydrochloride is an angiotensin-converting enzyme inhibitor. It suppresses the renal angiotensin-aldosterone system and reduces peripheral arterial resistance and blood pressure. It is used in the treatment of hypertension, either alone or in combination with other antihypertensive agents.

Test-Taking Strategy: Knowledge regarding this medication classification is necessary to answer this question. Eliminate options 2 and 3 first because they are similar. From the remaining options, recall that most ACE inhibitors end with "pril." This directs you to option 1. Review characteristics of this medication if you had difficulty with this question.

Level of Cognitive Ability: Comprehension
Client Needs: Physiological Integrity
Integrated Concept/Process: Nursing Process/Planning
Content Area: Pharmacology

Reference:
Hodgson, B., & Kizior, R. (2003). *Saunders nursing drug handbook 2003*. Philadelphia: W.B. Saunders, p. 954.

---

82. Quinidine gluconate (Duraquin) is prescribed for a client. Which of the following would the nurse specifically plan to monitor before administering this medication?

1 Temperature
2 Respirations
3 Blood pressure (BP)
4 Pulse oximetry

Answer: 3
Rationale: Quinidine gluconate is an antidysrhythmic medication. The BP should be monitored before administering the medication. Although pulse oximetry, temperature, and respirations may be components of the data collection, monitoring the BP is specific to the administration of this medication.

Test-Taking Strategy: Knowledge regarding the action and nursing interventions associated with the administration of this medication is necessary to answer this question. Review information about this medication if you had difficulty with this question.

Level of Cognitive Ability: Application
Client Needs: Physiological Integrity
Integrated Concept/Process: Nursing Process/Data Collection
Content Area: Pharmacology

Reference:
Hodgson, B., & Kizior, R. (2003). *Saunders nursing drug handbook 2003*. Philadelphia: W.B. Saunders, p. 954.

---

83. Quinine sulfate is prescribed for a client. The client asks the nurse about the purpose of this medication. The nurse bases the response on the information that this

Answer: 3
Rationale: Quinine sulfate is an antimalarial, antimyotonic medication. Its antimalarial effect elevates the pH in intracellular organelles of parasites, producing parasitic death. It relaxes the

medication is classified as which of the following?

1 Antidysrhythmic
2 Antimicrobial
3 Antimalarial
4 Antispasmodic

skeletal muscle by increasing the refractory period, decreasing excitability of motor end plates, and affecting distribution of calcium within muscle fiber. Options 1, 2, and 4 are incorrect.

Test-Taking Strategy: Knowledge regarding the action of this medication is necessary to answer this question. Review characteristics of this medication if you had difficulty with this question.

Level of Cognitive Ability: Comprehension
Client Needs: Physiological Integrity
Integrated Concept/Process: Nursing Process/Implementation
Content Area: Pharmacology

Reference:
Hodgson, B., & Kizior, R. (2003). *Saunders nursing drug handbook 2003.* Philadelphia: W.B. Saunders, p. 958.

---

84. A client has been given instructions for taking nitrofurantoin (Macrodantin) in the oral suspension form. The nurse determines that the client does not fully understand the medication information given if the client states which of the following?

1 "The medication discolors the urine to a brownish color."
2 "I should avoid driving while taking this medication."
3 "If a dose is missed, I should double the dose at the next scheduled time."
4 "I should rinse my mouth with water to avoid staining my teeth."

Answer: 3
Rationale: Doses should not be skipped or doubled. The medication does discolor the urine, which is not significant. The client should avoid driving until tolerance to the medication is known, because the medication causes dizziness and drowsiness. It is recommended that the client rinse the mouth with water after a dose because the oral suspension may stain teeth.

Test-Taking Strategy: Use the process of elimination and note the key words *does not fully understand.* Knowledge of general principles regarding client instructions related to medication therapy easily directs you to option 3. Review information about this medication if you had difficulty with this question.

Level of Cognitive Ability: Comprehension
Client Needs: Physiological Integrity
Integrated Concept/Process: Teaching/Learning
Content Area: Adult Health/Renal

Reference:
Hodgson, B., & Kizior, R. (2003). *Saunders nursing drug handbook 2003.* Philadelphia: W.B. Saunders, p. 814.

---

85. An LPN is assisting in developing a plan of care for a woman with an amniotic fluid embolism (AFE). The registered nurse has formulated a nursing diagnosis of impaired gas exchange related to blockage of the lungs from AFE. Which of the following outcomes should the LPN consider appropriate for this client?

1 The woman will verbalize an understanding of the complications of AFE
2 The woman will show no complications of hemorrhage, hypovolemia,

Answer: 4
Rationale: Option 4 identifies the appropriate outcome for the nursing diagnosis of impaired gas exchange. Option 1 relates to fear for self and baby, option 2 to risk for fluid volume deficit, and option 3 to altered tissue perfusion.

Test-Taking Strategy: Use the process of elimination. Focus on the key words *impaired gas exchange* and use the ABCs (airway, breathing, and circulation) to direct you to option 4. Also note the relationship between the words *impaired gas exchange* in the question and *normal gas exchange* in option 4. Review care to the client with AFE if you had difficulty with this question.

or disseminated intravascular coagulation

3 The woman will demonstrate normal cardiac rate, blood pressure, and skin color

4 The woman will demonstrate an effective respiratory rate and have a normal gas exchange

Level of Cognitive Ability: Analysis
Client Needs: Physiological Integrity
Integrated Concept/Process: Nursing Process/Planning
Content Area: Maternity

Reference:
Murray, S., McKinney, E., & Gorrie, T. (2002). *Foundations of maternal-newborn nursing* (3rd ed.). Philadelphia: W.B. Saunders, p. 768.

---

86. A mother is admitted to the postpartum unit after delivery of a healthy newborn. During the immediate postpartum period, how often does the nurse plan to take the mother's vital signs?

1 Every 15 minutes during the first hour after birth

2 Every 30 minutes during the first hour after birth

3 When the client arrives at the unit and 60 minutes later

4 When the client arrives at the unit and every 4 hours thereafter

Answer: 1
Rationale: During the immediate postpartum period, vital signs are taken every 15 minutes during the first hour after birth, every 30 minutes for the next 2 hours, and every hour for the next 2 to 6 hours. Vital signs are monitored thereafter every 4 hours for the first 24 hours and every 8 to 12 hours for the remainder of the hospital stay.

Test-Taking Strategy: Use the process of elimination. Note the key word *immediate* in the question. This should direct you to option 1, because this choice addresses the most frequent time frame for monitoring vital signs. If you had difficulty with this question, review postpartum assessments.

Level of Cognitive Ability: Application
Client Needs: Physiological Integrity
Integrated Concept/Process: Nursing Process/Planning
Content Area: Maternity

Reference:
Murray, S., McKinney, E., & Gorrie, T. (2002). *Foundations of maternal-newborn nursing* (3rd ed.). Philadelphia: W.B. Saunders, p. 438.

---

87. A nurse is monitoring the vital signs of a client after delivery of a healthy newborn. The nurse notes that the mother's apical pulse is 50 beats per minute (BPM). Which of the following nursing actions is most appropriate?

1 Document the finding

2 Notify the physician

3 Encourage the mother to ambulate, then reassess the apical pulse

4 Increase oral fluids

Answer: 1
Rationale: During the first week after birth, transient episodes of bradycardia are common. The woman's pulse may be as low as 40 to 50 BPM the first 1 to 2 days after delivery. It is not necessary to notify the physician. Options 2, 3, and 4 are not related to the issue of the question.

Test-Taking Strategy: Use the process of elimination. Knowledge regarding the normal findings in the postpartum period directs you to option 1. If you had difficulty with this question, review normal postpartum assessment findings.

Level of Cognitive Ability: Application
Client Needs: Physiological Integrity
Integrated Concept/Process: Nursing Process/Implementation
Content Area: Maternity

Reference:
Murray, S., McKinney, E., & Gorrie, T. (2002). *Foundations of maternal-newborn nursing* (3rd ed.). Philadelphia: W.B. Saunders, p. 440.

88. A nurse is caring for a woman in the post-partum unit. When the nurse checks the position of the fundus, the nurse notes that the fundus is displaced to one side. Which of the following nursing actions is most appropriate?
1 Notify the physician
2 Massage the fundus
3 Encourage fluids
4 Assist the client to empty the bladder

Answer: 4

Rationale: The position of the fundus should be midline. Displacement to the side indicates that the bladder may be full. It is not necessary to notify the physician. Fundal massage is performed when the uterus is soft and boggy. Administration of fluids is important in the postpartum period, but this action is unrelated to the issue of the question.

Test-Taking Strategy: Use the process of elimination. Knowledge regarding the normal findings in a woman in the postpartum period is necessary to answer this question. Focusing on the information provided in the question directs you to option 4. Review normal postpartum assessment findings if you had difficulty with this question.

Level of Cognitive Ability: Application
Client Needs: Physiological Integrity
Integrated Concept/Process: Nursing Process/Implementation
Content Area: Maternity

Reference:
Murray, S., McKinney, E., & Gorrie, T. (2002). *Foundations of maternal-newborn nursing* (3rd ed.). Philadelphia: W.B. Saunders, p. 441.

---

89. A nurse is assigned to care for a client with acquired immunodeficiency syndrome (AIDS). The nurse notes that a nursing diagnosis of Risk for Infection is documented in the client's care plan. The nurse evaluates that the client has not yet met expected outcomes if the client demonstrates which of the following?
1 Maintains a body temperature of less than 100° F
2 Has a shift to the left in white blood cells (WBCs)
3 Has negative urine and sputum cultures
4 Has a blood pressure (BP) of 128/86 mmHg with pulse rate of 82 breaths per minute

Answer: 2

Rationale: Signs of infection include fever (greater than 100° F); increased pulse and BP; high WBC count with a shift to the left (indicating rapid proliferation of WBCs); and positive cultures, such as for wounds, urine, sputum, or blood. If the client meets expected outcomes, the client is free of signs and symptoms of infection.

Test-Taking Strategy: Note the key words *has not yet met*. Use process of elimination to answer this question, remembering basic concepts related to infection. This allows you to eliminate each of the incorrect options. Review the indications of infection if you had difficulty with this question.

Level of Cognitive Ability: Analysis
Client Needs: Physiological Integrity
Integrated Concept/Process: Nursing Process/Evaluation
Content Area: Adult Health/Respiratory

Reference:
Ignatavicius, D., & Workman, M. (2002). *Medical-surgical nursing: critical thinking for collaborative care* (4th ed.). Philadelphia: W.B. Saunders, p. 301.

---

90. A client with chronic airflow limitation (CAL) is at risk for infection related to chronic respiratory disease. The nurse collects data regarding which of the following factors that predisposes the client to infection?
1 Controlled cough technique
2 Avoidance of crowds

Answer: 3

Rationale: A limited fluid intake can predispose the client to dehydration and respiratory infection because dehydration impairs the action of the cilia in the respiratory tree. Pursed lip breathing and controlled cough technique are taught to clients to help make breathing easier and assist with expectoration of secretions. Avoidance of crowds is an important measure to prevent infection in the client with CAL.

3 Limited fluid intake
4 Pursed lip breathing

Test-Taking Strategy: Use the process of elimination and knowledge of the risk factors that predispose the client with CAL to infection. Eliminate options 1 and 4 because these are breathing techniques. Recalling the effect of limiting fluid intake assists in directing you to option 3 from the remaining options. Review the predisposing risk factors for infection if you had difficulty with this question.

Level of Cognitive Ability: Comprehension
Client Needs: Physiological Integrity
Integrated Concept/Process: Nursing Process/Data Collection
Content Area: Adult Health/Respiratory

Reference:
Black, J., Hawks, J., & Keene, A. (2001). *Medical-surgical nursing: clinical management for positive outcomes* (6th ed.). Philadelphia: W.B. Saunders, p. 1702.

---

91. A client is diagnosed with polycythemia vera. The client asks the nurse about the disorder, and the nurse plans to base the response on which of the following characteristics of polycythemia vera?
1 It is classified as a myeloproliferative disorder
2 It is an anemia that occurs as the result of poor iron intake
3 It occurs as a result of a lack of the intrinsic factor
4 It occurs as a result of a hereditary factor

Answer: 1
Rationale: Polycythemia vera is defined as the increase in both the number of circulating erythrocytes and the concentration of hemoglobin within the blood. It is classified as a myeloproliferative disorder, meaning overgrowth of bone marrow. It usually develops in middle-aged people, particularly Jewish men. The cause remains unknown, although it is possibly a form of malignancy similar to leukemia and is often considered a premalignant condition, sometimes referred to as myeloproliferative dyscrasia. Iron deficiency anemia occurs as a result of poor intake of iron. The lack of the intrinsic factor produces pernicious anemia.

Test-Taking Strategy: Use the process of elimination. Focus on the name of the disorder to assist in answering the question. Note the relationship between *polycythemia* in the question and *myeloproliferative* in option 1. Review this disorder if you had difficulty with this question.

Level of Cognitive Ability: Comprehension
Client Needs: Physiological Integrity
Integrated Concept/Process: Teaching/Learning
Content Area: Fundamental Skills

Reference:
Black, J., Hawks, J., & Keene, A. (2001). *Medical-surgical nursing: clinical management for positive outcomes* (6th ed.). Philadelphia: W.B. Saunders, p. 2118.

---

92. A nurse is caring for a client with a diagnosis of suspected leukemia. The nurse prepares the client for which of the following diagnostic tests that will confirm this diagnosis?
1 Bone marrow aspiration biopsy
2 Lumbar puncture
3 Radiographic tests
4 Lymphangiogram

Answer: 1
Rationale: Bone marrow aspiration biopsy is a key diagnostic tool for confirming the diagnosis of leukemia and for identifying malignant cell types. Lumbar puncture may determine the presence of blast cells in the central nervous system. Radiographic tests may detect lesions and sites of infection. A lymphangiogram may be performed to locate malignant lesions and accurately classify the disease.

Test-Taking Strategy: Use the process of elimination. Focusing on the key word *confirm* in the question should direct you to option

1. If you had difficulty with this question, review the diagnostic tests for leukemia.

Level of Cognitive Ability: Application
Client Needs: Physiological Integrity
Integrated Concept/Process: Nursing Process/Planning
Content Area: Adult Health/Oncology

Reference:
Black, J., Hawks, J., & Keene, A. (2001). *Medical-surgical nursing: clinical management for positive outcomes* (6th ed.). Philadelphia: W.B. Saunders, p. 2168.

---

93. A nurse is caring for a client who is receiving chemotherapy for leukemia. The nurse reviews the laboratory results and notes that the neutrophil count is less than 500/mm³. Based on this laboratory result, the nurse implements which of the following?
  1 Using an electric shaver for shaving
  2 Providing meticulous skin decontamination before venipuncture
  3 Providing a soft tooth brush for oral care
  4 Avoiding overinflation of the blood pressure (BP) cuff and rotating the cuff to different sites when checking for BP

Answer: 2
Rationale: When the neutrophil count is less than 1000/mm³, the client is at risk for infection. Options 1, 3, and 4 address nursing interventions if the client is at risk for bleeding. Providing meticulous skin decontamination before venipuncture, maintaining sterile occlusion of IV and central venous catheters, and monitoring the oral temperature are critical nursing interventions for the client at risk for infection.

Test-Taking Strategy: Use the process of elimination. Recalling the relationship between a low neutrophil count and the risk for infection assists in directing you to option 2. If you had difficulty with this question, review the nursing plan of care for a client with leukemia.

Level of Cognitive Ability: Application
Client Needs: Physiological Integrity
Integrated Concept/Process: Nursing Process/Implementation
Content Area: Adult Health/Oncology

Reference:
Black, J., Hawks, J., & Keene, A. (2001). *Medical-surgical nursing: clinical management for positive outcomes* (6th ed.). Philadelphia: W.B. Saunders, p. 2170.

---

94. A nurse is caring for a client with cancer of the bowel who is receiving chemotherapy. When evaluating the laboratory findings, the nurse notes that the client's neutrophil count is 1000/mm³. Which of the following problems would be of most concern for this client based on this laboratory result?
  1 Alteration in nutrition
  2 Potential for infection
  3 Potential for hemorrhage
  4 Risk for ineffective individual coping

Answer: 2
Rationale: When the neutrophil count is less than 1000/mm³, the client is at risk for infection. A platelet count less than 20,000/mm³ places the client at risk for hemorrhage. There are no data in the question to support an alteration in nutrition or a risk for ineffective individual coping.

Test-Taking Strategy: Use the process of elimination. Knowledge regarding the normal neutrophil count and the relationship between a low neutrophil count and the risk for infection directs you to option 2. Review the risks associated with a low neutrophil count if you had difficulty with this question.

Level of Cognitive Ability: Analysis
Client Needs: Physiological Integrity
Integrated Concept/Process: Nursing Process/Evaluation
Content Area: Adult Health/Oncology

Reference:
Black, J., Hawks, J., & Keene, A. (2001). *Medical-surgical nursing: clinical management for positive outcomes* (6th ed.). Philadelphia: W.B. Saunders, pp. 392-393.

---

95. A pregnant client arrives at the prenatal clinic and is complaining that her breasts are very tender. The client is concerned about what is causing this discomfort. The nurse plans to base the response to the client on the fact that tender breasts during pregnancy occur as a result of which of the following?
1 Increased levels of estrogen and progesterone
2 Decreased levels of estrogen and progesterone
3 Increased levels of prolactin
4 Decreased levels of prolactin

Answer: 1
Rationale: The breasts become tender early in pregnancy because of increased levels of estrogen and progesterone. Self-care measures for breast tenderness include wearing a well-fitting brassiere that provides support for the breasts and decreases discomfort, and sleeping with a pillow.

Test-Taking Strategy: Knowledge regarding the physiological alterations that occur during pregnancy assists you in answering this question. If you had difficulty with this question, review the hormonal changes that occur as a result of pregnancy.

Level of Cognitive Ability: Comprehension
Client Needs: Physiological Integrity
Integrated Concept/Process: Nursing Process/Planning
Content Area: Maternity

Reference:
Murray, S., McKinney, E., & Gorrie, T. (2002). *Foundations of maternal-newborn nursing* (3rd ed.). Philadelphia: W.B. Saunders, p. 122.

---

96. A client has just been told by the physician that a cerebral angiogram will be obtained. The nurse then collects data from the client about which of the following conditions?
1 Claustrophobia
2 Excessive weight
3 Allergy to eggs
4 Allergy to iodine or shellfish

Answer: 4
Rationale: The client undergoing cerebral angiography is assessed for possible allergy to the contrast dye, which can be determined by questioning the client about allergies to iodine or shellfish. Allergy to eggs is irrelevant to the question. Claustrophobia and excessive weight are areas of concern with magnetic resonance imaging.

Test-Taking Strategy: Use the process of elimination. This concept is fundamental for angiography of any group of blood vessels. Remember that a primary concern is allergy to iodine or shellfish. Review this diagnostic test if you had difficulty with this question.

Level of Cognitive Ability: Application
Client Needs: Physiological Integrity
Integrated Concept/Process: Nursing Process/Data Collection
Content Area: Fundamental Skills

Reference:
Lewis, S., Heitkemper, M., & Dirksen, S. (2000). *Medical-surgical nursing: assessment and management of clinical problems* (5th ed.). St. Louis: Mosby, p. 1603.

---

97. A client is being prepared for a lumbar puncture (LP). The nurse assists the client into which of the following positions for the procedure?
1 Prone, in slight Trendelenburg position

Answer: 3
Rationale: The client undergoing LP is positioned lying on the side, with the legs pulled up against the abdomen and with the head bent down toward the chest. This position helps widen the spaces between the vertebrae.

2 Prone, with a pillow under the abdomen

3 Side-lying, with the legs pulled up and the head bent down onto the chest

4 Side-lying, with a pillow under the hip

Test-Taking Strategy: Use the process of elimination. Knowing that an LP is the introduction of a needle into the subarachnoid space, it is reasonable to assume that the position of the client must facilitate this. The correct option is the only position that flexes the vertebrae for easier needle insertion. Review this procedure if you had difficulty with this question.

Level of Cognitive Ability: Application
Client Needs: Physiological Integrity
Integrated Concept/Process: Nursing Process/Implementation
Content Area: Adult Health/Neurological

Reference:
Lewis, S., Heitkemper, M., & Dirksen, S. (2000). *Medical-surgical nursing: assessment and management of clinical problems* (5th ed.). St. Louis: Mosby, p. 1602.

---

98. A nurse notes fine involuntary eye movements a client's eyes. The nurse documents in the medical record that the client has which of the following?
1 Ataxia
2 Nystagmus
3 Pronator drift
4 Hyperreflexia

Answer: 2
Rationale: Nystagmus is characterized by fine involuntary eye movements. Ataxia is a disturbance in gait. Pronator drift occurs when a client cannot maintain the hands in a supinated position with the arms extended and eyes closed. This data collection technique may be done to detect small changes in muscle strength that might not otherwise be noted. Hyperreflexia is an excessive reflex action.

Test-Taking Strategy: To answer this question accurately, you must be familiar with abnormal findings of the neurological system. Review the description of nystagmus if you had difficulty with this question.

Level of Cognitive Ability: Application
Client Needs: Physiological Integrity
Integrated Concept/Process: Communication and Documentation
Content Area: Adult Health/Neurological

Reference:
Lewis, S., Heitkemper, M., & Dirksen, S. (2000). *Medical-surgical nursing: assessment and management of clinical problems* (5th ed.). St. Louis: Mosby, p. 1602.

---

99. A nurse is caring for a client with a cerebellar lesion. The nurse plans to obtain which of the following devices to assist the client in adapting to this problem?
1 Slider board
2 Raised toilet seat
3 Adaptive eating utensils
4 Walker

Answer: 4
Rationale: The cerebellum is responsible for balance and coordination. A walker provides stability for the client during ambulation. A slider board is useful in transferring a client who cannot move from a bed to a stretcher or wheelchair. A raised toilet seat is useful if the client does not have the mobility or ability to flex the hips. Adaptive eating utensils may be useful if the client has partial paralysis of the hand.

Test-Taking Strategy: Use the process of elimination. To answer this question correctly, you must know that the cerebellum controls balance and coordination. You then look for the option that will assist the client in one of these areas. This helps you to eliminate options 1 and 2. From the remaining options, recall that adaptive eating utensils are used when there is loss of fine motor coordination, such as with a cerebrovascular accident. The walker will help the client maintain balance. Review care to the client with a cerebellar lesion if you had difficulty with this question.

Level of Cognitive Ability: Application
Client Needs: Physiological Integrity
Integrated Concept/Process: Nursing Process/Planning
Content Area: Adult Health/Neurological

Reference:
Lewis, S., Heitkemper, M., & Dirksen, S. (2000). *Medical-surgical nursing: assessment and management of clinical problems* (5th ed.). St. Louis: Mosby, p. 1587.

---

100. A client with Bell's palsy has dysfunction of cranial nerve VII. The nurse monitors the client for which of the following signs and symptoms of this disorder?
1   Double vision and excessive tearing
2   Sharp facial pain and muscle twitching
3   Heightened taste and eye pain
4   Facial droop and excessive drooling

Answer: 4
Rationale: The facial nerve (cranial nerve VII) has both motor and sensory divisions. Common symptoms of dysfunction of this nerve include an inability to close the eye and blink automatically, facial asymmetry, drooling and inability to swallow secretions, loss of the ability to form tears, and possible loss of taste on the anterior two thirds of the tongue. Bell's palsy, fracture of the temporal bone, and parotid lacerations or contusions are often responsible for these symptoms.

Test-Taking Strategy: Questions related to cranial nerves are difficult unless you know the differences between them. If you remember that cranial nerve VII is the facial nerve, you can eliminate each of the incorrect options. Review Bell's palsy if you had difficulty with this question.

Level of Cognitive Ability: Analysis
Client Needs: Physiological Integrity
Integrated Concept/Process: Nursing Process/Data Collection
Content Area: Adult Health/Neurological

Reference:
Lewis, S., Heitkemper, M., & Dirksen, S. (2000). *Medical-surgical nursing: assessment and management of clinical problems* (5th ed.). St. Louis: Mosby, p. 1717.

---

101. A pregnant client arrives at a prenatal clinic for a regularly scheduled prenatal visit. The client tells the nurse that she has been having a clear and slightly whitish vaginal discharge. Which of the following actions by the nurse is most appropriate?
1   Obtain a culture of the vaginal discharge
2   Inform the client that she should see the physician immediately
3   Inform the client that this is a common occurrence in pregnancy
4   Inform the client that sexual intercourse should be avoided until the discharge has been further evaluated

Answer: 3
Rationale: Vaginal discharge called leukorrhea is common in pregnant women because of the increased mucus production by the endocervical gland. The mucus should be clear or slightly whitish and mucoid in appearance. Option 1 is unnecessary. Option 2 is unnecessary and may alarm the client. Option 4 is inaccurate based on the issue stated in the question.

Test-Taking Strategy: Use the process of elimination. Recalling that a clear or slightly whitish vaginal discharge is normal during pregnancy directs you to option 3. If you had difficulty with this question, review the physiological changes that occur in pregnancy.

Level of Cognitive Ability: Application
Client Needs: Physiological Integrity

Integrated Concept/Process: Nursing Process/Implementation
Content Area: Maternity

Reference:
Murray, S., McKinney, E., & Gorrie, T. (2002). *Foundations of maternal-newborn nursing* (3rd ed.). Philadelphia: W.B. Saunders, p. 122.

---

102. A pregnant woman is suspected of alcohol abuse, and the nurse checks the client for clinical manifestations associated with this practice. Which of the following would least likely be noted in the client?
1   Increased weight gain
2   Hypoglycemia
3   Sweating
4   Slurred speech

Answer: 1
Rationale: Clinical manifestations indicative of alcohol abuse during the prenatal period include poor weight gain, hypoglycemia, tremors at rest, nausea, weakness, anxiety, slurred speech, unsteady gait, obvious sweating of the palms and forehead, and generalized sweating.

Test-Taking Strategy: Use the process of elimination. Focusing on the key words *least likely* and the issue stated in the question should direct you to option 1. If you had difficulty with this question, review alcohol abuse during pregnancy.

Level of Cognitive Ability: Comprehension
Client Needs: Physiological Integrity
Integrated Concept/Process: Nursing Process/Data Collection
Content Area: Maternity

Reference:
Murray, S., McKinney, E., & Gorrie, T. (2002). *Foundations of maternal-newborn nursing* (3rd ed.). Philadelphia: W.B. Saunders, p. 207.

---

103. A nurse is checking for the presence of pitting edema in a prenatal client. The nurse presses the tips of the index and middle fingers against the skin of the client and holds pressure for 2 to 3 seconds. Upon releasing the pressure, the nurse notes a slight indentation. Which of the following determinations will the nurse make based on this finding?
1   1+ edema
2   2+ edema
3   3+ edema
4   4+ edema

Answer: 1
Rationale: After assessment of pitting edema, if the nurse notes a slight indentation, it is documented as a 1+ edema. A 2+ edema is an indentation approximately ¼-inch deep. A 3+ edema is an indentation approximately ½-inch deep, and a 4+ edema is an indentation approximately 1-inch deep.

Test-Taking Strategy: Use the process of elimination. Focusing on the key words *slight indentation* in the question should direct you to option 1. If you had difficulty with this question, review data collection and evaluation of pitting edema.

Level of Cognitive Ability: Comprehension
Client Needs: Physiological Integrity
Integrated Concept/Process: Nursing Process/Data Collection
Content Area: Maternity

Reference:
Murray, S., McKinney, E., & Gorrie, T. (2002). *Foundations of maternal-newborn nursing* (3rd ed.). Philadelphia: W.B. Saunders, p. 131.

---

104. A nurse is caring for a client with a diagnosis of chronic pancreatitis. The nurse collects data on the client knowing that which of the following symptoms indicates poor absorption of dietary fats?

Answer: 1
Rationale: The pancreas makes digestive enzymes that aid in the absorption of food and nutrients. Chronic pancreatitis interferes with the absorption of nutrients. Fat absorption is limited because of the lack of pancreatic lipase. Steatorrhea by definition

1   Steatorrhea
2   Bloody diarrhea
3   Electrolyte disturbances
4   Gastrointestinal reflux disease

means fatty stools and often results from malabsorption problems. Options 2, 3, and 4 are incorrect.

Test-Taking Strategy: Use the process of elimination and focus on the client's diagnosis. Recalling the definition of steatorrhea directs you to option 1. Additionally, options 2, 3, and 4 are rarely associated with chronic pancreatitis. Review the manifestations of this disorder if you had difficulty with this question.

Level of Cognitive Ability: Comprehension
Client Needs: Physiological Integrity
Integrated Concept/Process: Nursing Process/Data Collection
Content Area: Adult Health/Gastrointestinal

Reference:
Ignatavicius, D., & Workman, M. (2002). *Medical-surgical: critical thinking for collaborative care* (4th ed.). Philadelphia: W.B. Saunders, p. 1347.

---

105. A nurse is assigned to care for a client who is recovering from a burn injury affecting 60% of body surfaces. On the fourth hospital day, the nurse notes that the client's temperature is 102.8° F, pulse is 98 beats per minute, respirations are 24 breaths per minute, and blood pressure is 105/64 mmHg. Total parenteral nutrition (TPN) is infusing at 82 mL per hour. Which of the following initial nursing actions would be most appropriate?
1   Notify the RN
2   Check the client for signs of infection
3   Prepare to change the TPN solution and IV tubing
4   Prepare to discontinue the TPN and culture the tip of the catheter and the insertion site

Answer: 2
Rationale: The client is recovering from serious burns. The burn client is prone to several complications such as infection, dehydration, and sepsis. A temperature of 102.8° F is significant. On the fourth hospital day, infection may be the problem. The cause of the infection may be the burns, the TPN infusion or TPN site, or other problems. As an initial action, the nurse should check the client for signs of infection and then notify the RN. Options 3 and 4 may follow after notification of the RN.

Test-Taking Strategy: Use the process of elimination. Note the key words *on the fourth hospital day* and *initial nursing actions.* Use the steps of the nursing process, recalling that data collection is the first step. Only option 2 addresses data collection. Review the signs of infection in a client with a burn injury if you had difficulty with this question.

Level of Cognitive Ability: Application
Client Needs: Physiological Integrity
Integrated Concept/Process: Nursing Process/Implementation
Content Area: Fundamental Skills

Reference:
Ignatavicius, D., & Workman, M. (2002). *Medical-surgical: critical thinking for collaborative care* (4th ed.). Philadelphia: W.B. Saunders, pp. 1372; 1580.

---

106. A client has total parenteral nutrition (TPN) infusing per physician's order at 75 mL per hour. The nurse prepares to care for the client and plans to do which of the following?
1   Monitor the urine output hourly
2   Monitor the vital signs every hour
3   Monitor the blood glucose levels every 4 to 6 hours

Answer: 3
Rationale: Total parenteral nutrition delivers high concentrations of glucose. Because of the high concentrations of glucose, standard protocol for a client on TPN is to monitor blood glucose levels. The client may become hypoglycemic because of the addition of insulin to the TPN solution, or hyperglycemic and need supplemental insulin. Options 1, 2, and 4 may be parts of the plan, but the frequency noted in these options is not necessary unless a specific complication occurred.

4 Monitor the client for dependent edema every hour

Test-Taking Strategy: Use the process of elimination. Recalling the complications associated with TPN and noting the frequency in each of the options direct you to option 3. Review care to the client on TPN if you had difficulty with this question.

Level of Cognitive Ability: Application
Client Needs: Physiological Integrity
Integrated Concept/Process: Nursing Process/Planning
Content Area: Fundamental Skills

Reference:
Ignatavicius, D., & Workman, M. (2002). *Medical-surgical nursing: critical thinking for collaborative care* (4th ed.). Philadelphia: W.B. Saunders, p. 1372.

---

107. Magnesium sulfate by intramuscular injection is prescribed for a pregnant client. The nurse understands that this medication is most likely prescribed to do which of the following?
1 Control seizures caused by low magnesium levels
2 Increase the amount of water in feces
3 Increase sinoatrial (SA) node impulse formulation
4 Increase conduction time in the myocardium

Answer: 1
Rationale: Magnesium sulfate is administered to pregnant women to control seizures resulting from hypomagnesemia (as in eclampsia). A secondary effect of magnesium sulfate is that it acts as a laxative by increasing the water content of feces. Magnesium sulfate decreases SA node impulse formation and decreases myocardial conduction time.

Test-Taking Strategy: Use the process of elimination. Note the relationship between the name of the medication and option 1. Administering magnesium sulfate will most likely be necessary if the level is low. Review the action of this medication if you had difficulty with this question.

Level of Cognitive Ability: Comprehension
Client Needs: Physiological Integrity
Integrated Concept/Process: Nursing Process/Implementation
Content Area: Pharmacology

Reference:
Hodgson, B., & Kizior, R. (2003). *Saunders nursing drug handbook 2003.* Philadelphia: W.B. Saunders, p. 689.

---

108. A second-day postpartum client with diabetes mellitus has scant lochia with a foul odor and a temperature of 101.6° F. The physician suspects infection and writes orders to treat the client. Which of the following orders written by the physician should the nurse complete first?
1 Obtain a culture and sensitivity specimen of the lochia and urine
2 Administer ceftriaxone (Rocephin) as prescribed
3 Maintain bed rest in a supine position
4 Encourage an increased intake of oral fluids

Answer: 1
Rationale: A culture and sensitivity should be obtained before any antibiotic therapy is begun to avoid masking the microorganisms identified with the culture. Options 2 and 4 are standard parts of therapy for this type of infection but are not completed first. The nurse should question the order in option 3, because the client should be placed in a semi-Fowler's position to facilitate drainage.

Test-Taking Strategy: Use the process of elimination. Note the key word *first*. Remember that a culture and sensitivity specimen is always obtained before initiating antibiotic therapy. Review care to the client with a potential postpartum infection if you had difficulty with this question.

Level of Cognitive Ability: Application
Client Needs: Physiological Integrity

Integrated Concept/Process: Nursing Process/Implementation
Content Area: Maternity

Reference:
McKinney, E., Ashwill, J., Murray, S., James, S., Gorrie, T., & Droske, S. (2000). *Maternal-child nursing.* Philadelphia: W.B. Saunders, p. 730.

---

109. Sitz baths are prescribed for a postpartum client. The nurse understands that the purpose of the sitz baths is to assist with which of the following?
1 Reduce the edema and numb the tissue
2 Promote healing and provide comfort
3 Reduce infection and stimulate peristalsis
4 Cleanse the perineum and prevent hemorrhoids

Answer: 2
Rationale: Warm, moist heat is used during the first 24 hours postpartum after vaginal birth to provide comfort, promote healing, and reduce the incidence of infection. Ice is used to reduce the edema and numb the tissue. Stimulation of peristalsis is better achieved by ambulation. A sitz bath may provide comfort for hemorrhoids but does not prevent them.

Test-Taking Strategy: Use the process of elimination. Eliminate option 1 because heat from the sitz bath will not "numb." Eliminate option 4 because of the word "prevent." From the remaining options eliminate option 3 because a sitz bath will not necessarily "stimulate peristalsis." Review the purpose of a sitz bath if you had difficulty with this question.

Level of Cognitive Ability: Comprehension
Client Needs: Physiological Integrity
Integrated Concept/Process: Nursing Process/Implementation
Content Area: Maternity

Reference:
McKinney, E., Ashwill, J., Murray, S., James, S., Gorrie, T., & Droske, S. (2000). *Maternal-child nursing.* Philadelphia: W.B. Saunders, p. 492.

---

110. A nurse is preparing to administer a first dose of zalcitabine (HIVID) to a client. The nurse provides medication instructions to the client and tells the client about the need to have serial monitoring of which of the following tests to determine the effectiveness of therapy?
1 Enzyme-linked immunosorbent assay (ELISA)
2 Western blot
3 CD4 cell count
4 Complete blood cell (CBC) count with differential

Answer: 3
Rationale: This medication slows the progression of HIV disease by improving the CD4 cell count. The ELISA and Western blot are done to diagnose human immunodeficiency virus (HIV) initially. A CBC with differential may be done as part of an ongoing monitoring of the status of the client with HIV, and to detect adverse effects of other medications.

Test-Taking Strategy: Knowledge of the purpose and action of this medication is needed to answer this question. Review this medication if you had difficulty with this question.

Level of Cognitive Ability: Application
Client Needs: Physiological Integrity
Integrated Concept/Process: Nursing Process/Implementation
Content Area: Pharmacology

Reference:
Hodgson, B., & Kizior, R. (2003). *Saunders nursing drug handbook 2003.* Philadelphia: W.B. Saunders, p. 1174.

111. During the initial maternal–infant bonding period after the delivery of the placenta, the nurse's primary responsibility is which of the following?
  1 Make sure the infant stays warm and is in no danger of slipping from the parent's grasp
  2 Assist the mother to begin breastfeeding the infant immediately
  3 Protect the infant from infection by maintaining isolation of the infant
  4 Make sure the siblings are involved with the process

Answer: 1
Rationale: During the beginning of the interactions between the parents and the infant, the safety of the infant is the initial concern. Not all mothers breastfeed. Not all families have siblings. Protection of the infant is important but is not done by isolation of the infant.

Test-Taking Strategy: Focus on the issue of the question and use the process of elimination. Use Maslow's Hierarchy of Needs theory to assist in answering the question. Option 1 addresses both a physiological and a safety need. Review the concepts of maternal–infant bonding if you had difficulty with this question.

Level of Cognitive Ability: Application
Client Needs: Physiological Integrity
Integrated Concept/Process: Nursing Process/Implementation
Content Area: Maternity

Reference:
Burroughs, A., & Leifer, G. (2002). *Maternity nursing* (8th ed.). Philadelphia: W.B. Saunders, p. 116.

112. A nurse assigned to care for a lactating postpartum client plans to instruct the client to do which of the following?
  1 Resume the prepregnancy diet
  2 Increase caloric intake by 500 calories a day
  3 Limit fluid intake to 32 ounces of water a day to prevent engorgement
  4 Continue folate and iron supplements at the same dosage as during the pregnancy

Answer: 2
Rationale: Lactating women require at least 500 additional calories above that consumed during pregnancy to ensure an adequate milk supply. Women are encouraged to increase their normal fluid intake (six to eight 8-ounce glasses per day) to provide an additional 24 to 32 ounces of milk. Folate and iron requirements are lower than during pregnancy.

Test-Taking Strategy: Use the process of elimination. Focusing on the key word *lactating* tells you that additional calories are needed and directs you to option 2. Review the nutritional needs of a lactating postpartum client if you had difficulty with this question.

Level of Cognitive Ability: Application
Client Needs: Physiological Integrity
Integrated Concept/Process: Teaching/Learning
Content Area: Maternity

Reference:
McKinney, E., Ashwill, J., Murray, S., James, S., Gorrie, T., & Droske, S. (2000). *Maternal-child nursing.* Philadelphia: W.B. Saunders, p. 327.

113. A nurse determines that a breastfeeding mother is at risk of developing mastitis if the nurse observes the mother doing which of the following?
  1 Placing her finger in the infant's mouth to break suction on her nipple
  2 Offering one breast per feeding
  3 Manually expressing the remainder of breast milk after each feeding

Answer: 2
Rationale: Offering only one breast per feeding causes milk stasis, which is a risk factor for mastitis. The mother is encouraged to allow the infant to empty one breast completely, then to continue feeding the infant on the opposite breast. Newborns frequently tire and do not completely empty the second breast. The mother is instructed to express the remaining milk manually until an adequate milk supply is established and to offer the second breast first at the next feeding. A safety pin attached to the brassiere cup reminds the mother which breast should be offered

4   Gently pressing breast tissue away from the infant's nose while nursing

first each feeding. Breaking the infant's suction before removing the infant from the breast reduces nipple trauma (another risk factor for mastitis). Gentle pressure placed on the tissue does not influence the development of mastitis. It is recommended to allow the infant to breathe through the nose unobstructed while nursing.

Test-Taking Strategy: Use the process of elimination. Focus on the key words *at risk of developing mastitis.* Attempt to visualize each of the mother's actions and use knowledge regarding the risk factors for mastitis to assist in directing you to option 2. Review these risk factors if you had difficulty with this question.

Level of Cognitive Ability: Comprehension
Client Needs: Physiological Integrity
Integrated Concept/Process: Nursing Process/Data Collection
Content Area: Maternity

Reference:
Burroughs, A., & Leifer, G. (2002). *Maternity nursing* (8th ed.). Philadelphia: W.B. Saunders, p. 307.

---

114. Erythromycin base (Ilotycin) ophthalmic ointment is prescribed for the newborn. The nurse understands which of the following about this medication?
1.   It is more irritating to the newborn's eyes than silver nitrate
2.   It must be administered at room temperature to prevent side effects
3.   It may stain the infant's skin and must be wiped immediately
4.   It is useful to protect the newborn from both *Neisseria gonorrhoeae* and *Chlamydia*

Answer: 4
Rationale: Erythromycin base is effective against both *Neisseria gonorrhea* and *Chlamydia.* It is less irritating to the newborn's eyes than silver nitrate, does not stain, and may be administered at any safe temperature.

Test-Taking Strategy: Knowledge regarding this medication is necessary to answer this question. Review this newborn medication if you had difficulty with this question.

Level of Cognitive Ability: Comprehension
Client Needs: Physiological Integrity
Integrated Concept/Process: Nursing Process/Implementation
Content Area: Maternity

Reference:
Hodgson, B., & Kizior, R. (2003). *Saunders nursing drug handbook 2003.* Philadelphia: W.B. Saunders, p. 415.

---

115. A client who was tested for human immunodeficiency virus (HIV) after a recent exposure had a negative test result. Which of the following items should the nurse plan to include in posttest counseling?
1.   The test should be repeated in 6 months
2.   The test assures that the client is not infected with the HIV virus
3.   The client no longer needs to protect sexual partners
4.   The client probably has immunity to HIV

Answer: 1
Rationale: A negative test result indicates that no HIV antibodies were detected in the blood sample. A repeat test in 6 months is recommended because false-negative results can occur early in the infection. Options 2, 3, and 4 are incorrect.

Test-Taking Strategy: Use the process of elimination. Begin to answer this question by eliminating options 3 and 4 because they are false statements. Even without specific knowledge of the implications of test results, you should choose option 1 instead of option 2 because the words *assures* and *not* in option 2 are absolute; therefore, they are not likely to be correct. Review these testing procedures if you had difficulty with this question.

Level of Cognitive Ability: Application
Client Needs: Physiological Integrity
Integrated Concept/Process: Nursing Process/Implementation
Content Area: Fundamental Skills

Reference:

Black, J., Hawks, J., & Keene, A. (2001). *Medical-surgical nursing: clinical management for positive outcomes* (6th ed.). Philadelphia: W.B. Saunders, p. 2193.

---

116. A nurse notes signs of restlessness, dyspnea, anxiety, and a rapid pulse in a client at risk for adult respiratory distress syndrome. The priority nursing action is which of the following?

1 Stay with the client and position him or her to relieve dyspnea
2 Prepare to medicate the client with the PRN medication for anxiety
3 Reassure the client by checking the client's vital signs every 10 minutes
4 Check the client's medical record for a history of anxiety attacks

Answer: 1

Rationale: Signs of respiratory distress are often accompanied by fear of suffocation. In addition to immediate interventions to improve the client's respiratory status, the nurse's presence can provide reassurance and ease the client's anxiety. The vital signs should be monitored, but reassuring the client that this will be done will not relieve the anxiety. The client may receive medication if prescribed but this is not the priority. Option 4 will not relieve the distress.

Test-Taking Strategy: Use the process of elimination. Focus on the signs provided in the question and the need to reassure the client. Option 1 is the priority because it addresses both the client's dyspnea and the anxiety. Review care to the client suspected of fat embolism if you had difficulty with this question.

Level of Cognitive Ability: Application
Client Needs: Physiological Integrity
Integrated Concept/Process: Caring
Content Area: Adult Health/Musculoskeletal

Reference:

Phipps, W., Monahan, F., Sands, J. et al. (2003). *Medical-surgical nursing: health and illness perspective* (7th ed). St. Louis: Mosby, p. 565.

---

117. A nurse is teaching a client about care of the right leg cast that was just applied to treat a fracture. The nurse tells the client which of the following?

1 Elevation of the right leg above heart level should relieve foot swelling, which occurs while the leg is dependent
2 Foul odors coming from the cast should be reported only if there also is visible drainage on the outside of the cast
3 Swelling, blue-tinged toes, and pain of the right leg and foot with any movement are expected during the healing process
4 There is no danger of complications related to the cast after the cast has dried completely

Answer: 1

Rationale: Dependent edema may occur when the casted extremity is in the dependent position or when there is prolonged hip flexion while the client is sitting. Dependent edema caused by sluggish venous return should decrease when the leg is elevated above the level of the heart. If the edema is related to the potentially serious complication of compartment syndrome, pressure in the compartment is not decreased by elevating the leg above the heart; in fact, the pressure and swelling may increase with elevation. Therefore swelling that does not resolve after elevation of the extremity should be reported to the physician. Blue skin color and persistent pain are not typical and could be signs of compartment syndrome. Foul odors, with or without drainage, may indicate infection and should be reported to the physician.

Test-Taking Strategy: Use the process of elimination. Eliminate option 2 because of the words *only if there also is visible drainage.* Eliminate option 3 because these signs are not normal. Noting the key words *no danger* in option 4 assists in eliminating this option. Review care to the client with a cast if you had difficulty with this question.

Level of Cognitive Ability: Application
Client Needs: Physiological Integrity
Integrated Concept/Process: Teaching/Learning
Content Area: Adult Health/Musculoskeletal

Reference:
Black, J., Hawks, J., & Keene, A. (2001). *Medical-surgical nursing: clinical management for positive outcomes* (6th ed.). Philadelphia: W.B. Saunders, p. 606.

---

118. A nurse receives a telephone call from the parent of a toddler with acute lymphocytic leukemia (ALL). The parent tells the nurse that the child has developed epistaxis. The nurse advises the parent to do which of the following immediately?
1 Have the child lie down
2 Keep the child calm and quiet
3 Call 911
4 Apply a warm washcloth to the bridge of the nose

Answer: 2
Rationale: Keeping a child calm and quiet decreases blood flow. Laying the child down and applying a warm washcloth to the bridge of the nose increases blood flow. Additionally, the child should sit up and lean forward, not lie down. Even though bleeding for a child with ALL can be an emergency, steps should be taken immediately to resolve the nosebleed before calling 911.

Test-Taking Strategy: Use the process of elimination and note the key word *immediately*. Use principles related to gravity to assist in eliminating option 1. Use principles related to the effects of warmth to eliminate option 4. Focusing on the key word and recalling the steps that should be taken immediately to resolve the nosebleed assist in eliminating option 3. Review care to the child with epistaxis if you had difficulty with this question.

Level of Cognitive Ability: Application
Client Needs: Physiological Integrity
Integrated Concept/Process: Nursing Process/Implementation
Content Area: Child Health

Reference:
Schulte, E., Price, D., & Gwin, J. (2001). *Thompson's pediatric nursing* (8th ed.). Philadelphia: W.B. Saunders, p. 236.

---

119. A client recently diagnosed with tuberculosis (TB) is being admitted to the hospital. When collecting data from the client, a primary consideration is to identify which of the following?
1 Who the client contracted TB from so that the person can be reported for follow-up care
2 The names of close friends and family members
3 What medications are ordered, and what the client knows about their side effects
4 The religious affiliation or church of preference

Answer: 2
Rationale: Tuberculosis is a contagious disease that is spread through respiratory droplets. A primary consideration of the nurse is to identify the names of close friends and family members so that these individuals can be tested for exposure to TB. The client may not know from whom the disease was contracted. It is premature to determine knowledge about medications because treatment measures may not have been prescribed. The religious affiliation or church of preference is part of the data collection process but is not the primary consideration among the options provided.

Test-Taking Strategy: Use the process of elimination and note the key word *primary*. Recalling the route of transmission of TB assists in directing you to option 2. Review data collection techniques for the client recently diagnosed with TB if you had difficulty with this question.

Level of Cognitive Ability: Comprehension
Client Needs: Physiological Integrity
Integrated Concept/Process: Nursing Process/Data Collection
Content Area: Adult Health/Respiratory

Reference:
Lewis, S., Heitkemper, M., & Dirksen, S. (2000). *Medical-surgical nursing: assessment and management of clinical problems* (5th ed.). St. Louis: Mosby, p. 628.

---

120. The nurse in the prenatal clinic is taking a nutritional history from a 16-year-old adolescent. Which statement would suggest a possible problem if made by the client?

1 "I only want to gain 7 to 10 pounds because I want a small, petite baby girl."
2 "I will continue eating my afternoon snack of popcorn and coke."
3 "I don't like milk but I do like other dairy products."
4 "I should eat more foods that I am used to."

Answer: 1
Rationale: Pregnant adolescents are at higher risk for complications than are mature women. Adolescents are often concerned about their body image. If weight is a major focus, the client is more likely to restrict calories to avoid weight gain. Option 1 is the only option that suggests a possible problem. The client has no control over her fantasy of a small baby girl.

Test-Taking Strategy: Use the process of elimination. Note the key word *adolescent*. Recalling that body image is a concern of an adolescent directs you to option 1. Review pregnancy in the adolescent if you had difficulty with this question.

Level of Cognitive Ability: Analysis
Client Needs: Physiological Integrity
Integrated Concept/Process: Nursing Process/Data Collection
Content Area: Maternity

Reference:
McKinney, E., Ashwill, J., Murray, S., James, S., Gorrie, T., & Droske, S. (2000). *Maternal-child nursing.* Philadelphia: W.B. Saunders, p. 611.

---

121. A nurse is providing information to a client with hepatitis about the convalescence stage. Recognizing the need for psychosocial support for this client, the nurse suggests which of the following?

1 That the client stay in his or her room to facilitate resting
2 Diversionary activities that are not physically taxing
3 Joining an aerobic exercise class
4 That the client speak with his or her doctor about a prescription for antidepressant medications

Answer: 2
Rationale: The process of convalescence from hepatitis is long and slow. Physically, the client becomes easily fatigued and needs additional rest. However, as the client recovers, there is an equally important need for some diversion from the long days of bed rest. Option 1 socially isolates the client. Option 3 is a much too strenuous activity for the client. The use of antidepressant medications is contraindicated in a client with decreased liver function.

Test-Taking Strategy: Use the process of elimination, recalling that rest is needed to heal the liver of the client with hepatitis. Eliminate option 1 because this intervention socially isolates the client. Eliminate option 3 because this activity is strenuous. Eliminate option 4 because the use of antidepressant medications is contraindicated for a client with decreased liver function. Review care of the client with hepatitis if you had difficulty with this question.

Level of Cognitive Ability: Application
Client Needs: Physiological Integrity
Integrated Concept/Process: Nursing Process/Planning
Content Area: Adult Health/Gastrointestinal

Reference:
Lewis, S., Heitkemper, M., & Dirksen, S. (2000). *Medical-surgical nursing: assessment and management of clinical problems* (5th ed.). St. Louis: Mosby, p. 1201.

---

122. A client with diabetes mellitus who takes insulin tells the nurse, "I usually begin to feel sick late in the afternoon. Is there something wrong with me?" The most appropriate response by the nurse is which of the following?

1 "Don't worry about that. Most diabetics feel that way."
2 "Can you describe what you mean by 'feeling sick?'"
3 "Let me know if that happens today."
4 "Most people feel tired late in the afternoon."

Answer: 2

Rationale: An excess of insulin relative to the amount of blood glucose induces hypoglycemia. Depending on when the insulin is administered, the risk of hypoglycemia may be greatest in the late afternoon. The nurse should collect more data to determine if the client is actually experiencing hypoglycemia. Asking the client to describe the feeling provides the nurse with more data. Options 1, 3, and 4 are nontherapeutic communication techniques.

Test-Taking Strategy: Use the process of elimination and therapeutic communication techniques to answer the question. In addition, option 2 identifies data collection, the first step in the nursing process. Review the effects of insulin and hypoglycemic reactions if you had difficulty with this question.

Level of Cognitive Ability: Application
Client Needs: Physiological Integrity
Integrated Concept/Process: Nursing Process/Data Collection
Content Area: Adult Health/Endocrine

Reference:
Lewis, S., Heitkemper, M., & Dirksen, S. (2000). *Medical-surgical nursing: assessment and management of clinical problems* (5th ed.). St. Louis: Mosby, p. 1397.

---

123. A nurse is caring for a client with diabetes mellitus and is gathering data from the client about events leading to the client's request for medical attention. The nurse identifies which of the following as the major symptoms of diabetes mellitus?

1 Polydipsia, polyuria, polyphagia
2 Dyspepsia, polyuria, polyphagia
3 Hypoglycemia, polyuria, dysphagia
4 Hypoglycemia, polyuria, dysphasia

Answer: 1

Rationale: Polydipsia, polyuria, and polyphagia are the classic signs and symptoms of diabetes mellitus. Dyspepsia, dysphagia, and dysphasia are associated with other body systems (gastrointestinal and neurological).

Test-Taking Strategy: Remember the "three Ps" in diabetes mellitus: polydipsia, polyuria, and polyphagia. If you had difficulty with this question and are unfamiliar with the signs of diabetes mellitus, review this content.

Level of Cognitive Ability: Comprehension
Client Needs: Physiological Integrity
Integrated Concept/Process: Nursing Process/Data Collection
Content Area: Adult Health/Endocrine

Reference:
Lewis, S., Heitkemper, M., & Dirksen, S. (2000). *Medical-surgical nursing: assessment and management of clinical problems* (5th ed.). St. Louis: Mosby, p. 1371.

---

124. A client is being discharged from the hospital in 2 days. The physician tells the client to maintain a low-fat diet at home. The client demonstrates understanding of a low-fat diet by choosing which of the

Answer: 4

Rationale: Among the foods mentioned in the options, bread (toast without butter or margarine) contains the least amount of fat. Strawberry jelly contains calories but nominal fats. Bran muffins may be high in residue but are made with shortenings,

following foods from the hospital breakfast menu?
1   Bran muffin
2   Peanut butter sandwich
3   Bagel with cream cheese
4   Dry toast and strawberry jelly

which are high in fat. Peanut butter and cheese contain significant amounts of fat.

Test-Taking Strategy: Use the process of elimination and knowledge regarding those food items that are low in fat. This directs you to option 4. If you had difficulty with this question, review components of these food items.

Level of Cognitive Ability: Comprehension
Client Needs: Physiological Integrity
Integrated Concept/Process: Self-Care
Content Area: Fundamental Skills

Reference:
Williams, S. (2001) *Basic nutrition & diet therapy* (11th ed.). St. Louis: Mosby, pp. 35-37.

---

125. An LPN is assisting an RN is caring for a client receiving lidocaine (Xylocaine) for the treatment of ventricular tachycardia. The LPN assists in planning care knowing that this medication is classified as which of the following?
1   A diuretic
2   A calcium channel blocker
3   An antihypertensive
4   An antidysrhythmic

Answer: 4
Rationale: Lidocaine is classified as an antidysrhythmic and is used to treat cardiac dysrhythmias. It is not classified as a diuretic, calcium channel blocker, or antihypertensive.

Test-Taking Strategy: Use the process of elimination. Noting the diagnosis of the client, ventricular tachycardia, assists in directing you to the correct option. Review the action of this medication if you had difficulty with this question.

Level of Cognitive Ability: Comprehension
Client Needs: Physiological Integrity
Integrated Concept/Process: Nursing Process/Planning
Content Area: Pharmacology

Reference:
Hodgson, B., & Kizior, R. (2003). *Saunders nursing drug handbook 2003.* Philadelphia: W.B. Saunders, p. 662.

---

126. A nurse is interviewing a client with chronic obstructive pulmonary disease (COPD) who has a respiratory rate of 35 breaths per minute and is experiencing extreme dyspnea. Which of the following problems would the nurse identify as a barrier to collecting data?
1   Impaired verbal communication related to the physical condition
2   Ineffective individual coping related to client's inability to handle a crisis situation
3   Impaired verbal communication related to a neurological deficit
4   Ineffective individual coping related to COPD

Answer: 1
Rationale: A client may suffer physical or psychological alterations that impair communication. To speak spontaneously and clearly, a person must have an intact respiratory system. Extreme dyspnea is a physical condition affecting speech. Option 2 is judgmental and inappropriate. There is nothing to indicate that the client has a neurological deficit. Option 4 is a medical diagnosis.

Test-Taking Strategy: Use the process of elimination and focus on the data provided in the question. Option 1 clearly addresses the problem that the client is experiencing. Review care to the client with COPD and the barriers to communication if you had difficulty with this question.

Level of Cognitive Ability: Analysis
Client Needs: Physiological Integrity
Integrated Concept/Process: Nursing Process/Data Collection
Content Area: Adult Health/Respiratory

Reference:
Lewis, S., Heitkemper, M., & Dirksen, S. (2000). *Medical-surgical nursing: assessment and management of clinical problems* (5th ed.). St. Louis: Mosby, p. 707.

---

127. A client with late-stage emphysema complains of an occipital headache, drowsiness, and difficulty concentrating. The nurse interprets that these symptoms are compatible with which complication of emphysema?

1 Encephalopathy
2 Carbon dioxide narcosis
3 Carbon monoxide poisoning
4 Cerebral embolism

Answer: 2

Rationale: With late-stage emphysema, the retention of carbon dioxide can lead to carbon dioxide narcosis. This is manifested by occipital headache, drowsiness, and inability to concentrate. Other signs that may occur are bounding pulse, arterial carbon dioxide level greater than 75 mmHg, confusion, coma, and asterixis (flap tremor). Options 1, 3, and 4 are incorrect interpretations.

Test-Taking Strategy: To answer this question accurately, you must be familiar with the complications of emphysema. Recalling that emphysema is characterized by high carbon dioxide levels directs you to option 2. Review the manifestations associated with this disorder if you had difficulty with this question.

Level of Cognitive Ability: Analysis
Client Needs: Physiological Integrity
Integrated Concept/Process: Nursing Process/Data Collection
Content Area: Adult Health/Respiratory

Reference:
Lewis, S., Heitkemper, M., & Dirksen, S. (2000). *Medical-surgical nursing: assessment and management of clinical problems* (5th ed.). St. Louis: Mosby, p. 702.

---

128. A nurse witnesses an accident in which a pedestrian is hit by an automobile. The nurse stops at the scene and checks the victim, noting that the client is responsive and has possibly suffered a flail chest involving at least three ribs. The nurse should do which of the following to assist the victim's respiratory status until help arrives?

1 Assist the victim to sit up
2 Turn the victim onto the side with the flail chest
3 Remove the victim's shirt
4 Apply firm but gentle pressure with the hands to the flail segment

Answer: 4

Rationale: With a flail chest, the nurse applies firm yet gentle pressure to the flail segments of the ribs to stabilize the chest wall, which will ultimately help the victim's respiratory status. The nurse does not move an injured person for fear of worsening an undetected spinal injury. Removing the victim's shirt is of no value in this situation and could chill the victim, which is counterproductive. Injured persons should be kept warm until help arrives.

Test-Taking Strategy: Use knowledge of the principles of respiration and emergency nursing to answer this question. Eliminate option 3 first because this action is of no value to the victim. Next eliminate options 1 and 2 because a victim of injury should not be moved until the extent of injuries is determined. Review emergency care to the client with flail chest if you had difficulty with this question.

Level of Cognitive Ability: Application
Client Needs: Physiological Integrity
Integrated Concept/Process: Nursing Process/Implementation
Content Area: Adult Health/Respiratory

Reference:
Lewis, S., Heitkemper, M., & Dirksen, S. (2000). *Medical-surgical nursing: assessment and management of clinical problems* (5th ed.). St. Louis: Mosby, p. 645.

129. A nurse notes bilateral 2+ edema in the lower extremities of a client with known coronary artery disease who was admitted to the hospital 2 days ago. The nurse plans to do which of the following first?
1   Review the intake and output records for the last 2 days
2   Change the time of diuretic administration from morning to evening
3   Request a sodium restriction of 1 gram per day from the physician
4   Order daily weights starting on the following morning

Answer: 1
Rationale: Edema is the accumulation of excess fluid in the interstitial spaces, which can be determined by intake greater than output and by a sudden increase in weight. Diuretics should be given in the morning whenever possible to avoid nocturia. Strict sodium restrictions are reserved for clients with severe symptoms.

Test-Taking Strategy: Use the process of elimination and note the key word *first*. Note that option 1 can give the nurse immediate information about fluid balance. Review care to the client with coronary artery disease and edema if you had difficulty with this question.

Level of Cognitive Ability: Application
Client Needs: Physiological Integrity
Integrated Concept/Process: Nursing Process/Implementation
Content Area: Adult Health/Cardiovascular

Reference:
Lewis, S., Heitkemper, M., & Dirksen, S. (2000). *Medical-surgical nursing: assessment and management of clinical problems* (5th ed.). St. Louis: Mosby, p. 892.

---

130. A nurse is caring for a client in the emergency room who has chest pain. Which of the following observations by the nurse helps determine that this pain is caused by myocardial infarction (MI)?
1   The pain, unrelieved by nitroglycerin, was relieved with morphine sulfate
2   The pain was described as substernal and radiating to the left arm
3   The client experienced no nausea or vomiting
4   The client reports that the pain began while pushing a lawnmower

Answer: 1
Rationale: The pain of angina may radiate to the left arm, is often precipitated by exertion or stress, has few associated symptoms, and is relieved by rest and nitroglycerin. The pain of MI may radiate to the left arm, left shoulder, jaw, and neck. It typically begins spontaneously, lasts longer than 30 minutes, is frequently accompanied by associated symptoms (nausea, vomiting, dyspnea, diaphoresis, anxiety), and requires opioid analgesics for relief.

Test-Taking Strategy: Use the process of elimination. The question seeks to differentiate the pain of angina from that of MI, which may be similar at the onset. Remember that a classic hallmark of MI pain is that it rest and nitroglycerin provide no relief. Review the manifestations associated with MI if you had difficulty with this question.

Level of Cognitive Ability: Analysis
Client Needs: Physiological Integrity
Integrated Concept/Process: Nursing Process/Data Collection
Content Area: Adult Health/Cardiovascular

Reference:
Lewis, S., Heitkemper, M., & Dirksen, S. (2000). *Medical-surgical nursing: assessment and management of clinical problems* (5th ed.). St. Louis: Mosby, p. 853.

---

131. A nurse is assisting with positioning a client for pericardiocentesis to treat cardiac tamponade. The nurse places the client in which position?
1   Lying on the left side with a pillow under the chest wall

Answer: 3
Rationale: The client undergoing pericardiocentesis is positioned supine with the head of the bed raised to an angle of 45 to 60 degrees. This places the heart in close proximity to the chest wall for easier insertion of the needle into the pericardial sac.

2 Lying on the right side with a pillow under the head

3 Supine with the head of bed elevated at an angle of 45 to 60 degrees

4 Supine with slight Trendelenburg position

Test-Taking Strategy: If you are uncertain how to proceed with this question, visualize each of the positions described. Evaluate how the heart is sitting in the chest with each position and how easily the pericardial sac could be accessed with a needle. This should help you eliminate all the incorrect options to this question. Review this procedure if you had difficulty with this question.

Level of Cognitive Ability: Application
Client Needs: Physiological Integrity
Integrated Concept/Process: Nursing Process/Implementation
Content Area: Adult Health/Cardiovascular

Reference:
Lewis, S., Heitkemper, M., & Dirksen, S. (2000). *Medical-surgical nursing: assessment and management of clinical problems* (5th ed.). St. Louis: Mosby, p. 1878.

---

132. A nurse explains to a mother that her newborn is being admitted to the neonatal intensive care unit with a probable diagnosis of fetal alcohol syndrome (FAS). The nurse explains FAS to the mother and determines the effectiveness of the explanation when the mother states which of the following?

1 "Withdrawal symptoms will occur after 3 days."

2 "Mental retardation is unlikely to happen."

3 "Withdrawal symptoms are tremors, crying, and seizures."

4 "The reason the child is so large is because of the fetal alcohol syndrome."

Answer: 3
Rationale: The long-term prognosis for newborns with FAS is poor. Symptoms of withdrawal include tremors, sleeplessness, seizures, abdominal distention, hyperactivity, and uncontrollable crying. Central nervous system (CNS) disorders are the most common problems associated with FAS. Because of CNS disorders, children born with FAS are often hyperactive and have a high incidence of speech and language disorders. Symptoms of withdrawal often occur within 6 to 12 hours after birth or, at the latest, within 3 days of birth. Most newborns with FAS are mildly to severely mentally retarded. The newborn is usually growth-deficient at birth.

Test-Taking Strategy: Use the process of elimination. Thinking about the effects of FAS assists in eliminating options 2 and 4. From the remaining options, you must know that withdrawal symptoms can appear within 6 to 12 hours after birth or, at the latest, within 3 days of birth. Review the manifestations associated with FAS if you had difficulty with this question.

Level of Cognitive Ability: Comprehension
Client Needs: Physiological Integrity
Integrated Concept/Process: Nursing Process/Evaluation
Content Area: Maternity

Reference:
McKinney, E., Ashwill, J., Murray, S., James, S., Gorrie, T., & Droske, S. (2000). *Maternal-child nursing.* Philadelphia: W.B. Saunders, p. 616.

---

133. Ferrous sulfate (iron) is prescribed for a pregnant client. Before beginning this medication, the nurse reviews which of the following laboratory results that will provide the necessary baseline data for monitoring the therapeutic effect of the medication?

1 Hemoglobin level

2 Prothrombin time

Answer: 1
Rationale: Generally, a healthy diet provides adequate sources of iron. Because of the expansion of maternal blood volume and the production of fetal red blood cells, iron requirements increase in pregnancy. Hemoglobin measures the amount of oxygen in the blood. Options 2 and 4 identify tests performed for clients with bleeding disorders. Option 3 identifies a measurement test used to diagnose various anemias and blood diseases.

3 Iron binding levels
4 Clotting time

Test-Taking Strategy: Use the process of elimination and focus on the issue of the question. Recalling that the hemoglobin level identifies the presence of iron deficiency anemia directs you to this option. Review this laboratory test if you had difficulty with this question.

Level of Cognitive Ability: Application
Client Needs: Physiological Integrity
Integrated Concept/Process: Nursing Process/Data Collection
Content Area: Maternity

Reference:
Hodgson, B., & Kizior, R. (2003). *Saunders nursing drug handbook 2003.* Philadelphia: W.B. Saunders, p. 453.

---

134. A client is on warfarin sodium (Coumadin) therapy, and the nurse is monitoring the client for bleeding. The nurse understands that the antidote to this medication if an overdose occurred is which of the following?
1 Oral potassium supplements
2 Heparin sodium
3 Phytonadione (vitamin K)
4 Protamine sulfate

Answer: 3
Rationale: The effects of warfarin sodium overdose can be overcome with phytonadione (vitamin K). Vitamin K is an antagonist of warfarin sodium that can reverse warfarin-induced inhibition of clotting factor synthesis. Oral potassium is used for potassium deficiency. Heparin sodium is an anticoagulant. Protamine sulfate is the antidote for heparin sodium.

Test-Taking Strategy: Knowledge regarding the antidote for warfarin sodium is necessary to answer this question. Review the effects of this medication and the antidote if you had difficulty with this question.

Level of Cognitive Ability: Comprehension
Client Needs: Physiological Integrity
Integrated Concept/Process: Nursing Process/Planning
Content Area: Pharmacology

Reference:
Hodgson, B., & Kizior, R. (2003). *Saunders nursing drug handbook 2003.* Philadelphia: W.B. Saunders, p. 1170.

---

135. A client who takes aspirin every day reports to the nurse that dental surgery is recommended. The nurse most appropriately tells the client which of the following?
1 "Dental surgery can safely be done 48 hours after you stop taking your aspirin."
2 "Dental surgery is contraindicated."
3 "There is no risk to having such a minor surgery while continuing your aspirin therapy."
4 "Ask your pharmacist about the surgery."

Answer: 1
Rationale: Aspirin is an antiplatelet. For an elective procedure such as dental surgery, aspirin therapy should be stopped approximately 48 hours before the surgery to prevent bleeding complications. Options 2 and 3 are incorrect. Option 4 is an inappropriate response and places the client's concern on hold.

Test-Taking Strategy: Use the process of elimination and therapeutic communication techniques to answer the question. Eliminate options 2 and 3 first because of the words *no risk* and *contraindicated.* Next, eliminate option 4 because it is nontherapeutic and places the client's concerns on hold. Review the effects of aspirin if you had difficulty with this question.

Level of Cognitive Ability: Application
Client Needs: Physiological Integrity

Integrated Concept/Process: Communication and Documentation
Content Area: Pharmacology

Reference:
Ignatavicius, D., & Workman, M. (2002). *Medical-surgical nursing: critical thinking for collaborative care* (4th ed.). Philadelphia: W.B. Saunders, p. 241.

---

136. A nurse is monitoring a client who is at risk for developing acute renal failure (ARF). The nurse should become most concerned if which of the following is noted during data collection?

   1 Urine output 30 mL per hour for the last 3 hours, blood urea nitrogen (BUN) 10 mg/dL, creatinine 1.2 mg/dL

   2 Urine output 40 mL per hour for the last 3 hours, BUN 15 mg/dL, creatinine 0.8 mg/dL

   3 Urine output 20 mL per hour for the last 3 hours, BUN 35 mg/dL, creatinine 2.1 mg/dL

   4 Urine output 60 mL per hour for the last 3 hours, BUN 20 mg/dL, creatinine 1.1 mg/dL

Answer: 3

Rationale: The client is often oliguric or anuric with ARF, although the client may have nonoliguric renal failure. The BUN and serum creatinine levels also rise, indicating defective kidney function. Normal serum BUN levels are usually 5 to 20 mg/dL; normal creatinine levels range from 0.6 to 1.3 mg/dL. The greatest abnormality in urine output and laboratory values is described in option 3 and indicates the client who is most at risk for developing renal failure.

Test-Taking Strategy: To answer this question accurately, you must know that the client with ARF becomes oliguric or anuric and that serum BUN and creatinine levels rise. With this in mind, options 2 and 4 are eliminated first, because the urine output is above the minimum required level. From the remaining options, option 1 meets the minimum required hourly output, whereas option 3 falls below it. Also, recalling the normal serum BUN and creatinine levels helps you definitively choose option 3 instead of option 1. Review the findings in ARF if you had difficulty with this question.

Level of Cognitive Ability: Analysis
Client Needs: Physiological Integrity
Integrated Concept/Process: Nursing Process/Data Collection
Content Area: Adult Health/Renal

Reference:
Lewis, S., Heitkemper, M., & Dirksen, S. (2000). *Medical-surgical nursing: assessment and management of clinical problems* (5th ed.). St. Louis: Mosby, p. 1299.

---

137. A client with acute renal failure (ARF) has been treated with sodium polystyrene sulfonate (Kayexalate) and sorbitol by mouth. The nurse would evaluate this therapy as effective if which of the following values is noted on follow-up laboratory testing?

   1 Potassium 4.9 mEq/L

   2 Sodium 142 mEq/L

   3 Phosphorus 3.9 mg/dL

   4 Calcium 9.8 mg/dL

Answer: 1

Rationale: Of all the electrolyte imbalances that accompany renal failure, hyperkalemia is the most dangerous because it can lead to cardiac dysrhythmias and death. If the potassium level rises too high, sodium polystyrene sulfonate and sorbitol may be given to cause excretion of potassium through the gastrointestinal tract. Each of the electrolyte levels noted in the options falls within the normal reference range for that electrolyte. The potassium level is measured after administration of this medication to determine the extent of its effectiveness.

Test-Taking Strategy: To answer this question, you must know that the potassium level rises in ARF and that it is treated with medications identified in the question. This directs you to option 1. Review the therapeutic effects of these medications and care of the client with ARF if you had difficulty with this question.

Level of Cognitive Ability: Analysis
Client Needs: Physiological Integrity
Integrated Concept/Process: Nursing Process/Evaluation
Content Area: Adult Health/Renal

Reference:

Hodgson, B., & Kizior, R. (2003). *Saunders nursing drug handbook 2003.* Philadelphia: W.B. Saunders, p. 1022.

---

138. A nurse is caring for a client with chronic renal failure (CRF). The nurse monitors for which most frequent cardiovascular finding in the client with CRF?
1   Hypertension
2   Hypotension
3   Tachycardia
4   Bradycardia

Answer: 1

Rationale: Hypertension is the most common cardiovascular finding in the client with CRF. It is caused by a number of mechanisms, including volume overload, renin-angiotensin system stimulation, vasoconstriction from sympathetic stimulation, and absence of prostaglandins. Hypertension also may be the cause of the renal failure. It is important to monitor hypertension because it can lead to heart failure in the CRF client, resulting from increased cardiac workload in conjunction with fluid overload.

Test-Taking Strategy: Use the process of elimination. To answer this question accurately, you must know the pathophysiology of renal failure as well as its causes. Note that the options are broken into two sets: pulse and blood pressure. Knowing that BP is the key item to monitor helps you eliminate options 3 and 4. To choose correctly, you should recall that hypertension is associated with CRF, not hypotension. Review the cardiovascular signs in CRF if you had difficulty with this question.

Level of Cognitive Ability: Comprehension
Client Needs: Physiological Integrity
Integrated Concept/Process: Nursing Process/Data Collection
Content Area: Adult Health/Renal

Reference:

Black, J., Hawks, J., & Keene, A. (2001). *Medical-surgical nursing: clinical management for positive outcomes* (6th ed.). Philadelphia: W.B. Saunders, p. 882.

---

139. A client has sustained a closed fracture and has just had a cast applied to the affected arm. The client is complaining of intense pain. The nurse has elevated the limb, applied an ice bag, and administered an analgesic that has provided very little relief. The nurse interprets that this pain may be caused by which of the following?
1   Impaired tissue perfusion
2   The newness of the fracture
3   The anxiety of the client
4   Infection under the cast

Answer: 1

Rationale: Most pain associated with fractures can be minimized with rest, elevation, application of cold, and the administration of analgesics. Pain that is not relieved with these measures should be reported to the physician because it may result from impaired tissue perfusion, tissue breakdown, or necrosis. Because this is a new closed fracture and cast, infection would not have had time to set in.

Test-Taking Strategy: Use the process of elimination. Focusing on the data in the question assists in eliminating options 2 and 3. Because the fracture and cast are new, it is extremely unlikely that infection could have set in. The most likely option is impaired tissue perfusion, because pain from ischemia is not relieved by comfort measures and analgesics. Review the signs of impaired tissue perfusion in a client with a cast if you had difficulty with this question.

Level of Cognitive Ability: Analysis
Client Needs: Physiological Integrity
Integrated Concept/Process: Nursing Process/Data Collection
Content Area: Adult Health/Musculoskeletal

Reference:
Black, J., Hawks, J., & Keene, A. (2001). *Medical-surgical nursing: clinical management for positive outcomes* (6th ed.). Philadelphia: W.B. Saunders, p. 604.

---

140. A nurse is assisting in caring for a client who is receiving mannitol (Osmitrol) IV because of loss of consciousness from a closed head injury. The nurse determines that the medication was most effective if which of the following outcomes is noted?
  1 Diuresis of 500 mL in 4 hours and blood urea nitrogen (BUN) of 15 mg/dL
  2 Improved level of consciousness and normal intracranial pressure
  3 Weight loss of 1 kg and serum creatinine level of 0.8 mg/dL
  4 Serum creatinine level of 1.2 mg/dL and normal intracranial pressure

Answer: 2
Rationale: Mannitol is an osmotic diuretic that can be given parenterally to treat cerebral edema and secondary glaucoma when other methods have not been adequate or successful. Expected effects of the medication include rapid diuresis and fluid loss. For the client with cerebral edema (as in closed head injury), effectiveness is measured by neurological status and intracranial pressure readings. Lowering of intracranial pressure occurs within 15 minutes of administration, and diuresis occurs within 1 to 3 hours.

Test-Taking Strategy: Use the process of elimination. Note the key word *most* in the question. This tells you that more than one option is partially or totally correct. The client received the medication as treatment for a closed head injury, so the best parameters of successful treatment are the level of consciousness and intracranial pressure. Review this medication if you had difficulty with this question.

Level of Cognitive Ability: Analysis
Client Needs: Physiological Integrity
Integrated Concept/Process: Nursing Process/Evaluation
Content Area: Pharmacology

Reference:
Hodgson, B., & Kizior, R. (2003). *Saunders nursing drug handbook 2003.* Philadelphia: W.B. Saunders, p. 692.

---

141. A nurse is caring for a client with a history of renal insufficiency who is having captopril (Capoten) added to the medication regimen. Before administering the first dose, the nurse reviews the medical record for the results of urinalysis, especially noting the presence of which of the following?
  1 Casts
  2 Red blood cells (RBCs)
  3 Protein
  4 White blood cells (WBCs)

Answer: 3
Rationale: Captopril is an angiotensin-converting enzyme (ACE) inhibitor that is used for clients who do not respond to first-line antihypertensive agents. ACE inhibitors are used cautiously in clients with renal impairment. Before treatment is begun, baseline assessments of blood pressure, WBC count, and urine protein are done. The client with renal insufficiency may develop nephrotic syndrome, and may be monitored for proteinuria on a monthly basis for 9 months and periodically afterward.

Test-Taking Strategy: Use the process of elimination. The question tells you that the client has renal impairment and directs you to look at urinalysis results. RBCs and WBCs could be indications of trauma, infection, or both, so these options should be eliminated first. Casts are mineral deposits that form along the renal tubules and that occasionally appear in the urine. Normally, the kidneys conserve large protein molecules, which makes proteinuria abnormal. Therefore this is the best indicator and is the correct option. Review this medication if you had difficulty with this question.

Level of Cognitive Ability: Analysis
Client Needs: Physiological Integrity
Integrated Concept/Process: Nursing Process/Data Collection
Content Area: Pharmacology

Reference:
Hodgson, B., & Kizior, R. (2003). *Saunders nursing drug handbook 2003.* Philadelphia: W.B. Saunders, p. 167.

---

142. A nurse is caring for a client with chronic arterial insufficiency. The client complains of leg pain and cramping after walking three blocks, which is relieved when the client stops and rests. The nurse documents that the client is experiencing which of the following?

  1   Arterial-venous shunting
  2   Deep vein thrombosis
  3   Intermittent claudication
  4   Venous insufficiency

Answer: 3
Rationale: Intermittent claudication is a classic symptom of peripheral vascular disease. It is described as a cramplike pain that occurs with exercise and that is relieved by rest. Intermittent claudication is caused by ischemia and is very reproducible; that is, a predictable amount of exercise causes the pain each time.

Test-Taking Strategy: Use the process of elimination. The question tells you that this is an arterial disorder; therefore eliminate options 2 and 4 first. The word *intermittent* in option 3 is a clue that it is the correct option because it matches the timing cited in the question. Arterial venous shunting is not an intermittent type of problem. Review the manifestations of arterial disease and the definition of intermittent claudication if you had difficulty with this question.

Level of Cognitive Ability: Application
Client Needs: Physiological Integrity
Integrated Concept/Process: Communication and Documentation
Content Area: Adult Health/Cardiovascular

Reference:
Black, J., Hawks, J., & Keene, A. (2001). *Medical-surgical nursing: clinical management for positive outcomes* (6th ed.). Philadelphia: W.B. Saunders, p. 1400.

---

143. An LPN has been assigned to admit a 14-year-old female client to the family planning clinic. The client explains that she has missed several periods and has been gaining weight. To improve the client's nutritional status, the nurse gathers which of the following pieces of information?

  1   Date of last menstrual period, weight, blood pressure and urine test, resources available for proper diet
  2   The identity of the father and whether or not she is planning to keep the baby
  3   Type of insurance, whether she has had morning sickness, what her normal diet consists of

Answer: 1
Rationale: Because the client is several months pregnant and this is her first prenatal visit, the nurse's primary concern is her health status and her estimated date of delivery. Options 2 and 4 do not provide information that is helpful in planning prenatal care. The type of insurance coverage is information that a clinic or social worker may need, but it should not have any effect on the care provided to the client.

Test-Taking Strategy: Use the process of elimination. Note the key words *missed several periods.* Focus on the issue "to improve the client's nutritional status." Eliminate options 2 and 4 first because they are similar. From the remaining options, select option 1 because it elicits objective data as a baseline for planning and focuses on the issue of the question. Review care to the pregnant adolescent if you had difficulty with this question.

4 Is this her first pregnancy? What plans has she made for the baby?

Level of Cognitive Ability: Application
Client Needs: Physiological Integrity
Integrated Concept/Process: Nursing Process/Data Collection
Content Area: Maternity

Reference:
McKinney, E., Ashwill, J., Murray, S., James, S., Gorrie, T., & Droske, S. (2000). *Maternal-child nursing.* Philadelphia: W.B. Saunders, p. 611.

---

144. A client is admitted for elective surgery and lists the home medications that were taken that day. The nurse collects data about the medications taken and is most concerned if the client took which of the following?
   1 An antibiotic
   2 An anticoagulant
   3 A calcium channel blocker
   4 A beta-blocker

Answer: 2
Rationale: An anticoagulant suppresses coagulation by inhibiting clotting factors. A client admitted for elective surgery should have been instructed to discontinue the anticoagulant preoperatively as prescribed. The nurse should notify the physician even if this is unscheduled surgery. Vitamin K can be given to reverse the effects of the medication, but the client may still remain at risk for bleeding. The other medications listed in options 1, 3, and 4 do not place the client at risk.

Test-Taking Strategy: Use the process of elimination. Eliminate options 3 and 4 first because they are similar (both are cardiac medications). Next eliminate option 1 because antibiotics are often prescribed in the preoperative period. Review anticoagulant therapy and its associated risks if you had difficulty with this question.

Level of Cognitive Ability: Comprehension
Client Needs: Physiological Integrity
Integrated Concept/Process: Nursing Process/Data Collection
Content Area: Fundamental Skills

Reference:
Clark, J., Queener, S., & Karb, V. (2002). *Pharmacologic basis of nursing practice* (6th ed.). St Louis: Mosby, p. 258.

---

145. Streptokinase (Streptase) is administered to the client in the emergency room after diagnosis of an myocardial infarction. The nurse understands which of the following about this medication?
   1 Thrombolytics act to dissolve thrombi that have already formed
   2 Thrombolytics act to prevent thrombus formation
   3 Thrombolytics suppress the production of fibrin
   4 Streptokinase has been proved to reverse all detrimental effects of heart attacks

Answer: 1
Rationale: Thrombolytics such as streptokinase is most effective when started within 4 to 6 hours of symptom onset. Streptokinase acts to dissolve existing thrombi that are causing a blockage. Options 2, 3, and 4 are incorrect.

Test-Taking Strategy: Use the process of elimination and knowledge regarding the action of this medication. Eliminate option 4 because of the words *proved* and *all.* From the remaining options, recalling the action of this medication directs you to option 1. Review the action of this medication if you had difficulty with this question.

Level of Cognitive Ability: Analysis
Client Needs: Physiological Integrity
Integrated Concept/Process: Nursing Process/Planning
Content Area: Pharmacology

Reference:
Hodgson, B., & Kizior, R. (2003). *Saunders nursing drug handbook 2003.* Philadelphia: W.B. Saunders, p. 1033.

146. A nurse is assigned to care for a client who is receiving heparin intravenously. When planning care for the client, which of the following is the most important consideration?
1   Not allow the client to brush the teeth
2   Use an electric razor for shaving
3   Allow the client to sit only at the bedside
4   Provide complete care to the client

Answer: 2
Rationale: Clients receiving heparin should have extra considerations taken when planning care because these clients are at risk for bleeding. An electric shaver rather than a straight razor should be used for shaving. Options 1, 3, and 4 are not necessary.

Test-Taking Strategy: Use the process of elimination and knowledge regarding the side effects of this medication to assist in answering the question. Options 1 and 3 include the words *not* and *only* and should be eliminated. From the remaining options, select option 2 because this action will reduce the risk of bleeding. Additionally, it is best to allow the client to participate in care if possible. Review the characteristics of this medication if you had difficulty with this question.

Level of Cognitive Ability: Application
Client Needs: Physiological Integrity
Integrated Concept/Process: Nursing Process/Planning
Content Area: Pharmacology

Reference:
Hodgson, B., & Kizior, R. (2003). *Saunders nursing drug handbook 2003.* Philadelphia: W.B. Saunders, p. 545.

---

147. A client is to receive heparin 6,000 units subcutaneously. The medication label states heparin 10,000 units per 1 mL. The nurse prepares which of the following for administration?
1   1.66 mL
2   0.6 mL
3   0.06 mL
4   0.16 mL

Answer: 2
Rationale: Calculate the dosage by dividing the amount ordered by the amount available. The physician ordered 6000 units of heparin; therefore divide 6000 units by 10,000. Use the formula of dividing what is available by what is desired and multiply by 1 mL. This will calculate a dose of 0.6 mL.

Test-Taking Strategy: Read carefully to see that there are 10,000 units of heparin in 1 mL so less than 1 mL of solution is necessary for the prescribed dose. Recheck your calculation before selecting the option and be sure that the calculated dose makes sense. Review medication calculations if you had difficulty with this question.

Level of Cognitive Ability: Application
Client Needs: Physiological Integrity
Integrated Concept/Process: Nursing Process/Implementation
Content Area: Fundamental Skills

Reference:
deWit, S. (2001). *Fundamental concepts and skills for nursing.* Philadelphia: W.B. Saunders, p. 642.

---

148. A client taking an anticoagulant reports to the laboratory for scheduled follow-up laboratory work. The result indicates an International Normalized Ratio (INR) of 2.5. The nurse evaluates these results as:
1   Normal
2   Lower than normal and the anticoagulant dose should be increased

Answer: 1
Rationale: The normal INR is 2.0 to 3.0. A value of 2.5 indicates a normal value.

Test-Taking Strategy: Knowledge regarding the normal therapeutic value of the INR for a client on an anticoagulant is necessary to answer the question. Review this laboratory test if you had difficulty with this question.

3 Higher than normal and the antico-agulant dose should be decreased
4 Insignificant findings

Level of Cognitive Ability: Comprehension
Client Needs: Physiological Integrity
Integrated Concept/Process: Nursing Process/Evaluation
Content Area: Pharmacology

Reference:
Lehne, R. (2001). *Pharmacology for nursing care* (4th ed.). Philadelphia: W.B. Saunders, p. 568.

---

149. A nurse is collecting data from the client who is receiving weekly cyanocobalamin (vitamin B_{12}) injections. Which client statement indicates that the client is receiving the desired effects from the medication?
1 "I get dizzy when I stand up."
2 "I'm pain free now."
3 "I feel stronger and have an increased appetite."
4 "My nausea is better."

Answer: 3
Rationale: Cyanocobalamin is essential for DNA synthesis. It can take up to 3 years for the vitamin B_{12} stores to be depleted and symptoms of pernicious anemia to be noticed. Symptoms can include weakness, fatigue, anorexia, loss of taste, and diarrhea. To correct deficiencies, a crystalline form of vitamin B_{12} (cyanocobalamin) can be given intramuscularly. Options 1, 2, and 4 are unrelated to the use or effect of this medication.

Test-Taking Strategy: Use the process of elimination. Focus on the medication identified in the question, noting that it is a vitamin. With this in mind, eliminate options 1, 2, and 4. Review the desired effects of this vitamin injection if you had difficulty with this question.

Level of Cognitive Ability: Analysis
Client Needs: Physiological Integrity
Integrated Concept/Process: Nursing Process/Evaluation
Content Area: Pharmacology

Reference:
Hodgson, B., & Kizior, R. (2003). *Saunders nursing drug handbook 2003.* Philadelphia: W.B. Saunders, p. 289.

---

150. Ticlopidine (Ticlid), an antiplatelet, is prescribed for a client. The nurse reviews the client's record for documentation of which baseline data before administering the medication?
1 Most recent vital signs
2 Prothrombin level
3 White blood cell (WBC) differential results
4 A client history of stroke

Answer: 3
Rationale: Ticlopidine is an antiplatelet that is used to assist in the prevention of thrombotic stroke. Ticlopidine can cause neutropenia, which is an abnormally small number of mature white blood cells. Baseline data are necessary before initiating therapy. A complete blood count with WBC differential is necessary to determine neutropenia. Therapy may be stopped if this adverse effect occurs. The effects of neutropenia are reversible within 1 to 3 weeks after discontinuation of the medication.

Test-Taking Strategy: Knowledge regarding the adverse effects of this medication is necessary to answer this question. Review this medication if you had difficulty with this question.

Level of Cognitive Ability: Analysis
Client Needs: Physiological Integrity
Integrated Concept/Process: Nursing Process/Data Collection
Content Area: Pharmacology

Reference:
Hodgson, B., & Kizior, R. (2003). *Saunders nursing drug handbook 2003.* Philadelphia: W.B. Saunders, p. 1084.

151. A nurse is caring for a client who has had a transient ischemic attack. In the event that an ischemic stroke occurs, the nurse anticipates that which medication most likely will be prescribed initially?
1   An oral anticoagulant
2   A thrombolytic
3   An antiplatelet
4   A beta-blocker

Answer: 2

Rationale: Alteplase (Activase), a thrombolytic, may be prescribed for clients who experience ischemic strokes. For clients who are treated within 6 hours of the onset of symptoms, progression of the stroke frequently can be halted. Many of the symptoms present also can be reversed. A beta-blocker is used for cardiac and hypertensive conditions. An oral anticoagulant and an antiplatelet may be used to assist in preventing an ischemic stroke.

Test-Taking Strategy: Use the process of elimination focusing on the issue: a client who has had an ischemic stroke. Knowledge regarding the action of a beta-blocker assists in eliminating option 4. Focusing on the issue of the question assists in directing you to option 2 from the remaining options. Review pharmacological treatments for the client with a stroke if you had difficulty with this question.

Level of Cognitive Ability: Analysis
Client Needs: Physiological Integrity
Integrated Concept/Process: Nursing Process/Planning
Content Area: Pharmacology

Reference:
Hodgson, B., & Kizior, R. (2003). *Saunders nursing drug handbook 2003.* Philadelphia: W.B. Saunders, p. 35.

152. After receiving replacement surfactant therapy, the infant with respiratory distress syndrome (RDS) requires frequent arterial blood gas monitoring. Which of the following statements made by the infant's mother indicates that she understands the reason why frequent blood sampling is needed?
1   "Frequent blood gas tests help to monitor my baby's respiratory patterns."
2   "You just keep taking blood from my baby for all these tests."
3   "Taking blood samples is the hospital's policy after giving this medication."
4   "My baby will require frequent blood gas tests throughout the hospital stay."

Answer: 1

Rationale: Frequent monitoring may be necessary during the acute stages of RDS in the newborn, and especially after replacement surfactant therapy has occurred. This allows for trending of the respiratory status and assists decision making in further management. Options 2, 3, and 4 do not reflect an understanding of the purpose of the blood gases.

Test-Taking Strategy: Use the process of elimination and knowledge about surfactant replacement therapy and the associated procedures to answer this question. Note the relationship between the issue of the question and option 1. Review care to the infant with RDS if you had difficulty with this question.

Level of Cognitive Ability: Comprehension
Client Needs: Physiological Integrity
Integrated Concept/Process: Nursing Process/Evaluation
Content Area: Maternity

Reference:
McKinney, E., Ashwill, J., Murray, S., James, S., Gorrie, T., & Droske, S. (2000). *Maternal-child nursing.* Philadelphia: W.B. Saunders, p. 752.

153. A nurse reads the radiology report of the initial chest radiograph taken on the infant who is experiencing respiratory distress syndrome and has received replacement surfactant therapy. The report states that both lung fields have a

Answer: 3

Rationale: Chest radiographs in infants with respiratory distress related to hyaline membrane disease show a "ground-glass" appearance characteristic of the disease process. This finding is significant; it is not consistent with a diagnosis of bronchopulmonary dysplasia or indicative of a pneumothorax.

"ground-glass" appearance. How does the nurse evaluate this report?

1   Insignificant and unrelated to respiratory distress syndrome
2   Consistent with a diagnosis of bronchopulmonary dysplasia
3   Characteristic of respiratory distress syndrome secondary to hyaline membrane disease
4   Indicative of a pneumothorax

Test-Taking Strategy: Use the process of elimination. Focus on the issue of the question and note the relationship between *experiencing respiratory distress syndrome* in the question and *characteristic of respiratory distress syndrome* in the correct option. Review these findings if you had difficulty with this question.

Level of Cognitive Ability: Analysis
Client Needs: Physiological Integrity
Integrated Concept/Process: Nursing Process/Evaluation
Content Area: Maternity

Reference:
McKinney, E., Ashwill, J., Murray, S., James, S., Gorrie, T., & Droske, S. (2000). *Maternal-child nursing.* Philadelphia: W.B. Saunders, p. 752.

---

154. A nurse is caring for an infant with respiratory distress syndrome (RDS) secondary to hyaline membrane disease. The nurse is gathering data about the client and looks for a major finding associated with RDS when the nurse does which of the following?

1   Weighs the infant
2   Tests the infant's urine for glucose
3   Takes the infant's blood pressure
4   Reviews the results of the arterial blood gas test

Answer: 4
Rationale: Acidosis is a major manifestation of RDS that develops because of the hypoxemia associated with RDS. The results of the arterial blood gas test would indicate an acid-base imbalance. Options 1 and 3 may be components of the data collection, but they are not specifically associated with RDS. Option 2 is unrelated to RDS.

Test-Taking Strategy: Use the process of elimination. Focus on the disorder, RDS, to assist in directing you to the only option that addresses a respiratory assessment technique. Review the clinical manifestations associated with RDS and the data collection techniques if you had difficulty with this question.

Level of Cognitive Ability: Application
Client Needs: Physiological Integrity
Integrated Concept/Process: Nursing Process/Data Collection
Content Area: Maternity

Reference:
McKinney, E., Ashwill, J., Murray, S., James, S., Gorrie, T., & Droske, S. (2000). *Maternal-child nursing.* Philadelphia: W.B. Saunders, p. 752.

---

155. A nurse is reviewing laboratory results for a preterm infant with respiratory distress syndrome (RDS) and suspected hyaline membrane disease. The results of the lecithin-sphingomyelin (L/S) ratio drawn at 30 weeks gestation is reported as less than 2:1. The nurse evaluates these results as:

1   Normal
2   Higher than normal
3   Lower than normal
4   Insignificant

Answer: 3
Rationale: The presence of surfactant in amniotic fluid is an indicator of fetal lung maturity. Sampling may be done by amniocentesis or by removal of a fluid sample from the vagina after rupture of the membranes. Generally, pulmonary status is considered mature with an L/S ratio of at least 2:1.

Test-Taking Strategy: Use the process of elimination. Knowing that the L/S ratio can be an indicator of lung maturity, expect that the level would be less than normal in an infant with RDS. Additionally, select the option that is similar to the question. In this case *suspected hyaline membrane disease* and *indicating hyaline membrane disease* are similar. Review the L/S ratio if you had difficulty with this question.

Level of Cognitive Ability: Analysis
Client Needs: Physiological Integrity

Integrated Concept/Process: Nursing Process/Evaluation
Content Area: Maternity

Reference:
Murray, S., McKinney, E., & Gorrie, T. (2002). *Foundations of Maternals newborn nursing* (3rd ed.) Philadelphia: W.B. Saunders, pp. 227; 831.

---

156. A nurse caring for a small-for-gestational-age (SGA) infant reviews the results of a total serum calcium level. The results are reported as 5.9 mg/dL. How does the nurse evaluate these results?
1 Within normal limits
2 Less than normal
3 Greater than normal
4 Insignificant

Answer: 2
Rationale: SGA infants are at risk for developing hypocalcemia. The normal range for a total serum calcium is 7.0 mg/dL to 8.5 mg/dL. Options 1, 3, and 4 are incorrect.

Test-Taking Strategy: Knowledge regarding the normal total serum calcium level is necessary to answer this question. Review information about this laboratory test if you had difficulty with this question.

Level of Cognitive Ability: Comprehension
Client Needs: Physiological Integrity
Integrated Concept/Process: Nursing Process/Evaluation
Content Area: Maternity

Reference:
McKinney, E., Ashwill, J., Murray, S., James, S., Gorrie, T., & Droske, S. (2000). *Maternal-child nursing.* Philadelphia: W.B. Saunders, p. 755.

---

157. A nurse is caring for a small-for-gestational-age (SGA) infant. In evaluating growth and whether the infant is asymmetrically or symmetrically SGA, the nurse collects data regarding which of the following?
1 Temperature, pulse, and blood pressure
2 Head circumference, length, and weight
3 Weight, respiratory rate, and urine output
4 Chest circumference, hematocrit level, and blood glucose

Answer: 2
Rationale: Symmetrical versus asymmetrical growth determines whether the growth restriction began early or late in the pregnancy. It is determined by collecting information about head circumference, length, and weight. Options 1, 3 and 4 do not provide information about growth.

Test-Taking Strategy: Use the process of elimination, focusing on the issue of the question. Noting that the issue addresses growth assists you in choosing the option that addresses this issue. If you had difficulty with this question, review the techniques for determining growth factors in the SGA infant.

Level of Cognitive Ability: Comprehension
Client Needs: Physiological Integrity
Integrated Concept/Process: Nursing Process/Data Collection
Content Area: Maternity

Reference:
McKinney, E., Ashwill, J., Murray, S., James, S., Gorrie, T., & Droske, S. (2000). *Maternal-child nursing.* Philadelphia: W.B. Saunders, p. 755.

---

158. A nurse is monitoring a small-for-gestational-age (SGA) infant. Which of the following data indicate a potential complication in this infant?
1 A urinary output of less than 3 to 4 mL/kg per hour

Answer: 3
Rationale: One of the complications associated with SGA infants is intolerance of oral feedings. All the other options are values that are within normal limits and therefore are not complications. It is important to recognize that nutrition in the SGA infant is a primary consideration and if the infant is intolerant of oral

2 An axillary temperature of 99° F
3 Intolerance of oral feedings
4 Blood glucose level of 45 to 60 mg/dL

feedings, an alternate form of nutritional support should be implemented.

Test-Taking Strategy: Use the process of elimination and knowledge regarding the normal vital signs and laboratory values in an infant to assist in directing you to the correct option, which is option 3. Review the normal values and complications in an SGA infant if you had difficulty with this question.

Level of Cognitive Ability: Comprehension
Client Needs: Physiological Integrity
Integrated Concept/Process: Nursing Process/Evaluation
Content Area: Maternity

Reference:
McKinney, E., Ashwill, J., Murray, S., James, S., Gorrie, T., & Droske, S. (2000). *Maternal-child nursing.* Philadelphia: W.B. Saunders, p. 755.

---

159. A nurse is caring for a large-for-gestational-age (LGA) infant. The nurse is gathering data about the infant. A major symptom associated with LGA infants can be observed when the nurse does which of the following?
1 Takes the infant's blood pressure
2 Weighs the infant
3 Measures the infant's head circumference
4 Tests the infant's blood glucose

Answer: 4
Rationale: LGA infants are at risk for hypoglycemia, which is a major metabolic complication associated with LGA infants and can cause brain damage. Although options 1, 2, and 3 are components of data collection, they are not associated with a major complication.

Test-Taking Strategy: Use the process of elimination. Recalling that the LGA infant is at risk for hypoglycemia directs you to option 4. In addition, noting the key words *major symptom* assists in answering the question correctly. Options 1, 2, and 3 are data collection techniques for any infant. Review the complications associated with the LGA infant if you had difficulty with this question.

Level of Cognitive Ability: Comprehension
Client Needs: Physiological Integrity
Integrated Concept/Process: Nursing Process/Data Collection
Content Area: Maternity

Reference:
McKinney, E., Ashwill, J., Murray, S., James, S., Gorrie, T., & Droske, S. (2000). *Maternal-child nursing.* Philadelphia: W.B. Saunders, p. 756.

---

160. A nurse is caring for a large-for-gestational age infant who has polycythemia and hyperviscosity. The nurse anticipates that the physician will prescribe which of the following if the infant becomes symptomatic?
1 Radiographic kidney evaluation
2 Exchange transfusion
3 Ultrasound evaluation of the brain
4 Enteral feedings instead of oral feedings

Answer: 2
Rationale: The most likely intervention for an infant with symptomatic polycythemia and hyperviscosity is an exchange transfusion. This treatment improves cerebral blood flow, systemic blood flow, and oxygen transport. Options 1, 3, and 4 are not indicated in this situation.

Test-Taking Strategy: Use the process of elimination. Note the relationship between the words *polycythemia and hyperviscosity* in the question and *transfusion* in the correct option. Review the treatment for these disorders if you had difficulty with this question.

Level of Cognitive Ability: Comprehension
Client Needs: Physiological Integrity
Integrated Concept/Process: Nursing Process/Planning
Content Area: Maternity

Reference:
Wong, D., & Hockenberry-Eaton, M. (2001). *Wong's essentials of pediatric nursing.* St. Louis: Mosby, p. 304.

---

161. A physician informs a nurse that a large-for-gestational-age (LGA) infant who has polycythemia and hyperviscosity symptoms will undergo an exchange transfusion. The nurse knows that for this procedure to be implemented, the following fluid will be used for the exchange transfusion?
1   10% glucose
2   Lactated Ringer's solution
3   Pedialyte
4   Albumin

Answer: 4
Rationale: An exchange transfusion for polycythemia and hyperviscosity is primarily done with albumin. Normal saline is frequently used in a partial exchange. Options 1, 2, and 3 are not used for an exchange transfusion in this situation.

Test-Taking Strategy: Knowledge regarding the procedure for exchange transfusions for an LGA infant with polycythemia and hyperviscosity is necessary to answer the question. Review this content if you are unfamiliar with this procedure.

Level of Cognitive Ability: Analysis
Client Needs: Physiological Integrity
Integrated Concept/Process: Nursing Process/Planning
Content Area: Maternity

Reference:
Murray, S., McKinney, E., & Gorrie, T. (2002). *Foundations of maternal-newborn nursing.* Philadelphia: W.B. Saunders, p. 856.

---

162. During the exchange transfusion for a large-for-gestational-age infant who has polycythemia and hyperviscosity symptoms, the priority nursing action will be to monitor for which of the following?
1   Cardiac irregularities
2   Hypokalemia
3   Hyperglycemia
4   Hypercalcemia

Answer: 1
Rationale: Cardiac irregularities are a major complication of an exchange transfusion. Additionally, hyperkalemia, hypoglycemia, and hypocalcemia may occur.

Test-Taking Strategy: Knowledge regarding the complications associated with an exchange transfusion is necessary to answer the question. Use the ABCs (airway, breathing, and circulation) to direct you to option 1. Review the complications of this procedure if you had difficulty with this question.

Level of Cognitive Ability: Analysis
Client Needs: Physiological Integrity
Integrated Concept/Process: Nursing Process/Data Collection
Content Area: Maternity

Reference:
Wong, D., & Hockenberry-Eaton, M. (2001). *Wong's essentials of pediatric nursing.* St. Louis: Mosby, p. 294.

---

163. A nurse can best prevent a fluid volume deficit after the administration of a diuretic to a disoriented client by which of the following?

Answer: 1
Rationale: A disoriented client should be offered fluid by the caregiver to increase fluid intake and prevent dehydration. Options 2 and 3 do not ensure that the client will drink the

1   Frequently offering fluids
2   Advising the client to drink lots of fluids
3   Leaving water at the bedside
4   Keeping the client on bed rest

needed fluids. Option 4 is unrelated to the issue of the question.

Test-Taking Strategy: Use the process of elimination and focus on the issue of the question. Note the key words *disoriented client.* Eliminate option 4 because it is unrelated to the issue of the question. Eliminate options 2 and 3 because these actions cannot assure that the client will drink the needed fluids. Review care to the client with a fluid volume deficit if you had difficulty with this question.

Level of Cognitive Ability: Application
Client Needs: Physiological Integrity
Integrated Concept/Process: Nursing Process/Implementation
Content Area: Fundamental Skills

Reference:
Black, J., Hawks, J., & Keene, A. (2001). *Medical-surgical nursing: clinical management for positive outcomes* (6th ed.). Philadelphia: W.B. Saunders, p. 220.

---

164. A nurse is preparing to administer captopril (Capoten), an angiotensin-converting enzyme (ACE) inhibitor. Which of the following data would be most important to collect before administering the medication?
1   Blood pressure
2   Temperature
3   Lung sounds
4   Mental status

Answer: 1
Rationale: ACE inhibitors are potent antihypertensive medications. A baseline blood pressure is needed to evaluate the outcome of this therapy. Options 2, 3, and 4 are generally not affected by the action of ACE inhibitors.

Test-Taking Strategy: Use the process of elimination. Knowledge that ACE inhibitors are most often used to treat hypertension directs you to option 1. Review the actions and uses of ACE inhibitors if you had difficulty with this question.

Level of Cognitive Ability: Analysis
Client Needs: Physiological Integrity
Integrated Concept/Process: Nursing Process/Data Collection
Content Area: Pharmacology

Reference:
Hodgson, B., & Kizior, R. (2003). *Saunders nursing drug handbook 2003.* Philadelphia: W.B. Saunders, p. 167.

---

165. The nurse is preparing to administer an intramuscular (IM) injection to a toddler. The safest body site to administer the injection is which of the following?
1   Deltoid muscle
2   Vastus lateralis muscle
3   Ventrogluteal muscle
4   Dorsogluteal muscle

Answer: 2
Rationale: The vastus lateralis muscle is large enough to handle an IM injection in a toddler. Options 1, 3, and 4 are not appropriate sites to administer an IM injection because they are not large muscle groups.

Test-Taking Strategy: Use the process of elimination and knowledge regarding the administration of IM injections to a toddler to answer the question. Recalling the anatomy of muscle groups assists in directing you to the correct option. If you are unfamiliar with these administration techniques in the toddler, review this content.

Level of Cognitive Ability: Application
Client Needs: Physiological Integrity

Integrated Concept/Process: Nursing Process/Implementation
Content Area: Child Health

Reference:
Wong, D., & Hockenberry-Eaton, M. (2001). *Wong's essentials of pediatric nursing* (6th ed.). St. Louis: Mosby, p. 785.

---

166. A nurse is caring for a postmature infant who at 2 hours of age had a venous hematocrit of greater than 65%. The nurse reviews the results of the laboratory tests, knowing that during the next 24 hours the priority laboratory value to monitor is which of the following?
1 Blood urea nitrogen
2 Creatinine
3 Urine glucose
4 Bilirubin

Answer: 4
Rationale: Postmature infants are at risk for inadequate oxygen in utero, which predisposes the infant to polycythemia. Polycythemia then makes the infant prone to hyperbilirubinemia. In this infant, the priority is to monitor the bilirubin level.

Test-Taking Strategy: Use the process of elimination and knowledge regarding the care of the postmature infant. Note that options 1, 2, and 3 are similar and all relate to the renal system. Review care to the postmature infant if you had difficulty with this question.

Level of Cognitive Ability: Comprehension
Client Needs: Physiological Integrity
Integrated Concept/Process: Nursing Process/Data Collection
Content Area: Maternity

Reference:
McKinney, E., Ashwill, J., Murray, S., James, S., Gorrie, T., & Droske, S. (2000). *Maternal-child nursing.* Philadelphia: W.B. Saunders, p. 754.

---

167. An anticholinergic medication is prescribed for the preoperative client. The nurse prepares to administer the medication knowing that it does which of the following?
1 Relaxes the urinary bladder and helps to prevent urinary tract infections
2 Increases the heart rate and helps to prevent shock
3 Reduces respiratory tract secretions and helps to prevent aspiration
4 Prolongs blood clotting time and helps to prevent thrombophlebitis

Answer: 3
Rationale: Anticholinergics dry up secretions, which helps to prevent aspiration. Options 2 and 4 are inaccurate actions of the medication. Although the medication may relax the urinary bladder, this is not the purpose for administering the medication in the preoperative period. Additionally, this medication does not prevent urinary tract infections.

Test-Taking Strategy: Use the process of elimination, recalling that one of the risks associated with surgery is aspiration. This directs you to option 3. Review the actions of anticholinergics if you had difficulty with this question.

Level of Cognitive Ability: Comprehension
Client Needs: Physiological Integrity
Integrated Concept/Process: Nursing Process/Implementation
Content Area: Fundamental Skills

Reference:
Lehne, R. (2001). *Pharmacology for nursing care* (4th ed.). Philadelphia: W.B. Saunders, p. 118.

---

168. A nurse is caring for an infant with physiological jaundice. The nurse is gathering data and looks for a major symptom associated with physiological

Answer: 2
Rationale: The principal source of bilirubin is the hemolysis of erythrocytes. A cephalhematoma contains a large number of erythrocytes. As the red blood cells break down in the bruised area,

jaundice when doing which of the following?

1 Evaluating the infant's urine output
2 Noting the presence of a cephalhematoma
3 Determining the maternal blood type
4 Guaiacing the infant's meconium stool

they add to the bilirubin load. Maternal blood type, particularly in Rh incompatibility, is relevant to pathological jaundice. All meconium stools guaiac positive because meconium contains old red blood cells. Evaluating the urine output is not significant unless jaundice related to inadequate intake is suspected, which is primarily associated with breast milk jaundice.

Test-Taking Strategy: Knowledge regarding the differences between physiological jaundice and pathological jaundice is necessary to answer this question. Review these differences if you had difficulty with this question.

Level of Cognitive Ability: Analysis
Client Needs: Physiological Integrity
Integrated Concept/Process: Nursing Process/Data Collection
Content Area: Maternity

Reference:
McKinney, E., Ashwill, J., Murray, S., James, S., Gorrie, T., & Droske, S. (2000). *Maternal-child nursing.* Philadelphia: W.B. Saunders, p. 534.

---

169. A nurse is gathering data about a postterm infant born after the 42nd week of gestation. The most significant information is obtained when the nurse does which of the following?

1 Determines the maternal blood type
2 Obtains the Apgar scores
3 Obtains the infant's footprints
4 Carefully estimates the actual gestational age by recording the infant's weight, length, and head circumference on standard growth charts

Answer: 4
Rationale: The medical management of a postterm infant is different than that of a preterm or term infant. Documentation of the actual estimated gestational age is an important factor in determining management of the infant. Although options 1, 2, and 3 identify data that would be obtained, option 4 specifically identifies information necessary for the care of the postterm infant.

Test-Taking Strategy: Focus on the issue: postterm infant. Although all of the options identify information that would be collected, only option 4 identifies information related to the postterm infant. Review initial care to the postterm infant if you had difficulty with this question.

Level of Cognitive Ability: Comprehension
Client Needs: Physiological Integrity
Integrated Concept/Process: Nursing Process/Data Collection
Content Area: Maternity

Reference:
Wong, D., & Hockenberry-Eaton, M. (2001). *Wong's essentials of pediatric nursing* (6th ed.), St. Louis: Mosby, pp. 202-203.

---

170. A nurse is preparing to administer eye ointments to a newborn infant. The ointment is prescribed as prophylactic treatment to prevent ophthalmia neonatorum. The nurse anticipates that the most likely eye ointment or solution prescribed is which of the following?

1 Erythromycin ophthalmic ointment
2 Tetracycline ophthalmic ointment

Answer: 1
Rationale: The most likely medication to be prescribed to prevent ophthalmia neonatorum is Erythromycin ophthalmic ointment. Tetracycline ophthalmic ointment is used for prophylaxis against the organism *Neisseria gonorrhoeae.* Trifluridine ophthalmic solution is used for herpes simplex infections. Lacri-Lube is used to prevent drying of the eyes.

Test-Taking Strategy: Knowledge of the actions and uses of these medications is necessary to assist you in answering this question.

3   Lacri-Lube solution
4   Trifluridine ophthalmic solution

Review this content if you are unfamiliar with the medications addressed in the options and the prophylactic treatment for ophthalmia neonatorum.

Level of Cognitive Ability: Analysis
Client Needs: Physiological Integrity
Integrated Concept/Process: Nursing Process/Planning
Content Area: Pharmacology

Reference:
McKinney, E., Ashwill, J., Murray, S., James, S., Gorrie, T., & Droske, S. (2000). *Maternal-child nursing.* Philadelphia: W.B. Saunders, p. 563.

---

171. An infant born past 42 weeks gestation is considered postmature. One of the characteristics of a postmature infant is the decrease or absence of subcutaneous fat. When the nurse assists in preparing a nursing care plan, the nurse understands that the lack of subcutaneous fat requires which of the following for the infant?
1   Have supplemental calories added to the breast milk or formula
2   Be provided with a neutral thermal environment
3   Be offered feedings every 4 to 6 hours
4   Remain in the hospital for an extended period of time

Answer: 2
Rationale: Signs of postmaturity are noted during the initial data collection. Temperature regulation may be poor because fat stores have been used for nourishment in utero. The infant may need more time in a radiant warmer or incubator until thermoregulation is stable. Options 1, 3 and 4 will not affect temperature regulation.

Test-Taking Strategy: Use the process of elimination. Focus on the issue of the question: decrease or absence of subcutaneous fat. Recalling the relationship between this issue and thermal regulation directs you to option 2. Review thermal regulation in a newborn if you had difficulty with this question.

Level of Cognitive Ability: Comprehension
Client Needs: Physiological Integrity
Integrated Concept/Process: Nursing Process/Planning
Content Area: Maternity

Reference:
McKinney, E., Ashwill, J., Murray, S., James, S., Gorrie, T., & Droske, S. (2000). *Maternal-child nursing.* Philadelphia: W.B. Saunders, p. 754.

---

172. A client is admitted to the hospital with complications of celiac disease. Which of the following questions would be most helpful in obtaining information for the initial plan of care?
1   "What types of pasta can you eat?"
2   "What is your understanding of celiac disease?"
3   "Tell me about the types of foods that you like to eat."
4   "Have you eliminated whole wheat bread from your diet?"

Answer: 2
Rationale: Celiac disease also is known as gluten-induced enteropathy. It causes diseased intestinal villi, which results in fewer absorptive surfaces and malabsorption syndrome. Clients with celiac disease must maintain a gluten-free diet, which eliminates all products made from wheat, rye, barley, and oats. Beer, pasta, crackers, cereals, and many more substances contain gluten. To plan care, it is most important to determine the client's understanding of the disease.

Test-Taking Strategy: Use the process of elimination and the principles related to teaching and learning concepts. Option 2 focuses on the client's disorder and is the most global option. Review teaching–learning principles and this disorder if you had difficulty with this question.

Level of Cognitive Ability: Application
Client Needs: Physiological Integrity

Integrated Concept/Process: Nursing Process/Data Collection
Content Area: Fundamental Skills

Reference:
Williams, S. (2001). *Basic nutrition & diet therapy* (11th ed.). St. Louis: Mosby, p. 336.

---

173. A client with a duodenal ulcer asks the nurse why an antibiotic has been prescribed. The nurse responds by telling the client that this medication will do which of the following?
  1   Soothe the irritated mucosal surface
  2   Eliminate a germ that impairs mucosal function
  3   Reduce the inflammation
  4   Prevent secondary infections

Answer: 2
Rationale: Duodenal ulcers are strongly associated with *Helicobacter pylori* infection. It is believed that these bacteria colonize in the mucous cells and impair their function. Antibiotics are given to control this infection. Options 1 and 3 are not effects of antibiotics. Option 4 is a rare occurrence with duodenal ulcers.

Test-Taking Strategy: Use the process of elimination and knowledge regarding the actions of antibiotics to assist in eliminating options 1 and 3. Recalling the pathophysiology related to duodenal ulcers and their probable causes directs you to option 2 from the remaining options. Review this content if you had difficulty with this question.

Level of Cognitive Ability: Application
Client Needs: Physiological Integrity
Integrated Concept/Process: Nursing Process/Implementation
Content Area: Adult Health/Gastrointestinal

Reference:
Black, J., Hawks, J., & Keene, A. (2001). *Medical-surgical nursing: clinical management for positive outcomes* (6th ed.). Philadelphia: W.B. Saunders, p. 712.

---

174. A nurse is caring for a client who is receiving prednisone (Deltasone). The nurse plans to most closely monitor the client for the development of which of the following?
  1   Hypoglycemia
  2   Hyperglycemia
  3   Adrenal insufficiency
  4   Weight loss

Answer: 2
Rationale: Exogenously administered corticosteroids have profound systemic effects because they "mimic" naturally occurring adrenal hormones. Hyperglycemia occurs because of the stimulation of gluconeogenesis and the decreased use of glucose by the cells. Option 3 identifies a condition in which corticosteroids may be administered. Option 4 is an incorrect effect because weight gain is often experienced by clients receiving prednisone.

Test-Taking Strategy: Use the process of elimination. Knowledge regarding the side effects associated with the use of corticosteroids is necessary to answer this question. Review these side effects if you had difficulty with this question.

Level of Cognitive Ability: Application
Client Needs: Physiological Integrity
Integrated Concept/Process: Nursing Process/Planning
Content Area: Pharmacology

Reference:
Hodgson, B., & Kizior, R. (2003). *Saunders nursing drug handbook 2003.* Philadelphia: W.B. Saunders, p. 920.

175. A physician orders phenobarbital (Luminal) 25 mg PO every 6 hours. The medication label reads phenobarbital (Luminal) 20 mg per 5 mL. How many mL will the nurse prepare to administer one dose?
1   4 mL
2   6.25 mL
3   10 mL
4   15 mL

Answer: 2
Rationale: Follow the following formula for calculating medication doses.

$$\frac{Desired}{Available} \times mL = mL \ per \ dose$$

$$\frac{25 \ mg}{20 \ mg} \times 5 \ mL = 6.25 \ mL$$

Test-Taking Strategy: Knowledge of the formula for the calculation of a medication is necessary to answer this question. Follow the formula and ensure that the calculated dose makes sense. Review medication calculations if you had difficulty with this question.

Level of Cognitive Ability: Application
Client Needs: Physiological Integrity
Integrated Concept/Process: Nursing Process/Implementation
Content Area: Fundamental Skills

Reference:
deWit, S. (2001). *Fundamental concepts and skills for nursing.* Philadelphia: W.B. Saunders, p. 642.

176. A physician orders pentobarbital (Nembutal) 0.1 g PO at hour of sleep. The medication label reads pentobarbital 50-mg capsules. How many capsule(s) should the nurse administer to the client?
1   One capsule
2   Two capsules
3   Three capsules
4   Four capsules

Answer: 2
Rationale: Convert 0.1 g to mg. In the metric system, to convert larger to smaller multiply by 1000 or move the decimal three places to the right. Then, follow the following formula.

0.1 g = 100 mg

$$\frac{100 \ mg}{50 \ mg} \times 1 \ capsule = \frac{100 \ mg}{50 \ mg} = 2 \ capsules$$

Test-Taking Strategy: Knowledge of the formula for the calculation of a medication is necessary to answer this question. Remember to convert grams to milligrams. Follow the formula and ensure that the calculated dose makes sense. If you had difficulty with this question, review conversions and calculations.

Level of Cognitive Ability: Application
Client Needs: Physiological Integrity
Integrated Concept/Process: Nursing Process/Implementation
Content Area: Fundamental Skills

Reference:
deWit, S. (2001). *Fundamental concepts and skills for nursing.* Philadelphia: W.B. Saunders, p. 642.

177. A nurse visits a client at home. The client tells the nurse that the physician instructions state to take ibuprofen (Advil) 0.4 g for mild pain. The medication bottle

Answer: 3
Rationale: Convert 0.4 g to mg. In the metric system, to convert larger to smaller multiply by 1000 or move the decimal three places to the right. Then, follow the following formula.

states ibuprofen 200-mg tablets. How many tablet(s) should the nurse instruct the client to take?
1   ½ tablet
2   1 tablet
3   2 tablets
4   1.5 tablets

0.4 g = 400 mg

$$\frac{400 \text{ mg}}{200 \text{ mg}} \times 1 \text{ tablet} = 2 \text{ tablets}$$

Test-Taking Strategy: Knowledge of the formula for the calculation of a medication is necessary to answer this question. Remember to convert grams to milligrams. Follow the formula and ensure that the calculated dose makes sense. If you had difficulty with this question, review conversions and calculations.

Level of Cognitive Ability: Application
Client Needs: Physiological Integrity
Integrated Concept/Process: Teaching/Learning
Content Area: Fundamental Skills

Reference:
deWit, S. (2001). *Fundamental concepts and skills for nursing.* Philadelphia: W.B. Saunders, p. 642.

---

178. A nurse is admitting a client with a diagnosis of a nasal polyp to the surgical nursing unit. Which of the following would the nurse expect the client to describe when collecting data from the client?
1   A runny nose
2   Nasal obstruction
3   Headaches
4   Coryza

Answer: 2
Rationale: The primary symptom of a nasal polyp is nasal obstruction. A runny nose is suggestive of a cold or sinus drainage. Headache and coryza are not symptoms of a nasal tumor.

Test-Taking Strategy: Use the process of elimination. Focus on the diagnosis "nasal polyp." Visualize this disorder and the effect that it may have on the client to assist in directing you to option 2. Review the manifestations associated with this disorder if you had difficulty with this question.

Level of Cognitive Ability: Comprehension
Client Needs: Physiological Integrity
Integrated Concept/Process: Nursing Process/Data Collection
Content Area: Adult Health/Respiratory

Reference:
Black, J., Hawks, J., & Keene, A. (2001). *Medical-surgical nursing: clinical management for positive outcomes* (6th ed.). Philadelphia: W.B. Saunders, p. 1682.

---

179. An LPN is assisting an RN in preparing to insert a nasogastric (NG) tube into a client. The RN asks the LPN to assist in determining the appropriate length of the tube needed for insertion. The LPN does which of the following to provide the requested measurement?
1   Places the tube at the tip of the nose and measures by extending the tube to the earlobe and then down to the xiphoid process
2   Places the tube at the tip of the nose and measures by extending the tube to the sternum and then to the earlobe

Answer: 1
Rationale: The appropriate method of measuring the length of a tube needed for NG tube insertion is to place the tube at the tip of the nose and measure by extending the tube to the earlobe and then down to the xiphoid process. The tube should be marked at that length. Options 2, 3, and 4 are inaccurate measurement procedures.

Test-Taking Strategy: Use the process of elimination and knowledge regarding the appropriate procedure for measuring the length of an NG tube required for insertion to answer this question. Attempt to visualize the description in each of the options to help you answer the question correctly. Review this procedure if you had difficulty with this question.

3 Places the tube at the tip of the earlobe and measures by extending the tube to the nose and down to the umbilicus

4 Places the tube at the tip of the earlobe and measures by extending the tube to the nose and then to the xiphoid process

Level of Cognitive Ability: Application
Client Needs: Physiological Integrity
Integrated Concept/Process: Nursing Process/Implementation
Content Area: Adult Health/Gastrointestinal

Reference:
Perry, A., & Potter, P. (2002) *Clinical nursing Skills & techniques* (5th ed.). St. Louis: Mosby, p. 661.

---

180. A client is scheduled for percutaneous transhepatic cholangiography. The nurse is providing instructions regarding the procedure. Which of the following is an inaccurate description of the procedure?

1 A needle is inserted into the liver under fluoroscopic guidance

2 The client should hold the breath during insertion of the needle into the liver

3 Dye is injected into the liver as the needle is removed

4 The total time for the test is approximately 2 hours

Answer: 4
Rationale: During percutaneous transhepatic cholangiography, a needle is inserted into the liver under fluoroscopic guidance while the client holds the breath to stabilize the liver. The dye is injected as the needle is removed. The outline of the biliary tree is visualized under fluoroscopy. The total time for the test is approximately 30 minutes to 1 hour.

Test-Taking Strategy: Use the process of elimination. Note the key word "inaccurate" in the question. Noting the time period in option 4 helps direct you to this answer. Review this procedure if you are unfamiliar with it.

Level of Cognitive Ability: Comprehension
Client Needs: Physiological Integrity
Integrated Concept/Process: Nursing Process/Implementation
Content Area: Adult Health/Gastrointestinal

Reference:
Chernecky, C., & Berger, B. (2001). *Laboratory tests and diagnostic procedures* (3rd ed.). Philadelphia: W.B. Saunders, p. 806.

---

181. A client is scheduled for an endoscopic retrograde cholangiopancreatography. The nurse understands that which of the following is not a component in the client preparation for this test?

1 Obtain informed consent

2 Obtain baseline vital signs

3 Provide clear liquids on the morning of the test

4 Administer prescribed medications at least 30 minutes before the procedure

Answer: 3
Rationale: Client preparation for endoscopic retrograde cholangiopancreatography includes an NPO status for at least 6 to 8 hours before the procedure. An informed consent as well as baseline vital signs should be obtained. The nurse should administer prescribed medications at least 30 minutes before the procedure. Diazepam (Valium) may be ordered to calm the client. Atropine also may be ordered to dry secretions.

Test-Taking Strategy: Use the process of elimination. Note the key word *not* in the question. Noting that this test is an endoscopic examination assists in directing you to option 3. The client is kept NPO before endoscopic procedures. Review client preparation for this test if you had difficulty with this question.

Level of Cognitive Ability: Comprehension
Client Needs: Physiological Integrity
Integrated Concept/Process: Nursing Process/Planning
Content Area: Adult Health/Gastrointestinal

Reference:
Black, J., Hawks, J., & Keene, A. (2001). *Medical-surgical nursing: clinical management for positive outcomes* (6th ed.). Philadelphia: W.B. Saunders, p. 1086.

182. A nurse is monitoring a client after endoscopic retrograde cholangiopancreatography for complications of the procedure. Which of the following indicates a potential complication?
1. Lethargy
2. Lack of a gag reflex
3. Lack of a cough reflex
4. Abdominal pain

Answer: 4
Rationale: Postprocedural care after endoscopic retrograde cholangiopancreatography include monitoring vital signs and maintaining an NPO status until the gag reflex returns. The client probably received diazepam (Valium) before the procedure; consequently, lethargy is expected. A local anesthetic is sprayed into the client's throat; therefore it is possible that gag and cough reflexes will not be present. The client should be monitored for signs of cholangitis or perforation, which include signs of fever, abdominal pain (especially on the right upper quadrant), hypotension, and tachycardia.

Test-Taking Strategy: Use the process of elimination. Note the key words *potential complication*. You can eliminate options 2 and 3 first, noting that the test is endoscopic in nature and that with this type of test a local anesthetic is sprayed into the client's throat. Recalling that medication is administered before the procedure helps you to eliminate option 1. Review the complications of this diagnostic test if you had difficulty with this question.

Level of Cognitive Ability: Comprehension
Client Needs: Physiological Integrity
Integrated Concept/Process: Nursing Process/Data Collection
Content Area: Adult Health/Gastrointestinal

Reference:
Lewis, S., Heitkemper, M., & Dirksen, S. (2004). *Medical-Surgical nursing: assessment and management of clinical problems* (6th ed.). St. Louis: Mosby, p. 963.

183. A nurse is assisting a physician who is performing abdominal paracentesis on a client. The nurse should assist in placing the client into which of the following positions for this procedure?
1. Supine
2. Right lateral position
3. Left lateral position
4. Upright, or high-Fowler's position

Answer: 4
Rationale: During abdominal paracentesis, the nurse should support the client in an upright, or high-Fowler's position. This position allows the intestine to float posteriorly and helps prevent laceration during catheter insertion. Options 1, 2, and 3 are incorrect.

Test-Taking Strategy: Use the process of elimination. Eliminate options 1, 2, and 3 because they are similar. Additionally, attempting to visualize this procedure and each of the positions identified in the options directs you to option 4. If you had difficulty with this question, review the procedure for abdominal paracentesis.

Level of Cognitive Ability: Application
Client Needs: Physiological Integrity
Integrated Concept/Process: Nursing Process/Implementation
Content Area: Adult Health/Gastrointestinal

Reference:
Black, J., Hawks, J., & Keene, A. (2001). *Medical-surgical nursing: clinical management for positive outcomes* (6th ed.). Philadelphia: W.B. Saunders, p. 1086.

184. A client is seen in the health care clinic and a diagnosis of hypothyroidism is suspected. Which of the following findings does the nurse expect to note in the client?

Answer: 1
Rationale: Clinical manifestations associated with hypothyroidism include bradycardia; obesity; dry, sparse hair; flaky, dry, inelastic skin; and a lowered basal body temperature. The client's

1   Bradycardia
2   Exophthalmos
3   Profuse diaphoresis
4   Hyperactivity

ability to sweat also diminishes. Constipation and fecal impaction occur, and the client has an increased susceptibility to infection. The blood pressure may be normal or slightly elevated, and the temperature is normal to subnormal. Options 2, 3, and 4 are findings noted in hyperthyroidism.

Test-Taking Strategy: Use the process of elimination. Recalling that metabolic processes are decreased in hypothyroidism helps direct you to option 1. Options 2, 3, and 4 are findings noted in hyperthyroidism. Review the findings in hypothyroidism if you had difficulty with this question.

Level of Cognitive Ability: Comprehension
Client Needs: Physiological Integrity
Integrated Concept/Process: Nursing Process/Data Collection
Content Area: Adult Health/Endocrine

Reference:
Lewis, S., Heitkemper, M., & Dirksen, S. (2000). *Medical-surgical nursing: assessment and management of clinical problems* (5th ed.). St. Louis: Mosby, p. 1424.

---

185. A nurse is monitoring a client with hypothyroidism for neurological manifestations. Which of the following does the nurse expect to note in the client?
1   Fine tremors
2   Restlessness
3   Increased deep tendon reflexes
4   Slow, deliberate speech

Answer: 4
Rationale: In hypothyroidism, the client's neurological manifestations include decreased deep tendon reflexes, muscle sluggishness, fatigue, slow and deliberate speech, apathy, depression, impaired short-term memory, and lethargy. Options 1, 2, and 3 are signs of hyperthyroidism.

Test-Taking Strategy: Use the process of elimination. Recalling that metabolic processes are decreased in hypothyroidism helps direct you to option 4. Options 1, 2, and 3 are findings noted in hyperthyroidism. Review the findings in hypothyroidism if you had difficulty with this question.

Level of Cognitive Ability: Comprehension
Client Needs: Physiological Integrity
Integrated Concept/Process: Nursing Process/Data Collection
Content Area: Adult Health/Endocrine

Reference:
Lewis, S., Heitkemper, M., & Dirksen, S. (2000). *Medical-surgical nursing: assessment and management of clinical problems* (5th ed.). St. Louis: Mosby, p. 398.

---

186. A nurse is caring for a client with a diagnosis of thyrotoxicosis (thyroid storm). Which of the following would the nurse include in the plan of care for this client?
1   Use of a hypothermic blanket
2   Restriction of fluid intake
3   Administration of levothyroxine (Synthroid)
4   Administration of enemas and stool softeners

Answer: 1
Rationale: Thyroid storm is a potentially fatal acute episode of thyroid overactivity characterized by high fever, severe tachycardia, delirium, dehydration, and extreme irritability. Because thyroid storm is an emergency, it requires immediate interventions for control. The high fever is treated with hypothermic blankets, and dehydration is reversed with IV fluids. The other options are treatment measures for hypothyroidism.

Test-Taking Strategy: Use the process of elimination. Recalling that thyroid storm is an acute episode of thyroid overactivity helps you eliminate options 2, 3, and 4. Review this potentially fatal acute disorder if you had difficulty with this question.

Level of Cognitive Ability: Application
Client Needs: Physiological Integrity
Integrated Concept/Process: Nursing Process/Planning
Content Area: Adult Health/Endocrine

Reference:
Lewis, S., Heitkemper, M., & Dirksen, S. (2000). *Medical-surgical nursing: assessment and management of clinical problems* (5th ed.). St. Louis: Mosby, p. 1415.

---

187. A nurse is assisting to prepare a plan of care for a client with hyperthyroidism. The nurse is instructing the client regarding dietary measures. Which of the following foods are included in the plan of care?
1   Those high in bulk and fiber
2   Those low in calories
3   Those low in carbohydrates and fats
4   Those high in calories

Answer: 4
Rationale: The client with hyperthyroidism is usually extremely hungry because of increased metabolism. The client should be instructed to consume a high-calorie diet with six full meals a day. The client should be instructed to eat foods that are nutritious and that contain ample amounts of protein, carbohydrates, fats, and minerals. Clients should be discouraged from eating foods that increase peristalsis and thus result in diarrhea, such as highly seasoned, bulky, and fibrous foods.

Test-Taking Strategy: Use the process of elimination. Recalling that metabolic processes are increased in this condition assists you in eliminating options 1, 2, and 3. If you had difficulty with this question, review the dietary measures for the client with hyperthyroidism.

Level of Cognitive Ability: Application
Client Needs: Physiological Integrity
Integrated Concept/Process: Teaching/Learning
Content Area: Adult Health/Endocrine

Reference:
Lewis, S., Heitkemper, M., & Dirksen, S. (2000). *Medical-surgical nursing: assessment and management of clinical problems* (5th ed.). St. Louis: Mosby, p. 1415

---

188. The nurse is caring for a client after thyroidectomy and is monitoring for complications. Which of the following, if noted in the client, indicates a need for physician notification?
1   Surgical pain in the neck area
2   Voice hoarseness
3   Numbness and tingling around the mouth
4   Weakness of the voice

Answer: 3
Rationale: Hypocalcemia can develop after thyroidectomy if the parathyroid glands are accidentally removed or traumatized during surgery. The physician should be called immediately if the client develops numbness and tingling around the mouth or in the fingertips or toes, muscle spasms, or twitching. A hoarse or weak voice may occur temporarily if there has been unilateral injury to the laryngeal nerve during surgery. Pain is expected in the postoperative period. Calcium gluconate ampules should be available at the bedside, and the client should have a patent IV line in the event that hypocalcemic tetany occurs.

Test-Taking Strategy: Use the process of elimination. Eliminate options 2 and 4 first because they are similar. Noting that surgical pain is expected after thyroidectomy helps direct you to option 3. If you had difficulty with this question, review the complications associated with thyroidectomy.

Level of Cognitive Ability: Analysis
Client Needs: Physiological Integrity
Integrated Concept/Process: Nursing Process/Data Collection
Content Area: Adult Health/Endocrine

Reference:
Lewis, S., Heitkemper, M., & Dirksen, S. (2000). *Medical-surgical nursing: assessment and management of clinical problems* (5th ed.). St. Louis: Mosby, p. 1421.

---

189. A nurse is providing dietary instructions to a client with a diagnosis of hyperparathyroidism. Which statement by the client indicates a need for further instructions?
  1 "I should consume 3000 mL of fluid per day."
  2 "I should drink cranberry juice on a daily basis."
  3 "I should consume foods high in vitamin D."
  4 "I should consume foods high in fiber."

Answer: 3
Rationale: The client with hyperparathyroidism should consume at least 3000 mL of fluid per day. Dehydration is dangerous because it increases the serum calcium levels and promotes the formation of renal stones. Cranberry juice and prune juice help make the urine more acidic. A high urinary acidity helps prevent renal stone formation because calcium is more soluble in an acidic than in an alkaline urine. Clients should maintain a low-calcium, low-vitamin D diet. High-fiber foods are important to prevent constipation and fecal impaction resulting from the hypercalcemia that occurs with this disorder.

Test-Taking Strategy: Use the process of elimination and note the key words *need for further instructions.* Recalling the pathophysiology and dietary measures for the client with hyperparathyroidism assists you in answering this question. If you had difficulty with this question, review these important dietary measures.

Level of Cognitive Ability: Comprehension
Client Needs: Physiological Integrity
Integrated Concept/Process: Teaching/Learning
Content Area: Adult Health/Endocrine

Reference:
Lewis, S., Heitkemper, M., & Dirksen, S. (2000). *Medical-surgical nursing: assessment and management of clinical problems* (5th ed.). St. Louis: Mosby, p. 1428

---

190. A nurse is assisting in monitoring a client with acute hypoparathyroidism for signs of hypocalcemia. Which of the following would the nurse note on data collection if hypocalcemia is present?
  1 Hypoactive deep tendon reflexes
  2 Positive Homan's sign
  3 Positive Trousseau's sign
  4 Negative Chvostek's sign

Answer: 3
Rationale: Data collection findings from the client who is hypocalcemic include a positive Chvostek's sign and Trousseau's sign, hyperactive deep tendon reflexes, circumoral paresthesia, and numbness and tingling of the fingers. A positive Homan's sign is noted in thrombophlebitis.

Test-Taking Strategy: Use the process of elimination and focus on the issue: hypocalcemia. Recalling the findings from a hypocalcemic client directs you to option 3. Review these findings if you had difficulty with this question.

Level of Cognitive Ability: Comprehension
Client Needs: Physiological Integrity
Integrated Concept/Process: Nursing Process/Data Collection
Content Area: Adult Health/Endocrine

Reference:
Lewis, S., Heitkemper, M., & Dirksen, S. (2000). *Medical-surgical nursing: assessment and management of clinical problems* (5th ed.). St. Louis: Mosby, p. 1424.

191. A nurse is monitoring a client with hypoparathyroidism for signs of hypocalcemia. The nurse wraps a blood pressure (BP) cuff around the client's upper arm, fills the cuff, and monitors for spasms of the wrist and the hand. The nurse documents the findings, knowing that this test signifies the presence of which of the following?
1 Chvostek's sign
2 Homan's sign
3 Positive Allen's test
4 Trousseau's sign

Answer: 4
Rationale: Trousseau's sign occurs when spasms of the wrist and hand occur after compression of the upper arm by a BP cuff. Chvostek's sign is present when spasms of the facial muscles occur after a tap over a facial nerve, signifying facial hyperirritability. Homan's sign is the presence of pain in the calf area when the foot is dorsiflexed. The Allen's test indicates adequate circulation to the hand before arterial blood gases are obtained.

Test-Taking Strategy: Use the process of elimination. Eliminate option 2 because this sign is noted in the client with thrombophlebitis. Eliminate option 3 because this test is performed to determine adequacy of circulation before drawing arterial blood gases. Knowledge regarding the techniques for each of the remaining options assists in directing you to option 4. Review these techniques if you had difficulty with this question.

Level of Cognitive Ability: Comprehension
Client Needs: Physiological Integrity
Integrated Concept/Process: Nursing Process/Data Collection
Content Area: Adult Health/Endocrine

Reference:
Lewis, S., Heitkemper, M., & Dirksen, S. (2000). *Medical-surgical nursing: assessment and management of clinical problems* (5th ed.). St. Louis: Mosby, p. 1416.

192. A client reports to the health care clinic and tells the nurse that she felt a lump in her breast. The nurse prepares for further data collection, knowing that which of the following is a clinical manifestation of breast cancer?
1 A painful mass
2 A tender mass
3 A soft mobile mass
4 Nipple discharge

Answer: 4
Rationale: Clinical manifestations associated with breast cancer include a mass that is usually painless, nontender, hard, irregular in shape, and nonmobile. Nipple discharge and retraction, edema with peau d'orange skin, and dimpling may be present.

Test-Taking Strategy: Use the process of elimination. Eliminate options 1 and 2 first because they are similar. Recalling that breast cancer is most often associated with a mass that is hard assists in selecting option 4 from the remaining options. Review the clinical manifestations associated with breast cancer if you had difficulty with this question.

Level of Cognitive Ability: Comprehension
Client Needs: Physiological Integrity
Integrated Concept/Process: Nursing Process/Data Collection
Content Area: Adult Health/Oncology

Reference:
Lewis, S., Heitkemper, M., & Dirksen, S. (2000). *Medical-surgical nursing: assessment and management of clinical problems* (5th ed.). St. Louis: Mosby, p. 1480.

193. A client with breast cancer is scheduled for a simple mastectomy. The client asks the nurse what this type of surgery involves. The nurse plans to include which of the following in the response?

1   It involves the removal of the cancerous mass and some normal tissue to produce clean margins
2   It involves the removal of the breast, the axillary lymph nodes, and the overlying skin
3   It involves resection of breast tissue and some skin from the clavicle to the costal margin and from the midline to the latissimus dorsi
4   It involves the removal of the breast, the overlying skin, the pectoral muscles, and the axillary nodes

Answer: 3

Rationale: A simple mastectomy involves resection of breast tissue and some skin from the clavicle to the costal margin and from the midline to the latissimus dorsi. The axillary tail and pectoral fascia are also removed. Axillary nodes are not removed. Option 1 involves a lumpectomy. Option 2 involves a modified radical mastectomy, and option 4 involves a standard radical mastectomy.

Test-Taking Strategy: Use the process of elimination. Eliminate option 2 and 4 first because they are similar. Focusing on the words *simple mastectomy* assists in directing you to option 3 from the remaining options. Review the various types of mastectomies if you had difficulty with this question.

Level of Cognitive Ability: Comprehension
Client Needs: Physiological Integrity
Integrated Concept/Process: Nursing Process/Planning
Content Area: Adult Health/Oncology

Reference:
Lewis, S., Heitkemper, M., & Dirksen, S. (2000). *Medical-surgical nursing: assessment and management of clinical problems* (5th ed.). St. Louis: Mosby, p. 1491.

194. An emergency room nurse asks a licensed practical nurse to obtain the equipment needed to draw a blood sample for a blood alcohol level on a client. Which of the following supplies will not be needed for this procedure?

1   Tourniquet
2   Alcohol swabs
3   A blood-draw needle
4   A blood tube

Answer: 2

Rationale: Isopropyl alcohol or any antiseptic solution containing alcohol must not be used as a skin preparation before a blood alcohol specimen is drawn. These agents may falsely elevate the blood alcohol level and render the test invalid.

Test-Taking Strategy: Use the process of elimination. Note the key word *not* in the question. Focusing on the purpose for collecting the blood sample directs you to option 2. Review the procedure for obtaining a blood alcohol level if you had difficulty with this question.

Level of Cognitive Ability: Comprehension
Client Needs: Physiological Integrity
Integrated Concept/Process: Nursing Process/Implementation
Content Area: Fundamental Skills

Reference:
Chernecky, C., & Berger, B. (2001). *Laboratory tests and diagnostic procedures* (3rd ed.). Philadelphia: W.B. Saunders, p. 137.

195. A client is seen in the health care clinic because of complaints of lesions on the elbows and knees. The lesions are red raised papules, and large plaques covered by silvery scales are noticed on the elbows and knees. Psoriasis is diagnosed. The nurse understands that which of the following is not likely to be prescribed for the client?

1   Tar baths
2   Ultraviolet light treatments

Answer: 4

Rationale: Systemic corticosteroids are rarely used to treat psoriasis. Even though systemic corticosteroids quickly stop a flare-up, a rebound effect occurs after withdrawal of the steroids. This steroid rebound effect causes an immediate flare-up or converts the plaque or exfoliative type of psoriasis to pustular. Options 1, 2, and 3 are appropriate treatments for psoriasis.

Test-Taking Strategy: Use the process of elimination. Note the key word *not* in the question. Observe that options 1, 2, and 3 are similar. These options identify treatments that are local. Option 4 is

3 Topical lubricants
4 Systemic corticosteroids

different because it identifies a systemic treatment. Review treatment measures for psoriasis if you had difficulty with this question.

Level of Cognitive Ability: Comprehension
Client Needs: Physiological Integrity
Integrated Concept/Process: Nursing Process/Planning
Content Area: Adult Health/Integumentary

Reference:
Lewis, S., Heitkemper, M., & Dirksen, S. (2000). *Medical-surgical nursing: assessment and management of clinical problems* (5th ed.). St. Louis: Mosby, p. 511.

---

196. A client is diagnosed with herpes zoster (shingles). Which of the following pharmacological therapies does the nurse expect to be prescribed for the client?
1 Tetracycline hydrochloride (Achromycin)
2 Erythromycin base (E-Mycin)
3 Acyclovir (Zovirax)
4 Indomethacin (Indocin)

Answer: 3
Rationale: The goals of treatment are to relieve pain, prevent infection and scarring, and reduce the possibility of postherpetic neuralgia. Oral analgesics are prescribed to reduce the incidence of persistent pain. The lesions also may be injected with corticosteroids. Acyclovir is an antiviral agent; it may reduce the severity of herpes zoster if started early. Options 1 and 2 identify antibiotics that are not normally prescribed for this condition. Option 4 is a nonsteroidal antiinflammatory drug.

Test-Taking Strategy: Use the process of elimination. Recalling that herpes zoster is a virus directs you to option 3, the only option that identifies an antiviral medication. Review these medications if you are unfamiliar with them.

Level of Cognitive Ability: Analysis
Client Needs: Physiological Integrity
Integrated Concept/Process: Nursing Process/Planning
Content Area: Adult Health/Integumentary

Reference:
Lewis, S., Heitkemper, M., & Dirksen, S. (2000). *Medical-surgical nursing: assessment and management of clinical problems* (5th ed.). St. Louis: Mosby, p. 451.

---

197. A nurse is reviewing the nursing care plan of a client who has a stage 4 decubitus ulcer. Which of the following does the nurse expect to note on data collection of the client?
1 A reddened area that returns to normal skin color after 15 to 20 minutes of pressure relief
2 Intact skin
3 An area in which the top layer of skin is missing
4 A deep ulcer that extends into muscle and bone

Answer: 4
Rationale: A stage 4 decubitus ulcer is a deep ulcer that extends into muscle and bone. It has a foul smell, and the eschar is brown or black. Purulent drainage is common. In a stage 1 ulcer, the skin is intact, but the area may appear pale when pressure is first removed. A stage 1 ulcer also is identified by a reddened area that returns to normal skin color after 15 to 20 minutes of pressure relief. A stage 2 ulcer is an area in which the top layer of skin is missing.

Test-Taking Strategy: Use the process of elimination. Note the key words *stage 4 decubitus ulcer*. Recalling that a stage 4 decubitus ulcer is the most extensive type of ulcer directs you to option 4. Review the stages of decubitus ulcers if you had difficulty with this question.

Level of Cognitive Ability: Comprehension
Client Needs: Physiological Integrity

Integrated Concept/Process: Nursing Process/Data Collection
Content Area: Adult Health/Integumentary

Reference:
Lewis, S., Heitkemper, M., & Dirksen, S. (2000). *Medical-surgical nursing: assessment and management of clinical problems* (5th ed.). St. Louis: Mosby, p. 516.

---

198. A nurse notes documentation of a stage 3 pressure ulcer in a client's record. Which of the following does the nurse expect to note on data collection of the client?
1 A deep ulcer that extends into muscle and bone
2 A deep ulcer that extends into the dermis and the subcutaneous tissue
3 An area in which the top layer of skin is missing
4 A reddened area that returns to normal skin color after 15 to 20 minutes of pressure relief

Answer: 2
Rationale: A stage 3 pressure ulcer is a deep ulcer that extends into the dermis and subcutaneous tissue. White, gray, or yellow eschar usually is present at the bottom of the ulcer, and the ulcer crater may have a lip or edge. Purulent drainage is common. A stage 4 pressure ulcer is a deep ulcer that extends into muscle and bone. A stage 2 pressure ulcer is an area in which the top layer of skin is missing. A stage 1 pressure ulcer is a reddened area that returns to normal skin color after 15 to 20 minutes of pressure relief.

Test-Taking Strategy: Use the process of elimination, noting the key words *stage 3 pressure ulcer* and recalling that there are four stages of pressure ulcers. Think about the description of each stage. Eliminate option 4 first as indicative of a stage 1 pressure ulcer, identified by the absence of a break in the skin. Eliminate option 3 next, focusing on the words *top layer of skin is missing*, which indicates a stage 2 pressure ulcer. From the remaining options, select option 2 instead of option 1, knowing that option 1 describes the most extensive degree of altered skin integrity and therefore identifies a stage 4 pressure ulcer. Review these stages if you are unfamiliar with them.

Level of Cognitive Ability: Comprehension
Client Needs: Physiological Integrity
Integrated Concept/Process: Nursing Process/Data Collection
Content Area: Adult Health/Integumentary

Reference:
Lewis, S., Heitkemper, M., & Dirksen, S. (2000). *Medical-surgical nursing: assessment and management of clinical problems* (5th ed.). St. Louis: Mosby, p. 516.

---

199. A client is seen in the health care clinic, and a biopsy is performed on a skin lesion in which the physician suspects malignant melanoma. The nurse assists in preparing a plan of care based on which characteristic of this type of skin cancer?
1 It is an aggressive cancer that requires aggressive therapy to control its rapid spread
2 It is a slow-growing cancer and seldom metastasizes
3 It can grow so large that an entire area, such as the nose, lip, or ear, must be removed and reconstructed if it occurs on the face

Answer: 1
Rationale: Malignant melanoma, commonly called melanoma, is cancer of the melanocyte cells of the skin. It is an aggressive cancer that requires aggressive therapy to control its spread. Basal cell carcinoma, also known as basal cell epithelioma, is the most common form of skin cancer. It is a slow-growing cancer and seldom metastasizes, but it can grow so large that the entire area of the nose, lip, or ear must be removed and reconstructed.

Test-Taking Strategy: Knowledge regarding the various types of skin cancer is necessary to answer this question. If you had difficulty with this question, review this common type of cancer.

Level of Cognitive Ability: Comprehension
Client Needs: Physiological Integrity

4   It is the most common form of skin cancer

Integrated Concept/Process: Nursing Process/Planning
Content Area: Adult Health/Integumentary

Reference:
Lewis, S., Heitkemper, M., & Dirksen, S. (2000). *Medical-surgical nursing: assessment and management of clinical problems* (5th ed.). St. Louis: Mosby, p. 503.

---

200. A nurse is assisting in caring for a client brought to the emergency room after a burn injury that occurred in the basement of the home. The nurse would suspect an inhalation injury based on which of the following initial findings?
1   Expectoration of sputum tinged with blood
2   The presence of singed nasal hairs
3   Absent breath sounds in the lower lobes bilaterally
4   Tachycardia

Answer: 2
Rationale: Inhalation injuries are most common when a fire occurs in a closed space. The findings are facial burns, singed nasal hairs, and sputum tinged with carbon. In addition, auscultation of wheezing and rales suggests an inhalation injury.

Test-Taking Strategy: Use the process of elimination. Note the key word *initial* in the question. Think about each item in the options and focus on the key word. The first observation that the nurse would make is identified in option 2. If you had difficulty with this question, review the findings in an inhalation injury.

Level of Cognitive Ability: Analysis
Client Needs: Physiological Integrity
Integrated Concept/Process: Nursing Process/Data Collection
Content Area: Adult Health/Integumentary

Reference:
Lewis, S., Heitkemper, M., & Dirksen, S. (2000). *Medical-surgical nursing: assessment and management of clinical problems* (5th ed.). St. Louis: Mosby, p. 540.

---

201. A nurse is assisting in caring for a client who arrives at the emergency room with the emergency medical services team after a severe burn injury from an explosion. Once the initial assessment has been performed by the physician and life-threatening dysfunctions have been addressed, the nurse reviews the physician's orders anticipating that which pain medication will be prescribed?
1   Intravenous (IV) morphine sulfate
2   Aspirin with oxycodone (Percodan) via nasogastric tube
3   IV meperidine hydrochloride (Demerol)
4   Morphine sulfate by subcutaneous route

Answer: 1
Rationale: Once initial assessment has been made and the life-threatening dysfunctions have been addressed, pain medication can be administered. Narcotics administered IV are the initial medications of choice because absorption from the musculature is erratic and an ileus can be present in the burn client. The initial medication of choice is morphine sulfate, although other medications such as methadone, codeine, or hydromorphone also may be used. Narcotics are given IV until fluid resuscitation is complete and gastric motility is restored.

Test-Taking Strategy: Use the process of elimination and note the key words *severe burn injury*. This assists you in eliminating option 4. Recalling the potential complication of ileus associated with burn injuries helps you eliminate option 2. From the remaining options, you must know that morphine sulfate is the medication of choice. Review therapeutic management of a burn injury if you had difficulty with this question.

Level of Cognitive Ability: Analysis
Client Needs: Physiological Integrity
Integrated Concept/Process: Nursing Process/Planning
Content Area: Adult Health/Integumentary

Reference:
Lewis, S., Heitkemper, M., & Dirksen, S. (2000). *Medical-surgical nursing: assessment and management of clinical problems* (5th ed.). St. Louis: Mosby, p. 542,

---

202. A nurse is collecting data regarding the operative site in a client who underwent a breast reconstruction. The nurse is inspecting the flap and the areola of the nipple. The nurse notes that the areola is a deep red color around the edge. Which of the following nursing actions is most appropriate?

1   Document the findings
2   Elevate the breast
3   Encourage nipple massage
4   Notify the physician

Answer: 4

Rationale: After breast reconstruction, the flap is inspected for color, temperature, and capillary refill. Assessment of the nipple areola is made, and dressings are designed so this area can be observed. An areola that is deep red, purple, dusky, or black around the edge is reported to the physician immediately.

Test-Taking Strategy: Use the process of elimination. Noting the key words *deep red color* should assist in directing you to option 4. Review the complications associated with breast reconstruction if you had difficulty with this question.

Level of Cognitive Ability: Application
Client Needs: Physiological Integrity
Integrated Concept/Process: Nursing Process/Implementation
Content Area: Adult Health/Integumentary

Reference:
Lewis, S., Heitkemper, M., & Dirksen, S. (2000). *Medical-surgical nursing: assessment and management of clinical problems* (5th ed.). St. Louis: Mosby, p. 1491.

---

203. A nurse is caring for a client who has had intermaxillary fixation for mandibular fractures suffered during a motor vehicle accident. The client is complaining of a runny nose and asks the nurse for something to relieve this discomfort. Which of the following is the most appropriate nursing action?

1   Call the physician to obtain an antihistamine
2   Provide the client with additional Kleenex for the discharge from the nose
3   Check the discharge for the presence of glucose
4   Assure the client that this is a normal occurrence after surgery

Answer: 3

Rationale: When rhinorrhea (a thin, watery discharge from the nose) or otorrhea (ear inflammation with serum discharge) is noted, cerebrospinal fluid (CSF) may be leaking through the fractures. The nurse checks the fluid for glucose using a test tape or Ketostix. CSF contains glucose, whereas rhinorrhea does not. CSF dries on gauze as a concentric halolike ring and does not crust.

Test-Taking Strategy: Focusing on the anatomical location of this type of surgery assists in directing you to option 3. Remember drainage from a client's ears or nose after head surgery may indicate the presence of CSF. Also, option 3 is the only option that addresses data collection, the first step in the nursing process. Review the complications associated with this type of surgery if you had difficulty with this question.

Level of Cognitive Ability: Application
Client Needs: Physiological Integrity
Integrated Concept/Process: Nursing Process/Implementation
Content Area: Adult Health/Musculoskeletal

Reference:
Lewis, S., Heitkemper, M., & Dirksen, S. (2000). *Medical-surgical nursing: assessment and management of clinical problems* (5th ed.). St. Louis: Mosby, p. 1087.

---

204. A nurse is reinforcing teaching about the signs of peritonitis with a client who has begun peritoneal dialysis. The nurse

Answer: 1

Rationale: Typical symptoms of peritonitis include fever, nausea, malaise, rebound abdominal tenderness, and cloudy dialysate

instructs the client to report which of the following findings to the physician?
1 Cloudy dialysate output
2 Increased abdominal girth
3 Temperature of 99° F orally
4 Heartburn

output. The client does not need to measure abdominal girth. A low-grade temperature may or may not indicate that the client is developing peritonitis. The complaint of heartburn is too vague to be correct.

Test-Taking Strategy: Use the process of elimination. The key words in the question are *peritonitis* and *report.* This implies that the correct answer is a sign or symptom of peritonitis. This focus assists in eliminating options 2 and 4. From the remaining options, recall that infection would cause white blood cells to be present in the dialysate (yielding cloudy dialysate output) and that the fever would be high-grade rather than low-grade. Review the signs of peritonitis if you had difficulty with this question.

Level of Cognitive Ability: Application
Client Needs: Physiological Integrity
Integrated Concept/Process: Teaching/Learning
Content Area: Adult Health/Renal

Reference:
Lewis, S., Heitkemper, M., & Dirksen, S. (2000). *Medical-surgical nursing: assessment and management of clinical problems* (5th ed.). St. Louis: Mosby, p. 1320.

---

205. A nurse is assigned to assist in caring for a client receiving peritoneal dialysis. The nurse notes a brownish color to the dialysate output. The nurse interprets that this finding could result from which of the following conditions?
1 Early infection
2 Insufficient fluid instillation
3 Bladder perforation
4 Bowel perforation

Answer: 4
Rationale: Brown-colored or bloody drainage could indicate perforation of the bowel by the peritoneal dialysis catheter. If noted, this must be reported to the physician immediately. Early signs of infection include cloudy dialysate output or fever and, most likely, abdominal discomfort. Bladder perforation could yield yellow or bloody drainage. Insufficient fluid instillation is an incorrect option. The client would have no signs as a result of insufficient fluid instillation except outflow of smaller amounts of dialysate.

Test-Taking Strategy: Use the process of elimination. Focusing on the data in the question assists in directing you to option 4. Review the complications of peritoneal dialysis if you had difficulty with this question.

Level of Cognitive Ability: Analysis
Client Needs: Physiological Integrity
Integrated Concept/Process: Nursing Process/Data Collection
Content Area: Adult Health/Renal

Reference:
Lewis, S., Heitkemper, M., & Dirksen, S. (2000). *Medical-surgical nursing: assessment and management of clinical problems* (5th ed.). St. Louis: Mosby, p. 1321.

---

206. After reading the product literature about ofloxacin (Floxin), the nurse notes that the medication could cause crystalluria. The nurse tells the client taking the medication to do which of the following

Answer: 3
Rationale: To prevent crystalluria, the client should drink at least 1500 to 2000 mL of fluid per day. Milk interferes with the absorption of the medication. Consumption of carbonated beverages or mineral water is not harmful.

to decrease the likelihood of this adverse effect?

1   Avoid beverages that contain salts, such as mineral water

2   Avoid carbonated soft drink beverages

3   Drink at least 1500 to 2000 mL of fluid per day

4   Drink at least three glasses of milk per day

Test-Taking Strategy: Use the process of elimination. Recall that crystal formation results when there is excess solute load in relation to solvent (fluids). This knowledge guides you to select the option that increases the amount of body water, which in turn limits crystal formation. Use this line of reasoning to eliminate each of the incorrect options. Review this medication if you had difficulty with this question.

Level of Cognitive Ability: Application
Client Needs: Physiological Integrity
Integrated Concept/Process: Teaching/Learning
Content Area: Adult Health/Renal

Reference:
Clark, J., Queener, S., & Karb, V. (2002). *Pharmacologic basis of nursing practice* (6th ed.). St Louis: Mosby, p. 519.

---

207. A nurse is assisting in caring for a client receiving streptogramin (Synercid) by intravenous intermittent infusion for the treatment of a bone infection. The client develops diarrhea. Which of the following most appropriate nursing actions should the nurse implement?

1   Administer an antidiarrheal agent

2   Notify the RN

3   Stop the infusion

4   Monitor the client's temperature

Answer: 2
Rationale: Streptogramin is an antimicrobial agent. One adverse reaction to the medication is superinfection, including antibiotic-associated colitis, which may result from bacterial imbalance. The medication should be withheld if the client develops diarrhea. The nurse should not stop the infusion but notify the RN, who should then take the necessary actions and contact the physician.

Test-Taking Strategy: Use the process of elimination and knowledge regarding the side effects and nursing interventions related to this medication. From the options presented, the most appropriate is to notify the RN. Review the adverse effects of this medication if you had difficulty with this question.

Level of Cognitive Ability: Application
Client Needs: Physiological Integrity
Integrated Concept/Process: Nursing Process/Implementation
Content Area: Pharmacology

Reference:
Hodgson, B., & Kizior, R. (2003). *Saunders nursing drug handbook 2003.* Philadelphia: W.B. Saunders, p. 960.

---

208. A nurse is reviewing the record of a newborn in the nursery and notes that the physician has documented the presence of a suture split greater than 1 cm. On the basis of this documentation, the nurse expects to monitor for which of the following?

1   Swelling of the soft tissues of the head and scalp

2   Edema resulting from bleeding below the periosteum of the cranium

3   Increased intracranial pressure

4   Craniosynostosis

Answer: 3
Rationale: Normal suture lines may be approximated or overriding. They are also mobile. A split in the sutures as much as 1 cm is considered normal. Overriding suture lines are most often caused by the birthing process and resolve spontaneously. A suture split greater than 1 cm may indicate increased intracranial pressure. Option 1 describes a caput succedaneum. Option 2 describes a cephalhematoma. A hard, rigid, immobile suture line can be associated with premature closure or craniosynostosis and should be investigated further.

Test-Taking Strategy: Use the process of elimination. Focus on the data in the question and recall normal and abnormal newborn findings to answer this question. Review these findings if you had difficulty with this question.

Level of Cognitive Ability: Comprehension
Client Needs: Physiological Integrity
Integrated Concept/Process: Nursing Process/Data Collection
Content Area: Maternity

Reference:
McKinney, E., Ashwill, J., Murray, S., James, S., Gorrie, T., & Droske, S. (2000). *Maternal-child nursing.* Philadelphia: W.B. Saunders, p. 528.

---

209. A nurse is reviewing the laboratory results of an infant suspected of having hypertropic pyloric stenosis. Which of the following does the nurse most likely expect to note in this infant?
1 An elevated blood pH
2 A decreased blood pH
3 An elevated serum potassium
4 An elevated serum chloride

Answer: 1
Rationale: Laboratory findings for an infant with hypertropic pyloric stenosis include metabolic alkalosis caused by vomiting and decreased serum potassium, sodium, and chloride levels. Increased pH and bicarbonate level indicate metabolic alkalosis. Options 2, 3, and 4 are not typically noted in this disorder.

Test-Taking Strategy: Remember that metabolic alkalosis occurs from vomiting. Recalling that progressive projectile nonbilous vomiting occurs in hypertropic pyloric stenosis, the concepts related to acid-base balance, and the clinical manifestations of this disorder directs you to option 1. In metabolic alkalosis, the pH is elevated, as is the bicarbonate level. Option 1 identifies the elevation in pH. Review this disorder if you had difficulty with this question.

Level of Cognitive Ability: Analysis
Client Needs: Physiological Integrity
Integrated Concept/Process: Nursing Process/Data Collection
Content Area: Child Health

Reference:
McKinney, E., Ashwill, J., Murray, S., James, S., Gorrie, T., & Droske, S. (2000). *Maternal-child nursing.* Philadelphia: W.B. Saunders, p. 1140.

---

210. A nurse is preparing to administer an intramuscular (IM) injection to a 10-year-old child in the vastus lateralis muscle. The nurse understands that which of the following indicates the maximum volume of IM medication that can be safely administered into this muscle?
1 0.5 mL
2 1.5 mL
3 2.5 mL
4 3.0 mL

Answer: 2
Rationale: In a child aged 6 to 15 years, the maximum volume of IM medication that can be safely administered into the vastus lateralis muscle is 1.5 mL to 2.0 mL.

Test-Taking Strategy: Note the age of the child. Visualize each of the amounts in the options. Option 1 represents a small amount and options 3 and 4 represent large amounts of medication for IM injection into this muscle. Review IM administration techniques if you had difficulty with this question.

Level of Cognitive Ability: Comprehension
Client Needs: Physiological Integrity
Integrated Concept/Process: Nursing Process/Implementation
Content Area: Child Health

Reference:
Schulte, E., Price, D., & Gwin, J. (2001). *Thompson's pediatric nursing* (8th ed.). Philadelphia: W.B. Saunders, p. 363.

211. A nurse is monitoring a child with a head injury for signs of complications. Which of the following indicates to the nurse that physician notification is necessary?
1   A urine specific gravity of 1.015
2   A urine specific gravity of 1.020
3   A urine specific gravity of 1.030
4   A urine specific gravity of 1.035

Answer: 4
Rationale: Urine for specific gravity is normally 1.005 to 1.030. The nurse should monitor the specific gravity of a child with a head injury or brain tumor or at risk for increased intracranial pressure (ICP) every 4 to 6 hours. The physician should be notified if the urine for specific gravity is above 1.030 or less than 1.005. With increasing ICP, diabetes insipidus or syndrome of inappropriate antidiuretic hormone may occur.

Test-Taking Strategy: Recalling that the urine for specific gravity is normally 1.005 to 1.030 directs you to option 4. This is the only option that represents an abnormal value. Review this value or the care of a child with a head injury if you had difficulty with this question.

Level of Cognitive Ability: Analysis
Client Needs: Physiological Integrity
Integrated Concept/Process: Nursing Process/Data Collection
Content Area: Child Health

Reference:
Schulte, E., Price, D., & Gwin, J. (2001). *Thompson's pediatric nursing* (8th ed.). Philadelphia: W.B. Saunders, p. 355.

212. While collecting data from a client with trigeminal neuralgia, the nurse would expect the client to report which of the following?
1   Paralysis on one side of the face
2   Decreased pain after gentle massage
3   Sharp knifelike pain after brushing the teeth
4   Decreased pain after drinking cold beverages

Answer: 3
Rationale: Clients with trigeminal neuralgia report excruciating, sharp, knifelike facial pain (usually unilateral) after brushing their teeth and with exposure to extremes of hot or cold, touch, and chewing. Paralysis of one side of the face is seen with Bell's palsy. Massage and drinking cold beverages would not decrease the pain of trigeminal neuralgia.

Test-Taking Strategy: Use the process of elimination. The word *neuralgia* in the name of this disorder assists in directing you to the correct option. Review this disorder if you had difficulty with this question.

Level of Cognitive Ability: Comprehension
Client Needs: Physiological Integrity
Integrated Concept/Process: Nursing Process/Data Collection
Content Area: Adult Health/Neurological

Reference:
Lewis, S., Heitkemper, M., & Dirksen, S. (2000). *Medical-surgical nursing: assessment and management of clinical problems* (5th ed.). St. Louis: Mosby, p. 1713.

213. A nurse is caring for a client with a small venous stasis ulcer who has a new order to be out of bed. The nurse plans to

Answer: 4
Rationale: The client should have a reclining chair to allow the legs to be elevated when the client is not resting in bed.

obtain which of the following for use in the client's room to best enhance circulatory status of the affected area?
1   Warm, heavy blankets
2   Overbed trapeze
3   Bedside commode
4   Reclining chair

Positioning the client with the legs elevated allows gravity to drain the extremities while the client is at rest, thereby increasing venous drainage from the affected leg. An overbed trapeze is used for a client who needs assistance in repositioning himself or herself in bed. A bedside commode may be helpful for a client with limited mobility, but it does not increase circulation to the leg. Warm, heavy blankets could put extra weight on the ulcer and actually reduce venous drainage by causing added vasodilatation.

Test-Taking Strategy: Use the process of elimination and note the key words *best enhance circulatory status.* Recalling that the client with a venous problem has impaired venous drainage from the extremity helps you to eliminate each of the options that does not assist with venous drainage through leg elevation. Review care to the client with a venous problem if you had difficulty with this question.

Level of Cognitive Ability: Application
Client Needs: Physiological Integrity
Integrated Concept/Process: Nursing Process/Planning
Content Area: Adult Health/Cardiovascular

Reference:
Lewis, S., Heitkemper, M., & Dirksen, S. (2000). *Medical-surgical nursing: assessment and management of clinical problems* (5th ed.). St. Louis: Mosby, p. 1004.

---

214. A nurse inspects a client's right lower extremity and finds an open area that measures 3 by 4 cm in size. The area has a deep reddish base and is surrounded by skin that is edematous, with a brownish color to it. Pedal pulses are palpable in the right leg. The nurse interprets that the ulcerated area is due to which of the following predisposing conditions?
1   Venous insufficiency
2   Pulmonary embolism
3   Arterial insufficiency
4   Atrial fibrillation

Answer: 1
Rationale: The wound described in the question has the characteristics of a venous stasis ulcer. These ulcers are caused by conditions resulting in chronic venous congestion in the extremities. Examples of such conditions include venous insufficiency (varicose veins) and chronic deep vein thrombosis. Pulmonary embolism is a complication of deep vein thrombosis. Arterial insufficiency is accompanied by pain, and typical findings include pale, cool extremities that have diminished or absent pedal pulses. Atrial fibrillation may cause cardiac thrombi, which could break loose and travel to any area of the body, including the legs. This also would cause an acute onset of the classic symptoms found in clients with arterial insufficiency.

Test-Taking Strategy: To answer this question accurately, you must be able to discriminate among the findings that characterize arterial versus venous disease. Eliminate options 2 and 4 first, because they are not directly related to wound development. Recalling the differences in findings between arterial and venous disorders directs you to option 1 from the remaining options. Review these differences if you had difficulty with this question.

Level of Cognitive Ability: Analysis
Client Needs: Physiological Integrity
Integrated Concept/Process: Nursing Process/Data Collection
Content Area: Adult Health/Cardiovascular

Reference:
Lewis, S., Heitkemper, M., & Dirksen, S. (2000). *Medical-surgical nursing: assessment and management of clinical problems* (5th ed.). St. Louis: Mosby, p. 1004.

215. A client has just been admitted to the hospital with a nonhealing arterial leg ulcer. The nurse inspects the ulcer for which of the following characteristics?
1   Shallow, ruddy, and painless
2   Deep, pale, and painful
3   Deep, ruddy, and painless
4   Shallow, pale, and painful

Answer: 2
Rationale: Arterial ischemic leg ulcers are characteristically deep, pale, and painful. By contrast, venous stasis ulcers are more shallow, with a ruddy color to the ulcer. Venous ulcers are also painful, but less so than arterial ulcers. There is no ulcer that is characteristically painless.

Test-Taking Strategy: Use the process of elimination to answer this question. Eliminate options 1 and 3 first, knowing that ulcers are painful to clients. From the remaining options, select option 2 by recalling that arterial ulcers are deep because they are caused by tissue malnutrition. Review the characteristics of arterial ulcers if you had difficulty with this question.

Level of Cognitive Ability: Comprehension
Client Needs: Physiological Integrity
Integrated Concept/Process: Nursing Process/Data Collection
Content Area: Adult Health/Cardiovascular

Reference:
Lewis, S., Heitkemper, M., & Dirksen, S. (2000). *Medical-surgical nursing: assessment and management of clinical problems* (5th ed.). St. Louis: Mosby, p. 803.

216. A client returned from the postanesthesia care unit 8 hours ago after having a femoral-popliteal bypass graft to the left leg. The client exhibits increasing pallor and coolness in the left foot. Capillary refill time is 5 seconds, with a weakly palpable pedal pulse. The client complains of left leg pain that resembles the pain experienced before surgery. The nurse concludes which of the following about the client?
1   Is in need of immediate pain medication
2   Is experiencing graft occlusion
3   Has developed deep vein thrombosis
4   Has dislodged an embolus from the left atrium

Answer: 2
Rationale: The most frequent indication that a graft is occluding is the return of pain that is similar to that experienced preoperatively. Signs of impaired neurovascular status accompany the occlusion, including pallor, cool temperature, diminished capillary refill, and diminished or absent pedal pulses. If graft occlusion is suspected, the surgeon is notified. The symptoms do not resemble those of deep vein thrombosis. There is no indication that the client has a history of atrial fibrillation, which can result in arterial embolus caused by left atrial thrombus.

Test-Taking Strategy: Use the process of elimination. Eliminate option 1 first because the clinical manifestations indicate that a complication is occurring. Eliminate options 3 and 4 next because the problem is not venous in nature (option 3) and because there is no history of atrial fibrillation (predisposing to an embolus) mentioned in the question. Review the signs of graft occlusion if you had difficulty with this question.

Level of Cognitive Ability: Analysis
Client Needs: Physiological Integrity
Integrated Concept/Process: Nursing Process/Data Collection
Content Area: Adult Health/Cardiovascular

Reference:
Lewis, S., Heitkemper, M., & Dirksen, S. (2000). *Medical-surgical nursing: assessment and management of clinical problems* (5th ed.). St. Louis: Mosby, p. 990.

217. A nurse is assisting in delivering nursing care to an adult male client who has received tissue plasminogen activator

Answer: 4
Rationale: Tissue plasminogen activator is a thrombolytic medication that is used to dissolve thrombi or emboli caused by thrombus.

(t-PA, Activase). The nurse allows which of the following items to be used at the bedside by the client?

1   Dental floss
2   Firm-bristle toothbrush
3   Small nail trimming scissors
4   Electric razor

A frequent and potentially severe side effect of therapy is bleeding. The nurse manipulates the client's environment to reduce the hazard of bleeding associated with the use of sharp items at the bedside. The nurse provides soft Toothettes for mouth care and allows an electric razor for shaving. The nurse does not allow dental floss, a firm-bristle toothbrush, or scissors at the bedside; these items could cause minor trauma that results in bleeding.

Test-Taking Strategy: Use the process of elimination. Recalling that bleeding is a side effect of this therapy and knowing which common items used in personal care could cause bleeding directs you to option 4. Review the characteristics of this medication if you had difficulty with this question.

Level of Cognitive Ability: Application
Client Needs: Physiological Integrity
Integrated Concept/Process: Nursing Process/Implementation
Content Area: Pharmacology

Reference:
Hodgson, B., & Kizior, R. (2003). *Saunders nursing drug handbook 2003.* Philadelphia: W.B. Saunders, p. 35.

---

218. A nurse is assigned to assist in caring for a client who has just had insertion of an inferior vena cava (IVC) filter. In the first 24 hours after the procedure, the nurse plans to monitor the insertion site for which of the following?

1   Infection
2   Bleeding
3   Necrosis
4   Poor wound healing

Answer: 2
Rationale: The care of the client who has had insertion of an IVC filter is similar to that of any surgical client. In the first 24 hours after the procedure, the nurse is most concerned with signs of bleeding. Signs of infection or poor wound healing would not be apparent during this time frame. Option 3 is incorrect.

Test-Taking Strategy: Use the process of elimination. Note that the question contains the key words *monitor* and *first 24 hours.* This tells you that the correct answer is the option that poses the greatest risk to the client immediately after the procedure is completed. This directs you to option 2. Review basic postoperative care if you had difficulty with this question.

Level of Cognitive Ability: Application
Client Needs: Physiological Integrity
Integrated Concept/Process: Nursing Process/Implementation
Content Area: Adult Health/Cardiovascular

Reference:
Lewis, S., Heitkemper, M., & Dirksen, S. (2000). *Medical-surgical nursing: assessment and management of clinical problems* (5th ed.). St. Louis: Mosby, p. 999.

---

219. A client visits a physician's office for a yearly physical examination. The client tells the nurse that there has been a recent onset of sharp leg pain that begins after walking a distance of about 4 blocks and that stops when the client rests. The nurse interprets that the client is describing which of the following symptoms?

Answer: 3
Rationale: Intermittent claudication is the name given to leg pain that occurs with exercise and is relieved by rest. It is the classic symptom of peripheral arterial insufficiency. Rest pain is a sharp pain that occurs when the client is not exercising and indicates a worsening of peripheral arterial disease. Venous insufficiency is characterized by an achy type of leg pain that intensifies as the day progresses. Bone pain is not associated with the data in the question.

1   Bone pain
2   Rest pain
3   Intermittent claudication
4   Pain from venous insufficiency

Test-Taking Strategy: To answer this question correctly, it is necessary to know the common symptoms of peripheral arterial insufficiency. If this question was difficult, review the definition of intermittent claudication.

Level of Cognitive Ability: Comprehension
Client Needs: Physiological Integrity
Integrated Concept/Process: Nursing Process/Data Collection
Content Area: Adult Health/Cardiovascular

Reference:
Black, J., Hawks, J., & Keene, A. (2001). *Medical-surgical nursing: clinical management for positive outcomes* (6th ed.). Philadelphia: W.B. Saunders, p. 1368.

---

220. A client has been diagnosed with deep vein thrombosis (DVT) of the left leg. The nurse evaluates that the client's condition is improving if which of the following outcomes is noted?
1   Skin on the left leg is reddened and warm
2   Calf circumference is ½ inch greater than baseline
3   Homan's sign is positive
4   Edema is resolving

Answer: 4
Rationale: Symptoms of DVT include warm, reddened skin over the affected area, edema of the extremity, enlarged calf circumference, and a positive Homan's sign (pain with dorsiflexion of the foot). Indications that the condition is resolving are a reduction in these signs and symptoms.

Test-Taking Strategy: Use the process of elimination and note the key words "condition is improving." Recalling the signs and symptoms of DVT and focusing on the key words directs you to option 4. Review this disorder if you had difficulty with this question.

Level of Cognitive Ability: Comprehension
Client Needs: Physiological Integrity
Integrated Concept/Process: Nursing Process/Evaluation
Content Area: Adult Health/Cardiovascular

Reference:
Black, J., Hawks, J., & Keene, A. (2001). *Medical-surgical nursing: clinical management for positive outcomes* (6th ed.). Philadelphia: W.B. Saunders, p. 1424.

---

221. A nurse is planning to teach a client with angina pectoris about appropriate use of nitroglycerin sublingual tablets. Which of the following items should the nurse include in the plan?
1   Replace the medication 6 months after opening the bottle
2   Keep the tablets in a shirt pocket
3   Take up to five doses 5 minutes apart if chest pain occurs
4   Stop taking the medication if a headache occurs

Answer: 1
Rationale: Nitroglycerin is relatively unstable, and the medication should be replaced 6 months after the bottle is opened. The tablets should be kept away from heat, light, and moisture. The client may take up to three doses 5 minutes apart. If chest pain is not relieved, the client should seek emergency care. Headache is an expected side effect of the medication and usually diminishes as the client becomes accustomed to the medication.

Test-Taking Strategy: Knowledge of the proper use and storage of nitroglycerin sublingual tablets is needed to answer this question. Review these guidelines if you had difficulty with this question.

Level of Cognitive Ability: Application
Client Needs: Physiological Integrity
Integrated Concept/Process: Teaching/Learning
Content Area: Pharmacology

Reference:
Hodgson, B., & Kizior, R. (2003). *Saunders nursing drug handbook 2003.* Philadelphia: W.B. Saunders, p. 817.

---

222. A client is taking labetalol hydrochloride (Normodyne). The nurse monitors the client for which of the following frequent side effects of the medication?
  1 Tachycardia
  2 Impotence
  3 Increased energy level
  4 Night blindness

Answer: 2
Rationale: Impotence is a common side effect of labetalol and may be distressing to the client. Other side effects of this medication are bradycardia, weakness, and fatigue. Night blindness is unrelated to this medication, although this medication can cause blurred vision and dry eyes.

Test-Taking Strategy: Use the process of elimination. Recall that medications that end with *-lol* are beta-adrenergic blocking agents. Knowledge of the side effects associated with this classification of medications directs you to option 2. Review the side effects of this medication if you had difficulty with this question.

Level of Cognitive Ability: Application
Client Needs: Physiological Integrity
Integrated Concept/Process: Nursing Process/Data Collection
Content Area: Pharmacology

Reference:
Hodgson, B., & Kizior, R. (2003). *Saunders nursing drug handbook 2003.* Philadelphia: W.B. Saunders, p. 637

---

223. A client has a new prescription for nifedipine (Procardia). The nurse reinforces medication instructions and teaches the client which of the following?
  1 Expect urinary retention as a side effect
  2 Cut the dose in half if dizziness or syncope occurs
  3 Monitor own pulse daily
  4 Limit alcohol to 2 ounces per day

Answer: 3
Rationale: Nifedipine is a calcium-channel blocking agent, which can cause bradycardia as a side effect. For this reason, clients taking this medication are taught to monitor the pulse on a daily basis. Urinary frequency is a side effect, but urinary retention is not. Alcohol should not be used at all in the client taking a medication such as nifedipine because it could cause or worsen hypotension. Clients are not instructed to change medication doses on the basis of symptoms.

Test-Taking Strategy: Use the process of elimination. Recall that many of the calcium-channel blocking agents end with the suffix *-dipine.* This may be helpful in trying to remember the classification of this medication. From this point, knowledge of the side effects associated with this classification of medications directs you to option 3. Review this medication if you had difficulty with this question.

Level of Cognitive Ability: Application
Client Needs: Physiological Integrity
Integrated Concept/Process: Teaching/Learning
Content Area: Pharmacology

Reference:
Hodgson, B., & Kizior, R. (2003). *Saunders nursing drug handbook 2003.* Philadelphia: W.B. Saunders, p. 809.

224. The nurse is collecting data on a client taking aminophylline (Phyllocontin). The nurse notes that which of the following symptoms is a common side effect of the medication?
1   Nervousness
2   Urinary retention
3   Bradycardia
4   Diarrhea

Answer: 1
Rationale: Bronchodilators such as aminophylline commonly cause side effects such as nervousness, anxiety, nausea and vomiting, tachycardia, and palpitations. The nurse monitors for these symptoms in clients taking this type of medication. Urinary retention and diarrhea are not side effects of this medication.

Test-Taking Strategy: Focus on the name of the medication and recall that this medication is a bronchodilator. Knowledge of the side effects of this type of medication directs you to option 1. Review the characteristics of this medication if you had difficulty with this question.

Level of Cognitive Ability: Application
Client Needs: Physiological Integrity
Integrated Concept/Process: Nursing Process/Data Collection
Content Area: Pharmacology

Reference:
Hodgson, B., & Kizior, R. (2003). *Saunders nursing drug handbook 2003.* Philadelphia: W.B. Saunders, p. 49.

---

225. A client taking albuterol (Ventolin) experiences a severe episode of wheezing, which the nurse interprets as bronchospasm. A telephone call is made to the physician's office. The nurse tells the client to do which of the following while waiting for the physician to call?
1   Take the next dose as scheduled
2   Withhold the next dose
3   Take a double dose
4   Take half the dose

Answer: 2
Rationale: If bronchospasm occurs, the nurse instructs the client to withhold the medication. The physician is called immediately. This adverse effect is often caused by excessive use of adrenergic bronchodilators.

Test-Taking Strategy: Use the process of elimination. To answer this question correctly, it is necessary to know the expected and untoward effects of adrenergic bronchodilators such as albuterol. Noting the word *bronchospasm* in the question assists in directing you to option 2. Review the adverse effects of this medication if you had difficulty with this question.

Level of Cognitive Ability: Application
Client Needs: Physiological Integrity
Integrated Concept/Process: Nursing Process/Implementation
Content Area: Pharmacology

Reference:
Hodgson, B., & Kizior, R. (2003). *Saunders nursing drug handbook 2003.* Philadelphia: W.B. Saunders, p. 22.

---

226. A client has begun medication therapy with hydrochlorothiazide (Oretic). The nurse interprets that which of the following items reported by the client indicates that the client is experiencing a side effect of the medication?
1   Weight loss of 4 pounds
2   Decreased blood pressure
3   Photosensitivity
4   Hypoglycemia

Answer: 3
Rationale: Hydrochlorothiazide is a thiazide diuretic. It is used to promote fluid loss and reduce BP. These are intended effects of the medication. Photosensitivity and hyperglycemia are side effects. Hypoglycemia is not a side effect of this medication.

Test-Taking Strategy: To answer this question accurately, you must know that this medication is a potassium-wasting diuretic and be familiar with its associated side effects. This knowledge assists in eliminating options 1, 2, and 4. Review the side effects of this medication if you had difficulty with this question.

Level of Cognitive Ability: Comprehension
Client Needs: Physiological Integrity
Integrated Concept/Process: Nursing Process/Data Collection
Content Area: Pharmacology

Reference:
Hodgson, B., & Kizior, R. (2003). *Saunders nursing drug handbook 2003.* Philadelphia: W.B. Saunders, p. 552.

---

227. A nurse is evaluating the status of a client who is taking spironolactone (Aldactone). The nurse evaluates that this medication is not effective if the client demonstrates which of the following?
1 Decreased blood pressure
2 Increased urine output
3 Stable potassium level
4 Increased edema

Answer: 4
Rationale: Spironolactone is a potassium-sparing diuretic used to treat edema, high BP, and hyperaldosteronism. Thus it should decrease BP, increase urine output, maintain stable potassium levels, and decrease edema.

Test-Taking Strategy: Use the process of elimination and note the key words *not effective*. Recalling that this medication is a potassium-sparing diuretic directs you to option 4. Review characteristics of this medication if you had difficulty with this question.

Level of Cognitive Ability: Analysis
Client Needs: Physiological Integrity
Integrated Concept/Process: Nursing Process/Evaluation
Content Area: Pharmacology

Reference:
Hodgson, B., & Kizior, R. (2003). *Saunders nursing drug handbook 2003.* Philadelphia: W.B. Saunders, p. 1028.

---

228. An LPN says to the RN, "I think my client's closed chest drainage system has some kind of leak in it." The LPN bases this interpretation on which of the following observations of the closed chest drainage system?
1 Continuous bubbling in the water seal chamber
2 Intermittent bubbling in the water seal chamber
3 Continuous bubbling in the suction control chamber
4 Intermittent bubbling in the suction control chamber

Answer: 1
Rationale: Continuous bubbling in the water seal chamber through both inspiration and expiration indicates that there is an air leak in the system. A resolving pneumothorax indicates intermittent bubbling with respiration in the water seal chamber. Continuous bubbling in the suction control chamber indicates that suction is attached to the system and is working as expected. There cannot be intermittent bubbling in the suction control chamber; either the suction is turned on (bubbling) or off (no bubbling).

Test-Taking Strategy: To answer this question accurately, you must be familiar with closed chest drainage systems and indications of proper and improper function. Remember, continuous bubbling through both inspiration and expiration in the water seal chamber indicates that there is air leaking into the system. Review chest tube drainage systems if you had difficulty with this question.

Level of Cognitive Ability: Analysis
Client Needs: Physiological Integrity
Integrated Concept/Process: Nursing Process/Data Collection
Content Area: Adult Health/Respiratory

Reference:
Black, J., Hawks, J., & Keene, A. (2001). *Medical-surgical nursing: clinical management for positive outcomes* (6th ed.). Philadelphia: W.B. Saunders, p. 1732.

---

229. An LPN is asked by the RN to obtain the supplies necessary to initiate an IV line for a client who will receive peripheral fat infusions. Which of the following devices should the LPN select for initiation of the IV?

1   A 14-gauge needle
2   A 19-gauge needle
3   A 23-gauge needle
4   A 25-gauge needle

Answer: 2

Rationale: For peripheral fat infusions, a 19-gauge needle is used. A 14-, 16-, 18-, or 19-gauge needle is used for the administration of blood products. A 22- or 23-gauge needle is used for standard IV solutions. A 25-gauge needle is most often used to administer subcutaneous injections.

Test-Taking Strategy: Remember that the smaller the gauge number, the larger the needle. When answering questions similar to this one, specifically note the type of solution to be infused. It seems reasonable that an adequate-sized needle is necessary for administering a fat solution. Options 3 and 4 can be eliminated first because the needles described in these options are too small. Similarly, eliminate option 1, recalling that a 14-gauge needle is extremely large and is used primarily for blood products or for rapid emergency fluid administration. Review these concepts if you had difficulty with this question.

Level of Cognitive Ability: Application
Client Needs: Physiological Integrity
Integrated Concept/Process: Nursing Process/Implementation
Content Area: Fundamental Skills

Reference:
Perry, A., & Potter, P., (2002). *Clinical nursing skills & techniques* (5th ed.). St. Louis: Mosby, p. 696.

---

230. A nurse is caring for an elderly client receiving an IV infusion who is at risk for IV infiltration. The nurse inspects the IV site and plans care knowing that which of the following will not prevent the infiltration from occurring?

1   Use of an arm board
2   Anchoring the venipuncture cannula
3   Looping of the IV tubing
4   An IV placed in the antecubital area

Answer: 4

Rationale: Elderly clients are at an increased risk for infiltration because they have fragile veins. Preventive measures include avoiding venipuncture over an area of flexion, anchoring the venipuncture cannula, and looping the tubing securely. Use of an arm board or a splint is especially helpful for an active or restless person.

Test-Taking Strategy: Use the process of elimination. Note the key word *not* in the question. Visualize each of the options to identify the one that would not assist in preventing an infiltration. Noting the word *antecubital* in option 4 should direct you to this option. Review preventive measures related to infiltration if you had difficulty with this question.

Level of Cognitive Ability: Comprehension
Client Needs: Physiological Integrity
Integrated Concept/Process: Nursing Process/Planning
Content Area: Fundamental Skills

Reference:
Ignatavicius, D., & Workman, M. (2002). *Medical-surgical nursing: critical thinking for collaborative care* (4th ed.). Philadelphia: W.B. Saunders, p. 205.

231. A nurse is collecting data on a client with the diagnosis of Brown-Séquard syndrome. Which of the following findings does the nurse expect to note?

1 Loss of touch and vibration
2 Bilateral loss of pain and temperature sensation
3 Contralateral paralysis and loss of touch and vibration
4 Complete paraplegia or quadriplegia, depending on the level of injury

Answer: 1

Rationale: Brown-Séquard syndrome results from hemisection of the spinal cord, resulting in ipsilateral paralysis and loss of touch, pressure, vibration, and proprioception. Contralaterally, sensations of pain and temperature are lost because the fibers associated with them decussate after entering the cord.

Test-Taking Strategy: Knowledge of Brown-Séquard syndrome is necessary to answer this question correctly. If you are unfamiliar with this syndrome, review the findings and the nursing care.

Level of Cognitive Ability: Analysis
Client Needs: Physiological Integrity
Integrated Concept/Process: Nursing Process/Data Collection
Content Area: Adult Health/Neurological

Reference:
Black, J., Hawks, J., & Keene, A. (2001). *Medical-surgical nursing: clinical management for positive outcomes* (6th ed.). Philadelphia: W.B. Saunders, p. 2051.

232. A nurse is collecting data about a client who has a suspected spinal cord injury. Which of the following is the priority?

1 Pupillary response
2 Respiratory status
3 Mobility
4 Pain

Answer: 2

Rationale: All of the items in the options would be assessed with a suspected spinal cord injury client; however, respiratory status is the priority.

Test-Taking Strategy: Use the ABCs (airway, breathing, and circulation) to answer this question. Option 2 addresses airway. Review care to the client with a spinal cord injury if you had difficulty with this question.

Level of Cognitive Ability: Application
Client Needs: Physiological Integrity
Integrated Concept/Process: Nursing Process/Data Collection
Content Area: Adult Health/Neurological

Reference:
Black, J., Hawks, J., & Keene, A. (2001). *Medical-surgical nursing: clinical management for positive outcomes* (6th ed.). Philadelphia: W.B. Saunders, p. 2053.

233. A nurse is caring for a client who has recently been diagnosed with a spinal cord injury. The nurse reviews the client's record and anticipates that the most likely medication to be prescribed will be which of the following?

1 Propranolol (Inderal)
2 Methylprednisolone (Solu-Medrol)
3 Mannitol (Osmitrol)
4 Morphine sulfate

Answer: 2

Rationale: The most likely medication to be ordered for a recently diagnosed spinal cord injury is methylprednisolone. This medication is a glucocorticoid and is given to reduce traumatic edema. The use of propranolol, a beta-blocker; mannitol, an osmotic diuretic; or morphine sulfate, an opioid analgesic is not indicated based on the information in this question.

Test-Taking Strategy: Use the process of elimination. Note the words *recently been diagnosed* and the diagnosis *spinal cord injury*. Knowledge regarding the association between injury and edema assists you in answering the question. Review the medications or the treatment for spinal cord injury if you had difficulty with this question.

Level of Cognitive Ability: Analysis
Client Needs: Physiological Integrity
Integrated Concept/Process: Nursing Process/Planning
Content Area: Adult Health/Neurological

Reference:
Lewis, S., Heitkemper, M., & Dirksen, S. (2004). *Medical-surgical nursing: assessment and management of clinical problems* (6th ed.). St. Louis: Mosby, p. 1617.

---

234. A nurse is caring for a client with a diagnosis of acquired immunodeficiency syndrome (AIDS). The nurse plans care knowing that it is important to monitor for which of the following findings?
  1 Jaundiced skin
  2 White patches in the oral cavity
  3 Bradypnea
  4 Urine specific gravity of 1.010

Answer: 2
Rationale: Clients with AIDS frequently have opportunistic infections. *Candida albicans*, the causative organism of thrush, is a common opportunistic infection. Thrush presents as white patches in the oral cavity. Hairy leukoplakia also presents as white patches in the oral cavity. Jaundice is a symptom of hepatic disease. Clients with AIDS frequently develop pneumonia and thus may present with tachypnea not bradypnea. Clients with AIDS frequently have inadequate nutrition and hydration and thus may present with dehydration resulting in a high rather than low specific gravity.

Test-Taking Strategy: A knowledge of the pathophysiology of AIDS is important to answer this question correctly. If you understand the pathophysiology, you can eliminate options 1 and 4 because these are not associated with the disease. Clients with AIDS do have respiratory problems; however, the problem is an increased rather than decreased respiratory rate. Review the manifestations associated with AIDS if you had difficulty with this question.

Level of Cognitive Ability: Application
Client Needs: Physiological Integrity
Integrated Concept/Process: Nursing Process/Planning
Content Area: Fundamental Skills

Reference:
Black, J., Hawks, J., & Keene, A. (2001). *Medical-surgical nursing: clinical management for positive outcomes* (6th ed.). Philadelphia: W.B. Saunders, p. 2203.

---

235. A nurse is caring for a client who has been involved in a motor vehicle accident. The nurse monitors the client closely, knowing that the need to prepare for chest tube insertion will be necessary when the client exhibits which of the following symptoms?
  1 Shortness of breath and tracheal deviation
  2 Chest pain and shortness of breath
  3 Decreasing oxygen saturation on pulse oximetry and bradypnea
  4 Peripheral cyanosis and hypotension

Answer: 1
Rationale: Shortness of breath and tracheal deviation result when lung tissue and alveoli have collapsed. The trachea deviates to the unaffected side in the presence of a tension pneumothorax. Air entering the pleural cavity causes the lung to lose its normal negative pressure. The increasing pressure in the affected side displaces contents to the unaffected side. Shortness of breath results from decreased area available for diffusion of gases. Chest pain and shortness of breath are more commonly associated with myocardial ischemia or infarction. Clients requiring chest tubes exhibit decreasing oxygen saturation but will more likely experience tachypnea related to the hypoxia. Peripheral cyanosis is caused by circulatory disorders. Hypotension may be a result of tracheal shift and impedance of venous return to the heart. It also may be the result of other problems, such as a failing heart.

Test-Taking Strategy: Use the process of elimination. The clue that directs you to the correct option is shortness of breath and tracheal deviation. Tracheal deviation is a manifestation that indicates a tension pneumothorax, which is treated with closed chest drainage. Review the signs associated with tension pneumothorax, and the conditions that require closed chest drainage if you had difficulty with this question.

Level of Cognitive Ability: Analysis
Client Needs: Physiological Integrity
Integrated Concept/Process: Nursing Process/Data Collection
Content Area: Adult Health/Respiratory

Reference:
Black, J., Hawks, J., & Keene, A. (2001). *Medical-surgical nursing: clinical management for positive outcomes* (6th ed.). Philadelphia: W.B. Saunders, p. 1768.

---

236. A client has a serum sodium level of 129 mEq/L because of hypervolemia. The nurse reviews the physician's orders to determine whether which of the following most appropriate measures are prescribed?
1 Restrict intake to 2 grams of sodium per day
2 Restrict intake to 4 grams of sodium per day
3 Restrict fluids
4 Administer IV hypertonic saline

Answer: 3
Rationale: Hyponatremia is defined as a serum sodium level of less than 135 mEq/L. When it is caused by hypervolemia, it may be treated with fluid restriction. The low serum sodium level is caused by hemodilution. IV hypertonic saline is reserved for hyponatremia when the serum sodium level is lower than 125 mEq/L. A 4-gram sodium diet is a no-added-salt diet; a 2-gram sodium restriction would not raise the serum sodium level.

Test-Taking Strategy: Use the process of elimination. To answer this question accurately, you must know that the serum sodium level is low. With this in mind, you can eliminate option 1. Knowing that hypervolemia causes hemodilution of the serum sodium guides you to choose option 3 instead of options 2 and 4. Review treatment measures for hyponatremia if you had difficulty with this question.

Level of Cognitive Ability: Analysis
Client Needs: Physiological Integrity
Integrated Concept/Process: Nursing Process/Planning
Content Area: Fundamental Skills

Reference:
Black, J., Hawks, J., & Keene, A. (2001). *Medical-surgical nursing: clinical management for positive outcomes* (6th ed.). Philadelphia: W.B. Saunders, p. 227.

---

237. A nurse is preparing to apply a pulse oximeter to a client. To ensure accurate monitoring of the client's oxygenation status, the nurse implements which of the following?
1 Notifies the physician immediately of an oxygen saturation of less than 92%
2 Instructs the client not to move the sensor
3 Tapes the sensor to the client's finger

Answer: 2
Rationale: The pulse oximeter passes a beam of light through the tissue, and a sensor attached to the fingertip, toe, or earlobe measures the amount of light absorbed by the oxygen-saturated hemoglobin. The oximeter then gives a reading of the percentage of hemoglobin that is saturated with oxygen (SaO_2). Motion at the sensor site changes light absorption. The motion mimics the pulsatile motion of blood, and results can be inaccurate because the detector cannot distinguish between movement of blood and movement of the finger. The sensor should not be placed distal to BP cuffs, pressure dressings, arterial lines, or any invasive

4   Places the sensor on a finger below the blood pressure cuff

catheters. The sensor should not be taped to the client's finger because vasoconstriction may reduce arterial blood flow to the sensor. If values fall below preset norms (usually 90%) the client should be instructed to breathe deeply, if this is appropriate.

Test-Taking Strategy: Use the process of elimination. The issue of the question is *to ensure accurate monitoring.* Eliminate option 1 because although reporting low oxygen saturations to the physician is important, it is unrelated to ensuring accurate monitoring. Option 4 is unreasonable, so eliminate it also. When considering the remaining options, recalling that motion at the sensor site changes light absorption helps you select the correct option. Review the principles associated with pulse oximetry if you had difficulty with this question.

Level of Cognitive Ability: Application
Client Needs: Physiological Integrity
Integrated Concept/Process: Nursing Process/Implementation
Content Area: Adult Health/Respiratory

Reference:
Potter, A., & Perry, P. (2002). *Clinical nursing skills & techniques* (5th ed.). St. Louis: Mosby, pp. 250-253.

---

238. A nurse is working in a renal unit in a local hospital. The nurse interprets that which of the following clients in the unit is best suited for peritoneal dialysis as a treatment option?
1   A client with severe congestive heart failure
2   A client with a history of ruptured diverticuli
3   A client with a history of herniated lumbar disk
4   A client with a history of three previous abdominal surgeries

Answer: 1
Rationale: Peritoneal dialysis may be the treatment option of choice for clients with severe cardiovascular disease, which is worsened by the rapid shifts in fluid, electrolytes, urea, and glucose that occur with hemodialysis. For the same reason, peritoneal dialysis may be indicated for clients with diabetes mellitus. Relative contraindications to peritoneal dialysis include diseases of the abdomen, such as ruptured diverticuli or malignancies, extensive abdominal surgeries, history of peritonitis, obesity, and history of back problems, which could be aggravated by the fluid weight of the dialysate. Severe disease of the vascular system also may be a relative contraindication.

Test-Taking Strategy: Use the process of elimination. Note that the question asks you which of the clients presented is the best candidate for peritoneal dialysis. This implies that you must understand the advantages and disadvantages of peritoneal dialysis and use priority setting to eliminate each of the incorrect options. Therefore, options 2 and 4 can be eliminated easily. Knowledge of concepts related to fluid weight and fluid shifts in the body is needed to select between options 1 and 3. Review the indications for peritoneal dialysis if you had difficulty with this question.

Level of Cognitive Ability: Analysis
Client Needs: Physiological Integrity
Integrated Concept/Process: Nursing Process/Data Collection
Content Area: Adult Health/Renal

Reference:
Black, J., Hawks, J., & Keene, A. (2001). *Medical-surgical nursing: clinical management for positive outcomes* (6th ed.). Philadelphia: W.B. Saunders, p. 889.

239. A client undergoing long-term peritoneal dialysis is currently experiencing a problem with reduced outflow from the dialysis catheter. The nurse collecting data from the client most appropriately inquires whether the client has had a recent problem with which of the following?
  1 Vomiting
  2 Diarrhea
  3 Constipation
  4 Flatulence

Answer: 3
Rationale: Reduced outflow may be caused by catheter position and adherence to the omentum, infection, or constipation. Constipation may contribute to reduced outflow in part because peristalsis seems to aid in drainage. For this reason, bisacodyl suppositories sometimes are used prophylactically, even without a history of constipation. The other options are unrelated to impaired catheter drainage.

Test-Taking Strategy: Use the process of elimination. To discriminate among the options, evaluate them in terms of their effect on gut motility, which affects catheter outflow. Each of the incorrect options involves hypermotility of the gastrointestinal tract, which should facilitate outflow. Only the correct option, constipation, is related to decreased gut motility, which could impair fluid drainage. Review the factors that can cause reduced outflow if you had difficulty with this question.

Level of Cognitive Ability: Analysis
Client Needs: Physiological Integrity
Integrated Concept/Process: Nursing Process/Data Collection
Content Area: Adult Health/Renal

Reference:
Black, J., Hawks, J., & Keene, A. (2001). *Medical-surgical nursing: clinical management for positive outcomes* (6th ed.). Philadelphia: W.B. Saunders, p. 891.

240. A nurse is told that a client with a history of heart failure who is undergoing peritoneal dialysis has developed crackles in the lower lung fields. The nurse interprets that this finding is most likely related to which of the following?
  1 Compliance with dietary sodium restriction
  2 Adherence to digoxin (Lanoxin) therapy schedule
  3 Natural progression of the renal failure
  4 Intake greater than output on the dialysis record

Answer: 4
Rationale: Crackles in the lung fields of the peritoneal dialysis client result from overhydration or insufficient fluid removal during dialysis. An intake that is greater than the output of peritoneal dialysis fluid overhydrate the client, resulting in lung crackles. Adherence to medication and diet therapy should control this sign, not make it worse. If dialysis is effective, there is no connection between the progression of renal failure and the development of signs of overhydration.

Test-Taking Strategy: Use the process of elimination. Begin to answer this question by eliminating options 1 and 2. These options are incorrect because adherence to standard therapy should control the signs of heart failure, not make them worse. From the remaining options, knowing that crackles are caused by excess fluid in the body directs you to option 4. Review care to the client with peritoneal dialysis if you had difficulty with this question.

Level of Cognitive Ability: Analysis
Client Needs: Physiological Integrity
Integrated Concept/Process: Nursing Process/Data Collection
Content Area: Adult Health/Renal

Reference:
Black, J., Hawks, J., & Keene, A. (2001). *Medical-surgical nursing: clinical management for positive outcomes* (6th ed.). Philadelphia: W.B. Saunders, p. 891.

241. A nurse is teaching a client who is taking medications by inhalation about the advantages of a newly prescribed spacer. Which statement by the client identifies a need for further teaching?
1   "It reduces the frequency of medication to only once per day."
2   "It reduces the chance of yeast infection because large drops aren't deposited on mouth tissues."
3   "Medication is dispersed more deeply and uniformly."
4   "The need to coordinate timing between pressing the inhaler and inspiration is reduced."

Answer: 1

Rationale: There are key advantages to the use of a spacer for medications administered by inhalation. One is that it reduces the incidence of yeast infections, because large medication droplets are not deposited on oral tissues. The medication also is dispensed more deeply and uniformly than without a spacer. There is less need to coordinate the effort of inhalation with pressing on the canister of the inhaler. Finally, the use of a spacer may decrease either the number or volume of the puffs taken. Option 1 is too absolute and limiting by description.

Test-Taking Strategy: Use the process of elimination and note the key words *need for further teaching*. Note the use of the word *only* in option 1. The use of absolute words such as *only* in an option is likely to make that option incorrect. Review the principles related to the use of a spacer if you had difficulty with this question.

Level of Cognitive Ability: Comprehension
Client Needs: Physiological Integrity
Integrated Concept/Process: Teaching/Learning
Content Area: Adult Health/Respiratory

Reference:
Black, J., Hawks, J., & Keene, A. (2001). *Medical-surgical nursing: clinical management for positive outcomes* (6th ed.). Philadelphia: W.B. Saunders, p. 1696.

242. A nurse is caring for a client with a tentative diagnosis of pulmonary emphysema. The nurse monitors the client for which of the following signs that distinguishes emphysema from chronic bronchitis?
1   Copious sputum production
2   Marked dyspnea
3   Minimal weight loss
4   Cough that began before the onset of dyspnea

Answer: 2

Rationale: Key features of pulmonary emphysema include dyspnea that is often marked, late cough (after onset of dyspnea), scant mucus production, and marked weight loss. By contrast, chronic bronchitis is characterized by early onset of cough (before dyspnea), copious purulent mucus production, minimal weight loss, and milder severity of dyspnea.

Test-Taking Strategy: To answer this question accurately, you must understand the differences between these two respiratory disorders and their associated manifestations. Review the manifestations of emphysema if you had difficulty with this question.

Level of Cognitive Ability: Analysis
Client Needs: Physiological Integrity
Integrated Concept/Process: Nursing Process/Data Collection
Content Area: Adult Health/Respiratory

Reference:
Black, J., Hawks, J., & Keene, A. (2001). *Medical-surgical nursing: clinical management for positive outcomes* (6th ed.). Philadelphia: W.B. Saunders, p. 1692.

243. A client is diagnosed with vitamin K deficiency. The nurse should collect data from the client about which of the following that results from this deficiency?
1   Night blindness
2   Clotting problems

Answer: 2

Rationale: Vitamin K is associated with the production of prothrombin, which helps the blood properly clot. Vitamin A deficiency is associated with night blindness. Vitamin B_2 (riboflavin) deficiency is associated with scaly skin. Vitamin D deficiency is associated with skeletal pain.

3   Scaly skin
4   Skeletal pain

Test-Taking Strategy: Use the process of elimination. Recalling that vitamin K is associated with the production of prothrombin directs you to option 2. Review these vitamin deficiencies if you had difficulty with this question.

Level of Cognitive Ability: Comprehension
Client Needs: Physiological Integrity
Integrated Concept/Process: Nursing Process/Data Collection
Content Area: Fundamental Skills

Reference:
Williams, S. (2001). *Basic nutrition and diet therapy* (11th ed.). St. Louis: Mosby, p. 81.

---

244. A client has been diagnosed with goiter. The nurse would most likely note which of the following documented in the client's record?
1   Decreased wound healing
2   Chronic fatigue
3   Enlarged thyroid gland
4   Heart damage

Answer: 3
Rationale: Goiter is an enlargement of the thyroid gland. Enlargement occurs in an attempt to compensate for hormone deficiency. Decreased wound healing, chronic fatigue, and heart damage are not specifically associated with goiter.

Test-Taking Strategy: Consider the anatomical location of goiter. This easily directs you to option 3. Review this disorder if you had difficulty with this question.

Level of Cognitive Ability: Comprehension
Client Needs: Physiological Integrity
Integrated Concept/Process: Nursing Process/Data Collection
Content Area: Adult Health/Endocrine

Reference:
Black, J., Hawks, J., & Keene, A. (2001). *Medical-surgical nursing: clinical management for positive outcomes* (6th ed.). Philadelphia: W.B. Saunders, pp. 1089-1090.

---

245. During a wellness fair, a client admits to a nurse about not eating a well-balanced diet. According to the Food Guide Pyramid, which of the following statements is correct for the nurse to say?
1   "Your diet should consist of 6 to 11 servings of bread, cereal, pasta, and rice a day."
2   "Your diet should consist of 2 to 4 four servings of vegetables a day."
3   "Your diet should consist of 4 to 5 servings of milk, yogurt, and cheese a day."
4   "Your diet should consist of 4 to 6 servings of meat, poultry, fish, dry beans, and nuts a day."

Answer: 1
Rationale: The Food Guide Pyramid is a guide for healthy clients to get the proper amounts of nutrition. Carbohydrates should comprise 55% to 58% of a nutritious diet for a healthy client. Six to eleven servings of the bread, cereal, pasta, and rice is the correct amount. The correct serving for vegetables is 3 to 5. The correct servings of milk, yogurt, and cheese is 2 to 3. The correct serving of meat, poultry, fish, dry beans, and nuts is 2 to 3.

Test-Taking Strategy: Knowledge of the Food Guide Pyramid is necessary to answer this question. If you are unfamiliar with this nutrition guide, review this content.

Level of Cognitive Ability: Application
Client Needs: Physiological Integrity
Integrated Concept/Process: Teaching/Learning
Content Area: Fundamental Skills

Reference:
Potter, P., & Perry, A. (2001). *Fundamentals of nursing* (5th ed.). St. Louis: Mosby, p. 1336.

246. An 85-year-old client is hospitalized with a right fractured hip, and surgery is performed. The client refuses to get out of bed in the postoperative period. Which of the following statements is most appropriate for the nurse to make to the client?
1   "It is important for you to get out of bed so that calcium will go back into the bone."
2   "It is necessary to increase your calcium intake because you are spending too much time in bed."
3   "It is necessary to give you iodine to help in hemoglobin synthesis."
4   "You should remember to turn yourself in bed to keep from getting so stiff."

Answer: 1
Rationale: If a client does not increase activity, the bones will suffer from loss of calcium. Increasing calcium intake only leads to elevated amounts in the blood, which could cause kidney stones. Iron, not iodine, is recommended for hemoglobin synthesis because oxygen is necessary for wound healing. A client who is postoperative and is 85-years-old should be turned every two hours by the nursing staff.

Test-Taking Strategy: Focus on the issue and use the process of elimination. Recalling the effects of immobility assists in directing you to option 1. Review these effects if you had difficulty with this question.

Level of Cognitive Ability: Application
Client Needs: Physiological Integrity
Integrated Concept/Process: Nursing Process/Implementation
Content Area: Fundamental Skills

Reference:
Potter, P., & Perry, A. (2001). *Fundamentals of nursing* (5th ed.). St. Louis: Mosby, p. 1493.

---

247. A client is admitted to the hospital with a diagnosis of malnutrition. The client does not understand the results of the various prescribed laboratory tests. Which of the following statements to the client is accurate?
1   "Elevated creatinine levels indicate respiratory problems."
2   "Normal hemoglobin levels indicate that iron and protein intake is sufficient."
3   "Elevated albumin levels indicate dehydration."
4   "Normal red blood cell levels indicate adequate vitamin B_6 intake."

Answer: 2
Rationale: Normal hemoglobin levels indicate that iron and protein intake is sufficient. Elevated creatinine levels indicate kidney problems. Elevated albumin levels do not necessarily indicate dehydration. Normal red blood cell levels indicate adequate vitamin B_{12} intake.

Test-Taking Strategy: Use the process of elimination. Focus on the issue and seek the option that indicates an accurate statement. If you had difficulty with this question, review these blood tests and those that indicate malnutrition.

Level of Cognitive Ability: Comprehension
Client Needs: Physiological Integrity
Integrated Concept/Process: Nursing Process/Implementation
Content Area: Fundamental Skills

Reference:
Potter, P., & Perry, A. (2001). *Fundamentals of nursing* (5th ed.). St. Louis: Mosby, p. 1151.

---

248. A client has returned to the nursing unit after a gastroscopy procedure. Which of the following is an appropriate postprocedural nursing action?
1   Place the client in a supine position to provide comfort
2   Monitor the client's vital signs every hour for four hours
3   Provide saline gargles to aid in comfort as soon as the client returns

Answer: 4
Rationale: Before the procedure, medication is given to prevent a gag reflex. Upon return from the procedure, the nurse must check for the return of the gag reflex to prevent aspiration. After the procedure, the client must be placed in a side-lying or semi-Fowler's position to prevent aspiration. Vital signs should be taken every 30 minutes for 2 hours to detect abnormalities. Saline gargles must only be administered when the presence of the gag reflex has been confirmed.

4 Check the gag reflex by stroking the back of the client's throat

Test-Taking Strategy: Use the process of elimination and read each option carefully. Recall the importance of determining the presence of a gag reflex in the postprocedural period. Review postprocedural care after gastroscopy if you had difficulty with this question.

Level of Cognitive Ability: Application
Client Needs: Physiological Integrity
Integrated Concept/Process: Nursing Process/Implementation
Content Area: Adult Health/Gastrointestinal

Reference:
Black, J., Hawks, J., & Keene, A. (2001). *Medical-surgical nursing: clinical management for positive outcomes* (6th ed.). Philadelphia: W.B. Saunders, p. 658.

---

249. A client is on a regular diet and is a strict vegetarian. Which of the following food items on the diet menu will the client be willing to eat?
1 Chocolate milk shake
2 Buttered wheat toast
3 Stir-fried vegetables
4 Scrambled eggs

Answer: 3
Rationale: Stir-fried vegetables are allowed on a strict vegetarian diet. Milk shakes, butter, and eggs are dairy products and not eaten by a strict vegetarian.

Test-Taking Strategy: Use the process of elimination and note that options 1, 2, and 4 are similar in that they are all dairy products. Review this diet if you had difficulty with this question.

Level of Cognitive Ability: Comprehension
Client Needs: Physiological Integrity
Integrated Concept/Process: Nursing Process/Data Collection
Content Area: Fundamental Skills

Reference:
Potter, P., & Perry, A. (2001). *Fundamentals of nursing* (5th ed.). St. Louis: Mosby, p. 1344.

---

250. An elderly client has been complaining about suffering from heartburn. Which of the following statements about lessening the symptoms should the nurse provide to the client?
1 "After 20 to 30 minutes of eating, lie down to help the food digest."
2 "Eat a high-protein, low-fat diet on a daily basis."
3 "Drink at least three fruit juices a day as a main beverage."
4 "Try to eat more after you feel full to keep the stomach at full capacity."

Answer: 2
Rationale: A high-protein, low-fat diet is recommended for a client with heartburn. This type of diet allows the stomach valve to close and prevents gastric secretions from upsetting the stomach. At least 2 hours should pass before the client lies down to allow enough time for the stomach acid to decrease. Fruit juices should be avoided because their high level of acidity aggravates symptoms. Clients should not be encouraged to overeat, which increases acid production and causes stomach pressure.

Test-Taking Strategy: Note the key words *lessening the symptoms*. Use the process of elimination and knowledge about the factors that cause heartburn. Review these factors if you had difficulty with this question.

Level of Cognitive Ability: Application
Client Needs: Physiological Integrity
Integrated Concept/Process: Nursing Process/Implementation
Content Area: Fundamental Skills

Reference:
Potter, P., & Perry, A. (2001). *Fundamentals of nursing* (5th ed.). St. Louis: Mosby, p. 1374.

---

251. A nurse administers an antiemetic to a client who has vomited. Three hours later, the client tells the nurse that he or she is hungry and would like something to eat. Which of the following food items is best for the nurse to give the client?

1 Chicken broth
2 Buttered toast
3 Hot tea
4 Apple juice

Answer: 4

Rationale: Room temperature or cold foods are better tolerated by the client with episodes of nausea and vomiting. Hot items may increase the nausea because of the aromas emitted. Dry toast would be better tolerated by the client.

Test-Taking Strategy: Use the process of elimination. Eliminate options 1 and 3 because they are similar in that both are hot items. From the remaining options, recall that clear liquids are best tolerated after episodes of vomiting. Review care to the client with nausea and vomiting if you had difficulty with this question.

Level of Cognitive Ability: Application
Client Needs: Physiological Integrity
Integrated Concept/Process: Nursing Process/Implementation
Content Area: Fundamental Skills

Reference:
Potter, P., & Perry, A. (2001). *Fundamentals of nursing* (5th ed.). St. Louis: Mosby, p. 1709.

---

252. A nurse is caring for a client with a diagnosis of malnutrition. Which of the following is the most effective measure to monitor the client's status?

1 Intake and output
2 Skinfold measurements
3 Daily weights
4 Calorie count

Answer: 3

Rationale: Daily weights are the most accurate way to monitor the client's progress. It is important to weigh the client at the same time each day, have the same amount of clothes on, urinate beforehand, and use the same scale. It also is recommended that the client be weighed before breakfast. Options 1, 2, and 4 provide data about nutrition but are not the most effective measures.

Test-Taking Strategy: Focus on the client's diagnosis and the issue of the question. Recall that the client's weight most accurately provides data about the client's nutritional status. Review nutritional data collection measures if you had difficulty with this question.

Level of Cognitive Ability: Comprehension
Client Needs: Physiological Integrity
Integrated Concept/Process: Nursing Process/Data Collection
Content Area: Fundamental Skills

Reference:
Potter, P., & Perry, A. (2001). *Fundamentals of nursing* (5th ed.). St. Louis: Mosby, p. 1348.

---

253. A nurse plans to apply a moisturizer to an elderly client's dry skin. For maximum effectiveness, the nurse chooses which of the following?

1 A petrolatum-based ointment
2 An oil-based cream

Answer: 1

Rationale: Petrolatum provides the most effective moisturizing by forming an occlusive barrier on the skin and reducing water loss. Creams and lotions are mostly water-based, less occlusive, and less likely to reduce skin dryness than petrolatum-based products. Bath oils are not the most effective moisturizer.

3   A lotion moisturizer
4   An oil for the bath water

Test-Taking Strategy: Although all are products used for dry skin, note the key words, *maximum effectiveness*. Knowledge of skin preparation ingredients and how they work is necessary to answer this question correctly. Review these products if you had difficulty with this question.

Level of Cognitive Ability: Application
Client Needs: Physiological Integrity
Integrated Concept/Process: Nursing Process/Implementation
Content Area: Fundamental Skills

Reference:
Black, J., Hawks, J., & Keene, A. (2001). *Medical-surgical nursing: clinical management for positive outcomes* (6th ed.). Philadelphia: W.B. Saunders, p. 1283.

---

254. A nurse auscultates bowel sounds in a client and identifies an early sign of intestinal obstruction when which of the following is heard?
1   Absent bowel sounds
2   High-pitched tinkling sounds
3   Diminished sounds
4   Resonance

Answer: 2
Rationale: High-pitched tinkling sounds indicate an intestinal obstruction. Absent or diminished sounds may signify a paralytic ileus or later signs of an obstruction. Resonance is not a finding in auscultation.

Test-Taking Strategy: Use the process of elimination. Note key word *auscultates*. Eliminate option 4 because it does not deal with auscultation. Next eliminate options 1 and 3 (absent and diminished) because they are similar. Review findings in an intestinal obstruction if you had difficulty with this question.

Level of Cognitive Ability: Comprehension
Client Needs: Physiological Integrity
Integrated Concept/Process: Nursing Process/Data Collection
Content Area: Adult Health/Gastrointestinal

Reference:
Ignatavicius, D., & Workman, M. (2002). *Medical-surgical nursing: critical thinking for collaborative care* (4th ed.). Philadelphia: W.B. Saunders, p. 1256.

---

255. A nurse in a long-term care facility documents an apical pulse of 82 beats per minute (BPM), strong and irregular. The nurse notes that prior baseline data indicate that the client's apical pulse ranged from 60 to 90 BPM, strong and regular. The client complains of "feeling tired lately." A priority nursing action is which of the following?
1   Notify the client's physician
2   Place the client on bed rest
3   Schedule the client for a cardiac stress test
4   Initiate a fluid restriction of 1000 mL per 24 hours

Answer: 1
Rationale: Any change in the quality or character of the heart beat should be reported to the physician because this occurrence could be an indication of developing cardiac problems related to atherosclerosis, medications, or disease. With the data available, there is no need for bed rest or a fluid restriction. A physician's order must be obtained before scheduling the client for a stress test.

Test-Taking Strategy: Use the process of elimination. Note the key word *priority*. Options 2, 3, and 4 require a physician's order. Review the nursing interventions when a change of cardiac status occurs if you had difficulty with this question.

Level of Cognitive Ability: Application
Client Needs: Physiological Integrity
Integrated Concept/Process: Nursing Process/Implementation
Content Area: Fundamental Skills

Reference:

Black, J., Hawks, J., & Keene, A. (2001). *Medical-surgical nursing: clinical management for positive outcomes* (6th ed.). Philadelphia: W.B. Saunders, pp. 1451-1452.

---

256. A client with congestive heart failure has been receiving furosemide (Lasix) 40 mg PO, BID. The nurse understands that which of the following would not be an indicator of effective diuretic therapy?
1   Pitting pedal edema
2   A weight loss of 3 pounds in 24 hours
3   Clear lung sounds bilaterally
4   Decreased exertional dyspnea

Answer: 1
Rationale: Pitting pedal edema is a sign of excess fluid volume. Options 2, 3, and 4, are all signs of decreased edema, which is an indication that diuretic therapy has been effective in excreting excess fluid.

Test-Taking Strategy: Note the key word *not*. Use the process of elimination and select the option that would indicate the presence of edema. Review characteristics of this medication if you had difficulty with this question.

Level of Cognitive Ability: Analysis
Client Needs: Physiological Integrity
Integrated Concept/Process: Nursing Process/Evaluation
Content Area: Pharmacology

Reference:

Hodgson, B., & Kizior, R. (2003). *Saunders nursing drug handbook 2003.* Philadelphia: W.B. Saunders, p. 501.

---

257. A nurse is caring for an elderly client who has been prescribed bed rest and is concerned about the prevention of pneumonia. To detect early signs of pneumonia, the nurse monitors for which of the following?
1   Copious amounts of blood-tinged sputum
2   Diminished respiratory rate
3   A rectal temperature of 99° F and above
4   Poor skin turgor

Answer: 3
Rationale: The elderly may not present with the usual signs and symptoms of illness. Because of their lower than normal body temperature, an early sign of pneumonia would be a temperature of 99° F rectally. Blood-tinged sputum is usually a sign of congestive heart failure. In later stages of pneumonia, the respiratory rate increases in an attempt to compensate for poor oxygen exchange. Poor skin turgor is a sign of dehydration.

Test-Taking Strategy: Note the key word *early*. Focus on the issue, pneumonia, and use the process of elimination. Noting that the client is elderly directs you to option 3. Review the signs of pneumonia if you had difficulty with this question.

Level of Cognitive Ability: Application
Client Needs: Physiological Integrity
Integrated Concept/Process: Nursing Process/Implementation
Content Area: Adult Health/Respiratory

Reference:

Ebersole, P., & Hess, P. (2001). *Geriatric nursing & healthy aging.* St. Louis: Mosby, p. 431.

---

258. A client is receiving phenobarbital orally for treatment of a seizure disorder. The nurse monitors for which common side effect that can occur with the administration of this medication?
1   Drowsiness
2   Blurred vision

Answer: 1
Rationale: Drowsiness is a common side effect of phenobarbital. Blurred vision is not an associated side effect of this medication. Seizure activity could occur from abrupt withdrawal of medication therapy, or as a toxic reaction. Hypocalcemia is a rare toxic reaction.

3 Seizure activity
4 Hypocalcemia

Test-Taking Strategy: Note the key words *common side effect.* Use the process of elimination and knowledge regarding this medication to direct you to option 1. Review this medication if you are unfamiliar with it.

Level of Cognitive Ability: Application
Client Needs: Physiological Integrity
Integrated Concept/Process: Nursing Process/Implementation
Content Area: Pharmacology

Reference:
Hodgson, B., & Kizior, R. (2003). *Saunders nursing drug handbook 2003.* Philadelphia: W.B. Saunders, p. 883.

---

259. Many older clients experience changes in their activity and rest cycles. The nurse correctly identifies that an elderly client is having a sleep pattern disturbance when which of the following is noted on data collection?
1 Somnambulism
2 Apraxia
3 Nocturia
4 Verbal complaints of difficulty falling asleep

Answer: 4
Rationale: Somnambulism (sleepwalking), apraxia (inability to perform purposeful movements), and nocturia (excessive night-time urination) are not indicators of a disturbed sleep pattern.

Test-Taking Strategy: Focus on the issue *sleep pattern disturbance.* Note the relationship between this issue and option 4 to answer the question. Review these age-related changes if you had difficulty with this question.

Level of Cognitive Ability: Comprehension
Client Needs: Physiological Integrity
Integrated Concept/Process: Nursing Process/Data Collection
Content Area: Fundamental Skills

Reference:
Johnson, M., Bulechek, G., Dochterman, J. Maas, M., & Moorhead, S. (2001). *Nursing diagnoses, outcomes, and interventions.* St. Louis: Mosby, p. 309.

---

260. A nurse encourages an elderly client to perform deep breathing and coughing exercises. The nurse understands that which of the following normal age-related changes places the elderly at higher risk for respiratory infections?
1 Alveolar walls are destroyed
2 Lung tissue becomes less elastic and less rigid
3 Alveolar membrane thins
4 Reduced ciliary movement creates ineffective cough

Answer: 4
Rationale: Destruction of alveolar walls is a characteristic of chronic obstructive pulmonary disease, not a normal age-related change found in the elderly. As aging occurs, lung tissue becomes less elastic and more rigid (not less rigid), alveolar membranes thicken (not thin), and ciliary movement is reduced.

Test-Taking Strategy: Note the key words *normal age-related changes.* Read each option carefully and use knowledge of the aging process to answer the question. Review age-related changes if you had difficulty with this question.

Level of Cognitive Ability: Comprehension
Client Needs: Physiological Integrity
Integrated Concept/Process: Nursing Process/Implementation
Content Area: Fundamental Skills

Reference:
Ebersole, P., & Hess, P. (2001). *Geriatric nursing & healthy aging.* St. Louis: Mosby, p. 94.

261. A nurse is caring for an older client with the diagnosis of dehydration. The client also has diabetes mellitus. The client is alert but disoriented, pale, and slightly diaphoretic and the nurse suspects that the client is hypoglycemic. The most appropriate initial nursing intervention is to:

1 Administer oral glucose
2 Assist the client to bed, put the side rails up, and call the physician
3 Seat the client at the nurse's desk while checking the physician's orders
4 Obtain a fingerstick blood sample and test the glucose level

Answer: 4

Rationale: The nurse should confirm that the client is hypoglycemic by checking the blood glucose. Option 1 is incorrect because the hypoglycemia has not been determined. More information should be gathered before calling the physician; therefore, option 2 is incorrect. Option 3 does not meet the client's immediate needs.

Test-Taking Strategy: Note key word *suspects*. Focus on the information in the question to direct you to option 4. Review the nursing actions if hypoglycemia is suspected if you had difficulty with this question.

Level of Cognitive Ability: Application
Client Needs: Physiological Integrity
Integrated Concept/Process: Nursing Process/Implementation
Content Area: Adult Health/Endocrine

Reference:
Ebersole, P. , & Hess, P. (2001). *Geriatric nursing & healthy aging.* St. Louis: Mosby, pp. 183; 398.

---

262. A physician has ordered Regular insulin, 10 units, with NPH insulin 20 units subcutaneously, every morning. The nurse should:

1 Administer both Regular insulin and NPH insulin at 10 AM
2 Shake the NPH insulin vial to distribute the suspension
3 Draw up the Regular insulin first, then the NPH insulin in the same syringe
4 Draw up the NPH insulin first, then the Regular insulin in the same syringe

Answer: 3

Rationale: Regular insulin is always drawn up before the NPH insulin. Insulin is usually administered 15 to 30 minutes before a meal. To mix the NPH insulin suspension, the vial should be gently rotated. Shaking introduces air bubbles into the solution.

Test-Taking Strategy: Use the process of elimination. Remember "R" then "N" when drawing up both types of insulin in the same syringe. Review the technique for administering insulin if you had difficulty with this question.

Level of Cognitive Ability: Application
Client Needs: Physiological Integrity
Integrated Concept/Process: Nursing Process/Implementation
Content Area: Pharmacology

Reference:
Hodgson, B., & Kizior, R. (2003). *Saunders nursing drug handbook 2003.* Philadelphia: W.B. Saunders, p. 591.

---

263. A nurse is assigned to care for a client with a history of coronary artery disease (CAD). The nurse reviews the client's health record knowing that which of the following data documented in the record is related to CAD?

1 Hyperlipidemia
2 Edema
3 Decreased urinary output
4 Increased urinary output

Answer: 1

Rationale: CAD occurs because of accumulation of fatty plaque in the coronary arteries or as a result of arteriosclerotic changes. Elevated serum cholesterol and triglyceride levels (hyperlipidemia) play a major role in the development of CAD. Edema may be present if the client has congestive heart failure but edema and changes in urinary output are not significant contributors to the development of CAD.

Test-Taking Strategy: Use the process of elimination, recalling that hyperlipidemia is associated with CAD. Review these risk factors if you had difficulty with this question.

Level of Cognitive Ability: Comprehension
Client Needs: Physiological Integrity
Integrated Concept/Process: Nursing Process/Data Collection
Content Area: Fundamental Skills

Reference:

Black, J., Hawks, J., & Keene, A. (2001). *Medical-surgical nursing: clinical management for positive outcomes* (6th ed.). Philadelphia: W.B. Saunders, p. 1579.

---

264. A nurse is assigned to care for a client with a diagnosis of coronary artery disease (CAD). The nurse plans care knowing that:

1 Activity and stress improve coronary blood flow
2 Activity and stress are not related to coronary blood flow
3 Chest pain experienced only during exercise indicates necrosis
4 Chest pain experienced only during exercise indicates ischemia

Answer: 4

Rationale: CAD may go unrecognized for a period of time in persons with a sedentary lifestyle because adequate blood flow to the myocardium may be maintained despite the CAD. However, during times of emotional stress, increased physical activity, or both, the diseased coronary arteries may not be able to supply the myocardium with adequate blood. The inadequate perfusion of the myocardium, referred to as ischemia, causes pain yet no damage to the heart muscle occurs. Necrosis is a result of prolonged oxygen deprivation to the myocardium and tissue death (myocardial infarction).

Test-Taking Strategy: Use the process of elimination and knowledge about CAD to answer the question. Focusing on the issue, CAD, directs you to option 4. Review this content if you had difficulty with this question.

Level of Cognitive Ability: Application
Client Needs: Physiological Integrity
Integrated Concept/Process: Nursing Process/Planning
Content Area: Adult Health/Cardiovascular

Reference:

Black, J., Hawks, J., & Keene, A. (2001). *Medical-surgical nursing: clinical management for positive outcomes* (6th ed.). Philadelphia: W.B. Saunders, p. 1448.

---

265. A nurse is caring for a client diagnosed with coronary artery disease (CAD). Which of the following statements made by the client indicates the need for teaching?

1 "I can have someone from the office bring over my unfinished work so I can complete it as long as I do not get out of bed."
2 "I should conserve my energy and avoid stress."
3 "My diet should be low in salt and fat."
4 "I must keep these prongs in my nose to get the extra oxygen the doctor has prescribed."

Answer: 1

Rationale: Reducing the demands on the heart by encouraging rest and relaxation is important for the hospitalized client with CAD. Oxygen therapy frequently is ordered for cardiac clients to provide supplemental oxygen. A diet low in salt and fat is also prescribed.

Test-Taking Strategy: Note the key words *need for teaching*. Recalling that the goal of care for this client is to reduce the demands placed on the heart directs you to option 1. Review care of the client with CAD if you had difficulty with this question.

Level of Cognitive Ability: Comprehension
Client Needs: Physiological Integrity
Integrated Concept/Process: Nursing Process/Evaluation
Content Area: Adult Health/Cardiovascular

Reference:

Black, J., Hawks, J., & Keene, A. (2001). *Medical-surgical nursing: clinical management for positive outcomes* (6th ed.). Philadelphia: W.B. Saunders, p. 1582.

266. A nurse is assigned to care for a client with coronary artery disease (CAD) who is scheduled for a cardiac catheterization. After the catheterization, the priority nursing action is to monitor the:
1   Catheter insertion site
2   Temperature
3   Potassium level
4   Urine output

Answer: 1
Rationale: During the postcardiac catheterization period, priorities of nursing care include frequent monitoring of the blood pressure and pulse. The catheter insertion site is checked frequently for signs of bleeding and swelling. Distal pulses are also assessed. Potassium level, temperature, and urine output also should be monitored but are not the priority of the items identified in the options.

Test-Taking Strategy: Note the key word *priority*. Note the relationship between *catheterization* in the question and *catheter* in the correct option. Review postcardiac catheterization care if you had difficulty with this question.

Level of Cognitive Ability: Application
Client Needs: Physiological Integrity
Integrated Concept/Process: Nursing Process/Implementation
Content Area: Adult Health/Cardiovascular

Reference:
Black, J., Hawks, J., & Keene, A. (2001). *Medical-surgical nursing: clinical management for positive outcomes* (6th ed.). Philadelphia: W.B. Saunders, p. 198.

267. A client has a diagnosis of coronary artery disease. Blood samples are obtained to evaluate the client's serum cholesterol levels. Which of the following results should the nurse consider most desirable?
1   Elevated total lipoprotein levels
2   Decreased total lipoprotein levels
3   Increased low-density lipoproteins (LDL) and decreased high-density lipoproteins (HDL)
4   Decreased LDL and increased HDL

Answer: 4
Rationale: HDLs are considered to be the "good" cholesterol and LDLs are the "bad" cholesterol. LDLs come mainly from animal fats.

Test-Taking Strategy: Note the key words *most desirable*. Remember that LDL is "bad" and HDL is "good" to assist in answering questions similar to this one. Review these laboratory tests and their significance if you had difficulty with this question.

Level of Cognitive Ability: Analysis
Client Needs: Physiological Integrity
Integrated Concept/Process: Nursing Process/Evaluation
Content Area: Fundamental Skills

Reference:
Black, J., Hawks, J., & Keene, A. (2001). *Medical-surgical nursing: clinical management for positive outcomes* (6th ed.). Philadelphia: W.B. Saunders, p. 1517.

268. A pregnant client asks the nurse why tetracycline cannot be prescribed for her acne. The nurse responds by telling the client that the medication:
1   May cause premature labor
2   Is more likely to produce an allergic reaction
3   May cause deafness in the fetus
4   May darken the teeth and disrupt bone growth in the fetus

Answer: 4
Rationale: Tetracyclines are deposited in the teeth and bones of the fetus. These medications can cause permanent tooth enamel discoloration and can depress bone growth. This medication does not induce labor. Option 2 is incorrect because the allergic potential of any medication does not increase in pregnancy. Option 3 is incorrect.

Test-Taking Strategy: Knowledge about the effects of tetracycline on the fetus is necessary to answer this question. If you had difficulty with this question, review this medication classification.

Level of Cognitive Ability: Comprehension
Client Needs: Physiological Integrity

Integrated Concept/Process: Nursing Process/Implementation
Content Area: Pharmacology

Reference:
Hodgson, B., & Kizior, R. (2003). *Saunders nursing drug handbook 2003.* Philadelphia: W.B. Saunders, p. 1070.

---

269. A nurse is caring for a geriatric client who is receiving triazolam (Halcion). The nurse monitors the client closely knowing that this medication can cause:
1   Urinary retention
2   Impaired mobility
3   Constipation
4   Blood clots

Answer: 2
Rationale: Medications are metabolized and excreted more slowly in geriatric clients; therefore the risk of adverse effects is increased. Triazolam can cause confusion and dizziness leading to impaired mobility. Options 1, 3, and 4 are incorrect.

Test-Taking Strategy: Recalling that geriatric clients are more likely to experience adverse side effects of any medication directs you to option 2. Remember that safety is a priority concern with the elderly client. Review the adverse effects of this medication if you had difficulty with this question.

Level of Cognitive Ability: Application
Client Needs: Physiological Integrity
Integrated Concept/Process: Nursing Process/Implementation
Content Area: Pharmacology

Reference:
Hodgson, B., & Kizior, R. (2003). *Saunders nursing drug handbook 2003.* Philadelphia: W.B. Saunders, p. 1127.

---

270. When administering both cimetidine (Tagamet) and sucralfate (Carafate) to a client, the nurse should plan to give these medications:
1   At the same time
2   Only when the client complains of pain
3   2 hours apart
4   15 minutes apart

Answer: 3
Rationale: Because sucralfate forms a protective barrier at the stomach mucosal surface, it can prevent other medications from being absorbed. Sucralfate should be given 2 hours before or after other medications.

Test-Taking Strategy: Use the process of elimination. Recalling the action of sucralfate directs you to option 3. If you are unfamiliar with this medication, review this content.

Level of Cognitive Ability: Application
Client Needs: Physiological Integrity
Integrated Concept/Process: Nursing Process/Planning
Content Area: Pharmacology

Reference:
Hodgson, B., & Kizior, R. (2003). *Saunders nursing drug handbook 2003.* Philadelphia: W.B. Saunders, pp. 241, 1038.

---

271. A nurse is caring for a client receiving furosemide (Lasix). To evaluate the effectiveness of diuretic therapy, the nurse would monitor the:
1   Pulse
2   Potassium level

Answer: 3
Rationale: All diuretic medications result in an increased urinary output, thus reducing body weight. The pulse may be affected because of decreased circulating volume, but this is not an expected outcome of diuretic therapy. Potassium levels are monitored with some diuretics but this is for the purpose

3   Weight
4   Level of consciousness

of monitoring side effects not effective therapy. Option 4 is incorrect.

Test-Taking Strategy: Note the key word *effectiveness.* Knowledge about the effects of diuretic therapy easily directs you to the correct option. Review this classification of medications if you had difficulty with this question.

Level of Cognitive Ability: Analysis
Client Needs: Physiological Integrity
Integrated Concept/Process: Nursing Process/Evaluation
Content Area: Pharmacology

Reference:
Hodgson, B., & Kizior, R. (2003). *Saunders nursing drug handbook 2003.* Philadelphia: W.B. Saunders, p. 499.

---

272. A nurse is caring for a client who is taking warfarin sodium (Coumadin). To evaluate the effectiveness of therapy, the nurse monitors:
1   Daily weight
2   Blood pressure
3   Urinary output
4   Prothrombin time (PT) levels

Answer: 4
Rationale: Warfarin sodium is an anticoagulant that is given to maintain a PT of 1.5 times the normal level. Therefore, checking blood coagulation tests is an effective measure to determine effectiveness. Options 1, 2, and 3 are not affected by warfarin therapy.

Test-Taking Strategy: Knowledge about the purpose of warfarin sodium (Coumadin) is necessary to answer this question. Use this knowledge and the process of elimination to assist in directing you to option 4. Review this medication if you had difficulty with this question.

Level of Cognitive Ability: Analysis
Client Needs: Physiological Integrity
Integrated Concept/Process: Nursing Process/Evaluation
Content Area: Pharmacology

Reference:
Hodgson, B., & Kizior, R. (2003). *Saunders nursing drug handbook 2003.* Philadelphia: W.B. Saunders, p. 1170.

---

273. A nurse is caring for a client who is taking digoxin (Lanoxin). Before administering the medication, the nurse checks the client's:
1   Blood pressure
2   Temperature
3   Respiratory rate
4   Apical pulse rate

Answer: 4
Rationale: One of the adverse effects of digoxin is slowing of the pulse rate, which occurs because of a decreased conduction at the atrioventricular node. Therefore the nurse checks the client's apical pulse rate. Additionally, if the pulse is lower than 60 beats per minute, the medication is held and the physician is notified. Options 1, 2, and 3 are usually not affected by digoxin.

Test-Taking Strategy: Knowledge about the action and the effects of digoxin will assist in directing you to option 4. If you had difficulty with this question, review the nursing interventions related to this medication.

Level of Cognitive Ability: Application
Client Needs: Physiological Integrity

Integrated Concept/Process: Nursing Process/Implementation
Content Area: Pharmacology

Reference:
Hodgson, B., & Kizior, R. (2003). *Saunders nursing drug handbook 2003.* Philadelphia: W.B. Saunders, p. 349.

---

274. Chlorpromazine (Thorazine) has been prescribed for a client. The client returns to the physician's office for a follow-up examination and complains of restlessness and agitation. The nurse observes the client and collects additional data, knowing that which of the following signs may indicate a potentially serious complication related to this medication?
1   Blood pressure is slightly elevated
2   Weight has gone up one pound
3   The client is picking at skin sores
4   The client's lips smack repetitively

Answer: 4
Rationale: The most serious side effect of the phenothiazine antipsychotics is tardive dyskinesia. Early signs of this condition are lip sucking and smacking behaviors, tongue protrusion, facial grimacing, and choreiform movements. Options 1, 2, and 3 are not indicative of a complication related to this medication.

Test-Taking Strategy: Knowledge about the complications associated with the administration of chlorpromazine is necessary to answer this question. If you are unfamiliar with this medication and its adverse reactions, review this content.

Level of Cognitive Ability: Analysis
Client Needs: Physiological Integrity
Integrated Concept/Process: Nursing Process/Data Collection
Content Area: Pharmacology

Reference:
Hodgson, B., & Kizior, R. (2003). *Saunders nursing drug handbook 2003.* Philadelphia: W.B. Saunders, p. 232.

---

275. A school-aged child has history of upper respiratory infection accompanied by a sore throat. The physician explains to the LPN that the modified Jones criteria are being used to diagnose rheumatic fever. The nurse understands that the physician is looking for:
1   Evidence of streptococcal infection and the presence of two major manifestations or one major and two minor manifestations of rheumatic fever
2   A significant decrease in the child's sedimentation rate
3   An elevation in antistreptolysin-O antibodies
4   Emotional instability, purposeless movement, and muscular weakness

Answer: 1
Rationale: A high probability of rheumatic fever is indicated when there is evidence of at least two of the major or one major and two minor manifestations of the Jones criteria and evidence of a streptococcal infection. The sedimentation rate normally is increased in rheumatic fever. An elevation in antistreptolysin-O antibodies indicates a recent streptococcal infection, but does not alone diagnose rheumatic fever. Option 4 identifies clinical manifestations of chorea, which is one major manifestation. However, these alone are not enough to diagnose rheumatic fever according to the modified Jones criteria.

Test-Taking Strategy: Knowledge about the Jones criteria is necessary to answer this question. Note the relationship between rheumatic fever in the question and in the correct option. Review these criteria if you had difficulty with this question.

Level of Cognitive Ability: Analysis
Client Needs: Physiological Integrity
Integrated Concept/Process: Nursing Process/Data Collection
Content Area: Child Health

Reference:
Wong, D., & Hockenberry-Eaton, M. (2001). *Wong's essentials of pediatric nursing* (6th ed.). St. Louis: Mosby, p. 966.

276. A school-aged child sustains a fracture along the epiphyseal line of the femur after a fall from the garage roof. The nurse plans care knowing that a potential long-term effect of this type of injury likely is:
1 Osteomyelitis
2 Muscle atrophy
3 Paresthesias, paralysis, or both
4 Growth disturbance

Answer: 4
Rationale: Growth takes place at the epiphysis of the long bone. A fracture at this level can destroy the layer of germinal cells of the epiphysis resulting in growth disturbance. Osteomyelitis is an infection of the bone and is more likely to occur with a compound fracture rather than an epiphyseal fracture. Muscle atrophy may result from immobility or casting, but resolves as activity increases. Paresthesias and paralysis can result from edema and constriction of a cast, not specifically from fracture of the epiphysis.

Test-Taking Strategy: Note the key words *long-term effect*. Use the process of elimination. Focusing on the issue, epiphyseal line, directs you to option 4. Review the complications associated with a fractured femur if you had difficulty with this question.

Level of Cognitive Ability: Comprehension
Client Needs: Physiological Integrity
Integrated Concept/Process: Nursing Process/Planning
Content Area: Child Health

Reference:
Wong, D., & Hockenberry-Eaton, M. (2001). *Wong's essentials of pediatric nursing* (6th ed.). St. Louis: Mosby, p. 1211.

---

277. A nurse is reinforcing instructions to an 8-year-old child about measures to take to identify the early signs of an asthma episode. The nurse instructs the child to first:
1 Use a peak flow meter to measure for a drop in the expiratory flow rate
2 Deliver a dose of a bronchodilator by a metered-dose inhaler to see if it helps
3 Open the airway passages by using a hand-held nebulizer treatment
4 Perform chest percussion and postural drainage immediately

Answer: 1
Rationale: An asthmatic child over the age of 4 should be able to measure the expiratory flow. A drop in expiratory flow is the most reliable early sign of an asthma episode. Medications would be administered by a metered-dose inhaler or hand-held nebulizer if an asthma attack actually occurs. Chest percussion and postural drainage normally are used to clear air passages for children with cystic fibrosis, not asthma.

Test-Taking Strategy: Note the issue of the question and the key word *first*. The issue relates to identifying the presence of an asthma attack. Focusing on this issue easily directs you to option 1. Review child instructions about asthma if you had difficulty with this question.

Level of Cognitive Ability: Application
Client Needs: Physiological Integrity
Integrated Concept/Process: Self-Care
Content Area: Child Health

Reference:
McKinney, E., Ashwill, J., Murray, S. et al. (2000). *Maternal-child nursing.* Philadelphia: W.B. Saunders, p. 1229.

---

278. A nurse is caring for a client with a diagnosis of terminal cancer. In planning for the administration of a narcotic pain reliever, the nurse understands that:
1 Around-the-clock dosing gives better pain relief than PRN dosing

Answer: 1
Rationale: Administering around-the-clock dosing provides increased pain relief and decreases stressors associated with pain, such as anxiety and fear. Narcotic analgesics may be addictive but this is not the concern in a client with terminal cancer. Not all narcotic analgesics cause tachycardia. Although

2 Narcotic analgesics are highly addictive

3 Narcotic analgesics can cause tachycardia

4 Not all pain is real

option 4 may be accurate, this is not the concern in this situation.

Test-Taking Strategy: Use the process of elimination, knowledge about the effects of narcotic analgesics, and the client's diagnosis to answer the question. Review pain management and the administration of narcotic analgesics if you had difficulty with this question.

Level of Cognitive Ability: Comprehension
Client Needs: Physiological Integrity
Integrated Concept/Process: Caring
Content Area: Pharmacology

Reference:
Lehne, R. (2001). *Pharmacology for nursing care* (4th ed.). Philadelphia: W.B. Saunders, p. 270.

---

279. A pediatrician is evaluating a school-aged child after the teacher reports that the child is not paying attention during class. The teacher reports that the child appears to be daydreaming and staring off into space 40 or 50 times during the day, and that the child is alert and participates in classroom activity for the remainder of the day. The nurse assisting the pediatrician expects that the pediatrician will note which of the following on physical examination?

1 The child has attention deficit hyperactivity disorder (ADHD) and needs medication

2 The child has school phobia and the source of the problem should be determined

3 The child is probably experiencing absence seizures and will need to have an electroencephalography (EEG) to confirm this diagnosis

4 The child is a behavioral problem, and a referral to a special class may be necessary if things do not improve

Answer: 3
Rationale: Numerous, frequent episodes of a child staring off into space and then quickly returning to conversation or activities is a classic sign of absence seizures that can be confirmed by an EEG. Classic symptoms of ADHD include easy distraction, fidgeting, and problems following directions. School phobia includes physical symptoms that usually occur at home and may prevent the child from attending school. Severe behavior problems that necessitate special class placement have much more overt behavior than that described in the question.

Test-Taking Strategy: Focus on the description provided in the question and use knowledge about the symptoms associated with absence seizures to assist in directing you to option 3. If you had difficulty with this question, review the indicators of these types of seizures.

Level of Cognitive Ability: Analysis
Client Needs: Physiological Integrity
Integrated Concept/Process: Nursing Process/Data Collection
Content Area: Child Health

Reference:
Wong, D., & Hockenberry-Eaton, M. (2001). *Wong's essentials of pediatric nursing* (6th ed.). St. Louis: Mosby, p. 1099.

---

280. An adolescent female is admitted to the hospital for severe weight loss. During data collection the nurse notes that the client is suffering from a disturbed body image, amenorrhea, and appears to be depressed. A primary goal is to improve the client's nutritional status. Which of the following nursing actions will the nurse implement first?

Answer: 3
Rationale: Until the client begins to take adequate nutrition and is physiologically stable, the nurse cannot work with the client on other levels. Options 1, 2, and 4 are appropriate interventions that should be instituted once nutrition status has improved.

Test-Taking Strategy: Note the key word *first*. Use Maslow's Hierarchy of Needs theory, remembering that physiological needs are the priority. This easily directs you to option 3. Also note that option 3 is the only option that relates to data collection, the first

1 Establish a behavioral contract with the client in which she agrees to adhere to diet and a realistic exercise program

2 Weigh the client daily in the client's gown and without shoes, observing for any hidden objects that could alter weight

3 Observe the client during and after meals to be sure proper foods are eaten and that the client does not discard food after apparently consuming it

4 Involve the client and parents in family group sessions to work through psychological problems related to anorexia

step of the nursing process. Review interventions for the client with anorexia if you had difficulty with this question.

Level of Cognitive Ability: Application
Client Needs: Physiological Integrity
Integrated Concept/Process: Nursing Process/Implementation
Content Area: Child Health

Reference:
Wong, D., & Hockenberry-Eaton, M. (2001). *Wong's essentials of pediatric nursing* (6th ed.). St. Louis: Mosby, p. 562.

---

281. A client is placed on a magnesium-containing antacid. The nurse reviews the client's health record and determines that which of the following preexisting conditions require cautious use of this antacid?

1 Angina
2 Diabetes mellitus
3 Hypertension
4 Renal failure

Answer: 4

Rationale: The administration of magnesium-containing antacids can cause increased magnesium levels in the client with renal failure. Options 1, 2, and 3 identify disorders whose pathophysiology is not affected by magnesium.

Test-Taking Strategy: Knowledge about the contraindications associated with the use of magnesium-containing antacids is necessary to answer this question. Review these contraindications if you had difficulty with this question.

Level of Cognitive Ability: Analysis
Client Needs: Physiological Integrity
Integrated Concept/Process: Nursing Process/Data Collection
Content Area: Pharmacology

Reference:
Hodgson, B., & Kizior, R. (2003). *Saunders nursing drug handbook 2003.* Philadelphia: W.B. Saunders, p. 690.

---

282. A nurse is reviewing the health record of a client who is taking a daily dose of digoxin (Lanoxin). Which of the following would place the client at risk for toxicity if noted in the health record?

1 Hyperthyroidism, hyperthermia
2 Peptic ulcer disease
3 Hypothyroidism, loop diuretic use
4 Muscle spasms, ibuprofen (Motrin) use

Answer: 3

Rationale: Digitalis glycosides must be used cautiously in clients taking a loop diuretic because electrolyte imbalances such as hypokalemia can occur, increasing the risk of toxicity. The risk for toxicity also can occur in clients with an impaired ability to metabolize medication, such as occurs in hypothyroidism. Options 1, 2, and 4 are not associated with the risk for toxicity.

Test-Taking Strategy: Knowledge about the factors that increase the risk for digoxin toxicity is necessary to answer this question. Review this medication if you had difficulty with this question.

Level of Cognitive Ability: Analysis
Client Needs: Physiological Integrity

Integrated Concept/Process: Nursing Process/Data Collection
Content Area: Pharmacology

Reference:
Hodgson, B., & Kizior, R. (2003). *Saunders nursing drug handbook 2003.* Philadelphia: W.B. Saunders, p. 351.

---

283. A 5-year-old male child has a deficiency in factor VIII. An important goal is to relieve pain caused by bleeding into the joints. Which interventions does the nurse expect will be prescribed to achieve this goal?
1 Nonsteroidal antiinflammatory drugs (NSAIDs)
2 Joint immobilization
3 Hot packs to the affected joints
4 Physical therapy to help the child through the acute period

Answer: 2
Rationale: Joint immobilization assists in preventing bleeding and pain. NSAIDs can prolong bleeding time and increase the bleeding and pain caused by pressure of the confined fluid in the narrow joint space. Heat application increases blood flow to the area and promotes bleeding. Physical therapy can be helpful after the bleeding episode is under control, but therapy can increase bleeding during the acute period.

Test-Taking Strategy: Focus on the issue, to relieve pain caused by bleeding into the joints. Use principles related to the effects of heat and cold to eliminate option 3. Eliminate option 4 because of the word *acute* in this option. Recalling that NSAIDs present the risk of bleeding assists in directing you to option 2. Review these measures if you had difficulty with this question.

Level of Cognitive Ability: Comprehension
Client Needs: Physiological Integrity
Integrated Concept/Process: Nursing Process/Planning
Content Area: Child Health

Reference:
Wong, D., & Hockenberry-Eaton, M. (2001). *Wong's essentials of pediatric nursing* (6th ed.). St. Louis: Mosby, p. 998.

---

284. A 3-year-old child is admitted to the hospital with a diagnosis of acute lymphocytic leukemia (ALL). The nurse assigned to care for the child is concerned because the child is crying and stating, "My knees hurt." Which of the following interventions does the nurse plan for the child?
1 Administer 2.5 grains of aspirin
2 Apply cold packs to the knees
3 Apply heat to the knees
4 Attempt to involve the child in diversional activities so he or she will forget the discomfort

Answer: 2
Rationale: Bleeding into joints is a clinical manifestation of acute lymphocytic leukemia (ALL), and cold applications decrease joint discomfort. Aspirin has anticoagulant properties and should not be prescribed. Heat application will causes more blood circulation, which increases the pain and bleeding if present. Diversional activities do not relieve the pain.

Test-Taking Strategy: Focus on the child's diagnosis and use the process of elimination. Recalling that the associated risk of bleeding exists assists in eliminating options 1 and 3. From the remaining options, option 2 is the one that addresses the child's physiological need. Review care to the child with ALL if you had difficulty with this question.

Level of Cognitive Ability: Application
Client Needs: Physiological Integrity
Integrated Concept/Process: Nursing Process/Implementation
Content Area: Child Health

Reference:
Wong, D., & Hockenberry-Eaton, M. (2001). *Wong's essentials of pediatric nursing* (6th ed.). St. Louis: Mosby, p. 1011.

285. A 30-month-old male child is brought to the urgent care clinic. The mother is concerned because the child is difficult to awaken, complains of a "tummy ache," and is irritable. Of the following questions, which one does the nurse expect the physician to ask the mother if lead poisoning is suspected?
   1   "Has your child been breathing rapidly and sweating profusely?"
   2   "Does your child's breath have a sweet, fruity odor?"
   3   "Do you live in a house more than 25 years old or very close to a freeway?"
   4   "Does you child chew on pencils or crayons while drawing?"

Answer: 3
Rationale: Homes that are older than 25 years may have lead paint and will most likely have lead pipes. Living close to high traffic areas also can contribute to lead poisoning, which may result from breathing exhaust. Hyperventilation and diaphoresis are signs of salicylate not lead poisoning. A fruity breath odor is a symptom of ketoacidosis. Pencil lead is made of graphite so it does not present a hazard. Crayons are not toxic.

Test-Taking Strategy: Knowledge about the contributing factors of lead poisoning is necessary to answer this question. Noting the words *house more than 25 years old* directs you to option 3. If you are unfamiliar with these factors, review this content

Level of Cognitive Ability: Analysis
Client Needs: Physiological Integrity
Integrated Concept/Process: Nursing Process/Data Collection
Content Area: Child Health

Reference:
Wong, D., & Hockenberry-Eaton, M. (2001). *Wong's essentials of pediatric nursing* (6th ed.). St. Louis: Mosby, p. 478.

---

286. A client is diagnosed with acute inferior myocardial infarction (MI) and is receiving heparin therapy. The nurse monitors for which of the following associated complications of this therapy?
   1   Decreased urine output
   2   Infection
   3   Constipation
   4   Bleeding

Answer: 4
Rationale: Heparin is an anticoagulant, which decreases clotting time. The nurse monitors the client for signs of bleeding such as bleeding gums, petechiae, hematoma formation, and blood in stool and urine. Infection, constipation, and decreased urine output are not related to heparin therapy.

Test-Taking Strategy: Recalling that heparin is an anticoagulant easily directs you to option 4. If you are unfamiliar with the nursing care involved when a client is on heparin therapy, review this content.

Level of Cognitive Ability: Application
Client Needs: Physiological Integrity
Integrated Concept/Process: Nursing Process/Implementation
Content Area: Pharmacology

Reference:
Hodgson, B., & Kizior, R. (2003). *Saunders nursing drug handbook 2003.* Philadelphia: W.B. Saunders, p. 545.

---

287. A client is preparing for discharge after coronary artery bypass graft surgery (CABG). The client asks the nurse if sexual activity is permitted after discharge. Which of the following is the most appropriate nursing response?
   1   "No. Sexual activity is not recommended after open heart surgery."
   2   "I do not know. Wait and discuss this with your physician."

Answer: 3
Rationale: Activity restrictions are often a concern of clients after CABG. Resuming normal sexual relations will be allowed, but the physician decides when the client can safely resume this activity. Options 1, 2, and 4 are incorrect.

Test-Taking Strategy: Use knowledge about client instructions after CABG and therapeutic communication techniques to answer this question. Eliminate options 1 and 4 first because they are similar and could cause increased anxiety in the client. Next,

3 "Sexual activity will be allowed. The physician will inform you when you can resume sexual activity."

4 "No. Sexual activity can cause rupture of your cardiac suture lines."

eliminate option 2 because it places the client's feelings on hold. Review client instructions following this type of surgery if you had difficulty with this question.

Level of Cognitive Ability: Application
Client Needs: Physiological Integrity
Integrated Concept/Process: Nursing Process/Implementation
Content Area: Adult Health/Cardiovascular

Reference:
Ignatavicius, D., & Workman, M. (2002). *Medical-surgical nursing: critical thinking for collaborative care* (4th ed.). Philadelphia: W. B. Saunders, p. 813.

---

288. A 4-week-old infant is brought to the pediatrician for the first well-baby appointment. The mother is concerned because the child has been vomiting after meals and the vomiting is becoming more frequent and forceful. The physician suspects pyloric stenosis. Which of the following clinical manifestations help to establish the diagnosis?

1 The infant cries loudly and continuously during the evening hours, appears to be in considerable pain, but otherwise nurses or takes formula well

2 A previously happy healthy infant suddenly becomes pale, cries out, and draws up the legs to the chest

3 Vomitus contains sour undigested food, but no bile. The child is constipated and visible peristaltic waves move from left to right across the abdomen

4 Ribbonlike stool, bile-stained emesis, and the absence of peristalsis and abdominal distention are apparent

Answer: 3
Rationale: Option 3 identifies the classic symptoms of pyloric stenosis. Crying during the evening hours, appearing to be in pain, but otherwise eating well are clinical manifestations of colic. An infant who suddenly becomes pale, cries out, and draws the legs up to the chest is demonstrating physical signs of intussusception. Ribbonlike stool, bile-stained emesis, with the absence of peristalsis and abdominal distention are symptoms of congenital megacolon (Hirschsprung's disease).

Test-Taking Strategy: Knowledge about the clinical manifestations associated with pyloric stenosis is necessary to answer this question. If you are unfamiliar with these manifestations, review this content.

Level of Cognitive Ability: Analysis
Client Needs: Physiological Integrity
Integrated Concept/Process: Nursing Process/Data Collection
Content Area: Child Health

Reference:
Wong, D., & Hockenberry-Eaton, M. (2001). *Wong's essentials of pediatric nursing* (6th ed.). St. Louis: Mosby, p. 921.

---

289. A nurse is caring for a child with *Haemophilus influenzae* meningitis. As a part of the nursing care plan, the nurse will monitor the child for the complication of nerve deafness. The nurse anticipates that the most likely medication to be prescribed to decrease the incidence of nerve deafness will be:

1 Ceftriaxone sodium (Rocephin)
2 Furosemide (Lasix)
3 Ceftazidime (Fortaz)
4 Hydrocortisone (Solu-Cortef)

Answer: 4
Rationale: Ceftriaxone sodium and ceftazidime are third-generation cephalosporins and are prescribed as the antibiotic of choice for *Haemophilus influenzae* meningitis, but do not specifically decrease the incidence of nerve deafness. Furosemide is a diuretic. The administration of an intravenous corticosteroid early in the course of the disease has decreased the incidence of nerve deafness as a complication.

Test-Taking Strategy: Focus on the issue, which is to decrease the incidence of nerve deafness. Knowledge about the medication to be prescribed is necessary to answer the question. Review the care to the child with meningitis if you had difficulty with this question.

Level of Cognitive Ability: Analysis
Client Needs: Physiological Integrity
Integrated Concept/Process: Nursing Process/Planning
Content Area: Child Health

Reference:
Wong, D., & Hockenberry-Eaton, M. (2001). *Wong's essentials of pediatric nursing* (6th ed.). St. Louis: Mosby, p. 1092.

---

290. A client is hospitalized with chest pain and a myocardial infarction is suspected. The client tells the nurse that the chest pain has returned and the nurse administers one 0.4-mg nitroglycerin tablet sublingually as prescribed. If the pain is not relieved, what should the nurse do next?
1 Notify the physician
2 Administer another sublingual nitroglycerin tablet in 5 minutes
3 Place the client in the Trendelenburg position
4 Increase the oxygen flow rate

Answer: 2
Rationale: Nitroglycerin tablets are administered one every 5 minutes, not exceeding three tablets, for chest pain as long as the client maintains a systolic blood pressure of 100 mmHg or above. The physician is notified if the chest pain is not relieved after administering the three tablets. Placing the client in the Trendelenburg (head-lowered) position may be necessary with sudden drops in blood pressure, at which time the physician should be notified. Increasing oxygen flow rates are done with an order from a physician.

Test-Taking Strategy: Knowledge about the administration procedure for nitroglycerin when a client is experiencing chest pain is necessary to answer this question. If you had difficulty with this question, review the procedure for the administration of nitroglycerin.

Level of Cognitive Ability: Application
Client Needs: Physiological Integrity
Integrated Concept/Process: Nursing Process/Implementation
Content Area: Pharmacology

Reference:
Hodgson, B., & Kizior, R. (2003). *Saunders nursing drug handbook 2003.* Philadelphia: W.B. Saunders, p. 817.

---

291. An LPN is assisting in the care of a client who has a diagnosis of suspected myocardial infarction. The client has been experiencing chest pain that is unrelieved by nitroglycerin. The RN administers morphine sulfate 5 mg IV as prescribed by the physician. After the administration of the morphine sulfate, the LPN should:
1 Increase the oxygen flow rate
2 Monitor respirations and blood pressure
3 Monitor urinary output
4 Place the client in the Trendelenburg position

Answer: 2
Rationale: Morphine sulfate is administered to control pain in cardiac clients. The LPN must monitor the client's heart rhythm and vital signs, especially the client's respirations. Signs of morphine sulfate toxicity include respiratory depression and hypotension. The client will be placed in the Trendelenburg position if a sudden drop in blood pressure occurs. Urinary output is not directly related to the administration of this medication. The oxygen flow rate is not increased without a physician's order to do so.

Test-Taking Strategy: Focus on the issue of the question and recall the side effects associated with the administration of morphine sulfate. Remembering that this medication affects the respiratory status easily directs you to the correct option. Review the side effects of this medication if you had difficulty with this question.

Level of Cognitive Ability: Application
Client Needs: Physiological Integrity

Integrated Concept/Process: Nursing Process/Implementation
Content Area: Pharmacology

Reference:
Hodgson, B., & Kizior, R. (2003). *Saunders nursing drug handbook 2003.* Philadelphia: W.B. Saunders, p. 767.

---

292. A nurse is caring for a client with a diagnosis of chest pain and is suspected of having myocardial infarction (MI). The physician has ordered laboratory studies to evaluate the client's progress. Which of the following laboratory data reports is significant to the diagnosis of an MI?
1 Decreased white blood cell (WBC) count
2 Increased hematocrit (HCT)
3 Increased creatine kinase (CK-MB)
4 Increased creatine kinase (CK-MM)

Answer: 3
Rationale: Cardiac enzymes and isoenzymes are used to confirm MI. CK-MB is specific for the heart tissue, CK-MM reflects injury to general skeletal muscle, and CK-BB reflects brain tissue injury. The WBCs tend to increase during acute myocardial infarction. The HCT is not specifically related to an MI.

Test-Taking Strategy: Knowledge about the specific cardiac isoenzymes is necessary to answer this question. Remember that CK-MB is specific to the cardiac muscle. Review these isoenzymes if you had difficulty with this question.

Level of Cognitive Ability: Comprehension
Client Needs: Physiological Integrity
Integrated Concept/Process: Nursing Process/Data Collection
Content Area: Adult Health/Cardiovascular

Reference:
Black, J., Hawks, J., & Keene, A. (2001). *Medical-surgical nursing: clinical management for positive outcomes* (6th ed.). Philadelphia: W.B. Saunders, p. 1464.

---

293. A client is diagnosed with acute inferior myocardial infarction and is placed on bed rest. The nurse plans care understanding that a potential complication related to complete bed rest is:
1 Increased chest pain
2 Constipation
3 Diarrhea
4 Arthritis

Answer: 2
Rationale: Constipation occurs as a result of inactivity and is an undesirable complication for cardiac clients because straining or bearing down triggers the Valsalva maneuver, which increases cardiac workload. Options 1, 3, and 4 are unrelated to bed rest.

Test-Taking Strategy: Use the process of elimination. Recalling the complications that are related to bed rest directs you to the correct option. If you had difficulty with this question, review the complications associated with bed rest.

Level of Cognitive Ability: Comprehension
Client Needs: Physiological Integrity
Integrated Concept/Process: Nursing Process/Planning
Content Area: Fundamental Skills

Reference:
Black, J., Hawks, J., & Keene, A. (2001). *Medical-surgical nursing: clinical management for positive outcomes* (6th ed.). Philadelphia: W.B. Saunders, p. 615.

---

294. A client is diagnosed with myocardial infarction. The cardiac catheterization reveals 99% occlusion of the left anterior descending (LAD) coronary artery. What

Answer: 2
Rationale: The LAD perfuses most of the left ventricular muscle mass and the septum. Options 1, 3, and 4 are not affected by the LAD.

side of the heart does the nurse expect to be affected?

1 Right ventricle and septum
2 Left ventricle and septum
3 Right ventricle
4 Left atrium

Test-Taking Strategy: Noting the key word *left* in the question assists in eliminating options 1 and 3. Recalling that the left ventricle is primarily responsible for pumping the blood to the body assists in directing you to option 2. Review the anatomy of the coronary arteries if you had difficulty with this question.

Level of Cognitive Ability: Knowledge
Client Needs: Physiological Integrity
Integrated Concept/Process: Nursing Process/Data Collection
Content Area: Fundamental Skills

Reference:
Ignatauicius, D., & Workman, M. (2002). *Medical Surgical Nursing: critical thinking for collaborative care* (4th ed). Philadelphia: W. B. Saunders, p. 621.

---

295. A client diagnosed with unstable angina is returning to the nursing unit after an angioplasty. The nurse observes the client for what mental status changes, knowing that a change could indicate a complication of this procedure?

1 Reactions from the contrast medium
2 Cerebral hemorrhage
3 Cerebral emboli
4 Increased intraocular pressure

Answer: 3
Rationale: Angioplasty involves using a balloon-tipped catheter to displace or flatten the plaque built up along the arterial walls, thereby enlarging the diameter of the vessel. There is a chance for a small piece of the plaque to become dislodged, which could create an embolus. Reactions from the contrast most likely will occur immediately, not when the client returns to the nursing unit. Cerebral hemorrhage and increased intraocular pressure are not directly related to postangioplasty complications.

Test-Taking Strategy: Note the key words *returning to the nursing unit* and *mental status changes*. Knowledge about what is involved in an angioplasty and the associated complications directs you to option 3. Review these complications if you had difficulty with this question.

Level of Cognitive Ability: Analysis
Client Needs: Physiological Integrity
Integrated Concept/Process: Nursing Process/Data Collection
Content Area: Adult Health/Cardiovascular

Reference:
Black, J., Hawks, J., & Keene, A. (2001). *Medical-surgical nursing: clinical management for positive outcomes* (6th ed.). Philadelphia: W.B. Saunders, pp. 1954; 1956.

---

296. A client is diagnosed with angina. The nurse reviews the client's diagnostic and laboratory results, knowing that which of the following findings are indicative of ischemia?

1 S-T wave depression on electrocardiogram (ECG)
2 Electroencephalogram (EEG) wave increases
3 Increased serum potassium levels
4 Decreased serum potassium levels

Answer: 1
Rationale: Ischemia may be detected on an ECG by changes in the S-T wave or by T-wave inversion. Ischemia represents a decreased amount of oxygen to the myocardium. EEG and potassium level findings are not directly related to coronary ischemia.

Test-Taking Strategy: Knowledge about the findings in myocardial ischemia is necessary to answer this question. Focusing on the client's diagnosis assists in directing you to option 1. If you are unfamiliar with these diagnostic findings, review this content.

Level of Cognitive Ability: Analysis
Client Needs: Physiological Integrity

Integrated Concept/Process: Nursing Process/Data Collection
Content Area: Adult Health/Cardiovascular

Reference:
Black, J., Hawks, J., & Keene, A. (2001). *Medical-surgical nursing: clinical management for positive outcomes* (6th ed.). Philadelphia: W.B. Saunders, p. 1581.

---

297. A nurse is caring for a client with a diagnosis of angina. The client requests something to drink. Which of the following beverages would the nurse give to the client?
1   Coffee
2   Tea
3   Cola
4   Lemonade

Answer: 4
Rationale: Clients experiencing angina should not consume caffeinated beverages because of the vasoconstriction effect associated with caffeine. Options 1, 2, and 3 are items that contain caffeine.

Test-Taking Strategy: Use the process of elimination. Note that options 1, 2, and 3 are similar because they all contain caffeine. If you are unfamiliar with the food items that contain caffeine, review this information.

Level of Cognitive Ability: Application
Client Needs: Physiological Integrity
Integrated Concept/Process: Nursing Process/Implementation
Content Area: Fundamental Skills

Reference:
Black, J., Hawks, J., & Keene, A. (2001). *Medical-surgical nursing: clinical management for positive outcomes* (6th ed.). Philadelphia: W.B. Saunders, p. 1582.

---

298. A client is admitted to the hospital with unstable angina. As the nurse assists to plan care for the client, it is imperative that:
1   Plenty of time is allotted for rest and relaxation
2   Large meals are served three times a day
3   Visitors are permitted liberal visiting hours
4   The client performs all activities of daily living

Answer: 1
Rationale: The client requires plenty of rest and relaxation to prevent decreased blood supply to the myocardium as a result of increased demands. Large meals are contraindicated because of the increased metabolic requirement for digestion and consumption. Visitors are limited to ensure proper rest. The client needs assistance with activities of daily living because rest is important.

Test-Taking Strategy: Focus on the client's diagnosis and use the process of elimination. Remembering that clients with angina require rest easily directs you to option 1. Review care of the client with angina if you had difficulty with this question.

Level of Cognitive Ability: Application
Client Needs: Physiological Integrity
Integrated Concept/Process: Nursing Process/Planning
Content Area: Adult Health/Cardiovascular

Reference:
Black, J., Hawks, J., & Keene, A. (2001). *Medical-surgical nursing: clinical management for positive outcomes* (6th ed.). Philadelphia: W.B. Saunders, p. 1582.

---

299. A nurse is caring for a client diagnosed with angina. The client receives nitroglycerin sublingually, PRN for chest pain. Which vital sign must the nurse monitor closely when administering nitroglycerin?

Answer: 3
Rationale: Nitroglycerin is a vasodilator used to increase coronary artery blood flow. The side effects of nitroglycerin include postural hypotension, flushing, headache, dizziness, and rash. Monitoring blood pressure is most important.

1 Respirations
2 Heart rate
3 Blood pressure
4 Temperature

Test-Taking Strategy: Use the process of elimination. Recalling that nitroglycerin is a vasodilator directs you to option 3. Review the side effects of nitroglycerin if you had difficulty with this question.

Level of Cognitive Ability: Application
Client Needs: Physiological Integrity
Integrated Concept/Process: Nursing Process/Implementation
Content Area: Pharmacology

Reference:
Hodgson, B., & Kizior, R. (2003). *Saunders nursing drug handbook 2003.* Philadelphia: W.B. Saunders, p. 815.

---

300. A nurse is caring for a client admitted to the hospital with a diagnosis of angina. While caring for the client, the client begins to experience chest pain. Which of the following data should be obtained by the nurse immediately?
1 Location and intensity of pain
2 Symptoms of nausea
3 Presence of a fever
4 Blood pressure

Answer: 1
Rationale: The nurse must assess the pain by requesting a description of pain intensity, location, duration, and quality. Assessment of the pain is the priority, although the nurse may check the client's vital signs and for symptoms of nausea.

Test-Taking Strategy: Note the key word *immediately.* Focus on the issue of the question and note the relationship between the issue and option 1. Review immediate care of the client experiencing chest pain if you had difficulty with this question.

Level of Cognitive Ability: Application
Client Needs: Physiological Integrity
Integrated Concept/Process: Nursing Process/Data Collection
Content Area: Adult Health/Cardiovascular

Reference:
Black, J., Hawks, J., & Keene, A. (2001). *Medical-surgical nursing: clinical management for positive outcomes* (6th ed.). Philadelphia: W.B. Saunders, p. 1448.

---

301. A client has been placed in seclusion. The nurse is responsible for assisting in providing and documenting care for the client. Which of the following most completely identifies the components requiring documentation?
1 Vital signs, toileting, and checking the client based on protocol time frame, such as every 15 minutes
2 Ambulating, toileting, and checking the client based on protocol time frame, such as every 15 minutes
3 Vital signs, toileting, feeding or fluid intake, and checking client based on protocol time frame, such as every 15 minutes
4 Vital signs, reason for the seclusion, date and time

Answer: 3
Rationale: Option 3 addresses the client's basic needs during seclusion. Options 1 and 2 are not complete in terms of identification of physiological needs. Option 4 contains data that are documented at the time seclusion is initiated.

Test-Taking Strategy: Use the process of elimination. Eliminate option 4 first because these data are documented at the time seclusion is initiated. From the remaining options, use Maslow's Hierarchy of Needs theory to prioritize. Option 3 most completely addresses the client's basic needs. Review care of the client in seclusion if you had difficulty with this question.

Level of Cognitive Ability: Comprehension
Client Needs: Physiological Integrity
Integrated Concept/Process: Communication and Documentation
Content Area: Mental Health

Reference:
Varcarolis, E. (2002). *Foundations of psychiatric mental health nursing* (4th ed.). Philadelphia: W.B. Saunders, p. 175.

302. A client with a Sengstaken-Blakemore tube in place is admitted to the hospital from the emergency room. The nurse assigned to assist in caring for the client plans care understanding that the purpose of this tube is to:
1 Control bleeding from gastritis
2 Apply pressure to esophageal varices
3 Control ascites
4 Remove ammonia-forming bacteria from the gastrointestinal tract

Answer: 2
Rationale: A Sengstaken-Blakemore tube is inserted in cirrhosis clients with ruptured esophageal varices. It has esophageal and gastric balloons. The esophageal balloon exerts pressure on the ruptured esophageal varices and stops the bleeding. The gastric balloon holds the tube in correct position and prevents migration of the esophageal balloon, which would harm the client.

Test-Taking Strategy: Focus on the issue and use the process of elimination. Option 2 correctly defines the purpose of the tube. All of the other options identify treatment goals for clients with ruptured esophageal varices. Review the purpose of this tube if you had difficulty with this question.

Level of Cognitive Ability: Comprehension
Client Needs: Physiological Integrity
Integrated Concept/Process: Nursing Process/Planning
Content Area: Adult Health/Gastrointestinal

Reference:
Ignatavicius, D., & Workman, M. (2002). *Medical-surgical nursing: critical thinking for collaborative care* (4th ed.). Philadelphia: W.B. Saunders, p. 1308.

303. A nurse is instructing a client with chronic obstructive pulmonary disease (COPD) about breathing techniques. The nurse teaches the client breathing techniques that incorporate which of the following modalities?
1 Pursed-lip breathing
2 Intercostal chest expansion
3 Inspiratory breathing
4 Chest physical therapy

Answer: 1
Rationale: Pursed-lip breathing allows the client to slowly exhale carbon dioxide while keeping the airways open. Intercostal chest expansion, inspiratory breathing, and chest physical therapy are not breathing techniques.

Test-Taking Strategy: Use the process of elimination. Eliminate options 2, 3, and 4 first because these are not breathing techniques. Remembering that pursed-lip breathing is associated with the COPD client assists in directing you to the correct option. Review breathing techniques for the client with COPD if you had difficulty with this question.

Level of Cognitive Ability: Application
Client Needs: Physiological Integrity
Integrated Concept/Process: Teaching/Learning
Content Area: Adult Health/Respiratory

Reference:
Ignatavicius, D., & Workman, M. (2002). *Medical-surgical nursing: critical thinking for collaborative care* (4th ed.). Philadelphia: W.B. Saunders, p. 547.

304. A physician has ordered a partial rebreathing face mask for the client who has terminal lung cancer. The nurse plans care knowing that the mask:
1 Delivers accurate fraction of inspired oxygen (FiO_2) to the client
2 Conserves oxygen by having the client rebreathe some of his or her own exhaled air

Answer: 2
Rationale: Rebreathing masks have a reservoir bag that conserves oxygen and requires a high liter flow to achieve concentrations of 40% to 60%. It does not deliver accurate (FiO_2) to the client. The bag should not deflate during inspiration. A rebreathing bag conserves oxygen by having the client rebreathe his or her own exhaled air.

Test-Taking Strategy: Use the process of elimination. Note the relationship of the phrase *partial rebreathing* in the question and *rebreathe*

3 Requires that the reservoir bag be deflated during inspiration to work effectively

4 Requires a low liter flow to prevent rebreathing of carbon dioxide

some of his or her own exhaled air in the correct option. Review oxygen delivery systems if you had difficulty with this question.

Level of Cognitive Ability: Comprehension
Client Needs: Physiological Integrity
Integrated Concept/Process: Nursing Process/Planning
Content Area: Adult Health/Respiratory

Reference:
Potter, P., & Perry, A. (2001). *Fundamentals of nursing* (5th ed.). St. Louis: Mosby, p. 1177.

---

305. A 48-year-old man is brought to the emergency room complaining of chest pain. His vital signs are blood pressure (BP) 150/90 mmHg, pulse (P) 88 beats per minute (BPM), and respirations (R) 20 breaths per minute. The nurse administers nitroglycerin 0.4 mg sublingually. To evaluate the effectiveness of this medication, the nurse should expect which of the following changes in the vital signs?

1 BP 160/100 mmHg, P 120 BPM, R 16 breaths per minute
2 BP 150/90 mmHg, P 70 BPM, R 24 breaths per minute
3 BP 100/60 mmHg, P 96 BPM, R 20 breaths per minute
4 BP 100/60 mmHg, P 70 BPM, R 24 breaths per minute

Answer: 3
Rationale: Nitroglycerin dilates both arteries and veins causing blood to pool in the periphery. This causes a reduced preload and therefore a drop in cardiac output. This vasodilation causes the blood pressure to fall. The drop in cardiac output causes the sympathetic nervous system to respond and attempt to maintain cardiac output by increasing the pulse. Beta-blockers such as propranolol (Inderal) often are used in conjunction with nitroglycerin to prevent this rise in heart rate.

Test-Taking Strategy: Use the process of elimination. Knowing that nitroglycerin is a vasodilator and that it causes the BP to drop assists in eliminating option 1 and 2. Also, if chest pain is reduced and cardiac workload is reduced, the client will be more comfortable; therefore a rise in respirations should not be seen. This assists in directing you to option 3. If you had difficulty with this question, review the effects of nitroglycerin.

Level of Cognitive Ability: Analysis
Client Needs: Physiological Integrity
Integrated Concept/Process: Nursing Process/Evaluation
Content Area: Pharmacology

Reference:
Hodgson, B., & Kizior, R. (2002). *Saunders nursing drug handbook 2002.* Philadelphia: W.B. Saunders, p. 802.

---

306. A client who had abdominal surgery is 1 day postoperative and has a nasogastric tube. The nurse assisting in caring for the client notes the absence of bowel sounds. The nurse's best action is to:

1 Contact the RN immediately
2 Remove the nasogastric tube
3 Feed the client
4 Continue to monitor for bowel sounds

Answer: 4
Rationale: Bowel sounds may be absent for 2 to 3 days after surgery because of bowel manipulation during surgery. The nurse should continue to monitor the client. If present, the nasogastric tube should stay in place and the client kept NPO until after the onset of bowel sounds. Additionally, the nurse should not remove the nasogastric tube. There is no need to contact the RN immediately, although the finding should be reported.

Test-Taking Strategy: Use the process of elimination. Note the key words *1 day postoperative.* Knowledge that bowel sounds may not return for 2 to 3 days postoperative assists in answering this question. If you had difficulty with this question, review normal postoperative findings after abdominal surgery.

Level of Cognitive Ability: Application
Client Needs: Physiological Integrity
Integrated Concept/Process: Nursing Process/Implementation
Content Area: Adult Health/Gastrointestinal

Reference:
Ignatavicius, D., & Workman, M. (2002). *Medical-surgical nursing: critical thinking for collaborative care* (4th ed.). Philadelphia: W.B. Saunders, p. 290.

---

307. Which complication should the nurse be particularly alert for when monitoring a client with pregnancy-induced hypertension (PIH) during labor?
1 Seizures
2 Placenta previa
3 Hallucinations
4 Altered respiratory status

Answer: 1
Rationale: The major complication of PIH is seizures. Placenta previa, hallucinations, or altered respiratory status are not directly associated with PIH.

Test-Taking Strategy: Use the process of elimination. Recalling that seizures are a concern with PIH assists in directing you to the correct option. If you had difficulty with this question, review the complications of PIH.

Level of Cognitive Ability: Comprehension
Client Needs: Physiological Integrity
Integrated Concept/Process: Nursing Process/Data Collection
Content Area: Maternity

Reference:
Burroughs, A., & Leifer, G. (2002). *Maternity nursing* (8th ed.). Philadelphia: W.B. Saunders, p. 231.

---

308. Which statement by the mother of a newly circumcised infant indicates knowledge of necessary postcircumcision care?
1 "I should check for bleeding every hour for the first 12 hours."
2 "I should clean his penis every hour with baby wipes."
3 "I should wrap his penis completely in dry sterile gauze, making sure it is dry when I change his diaper."
4 "My baby will not urinate for the next 24 hours because of swelling."

Answer: 1
Rationale: The mother should be taught to watch for bleeding, checking the site hourly for 8 to 12 hours. Voiding should be monitored. The mother should call the physician if the baby has not urinated within 24 hours. Swelling or damage may obstruct urine output. When the diaper is changed, Vaseline gauze should be reapplied. Frequent diaper changes prevent contamination of the site. Water is used for cleaning because soap or baby wipes may irritate the area and cause discomfort.

Test-Taking Strategy: Use the process of elimination. Eliminate option 2 because baby wipes cause stinging in the newly circumcised penis. Eliminate option 3 because dry gauze sticks to the penis if the gauze is completely dry. Eliminate option 4 because penile swelling prevents voiding, and this should be reported to the physician. Review postcircumcision care if you had difficulty with this question.

Level of Cognitive Ability: Comprehension
Client Needs: Physiological Integrity
Integrated Concept/Process: Nursing Process/Evaluation
Content Area: Maternity

Reference:
Burroughs, A., & Leifer, G. (2002). *Maternity nursing* (8th ed.). Philadelphia: W.B. Saunders, pp. 177-178.

309. A nurse plans to reinforce which of the following essential discharge instructions to the client with testicular cancer after testicular surgery?
1 "Report any elevation in temperature to your physician."
2 "You cannot drive for 6 weeks."
3 "You cannot be fitted for a prosthesis for 6 months."
4 "Refrain from sitting for long periods."

Answer: 1
Rationale: For the client who has had testicular surgery, the nurse should emphasize the importance of notifying the physician if chills, fever, drainage, redness, or discharge occurs. These symptoms may indicate the presence of an infection. The client may drive 1 week after testicular surgery; often, a prosthesis is inserted during surgery. Sitting should be avoided with prostrate surgery because of the risk of hemorrhage; however, the risk is not as high with testicular surgery.

Test-Taking Strategy: Use Maslow's Hierarchy of Needs theory. Infection is the priority. Elevation of temperature could signal an infection after any surgical procedure and should be reported. Review care of the client after this type of surgery if you had difficulty with this question.

Level of Cognitive Ability: Comprehension
Client Needs: Physiological Integrity
Integrated Concept/Process: Teaching/Learning
Content Area: Adult Health/Oncology

Reference:
Ignatavicius, D., & Workman, M. (2002). *Medical-surgical nursing: critical thinking for collaborative care* (4th ed.). Philadelphia: W.B. Saunders, p. 1799.

310. A nurse is caring for a client with Parkinson's disease. The client is taking benztropine mesylate (Cogentin) 6 mg PO daily. The nurse understands that the priority nursing action for caring for clients on this medication is to monitor:
1 Pupil response
2 Respiratory status
3 Intake and output
4 Pulse

Answer: 3
Rationale: Urinary retention is a side effect of benztropine mesylate. The nurse should observe for dysuria, distended abdomen, infrequent voiding of small amounts, and overflow incontinence. Options 1, 2, and 4 are not related to this medication.

Test-Taking Strategy: Use the process of elimination. Recalling that urinary retention is a concern with this medication directs you to option 3. Review this medication and its side effects if you had difficulty with this question.

Level of Cognitive Ability: Application
Client Needs: Physiological Integrity
Integrated Concept/Process: Nursing Process/Data Collection
Content Area: Pharmacology

Reference:
Hodgson, B., & Kizior, R. (2002). *Saunders nursing drug handbook 2002.* Philadelphia: W.B. Saunders, p. 113.

311. A nurse is teaching a client with chronic obstructive pulmonary disease (COPD) how to purse lip breath. The nurse instructs the client:
1 That inhalation should be twice as long as exhalation
2 To loosen the abdominal muscles while breathing out

Answer: 3
Rationale: Prolonging the time for exhaling reduces air trapping caused by airway narrowing or collapse in COPD. Tightening the abdominal muscles aids in expelling air. Exhaling through pursed lips increases the intraluminal pressure and prevents the airways from collapsing.

3 That exhalation should be twice as long as inhalation
4 To inhale with pursed lips and exhale with the mouth open wide

Test-Taking Strategy: Use the process of elimination. Recalling that the major purpose of pursed-lip breathing is to prevent air trapping during exhalation directs you to the correct option. Review the principles of pursed-lip breathing if you are unfamiliar with this technique.

Level of Cognitive Ability: Application
Client Needs: Physiological Integrity
Integrated Concept/Process: Teaching/Learning
Content Area: Adult Health/Respiratory

Reference:
Potter, P., & Perry, A. (2001). *Fundamentals of nursing* (5th ed.). St. Louis: Mosby, p. 1189.

---

312. A 44-year-old client is taking lithium carbonate (Eskalith) for treatment of bipolar disorder. Which of the following questions should the nurse ask the client when collecting data to determine signs of early drug toxicity?
1 "Have you been experiencing seizures over the past few days?"
2 "Do you frequently have headaches?"
3 "Have you been experiencing any nausea, vomiting, or diarrhea?"
4 "Have you noted excessive urination?"

Answer: 3
Rationale: Common early signs of lithium toxicity are gastrointestinal (GI) disturbances such as nausea, vomiting, or diarrhea. The questions identified in options 1, 2, and 4 are unrelated to lithium toxicity.

Test-Taking Strategy: Use the process of elimination and focus on the issue. The question asks for the early signs of lithium toxicity. Recalling that GI disturbances occur early in toxicity assists in directing you to option 3. Review these signs if you had difficulty with this question.

Level of Cognitive Ability: Application
Client Needs: Physiological Integrity
Integrated Concept/Process: Nursing Process/Data Collection
Content Area: Pharmacology

Reference:
Hodgson, B., & Kizior, R. (2002). *Saunders nursing drug handbook 2002.* Philadelphia: W.B. Saunders, p. 672.

---

313. A client is admitted to the hospital for repair of an unruptured cerebral aneurysm. The nurse assigned to care for the client monitors the client for signs of aneurysm rupture. Which finding will the nurse note first if the aneurysm ruptures?
1 Widened pulse pressure
2 Unilateral slowing of pupil response
3 Unilateral motor weakness
4 A decline in the level of consciousness

Answer: 4
Rationale: Rupture of a cerebral aneurysm usually results in increased intracranial pressure. The first sign of increased intracranial pressure is a change in the level of consciousness caused by compression of the reticular formation. This change in consciousness can be as subtle as drowsiness or restlessness. Because centers that control blood pressure are located lower in the brain stem than those that control consciousness, a pulse pressure alteration is a later sign. Options 1, 2, and 3 are not early signs of increased intracranial pressure.

Test-Taking Strategy: Use the process of elimination and note the key word *first*. Remember that changes in level of consciousness are the first indication of increased intracranial pressure. Review the clinical manifestations associated with increased intracranial pressure and aneurysm rupture if you had difficulty with this question.

Level of Cognitive Ability: Comprehension
Client Needs: Physiological Integrity
Integrated Concept/Process: Nursing Process/Data Collection
Content Area: Adult Health/Neurological

Reference:
Black, J., Hawks, J., & Keene, A. (2001). *Medical-surgical nursing: clinical management for positive outcomes* (6th ed.). Philadelphia: W.B. Saunders, p. 1942.

---

314. A client has not eaten or had anything to drink for 4 hours after two episodes of nausea and vomiting. Which of the following items is best to offer the client who is ready to try resuming oral intake?
1 Ginger ale
2 Gelatin
3 Toast
4 Dry cereal

Answer: 1
Rationale: Clear liquids are tolerated first after episodes of nausea and vomiting. If the client tolerates sips (20 to 30 mL at a time) of clear liquids, such as water or ginger ale, then the amounts may be increased and gelatin, tea, and broth may be added. Once these are tolerated, solid foods such as toast, cereal, chicken, and other easily digested foods may be tried.

Test-Taking Strategy: Use the process of elimination. Begin to answer this question by eliminating options 3 and 4, which identify solid foods and are less well tolerated than liquids. Choose ginger ale over gelatin because it is a liquid at all temperatures. Review care of the client with nausea and vomiting if you had difficulty with this question.

Level of Cognitive Ability: Application
Client Needs: Physiological Integrity
Integrated Concept/Process: Nursing Process/Implementation
Content Area: Adult Health/Gastrointestinal

Reference:
Williams, S. (2001) *Basic nutrition & diet therapy* (11th ed.). St. Louis: Mosby, pp. 451.

---

315. A client has just undergone an upper gastrointestinal (GI) series. The nurse plans which of the following upon the client's return to the unit, which is an important part of routine postprocedural care?
1 Liquid diet
2 Bland diet
3 NPO status
4 Laxative

Answer: 4
Rationale: Barium sulfate, which is used as contrast material during an upper GI series, is a constipating material. If it is not eliminated from the GI tract, it can cause obstruction. Therefore, laxatives or cathartics are administered as part of routine postprocedural care. Options 2 and 4 are unnecessary. Increased fluids are helpful but a liquid diet is not necessary.

Test-Taking Strategy: Use the process of elimination. Recalling that barium is administered during this test and its side effects directs you to the correct option. Review postprocedural care after an upper GI series if you had difficulty with this question.

Level of Cognitive Ability: Application
Client Needs: Physiological Integrity
Integrated Concept/Process: Nursing Process/Planning
Content Area: Adult Health/Gastrointestinal

Reference:
Chernecky, C., & Berger, B. (2001). *Laboratory tests and diagnostic procedures* (3rd ed.). Philadelphia: W.B. Saunders, p. 202.

316. A nurse is administering continuous nasogastric tube feedings to a client. The nurse takes which of the following actions as part of routine care for this client?

   1   Checks the residual every 4 hours

   2   Changes the feeding bag and tubing every 12 hours

   3   Pours additional feeding into the bag when 25 mL is left

   4   Holds the feeding if greater than 200 mL of residual is aspirated

Answer: 1

Rationale: The placement of a nasogastric feeding tube is checked at least every 4 hours for residual when administering continuous tube feedings. It is checked before each bolus with intermittent feedings. The feeding should be withheld for 30 to 60 minutes if the residual is greater than 100 mL or is an amount greater than that prescribed by the physician or designated by agency protocol. The bag and tubing are completely changed every 24 hours. The bag should be rinsed before adding new formula to the bag that is hanging.

Test-Taking Strategy: Note the key words *continuous nasogastric tube feedings*. Use the Nursing Process to answer the question. Option 1 is the only option that addresses data collection. If you had difficulty with this question, review the nursing care associated with this procedure.

Level of Cognitive Ability: Application
Client Needs: Physiological Integrity
Integrated Concept/Process: Nursing Process/Implementation
Content Area: Fundamental Skills

Reference:
Black, J., Hawks, J., & Keene, A. (2001). *Medical-surgical nursing: clinical management for positive outcomes* (6th ed.). Philadelphia: W.B. Saunders, p. 676.

---

317. A nurse is asked to obtain dressing supplies for a client who is scheduled to have a chest tube inserted by the physician. The nurse selects which of the following materials to be used as the first layer of the dressing at the chest tube insertion site?

   1   Sterile 4 × 4 gauze pad

   2   Absorbent Kerlix dressing

   3   Gauze impregnated with povidone-iodine

   4   Petrolatum jelly gauze

Answer: 4

Rationale: The first layer of the chest tube dressing is petrolatum jelly gauze, which allows for an occlusive seal at the chest tube insertion site. Additional layers of gauze cover this layer, and the dressing is secured with a strong adhesive tape or Elastoplast tape.

Test-Taking Strategy: Use the process of elimination. The key words are *first layer*. Recalling that it is imperative to have an occlusive seal at the site and knowing which dressing material to use to help achieve that occlusive seal direct you to the correct option. Review preparation for this procedure if you had difficulty with this question.

Level of Cognitive Ability: Application
Client Needs: Physiological Integrity
Integrated Concept/Process: Nursing Process/Implementation
Content Area: Adult Health/Respiratory

Reference:
Black, J., Hawks, J., & Keene, A. (2001). *Medical-surgical nursing: clinical management for positive outcomes* (6th ed.). Philadelphia: W.B. Saunders, p. 1739.

---

318. A client being seen in the physician's office for follow-up 2 weeks after pneumonectomy complains of numbness and tenderness at the surgical site. The nurse tells the client that this is:

   1   A severe problem, and the client probably will be rehospitalized

Answer: 4

Rationale: Clients who undergo pneumonectomy may experience numbness, altered sensation, or tenderness in the area that surrounds the incision. These sensations may last for months. It is not considered to be a severe problem and is not indicative of wound infection.

2   Often the first sign of wound infection, and checks the client's temperature

3   Probably caused by permanent nerve damage as a result of surgery

4   Not likely to be permanent, but may last for some months

Test-Taking Strategy: Use the process of elimination. Eliminate option 1 because of the word *severe*. Eliminate option 2 because numbness and tenderness are not signs of infection. Eliminate option 3 because of the word *permanent*. Review the effects of this surgical procedure if you had difficulty with this question.

Level of Cognitive Ability: Application
Client Needs: Physiological Integrity
Integrated Concept/Process: Nursing Process/Implementation
Content Area: Adult Health/Respiratory

Reference:
Ignatavicius, D., & Workman, M. (2002). *Medical-surgical nursing: critical thinking for collaborative care* (4th ed.). Philadelphia: W.B. Saunders, p. 291.

---

319. A client scheduled for pneumonectomy tells the nurse that a friend had chest surgery, and asks how long the chest tubes will be in place. The nurse responds that:
1   They will be in for 24 to 48 hours
2   They will be removed after 3 to 4 days
3   They usually function for a full week after surgery
4   It is likely that there will be no chest tubes in place after surgery

Answer: 4
Rationale: Pneumonectomy involves removal of the entire lung, usually because of extensive disease such as bronchogenic carcinoma, unilateral tuberculosis, or lung abscess. Chest tubes are not inserted because the cavity is left to fill with serosanguinous fluid, which later solidifies. The phrenic nerve is severed or crushed to elevate the diaphragm, further decreasing the size of the chest cavity on the operative side.

Test-Taking Strategy: Use the process of elimination. Recall that the entire lung is removed with this procedure. This guides you to reason that chest tubes are unnecessary, because there is no lung remaining to reinflate to fill the pleural space. Review this surgical procedure if you had difficulty with this question.

Level of Cognitive Ability: Application
Client Needs: Physiological Integrity
Integrated Concept/Process: Nursing Process/Implementation
Content Area: Adult Health/Respiratory

Reference:
Black, J., Hawks, J., & Keene, A. (2001). *Medical-surgical nursing: clinical management for positive outcomes* (6th ed.). Philadelphia: W.B. Saunders, p. 1731.

---

320. A nurse is assigned to assist in caring for the client with a diagnosis of a dissecting abdominal aortic aneurysm. The nurse avoids doing which of the following while caring for this client?
1   Turn the client to the side to look for ecchymosis on the lower back
2   Monitor vital signs
3   Perform deep palpation of the abdomen
4   Tell the client to report back, shoulder, or neck pain

Answer: 3
Rationale: The nurse avoids deep palpation in the client in which a dissecting aneurysm is known or suspected. Doing so could place the client at risk for rupture. The nurse looks for ecchymosis on the lower back to determine aneurysm leaking, and tells the client to report back, neck, shoulder, or extremity pain. An important nursing action is monitoring for changes in vital signs that may indicate signs of a worsening of the condition.

Test-Taking Strategy: Use the process of elimination and note the key word *avoids*. With the diagnosis presented, the only option that could cause harm is the option related to deep palpation. Review care of the client with a dissecting abdominal aortic aneurysm if you had difficulty with this question.

Level of Cognitive Ability: Application
Client Needs: Physiological Integrity
Integrated Concept/Process: Nursing Process/Implementation
Content Area: Adult Health/Cardiovascular

Reference:

Black, J., Hawks, J., & Keene, A. (2001). *Medical-surgical nursing: clinical management for positive outcomes* (6th ed.). Philadelphia: W.B. Saunders, p. 1416.

---

321. A client has an abdominal aortic aneurysm. The nurse best detects bleeding from the aneurysm by:
1   Measuring abdominal girth every 4 hours
2   Checking the pulses with a Doppler every 4 hours
3   Asking the client about mild pain in the area PRN
4   Palpating the pedal pulses every 4 hours

Answer: 1
Rationale: Bleeding from an aneurysm causes blood to accumulate in the retroperitoneal area. This can most directly be detected by measuring abdominal girth. Palpation and auscultation of pulses determines patency, and may be of some use with detecting bleeding if the pulses are diminished because of reduced circulating volume. However, other signs of hypovolemic shock also may be apparent by that time. Assessment of pain is done routinely, and mild regional discomfort is expected.

Test-Taking Strategy: The key words are *bleeding, aneurysm,* and *best detects.* You could select the correct option by looking for an abdominal assessment, because the aneurysm is located in the peritoneal cavity. This should direct you to option 1. Review postprocedural care if you had difficulty with this question.

Level of Cognitive Ability: Application
Client Needs: Physiological Integrity
Integrated Concept/Process: Nursing Process/Data Collection
Content Area: Adult Health/Cardiovascular

Reference:

Lewis, S., Heitkemper, M., & Dirksen, S. (2004). *Medical-surgical nursing: assessment and management of clinical problems* (6th ed.). St. Louis: Mosby, p. 914.

---

322. A nurse is assigned to care for a client who underwent peripheral arterial bypass surgery 16 hours previously. When collecting data from the client, the client complains of increasing pain in the leg at rest that worsens with movement and is accompanied by paresthesias. The nurse should take which of the following actions?
1   Administer a prescribed narcotic analgesic
2   Apply warm moist heat for comfort
3   Apply ice to minimize any developing swelling
4   Notify the RN

Answer: 4
Rationale: Compartment syndrome can occur after this procedure. Compartment syndrome is characterized by increased pressure within a muscle compartment caused by bleeding or excessive edema. It compresses the nerves in the area and can cause vascular compromise. The classic signs are pain at rest that intensifies with movement and the development of paresthesias. The RN is notified immediately. The RN then contacts the physician, because the client could require an emergency fasciotomy.

Test-Taking Strategy: Use the process of elimination and note the key words *increasing pain.* The signs and symptoms described in the case situation indicate a new problem, about which the RN needs to be notified. Review the complications of this procedure if you had difficulty with this question.

Level of Cognitive Ability: Application
Client Needs: Physiological Integrity
Integrated Concept/Process: Nursing Process/Implementation
Content Area: Adult Health/Cardiovascular

Reference:
Black, J., Hawks, J., & Keene, A. (2001). *Medical-surgical nursing: clinical management for positive outcomes* (6th ed.). Philadelphia: W.B. Saunders, p. 1409.

323. A nurse who is assisting in an ambulatory care clinic takes a client's blood pressure in the left arm and notes that it is 200/118 mmHg. The first action of the nurse is to:
1. Report the elevation to the RN
2. Inquire about the presence of kidney disorders
3. Check the blood pressure in the right arm
4. Recheck the blood pressure in the same arm within 30 seconds

Answer: 3

Rationale: Upon getting an initially high reading, the nurse takes the pressure in the opposite arm to see if the blood pressure is elevated in one extremity only. The nurse also rechecks the blood pressure in the same arm, but waits at least 2 minutes between readings. The nurse inquires about the presence of kidney disorders, which could contribute to elevated blood pressure. The nurse notifies the RN, who contacts the physician because immediate treatment is necessary. However, this should not be done without obtaining verification of the elevation.

Test-Taking Strategy: Use the process of elimination and note the key word *first*. This tells you that more than one or all of the options may be partially or totally correct. In this instance, eliminate option 4 first because it is incorrect. Choose option 3 over the other options because it provides verification of the initial reading. Review the procedures for taking a blood pressure if you had difficulty with this question.

Level of Cognitive Ability: Application
Client Needs: Physiological Integrity
Integrated Concept/Process: Nursing Process/Implementation
Content Area: Adult Health/Cardiovascular

Reference:
Black, J., Hawks, J., & Keene, A. (2001). *Medical-surgical nursing: clinical management for positive outcomes* (6th ed.). Philadelphia: W.B. Saunders, p. 184.

324. A hospitalized client has been diagnosed with thrombophlebitis. The nurse avoids doing which of the following during the care of this client?
1. Maintaining the client on bed rest
2. Applying moist heat to the leg
3. Elevating the feet above heart level
4. Placing a pillow under the client's knees

Answer: 4

Rationale: The nurse avoids placing a pillow under the knees of a client with thrombophlebitis because it obstructs venous return to the heart and exacerbates impairment of blood flow. The client is maintained on bed rest for 3 to 7 days after a diagnosis of thrombophlebitis is made to prevent the occurrence of pulmonary embolus. The feet are elevated above heart level to aid in venous return, and warm moist heat may be used to aid in comfort and reduce venospasm.

Test-Taking Strategy: Use the process of elimination and note the key word *avoids*. Use principles related to gravity and relief of inflammation to answer this question. This should direct you to the action to avoid. Review care of the client with thrombophlebitis if you had difficulty with this question.

Level of Cognitive Ability: Application
Client Needs: Physiological Integrity
Integrated Concept/Process: Nursing Process/Implementation
Content Area: Adult Health/Cardiovascular

Reference:
Black, J., Hawks, J., & Keene, A. (2001). *Medical-surgical nursing: clinical management for positive outcomes* (6th ed.). Philadelphia: W.B. Saunders, p. 1425.

---

325. A new prenatal client is 6 months pregnant. On the first prenatal visit, the nurse notes that the client is gravida 4, para 0, aborta 3. The client is 5'6" tall, weighs 130 pounds, and is 25 years old. The client states, "I get really tired after working all day and I can't keep up with my housework." Which factor in the preceding data leads the nurse to suspect gestational diabetes?

1 Fatigue
2 Obesity
3 Maternal age
4 Previous fetal demise

Answer: 4

Rationale: Fatigue is a normal occurrence during pregnancy. The client is not obese, based on the height and weight of the client. To be at high risk for gestational diabetes, the maternal age should be greater than 30 years. A previous history of unexplained stillbirths or miscarriages puts the client at high risk for gestational diabetes.

Test-Taking Strategy: Use the process of elimination. Option 1 can be eliminated by recalling that fatigue normally occurs during pregnancy. Options 2, 3, and 4 are all risk factors for gestational diabetes. However, options 2 and 3 do not apply to this client. If you had difficulty with this question, review the risk factors associated with gestational diabetes.

Level of Cognitive Ability: Comprehension
Client Needs: Physiological Integrity
Integrated Concept/Process: Nursing Process/Data Collection
Content Area: Maternity

Reference:
Burroughs, A., & Leifer, G. (2002). *Maternity nursing* (8th ed.). Philadelphia: W.B. Saunders, p. 239.

---

326. A nurse in the emergency room is caring for a client who is bleeding from a scalp laceration obtained during a fall from a stepladder. The nurse takes which of the following actions first in the care of the wound?

1 Ask the client about timing of the last tetanus vaccination
2 Cleanse the wound with sterile normal saline
3 Prepare for suturing the area
4 Administer a prophylactic antibiotic

Answer: 2

Rationale: The initial nursing action is to cleanse the wound thoroughly with sterile normal saline. This removes dirt or foreign matter in the wound, and allows visualization of the size of the wound. Direct pressure is also applied initially as needed to control bleeding. If suturing is necessary, the surrounding hair may be shaved. Prophylactic antibiotics often are ordered. The date of the client's last tetanus shot are determined, and prophylaxis is given if needed as prescribed.

Test-Taking Strategy: Use the process of elimination. Note the key words *care of the wound* and *first*. The first action that focuses on actual care of the wound is option 2. Review care of the client with a laceration if you had difficulty with this question.

Level of Cognitive Ability: Application
Client Needs: Physiological Integrity
Integrated Concept/Process: Nursing Process/Implementation
Content Area: Adult Health/Integumentary

Reference:
Black, J., Hawks, J., & Keene, A. (2001). *Medical-surgical nursing: clinical management for positive outcomes* (6th ed.). Philadelphia: W.B. Saunders, p. 2280.

327. A nurse is assigned to assist in caring for a client who sustained a closed head injury 6 hours previously. After report, the nurse finds that the client has vomited, is confused, and complains of dizziness and a headache. Which of the following is the most important first nursing action?

1   Administer an antiemetic
2   Change the client's gown and bed linens
3   Reorient the client to surroundings
4   Notify the RN

Answer: 4

Rationale: The client with a closed head injury is at risk of developing increased intracranial pressure. This is evidenced by symptoms such as headache, dizziness, confusion, weakness, and vomiting. Because of the implications of the symptoms, the most important nursing action is to notify the RN, who then contacts the physician. Other nursing actions that are appropriate include physical care of the client and reorientation to surroundings.

Test-Taking Strategy: Use the process of elimination. Note the key words *most important first nursing action*. This directs you to prioritize nursing actions. Considering the closed head injury and the developing signs and symptoms, the nurse should suspect increased intracranial pressure. This should direct you to option 4. Review care of the client with a closed head injury if you had difficulty with this question.

Level of Cognitive Ability: Application
Client Needs: Physiological Integrity
Integrated Concept/Process: Nursing Process/Implementation
Content Area: Adult Health/Neurological

Reference:
Black, J., Hawks, J., & Keene, A. (2001). *Medical-surgical nursing: clinical management for positive outcomes* (6th ed.). Philadelphia: W.B. Saunders, p. 2038.

---

328. A client is brought into the emergency department after suffering a head injury. The first action by the nurse is to determine the client's:

1   Respiratory rate and depth
2   Pulse and blood pressure
3   Level of consciousness
4   Ability to move extremities

Answer: 1

Rationale: The first action of the nurse is to ensure that the client has an adequate airway and respiratory status. In rapid sequence, the client's circulatory status is evaluated, followed by evaluation of the neurological status.

Test-Taking Strategy: Use the ABCs (airway, breathing, and circulation). The correct option deals with the client's airway. Respiratory rate and depth support this action. Review initial care of the client with a head injury if you had difficulty with this question.

Level of Cognitive Ability: Application
Client Needs: Physiological Integrity
Integrated Concept/Process: Nursing Process/Implementation
Content Area: Adult Health/Neurological

Reference:
Black, J., Hawks, J., & Keene, A. (2001). *Medical-surgical nursing: clinical management for positive outcomes* (6th ed.). Philadelphia: W.B. Saunders, p. 2030.

---

329. A client with a spinal cord injury is at risk of developing foot drop. The nurse utilizes which of the following as the most effective preventive measure?

1   Heel protectors
2   Posterior splints
3   Pneumatic boots
4   Foot board

Answer: 2

Rationale: The most effective means of preventing foot drop are the use of posterior splints or high top sneakers. A foot board prevents plantar flexion, but also places the client more at risk for developing pressure ulcers of the feet. Pneumatic boots prevent deep vein thrombosis, but not foot drop. Heel protectors protect the skin but do not prevent foot drop.

Test-Taking Strategy: Use the process of elimination. Focus on the issue "prevention" of foot drop. This guides you to select the option that immobilizes the foot in a functional position while protecting the skin of the extremities. Review the purposes of these devices if you had difficulty with this question.

Level of Cognitive Ability: Application
Client Needs: Physiological Integrity
Integrated Concept/Process: Nursing Process/Implementation
Content Area: Fundamental Skills

Reference:
Black, J., Hawks, J., & Keene, A. (2001). *Medical-surgical nursing: clinical management for positive outcomes* (6th ed.). Philadelphia: W.B. Saunders, p. 1973.

---

330. A client is ambulatory and wearing a halo vest after cervical spine fracture. The nurse tells the client to avoid which of the following because it will present a risk for injury?
1 Bending at the waist
2 Using a walker
3 Wearing rubber-soled shoes
4 Scanning the environment

Answer: 1
Rationale: The client with a halo vest should avoid bending at the waist because the halo vest is heavy, and the client's trunk is limited in flexibility. It is helpful for the client to scan the environment visually because the client's peripheral vision is diminished from keeping the neck in a stationary position. Use of a walker and rubber-soled shoes may help prevent falls and injury; therefore, they are helpful also.

Test-Taking Strategy: Use the process of elimination and note the key word *avoid*. This guides you to look for an action that could put the client at risk for injury. Attempt to visualize this device and each of the items or actions in the options to assist in identifying how injury could be prevented. Review care of the client with a halo vest if you had difficulty with this question.

Level of Cognitive Ability: Application
Client Needs: Physiological Integrity
Integrated Concept/Process: Nursing Process/Implementation
Content Area: Adult Health/Neurological

Reference:
Black, J., Hawks, J., & Keene, A. (2001). *Medical-surgical nursing: clinical management for positive outcomes* (6th ed.). Philadelphia: W.B. Saunders, p. 2054.

---

331. A nurse is assisting in caring for the client who has undergone transphenoidal resection of a pituitary adenoma. The nurse measures which of the following to detect occurrence of the most common complication of this surgery?
1 Pulse rate
2 Temperature
3 Urine output
4 Oxygen saturation

Answer: 3
Rationale: The most common complication of surgery on the pituitary gland is temporary diabetes insipidus. This results from deficiency in antidiuretic hormone (ADH) secretion as a result of surgical trauma. The nurse measures the client's urine output to determine whether this complication is occurring.

Test-Taking Strategy: Use the process of elimination. Note the key words *most common complication*. Recall that the pituitary gland is responsible for the production of ADH. This allows you to eliminate each of the incorrect options and directs you to option 3. Review the complications of this surgical procedure if you had difficulty with this question.

Level of Cognitive Ability: Application
Client Needs: Physiological Integrity
Integrated Concept/Process: Nursing Process/Data Collection
Content Area: Adult Health/Neurological

Reference:
Black, J., Hawks, J., & Keene, A. (2001). *Medical-surgical nursing: clinical management for positive outcomes* (6th ed.). Philadelphia: W.B. Saunders, p. 1937.

---

332. A nurse is asked to prepare the laboratory requisition that will accompany an arterial blood gas specimen being sent to the laboratory for analysis. The nurse does not need to write which of the following pieces of information on the requisition?

1   The date and time the specimen was drawn
2   A list of client allergies
3   Any supplemental oxygen the client is receiving
4   The client's temperature

Answer: 2

Rationale: An arterial blood gas requisition usually contains information about the date and time the specimen was drawn, the client's temperature, whether the specimen was drawn on room air or using supplemental oxygen, and the ventilator settings (if the client is on a mechanical ventilator). A list of allergies is not needed because this will not affect the analysis of the results.

Test-Taking Strategy: Use the process of elimination. Note the key word *not*. Review the options from the viewpoint of the relevance of the item to the client's airway status or oxygen utilization. The client's allergies do not have a direct bearing on the laboratory results. Review this test if you had difficulty with this question.

Level of Cognitive Ability: Application
Client Needs: Physiological Integrity
Integrated Concept/Process: Nursing Process/Implementation
Content Area: Adult Health/Respiratory

Reference:
Chernecky, C., & Berger, B. (2001). *Laboratory tests and diagnostic procedures* (3rd ed.). Philadelphia: W.B. Saunders, p. 230.

---

333. To promote a successful postoperative recovery for a client who had one adrenal gland removed, the nurse plans to reinforce which of the following instructions?

1   The need for lifelong replacement of all adrenal hormones
2   Instructions about early signs of a wound infection
3   The reason for maintaining a diabetic diet
4   The proper application of an ostomy pouch

Answer: 2

Rationale: A client who is undergoing a unilateral adrenalectomy will be placed on corticosteroids temporarily to avoid a cortisol deficiency. These medications will be gradually weaned in the postoperative period until discontinued. Because of the antiinflammatory properties of corticosteroids, clients who undergo adrenalectomies are at increased risk of developing wound infections. Because of this increased risk of infection, it is important for the client to know measures to prevent infection, early signs of infection, and what to do if an infection seems to be present. Options 1, 3, and 4 are unnecessary after this surgical procedure.

Test-Taking Strategy: Use the process of elimination. Recalling that the hormones from the adrenal glands are needed for proper immune system function should assist in eliminating options 3 and 4. From this point, note that the question states that only one adrenal gland was removed. Remember that one gland can take over the function of two adrenal glands. This directs you to option 2. Review the function of the adrenal glands if you had difficulty with this question.

Level of Cognitive Ability: Application
Client Needs: Physiological Integrity
Integrated Concept/Process: Nursing Process/Planning
Content Area: Adult Health/Endocrine

Reference:
Black, J., Hawks, J., & Keene, A. (2001). *Medical-surgical nursing: clinical management for positive outcomes* (6th ed.). Philadelphia: W.B. Saunders, p. 1133.

---

334. A client has undergone transphenoidal surgery for a pituitary adenoma. The nurse plans to reinforce teaching and tells the client to:

1 Remove the nasal packing after 48 hours
2 Cough and deep breathe hourly
3 Take acetaminophen (Tylenol) for severe headache
4 Report frequent swallowing or post-nasal drip

Answer: 4

Rationale: The client should report frequent swallowing or postnasal drip after transphenoidal surgery because it could indicate cerebrospinal fluid (CSF) leakage. The surgeon removes the nasal packing, usually after 24 hours. The client should deep breathe, but coughing is contraindicated because it could cause increased intracranial pressure. The client also should report a severe headache because it could indicate increased intracranial pressure.

Test-Taking Strategy: Use the process of elimination. Recalling the anatomical location related to this surgery assists in providing the clue that the concern is increased intracranial pressure and the symptoms of CSF leak. This directs you to option 4. Review this surgical procedure if you had difficulty with this question.

Level of Cognitive Ability: Application
Client Needs: Physiological Integrity
Integrated Concept/Process: Nursing Process/Implementation
Content Area: Adult Health/Neurological

Reference:
Black, J., Hawks, J., & Keene, A. (2001). *Medical-surgical nursing: clinical management for positive outcomes* (6th ed.). Philadelphia: W.B. Saunders, p. 1937.

---

335. A client is receiving desmopressin (DDAVP) intranasally. The nurse would not use which of the following measurements to determine the effectiveness of this medication?

1 Urine output
2 Pupillary response
3 Presence of edema
4 Daily weight

Answer: 2

Rationale: DDAVP is an analog of vasopressin (antidiuretic hormone). It is used in the management of diabetes insipidus. The nurse monitors the client's fluid balance to determine the effectiveness of the medication. Fluid status can be evaluated by noting intake and urine output, daily weight, and presence of edema.

Test-Taking Strategy: Use the process of elimination and note the key word *not*. Remember that options that are similar are not likely to be correct. In this case, each of the incorrect options relates to fluid balance. The option that is different, the pupillary response, is the answer to the question as stated. Review this medication if you had difficulty with this question.

Level of Cognitive Ability: Analysis
Client Needs: Physiological Integrity
Integrated Concept/Process: Nursing Process/Evaluation
Content Area: Pharmacology

Reference:
Hodgson, B., & Kizior, R. (2003). *Saunders nursing drug handbook 2003.* Philadelphia: W.B. Saunders, p. 323.

336. As the nurse brings the 10:00 AM doses of furosemide (Lasix) and nifedipine (Procardia) into the room of an assigned client, the client asks the nurse for a dose of aluminum hydroxide gel, which is ordered on a PRN basis for dyspepsia. Which of the following actions by the nurse is most appropriate?
1 Administer all three medications at this time
2 Ask the client if it is possible to wait 1 hour for the aluminum hydroxide gel
3 Give the nifedipine, aluminum hydroxide, and furosemide in 1 hour
4 Give the furosemide, aluminum hydroxide, and nifedipine in 1 hour

Answer: 2
Rationale: Antacids such as aluminum hydroxide often interfere with the absorption of other medications. For this reason, antacids should be separated from other medications by at least 1 hour. Because of the diuretic action of the furosemide, and the antihypertensive action of the nifedipine, it is more important to receive them on time, if the client can tolerate waiting for the aluminum hydroxide gel.

Test-Taking Strategy: Use the process of elimination. To answer this question accurately, it is necessary to understand that antacids interfere with absorption of other medications. With this in mind, option 1 can be eliminated. From the remaining options, recalling that the diuretic and antihypertensive medication should be administered on time assists in directing you to option 2. Review the effects of antacids on medications if you had difficulty with this question.

Level of Cognitive Ability: Application
Client Needs: Physiological Integrity
Integrated Concept/Process: Nursing Process/Implementation
Content Area: Pharmacology

Reference:
Hodgson, B., & Kizior, R. (2003). *Saunders nursing drug handbook 2003.* Philadelphia: W.B. Saunders, p. 38.

337. A client has been placed on medication therapy with amitriptyline (Elavil). The nurse monitors the client for which common side effect of this medication?
1 Drowsiness and fatigue
2 Diarrhea
3 Hypertension
4 Polyuria

Answer: 1
Rationale: Common side effects of medication therapy with amitriptyline (a tricyclic antidepressant) are the central nervous system effects of drowsiness, fatigue, lethargy, and sedation. Other common side effects include dry mouth or eyes, blurred vision, hypotension, and constipation.

Test-Taking Strategy: Use the process of elimination. Recalling that this medication is an antidepressant directs you to option 1. Review the side effects of this medication if you had difficulty with this question.

Level of Cognitive Ability: Application
Client Needs: Physiological Integrity
Integrated Concept/Process: Nursing Process/Implementation
Content Area: Pharmacology

Reference:
Hodgson, B., & Kizior, R. (2003). *Saunders nursing drug handbook 2003.* Philadelphia: W.B. Saunders, p. 54.

338. A client with a 5-year history of depression has been admitted to the nursing unit on a voluntary basis. When collecting data from the client, which of the following comments by the nurse would best obtain data about the recent sleeping patterns of the client?

Answer: 3
Rationale: Option 3 is open-ended and allows the client to say what is most relevant and important at the time. Option 1 could lead to a one-word answer, and that is not the desired response for adequate data collection. One night of sleep does not tell the nurse how the pattern has been over time. Anyone may or may not sleep well for one night, and that sleep or loss of sleep does

1   "Have you been having trouble sleeping at home?"
2   "How did you sleep last night?"
3   "Tell me about your sleeping patterns."
4   "You look as if you could use some sleep."

not indicate a problem. Option 4 could be interpreted by the depressed person as a negative statement and could close further communication needed for thorough data collection.

Test-Taking Strategy: Use therapeutic communication techniques. Select the option that allows the client to take the lead in the conversation. Also, note that option 3 is the only open-ended question. Review therapeutic communication techniques if you had difficulty with this question.

Level of Cognitive Ability: Application
Client Needs: Physiological Integrity
Integrated Concept/Process: Nursing Process/Data Collection
Content Area: Mental Health

Reference:
Varcarolis, E. (2002). *Foundations of psychiatric mental health nursing* (4th ed.). Philadelphia: W.B. Saunders, p. 254.

---

339. When administering an intramuscular (IM) injection in the gluteal muscle, the best position for the client to assume to relax the muscle is:
1   On the side with the knee of the uppermost leg flexed
2   On the side with the knee of the lowermost leg flexed
3   Prone with a toe-in position
4   In the Sims' position with a toe-in position

Answer: 3
Rationale: A prone toe-in position promotes internal rotation of the hips, which relaxes the muscle and makes the injection less painful. Options 1, 2, and 4 will not relax the muscle.

Test-Taking Strategy: Use the process of elimination. The key words are *relax the muscle.* Visualize each position described in the options to direct you to option 3. If you are unfamiliar with the position for administering IM medications, review this procedure.

Level of Cognitive Ability: Application
Client Needs: Physiological Integrity
Integrated Concept/Process: Nursing Process/Implementation
Content Area: Fundamental Skills

Reference:
Potter, P., & Perry, A. (2001). *Fundamentals of nursing* (5th ed.). St. Louis: Mosby, p. 944.

---

340. Which nursing intervention is appropriate when caring for a child after a tepid tub bath to treat hyperthermia?
1   Place the child in bed and cover with a blanket
2   Leave the child uncovered for 15 minutes
3   Help the child put on a cotton sleep shirt
4   Take the child's axillary temperature in 2 hours

Answer: 3
Rationale: Cotton is a lightweight material that protects the child from becoming chilled after the bath. Option 1 is incorrect because a blanket is heavy and may increase the child's body temperature and further increase metabolism. Option 2 is incorrect because the child should not be left uncovered. Option 4 is incorrect because the child's temperature should be reassessed a half-hour after the bath.

Test-Taking Strategy: Use the process of elimination. Eliminate option 1 because of the word *blanket.* Eliminate option 2 because the child should not be left uncovered. Eliminate option 4 because the child's temperature should be reassessed in a half-hour. If you had difficulty with this question, review care to a child with hyperthermia.

Level of Cognitive Ability: Application
Client Needs: Physiological Integrity
Integrated Concept/Process: Nursing Process/Implementation
Content Area: Child Health

Reference:
Schulte, E., Price, D., & Gwin, J. (2001). *Thompson's pediatric nursing* (8th ed.). Philadelphia: W.B. Saunders, p. 352.

---

341. A nurse is caring for an infant who has diarrhea. Which of these clinical manifestations should a nurse recognize as the earliest symptom of dehydration?
1 Apical pulse rate of 160 beats per minute
2 Capillary refill of 2 seconds
3 Gray, mottled skin
4 Cool extremities

Answer: 1
Rationale: Dehydration causes interstitial fluid to shift to the vascular compartment in an attempt to maintain fluid volume. Circulatory failure occurs when the body is unable to compensate for fluid lost. The blood pressure decreases, and the pulse increases. This is followed by peripheral symptoms. Options 2, 3, and 4 are incorrect. These findings reflect diminished peripheral circulation.

Test-Taking Strategy: Use the process of elimination. Focus on the key word *earliest*. Option 1 is most directly relates to the ABCs (airway, breathing, and circulation). If you had difficulty with this question, review the early signs of dehydration.

Level of Cognitive Ability: Comprehension
Client Needs: Physiological Integrity
Integrated Concept/Process: Nursing Process/Data Collection
Content Area: Child Health

Reference:
McKinney, E., Ashwill, J., Murray, S. et al. (2000). *Maternal-child nursing.* Philadelphia: W.B. Saunders, pp. 831; 1094.

---

342. A nurse administers acetylsalicylic acid (Aspirin) as prescribed before a percutaneous transluminal coronary angioplasty (PTCA) for coronary artery disease to:
1 Prevent postprocedural hyperthermia
2 Relieve postprocedural pain
3 Prevent thrombus formation
4 Prevent inflammation of the puncture site

Answer: 3
Rationale: Before PTCA, the client is usually given an anticoagulant, commonly aspirin, to help reduce the risk of occlusion of the artery during the procedure. Options 1, 2, and 4 are unrelated to the purpose of administering aspirin to this client.

Test-Taking Strategy: Use the process of elimination. Recalling the action and properties of aspirin assists in directing you to the correct option. Additionally, awareness of the potential complications of a PTCA and nursing measures to prevent these complications assists in answering the question. If you had difficulty with this question, review the action and uses of aspirin and the complications associated with PTCA.

Level of Cognitive Ability: Application
Client Needs: Physiological Integrity
Integrated Concept/Process: Nursing Process/Implementation
Content Area: Adult Health/Cardiovascular

Reference:
Black, J., Hawks, J., & Keene, A. (2001). *Medical-surgical nursing: clinical management for positive outcomes* (6th ed.). Philadelphia: W.B. Saunders, p. 1524.

343. A nurse administers acetaminophen (Tylenol) as prescribed before the administration of topical nitrates because:
1 Headache is a common side effect of nitrates
2 Acetaminophen potentiates the therapeutic effects of nitrates
3 Acetaminophen does not interfere with platelet action as aspirin (acetylsalicylic acid) does
4 Fever usually accompanies myocardial infarction

Answer: 1
Rationale: Headache occurs as a side effect of nitrates. Acetaminophen may be given before nitrates to prevent headaches or minimize the discomfort from the headaches. Options 2, 3, and 4 do not identify the purpose for administering acetaminophen.

Test-Taking Strategy: Use the process of elimination. Focusing on the issue of the question and recalling that headache is a common side effect of nitrates assists in directing you to the correct option. If you had difficulty with this question, review the side effects of nitrates and the purpose of administering acetaminophen before these medications.

Level of Cognitive Ability: Application
Client Needs: Physiological Integrity
Integrated Concept/Process: Nursing Process/Implementation
Content Area: Pharmacology

Reference:
Clark, J., Quiena, S., & Karb, V. (2002). *Pharmacologic basis of nursing practice* (6th ed.). St Louis: Mosby, p. 188.

344. A nurse is caring for a male client with urolithiasis. Important care and teaching includes which of the following?
1 Turn, cough, and deep breathe every 2 hours
2 Restrict physical activities
3 Strain all urine from each voiding
4 Weight the client daily

Answer: 3
Rationale: Obstruction of the urinary tract is the primary problem associated with urolithiasis. Stones recovered from straining urine can be analyzed and can provide direction for prevention of further stone formation. Activities should not be restricted. Options 1 and 4 are not specifically related to the issue of the question.

Test-Taking Strategy: Use the process of elimination and select the option that is associated most commonly with the client with urolithiasis. In this situation, straining all urine is the most common or typical intervention. If you had difficulty with this question, review care of the client with urolithiasis.

Level of Cognitive Ability: Application
Client Needs: Physiological Integrity
Integrated Concept/Process: Nursing Process/Implementation
Content Area: Adult Health/Renal

Reference:
Black, J., Hawks, J., & Keene, A. (2001). *Medical-surgical nursing: clinical management for positive outcomes* (6th ed.). Philadelphia: W.B. Saunders, p. 825.

345. A nurse is assigned to assist in caring for a newly delivered breastfeeding infant. Which of the following interventions performed by the nurse best prevents jaundice in this infant?
1 Encouraging the mother to offer a formula supplement after each breastfeeding session
2 Keeping the infant NPO until the second period of reactivity

Answer: 4
Rationale: To help facilitate a decrease in jaundice, the mother should breastfeed the infant frequently in the immediate birth period, because colostrum is a natural laxative and helps promote the passage of meconium. Offering the infant a formula supplement will cause nipple confusion and decrease the amount of milk produced by the mother. Breastfeeding should begin as soon as possible after birth while the infant is in the first period of reactivity. Delaying breastfeeding decreases the production of prolactin, which decreases the mother's milk production. Phototherapy requires a

3 Placing the infant under phototherapy

4 Requesting that the mother breast-feed the infant every 2 to 3 hours

physician's order and is not implemented until bilirubin levels are 12 mg/dL or higher in the healthy term infant.

Test-Taking Strategy: Use the process of elimination. Recalling the pathophysiology related to jaundice and the nursing interventions used to prevent jaundice in the breastfeeding infant directs you to option 4. If you had difficulty with this question, review these important nursing interventions.

Level of Cognitive Ability: Application
Client Needs: Physiological Integrity
Integrated Concept/Process: Nursing Process/Implementation
Content Area: Maternity

Reference:
Murray, S., McKinney, E. & Gorrie, T. (2002). *Foundations of maternal members nursing* (3rd ed). Philadelphia: W. B. Saunders, p. 592.

---

346. A nurse is caring for a client scheduled for arthroscopy. In the postoperative period, the priority nursing action is which of the following?

1 Monitor intake and output

2 Monitor for numbness or tingling

3 Check the complete blood count results

4 Check the dressing at the surgical site

Answer: 2
Rationale: The priority nursing action is to monitor the affected area for numbness or tingling. Options 1, 3, and 4 are also components of postoperative care but considering the options presented, are not the priority.

Test-Taking Strategy: Note the key word *priority*. Use the ABCs (airway, breathing, and circulation) to answer the question. This assists in directing you to option 2. If you had difficulty with this question, review nursing care after arthroscopy.

Level of Cognitive Ability: Application
Client Needs: Physiological Integrity
Integrated Concept/Process: Nursing Process/Implementation
Content Area: Adult Health/Musculoskeletal

Reference:
Ignatauicius, D., & Workman, M. (2002). *Medical surgical nursing: critical thinking for collaborative care* (4th ed.). Philadelphia: W. B. Saunders, p. 1091.

---

347. A nurse is caring for a client with active tuberculosis who has started medication therapy that includes rifampin (Rifadin). Which of the following is an expected observation?

1 Orange-colored body secretions

2 Bilious urine

3 Yellow sclera

4 Clay-colored stools

Answer: 1
Rationale: Secretions are orange in color when the client is taking rifampin. The client should be instructed that the secretions will be orange in color and can permanently discolor soft contact lenses. Options 2, 3, and 4 are not expected observations.

Test-Taking Strategy: Use the process of elimination. Options 2, 3, and 4 are not expected observations. Also, note that these options are similar in that they are all symptoms of intrahepatic obstruction as seen in viral hepatitis. If you had difficulty with this question, review this important medication.

Level of Cognitive Ability: Comprehension
Client Needs: Physiological Integrity
Integrated Concept/Process: Nursing Process/Data Collection
Content Area: Adult Health/Respiratory

Reference:
Hodgson, B., & Kizior, R. (2003). *Saunders nursing drug handbook 2003.* Philadelphia: W.B. Saunders, p. 979.

---

348. A nurse sends a sputum specimen for culture to the laboratory from a client with suspected active tuberculosis (TB). The nurse is told that the results report that *Mycobacterium tuberculosis* is cultured. The nurse determines that these results are:
1   Positive for active tuberculosis
2   Inconclusive until a repeat sputum is sent
3   Not reliable unless the client has also had a positive Mantoux test
4   Positive for a less virulent strain of tuberculosis

Answer: 1
Rationale: Culture of *Mycobacterium tuberculosis* from sputum or other body secretions or tissue is the only method of confirming the diagnosis. Options 2 and 4 are incorrect statements. The Mantoux test is used in supporting the diagnosis, but does not confirm active disease.

Test-Taking Strategy: Recalling that *Mycobacterium tuberculosis* is the bacteria responsible for tuberculosis and that culture of the bacteria from sputum confirms the diagnosis directs you to option 1. Because tuberculosis affects the respiratory system, it makes sense that the bacteria will be found in the sputum if the client has active disease, therefore confirming the diagnosis. If you had difficulty with this question, review the diagnostic tests associated with active TB.

Level of Cognitive Ability: Analysis
Client Needs: Physiological Integrity
Integrated Concept/Process: Nursing Process/Data Collection
Content Area: Adult Health/Respiratory

Reference:
Black, J., Hawks, J., & Keene, A. (2001). *Medical-surgical nursing: clinical management for positive outcomes* (6th ed.). Philadelphia: W.B. Saunders, p. 1719.

---

349. Which of the following nursing interventions should receive highest priority in caring for the client with applied wrist restraints?
1   Providing range of motion exercises
2   Removing the restraints periodically
3   Applying lotion to the skin under the restraints
4   Assessing the color, sensation, and pulses distal to the restraint

Answer: 4
Rationale: Assessing the color, sensation, and pulses distal to the restraint provides data about the potential complication of neurovascular compromise that is associated with the use of restraints. Of the options presented, this is the priority. All of the other interventions should be implemented as well. Remember that restraints, if used, should be removed at least every 2 hours or as specified by the agency policy and procedure.

Test-Taking Strategy: Use the ABCs (airway, breathing, and circulation). Assessing color, sensation, and pulses is the highest priority because it determines circulation. Review care of the client with wrist restraints if you had difficulty with this question.

Level of Cognitive Ability: Application
Client Needs: Physiological Integrity
Integrated Concept/Process: Nursing Process/Implementation
Content Area: Fundamental Skills

Reference:
Potter, P., & Perry, A. (2001). *Fundamentals of nursing* (5th ed.). St. Louis: Mosby, p. 1035.

350. A nurse is preparing to administer betamethasone (Celestone) by the IM route as prescribed to a 30-week gestation client in preterm labor. The client asks the nurse why she is receiving steroids. The nurse responds by telling the client that the betamethasone will:

1   "Help your baby's lungs mature faster."
2   "Prevent your membranes from rupturing."
3   "Decrease the incidence of fetal infection."
4   "Help stop your labor contractions."

Answer: 1

Rationale: Respiratory distress syndrome is the most common cause of morbidity and mortality in preterm infants. Betamethasone, a corticosteroid, is given to enhance fetal lung maturity. The medication's optimal benefits begin 24 hours after initial therapy. Options 2 and 3 are incorrect. Also, betamethasone can actually mask signs of infection. Betamethasone does not prevent rupture of the membranes. Even though betamethasone may be given during the time that tocolytic agents are administered, it does not inhibit preterm labor.

Test-Taking Strategy: Use the process of elimination. The word *preterm* may assist you in recalling that this medication is given to enhance fetal lung maturity. Review the action of this medication if you had difficulty with this question.

Level of Cognitive Ability: Application
Client Needs: Physiological Integrity
Integrated Concept/Process: Nursing Process/Implementation
Content Area: Maternity

Reference:
McKinney, E., Ashwill, J., & Murray, S. et al. (2000). *Maternal-child nursing.* Philadelphia: W.B. Saunders, p. 702.

---

351. A nurse is caring for a client with a history of congestive heart failure. The physician has ordered furosemide (Lasix) 40 mg daily to prevent fluid overload. Which laboratory value should be closely monitored by the nurse?

1   Glucose
2   Sodium
3   Potassium
4   Magnesium

Answer: 3

Rationale: Furosemide is a non–potassium-sparing diuretic and insufficient replacement may lead to hypokalemia. Options 1, 2, and 4 are not a concern when administering this medication.

Test-Taking Strategy: Note that the question states that furosemide (Lasix) is ordered to prevent fluid overload. This indicates that this medication is a diuretic. Remember, with a non–potassium-sparing diuretic, the most critical laboratory value to monitor is the potassium level. Review this medication if you had difficulty with this question.

Level of Cognitive Ability: Comprehension
Client Needs: Physiological Integrity
Integrated Concept/Process: Nursing Process/Data Collection
Content Area: Pharmacology

Reference:
Hodgson, B., & Kizior, R. (2003). *Saunders nursing drug handbook 2003.* Philadelphia: W.B. Saunders, p. 501.

---

352. A nurse is reinforcing teaching to a client who is being discharged and going home with orders for self-administration of enoxaparin (Lovenox) 30 mg BID SC. The nurse plans to tell the client to monitor for which of the following highest priority items?

Answer: 2

Rationale: Enoxaparin is an anticoagulant. A common side effect of anticoagulant therapy is bleeding. Because of this, the nurse instructs the client to monitor for signs that could indicate bleeding, such as bleeding gums, bruising, hematuria, or dark tarry stools. Options 1, 3, and 4 are not associated with the use of this medication.

1	Headaches
2	Bleeding gums or bruising
3	Constipation
4	Nausea or vomiting

Test-Taking Strategy: Use the process of elimination. Note the key words *highest priority*. Recalling that this medication is an anticoagulant directs you to option 2. Review this medication if you had difficulty with this question.

Level of Cognitive Ability: Application
Client Needs: Physiological Integrity
Integrated Concept/Process: Nursing Process/Planning
Content Area: Pharmacology

Reference:
Hodgson, B., & Kizior, R. (2003). *Saunders nursing drug handbook 2003.* Philadelphia: W.B. Saunders, p. 399.

---

353. A client has been given a prescription for sulfasalazine (Azulfidine) for the treatment of ulcerative colitis. While conducting medication teaching, the nurse asks the client if the client has a history of allergy to:
1 Salicylates or acetaminophen
2 Sulfonamides or salicylates
3 Shellfish or calcium channel blockers
4 Histamine receptor antagonists or beta-blockers

Answer: 2
Rationale: The client who has been prescribed sulfasalazine should be checked for a history of allergy to either sulfonamides or salicylates, because of the chemical composition of the medication. The other options are incorrect.

Test-Taking Strategy: Use the process of elimination. Note the relationship of *sulfasalazine* in the question and *sulfonamides* in the correct option. Review the contraindications associated with the use of this medication if you had difficulty with this question.

Level of Cognitive Ability: Application
Client Needs: Physiological Integrity
Integrated Concept/Process: Nursing Process/Data Collection
Content Area: Pharmacology

Reference:
Hodgson, B., & Kizior, R. (2003). *Saunders nursing drug handbook 2003.* Philadelphia: W.B. Saunders, p. 1041.

---

354. A nurse is caring for a client who is experiencing an alteration in the oral mucous membranes. The nurse avoids using which of the following items when giving mouth care to this client?
1 Nonalcoholic mouthwash
2 Soft toothbrush
3 Lip moistener
4 Lemon-glycerin swabs

Answer: 4
Rationale: The nurse avoids using lemon-glycerin swabs for the client with altered oral mucous membranes because they dry the membranes further and could cause pain. Items that are helpful include a soft toothbrush to prevent trauma, lip moistener to prevent lip cracking, and soothing cleansing rinses, such as nonalcoholic mouthwash.

Test-Taking Strategy: Use the process of elimination and note the key word *avoids*. Evaluate each of the options in terms of the likelihood of causing trauma to at-risk tissue. Review the principles of mouth care if you had difficulty with this question.

Level of Cognitive Ability: Application
Client Needs: Physiological Integrity
Integrated Concept/Process: Nursing Process/Implementation
Content Area: Fundamental Skills

Reference:
deWit, S. (2001). *Fundamental concepts and skills for nursing.* Philadelphia: W.B. Saunders, p. 300.

---

355. A client has asymptomatic hypocalcemia from decreased dietary intake. The nurse giving the client an oral calcium supplement should administer this medication with:

1 Water
2 A carbonated beverage
3 Fruit juice
4 Any lactose-free product

Answer: 1
Rationale: Calcium supplements should be taken with a large glass of water. Administration with or after meals promotes absorption. Options 2, 3, and 4 are incorrect.

Test-Taking Strategy: Use the process of elimination. Recalling absorption factors associated with the administration of calcium will direct you to option 1. Review the administration of oral calcium if you had difficulty with this question.

Level of Cognitive Ability: Application
Client Needs: Physiological Integrity
Integrated Concept/Process: Nursing Process/Implementation
Content Area: Pharmacology

Reference:
Lehore, R. (2001). *Pharmacology for nursing care* (4th ed.). Philadelphia: W.B. Saunders, p. 818.

---

356. A nurse has an order to administer two ophthalmic medications to the client who has undergone eye surgery. The nurse waits for how many minutes after the first medication before giving the second?

1 One
2 Two
3 Five
4 Ten

Answer: 3
Rationale: The nurse waits for 5 minutes between administration of the two separate ophthalmic medications. This allows for adequate ocular absorption of the medication, and prevents the second medication from flushing out the first.

Test-Taking Strategy: Specific knowledge of time frames for administration of ocular medications is needed to answer this question. Review the principles of ocular medication administration if you had difficulty with this question.

Level of Cognitive Ability: Application
Client Needs: Physiological Integrity
Integrated Concept/Process: Nursing Process/Implementation
Content Area: Adult Health/Eye

Reference:
Gutierrez, K., & Queener, S. (2003). *Pharmacology for nursing practice.* St. Louis & Mosby, p. 1091.

---

357. Serum calcium levels indicate that the client has hypercalcemia. The nurse avoids doing which of the following, which would aggravate the condition?

1 Limit sodium intake
2 Encourage increased fluid intake
3 Withhold calcium carbonate antacids
4 Limit calcium containing foods

Answer: 1
Rationale: Sodium should not be limited for the client with hypercalcemia, unless sodium is contraindicated, such as with heart failure. Retention of sodium promotes loss of calcium by the kidneys. Fluid intake is increased to help flush calcium from the body, and calcium-containing medications and foods are withheld or limited, respectively.

Test-Taking Strategy: Use the process of elimination. Note the key word *avoids.* Focusing on the client's diagnosis assists in eliminating options 2, 3, and 4. Review the treatment for hypercalcemia if you had difficulty with this question.

Level of Cognitive Ability: Application
Client Needs: Physiological Integrity
Integrated Concept/Process: Nursing Process/Implementation
Content Area: Fundamental Skills

Reference:
deWit, S. (2001). *Fundamental concepts and skills for nursing.* Philadelphia: W.B. Saunders, p. 448.

---

358. A client receiving lithium (Eskalith) is noted to be drowsy, has slurred speech, and is experiencing muscle twitching and impaired coordination. Which of the following actions should the nurse take?
1 Double the next lithium dose
2 Increase fluids to 2000 mL per day
3 Hold one dose of lithium
4 Contact the physician

Answer: 4
Rationale: Signs and symptoms of lithium toxicity include vomiting and diarrhea, and nervous system changes such as slurred speech, incoordination, drowsiness, muscle weakness, or twitching. The physician should be notified before administering any further doses. As long as there are no contraindications, the client should routinely take in between 2000 to 3000 mL of fluid per day while taking this medication.

Test-Taking Strategy: Use the process of elimination. Eliminate options 1 and 3 first recalling that it is not common practice to either hold one dose or double a medication dose without a specific order. From the remaining options, recalling the signs of lithium toxicity directs you to option 4. Review the signs of toxicity of this medication if you had difficulty with this question.

Level of Cognitive Ability: Application
Client Needs: Physiological Integrity
Integrated Concept/Process: Nursing Process/Implementation
Content Area: Pharmacology

Reference:
Hodgson, B., & Kizior, R. (2003). *Saunders nursing drug handbook 2003.* Philadelphia: W.B. Saunders, p. 672.

---

359. A client has started medication therapy with metoclopramide (Reglan). The nurse monitors which of the following items to determine the effectiveness of therapy?
1 Urine output
2 Breath sounds
3 Complaints of headache
4 Episodes of vomiting

Answer: 4
Rationale: Metoclopramide is an antiemetic. The nurse monitors to see whether the client has experienced a decrease or absence of vomiting to determine the effectiveness of therapy. Options 1, 2, and 3 are not associated with the use of this medication.

Test-Taking Strategy: Use the process of elimination. Knowledge that this medication is an antiemetic directs you to the correct option. Review this medication if you had difficulty with this question.

Level of Cognitive Ability: Application
Client Needs: Physiological Integrity
Integrated Concept/Process: Nursing Process/Implementation
Content Area: Pharmacology

Reference:
Hodgson, B., & Kizior, R. (2003). *Saunders nursing drug handbook 2003.* Philadelphia: W.B. Saunders, p. 732.

---

360. When checking the height of a cane before ambulating a client, the nurse checks to be sure that the top of the cane is parallel to the:
1   Greater trochanter of the femur
2   Midline between the greater trochanter and the waist
3   Waistline
4   Uppermost level of the thigh

Answer: 1

Rationale: The top of the cane should reach the level of the greater trochanter of the client's femur. Options 2, 3, and 4 are incorrect.

Test-Taking Strategy: Use the process of elimination. Visualize each of the positions described in the options. Eliminate options 2 and 3 because these positions are too high. Conversely, eliminate option 4 because this position is too low. Review safe procedures for ambulation with a cane if you had difficulty with this question.

Level of Cognitive Ability: Application
Client Needs: Physiological Integrity
Integrated Concept/Process: Nursing Process/Implementation
Content Area: Fundamental Skills

Reference:
Potter, P., & Perry, A. (2001). *Fundamentals of nursing* (5th ed.). St. Louis: Mosby, p. 1008.

---

361. When ambulating a client, the best position for the nurse in assisting the client is to stand:
1   Behind the client
2   In front of the client
3   On the unaffected side of the client
4   On the affected side of the client

Answer: 4

Rationale: When walking with the client, the nurse should stand on the affected side. The nurse should position the free hand at the shoulder area so that the client can be pulled toward the nurse in the event that the client falls forward. The client is instructed to look up and outward rather than at his or her feet.

Test-Taking Strategy: Use the process of elimination. Eliminate options 1 and 2 because neither position places the nurse in a strategic position should the client lose balance and begin to fall forward or backward. Recalling that support is needed on the affected side assists in directing you to the correct option from those remaining. Review ambulation procedures if you had difficulty with this question.

Level of Cognitive Ability: Application
Client Needs: Physiological Integrity
Integrated Concept/Process: Nursing Process/Implementation
Content Area: Fundamental Skills

Reference:
Potter, P., & Perry, A. (2001). *Fundamentals of nursing* (5th ed.). St. Louis: Mosby, p. 1006.

---

362. A nurse is preparing to administer an intramuscular injection as prescribed to a 2-year-old child. The nurse selects which best site to administer the medication?
1   Ventral gluteal muscle
2   Dorsal gluteal muscle

Answer: 4

Rationale: The vastus lateralis muscle is well developed at birth. It is the best choice for all age groups, but should always be used in children younger than 3 years. This muscle is able to tolerate larger volumes and is not located near vital structures such as nerves and blood vessels.

| 3 | Deltoid muscle |
| 4 | Vastus lateralis muscle |

Test-Taking Strategy: The key word *best* requires prioritizing. Because options 1 and 2 are similar, neither are likely to be correct. Remember that the deltoid is a smaller muscle near important nerves and is generally not a preferred site for an IM injection. If you had difficulty with this question, review the procedure for administering IM injections in a 2-year-old.

Level of Cognitive Ability: Application
Client Needs: Physiological Integrity
Integrated Concept/Process: Nursing Process/Implementation
Content Area: Child Health

Reference:
Wong, D., & Hockenberry-Eaton, M. (2001). *Wong's essentials of pediatric nursing* (6th ed.). St. Louis: Mosby, p. 786.

---

363. Which statement by an adolescent indicates a need for follow-up data collection and intervention?
1 "I find myself very moody; I'm happy one minute and crying the next."
2 "I can't seem to wake up in the morning. I would sleep until noon if I could."
3 "I don't eat anything with fat in it and I've lost 8 pounds in 2 weeks!"
4 "When I get stressed out about school, I just like to be alone."

Answer: 3
Rationale: Undereating is a common problem in teenagers who have heightened awareness of body image and receive peer pressure to try excessively restrictive diets. Omitting all fat and major weight loss during a time of growth suggest inadequate nutrition and a possible eating disorder.

Test-Taking Strategy: Use the process of elimination and note the words *need for follow-up.* Select the option that indicates a problem or abnormality. Options 1, 2, and 4 are common and normal behaviors or feelings during adolescence. If you had difficulty with this question, review the development stage of the adolescent.

Level of Cognitive Ability: Comprehension
Client Needs: Physiological Integrity
Integrated Concept/Process: Nursing Process/Data Collection
Content Area: Child Health

Reference:
Wong, D., & Hockenberry-Eaton, M. (2001). *Wong's essentials of pediatric nursing* (6th ed.). St. Louis: Mosby, p. 524.

---

364. A nurse is caring for a client who has bipolar disorder and is having a manic episode. The most appropriate menu choice for this client would be which of the following?
1 Scrambled eggs, orange juice, coffee with cream and sugar
2 Cheeseburger, banana, milk
3 Beef stew, fruit salad, tea
4 Macaroni and cheese, apple, milk

Answer: 2
Rationale: The client in a manic state often has inadequate food and fluid intake because of physical agitation. Foods that the client can eat "on the run" are best because the client is too active to sit at meals and use utensils.

Test-Taking Strategy: Use the process of elimination and focus on the client's diagnosis. Recall that the client in a manic state should not have caffeine-containing products; therefore eliminate options 1 and 3. From the remaining options, note that option 2 identifies finger foods. Remember the concept of "finger foods" with these clients. Review the nutritional needs of the client with mania if you had difficulty with this question.

Level of Cognitive Ability: Application
Client Needs: Physiological Integrity

Integrated Concept/Process: Nursing Process/Implementation
Content Area: Mental Health

Reference:
Bauer, B., & Hill, S. (2000). *Mental health nursing.* Philadelphia: W.B. Saunders, p. 270.

---

365. A nurse is caring for a client who is receiving lithium carbonate (Eskalith). The nurse is told that the results of the lithium level is 1.8 mEq /L. The nurse determines these results as:
1   Within normal limits
2   Higher than normal limits indicating toxicity
3   Lower than normal limits
4   Insignificant

Answer: 2
Rationale: The therapeutic level for lithium is 0.6 to 1.2 mEq/L. A level of 1.8 indicates toxicity and requires that the medication be withheld and the blood work repeated. The physician is also notified.

Test-Taking Strategy: Knowledge of the therapeutic lithium level is necessary to answer this question. Review this therapeutic level if you had difficulty with this question.

Level of Cognitive Ability: Comprehension
Client Needs: Physiological Integrity
Integrated Concept/Process: Nursing Process/Evaluation
Content Area: Pharmacology

Reference:
Hodgson, B., & Kizior, R. (2003). *Saunders nursing drug handbook 2003.* Philadelphia: W.B. Saunders, p. 672.

---

366. A client calls the physician's office and tells the nurse that she found an area that looks like the peel of an orange when performing breast self-examination and that she found no other changes. The nurse should:
1   Tell the client there is nothing to worry about
2   Arrange for the client to be seen by the physician as soon as possible
3   Tell the client to take her temperature and call back if she has a fever
4   Tell the client to point the area out to the physician at her next regularly scheduled appointment

Answer: 2
Rationale: Peau d'orange or the orange peel appearance of the skin over the breast is associated with late breast cancer. Realizing that this is what the client is describing, you should arrange for the client to be seen by the physician as soon as possible. Peau d'orange is not indicative of an infection; therefore it is not necessary to have the client take her temperature.

Test-Taking Strategy: Use the process of elimination. Recalling that Peau d'orange is a sign of breast cancer assists in directing you to option 2. If you had difficulty with this question, review the signs of breast cancer.

Level of Cognitive Ability: Application
Client Needs: Physiological Integrity
Integrated Concept/Process: Nursing Process/Implementation
Content Area: Adult Health/Oncology

Reference:
Lewis, S., Heitkemper, M., & Dirksen, S. (2004). *Medical surgical nursing: assessment and management of clinical problems* (6th ed). St Louis: Mosby, p. 1368.

---

367. A client with Cushing's syndrome is being instructed by the nurse about follow-up care. Which statement by the client indicates a need for further instruction?

Answer: 2
Rationale: Hypokalemia is associated with this condition and the client should consume foods high in potassium. Clients experience activity intolerance, osteoporosis, and frequent bruising. Fluid volume excess results from water and sodium

1   "I should avoid contact sports."
2   "I should avoid foods rich in potassium."
3   "I should check my ankles for swelling."
4   "I should check my blood sugar regularly."

retention. Hyperglycemia is caused by an increased cortisol secretion.

Test-Taking Strategy: Use the process of elimination. Note the key words *need for further instruction.* Recalling the pathophysiology associated with this disorder directs you to option 2. If you had difficulty with this question, review this disorder.

Level of Cognitive Ability: Comprehension
Client Needs: Physiological Integrity
Integrated Concept/Process: Nursing Process/Evaluation
Content Area: Adult Health/Endocrine

Reference:
Black, J., Hawks, J., & Keene, A. (2001). *Medical-surgical nursing: clinical management for positive outcomes* (6th ed.). Philadelphia: W.B. Saunders, p. 1126.

---

368. A client with aldosteronism is being treated with spironolactone (Aldactone). Which of the following parameters indicates to the nurse that the treatment is effective?
1   A decrease in blood pressure
2   A decrease in sodium excretion
3   A decrease in plasma potassium
4   A decrease in body metabolism

Answer: 1
Rationale: Spironolactone antagonizes the effect of aldosterone and decreases circulating volume by inhibiting tubular reabsorption of sodium and water. It lowers the blood pressure. It increases excretion of sodium and plasma potassium. It has no effect on body metabolism.

Test-Taking Strategy: Use the process of elimination. Note the key word *effective.* Recalling that this medication is also used in hypertensive conditions directs you to the correct option. Review the effects of this medication if you had difficulty with this question.

Level of Cognitive Ability: Comprehensive
Client Needs: Physiological Integrity
Integrated Concept/Process: Nursing Process/Evaluation
Content Area: Pharmacology

Reference:
Hodgson, B., & Kizior, R. (2003). *Saunders nursing drug handbook 2003.* Philadelphia: W.B. Saunders, p. 1028.

---

369. A client with cancer tells the nurse that the food on the meal tray tastes "funny." Which intervention by the nurse is appropriate?
1   Keep the client NPO
2   Administer an antiemetic as ordered
3   Provide oral hygiene care
4   Ask for an order for total parenteral nutrition (TPN)

Answer: 3
Rationale: Cancer treatments may cause distortion of taste. Frequent oral hygiene aids in preserving taste function. Keeping a client NPO increases nutritional risks. Antiemetics are used when nausea and vomiting are a problem. TPN is used when oral intake is not possible.

Test-Taking Strategy: Use the process of elimination and focus on the issue, taste sensation. Only option 3 addresses this issue. If you had difficulty with this question, review the effects of cancer treatments.

Level of Cognitive Ability: Application
Client Needs: Physiological Integrity
Integrated Concept/Process: Nursing Process/Implementation
Content Area: Adult Health/Oncology

Reference:
Black, J., Hawks, J., & Keene, A. (2001). *Medical-surgical nursing: clinical management for positive outcomes* (6th ed.). Philadelphia: W.B. Saunders, p. 394.

---

370. A common finding in the health history of a client with chronic pancreatitis that the nurse expects to note is:

1   Abdominal pain relieved with food or antacids
2   Exposure to occupational chemicals
3   Weight gain
4   Use of alcohol

Answer: 4

Rationale: Chronic pancreatitis is found most often in alcoholics. Abstinence from alcohol is important to prevent the client from developing chronic pancreatitis. Clients usually have malabsorption with weight loss. Pain is not relieved with food or antacids. Chemical exposure is associated with cancer of the pancreas.

Test-Taking Strategy: Use the process of elimination. Focusing on the words *chronic pancreatitis* assists in directing you to option 4. Review the causes of pancreatitis if you had difficulty with this question.

Level of Cognitive Ability: Comprehension
Client Needs: Physiological Integrity
Integrated Concept/Process: Nursing Process/Data Collection
Content Area: Adult Health/Gastrointestinal

Reference:
Black, J., Hawks, J., & Keene, A. (2001). *Medical-surgical nursing: clinical management for positive outcomes* (6th ed.). Philadelphia: W.B. Saunders, p. 1200.

---

371. A client has been taking corticosteroids to control rheumatoid arthritis. What abnormal laboratory value most likely will be noted as a result of taking this medication?

1   Elevated serum potassium
2   Decreased serum sodium
3   Increased serum glucose
4   Increased white blood cells

Answer: 3

Rationale: Glucocorticoid (corticosteroid) medications have three primary uses: replacement therapy for adrenal insufficiency, immunosuppressive therapy, and antiinflammatory therapy. Exogenous glucocorticoids cause the same effects on cellular activity as the naturally produced glucocorticoids; however, exogenous glucocorticoids may produced undesired clinical outcomes. The glucocorticoids stimulate appetite and increase caloric intake. They also increase the availability of glucose for energy. These combined effects cause the blood glucose levels to rise, making clients prone to hyperglycemia. Options 1, 2, and 4 are not associated with the use of glucocorticoids.

Test-Taking Strategy: Knowledge of the side effects of glucocorticoids helps to answer this question. If you are unfamiliar with these medications and their uses, side effects, and contraindications, review this content.

Level of Cognitive Ability: Analysis
Client Needs: Physiological Integrity
Integrated Concept/Process: Nursing Process/Data Collection
Content Area: Pharmacology

Reference:
Lehne, R. (2001). *Pharmacology for nursing care* (4th ed.). Philadelphia: W.B. Saunders, p. 660.

372. A nurse is assigned to care for a group of clients on the clinical nursing unit. The nurse determines that which of them is most at risk for development of pulmonary embolism?
1   A 65-year-old man out of bed 1 day after prostate resection
2   A 73-year-old woman who has just had pinning of a hip fracture
3   A 25-year-old woman with diabetic ketoacidosis
4   A 38-year-old man with pulmonary contusion after an auto accident

Answer: 2
Rationale: Clients frequently at risk for pulmonary embolism include clients who are immobilized. This is especially true in the immobilized postoperative client. Other causes include those with conditions that are characterized by hypercoagulability, endothelial disease, and advancing age.

Test-Taking Strategy: Use the process of elimination. These options can be compared best by evaluating the degree of immobility that each client has and the age of the client, which is given in each option. The clients in options 1 and 3 have the least long-term anticipated immobility; therefore they should be eliminated first. From the remaining options, the younger client with the lung contusion is expected to be more mobile than the elderly woman with hip fracture, leaving option 2 as the answer. Review the causes of pulmonary embolism if you had difficulty with this question.

Level of Cognitive Ability: Comprehension
Client Needs: Physiological Integrity
Integrated Concept/Process: Nursing Process/Data Collection
Content Area: Fundamental Skills

Reference:
deWit, S. (2001). *Fundamental concepts and skills for nursing.* Philadelphia: W.B. Saunders, p. 773.

373. A physician has inserted a nasoenteric tube for the treatment of intestinal obstruction. The nurse tells the client to lie in which position to help the tube advance into the duodenum through the pyloric sphincter?
1   Supine with the head of the bed flat
2   Supine with the head elevated 30 degrees
3   On the right side
4   On the left side

Answer: 3
Rationale: The client is instructed to lie on the right side to aid in passage of the tube from the stomach into the duodenum, past the pyloric sphincter.

Test-Taking Strategy: Use knowledge of basic anatomy and the position of the stomach to assist in answering this question. Knowledge of this position can be applied to the management of a client with any type of nasoenteric tube. Review the anatomy of the gastrointestinal tract if you had difficulty with this question.

Level of Cognitive Ability: Application
Client Needs: Physiological Integrity
Integrated Concept/Process: Nursing Process/Implementation
Content Area: Adult Health/Gastrointestinal

Reference:
Perry, A., & Potter, P., (2002). *Clinical nursing skills & techniques* (5th ed.). St. Louis: Mosby, p. 663.

374. A nurse is monitoring the renal function of the client. After directly noting urine volume and characteristics, the nurse checks which of the following items as the best indirect indicator of renal status?
1   Bladder distention
2   Level of consciousness

Answer: 4
Rationale: The kidneys normally receive 20% to 25% of the cardiac output, even under conditions of rest. Adequate renal perfusion is necessary for kidney function to be optimal. Perfusion can be estimated best by the blood pressure, which is an indirect reflection of the adequacy of cardiac output. The pulse rate affects the cardiac output, but can be altered by factors unrelated to

3   Pulse rate
4   Blood pressure

kidney function. Bladder distention reflects a problem or obstruction that is most often distal to the kidneys. Level of consciousness is an unrelated item.

Test-Taking Strategy: Use the process of elimination. Eliminate level of consciousness first as the item most unrelated to kidney function. Because bladder distention can be affected by a number of other factors besides renal function, this is eliminated next. To choose between pulse and blood pressure, remember that the cardiac output overall helps determine the blood pressure and renal perfusion. Thus, blood pressure is the more global option, and the one more directly related to kidney perfusion. Review the factors that affect renal perfusion if you had difficulty with this question.

Level of Cognitive Ability: Application
Client Needs: Physiological Integrity
Integrated Concept/Process: Nursing Process/Implementation
Content Area: Adult Health/Renal

Reference:
Black, J., Hawks, J., & Keene, A. (2001). *Medical-surgical nursing: clinical management for positive outcomes* (6th ed.). Philadelphia: W. B. Saunders, p. 852.

---

375. A client with ascites and slight jaundice is seen in the ambulatory care clinic. The nurse collecting data from the client asks the client about a history of chronic use of which of the following medications?
1   Acetaminophen (Tylenol)
2   Acetylsalicylic acid (Aspirin)
3   Ibuprofen (Advil)
4   Ranitidine (Zantac)

Answer: 1
Rationale: Acetaminophen is a potentially hepatotoxic medication. Use of this medication and other hepatotoxic agents should be investigated whenever a client presents with symptoms compatible with liver disease (such as ascites and jaundice). Options 2, 3, and 4 are not as toxic to the liver.

Test-Taking Strategy: To answer this question, it is first necessary to know that the symptoms identified in the question are compatible with liver disease. With this in mind, evaluate each of the options for their relative ability to be toxic to the liver. Review the medications that are hepatotoxic if you are unfamiliar with them.

Level of Cognitive Ability: Application
Client Needs: Physiological Integrity
Integrated Concept/Process: Nursing Process/Data Collection
Content Area: Adult Health/Gastrointestinal

Reference:
Hodgson, B., & Kizior, R. (2003). *Saunders nursing drugs handbook 2003.* Philadelphia: W. B. Saunders, p. 9.

---

376. A nurse is assigned to care for a client who has just undergone eye surgery. The nurse plans to instruct the client that which of the following activities is permitted in the postoperative period?
1   Reading
2   Watching television
3   Bending over
4   Lifting objects

Answer: 2
Rationale: The client is taught to avoid doing activities that raise intraocular pressure and could cause complications in the postoperative period. The client is also taught to avoid activities that cause rapid eye movements that are irritating in the presence of postoperative inflammation. For these reasons, the client is taught to avoid bending over, lifting heavy objects, straining, sneezing, making sudden movements, or reading. Watching television is permissible because the eye does not need to move rapidly with

this activity, and this activity does not increase intraocular pressure.

Test-Taking Strategy: Think about the issue of intraocular pressure when answering this question. Eliminate options 3 and 4 first, because they obviously increase intraocular pressure. Choose option 2 instead of option 1 because it is less taxing to the eyes. Review care of the client after eye surgery if you had difficulty with this question.

Level of Cognitive Ability: Application
Client Needs: Physiological Integrity
Integrated Concept/Process: Nursing Process/Planning
Content Area: Adult Health/Eye

Reference:
Black, J., Hawks, J., & Keene, A. (2001). *Medical-surgical nursing: clinical management for positive outcomes* (6th ed.). Philadelphia: W.B. Saunders, p. 1817.

---

377. A female client with a history of chronic infection in the urinary system complains of burning and urinary frequency. To determine whether the current problem is of renal origin, the nurse asks the client if the client is experiencing pain or discomfort in the:
1 Suprapubic area
2 Flank area
3 Urinary meatus
4 Labium

Answer: 2
Rationale: Pain or discomfort from a problem that originates in the kidney is felt at the costovertebral angle (flank area) on the affected side. Ureteral pain is felt in the ipsilateral labium in the female client, or the ipsilateral scrotum in the male client. Bladder infection often is accompanied by suprapubic pain, and pain or burning at the urinary meatus when voiding.

Test-Taking Strategy: Use the process of elimination and focus on the issue, which is renal origin. Recalling that the kidneys sit higher than the level of the bladder and retroperitoneally assists in eliminating the incorrect options. Review the effects of a renal disorder if you had difficulty with this question.

Level of Cognitive Ability: Application
Client Needs: Physiological Integrity
Integrated Concept/Process: Nursing Process/Data Collection
Content Area: Adult Health/Renal

Reference:
Black, J., Hawks, J., & Keene, A. (2001). *Medical-surgical nursing: clinical management for positive outcomes* (6th ed.). Philadelphia: W.B. Saunders, pp. 747-748.

---

378. During a routine visit to the physician's office, an elderly client with diabetes mellitus complains of vision changes. The client describes vision blurring, with difficulty reading and driving at night. Given the client's history, the nurse interprets that the client is probably developing:
1 Detached retina
2 Papilledema
3 Glaucoma
4 Cataracts

Answer: 4
Rationale: Although the incidence of cataracts increases with age, the elderly client with diabetes mellitus is at greater risk for developing cataracts. The most frequent complaint is of blurred vision that is not accompanied by pain. The client also may experience difficulty when reading, night driving, and glare.

Test-Taking Strategy: Use the process of elimination and focus on the information in the question. Recalling the signs and symptoms of cataracts directs you to option 4. Review the signs and symptoms of cataracts if you had difficulty with this question.

Level of Cognitive Ability: Comprehension
Client Needs: Physiological Integrity
Integrated Concept/Process: Nursing Process/Data Collection
Content Area: Adult Health/Eye

Reference:
Black, J., Hawks, J., & Keene, A. (2001). *Medical-surgical nursing: clinical management for positive outcomes* (6th ed.). Philadelphia: W.B. Saunders, p. 1814.

---

379. A nurse inquires about a smoking history when collecting data from a client with coronary artery disease (CAD). The most important item for the nurse to identify is the:
1 Number of pack-years
2 Brand of cigarettes used
3 Desire to quit smoking
4 Number of past attempts to quit smoking

Answer: 1
Rationale: The number of cigarettes smoked daily and the duration of the habit are used to calculate the number of pack years, which is the standard method of documenting smoking history. The brand of cigarettes may give a general indication of tar and nicotine levels, but the information has no immediate clinical use. Desire to quit and number of past attempts to quit smoking may be useful when the nurse develops a smoking cessation plan with the client.

Test-Taking Strategy: Use the process of elimination. The question directs you to identify the most important item. This indicates that more than one option is correct. The option that most closely predicts the degree of added risk of CAD is the number of pack years. Review the risks associated with CAD if you had difficulty with this question.

Level of Cognitive Ability: Comprehension
Client Needs: Physiological Integrity
Integrated Concept/Process: Nursing Process/Data Collection
Content Area: Adult Health/Cardiovascular

Reference:
Black, J., Hawks, J., & Keene, A. (2001). *Medical-surgical nursing: clinical management for positive outcomes* (6th ed.). Philadelphia: W.B. Saunders, p. 1455.

---

380. A client with primary open angle glaucoma has been prescribed timolol maleate (Timoptic) ophthalmic drops. The client asks the nurse how this medication works. The nurse tells the client that the medication lowers intraocular pressure by:
1 Reducing intracranial pressure
2 Increasing contractions of the ciliary muscle
3 Constricting the pupil
4 Reducing production of aqueous humor

Answer: 4
Rationale: Beta–adrenergic-blocking agents such as timolol reduce intraocular pressure by decreasing the production of aqueous humor. Miotic agents (such as pilocarpine) increase contractions of the ciliary muscle and constrict the pupil, thereby increasing the outflow of aqueous humor.

Test-Taking Strategy: Use the process of elimination. Eliminate option 1 because this medication is unrelated to intracranial pressure. Next eliminate options 2 and 3 because these are both actions of miotic agents. Review the action of this medication if you had difficulty with this question.

Level of Cognitive Ability: Application
Client Needs: Physiological Integrity
Integrated Concept/Process: Nursing Process/Implementation
Content Area: Pharmacology

Reference:
Hodgson, B., & Kizior, R. (2003). *Saunders nursing drug handbook 2003.* Philadelphia: W.B. Saunders, p. 1086.

381. A client is complaining of knee pain. The knee is swollen, reddened, and warm to the touch. The nurse interprets that the client's signs and symptoms are not compatible with:
1   Inflammation
2   Degenerative disease
3   Infection
4   Recent injury

Answer: 2
Rationale: Redness and heat are associated with musculoskeletal inflammation, infection, or a recent injury. Degenerative disease is accompanied by pain, but there is no redness. Swelling may or may not occur.

Test-Taking Strategy: Use the process of elimination and note the key word *not*. Swelling, redness, and warmth are signs of inflammation. The body's inflammatory response is triggered by inflammation, infection, and injury. This should easily direct you to the correct option. Review the signs of inflammation if you had difficulty with this question.

Level of Cognitive Ability: Comprehension
Client Needs: Physiological Integrity
Integrated Concept/Process: Nursing Process/Data Collection
Content Area: Adult Health/Musculoskeletal

Reference:
Black, J., Hawks, J., & Keene, A. (2001). *Medical-surgical nursing: clinical management for positive outcomes* (6th ed.). Philadelphia: W.B. Saunders, p. 552.

---

382. A client seeks treatment in the emergency room for a lower leg injury. There is a visible deformity to the lower aspect of the leg, and the injured leg appears shorter than the other. The area is painful, swollen, and beginning to become ecchymotic. The nurse interprets that this client has experienced a:
1   Contusion
2   Fracture
3   Sprain
4   Strain

Answer: 2
Rationale: Typical signs and symptoms of a fracture include pain, loss of function in the area, deformity, shortening of the extremity, crepitus, swelling, and ecchymosis. Not all fractures lead to the development of every sign. A contusion results from a blow to soft tissue and causes pain, swelling, and ecchymosis. A sprain is an injury to a ligament caused by a wrenching or twisting motion. Symptoms include pain, swelling, and inability to use the joint or bear weight normally. A strain results from a pulling force on the muscle. Symptoms include soreness and pain with muscle use.

Test-Taking Strategy: Use the process of elimination. Within the list of signs and symptoms in the question, note the one that states one leg is shorter than the other. Only a fractured bone (which shortens with displacement) could cause this sign. Review the signs of a fracture if you had difficulty with this question.

Level of Cognitive Ability: Comprehension
Client Needs: Physiological Integrity
Integrated Concept/Process: Nursing Process/Data Collection
Content Area: Adult Health/Musculoskeletal

Reference:
Black, J., Hawks, J., & Keene, A. (2001). *Medical-surgical nursing: clinical management for positive outcomes* (6th ed.). Philadelphia: W.B. Saunders, pp. 589-590.

---

383. A client presents to the emergency department with a chemical burn of the left eye. The first action of the nurse is to immediately:
1   Flush the eye continuously with a sterile solution

Answer: 1
Rationale: When the client has suffered a chemical burn of the eye, the nurse immediately flushes the eye with a sterile solution continuously for 15 minutes. If a sterile eye irrigation solution is not available, running water may be used. Determining the nature of the chemical is helpful, but is not

2 Apply a cold compress to the injured eye

3 Apply a nonocclusive bandage to the eye

4 Determine the nature of the chemical agent

the priority action. Applying compresses or bandages are incorrect, because they do not rid the eye of the damaging chemical. Cold compresses are used for blows to the eye, whereas light bandages may be placed over cuts of the eye or eyelid.

Test-Taking Strategy: Use the process of elimination. Focusing on the type of eye injury and noting the key word *chemical* directs you to option 1. Review emergency care related to chemical burns to the eye if you had difficulty with this question.

Level of Cognitive Ability: Application
Client Needs: Physiological Integrity
Integrated Concept/Process: Nursing Process/Implementation
Content Area: Adult Health/Eye

Reference:
Black, J., Hawks, J., & Keene, A. (2001). *Medical-surgical nursing: clinical management for positive outcomes* (6th ed.). Philadelphia: W.B. Saunders, p. 2278.

---

384. A client tells the nurse about a pattern of getting a strong urge to void, which is followed by incontinence before the client can get to the bathroom. The nurse determines that the client is experiencing which problem?

1 Reflex incontinence

2 Stress incontinence

3 Urge incontinence

4 Total incontinence

Answer: 3
Rationale: Urge incontinence occurs when the client has urinary incontinence soon after experiencing urgency. Reflex incontinence occurs when incontinence occurs at rather predictable times that correspond to attainment of a certain bladder volume. Stress incontinence occurs when the client voids in increments that are less than 50 mL, and has increased abdominal pressure. Total incontinence occurs when there is an unpredictable and continuous loss of urine.

Test-Taking Strategy: Use the process of elimination. Focus on the data in the question and note the words *strong urge to void*. Note the relationship between these words and option 3. Review the types of incontinence if you had difficulty with this question.

Level of Cognitive Ability: Comprehension
Client Needs: Physiological Integrity
Integrated Concept/Process: Nursing Process/Data Collection
Content Area: Adult Health/Renal

Reference:
Black, J., Hawks, J., & Keene, A. (2001). *Medical-surgical nursing: clinical management for positive outcomes* (6th ed.). Philadelphia: W.B. Saunders, p. 749.

---

385. A nurse is instilling an otic solution into the adult client's left ear. The nurse avoids doing which of the following as part of this procedure?

1 Warming the solution to room temperature

Answer: 4
Rationale: The dropper is not allowed to touch any object or any part of the client's skin. The solution is warmed before use. The client is placed on the side with the affected ear directed upward. The nurse pulls the auricle backward and upward, and instills the medication by holding the dropper about 1 cm above the ear canal.

2   Placing the client in a side-lying position with the ear facing up
3   Pulling the auricle backward and upward
4   Placing the tip of the dropper on the edge of the ear canal

Test-Taking Strategy: Use the process of elimination and note the key word *avoids*. Visualizing this procedure assists in directing you to option 4. Review this basic nursing procedure if you had difficulty with this question.

Level of Cognitive Ability: Application
Client Needs: Physiological Integrity
Integrated Concept/Process: Nursing Process/Implementation
Content Area: Adult Health/Ear

Reference:
deWit, S. (2001). *Fundamental concepts and skills for nursing.* Philadelphia: W.B. Saunders, p. 668.

---

386. Catatonic excitement has been diagnosed in a client who has been pacing rapidly nonstop for several hours and is not eating or drinking. The nurse recognizes that in this situation:
1   There is an urgent need for physical and medical control
2   There is an urgent need for restraint
3   There is a need to encourage verbalization of feelings
4   The client will soon become catatonic stuporous

Answer: 1
Rationale: Catatonic excitement is manifested by a state of extreme psychomotor agitation. Clients urgently require physical and medical control because they are often destructive and violent to others, and their excitement can cause them to injure themselves or collapse from complete exhaustion.

Test-Taking Strategy: Focus on the data in the question. Use Maslow's Hierarchy of Needs theory to answer the question. Remember, physiological needs come first. This directs you to option 1. Review the priority needs for the client with catatonic excitement if you had difficulty with this question.

Level of Cognitive Ability: Comprehension
Client Needs: Physiological Integrity
Integrated Concept/Process: Nursing Process/Data Collection
Content Area: Mental Health

Reference:
Varcarolis, E. (2002). *Foundations of psychiatric mental health nursing* (4th ed.). Philadelphia: W.B. Saunders, p. 534.

---

387. Which of the following laboratory data indicate a potential complication associated with type 1 diabetes mellitus?
1   Blood glucose 112 mg/dL
2   Ketonuria
3   Blood urea nitrogen (BUN) 18 mg/dL
4   Potassium 4.2 mEq

Answer: 2
Rationale: Ketonuria is an abnormal finding in the diabetic client that indicates ketosis. Ketosis is a metabolic effect from the lack of insulin on fat metabolism and occurs in type 1 diabetes mellitus. It is associated with severe complications of diabetic ketoacidosis (hyperglycemia, ketosis, and acidosis). Option 1, 3, and 4 are all normal laboratory findings.

Test-Taking Strategy: Use the process of elimination and focus on the client's diagnosis and the issue of the question: a complication. Recalling the normal range of the laboratory values listed in the options directs you to option 2. Remember that ketonuria is an abnormal finding. Review the complications of diabetes mellitus if you had difficulty with this question.

Level of Cognitive Ability: Comprehension
Client Needs: Physiological Integrity

Integrated Concept/Process: Nursing Process/Data Collection
Content Area: Adult Health/Endocrine

Reference:
Black, J., Hawks, J., & Keene, A. (2001). *Medical-surgical nursing: clinical management for positive outcomes* (6th ed.). Philadelphia: W.B. Saunders, p. 1172.

---

388. A nurse is collecting data from a male client with diabetes mellitus who has been taking insulin for many years. The client states that currently he is experiencing periods of hypoglycemia followed by periods of hyperglycemia. The nurse determines that the most likely cause for this occurrence is:

1 Injecting insulin at the site of lipodystrophy
2 Adjusting insulin according to the blood glucose level
3 Eating snacks between meals
4 Initiating the use of the insulin pump

Answer: 1
Rationale: Tissue hypertrophy (lipodystrophy) involves thickening of the subcutaneous tissue at the injection sites. This can interfere with the absorption of insulin, resulting in erratic blood glucose levels. Because the client has been on insulin for many years, this is the most likely cause of poor control.

Test-Taking Strategy: Use the process of elimination. The key words *taking insulin for many years* indicate that you must consider a long-term complication of insulin administration, such as lipodystrophy. Options 2, 3, and 4 are actually appropriate techniques to use to regulate blood glucose levels. Review this complication of insulin injections if you had difficulty with this question.

Level of Cognitive Ability: Comprehension
Client Needs: Physiological Integrity
Integrated Concept/Process: Nursing Process/Data Collection
Content Area: Adult Health/Endocrine

Reference:
Lewis, S., Heitkemper, M., & Dirksen, S. (2004). *Medical-surgical nursing: assessment and management of clinical problems* (6th ed.). St. Louis: Mosby, p. 1276.

---

389. A nurse is assisting in caring for a client after a suprapubic prostatectomy. The nurse monitors the continuous bladder irrigation to detect which of the following signs of catheter blockage?

1 Drainage that is pale pink
2 Drainage that is bright red
3 Urine leakage around the three-way catheter at the meatus
4 True urine output of 50 mL per hour

Answer: 3
Rationale: Catheter blockage or occlusion by clots after prostatectomy can result in urine back-up and leakage around the catheter at the urethral meatus. This is accompanied by a stoppage of outflow through the catheter into the drainage bag. Bright red drainage indicates that the irrigant is running too slowly; pale pink drainage indicates sufficient flow. A true urine output of 50 mL per hour indicates catheter patency.

Test-Taking Strategy: Use the process of elimination and focus on the issue, which is catheter blockage. Eliminate options 1 and 2 first because of the word *drainage*. This implies catheter patency. Apply basic principles related to Foley catheter management to select the correct option from those remaining. A leakage around the catheter at the meatus indicates blockage. Review the signs of catheter blockage if you had difficulty with this question.

Level of Cognitive Ability: Application
Client Needs: Physiological Integrity
Integrated Concept/Process: Nursing Process/Data Collection
Content Area: Adult Health/Renal

Reference:
Black, J., Hawks, J., & Keene, A. (2001). *Medical-surgical nursing: clinical management for positive outcomes* (6th ed.). Philadelphia: W.B. Saunders, p. 956.

390. A nurse is assigned to assist in caring for a client after transurethral prostatectomy. The nurse avoids doing which of the following after this procedure?
1   Reporting signs of confusion
2   Administering belladonna and opium (B&O) suppositories at room temperature as prescribed
3   Removing the traction tape on the three-way catheter
4   Monitoring hourly urine output

Answer: 3
Rationale: The nurse avoids removing the traction tape applied by the surgeon in the operating room. The purpose of this tape is to place pressure on the prostate and reduce hemorrhage. B&O suppositories, ordered on a PRN basis for bladder spasm, should be warmed to room temperature before administration. The nurse routinely monitors hourly urine output because the client has a three-way bladder irrigation running. The nurse also monitors for confusion, which could result from hyponatremia secondary to the hypotonic irrigant used during the surgical procedure.

Test-Taking Strategy: Use the process of elimination. Note the key word *avoids*. Eliminate options 1 and 4 first because they are part of routine nursing care and are not contraindicated in the care of this client. Choose correctly between the remaining options either through knowledge of the use of bladder antispasmodics or knowledge of this specific surgical procedure. Review this procedure if you had difficulty with this question.

Level of Cognitive Ability: Application
Client Needs: Physiological Integrity
Integrated Concept/Process: Nursing Process/Implementation
Content Area: Adult Health/Renal

Reference:
Black, J., Hawks, J., & Keene, A. (2001). *Medical-surgical nursing: clinical management for positive outcomes* (6th ed.). Philadelphia: W.B. Saunders, p. 957.

391. A client is due for a dose of bumetanide (Bumex). The nurse temporarily withholds the dose and notifies the physician if which of the following laboratory results is noted?
1   Sodium 137 mEq/L
2   Potassium 2.9 mEq/L
3   Magnesium 2.5 mg/dL
4   Chloride 106 mEq/L

Answer: 2
Rationale: Bumetanide is a loop diuretic, which is not potassium sparing. The value given for potassium is below the therapeutic range of 3.5 to 5.1 mEq/L for this electrolyte. The nurse should notify the physician before giving the dose so that potassium may be ordered. Options 1, 3, and 4 are normal laboratory values.

Test-Taking Strategy: Use the process of elimination and focus on the issue: withholding the dose and notifying the physician. Eliminate options 1, 3, and 4 because they are normal laboratory values. Review this medication and the normal potassium level if you had difficulty with this question.

Level of Cognitive Ability: Application
Client Needs: Physiological Integrity
Integrated Concept/Process: Nursing Process/Implementation
Content Area: Pharmacology

Reference:
Hodgson, B., & Kizior, R. (2003). *Saunders nursing drug handbook 2003.* Philadelphia: W.B. Saunders, p. 145.

392. A client with heart failure is receiving furosemide (Lasix) and digoxin (Lanoxin) daily. When the nurse enters the client's room to administer the morning medication doses the client complains of anorexia, nausea, and yellow vision. The nurse should plan to do which of the following first?

1 Administer the medications
2 Give the digoxin only
3 Check the morning serum potassium level
4 Check the morning serum digoxin level

Answer: 4

Rationale: The nurse should check for the result of the digoxin level that was drawn, because the symptoms described by the client are compatible with toxicity. Knowing that a low potassium level may contribute to toxicity, checking the serum potassium level may give useful additive information but is not the first action. The digoxin should be withheld until the level is known, making options 1 and 2 incorrect.

Test-Taking Strategy: Use the process of elimination. Note the key word *first*. Eliminate options 1 and 2 because it is inappropriate to administer the medication(s) without investigating further. From the remaining options, noting that the client's complaints indicate toxicity directs you to option 4. Review the signs of digoxin toxicity if you had difficulty with this question.

Level of Cognitive Ability: Application
Client Needs: Physiological Integrity
Integrated Concept/Process: Nursing Process/Implementation
Content Area: Pharmacology

Reference:
Hodgson, B., & Kizior, R. (2003). *Saunders nursing drug handbook 2003.* Philadelphia: W.B. Saunders, p. 350.

393. A nurse is administering an oral dose of erythromycin (E-Mycin) to an assigned client. The nurse most appropriately gives this medication with a:

1 Full glass of milk
2 Full glass of water
3 Sip of orange juice
4 Any noncitrus beverage

Answer: 2

Rationale: Erythromycin is a macrolide antibiotic that should be taken with a full glass of water. Sufficient volume is needed to obtain maximal effect of the medication. Depending on the specific type of erythromycin, it may need to be administered on an empty stomach, with meals, or regardless of timing of meals. The nurse should verify the best method of administration for the type ordered.

Test-Taking Strategy: Use the process of elimination and note the key words *most appropriately*. Eliminate options 1, 3, and 4 because they indicate administering the medication with some type of liquid food substance. Review this medication if you had difficulty with this question.

Level of Cognitive Ability: Application
Client Needs: Physiological Integrity
Integrated Concept/Process: Nursing Process/Implementation
Content Area: Pharmacology

Reference:
Hodgson, B., & Kizior, R. (2003). *Saunders nursing drug handbook 2003.* Philadelphia: W.B. Saunders, p. 416.

394. A client with a fractured femur who has had an open reduction-internal fixation is receiving ketorolac (Toradol). The nurse evaluates the effectiveness of the medication by monitoring the client's:

1 Serum calcium level
2 White blood cell count

Answer: 4

Rationale: Ketorolac is a nonopioid analgesic and nonsteroidal antiinflammatory drug. It acts by inhibiting prostaglandin synthesis and produces analgesia that is peripherally mediated. The nurse evaluates the effectiveness of this medication by using the pain rating scale with the client.

3 Temperature
4 Pain rating

Test-Taking Strategy: Use the process of elimination. The diagnosis of the client, fractured femur, may provide you with the clue that this medication is an analgesic. This directs you to option 4. Review this medication if you had difficulty with this question.

Level of Cognitive Ability: Analysis
Client Needs: Physiological Integrity
Integrated Concept/Process: Nursing Process/Evaluation
Content Area: Pharmacology

Reference:
Hodgson, B., & Kizior, R. (2003). *Saunders nursing drug handbook 2003.* Philadelphia: W.B. Saunders, p. 633.

---

395. A client has an order for beclomethasone dipropionate (Beclovent) to be given by the intranasal route. The client also has an order for a nasal decongestant. Which of the following methods of administration by the nurse is correct?
1 Administer the beclomethasone dipropionate 15 minutes before the decongestant
2 Administer the decongestant 15 minutes before the beclomethasone dipropionate
3 Administer the beclomethasone dipropionate immediately before the decongestant
4 Administer the decongestant immediately before the beclomethasone dipropionate

Answer: 2
Rationale: The nasal decongestant should be administered 15 minutes before the beclomethasone (a glucocorticoid) to clear the nasal passages and enhance absorption of the medication. Options 1, 3, and 4 are incorrect.

Test-Taking Strategy: Use the same principles in answering this question that you would use when administering bronchodilators and corticosteroids together. This helps you choose the correct option. Review these types of medication and their appropriate method of administration if you had difficulty with this question.

Level of Cognitive Ability: Application
Client Needs: Physiological Integrity
Integrated Concept/Process: Nursing Process/Implementation
Content Area: Pharmacology

Reference:
Clark, J., Quiena, S., & Karb, V. (2002). *Pharmacologic basis of nursing practice* (6th ed.). St Louis: Mosby, p. 357.

---

396. A client is receiving tobramycin (Tobrex). The nurse evaluates that the client is responding well to the medication therapy if which of the following laboratory results is noted?
1 White blood cell (WBC) count 8000/mm^3 and creatinine level 0.9 mg/dL
2 WBC count 15,000/mm^3 and blood urea nitrogen (BUN) 38 mg/dL
3 Sodium 140 mEq/L and potassium 3.9 mEq/L
4 Sodium 145 mEq/L and chloride 106 mEq/L

Answer: 1
Rationale: Tobramycin is an antibiotic (aminoglycoside) that causes nephrotoxicity and ototoxicity. The medication is effective if the WBC count drops back into the normal range and kidney function remains normal. Option 2 indicates an abnormal WBC count and an elevated BUN, and options 3 and 4 are unrelated to this medication.

Test-Taking Strategy: Use the process of elimination and note the key words *responding well.* Begin to answer this question by eliminating options 3 and 4 first knowing that tobramycin is an antibiotic. Recalling that aminoglycosides cause nephrotoxicity, you would then choose option 1 over option 2 as correct, using laboratory values as your guide. Review this medication and normal laboratory values if you had difficulty with this question.

Level of Cognitive Ability: Analysis
Client Needs: Physiological Integrity

Integrated Concept/Process: Nursing Process/Evaluation
Content Area: Pharmacology

Reference:
Hodgson, B., & Kizior, R. (2003). *Saunders nursing drug handbook 2003.* Philadelphia: W.B. Saunders, p. 1096.

---

397. A nursing intervention for the client taking maintenance dosages of lithium carbonate (Eskalith) include:
1 Monitoring daily serum lithium levels
2 Performing a weekly electrocardiogram (ECG)
3 Observing for remission of depressive states
4 Monitoring intake and output

Answer: 4
Rationale: Lithium is used to treat manic disorders, not depression. Side effects of lithium are nausea, tremors, polyuria, and polydipsia. The serum lithium concentration is checked approximately every 2 to 4 days during initial therapy, and at longer intervals thereafter. Toxic levels of lithium may induce ECG changes; however, there is no need to perform weekly ECGs if maintenance levels are maintained.

Test-Taking Strategy: Use the process of elimination. Eliminate options 1 and 2 first because of the words *daily* and *weekly.* From the remaining options, use knowledge of the side effects and the use of the medication to direct you to the correct option. If you had difficulty with this question, review nursing interventions related to the administration of lithium.

Level of Cognitive Ability: Application
Client Needs: Physiological Integrity
Integrated Concept/Process: Nursing Process/Implementation
Content Area: Pharmacology

Reference:
Hodgson, B., & Kizior, R. (2003). *Saunders nursing drug handbook 2003.* Philadelphia: W.B. Saunders, p. 672.

---

398. A nurse is collecting data from a client admitted to the hospital with a diagnosis of Raynaud's disease. The nurse accurately checks for the symptoms associated with Raynaud's disease when the nurse:
1 Observes for softening of the nails or nail beds
2 Palpates for diminished or absent peripheral pulses
3 Checks for rash on the digits
4 Palpates for a rapid or irregular peripheral pulse

Answer: 2
Rationale: Raynaud's disease produces closure of the small arteries in the distal extremities in response to cold, vibration, or external stimuli. Palpation for diminished or absent peripheral pulses checks for interruption of circulation. The nails grow slowly, become brittle or deformed, and heal poorly around the nail beds when infected. Skin changes include hair loss, thinning or tightening of the skin, and delayed healing of cuts or injuries. Although palpation of peripheral pulses is correct, it is incorrect to find a rapid or irregular pulse. Peripheral pulses may be normal, absent, or diminished.

Test-Taking Strategy: Use the ABCs (airway, breathing, and circulation). This directs you to option 2. Review the manifestations associated with this disorder if you had difficulty with this question.

Level of Cognitive Ability: Application
Client Needs: Physiological Integrity
Integrated Concept/Process: Nursing Process/Data Collection
Content Area: Pharmacology

Reference:
Black, J., Hawks, J., & Keene, A. (2001). *Medical-surgical nursing: clinical management for positive outcomes* (6th ed.). Philadelphia: W.B. Saunders, p. 1421.

399. A nurse monitors the respiratory status of the client being treated for acute exacerbation of chronic obstructive pulmonary disease (COPD). Which of the following initial findings indicates a deterioration in ventilation?
1 Cyanosis
2 Rapid, shallow respirations
3 Hyperinflated chest
4 Barrel chest

Answer: 2

Rationale: An increase in the rate of respirations and a decrease in the depth of respirations indicates a deterioration in ventilation. Cyanosis is not a good indicator of oxygenation in the client with COPD and may be present with some but not all clients. A hyperinflated chest (barrel chest) and hypertrophy of the accessory muscles of the upper chest and neck normally may be found in clients with severe COPD.

Test-Taking Strategy: Use the process of elimination. Note the key words *initial* and *deterioration in ventilation.* Eliminate options 3 and 4 first because they are similar. Because cyanosis is not a good indicator of oxygenation in the client with COPD, eliminate option 1. Review the clinical manifestations associated with COPD if you had difficulty with this question.

Level of Cognitive Ability: Comprehension
Client Needs: Physiological Integrity
Integrated Concept/Process: Nursing Process/Data Collection
Content Area: Adult Health/Respiratory

Reference:
Black, J., Hawks, J., & Keene, A. (2001). *Medical-surgical nursing: clinical management for positive outcomes* (6th ed.). Philadelphia: W.B. Saunders, p. 1696.

400. Which of the following data-collection findings most appropriately determines the effectiveness of postural drainage and chest physiotherapy in the client with chronic obstructive pulmonary disease (COPD)?
1 The client expectorates large amounts of sputum
2 The client's cough is suppressed
3 The client is able to maintain the necessary position for postural drainage and chest physiotherapy
4 The client's expiration time becomes less prolonged

Answer: 1

Rationale: Postural drainage and chest physiotherapy (CPT) aid in improving airway clearance by mobilizing secretions to make them easier to expectorate. It is necessary for the client to cough effectively to expectorate secretions. The ability to maintain the necessary position for these respiratory treatment does not evaluate the effectiveness of the treatment. It is a normal expectation that clients with even stable COPD will demonstrate a prolonged expiration time that exceeds 4 seconds.

Test-Taking Strategy: Use the process of elimination. Note the key words *determines the effectiveness.* Keeping this in mind as well as the purpose of CPT and postural drainage assists in directing you to the correct option. Options 2 and 3 do not determine effectiveness. A prolonged expiration time is a normal expectation in this disorder and has no relationship to these respiratory treatments. Review the purpose of these respiratory treatments if you had difficulty with this question.

Level of Cognitive Ability: Analysis
Client Needs: Physiological Integrity
Integrated Concept/Process: Nursing Process/Evaluation
Content Area: Adult Health/Respiratory

Reference:
Black, J., Hawks, J., & Keene, A. (2001). *Medical-surgical nursing: clinical management for positive outcomes* (6th ed.). Philadelphia: W.B. Saunders, p. 1698.

401. Diazepam (Valium) is prescribed for the client with anxiety. The nurse reinforces instructions to the client and tells the client to expect which side effect?
1 Incoordination
2 Cough
3 Tinnitus
4 Hypertension

Answer: 1

Rationale: Diazepam, a benzodiazepine, can cause motor incoordination and ataxia; safety precautions should be instituted for clients taking this medication. Options 2, 3, and 4 are unrelated to this medication.

Test-Taking Strategy: Use the process of elimination. Recalling that many of the medications used to treat anxiety can cause incoordination assists in answering the question. Review the side effects of this medication if you had difficulty with this question.

Level of Cognitive Ability: Application
Client Needs: Physiological Integrity
Integrated Concept/Process: Teaching/Learning
Content Area: Pharmacology

Reference:
Hodgson, B., & Kizior, R. (2003). *Saunders nursing drug handbook 2003.* Philadelphia: W.B. Saunders, p. 336.

402. A nurse is assisting in caring for a client receiving oxytocin (Pitocin) to induce labor. During the administration of oxytocin, it is most important for the nurse to monitor the:
1 Urinary output
2 Fetal heart rate
3 Maternal temperature
4 Maternal blood glucose

Answer: 2

Rationale: Oxytocin produces uterine contractions. Uterine contractions can cause fetal anoxia; therefore, it is most important to monitor the fetal heart rate. Options 1, 3, and 4 are unrelated to the administration of this medication.

Test-Taking Strategy: Use the ABCs (airway, breathing, and circulation) to answer the question. This directs you to option 2. Review the action and nursing implications associated with the administration of this medication if you had difficulty with this question.

Level of Cognitive Ability: Application
Client Needs: Physiological Integrity
Integrated Concept/Process: Nursing Process/Data Collection
Content Area: Pharmacology

Reference:
Hodgson, B., & Kizior, R. (2003). *Saunders nursing drug handbook 2003.* Philadelphia: W.B. Saunders, p. 853.

403. A nursing instructor asks a nursing student about the reason for medication toxicity occurring in the neonate. The student understands the reason for this occurrence when the student verbalizes that in the neonate:
1 The lungs are immature
2 The kidneys are smaller
3 Cerebral function is not fully developed
4 The liver is not fully developed

Answer: 4

Rationale: The liver is not fully developed in the neonate and cannot detoxify many medications. Options 1, 2, and 3 are incorrect.

Test-Taking Strategy: Use the process of elimination and knowledge about the normal physiological maturity associated with the neonate. Recalling that the liver is associated with the detoxification of medications assists in directing you to the correct option. Review the normal physiological findings in the neonate if you had difficulty with this question.

Level of Cognitive Ability: Comprehension
Client Needs: Physiological Integrity

Integrated Concept/Process: Teaching/Learning
Content Area: Maternity

Reference:
McKinney, E., Ashwill, J., Murray, S., James, S., Gorrie, T., & Droske, S. (2000). *Maternal-child nursing.* Philadelphia: W.B. Saunders, p. 524.

---

404. A client is hospitalized for ingesting an overdose of acetaminophen (Tylenol). The nurse prepares to administer which specific antidote as prescribed for this medication overdose?
1   Protamine sulfate
2   Naloxone hydrochloride (Narcan)
3   Acetylcysteine (Mucomyst)
4   Phytonadione (Vitamin K)

Answer: 3
Rationale: Acetylcysteine restores sulfhydryl groups that are depleted by acetaminophen metabolism. Vitamin K is the antidote for warfarin sodium (Coumadin). Naloxone hydrochloride reverses respiratory depression. Protamine sulfate is the antidote for heparin.

Test-Taking Strategy: Use the process of elimination. Recalling the specific antidotes for both heparin and warfarin sodium (Coumadin) assists in eliminating options 1 and 4. Recalling that naloxone hydrochloride reverses respiratory depression assists in eliminating option 2. Review these antidotes if you had difficulty with this question.

Level of Cognitive Ability: Application
Client Needs: Physiological Integrity
Integrated Concept/Process: Nursing Process/Planning
Content Area: Pharmacology

Reference:
Hodgson, B., & Kizior, R. (2003). *Saunders nursing drug handbook 2003.* Philadelphia: W.B. Saunders, p. 9.

---

405. A nurse is observing a client to determine that the client is correctly using a walker. When evaluating the client's use of a walker, the nurse expects to note which of the following?
1   The client puts all four points of the walker flat on the floor, puts weight on the hand pieces, and then walks into it
2   The client puts weight on the hand pieces, moves the walker forward, and then walks into it
3   The client puts weight on the hand pieces, slides the walker forward, and then walks into it
4   The client walks into the walker, puts weight on the hand pieces, and then puts all four points of the walker flat on the floor

Answer: 1
Rationale: When the client uses a walker, the nurse stands adjacent to the affected side. The client is instructed to put all four points of the walker 2 feet forward flat on the floor before putting weight on the hand pieces. This ensures client safety and prevents stress cracks in the walker. The client is then instructed to move the walker forward and walk into it.

Test-Taking Strategy: Attempt to visualize this procedure. Options 2 and 3 can be eliminated because putting weight on the hand pieces initially will cause an unsafe situation. From the remaining options, recalling that the walker is placed on all four points first assists in directing you to option 1. Review this procedure if you had difficulty with this question.

Level of Cognitive Ability: Comprehension
Client Needs: Physiological Integrity
Integrated Concept/Process: Nursing Process/Evaluation
Content Area: Fundamental Skills

Reference:
deWit, S. (2001). *Fundamental concepts and skills for nursing.* Philadelphia: W.B. Saunders, p. 827.

406. When evaluating a client for the correct height of crutches, the nurse expects to note which of the following?

1 The client is able to rest the axillae on the axillary bars
2 The nurse is able to place two fingers comfortably between the axillae and the axillary bars
3 The client is able to maintain the arms in a straight position when standing with the crutches
4 The nurse is able to place four fingers comfortably between the axillae and the axillary bars

Answer: 2

Rationale: With the client's elbows flexed 20 to 30 degrees, the shoulders in a relaxed position, and the crutches placed approximately 15 cm (6 inches) anterolateral from the toes, the nurse should be able to place two fingers comfortably between the axillae and axillary bars. The crutches are adjusted if there is too much or too little space at the axillary area. The client is advised never to rest the axillae on the axillary bars because this could injure the brachial plexus (the nerve in the axillae that supplies the arm and shoulder area). Ambulation is stopped if the client complains of numbness or tingling in the hands or arms.

Test-Taking Strategy: Use the process of elimination. Attempt to visualize each of the options and eliminate those that are not reasonable and will not provide safety. Review this procedure if you had difficulty with this question.

Level of Cognitive Ability: Comprehension
Client Needs: Physiological Integrity
Integrated Concept/Process: Nursing Process/Evaluation
Content Area: Fundamental Skills

Reference:
deWit, S. (2001). *Fundamental concepts and skills for nursing.* Philadelphia: W.B. Saunders, p. 827.

---

407. A client with myasthenia gravis is admitted to the hospital. The nurse reviews the health record and notes that the client is taking pyridostigmine (Mestinon). The nurse checks the client for adverse effects of the medication, which include:

1 Abdominal cramps
2 Mouth ulcers
3 Depression
4 Unexplained weight gain

Answer: 1

Rationale: Pyridostigmine is an acetylcholinesterase inhibitor. Abdominal discomfort and cramps is an adverse reaction to the medication. Options 2, 3, and 4 are not specific adverse effects associated with the use of this medication.

Test-Taking Strategy: Recall that myasthenia gravis is a neuromuscular disorder. Use knowledge of the adverse effects of this medication to direct you to option 1. Review the side effects associated with this medication, if you had difficulty with this question.

Level of Cognitive Ability: Application
Client Needs: Physiological Integrity
Integrated Concept/Process: Nursing Process/Data Collection
Content Area: Pharmacology

Reference:
Hodgson, B., & Kizior, R. (2003). *Saunders nursing drug handbook 2003.* Philadelphia: W.B. Saunders, p. 950.

---

408. A client with a fractured right ankle has a short leg plaster cast applied. During discharge teaching, the nurse reinforces which of the following information to prevent complications?

Answer: 1

Rationale: Leg elevation is important to increase venous return and decrease edema, which can cause compartment syndrome, a major complication of fractures and casting. Option 2 is incorrect because weight bearing on a fractured extremity is determined by the physician during follow-up examination

1 Keep the right ankle elevated with pillows above the heart for 24 to 48 hours
2 Weight bear on the right leg only after the cast is dry
3 Expect burning and tingling sensations under the cast for 3 to 4 days
4 Trim the rough edges of the cast after it is dry

after radiograph. Although the client may feel heat after the cast is applied, a burning or tingling sensation or both indicate nerve damage and ischemia and is not expected; it should be reported immediately. Option 4 is incorrect because any cast modifications should be done by trained personnel under medical supervision, although the client, family, or both may be taught how to "petal" the cast to prevent skin irritation and breakdown.

Test-Taking Strategy: Remember, skin breakdown, compartment syndrome, cast damage, and venous thrombosis are all potential complications associated with casting. Use the ABCs (airway, breathing, and circulation). Option 1 is associated with maintenance of circulation. Review client instructions about cast care if you had difficulty with this question.

Level of Cognitive Ability: Application
Client Needs: Physiological Integrity
Integrated Concept/Process: Teaching/Learning
Content Area: Adult Health/Musculoskeletal

Reference:
deWit, S. (2001). *Fundamental concepts and skills for nursing.* Philadelphia: W.B. Saunders, p. 810.

---

409. An older adult female client with a fractured left tibia has a long leg cast and is using crutches to ambulate. In caring for the client, the nurse should be alert for which sign that indicates a complication associated with crutch walking?
1 Forearm muscle weakness
2 Left leg paresthesias
3 Triceps muscle spasms
4 Weak biceps brachii

Answer: 1
Rationale: Forearm muscle weakness is a sign of radial nerve injury caused by crutch pressure on the axillae. When clients lack upper body strength, especially in the flexor and extensor muscles of the arms, they frequently allow their weight to rest on their axillae instead of their arms while ambulating with crutches. Older adult women tend to have poor upper body strength. Option 2 is a sign of compartment syndrome, a complication of fractures, not crutch walking. Option 3 might occur as a result of increased muscle use, but is not a complication of crutch walking. Option 4 is a common physical finding in older adults, especially women, and is not a complication of crutch walking.

Test-Taking Strategy: Use the process of elimination. When asked about a complication of the use of crutches, think about nerve injury caused by crutch pressure on the axillae. This assists in directing you to option 1. Review the complications of crutch walking if you had difficulty with this question.

Level of Cognitive Ability: Comprehension
Client Needs: Physiological Integrity
Integrated Concept/Process: Nursing Process/Data Collection
Content Area: Adult Health/Musculoskeletal

Reference:
deWit, S. (2001). *Fundamental concepts and skills for nursing.* Philadelphia: W.B. Saunders, p. 827.

410. A nurse is caring for a client admitted to the hospital with a diagnosis of active tuberculosis (TB). This nurse understands that this diagnosis was confirmed by a:
1 Mantoux test
2 Sputum culture
3 Tine test
4 Chest radiograph

Answer: 2

Rationale: Sputum culture of *Mycobacterium tuberculosis* confirms the diagnosis of TB. Usually three sputum samples are obtained for the acid-fast smear. After the start of therapy, sputum samples are obtained again to determine the effectiveness of therapy. A positive Tine or Mantoux test indicates exposure to TB but does not confirm the presence of *Mycobacterium tuberculosis*. A positive chest radiograph may indicate the presence of tuberculosis lesions, but again does not confirm active disease.

Test-Taking Strategy: Use the process of elimination and note the key word *confirmed*. Active TB can be confirmed only by the presence of acid-fast bacilli. The sputum culture is the only method of determining the presence of this organism. Review the diagnostic tests for TB if you had difficulty with this question.

Level of Cognitive Ability: Comprehension
Client Needs: Physiological Integrity
Integrated Concept/Process: Nursing Process/Data Collection
Content Area: Adult Health/Respiratory

Reference:
Black, J., Hawks, J., & Keene, A. (2001). *Medical-surgical nursing: clinical management for positive outcomes* (6th ed.). Philadelphia: W.B. Saunders, p. 1719.

411. A nurse employed in an obstetrician's office checks the fundal height in a client in the second trimester of pregnancy. When measuring this, the nurse most likely expects the measurement:
1 To correlate with gestational age
2 To be greater than gestational age
3 To be lesser than gestational age
4 To have no correlation to gestational age

Answer: 1

Rationale: Up to the third trimester, the measurement of fundal height correlates with gestational age, on average.

Test-Taking Strategy: Note the key words *second trimester*. Use these key words and knowledge about fundal height and gestational age to answer the question. If you had difficulty with this question, review data collection findings in the prenatal period.

Level of Cognitive Ability: Comprehension
Client Needs: Physiological Integrity
Integrated Concept/Process: Nursing Process/Data Collection
Content Area: Maternity

Reference:
McKinney, E., Ashwill, J., Murray, S., James, S., Gorrie, T., & Droske, S. (2000). *Maternal-child nursing.* Philadelphia: W.B. Saunders, p. 486.

412. A nurse is reviewing the health record of a neonate admitted to the nursery. The nurse notes documentation that the anterior fontanel of the neonate is soft. The nurse interprets this finding as indicative of:
1 Increased intracranial pressure
2 Dehydration
3 Decreased intracranial pressure
4 A normal finding

Answer: 4

Rationale: The anterior fontanel is normally 2 to 3 cm in width, 3 to 4 cm in length, and diamondlike in shape. It can be described as soft, which is normal, or full and bulging, which can indicate increased intracranial pressure. Conversely, a depressed fontanel can mean that the neonate is dehydrated.

Test-Taking Strategy: Knowledge of the normal findings in a neonate is necessary to answer this question. Review the findings related to the fontanels if you had difficulty with this question.

Level of Cognitive Ability: Comprehension
Client Needs: Physiological Integrity
Integrated Concept/Process: Nursing Process/Data Collection
Content Area: Maternity

Reference:
McKinney, E., Ashwill, J., Murray, S., James, S., Gorrie, T., & Droske, S. (2000). *Maternal-child nursing.* Philadelphia: W.B. Saunders, p. 358.

---

413. A nurse is caring for a client who had a pelvic exenteration. While caring for the client, the client complains of pain in the calf. The nurse:

1 Administers PRN meperidine hydrochloride (Demerol) as ordered
2 Observes the calf for temperature, color, and size
3 Lightly massages the area to relieve muscle pain
4 Asks the client to walk and observe the gait

Answer: 2
Rationale: The nurse monitors for postoperative complications such as deep vein thrombosis (DVT), pulmonary emboli, and wound infection. Pain in the calf may indicate DVT. Change in color, temperature, or size of client's calf also may indicate this complication. Options 3 and 4 may result in an embolus if in fact this client has DVT. Pain medication for this client's complaint is not the appropriate nursing action.

Test-Taking Strategy: Use the process of elimination. Remember that data collection is the first step of the Nursing Process. Only option 2 specifically addresses data collection. Review postoperative complications and appropriate interventions if you had difficulty with this question.

Level of Cognitive Ability: Application
Client Needs: Physiological Integrity
Integrated Concept/Process: Nursing Process/Implementation
Content Area: Fundamental Skills

Reference:
Black, J., Hawks, J., & Keene, A. (2001). *Medical-surgical nursing: clinical management for positive outcomes* (6th ed.). Philadelphia: W.B. Saunders, pp. 308; 997.

---

414. A nurse is checking the patency of a peripheral IV site and suspects an infiltration. The nurse performs which of the following actions to determine if the IV has infiltrated?

1 Checks the surrounding tissue for edema and coolness
2 Strips the tubing quickly while checking for a rapid blood return
3 Increases the IV flow rate and observes the site for immediate tightening of tissue
4 Checks the area around the IV site for discomfort, redness, and warmth

Answer: 1
Rationale: When checking an IV site for signs of infiltration, it is important to check the site for edema and coolness, which signify leakage of the IV fluid into the surrounding tissues. Stripping the tubing does not cause a blood return but forces IV fluids into the vein or surrounding tissues, which could cause more tissue damage. Increasing the flow rate may be damaging to the tissues if the IV has infiltrated. The IV site feels cool if the IV fluid has infiltrated into the surrounding tissues.

Test-Taking Strategy: Use the process of elimination and focus on the issue, which is infiltration. Recalling that edema and coolness occur with an infiltration directs you to option 1. Review the signs of infiltration if you had difficulty with this question.

Level of Cognitive Ability: Application
Client Needs: Physiological Integrity
Integrated Concept/Process: Nursing Process/Implementation
Content Area: Fundamental Skills

Reference:
Potter, P., & Perry, A. (2001). *Fundamentals of nursing* (5th ed.). St. Louis: Mosby, p. 1234.

415. A client is brought into the emergency room after a car accident. A neck injury is suspected. The client is unresponsive, not breathing, and pulseless. The nurse prepares to open the client's airway by which of the following methods?

1 Tilt the head and lift the chin
2 Lift the head up, put it on two pillows, and attempt to ventilate
3 Use the jaw-thrust maneuver
4 Keep the client flat and grasp the tongue

Answer: 3

Rationale: The most appropriate way to open the airway in suspected neck injuries is the jaw thrust maneuver. This maneuver will prevent further injury if a neck injury is present. Options 1, 2, and 4 are incorrect actions.

Test-Taking Strategy: Use the process of elimination. The key words are *neck injury is suspected*. Knowledge about airway management should assist in eliminating options 2 and 4. From the remaining options, eliminate option 1 because this method will cause further damage to a neck injury. Review basic life support measures if you had difficulty with this question.

Level of Cognitive Ability: Application
Client Needs: Physiological Integrity
Integrated Concept/Process: Nursing Process/Implementation
Content Area: Fundamental Skills

Reference:
Potter, P., & Perry, A. (2001). *Fundamentals of nursing* (5th ed.). St. Louis: Mosby, p. 1184.

416. A nurse is caring for a child with Reye syndrome. The nurse identifies that a major symptom associated with Reye syndrome is present when the nurse notes:

1 Persistent vomiting
2 Protein in the urine
3 A history of a staphylococcus infection in the record
4 Symptoms of hyperglycemia

Answer: 1

Rationale: Persistent vomiting is a major symptom associated with intracranial pressure. Intracranial pressure and encephalopathy are major symptoms of Reye syndrome. Options 2, 3, and 4 are incorrect. Protein is not present in the urine. Reye syndrome is related to a history of viral infections, and hypoglycemia is a symptom of this disease.

Test-Taking Strategy: Use the process of elimination, recalling that intracranial pressure is associated with Reye syndrome. This directs you to option 1. Review the symptoms of Reye syndrome and the signs of intracranial pressure if you had difficulty with this question.

Level of Cognitive Ability: Comprehension
Client Needs: Physiological Integrity
Integrated Concept/Process: Nursing Process/Data Collection
Content Area: Child Health

Reference:
Wong, D., & Hockenberry-Eaton, M. (2001). *Wong's essentials of pediatric nursing* (6th ed.). St. Louis: Mosby, p. 1096.

417. A nurse is caring for an adolescent client with conjunctivitis and is planning to reinforce home care instructions. Which of the following instructions should the nurse include in the plan of care?

Answer: 3

Rationale: Eye makeup should be replaced, but can still be worn. Cool compresses decrease pain and irritation. Isolation for 24 hours after antibiotics are initiated is necessary. All contact lenses should be replaced.

1 Avoid using all eye makeup to prevent possible reinfection
2 Apply warm compresses to lessen irritation
3 Replace contact lenses when the infection clears
4 Stay home for 3 days after starting antibiotic eye drops to avoid the spread of infection

Test-Taking Strategy: Use the process of elimination. Eliminate option 1 because of the absolute word *all*. Eliminate option 4 because 3 days is a lengthy period to remain isolated, particularly if antibiotics have been initiated. Select option 3 over option 2 knowing that cool, not warm, compresses decrease pain and irritation. Review home care instructions for the client with conjunctivitis if you had difficulty with this question.

Level of Cognitive Ability: Application
Client Needs: Physiological Integrity
Integrated Concept/Process: Nursing Process/Planning
Content Area: Child Health

Reference:
Wong, D., & Hockenberry-Eaton, M. (2001). *Wong's essentials of pediatric nursing* (6th ed.). St. Louis: Mosby, p. 466.

418. A child is admitted to the hospital with a suspected diagnosis of pneumococcus pneumonia. The nurse initially prepares:
1 For a chest x-ray to be done to determine how much consolidation there is in the lungs
2 To allow the child to go to the playroom to play with other children
3 To monitor the child's respiratory rate and breath sounds
4 To start antibiotic therapy immediately

Answer: 3
Rationale: A complication of pneumococcus pneumonia can be a pleural effusion, so the respiratory status of the child should be monitored. Option 1 is medical management, not nursing care. Antibiotic therapy is not started until cultures are obtained. The child should not be allowed in the playroom at this time.

Test-Taking Strategy: Use the process of elimination. Note the key word *initially*. Option 3 addresses data collection, the first step of the nursing process. This option also addresses the ABCs (airway, breathing, and circulation). It is also the option that is directly related to the child's diagnosis. Review care of the client with pneumococcus pneumonia if you had difficulty with this question.

Level of Cognitive Ability: Application
Client Needs: Physiological Integrity
Integrated Concept/Process: Nursing Process/Implementation
Content Area: Child Health

Reference:
Wong, D., & Hockenberry-Eaton, M. (2001). *Wong's essentials of pediatric nursing* (6th ed.). St. Louis: Mosby, p. 844.

419. A nurse is assigned to care for a client suspected of bulimia nervosa. When collecting data from the client, the nurse is aware that a characteristic of bulimia is that the client:
1 Overeats for the enjoyment of food
2 Binge eats, then purges
3 Overeats in response to losing control over a weight loss diet
4 Is accepting of body size

Answer: 2
Rationale: Options 1, 3, and 4 are true of the obese person who may binge eat. Individuals with bulimia nervosa develop cycles of binge eating followed by purging. They seldom attempt to diet and have no sense of loss of control.

Test-Taking Strategy: Use the process of elimination. Eliminate options 1 and 3 because they are similar. From the remaining options, recalling the definition of bulimia directs you to option 2. If you had difficulty with this question, review the characteristics associated with this disorder.

Level of Cognitive Ability: Comprehension

Client Needs: Physiological Integrity
Integrated Concept/Process: Nursing Process/Data Collection
Content Area: Mental Health

Reference:
Varcarolis, E. (2002). *Foundations of psychiatric mental health nursing* (4th ed.). Philadelphia: W.B. Saunders, p. 425.

---

420. A client who has experienced a cerebrovascular accident has partial hemiplegia of the left leg. The straight leg cane formerly used by the client is not quite sufficient now. The nurse determines that the client could benefit from the somewhat greater support and stability provided by a:
1 Quad-cane
2 Wooden crutch
3 Lofstrand crutch
4 Wheelchair

Answer: 1
Rationale: A quad-cane may be used by the client requiring greater support and stability than is provided by a straight leg cane. The quad-cane provides a four-point base of support and is indicated for use by clients with partial or complete hemiplegia. Neither crutches nor a wheelchair is indicated for use with a client such as described in the question. A Lofstrand crutch is useful for clients with bilateral weakness.

Test-Taking Strategy: Use the process of elimination. Giving a wheelchair to a client with partial hemiplegia is excessive and is eliminated first. Wooden crutches are not indicated because there is no restriction in weight bearing. A Lofstrand crutch is useful with bilateral weakness. Review each of these assistive devices if you had difficulty with this question.

Level of Cognitive Ability: Comprehension
Client Needs: Physiological Integrity
Integrated Concept/Process: Nursing Process/Planning
Content Area: Adult Health/Neurological

Reference:
Potter, P., & Perry, A. (2001). *Fundamentals of nursing* (5th ed.). St. Louis: Mosby, p. 1008.

---

421. A nurse is caring for a client who has developed compartment syndrome from a severely fractured arm. The client asks the nurse how this can happen. The nurse's response is based on the understanding that:
1 An injured artery causes impaired arterial perfusion through the compartment
2 The fascia expands with injury, causing pressure on underlying nerves and muscles
3 A bone fragment has injured the nerve supply in the area
4 Bleeding and swelling cause increased pressure in an area that cannot expand

Answer: 4
Rationale: Compartment syndrome is caused by bleeding and swelling within a compartment, which is lined by fascia that does not expand. The bleeding and swelling put pressure on the nerves, muscles, and blood vessels in the compartment, which trigger the symptoms.

Test-Taking Strategy: Use the process of elimination. Option 1 should be eliminated first because compartment syndrome is not caused by an arterial injury. Knowing that the fascia itself cannot expand helps to eliminate option 2. To select from the remaining options, it is necessary to know that bleeding and swelling, and not a nerve injury, cause the symptoms. Review the cause of this disorder if you had difficulty with this question.

Level of Cognitive Ability: Comprehension
Client Needs: Physiological Integrity
Integrated Concept/Process: Nursing Process/Implementation
Content Area: Adult Health/Musculoskeletal

Reference:
Black, J., Hawks, J., & Keene, A. (2001). *Medical-surgical nursing: clinical management for positive outcomes* (6th ed.). Philadelphia: W.B. Saunders, p. 599.

422. A client has undergone fasciotomy to treat compartment syndrome of the leg. The nurse plans to provide which type of prescribed wound care to the fasciotomy site?
1   Dry sterile dressings
2   Moist sterile saline dressings
3   Hydrocolloid dressings
4   One-half strength Betadine dressings

Answer: 2
Rationale: The fasciotomy site is not sutured but is left open to relieve pressure and edema. The site is covered with moist, not dry, sterile saline dressings. After 3 to 5 days, when perfusion is adequate and edema subsides, the wound is debrided and closed. A hydrocolloid dressing is not used with clean, open incisions. The incision is clean, not dirty; therefore there should be no reason to use Betadine.

Test-Taking Strategy: Use the process of elimination, recalling what a fasciotomy involves and knowing the basics of wound care. With fasciotomy, the skin is not sutured closed but left open for pressure relief. Moist tissue must remain moist, which eliminates option 1. A hydrocolloid dressing is not indicated for use with clean, open incisions, which eliminates option 3. The incision is clean, not dirty, so there should be no reason to require Betadine. Knowing that Betadine can be irritating to normal tissues is an additional reason to choose option 2 instead of option 4. Review care after this procedure if you had difficulty with this question.

Level of Cognitive Ability: Application
Client Needs: Physiological Integrity
Integrated Concept/Process: Nursing Process/Planning
Content Area: Adult Health/Musculoskeletal

Reference:
Ignatavicius, D., & Workman, M. (2002) *Medical-surgical nursing: critical thinking for collaborative care* (4th ed). Philadelphia: W. B. Saunders, pp. 1128; 1159; 1172.

423. The most appropriate method to administer eardrops to the infant is to:
1   Pull up and back on the auricle and direct the solution toward the wall of the ear canal
2   Pull down and back on the auricle and direct the solution onto the eardrum
3   Pull down and back on the ear lobe and direct the solution toward the wall of the canal
4   Pull up and back on the ear lobe and direct the solution toward the wall of the canal

Answer: 3
Rationale: The infant should be turned on the side with the affected ear uppermost. With the nondominant hand, the earlobe is pulled down and back. The medication is administered by aiming it at the wall of the canal rather than directly onto the eardrum. The infant should be held or positioned with the affected ear uppermost for 10 to 15 minutes to retain the solution. In the adult, the ear is pulled up and back to straighten the auditory canal.

Test-Taking Strategy: Use the process of elimination and note that the question addresses an infant. Eliminate option 2 because the solution should not be directed onto the eardrum. Visualize each remaining options. Option 1 is eliminated because it is the adult procedure. It would be difficult to pull up and back on an earlobe; therefore eliminate option 4. Review the procedure for administering ear medications in an infant and adult if you had difficulty with this question.

Level of Cognitive Ability: Application
Client Needs: Physiological Integrity

Integrated Concept/Process: Nursing Process/Implementation
Content Area: Child Health

Reference:
Schulte, E., Price, D., & Gwin, J. (2001). *Thompson's pediatric nursing* (8th ed.). Philadelphia: W.B. Saunders, p. 362.

---

424. A nurse is asked to assist the physician with the removal of a chest tube. During removal of the chest tube, the nurse plans to instruct the client to:
1   Breathe out forcefully
2   Breathe in deeply
3   Hold their breath
4   Breathe normally

Answer: 3
Rationale: The client is instructed in the Valsalva maneuver so that the client can hold his or her breath and bear down as the physician removes the tube. This increases intrathoracic pressure, thereby lessening the potential for air to enter the pleural space.

Test-Taking Strategy: Use the process of elimination. Eliminate options 2 and 4 because they are similar because breathing causes air to enter the pleural space. From the remaining options, eliminate option 1 because of the word *forcefully*. Review the procedure for the removal of chest tubes if you had difficulty with this question.

Level of Cognitive Ability: Application
Client Needs: Physiological Integrity
Integrated Concept/Process: Nursing Process/Implementation
Content Area: Adult Health/Respiratory

Reference:
Lewis, S., Heitkemper, M., & Dirksen, S. (2004). *Medical-surgical nursing: assessment and management of clinical problems.* (6th ed.). St Louis: Mosby, p. 625.

---

425. An older client recently admitted to the hospital with a hip fracture is placed in Buck's traction. The nurse assigned to care for the client should frequently monitor the client's:
1   Vital signs
2   Mental state
3   Ability to perform range of motion
4   Neurovascular status

Answer: 4
Rationale: The neurovascular status of the extremity of the client in Buck's traction must be checked every 2 hours for the first 24 hours. Older clients are especially at risk for neurovascular compromise because many of these clients already have disorders that affect the peripheral vascular system. The client's physiological status determines the frequency of vital signs, not the presence or absence of Buck's traction. Although clients in some types of traction do become depressed after a few days or weeks, Buck's traction usually is used preoperatively, which typically involves a few hours or 1 to 2 days at the most. Range of motion of the involved leg is contraindicated in hip fractures.

Test-Taking Strategy: Use the process of elimination. Eliminate option 3 first because range of motion is contraindicated in a hip fracture. From the remaining options, focus on the issue, which is Buck's traction, and visualize this type of device. Although determining vital signs is the most global option, neurovascular status is specific to the use of traction. Review nursing care of the client in traction if you had difficulty with this question.

Level of Cognitive Ability: Application
Client Needs: Physiological Integrity
Integrated Concept/Process: Nursing Process/Implementation
Content Area: Adult Health/Musculoskeletal

Reference:
Black, J., Hawks, J., & Keene, A. (2001). *Medical-surgical nursing: clinical management for positive outcomes* (6th ed.). Philadelphia: W.B. Saunders, p. 599.

426. A client who has a renal mass asks the nurse why an ultrasound has been scheduled as opposed to other diagnostic tests that may be ordered. The nurse most appropriately formulates a response based on the understanding that:
1   An ultrasound can differentiate a solid mass from a fluid-filled cyst
2   An ultrasound is much more cost effective than other diagnostic tests
3   All other tests are more invasive than an ultrasound
4   All other tests require more elaborate postprocedural care

Answer: 1
Rationale: A significant advantage of an ultrasound is that it can differentiate a solid mass from a fluid-filled mass. It is noninvasive and does not require any special after care. There are other diagnostic tests, such as MRI and CT scanning, which are also noninvasive (unless contrast is used), that require no special after care either. However, it is the ultrasound that can discriminate between solid and fluid masses most optimally.

Test-Taking Strategy: Use the process of elimination. Eliminate options 3 and 4 first because it is unlikely that any response with the word *all* in it is likely to be true. From the remaining options, recalling that ultrasonography uses sound waves reflected back from tissues of different densities directs you to option 1. Review the purpose of ultrasonography if you had difficulty with this question.

Level of Cognitive Ability: Comprehension
Client Needs: Physiological Integrity
Integrated Concept/Process: Nursing Process/Implementation
Content Area: Adult Health/Renal

Reference:
Black, J., Hawks, J., & Keene, A. (2001). *Medical-surgical nursing: clinical management for positive outcomes* (6th ed.). Philadelphia: W.B. Saunders, p. 657.

427. A client has been admitted to the hospital with acute glomerulonephritis. The nurse plans to collect data and initially asks the client about a recent history of:
1   Bleeding ulcer
2   Hypertension
3   Fungal infection
4   Streptococcal infection

Answer: 4
Rationale: The predominant cause of acute glomerulonephritis is infection with beta-hemolytic streptococcus 3 weeks before the onset of symptoms. Other infectious agents besides bacteria that could trigger the disorder include viruses or parasites. Hypertension and bleeding ulcer are not precipitating causes.

Test-Taking Strategy: Use the process of elimination. Knowing that infection is a common trigger for glomerulonephritis helps you to eliminate options 1 and 2 first. From the remaining options, it is necessary to know that streptococcal infections are a common cause of this problem. Review the causes of this disorder if you had difficulty with this question.

Level of Cognitive Ability: Application
Client Needs: Physiological Integrity
Integrated Concept/Process: Nursing Process/Data Collection
Content Area: Adult Health/Renal

Reference:
Black, J., Hawks, J., & Keene, A. (2001). *Medical-surgical nursing: clinical management for positive outcomes* (6th ed.). Philadelphia: W.B. Saunders, p. 863.

428. A nurse is caring for a client receiving bolus feedings via a nasogastric tube. As the nurse is finishing the feeding, the client asks for the head of the bed to be positioned flat to sleep. Which of the following positions is the most appropriate choice for this client at this time?

1 Head of bed flat with the client in the supine position for at least 30 minutes
2 Head of bed elevated 35 to 40 degrees with the client in the right lateral position for at least 30 minutes
3 Head of bed elevated 45 to 60 degrees with the client in the supine position for at least 60 minutes
4 Head of bed in semi-Fowler's position with the client in the left lateral position for at least 60 minutes

Answer: 2
Rationale: Aspiration is a possible complication associated with nasogastric tube feeding. The head of the bed is elevated 35 to 40 degrees for at least 30 minutes after bolus tube feeding to prevent vomiting and aspiration. The right lateral position uses gravity to facilitate gastric retention to prevent vomiting. The flat supine position is avoided for the first 30 minutes after a tube feeding.

Test-Taking Strategy: Use the process of elimination. Eliminate options 1 and 3 first because a supine position places the client at risk for aspiration. From the remaining options, think about the anatomy of the gastrointestinal system. Option 2 and 4 indicate the same head elevation, but the right lateral position uses gravity to facilitate gastric retention to prevent vomiting. Review care of the client receiving nasogastric tube feedings if you had difficulty with this question.

Level of Cognitive Ability: Application
Client Needs: Physiological Integrity
Integrated Concept/Process: Nursing Process/Implementation
Content Area: Fundamental Skills

Reference:
Black, J., Hawks, J., & Keene, A. (2001). *Medical-surgical nursing: clinical management for positive outcomes* (6th ed.). Philadelphia: W.B. Saunders, p. 676.

429. A nurse is caring for a client with acute pancreatitis and a history of alcoholism. Which of the following data would be a sign of paralytic ileus, a complication of acute pancreatitis?

1 Firm, nontender mass palpable at the lower right costal margin
2 Severe, constant pain with rapid onset
3 Inability to pass flatus
4 Loss of anal sphincter control

Answer: 3
Rationale: An inflammatory reaction such as acute pancreatitis can cause paralytic ileus, the most common form of nonmechanical obstruction. Inability to pass flatus is a clinical manifestation of paralytic ileus. Option 1 is the description of the physical finding of liver enlargement. The liver is usually enlarged in cases of cirrhosis or hepatitis. Although this client may have an enlarged liver, an enlarged liver is not a sign of paralytic ileus or intestinal obstruction. Pain is associated with paralytic ileus, but the pain usually presents as a more constant generalized discomfort. Pain that is severe, constant, and rapid in onset is more likely caused by strangulation of the bowel. Loss of sphincter control is not a sign of paralytic ileus.

Test-Taking Strategy: Use the process of elimination and focus on the issue, paralytic ileus. Recalling the pathophysiology related to this complication and noting the word *paralytic* assists in directing you to option 3. Review the signs of paralytic ileus if you had difficulty with this question.

Level of Cognitive Ability: Comprehension
Client Needs: Physiological Integrity
Integrated Concept/Process: Nursing Process/Data Collection
Content Area: Adult Health/Gastrointestinal

Reference:
Black, J., Hawks, J., & Keene, A. (2001). *Medical-surgical nursing: clinical management for positive outcomes* (6th ed.). Philadelphia: W.B. Saunders, pp. 1195; 1511.

430. After collecting data on a client with a diagnosis of cholelithiasis, the nurse reports that the bowel sounds are normal. The nurse documents which of the following best descriptions of normal bowel sounds?
1 Waves of loud gurgles auscultated in all four quadrants
2 Very high-pitched loud rushes auscultated, especially in one or two quadrants
3 Relatively high-pitched clicks or gurgles auscultated in all four quadrants
4 Low-pitched swishing auscultated in one or two quadrants

Answer: 3
Rationale: Although frequency and intensity of bowel sounds vary depending on the phase of digestion, normal bowel sounds are relatively high-pitched clicks or gurgles. Loud gurgles (borborygmi) indicate hyperperistalsis. Bowel sounds are higher-pitched and loud (hyperresonance) when the intestines are under tension, such as in intestinal obstruction. A swishing or buzzing sound represents turbulent blood flow that may be associated with a bruit.

Test-Taking Strategy: Use the process of elimination. Normally, bowel sounds should be audible in all four quadrants; therefore options 2 and 4 can be eliminated. Focusing on the issue, normal bowel sounds, directs you to option 3 from the remaining choices. Review these characteristics of bowel sounds if you had difficulty with this question.

Level of Cognitive Ability: Application
Client Needs: Physiological Integrity
Integrated Concept/Process: Communication and Documentation
Content Area: Adult Health/Gastrointestinal

Reference:
deWit, S. (2001). *Fundamental concepts and skills for nursing.* Philadelphia: W.B. Saunders, p. 383.

431. A nurse is assigned to care for a client with nephrotic syndrome. The nurse checks which of the following most important parameters on a daily basis?
1 Albumin level
2 Weight
3 Blood urea nitrogen (BUN) level
4 Activity tolerance

Answer: 2
Rationale: The client with nephrotic syndrome typically presents with edema, hypoalbuminemia, and proteinuria. The nurse carefully checks the fluid balance of the client, which includes daily monitoring of weight, intake and output, edema, and girth measurements. Albumin levels are monitored as they are prescribed, as are the BUN and creatinine levels. The client's activity level is adjusted according to the amount of edema and water retention. The client's activity level should be restricted as edema increases.

Test-Taking Strategy: Use the process of elimination. Recalling that the activity level is adjusted according to the volume of fluid retention helps you to eliminate option 4. From the remaining options, recall that edema is a significant clinical manifestation and note the word *daily* in the stem of the question. This directs you to option 2. Review nursing interventions for the client with nephrotic syndrome if you had difficulty with this question.

Level of Cognitive Ability: Application
Client Needs: Physiological Integrity
Integrated Concept/Process: Nursing Process/Data Collection
Content Area: Adult Health/Renal

Reference:
Black, J., Hawks, J., & Keene, A. (2001). *Medical-surgical nursing: clinical management for positive outcomes* (6th ed.). Philadelphia: W.B. Saunders, p. 863.

432. A client is being admitted to the nursing unit with urolithiasis and ureteral colic. The nurse checks the client for pain that is:

1 Dull and aching in the costovertebral area
2 Sharp and radiating posteriorly to the spinal column
3 Excruciating, wavelike, and radiating toward the genitalia
4 Aching and cramplike throughout the abdomen

Answer: 3

Rationale: The pain of ureteral colic is caused by movement of a stone through the ureter, and is sharp, excruciating, and wavelike, radiating to the genitalia and thigh. The stone causes reduced flow of urine, and the urine also contains blood because of the stone's abrasive action on urinary tract mucosa. Stones in the renal pelvis cause pain that is a deep ache in the costovertebral area. Renal colic is characterized by pain that is acute, with nausea and vomiting, and tenderness over the costovertebral area.

Test-Taking Strategy: Use the process of elimination. Begin to answer this question by eliminating option 4 because this pattern of pain is nonspecific and is the least likely to be the correct option. From the remaining options, recall the anatomical location of the kidneys and ureters. Because the kidneys are located in the posterior abdomen near the ribcage, pain in the costovertebral area is more likely to be associated with stones in the renal pelvis. On the other hand, sharp wavelike pain that radiates toward the genitalia is more consistent with the location of the ureters. Review the characteristics of pain associated with urolithiasis and ureteral colic if you had difficulty with this question.

Level of Cognitive Ability: Comprehension
Client Needs: Physiological Integrity
Integrated Concept/Process: Nursing Process/Data Collection
Content Area: Adult Health/Renal

Reference:
Black, J., Hawks, J., & Keene, A. (2001). *Medical-surgical nursing: clinical management for positive outcomes* (6th ed.). Philadelphia: W.B. Saunders, p. 750.

433. A nurse is collecting data from a client with left-sided heart failure. The client states that it is necessary to use three pillows under the head and chest at night to be able to breathe comfortably while sleeping. The nurse documents that the client is experiencing:

1 Dyspnea on exertion
2 Dyspnea at rest
3 Orthopnea
4 Paroxysmal nocturnal dyspnea

Answer: 3

Rationale: Dyspnea is a subjective problem that can range from an awareness of breathing to physical distress, and does not necessarily correlate with the degree of heart failure. Dyspnea can be exertional or at rest. Orthopnea is a more severe form of dyspnea, requiring the client to use pillows to support the head and thorax at night. Paroxysmal nocturnal dyspnea is a severe form of dyspnea occurring suddenly at night because of rapid fluid reentry into the vasculature from the interstitium during sleep.

Test-Taking Strategy: Use the process of elimination. Eliminate options 1 and 4 because the question mentions nothing about exertion or a sudden (paroxysmal) event. Select option 3 instead of 2 because the client is breathing "comfortably" with the use of pillows. Review the characteristics associated with orthopnea if you had difficulty with this question.

Level of Cognitive Ability: Application
Client Needs: Physiological Integrity
Integrated Concept/Process: Communication and Documentation
Content Area: Adult Health/Cardiovascular

Reference:
Black, J., Hawks, J., & Keene, A. (2001). *Medical-surgical nursing: clinical management for positive outcomes* (6th ed.). Philadelphia: W.B. Saunders, p. 1452.

---

434. A client with renal cancer is being treated preoperatively with radiation therapy. The nurse evaluates that the client has an understanding of proper care of the skin over the treatment field if the client states to:
1 Avoid skin exposure to direct sunlight and chlorinated water
2 Use lanolin-based cream on the affected skin on a daily basis
3 Remove the lines or ink marks using a gentle soap after each treatment
4 Use the hottest water possible to wash the treatment site twice daily

Answer: 1
Rationale: The client undergoing radiation therapy should avoid washing the site until instructed to do so. The client should then wash using mild soap and warm or cool water, and pat the area dry. No lotions, creams, alcohol, or deodorants should be placed on the skin over the treatment site. Lines or ink marks that are placed on the skin to guide the radiation therapy should be left in place. The affected skin should be protected from temperature extremes, direct sunlight, and chlorinated water (as from swimming pools).

Test-Taking Strategy: Use the process of elimination. Begin to answer this question by eliminating options 2 and 4 because of the words *lanolin* and *hottest* in these options. Recalling that markings used to guide therapy are to be left in place helps you to choose option 1 instead of option 3 from the remaining options. Review skin care for the client receiving radiation therapy if you had difficulty with this question.

Level of Cognitive Ability: Comprehension
Client Needs: Physiological Integrity
Integrated Concept/Process: Self-Care
Content Area: Adult Health/Oncology

Reference:
Black, J., Hawks, J., & Keene, A. (2001). *Medical-surgical nursing: clinical management for positive outcomes* (6th ed.). Philadelphia: W.B. Saunders, p. 380.

---

435. Which of the following sites is best for checking the pulse during cardiopulmonary resuscitation (CPR) in a 6-month-old infant?
1 Femoral
2 Carotid
3 Radial
4 Brachial

Answer: 4
Rationale: The carotid is the most central and accessible artery in children older than 1 year of age. However, the very short and often flat neck of the infant renders the carotid pulse difficult to palpate. Therefore it is preferable to use the brachial pulse, located on the inner side of the upper arm midway between the elbow and shoulder.

Test-Taking Strategy: Use the process of elimination and focus on the age of the infant. Recall the principles related to CPR to answer this question. Review these principles if you had difficulty with this question.

Level of Cognitive Ability: Comprehension
Client Needs: Physiological Integrity
Integrated Concept/Process: Nursing Process/Data Collection
Content Area: Child Health

Reference:
Wong, D., & Hockenberry-Eaton, M. (2001). *Wong's essentials of pediatric nursing* (6th ed.). St. Louis: Mosby, p. 871.

436. A client with renal failure is receiving epoetin alfa (Epogen) to support erythropoiesis. The nurse questions the client about compliance with taking which of the following medications, which supports red blood cell (RBC) production?
1 Calcium supplement
2 Iron supplement
3 Magnesium supplement
4 Zinc supplement

Answer: 2
Rationale: Iron is needed for RBC production. Otherwise, the body cannot produce sufficient erythrocytes. The client is not receiving the full benefit of this costly therapy with epoetin alfa if iron is not taken.

Test-Taking Strategy: Use the process of elimination. Note the relationship of RBC production in the question and iron in the correct option. Review the concepts related to epoetin alfa and RBC production if you had difficulty with this question.

Level of Cognitive Ability: Application
Client Needs: Physiological Integrity
Integrated Concept/Process: Nursing Process/Data Collection
Content Area: Adult Health/Renal

Reference:
Clark, J., Queener, S., & Karb, V. (2002). *Pharmacologic basis of nursing practice* (6th ed.). St Louis: Mosby, p. 281.

---

437. A client who just underwent tonsillectomy has become restless. The nurse notes an increasing pulse rate, slight pallor, and frequent swallowing. The nurse most appropriately interprets that:
1 The client needs pain medication
2 The client may have postoperative bleeding or hemorrhage
3 This is an expected postoperative finding
4 The client most likely has some mild postoperative edema

Answer: 2
Rationale: Signs of postoperative hemorrhage include pallor, restlessness, frequent swallowing, large amounts of bloody drainage or vomitus, increasing pulse rate, and a falling blood pressure. These signs should be reported to the surgeon. Although some of the signs and symptoms exhibited by the client could also result from pain (such as restlessness and increasing pulse), the presence of the others indicates bleeding.

Test-Taking Strategy: Use the process of elimination. Recalling the concepts related to hemorrhage and shock and focusing on the signs presented in the question direct you to option 2. Review postoperative complications after tonsillectomy if you had difficulty with this question.

Level of Cognitive Ability: Analysis
Client Needs: Physiological Integrity
Integrated Concept/Process: Nursing Process/Evaluation
Content Area: Adult Health/Respiratory

Reference:
Black, J., Hawks, J., & Keene, A. (2001). *Medical-surgical nursing: clinical management for positive outcomes* (6th ed.). Philadelphia: W.B. Saunders, p. 1679.

---

438. A nurse is reviewing the results of a sweat test performed on a child with cystic fibrosis (CF). The nurse would expect to note which of the following?
1 A sweat bicarbonate concentration less than 40 mEq/L
2 A sweat potassium concentration less than 40 mEq/L
3 A sweat potassium concentration less than 60 mEq/L

Answer: 4
Rationale: The consistent finding of abnormally high chloride concentrations in the sweat is a unique characteristic of CF. Normally the sweat chloride concentration is less than 40 mEq/L. A chloride concentration greater than 60 mEq/L is diagnostic of CF. Bicarbonate and potassium concentration is unrelated to the sweat test.

Test-Taking Strategy: Use the process of elimination. Eliminate options 1, 2, and 3 because the bicarbonate and the potassium

4   A sweat chloride concentration greater than 60 mEq/L

level are unrelated to the sweat test. Also, note that option 4 is different, indicating a "greater" value. Review this test if you had difficulty with this question.

Level of Cognitive Ability: Comprehension
Client Needs: Physiological Integrity
Integrated Concept/Process: Nursing Process/Data Collection
Content Area: Child Health

Reference:
Schulte, E., Price, D., & Gwin, J. (2001). *Thompson's pediatric nursing* (8th ed.). Philadelphia: W.B. Saunders, p. 142.

---

439. A nurse performs a neurovascular check on a client with a newly applied cast. Close observation and further evaluation will be necessary if the nurse notes:
1   Capillary refill less than 6 seconds
2   Palpable pulses distal to the cast
3   Sensation when the area distal to the cast is pinched
4   Blanching of the nail bed when depressed

Answer: 1
Rationale: To check for adequate circulation (capillary refill), the nail bed of each finger or toe is depressed until it blanches and then the pressure is released. Optimally, the color will change from white to pink rapidly (less than 3 seconds). If this does not occur, the toes or fingers require close observation and further evaluation. Palpable pulses and sensations distal to the cast is expected. However, the physician must be notified if pulses cannot be palpated or the client complains of numbness or tingling.

Test-Taking Strategy: Use the process of elimination. Note the key words *close observation and further evaluation*. Eliminate options 2, 3, and 4 because these options identify normal expected findings. Option 1 identifies an abnormal or unexpected finding. Review the technique for checking capillary refill if you had difficulty with this question.

Level of Cognitive Ability: Comprehension
Client Needs: Physiological Integrity
Integrated Concept/Process: Nursing Process/Data Collection
Content Area: Adult Health/Neurological

Reference:
deWit, S. (2001). *Fundamental concepts and skills for nursing.* Philadelphia: W.B. Saunders, pp. 815; 818.

---

440. A client undergoes a cholecystectomy and returns from surgery with a T tube in place. The nurse is assigned to assist in caring for the client and is instructed to monitor the drainage from the T tube. During the first 24 hours after surgery, the nurse expects how much bile to drain from the T tube?
1   50 to 100 mL
2   100 to 150 mL
3   300 to 500 mL
4   800 to 1100 mL

Answer: 3
Rationale: In the initial postoperative period, bloody drainage is expected, which changes to green-brown bile. Bile output is 400 mL a day with a gradual decrease in amount. Bile drainage amounts in excess of 1000 mL a day should be reported to the physician.

Test-Taking Strategy: Use the process of elimination and note the key words *during the first 24 hours*. This provides you with the clue that the output will be on the higher side and assist in eliminating options 1 and 2. Attempt to visualize the amounts identified in the remaining options. Option 4 identifies an excessive amount and should be eliminated. Review postoperative expectations after cholecystectomy if you had difficulty with this question.

Level of Cognitive Ability: Comprehension
Client Needs: Physiological Integrity
Integrated Concept/Process: Nursing Process/Evaluation
Content Area: Adult Health/Gastrointestinal

Reference:

Black, J., Hawks, J., & Keene, A. (2001). *Medical-surgical nursing: clinical management for positive outcomes* (6th ed.). Philadelphia: W.B. Saunders, p. 1215

---

441. A client with Crohn's disease is admitted to the hospital for creation of a Kock pouch, and the client asks the nurse about this type of pouch. Which of the following is not a part of the nurse's description?

1   The reservoir gradually increases in size and may attain a capacity of 500 mL

2   The adjustment to body image is usually less traumatic than for clients with conventional ileostomies

3   The intraabdominal pouch is created from the looped sigmoid colon

4   The stoma is covered with a bandage between intubations to absorb leaks or mucus

Answer: 3

Rationale: The intraabdominal pouch (reservoir) is created from the looped ileum not the sigmoid. It collects feces, making external collection pouches unnecessary. The stoma is covered with a bandage or gauze pad between intubations to absorb leaks or mucus. The reservoir gradually increases in size and may attain a capacity of 500 mL. The adjustment to the body change is usually less traumatic for these clients than for those with conventional ileostomies.

Test-Taking Strategy: Use the process of elimination and note the key word *not.* Recalling the anatomical location of the creation of this type of pouch directs you to option 3. Review this procedure if you had difficulty with this question.

Level of Cognitive Ability: Comprehension
Client Needs: Physiological Integrity
Integrated Concept/Process: Nursing Process/Implementation
Content Area: Adult Health/Gastrointestinal

Reference:

Black, J., Hawks, J., & Keene, A. (2001). *Medical-surgical nursing: clinical management for positive outcomes* (6th ed.). Philadelphia: W.B. Saunders, p. 775.

---

442. A nurse is assisting in collecting assessment data on a newborn suspected of having Down syndrome. When checking the newborn's skin, which of the following does the nurse expect to note if this syndrome is present?

1   Several creases noted across the palm

2   A single crease across the palm

3   The absence of creases across the palm

4   Two large creases across the palm

Answer: 2

Rationale: A single crease across the palm (simian crease) is most often associated with chromosomal abnormalities, notably Down syndrome.

Test-Taking Strategy: Knowledge about the characteristics associated with Down syndrome is needed to answer this question. Review the characteristics of this disorder if you had difficulty with this question.

Level of Cognitive Ability: Comprehension
Client Needs: Physiological Integrity
Integrated Concept/Process: Nursing Process/Data Collection
Content Area: Maternity

Reference:

Burroughs, A., & Leifer, G. (2002). *Maternity nursing* (8th ed.). Philadelphia: W.B. Saunders, p. 283.

---

443. A nurse is caring for a client admitted to the surgical nursing unit after a right modified radical mastectomy. The nurse

Answer: 4

Rationale: If there is drainage or bleeding from the surgical site after mastectomy, gravity causes the drainage to seep down and

would include which of the following when caring for this client?

1 Position the client supine with the right arm elevated on a pillow
2 Take blood pressures in the right arm only
3 Have serum laboratory samples drawn from the right arm only
4 Check the right posterior axilla area when checking the surgical dressing

soak the posterior axillary portion of the dressing first. The nurse checks this area to detect early bleeding. The client should be positioned with the head in semi-Fowler's position and the arm elevated on pillows to decrease edema. Edema is likely to occur because lymph drainage channels have been resected during the surgical procedure. Blood pressure, venipunctures, and IV sites should not involve the use of the operative arm.

Test-Taking Strategy: Use the process of elimination. Remember that options that are similar are not likely to be correct. This guides you to eliminate options 2 and 3 first. Also, note the absolute word *only* in these options. From the remaining options, use knowledge of the effects of gravity to direct you to option 4. Review care of the client after this surgical procedure if you had difficulty with this question.

Level of Cognitive Ability: Application
Client Needs: Physiological Integrity
Integrated Concept/Process: Nursing Process/Implementation
Content Area: Adult Health/Oncology

Reference:
Lewis, S., Heitkemper, M., & Dirksen, S. (2004). *Medical-surgical nursing: assessment and management of clinical problems.* (6th ed.). St Louis: Mosby, p. 1374.

---

444. A client is at risk for infection after radical vulvectomy. The nurse avoids doing which of the following when giving perineal care to this client?

1 Cleanse using warm tap water and a bulb syringe
2 Intermittently expose the wound to air
3 Provide perineal care after each voiding and bowel movement
4 Provide prescribed sitz baths after the sutures are removed

Answer: 1
Rationale: A sterile solution such as normal saline should be used for perineal care using an aseptic syringe or a water pick. This should be done regularly twice a day and after each voiding and bowel movement. The wound is intermittently exposed to air to permit drying and prevent maceration. Once sutures are removed, sitz baths may be prescribed to stimulate healing and soothe the area.

Test-Taking Strategy: Use the process of elimination. Note the key word *avoids*. Begin to answer this question by eliminating options 3 and 4, which are accepted practices. From the remaining options, note the words *tap water* in option 1. Using principles of asepsis and knowledge of the conditions that cause a wound infection directs you to option 1. Review the principles of asepsis and preventing wound infections if you had difficulty with this question.

Level of Cognitive Ability: Application
Client Needs: Physiological Integrity
Integrated Concept/Process: Nursing Process/Implementation
Content Area: Adult Health/Oncology

Reference:
Black, J., Hawks, J., & Keene, A. (2001). *Medical-surgical nursing: clinical management for positive outcomes* (6th ed.). Philadelphia: W.B. Saunders, p. 1007.

---

445. A nurse is assisting a client with hepatic encephalopathy to fill out the dietary menu. The nurse advises the client to avoid which of the following entree

Answer: 4
Rationale: Clients with hepatic encephalopathy have impaired ability to convert ammonia to urea and must limit the intake of protein and ammonia-containing foods in the diet. The client

items, which could aggravate the client's condition?

1   Fresh fruit plate
2   Tomato soup
3   Vegetable lasagna
4   Ground beef patty

should avoid foods such as chicken, beef, ham, cheese, buttermilk, potatoes, onions, peanut butter, and gelatin.

Test-Taking Strategy: Use the process of elimination. Recalling that clients with hepatic encephalopathy must limit the intake of protein assists in directing you to the correct option. Note that options 1, 2, and 3 are similar in that they address food items of a fruit and vegetable nature. Option 4 is the option that is different. Review dietary measures for the client with hepatic encephalopathy if you had difficulty with this question.

Level of Cognitive Ability: Application
Client Needs: Physiological Integrity
Integrated Concept/Process: Nursing Process/Implementation
Content Area: Adult Health/Gastrointestinal

Reference:
Black, J., Hawks, J., & Keene, A. (2001). *Medical-surgical nursing: clinical management for positive outcomes* (6th ed.). Philadelphia: W.B. Saunders, p. 1252.

---

446. A client with a colostomy is complaining of gas building up in the colostomy bag. The nurse tells the client that which of the following food items will not aggravate this problem?

1   Beans
2   Cauliflower
3   Potatoes
4   Corn

Answer: 3
Rationale: Gas forming foods include corn, cauliflower, onions, beans, and cabbage. These should be avoided by the client with a colostomy until tolerance to them is determined.

Test-Taking Strategy: Use the process of elimination and note the key word *not*. Use knowledge of the basic principles related to nutrition and focus on the issue, gas-forming foods, to direct you to the correct option. Review those food items that are gas forming if you had difficulty with this question.

Level of Cognitive Ability: Application
Client Needs: Physiological Integrity
Integrated Concept/Process: Nursing Process/Implementation
Content Area: Adult Health/Gastrointestinal

Reference:
Black, J., Hawks, J., & Keene, A. (2001). *Medical-surgical nursing: clinical management for positive outcomes* (6th ed.). Philadelphia: W.B. Saunders, p. 786.

---

447. A client admitted to the hospital with a diagnosis of cirrhosis has massive ascites and difficulty breathing. The nurse performs which of the following interventions as a priority measure to assist the client with breathing?

1   Checks respirations every 4 hours
2   Repositions side to side every 2 hours
3   Encourages deep breathing every 2 hours
4   Elevates the head of the bed 60 degrees

Answer: 4
Rationale: The client is having difficulty breathing because of upward pressure on the diaphragm from the ascitic fluid. Elevating the head of the bed enlists the aid of gravity in relieving pressure on the diaphragm. The other options are appropriate general measures for the client with ascites, but the priority measure is the one that relieves diaphragmatic pressure.

Test-Taking Strategy: Use the process of elimination. Note the key words *priority measure*. This tells you that more than one or all of the questions may be partially or totally correct. In this case, every option is a correct nursing action, but elevating the head of the bed takes highest priority in providing immediate relief of symptoms. Review care of the client with ascites if you had difficulty with this question.

Level of Cognitive Ability: Application
Client Needs: Physiological Integrity
Integrated Concept/Process: Nursing Process/Implementation
Content Area: Adult Health/Gastrointestinal

Reference:
Black, J., Hawks, J., & Keene, A. (2001). *Medical-surgical nursing: clinical management for positive outcomes* (6th ed.). Philadelphia: W.B. Saunders, p. 1246.

---

448. A client with acute diverticulitis has just been advanced from a liquid diet to solids. The nurse encourages the client to take in foods that are:
1 Low fiber
2 High protein
3 Moderate in fat
4 High carbohydrate

Answer: 1
Rationale: The purpose of a low-fiber diet in a client with diverticulitis is to allow the bowel to rest while the inflammation subsides. The client should also avoid foods such as nuts, corn, popcorn, and raw celery, which are high in roughage.

Test-Taking Strategy: Use the process of elimination. Recalling that diverticulitis indicates inflammation assists in directing you to the correct option. If this question was difficult, review the diet prescribed for this disorder.

Level of Cognitive Ability: Application
Client Needs: Physiological Integrity
Integrated Concept/Process: Nursing Process/Implementation
Content Area: Adult Health/Gastrointestinal

Reference:
Black, J., Hawks, J., & Keene, A. (2001). *Medical-surgical nursing: clinical management for positive outcomes* (6th ed.). Philadelphia: W.B. Saunders, p. 789.

---

449. A nurse caring for the client with hepatic encephalopathy checks the client for asterixis. To appropriately check for asterixis the nurse:
1 Asks the client to extend an arm, dorsiflex the wrist, and extend the fingers
2 Checks the stools for clay-colored pigmentation
3 Asks the client to sign own name and notes any difficulty with writing
4 Reviews serum levels of bilirubin and alkaline phosphatase for elevation

Answer: 1
Rationale: Asterixis is an abnormal muscle tremor often associated with hepatic encephalopathy. The nurse asks the client to extend an arm, dorsiflex the wrist, and extend the fingers. The nurse then checks for muscle tremors. Asterixis is sometimes called "liver flap." Options 2, 3, and 4 are associated with hepatitis but are not signs of asterixis.

Test-Taking Strategy: Specifically, knowledge of how to test for asterixis is needed to answer this question. Review the technique for testing for asterixis if you had difficulty with this question.

Level of Cognitive Ability: Application
Client Needs: Physiological Integrity
Integrated Concept/Process: Nursing Process/Data Collection
Content Area: Adult Health/Gastrointestinal

Reference:
Black, J., Hawks, J., & Keene, A. (2001). *Medical-surgical nursing: clinical management for positive outcomes* (6th ed.). Philadelphia: W.B. Saunders, p. 1227.

---

450. A nurse instructs a preoperative client in the proper use of an incentive spirometer. In the postoperative period, the nurse

Answer: 1
Rationale: Incentive devices have many desired and positive effects. Incentive devices provide the stimulus for a spontaneous

determines that the incentive spirometer was effective if the client exhibits:

1   Coughing
2   Shallow breaths
3   Audible wheezing
4   Unilateral chest expansion

deep breath. Through use of the sustained maximal inspiration concept, spontaneous deep breathing reduces atelectasis, opens airways, stimulates coughing, and actively encourages individual participation in recovery. Shallow breaths, wheezing, and unilateral chest expansion indicate that the incentive spirometry was not effective. Wheezing indicates narrowing or obstruction of the airway, and unilateral chest expansion could indicate atelectasis.

Test-Taking Strategy: Use the process of elimination and focus on the issue: the incentive spirometer was effective. Options 2, 3, and 4 indicate abnormal findings. Therefore, eliminate these options. Review the purpose of an incentive spirometer if you had difficulty with this question.

Level of Cognitive Ability: Comprehension
Client Needs: Physiological Integrity
Integrated Concept/Process: Nursing Process/Evaluation
Content Area: Fundamental Skills

Reference:
deWit, S. (2001). *Fundamental concepts and skills for nursing.* Philadelphia: W.B. Saunders, p. 535.

---

451. A client is to be started on prazosin (Minipress). The client asks the nurse why the first three doses must be taken at bedtime. The nurse's response is based on the understanding that during early use, prazosin:

1   Can cause dizziness, lightheadedness, or possible syncope
2   Results in extreme drowsiness
3   Should be taken when the stomach is empty
4   Can cause significant dependent edema

Answer: 1
Rationale: Prazosin is an alpha-adrenergic blocking agent. "First-dose hypotensive reaction" may occur during early therapy, which is characterized by dizziness, lightheadedness, and possible syncope. This also can occur during periods when the dosage is increased. This effect usually disappears with continued use or when the dosage is decreased. Options 2, 3, and 4 are incorrect.

Test-Taking Strategy: Use the process of elimination. Recalling that prazosin is an antihypertensive agent assists in directing you to option 1. Remember, orthostatic hypotension, which causes dizziness, lightheadedness, and possible syncope, can occur with the use of antihypertensives. Review this medication if you had difficulty with this question.

Level of Cognitive Ability: Comprehension
Client Needs: Physiological Integrity
Integrated Concept/Process: Nursing Process/Implementation
Content Area: Pharmacology

Reference:
Hodgson, B., & Kizior, R. (2003). *Saunders nursing drug handbook 2003.* Philadelphia: W.B. Saunders, p. 916.

---

452. A nurse has applied the prescribed dressing to the leg of a client with an ischemic arterial leg ulcer. The nurse uses which of the following methods of covering the dressing?

1   Apply a sterile pad, and tape it to the skin

Answer: 4
Rationale: With an arterial ulcer, the nurse applies tape only to the bandage itself. Tape is never used directly on the skin because it could cause further tissue damage. For the same reason, Montgomery straps are not applied to the skin (although these are generally intended for use on abdominal wounds). Standard dressing technique includes the use of Kling rolls on circumferential dressings.

2 Apply a Kling roll, and tape it to the skin

3 Apply small Montgomery straps, and tie the edges together

4 Apply a Kling roll, and tape the edge of the roll onto the bandage

Test-Taking Strategy: Use the process of elimination. Recalling that tape is not applied to the skin assists in eliminating options 1 and 2. For the same reason, eliminate option 3 because the Montgomery straps also must adhere to the skin. Review care of the client with an arterial ulcer if you had difficulty with this question.

Level of Cognitive Ability: Application
Client Needs: Physiological Integrity
Integrated Concept/Process: Nursing Process/Implementation
Content Area: Adult Health/Cardiovascular

Reference:
deWit, S. (2001). *Fundamental concepts and skills for nursing.* Philadelphia: W.B. Saunders, p. 787.

---

453. Breathing exercises and postural drainage are ordered for a child with cystic fibrosis (CF). The most appropriate plan to implement these procedures include which of the following?

1 Perform the postural drainage, then the breathing exercises

2 Perform the breathing exercises, then the postural drainage

3 Plan the breathing exercises and the postural drainage so they are scheduled 4 hours apart

4 Perform postural drainage in the morning and breathing exercises in the evening

Answer: 1
Rationale: Breathing exercises are recommended for the majority of children with CF, even for those with minimal pulmonary involvement. The exercises are usually performed twice daily, and they are preceded with postural drainage. The postural drainage mobilizes secretions and the breathing exercises then assist with expectoration. Exercises to assist with posture and to mobilize the thorax are included, such as swinging the arms, and bending and twisting the trunk. The ultimate aim of these exercises is to establish a good habitual breathing pattern.

Test-Taking Strategy: Use the process of elimination. Recalling that postural drainage and breathing exercises are most effective when performed together assists in eliminating options 3 and 4. From the remaining options, consider the effectiveness that each procedure will have on the mobilization of secretions. This directs you to option 1. Review the effects of these procedures if you had difficulty with this question.

Level of Cognitive Ability: Application
Client Needs: Physiological Integrity
Integrated Concept/Process: Nursing Process/Planning
Content Area: Child Health

Reference:
Schulte, E., Price, D., & Gwin, J. (2001). *Thompson's pediatric nursing* (8th ed.). Philadelphia: W.B. Saunders, p. 142.

---

454. A child is admitted to the pediatric unit with a diagnosis of celiac disease. Based on this diagnosis, the nurse expects that the child's stools will be:

1 Dark in color
2 Abnormally small in amount
3 Unusually hard
4 Particularly offensive in odor

Answer: 4
Rationale: The stools of a child with celiac disease are characteristically malodorous, pale, large (bulky), and soft (loose). Excessive flatus is common, and bouts of diarrhea may occur. Options 1, 2, and 3 are not characteristics of this disorder.

Test-Taking Strategy: Knowledge about the manifestations that occur in celiac disease is necessary to answer this question. Review these manifestations if you had difficulty with this question.

Level of Cognitive Ability: Comprehension
Client Needs: Physiological Integrity
Integrated Concept/Process: Nursing Process/Data Collection
Content Area: Child Health

Reference:
Wong, D., & Hockenberry-Eaton, M. (2001). *Wong's essentials of pediatric nursing* (6th ed.). St. Louis: Mosby, p. 927.

---

455. A nurse is assigned to care for a client with suspected pregnancy-induced hypertension (PIH). The nurse understands that the significant findings in the client with PIH include:
1 Glycosuria, hypertension, and obesity
2 Edema, ketonuria, and obesity
3 Edema, tachycardia, and ketonuria
4 Hypertension, edema, and proteinuria

Answer: 4
Rationale: PIH is the most common hypertensive disorder in pregnancy. It is characterized by the development of hypertension, proteinuria, and edema. Glycosuria and ketonuria occur in diabetes mellitus. Tachycardia and obesity are not specifically related to PIH.

Test-Taking Strategy: Use the process of elimination and focus on the name of the disorder identified in the question. Eliminate options 2 and 3 because they do not address hypertension. From the remaining options, recalling that glycosuria is an indication of diabetes assists in directing you to option 4. Review the clinical manifestations associated with PIH if you had difficulty with this question.

Level of Cognitive Ability: Comprehension
Client Needs: Physiological Integrity
Integrated Concept/Process: Nursing Process/Data Collection
Content Area: Maternity

Reference:
Burroughs, A., & Leifer, G. (2002). *Maternity nursing* (8th ed.). Philadelphia: W.B. Saunders, p. 231.

---

456. A client who undergoes a gastric resection is at risk for developing dumping syndrome. The nurse monitors for which of the following that is a symptom of this syndrome?
1 Extreme thirst
2 Bradycardia
3 Dizziness
4 Constipation

Answer: 3
Rationale: The clinical manifestations of dumping syndrome occur 5 to 30 minutes after eating. Symptoms include vasomotor disturbances such as vertigo, tachycardia, syncope, sweating, pallor, palpations, and the desire to lie down. Options 1, 2, and 4 are not associated with dumping syndrome.

Test-Taking Strategy: Use the process of elimination. Recalling that the symptoms associated with dumping syndrome are vasomotor in nature directs you to option 3. Review this disorder and the appropriate treatment measures if you had difficulty with this question.

Level of Cognitive Ability: Application
Client Needs: Physiological Integrity
Integrated Concept/Process: Nursing Process/Data Collection
Content Area: Adult Health/Gastrointestinal

Reference:
Black, J., Hawks, J., & Keene, A. (2001). *Medical-surgical nursing: clinical management for positive outcomes* (6th ed.). Philadelphia: W.B. Saunders, p. 721.

457. When assessing a client for the major postoperative complication after a craniotomy, the nurse monitors for:
1 Restlessness
2 Bleeding
3 Hypotension
4 Bradycardia

Answer: 1
Rationale: The major postoperative complication after craniotomy is increased intracranial pressure (ICP) from cerebral edema, hemorrhage, or obstruction of the normal flow of cerebrospinal fluid. Symptoms of increased ICP include severe headache, deteriorating level of consciousness, restlessness, irritability, and dilated or pinpoint pupils that are slow to react or are nonreactive to light.

Test-Taking Strategy: Use the process of elimination. Remember, always monitor the neurological client for increased ICP. Recall that changes in the level of consciousness (LOC) is the first indicator of increased ICP. Option 1 is the only option that addresses LOC. Review the signs of increased ICP and postoperative complications after craniotomy if you had difficulty with this question.

Level of Cognitive Ability: Application
Client Needs: Physiological Integrity
Integrated Concept/Process: Nursing Process/Data Collection
Content Area: Adult Health/Neurological

Reference:
Black, J., Hawks, J., & Keene, A. (2001). *Medical-surgical nursing: clinical management for positive outcomes* (6th ed.). Philadelphia: W.B. Saunders, p. 1938.

458. Buck's traction is applied to an elderly client after a hip fracture. The client asks the nurse about the traction. The nurse responds knowing that Buck's traction is a:
1 Skin traction involving the use of traction attached to the skin and soft tissues
2 Skeletal traction involving the use of surgically inserted pins
3 Circumferential traction involving the use of a belt around the body
4 Plaster traction involving the use of a cast

Answer: 1
Rationale: Buck's traction is a form of skin traction and involves the use of a belt or halter that is attached to the skin and soft tissues. The purpose of this type of traction is to decrease painful muscle spasms that accompany fractures. The weight that is used as a pulling force is limited (5 to 10 lb), to prevent injury to the skin. Pins, a belt around the body, or plaster is not used in this type of traction.

Test-Taking Strategy: Use the process of elimination. Recalling that Buck's traction is a skin traction assists in eliminating options 2, 3, and 4. Review the purpose and principles related to this type of traction if you had difficulty with this question.

Level of Cognitive Ability: Comprehension
Client Needs: Physiological Integrity
Integrated Concept/Process: Nursing Process/Implementation
Content Area: Adult Health/Musculoskeletal

Reference:
deWit, S. (2001). *Fundamental concepts and skills for nursing*. Philadelphia: W.B. Saunders, p. 809.

459. A client arrives in the emergency unit with burns to both legs and perineal areas. Using the Rule of Nines, the nurse determines that approximately what percentage of the client's body surface has been burned?

Answer: 3
Rationale: The most rapid method used to calculate the size of a burn injury in adult clients whose weights are in normal proportion to their heights is the Rule of Nines. This method divides the body into areas that are in multiples of 9%. Each leg is 18%, each arm is 9%, and the head is 9%. The trunk is 36%

1	19%
2	46%
3	37%
4	65%

and the perineal area is 1%. Both legs and perineal area equal 37%.

Test-Taking Strategy: Knowledge about the percentages associated with this method of calculating burn injuries is necessary to answer this question. Memorize these percentages if you had difficulty with this question.

Level of Cognitive Ability: Comprehension
Client Needs: Physiological Integrity
Integrated Concept/Process: Nursing Process/Data Collection
Content Area: Adult Health/Integumentary

Reference:
Black, J., Hawks, J., & Keene, A. (2001). *Medical-surgical nursing: clinical management for positive outcomes* (6th ed.). Philadelphia: W.B. Saunders, p. 1339.

---

460. Skin closure with heterograft is performed on a burn client. The client asks the nurse about the meaning of a heterograft. The nurse bases the response on the knowledge that a heterograft can best be described as:
1 Skin from another species
2 Skin from a cadaver
3 Skin from the burned client
4 Skin from a skin bank

Answer: 1
Rationale: Biologic dressings are usually heterograft or homograft material. Heterograft is skin from another species. The most commonly used type of heterograft is pigskin because of its availability and its relative compatibility with human skin. Homograft is skin from another human, which is usually obtained from a cadaver and is provided through a skin bank. Autograft is skin from the client.

Test-Taking Strategy: Use the process of elimination. Options 2, 3, and 4 all relate to grafts from human skin. Option 1 is the option that is different. Review the various types of skin closure grafts if you had difficulty with this question.

Level of Cognitive Ability: Comprehension
Client Needs: Physiological Integrity
Integrated Concept/Process: Nursing Process/Implementation
Content Area: Adult Health/Integumentary

Reference:
Lewis, S., Heitkemper, M., & Dirksen, S. (2004). *Medical-surgical nursing: assessment and management of clinical problems* (6th ed.). St. Louis: Mosby, p. 529.

---

461. A nurse is assigned to assist in caring for a hospitalized client who sustained a head injury. The nurse positions this client:
1 With the head elevated on a pillow
2 In left Sims'
3 In reverse Trendelenburg
4 With the head of the bed elevated 30 degrees to 45 degrees

Answer: 4
Rationale: The client is positioned to avoid extreme flexion or extension of the neck and to maintain the head in the midline, neutral position. The client is logrolled when turned to avoid extreme hip flexion. The head of the bed is elevated 30 degrees to 45 degrees. All of these measures are used to enhance venous drainage, which helps prevent increased intracranial pressure (ICP).

Test-Taking Strategy: Use the process of elimination and focus on the issue, the concern about increased ICP. Bearing this in mind, and considering the principles of gravity, you should be able to eliminate options 1, 2, and 3. Review care of the client after a head injury if you had difficulty with this question.

Level of Cognitive Ability: Application
Client Needs: Physiological Integrity
Integrated Concept/Process: Nursing Process/Implementation
Content Area: Adult Health/Neurological

Reference:
Black, J., Hawks, J., & Keene, A. (2001). *Medical-surgical nursing: clinical management for positive outcomes* (6th ed.). Philadelphia: W.B. Saunders, p. 2038.

---

462. An infant is admitted to the pediatric unit with a diagnosis of esophageal atresia. The nurse reviews the health history and expects to note which typical finding of this disorder documented in the record?
1 Continuous drooling
2 Diaphragmatic breathing
3 Slowed reflexes
4 Passage of large amounts of frothy stool

Answer: 1
Rationale: Esophageal atresia prevents the passage of swallowed mucus and saliva into the stomach. After fluid has accumulated in the pouch, it flows from the mouth and the infant then drools continuously. Options 2, 3, and 4 are not associated with this disorder.

Test-Taking Strategy: Use the process of elimination. Eliminate options 3 and 4 by considering the anatomical location of the disorder. From the remaining options, focusing on the word *atresia* assists in directing you to the correct option. Review the manifestations associated with this disorder, if you had difficulty with this question.

Level of Cognitive Ability: Comprehension
Client Needs: Physiological Integrity
Integrated Concept/Process: Nursing Process/Data Collection
Content Area: Child Health

Reference:
Murray, S., McKinney, E., & Gorrie, T. (2002). *Foundations of maternal-newborn nursing* (3rd ed.). Philadelphia: W.B. Saunders, 864.

---

463. A nurse is monitoring a client with acquired immunodeficiency syndrome (AIDS) for early signs of Kaposi's sarcoma. The nurse observes the client for lesion(s) that are:
1 Unilateral, raised, and bluish-purple in color
2 Bilateral, flat, and pink, turning to dark violet or black in color
3 Unilateral, red, raised, and resembling a blister
4 Bilateral, flat, and brownish and scaly in appearance

Answer: 2
Rationale: Kaposi's sarcoma generally starts with an area that is flat and pink and changes to a dark violet or black color. The lesions usually are present bilaterally. They may appear in many areas of the body and are treated with radiation, chemotherapy, and cryotherapy. Options 1, 3, and 4 are incorrect descriptions.

Test-Taking Strategy: Use the process of elimination. Knowing that Kaposi's sarcoma occurs in a bilateral pattern helps you to eliminate options 1 and 3. Knowledge of the character of the lesions is necessary to discriminate between options 2 and 4. Review the characteristics of this disorder if you had difficulty with this question.

Level of Cognitive Ability: Application
Client Needs: Physiological Integrity
Integrated Concept/Process: Nursing Process/Data Collection
Content Area: Adult Health/Respiratory

Reference:
Black, J., Hawks, J., & Keene, A. (2001). *Medical-surgical nursing: clinical management for positive outcomes* (6th ed.). Philadelphia: W.B. Saunders, p. 2205.

464. A nurse is told that a client is suspected of having pleural effusion. The nurse monitors the client for typical manifestations, including:

1 Dyspnea at rest and moist, productive cough
2 Dyspnea on exertion and moist, productive cough
3 Dyspnea at rest and dry, nonproductive cough
4 Dyspnea on exertion and dry, nonproductive cough

Answer: 4
Rationale: Typical findings in the client with a pleural effusion include dyspnea that usually occurs with exertion and a dry, nonproductive cough. The cough is caused by bronchial irritation and possible mediastinal shift.

Test-Taking Strategy: Use the process of elimination. Recalling that a pleural effusion is in the pleural space and not the airways may help you to eliminate options 1 and 2, the options that address the productive cough. Knowing that dyspnea occurs on exertion before it occurs at rest helps you to choose option 4 over option 3. Review the manifestations associated with pleurisy if you had difficulty with this question.

Level of Cognitive Ability: Application
Client Needs: Physiological Integrity
Integrated Concept/Process: Nursing Process/Data Collection
Content Area: Adult Health/Respiratory

Reference:
Black, J., Hawks, J., & Keene, A. (2001). *Medical-surgical nursing: clinical management for positive outcomes* (6th ed.). Philadelphia: W.B. Saunders, p. 1742.

465. A nurse explains to the mother of a newborn the purpose of giving the vitamin K injection to her newborn. The nurse determines that the mother understands the purpose of the vitamin K when the mother states:

1 "The newborn's blood levels are low."
2 "The newborn's liver can't produce vitamin K."
3 "The newborn lacks vitamins."
4 "The newborn lacks intestinal bacteria."

Answer: 4
Rationale: The absence of normal flora needed to synthesize vitamin K in the normal newborn gut results in low levels of vitamin K and creates a transient blood coagulation deficiency between the second and fifth day of life. From a low point at about 2 to 3 days after birth, these coagulation factors rise slowly, but do not approach normal adult levels until 9 months of age or later. Increasing levels of these vitamin K dependent factors indicate a response to dietary intake and bacterial colonization of the intestines. An injection of vitamin K is given prophylactically on the day of birth to combat the deficiency. Options 1, 2, and 3 are incorrect.

Test-Taking Strategy: Knowledge about the synthesis of vitamin K is necessary to answer this question. Review the purpose of administering vitamin K in the newborn if you had difficulty with this question.

Level of Cognitive Ability: Comprehension
Client Needs: Physiological Integrity
Integrated Concept/Process: Nursing Process/Evaluation
Content Area: Maternity

Reference:
McKinney, E., Ashwill, J., Murray, S., James, S., Gorrie, T., & Droske, S. (2000). *Maternal-child nursing.* Philadelphia: W.B. Saunders, p. 563.

466. A nurse notes that a client's urinalysis report contains a notation of positive red blood cells (RBCs). The nurse interprets that this finding is unrelated to which of

Answer: 1
Rationale: Hematuria can be caused by trauma to the kidney, such as with blunt trauma to the lower posterior trunk or flank. Kidney stones can cause hematuria as they scrape the endothelial lining

the following items that is part of the client's clinical picture?

1 Diabetes mellitus
2 Concurrent anticoagulant therapy
3 History of kidney stones
4 History of recent blow to the right flank

of the urinary system. Anticoagulant therapy can cause hematuria as a side effect. Diabetes mellitus does not cause hematuria, although it can lead to renal failure from prerenal causes.

Test-Taking Strategy: Use the process of elimination and note the key word *unrelated*. Begin to answer this question by eliminating options 2 and 4, which are most obviously likely to cause RBCs to be found in the urine. From the remaining options, recalling that the scraping of the stones against mucosa could cause minor trauma and bleeding helps you to eliminate this option as well. Thus diabetes mellitus is the item unrelated to positive RBCs in the urine. Review the causes of hematuria if you had difficulty with this question.

Level of Cognitive Ability: Comprehension
Client Needs: Physiological Integrity
Integrated Concept/Process: Nursing Process/Data Collection
Content Area: Adult Health/Renal

Reference:
Black, J., Hawks, J., & Keene, A. (2001). *Medical-surgical nursing: clinical management for positive outcomes* (6th ed.). Philadelphia: W.B. Saunders, pp. 859; 868.

---

467. A nurse is instructed to ambulate a client with a Foley catheter four times a day in the hall. The nurse understands that the safest way to accomplish this while maintaining the integrity of the catheter is to:

1 Tie the drainage bag to the client's waist while ambulating
2 Use a walker to hang the drainage bag from while ambulating
3 Tell the client to hold the drainage bag lower than the level of the bladder
4 Change the drainage bag to a leg collection bag

Answer: 4
Rationale: The safest way to protect the integrity of the catheter with a mobile client is to attach the tube to a leg collection bag. This allows for greater freedom of movement, while alleviating worry over accidental disconnection or dislodgment. The drainage bag should be maintained below the level of the bladder; therefore options 1 and 2 are incorrect. Options 1, 2, and 3 all present the potential risk of tension or pulling on the catheter by the client during ambulation.

Test-Taking Strategy: Use the process of elimination. Eliminate options 1 and 2, recalling that the drainage bag should be maintained below the level of the bladder. Also note that options 1, 2, and 3 all present the risk of tension or pulling on the catheter by the client during ambulation. Review care of the client with a Foley catheter if you had difficulty with this question.

Level of Cognitive Ability: Comprehension
Client Needs: Physiological Integrity
Integrated Concept/Process: Nursing Process/Implementation
Content Area: Adult Health/Renal

Reference:
Potter, P., & Perry, A. (2001). *Fundamentals of nursing* (5th ed.). St. Louis: Mosby, p. 1424.

---

468. A client recently diagnosed with polycystic kidney disease has just finished speaking with the physician about the disorder. The client asks the nurse to explain again what the most serious complication of

Answer: 3
Rationale: The most serious complication of polycystic kidney disease is ESRD, which would be managed with dialysis or transplant. Chronic UTIs are the most common complication, because of the altered anatomy of the kidney and from the development

the disorder might be. In formulating a response, the nurse incorporates the understanding that the most serious complication is:

1　Diabetes insipidus
2　Syndrome of inappropriate antidiuretic hormone (SIADH) secretion
3　End-stage renal disease (ESRD)
4　Chronic urinary tract infection (UTI)

of resistant strains of bacteria. Diabetes insipidus and SIADH secretion are unrelated disorders.

Test-Taking Strategy: Use the process of elimination and note the key words *most serious*. Note the relationship between these words and the words *end-stage* in option 3. This assists in directing you to this option. Review the complications of polycystic kidney disease if you had difficulty with this question.

Level of Cognitive Ability: Comprehension
Client Needs: Physiological Integrity
Integrated Concept/Process: Nursing Process/Implementation
Content Area: Adult Health/Renal

Reference:
Black, J., Hawks, J., & Keene, A. (2001). *Medical-surgical nursing: clinical management for positive outcomes* (6th ed.). Philadelphia: W.B. Saunders, p. 871.

---

469. It has been 12 hours since the client's delivery of a healthy newborn. The nurse checks the mother's uterus for the process of involution and documents that it is progressing normally when palpation of the client's fundus is noted:

1　At the level of the umbilicus
2　Midway between the umbilicus and the symphysis pubis
3　One finger-breadth below the umbilicus
4　Two finger-breadths below the umbilicus

Answer: 1

Rationale: The term involution is used to describe the rapid reduction in size and the return of the uterus to a normal condition similar to its nonpregnant state. Immediately after the delivery of the placenta, the uterus contracts to the size of a large grapefruit. The fundus is situated in the midline between the symphysis pubis and the umbilicus. Within 6 to 12 hours after birth, the fundus of the uterus rises to the level of the umbilicus. The top of the fundus remains at the level of the umbilicus for a day or so and then descends into the pelvis approximately one finger-breadth on each succeeding day.

Test-Taking Strategy: Knowledge about the normal process of involution is necessary to answer the question. The key words *12 hours after birth* should assist in selecting the correct option. Attempt to visualize the process of involution and the expected finding to direct you to option 1. Review this process if you had difficulty with this question.

Level of Cognitive Ability: Comprehension
Client Needs: Physiological Integrity
Integrated Concept/Process: Nursing Process/Data Collection
Content Area: Maternity

Reference:
McKinney, E., Ashwill, J., Murray, S., James, S., Gorrie, T., & Droske, S. (2000). *Maternal-child nursing.* Philadelphia: W.B. Saunders, p. 325.

---

470. A client with a gastric tumor is scheduled for a subtotal gastrectomy (Billroth II procedure). The client asks the nurse about the procedure. The nurse explains the procedure knowing that the best description is that:

1　The proximal end of the distal stomach is anastomosed to the duodenum

Answer: 4

Rationale: In the Billroth II procedure, the lower portion of the stomach is removed and the remainder is anastomosed to the jejunum. This technique is preferred for the treatment of duodenal ulcer because recurrent ulceration develops less frequently. The duodenal stump is preserved to permit bile flow to the jejunum.

Test-Taking Strategy: Use the process of elimination. The word *gastrectomy* indicates removal of the stomach. This should assist in

2   The antrum of the stomach is removed with the remaining portion anastomosed to the duodenum

3   The entire stomach is removed and the esophagus is anastomosed to the duodenum

4   The lower portion of the stomach is removed and the remainder is anastomosed to the jejunum

eliminating option 1. The word *subtotal* indicates lower and a part of. This should easily direct you to option 4. If you had difficulty with this question, review this surgical procedure.

Level of Cognitive Ability: Comprehension
Client Needs: Physiological Integrity
Integrated Concept/Process: Nursing Process/Implementation
Content Area: Adult Health/Gastrointestinal

Reference:
Black, J., Hawks, J., & Keene, A. (2001). *Medical-surgical nursing: clinical management for positive outcomes* (6th ed.). Philadelphia: W.B. Saunders, p. 720.

---

471. A client with diabetes mellitus receives Humulin Regular insulin 8 units subcutaneously at 7:30 AM. The nurse would be most alert for signs of hypoglycemia at what time during the day?
1.   9:30 AM to 11:30 AM
2.   11:30 AM to 1:30 PM
3.   1:30 PM to 3:30 PM
4.   3:30 PM to 5:30 PM

Answer: 1
Rationale: Humulin Regular insulin is a short-acting insulin. Its onset of action occurs in a half hour and it peaks in 2 to 4 hours. Its duration of action is 4 to 6 hours. A hypoglycemia reaction will most likely occur at peak time, and in this situation, between 9:30 AM and 11:30 AM.

Test-Taking Strategy: Use the process of elimination. Recalling that Regular insulin is a short-acting insulin assists in directing you to option 1. Review both NPH and Regular insulin if you had difficulty with this question.

Level of Cognitive Ability: Comprehension
Client Needs: Physiological Integrity
Integrated Concept/Process: Nursing Process/Data Collection
Content Area: Pharmacology

Reference:
Hodgson, B., & Kizior, R. (2003). *Saunders nursing drug handbook 2003.* Philadelphia: W.B. Saunders, p. 590.

---

472. A nurse assists in developing a postoperative plan of care for the client scheduled for hypophysectomy. The nurse understands that which of the following would not be a component of the postoperative plan of care?
1   Mouth care
2   Coughing and deep breathing
3   Monitoring I&O
4   Daily weights

Answer: 2
Rationale: Toothbrushing, sneezing, coughing, nose blowing, and bending are activities that should be avoided postoperatively in the client who underwent a hypophysectomy. These activities interfere with the healing of the incision and can disrupt the graft.

Test-Taking Strategy: Use the process of elimination and note the key word *not*. Consider the anatomical location of the surgical procedure when answering this question. Although coughing and deep breathing are usually a normal component of postoperative care, in this situation, coughing is contraindicated. Review care after a hypophysectomy if you had difficulty with this question.

Level of Cognitive Ability: Comprehension
Client Needs: Physiological Integrity
Integrated Concept/Process: Nursing Process/Planning
Content Area: Adult Health/Endocrine

Reference:
Lewis, S., Heitkemper, M., & Dirksen, S. (2004). *Medical-surgical nursing: assessment and management of clinical problems* (6th ed.). St. Louis: Mosby, p. 1305.

473. A nurse is assigned to care for a client who underwent a thyroidectomy. The nurse is instructed to monitor the client for signs of damage to the parathyroid glands. Which of the following indicates that the client has experienced damage to the parathyroid glands?
1   Hoarseness
2   Tingling around the mouth
3   Respiratory distress
4   Neck pain

Answer: 2
Rationale: The parathyroid glands can be damaged or their blood supply impaired during thyroid surgery. Hypocalcemia and tetany result when parathyroid levels decrease. The nurse monitors for complaints of tingling around the mouth or of the toes or fingers and muscular twitching because these are signs of calcium deficiency. Additional later signs of hypocalcemia are positive Chvostek's and Trousseau's signs. Options 1, 3, and 4 are not signs that indicate damage to the parathyroid glands.

Test-Taking Strategy: Use the process of elimination. Recalling that hypocalcemia results when parathyroid levels decrease and remembering the signs of a calcium deficiency assist in directing you to the correct option. Review postoperative care after thyroidectomy and the signs of parathyroid damage if you had difficulty with this question.

Level of Cognitive Ability: Analysis
Client Needs: Physiological Integrity
Integrated Concept/Process: Nursing Process/Data Collection
Content Area: Adult Health/Endocrine

Reference:
Black, J., Hawks, J., & Keene, A. (2001). *Medical-surgical nursing: clinical management for positive outcomes* (6th ed.). Philadelphia: W.B. Saunders, p. 1105.

474. A nurse is caring for a client who is comatose. The nurse notes in the chart that the client is exhibiting decerebrate posturing. The nurse monitors the client knowing that decerebrate posturing can best be described as:
1   The extension of the extremities after a stimulus
2   The flexion of the extremities after a stimulus
3   Upper extremity flexion with lower extremity extension
4   Upper extremity extension with lower extremity flexion

Answer: 1
Rationale: Decerebrate posturing, which can occur with upper brain stem injury, is the extension of the extremities after a stimulus. Options 2, 3, and 4 are incorrect descriptions.

Test-Taking Strategy: Use the process of elimination. Remember, decerebrate also may be known as extension. Recalling this concept assists in directing you to option 1. Review posturing and its relationship to neurological disorders if you had difficulty with this question.

Level of Cognitive Ability: Comprehension
Client Needs: Physiological Integrity
Integrated Concept/Process: Nursing Process/Data Collection
Content Area: Adult Health/Neurological

Reference:
Black, J., Hawks, J., & Keene, A. (2001). *Medical-surgical nursing: clinical management for positive outcomes* (6th ed.). Philadelphia: W.B. Saunders, p. 1888.

475. A nurse reinforces instructions to the postpartum client about observation of lochia. The nurse evaluates that the client

Answer: 4
Rationale: The uterus rids itself of the debris remaining after birth through a discharge called lochia, which is classified according to

understands what to expect when the client states that on the second day postpartum, the lochia should be:

1 Yellow
2 White
3 Pink
4 Red

its appearance and contents. Lochia rubra is dark red in color. It occurs for the first 2 to 3 days and contains epithelial cells, erythrocytes, leukocytes, shreds of decidua, and occasionally fetal meconium, lanugo, and vernix caseosa. Lochia should not contain large clots; if it does the cause should be investigated without delay. Lochia serosa is a brownish-pink discharge that normally occurs from days 4 to 10 postpartum. Lochia alba is the whitish discharge that normally occurs from days 10 to 14 postpartum.

Test-Taking Strategy: Use the process of elimination. Noting the key words *second day postpartum* should direct you to option 4. If you had difficulty with this question, review the normal postpartum findings.

Level of Cognitive Ability: Comprehension
Client Needs: Physiological Integrity
Integrated Concept/Process: Teaching/Learning
Content Area: Maternity

Reference:
Burroughs, A., & Leifer, G. (2002). *Maternity nursing* (8th ed.). Philadelphia: W.B. Saunders, p. 202.

---

476. A nurse is collecting data about a client's cigarette smoking habit. The client admits to smoking three fourths of a pack per day for the last 10 years. The nurse would determine that the client has a smoking history of how many pack-years?

1 0.75 pack-years
2 7.5 pack-years
3 15 pack-years
4 30 pack-years

Answer: 2
Rationale: The standard method for quantifying the smoking history is to multiply the number of packs smoked per day by the number of years of smoking. The number is recorded as the number of pack-years. The calculation for the number of pack-years for the client who has smoked three fourths of a pack per day for 10 years is: 0.75 (three fourths) packs × 10 years = 7.5 pack-years.

Test-Taking Strategy: This question tests a fundamental concept related to history taking related to smoking. Review the method for determining pack years if you had difficulty with this question.

Level of Cognitive Ability: Comprehension
Client Needs: Physiological Integrity
Integrated Concept/Process: Nursing Process/Data Collection
Content Area: Adult Health/Respiratory

Reference:
Black, J., Hawks, J., & Keene, A. (2001). *Medical-surgical nursing: clinical management for positive outcomes* (6th ed.). Philadelphia: W.B. Saunders, p. 355.

---

477. An LPN is assigned to care for a client with cancer. The LPN reviews the plan of care developed by the RN and notes that the client has a nursing diagnosis of Risk for Injury related to thrombocytopenia secondary to the side effects of chemotherapy. Based on the plan of care, the LPN plans to monitor the results of which of the following laboratory studies closely?

Answer: 1
Rationale: The client with thrombocytopenia has an insufficient number of platelets. This puts the client at risk for bleeding. Other related studies that should be monitored include hemoglobin, hematocrit, and coagulation studies. The WBC count is a test that indicates the risk for or the presence of infection, whereas the ESR is a nonspecific test indicating inflammation. The ANA titer is a test of immune function and can indicate the presence of certain autoimmune disorders.

1 Platelet count
2 White blood cell (WBC) count
3 Erythrocyte sedimentation rate (ESR)
4 Antinuclear antibody (ANA) titer

Test-Taking Strategy: Use the process of elimination. Recalling the definition of thrombocytopenia directs you to option 1. Review the common side effects of chemotherapy if you had difficulty with this question.

Level of Cognitive Ability: Analysis
Client Needs: Physiological Integrity
Integrated Concept/Process: Nursing Process/Data Collection
Content Area: Adult Health/Oncology

Reference:
Black, J., Hawks, J., & Keene, A. (2001). *Medical-surgical nursing: clinical management for positive outcomes* (6th ed.). Philadelphia: W.B. Saunders, p. 393.

---

478. An LPN is assigned to care for a client with a diagnosis of bladder cancer who recently received chemotherapy. The RN tells the LPN that the client's platelet count is 20,000/mm³. Based on this laboratory value, the LPN would most appropriately plan to do which of the following?
  1 Tell the client that if anyone delivers fresh flowers that they should be returned to the florist
  2 Tell the client not to eat any fresh fruits
  3 Monitor for signs of infection in the client
  4 Monitor the client's skin for the presence of petechiae

Answer: 4
Rationale: When the platelet count is decreased, the client is at risk for bleeding. A high risk of hemorrhage exists when the platelet count is less than 20,000/mm³. Fatal central nervous system hemorrhage or massive gastrointestinal hemorrhage can occur when the platelet count is less than 10,000/mm³. The client should be monitored for signs of bleeding. Options 1, 2, and 3 are specific interventions related to the risk of infection and although they may be a component of the plan of care, they are not specific to the risk for bleeding. Additionally, option 1 is not a therapeutic statement to the client.

Test-Taking Strategy: Use the process of elimination. Recalling the normal platelet count and determining that a low count places the client at risk for bleeding assists in eliminating options 1, 2, and 3. Review the normal platelet count and the plan of care for a client with a low count if you had difficulty with this question.

Level of Cognitive Ability: Analysis
Client Needs: Physiological Integrity
Integrated Concept/Process: Nursing Process/Planning
Content Area: Adult Health/Oncology

Reference:
Black, J., Hawks, J., & Keene, A. (2001). *Medical-surgical nursing: clinical management for positive outcomes* (6th ed.). Philadelphia: W.B. Saunders, p. 393.

---

479. An LPN is assigned to care for a client who is scheduled for keratoplasty. The nurse reviews the plan of care formulated by the RN before caring for the client. The LPN understands that which of the following will not be a component of the plan of care for the client?
  1 Obtaining a culture and sensitivity with conjunctival swabs
  2 Instilling antibiotic ophthalmic medication as prescribed
  3 Check eyes for signs of infection

Answer: 4
Rationale: Keratoplasty is done by removing damaged corneal tissue and replacing it with corneal tissue from a human donor (live or cadaver). Preoperative preparation of the recipient's eye may include obtaining a culture and sensitivity with conjunctival swabs, instilling antibiotic ophthalmic medication, and checking for signs of infection. Some ophthalmologists order medications such as 2% pilocarpine to constrict the pupil before surgery.

Test-Taking Strategy: Use the process of elimination. Note the key word *not* in the stem of the question. Recall that in this type of eye surgery, the eye is constricted before surgery. This directs you to

4 Administering medications that dilate the pupil

option 4. Review this preoperative preparation if you had difficulty with this question.

Level of Cognitive Ability: Comprehension
Client Needs: Physiological Integrity
Integrated Concept/Process: Nursing Process/Planning
Content Area: Adult Health/Eye

Reference:
Ignatavicius, D., & Workman, M. (2002). *Medical-surgical nursing: critical thinking for collaborative care* (4th ed.). Philadelphia: W.B. Saunders, p. 1030.

---

480. A nurse reviews the chart of an assigned client and notes that the physician has documented that the client is legally blind. The nurse plans care knowing that this condition is characterized as:
1 The client can perform some work that requires visual ability
2 The client retains some perception of light and movement
3 The client has no light perception at all
4 The client has a severe vision impairment with some visual ability

Answer: 2
Rationale: Legal blindness implies that the person cannot perform work that requires visual ability. The person who is legally blind usually retains some perception of light and movement. Total blindness means the absence of all light perception. Low vision is a term that is used to refer to a legally blind person or persons with severe vision impairment who still have some visual ability.

Test-Taking Strategy: Knowledge about the definition of legal blindness is necessary to answer this question. If you are unfamiliar with this definition and disorder, review this content.

Level of Cognitive Ability: Comprehension
Client Needs: Physiological Integrity
Integrated Concept/Process: Nursing Process/Planning
Content Area: Adult Health/Eye

Reference:
Lewis, S., Heitkemper, M., & Dirksen, S. (2004). *Medical-surgical nursing: assessment and management of clinical problems* (6th ed.). St. Louis: Mosby, p. 443.

---

481. A nurse is assigned to care for a client with a diagnosis of angina pectoris. While giving care, the client develops acute anginal chest discomfort. The nurse prepares to immediately administer:
1 Morphine sulfate
2 Propanolol (Inderal)
3 Nifedipine (Procardia)
4 Nitroglycerin (Nitrostat)

Answer: 4
Rationale: Angina usually responds to sublingual nitroglycerin. Pain relief usually begins within 1 or 2 minutes after the administration of sublingual nitroglycerin. Morphine sulfate is usually administered if the sublingual route has failed to relieve the pain. Nifedipine is often used in the maintenance treatment of angina rather than for acute episodes. Propanolol is used to treat certain cardiac disorders and also may be used to treat hypertension.

Test-Taking Strategy: Knowledge about the actions to take and the medication used to treat an acute episode of angina is necessary to answer this question. If you are unfamiliar with the treatment measure and the medication nitroglycerin, review this content.

Level of Cognitive Ability: Application
Client Needs: Physiological Integrity
Integrated Concept/Process: Nursing Process/Implementation
Content Area: Adult Health/Cardiovascular

Reference:
Black, J., Hawks, J., & Keene, A. (2001). *Medical-surgical nursing: clinical management for positive outcomes* (6th ed.). Philadelphia: W.B. Saunders, p. 1582.

482. A nurse is caring for a client after a radical mastectomy. The nurse implements which of the following measures to prevent lymphedema of the affected arm, a complication of this surgery?
1   Placing the affected arm in a dependent position
2   Placing a cool compress on the affected arm
3   Placing the affected arm on a pillow
4   Telling the client to avoid arm exercises in the affected arm

Answer: 3
Rationale: After mastectomy, the arm should be elevated above the level of the heart. Arm exercises should be encouraged as prescribed. No blood pressure readings, injections, IV lines, or blood draws should be performed on the affected arm. Cool compresses are not a suggested measure to prevent lymphedema from occurring.

Test-Taking Strategy: Note the key word *prevent.* Use the process of elimination and the principles related to gravity to assist in directing you to option 3. Remember, elevation assists in preventing edema. Review these measures if you had difficulty with this question.

Level of Cognitive Ability: Application
Client Needs: Physiological Integrity
Integrated Concept/Process: Nursing Process/Implementation
Content Area: Adult Health/Oncology

Reference:
Ignatavicius, D., & Workman, M. (2002). *Medical-surgical: critical thinking for collaborative care* (4th ed.). Philadelphia: W.B. Saunders, p. 1744.

483. A client with chronic renal failure (CRF) did not receive any juice on the breakfast meal tray. The nurse obtains a cup of which of the following juices from the unit kitchen?
1   Grape
2   Grapefruit
3   Orange
4   Prune

Answer: 1
Rationale: Apple juice and grape juice are low in potassium, and are the better choices of juice for the client with CRF. Prune, orange, and grapefruit juice are high in potassium, and should be used cautiously or avoided in these clients.

Test-Taking Strategy: Use the process of elimination and remember that potassium is limited in the client with CRF. Next, use basic nutritional principles to recall the potassium content of the various juices listed. This directs you to option 1. Review dietary measures for the client with renal failure if this question was difficult.

Level of Cognitive Ability: Application
Client Needs: Physiological Integrity
Integrated Concept/Process: Nursing Process/Implementation
Content Area: Adult Health/Renal

Reference:
Lewis, S., Heitkemper, M., & Dirksen, S. (2000). *Medical-surgical nursing: assessment and management of clinical problems* (5th ed.). St. Louis: Mosby, p. 1307.

484. A nurse is assisting in preparing a plan of care for the client scheduled for an abdominal perineal resection. Which of the following nursing interventions should the nurse suggest be included in the plan?

Answer: 2
Rationale: Immediately after surgery, profuse serosanguineous drainage from the perineal wound is expected. There is no need to notify the physician at this time. A Penrose drain should not be clamped because this action will cause the accumulation of fluid

1 Notify the physician if serosanguineous drainage from the wound is present
2 Change the wound dressing
3 Clamp the Penrose drain
4 Remove and replace the perineal packing 12 hours after the procedure

within the tissue. Both Penrose drains and packing are removed gradually over a period of 5 to 7 days. The nurse should not remove the perineal packing.

Test-Taking Strategy: Use the process of elimination. Eliminate options 3 and 4 knowing that these are inappropriate interventions. From the remaining options, recalling the normal expectations after this type of surgery assists in directing you to option 2 as the most appropriate action. Review postoperative expectations after abdominal perineal resection if you had difficulty with this question.

Level of Cognitive Ability: Application
Client Needs: Physiological Integrity
Integrated Concept/Process: Nursing Process/Planning
Content Area: Adult Health/Oncology

Reference:
Lewis, S., Heitkemper, M., & Dirksen, S. (2000). *Medical-surgical nursing: assessment and management of clinical problems* (5th ed.). St. Louis: Mosby, p. 981.

---

485. A nurse is assisting in planning care for the client with aldosteronism. The nurse plans to monitor for which of the following in the client?
1 Gastrointestinal bleeding
2 Hypoglycemia
3 Fluid overload
4 Urinary retention

Answer: 3
Rationale: Aldosterone plays a major role in fluid and electrolyte balance. Hypersecretion of aldosterone leads to sodium and water retention, which can lead to fluid overload. The other options are not part of the clinical picture that occurs with this health problem.

Test-Taking Strategy: Use the process of elimination recalling the pathophysiology of aldosteronism and its effects on the status of the client. Recalling that hypersecretion of aldosterone leads to sodium and water retention directs you to option 3. Review this disorder if you had difficulty with this question.

Level of Cognitive Ability: Application
Client Needs: Physiological Integrity
Integrated Concept/Process: Nursing Process/Planning
Content Area: Adult Health/Endocrine

Reference:
Lewis, S., Heitkemper, M., & Dirksen, S. (2000). *Medical-surgical nursing: assessment and management of clinical problems* (5th ed.). St. Louis: Mosby, p. 1444.

---

486. A client with chronic renal failure has a new medication order for epoetin alfa (Epogen). The nurse plans to give this medication by which of the following ways?
1 With a full glass of water
2 Diluted in juice to enhance taste
3 Subcutaneously
4 Intramuscularly

Answer: 3
Rationale: Epoetin alfa is erythropoietin that has been manufactured through the use of recombinant DNA technology. It is used to treat anemia in the client with chronic renal failure. The medication may be administered subcutaneously or intravenously.

Test-Taking Strategy: Specific knowledge of epoetin alfa is necessary to answer this question. If this medication or its methods of administration are unfamiliar to you, review this content.

Level of Cognitive Ability: Application
Client Needs: Physiological Integrity

Integrated Concept/Process: Nursing Process/Planning
Content Area: Adult Health/Renal

Reference:
Hodgson, B., & Kizior, R. (2003). *Saunders nursing drug handbook 2003.* Philadelphia: W.B. Saunders. p. 406.

---

487. A nurse is asked to reinforce teaching with a client with chronic renal failure who has been started on hemodialysis. The nurse includes which of the following pieces of information in discussions with the client?

1   It is unnecessary to stay within the fluid restriction on the day before hemodialysis
2   It is all right to eat unlimited protein on the day before hemodialysis
3   Most daily medications should be taken after hemodialysis, not before
4   Most daily medications should be double-dosed if going for hemodialysis that day

Answer: 3

Rationale: Many medications are dialyzable, which means they are removed from the bloodstream during dialysis. Because of this, many medications are withheld on the day of dialysis until after the procedure. It is not typical for medications to be *double-dosed* because there is no way to be certain how much of each medication is cleared by dialysis. Clients receiving hemodialysis are not told that it is acceptable to disregard dietary and fluid restrictions.

Test-Taking Strategy: Use the process of elimination. Remember that options that are similar are not likely to be correct. With this in mind, eliminate options 1 and 2 first. From the remaining options, use general principles related to medication administration. Remember, medications should not be *double-dosed.* Review preprocedural measures for dialysis if you had difficulty with this question.

Level of Cognitive Ability: Application
Client Needs: Physiological Integrity
Integrated Concept/Process: Nursing Process/Implementation
Content Area: Adult Health/Renal

Reference:
Lewis, S., Heitkemper, M., & Dirksen, S. (2004). *Medical-surgical nursing: assessment and management of clinical problems* (6th ed.). St. Louis: Mosby, p. 1236.

---

488. A client with acquired immunodeficiency syndrome (AIDS) is experiencing shortness of breath because of *Pneumocystis carinii* pneumonia. The nurse plans to do which of the following to assist the client in performing activities of daily living?

1   Provide supportive care
2   Provide meals and snacks with high-protein, high-calorie, and high-nutritional value
3   Provide small frequent meals
4   Offer food with low microbial content

Answer: 1

Rationale: Providing supportive care as needed reduces the client's physical and emotional energy demands and conserves energy resources for other functions such as breathing. Options 2, 3, and 4 are important interventions for the client with AIDS, but do not address the issue of the question. Option 2 assists the client in maintaining appropriate weight and proper nutrition. Option 3 assists the client in tolerating meals better. Option 4 decreases the client's risk for infection.

Test-Taking Strategy: Use the process of elimination. Focusing on the issue, shortness of breath, assists in directing you to option 1. Also, note that options 2, 3, and 4 are similar in that they are all dietary interventions. Option 1 is the one that is different. Review care of the client with AIDS if you had difficulty with this question.

Level of Cognitive Ability: Application
Client Needs: Physiological Integrity
Integrated Concept/Process: Nursing Process/Planning
Content Area: Adult Health/Respiratory

Reference:
Black, J., Hawks, J., & Keene, A. (2001). *Medical-surgical nursing: clinical management for positive outcomes* (6th ed.). Philadelphia: W.B. Saunders, p. 2202.

---

489. A client is admitted to the nursing unit after a fall from a roof. The client has multiple lacerations and a right leg fracture, which has been treated with a plaster cast. The nurse positions the right leg in which manner to promote optimal circulation?
  1 Elevated on pillows continuously for 24 to 48 hours
  2 Elevated for 3 hours, and then placed flat for 1 hour
  3 In a flat or level position
  4 Flat for 3 hours, and then elevated for 1 hour

Answer: 1
Rationale: A casted extremity is elevated continuously for the first 24 to 48 hours to minimize swelling and promote venous drainage. The other options are not part of standard positioning of the newly casted extremity.

Test-Taking Strategy: Use the process of elimination. Remember that edema sets in after fracture and can be increased by casting. Using the concepts related to gravity assists in eliminating options 2, 3, and 4. Review appropriate positioning after casting of an extremity if you had difficulty with this question.

Level of Cognitive Ability: Application
Client Needs: Physiological Integrity
Integrated Concept/Process: Nursing Process/Implementation
Content Area: Adult Health/Musculoskeletal

Reference:
Black, J., Hawks, J., & Keene, A. (2001). *Medical-surgical nursing: clinical management for positive outcomes* (6th ed.). Philadelphia: W.B. Saunders, p. 602.

---

490. A client has had a repair of an abdominal aortic aneurysm (AAA). The nurse assigned to assist in caring for the client places highest priority on which of the following nursing activities immediately after surgery?
  1 Checking peripheral pulses
  2 Administration of oral narcotic analgesics
  3 Pulmonary hygiene measures
  4 Application of pneumatic boots

Answer: 1
Rationale: Checking the peripheral pulses are the highest priority immediately after repair of AAA. This indicates whether the graft is patent and perfusing the lower extremities. The client would receive parenteral narcotics immediately after surgery. Prevention of respiratory and circulatory complications (options 3 and 4) is also important but does not supersede determining graft patency.

Test-Taking Strategy: Note the key words *highest priority*. Recalling that this surgical procedure is vascular in nature, look for the option that most directly addresses prevention or treatment of a vascular complication. Also, use of the ABCs (airway, breathing, and circulation) directs you to option 1. Review care of the client after this type of surgery if you had difficulty with this question.

Level of Cognitive Ability: Application
Client Needs: Physiological Integrity
Integrated Concept/Process: Nursing Process/Implementation
Content Area: Adult Health/Cardiovascular

Reference:
Black, J., Hawks, J., & Keene, A. (2001). *Medical-surgical nursing: clinical management for positive outcomes* (6th ed.). Philadelphia: W.B. Saunders, p. 1417.

---

491. A client scheduled for annuloplasty asks the nurse to explain again what the surgical procedure entails. In planning a

Answer: 2
Rationale: Annuloplasty is used for mitral or tricuspid regurgitation, and involves reconstruction of the annulus and the valve

response, the nurse would incorporate which of the following points?

1 The stenotic valve leaflets are separated, and any calcium deposits are removed
2 The valve leaflets are repaired with possible implantation of a prosthetic ring
3 The valve is replaced with a mechanical valve
4 The valve is replaced with a biologic valve

leaflets. Annulus repair may or may not involve insertion of a prosthetic ring. Option 1 describes commissurotomy, whereas options 3 and 4 are types of valve replacement.

Test-Taking Strategy: It is necessary to be familiar with the different types of cardiac valvular surgery to answer this question correctly. The word *possible* in option 2 indicates that it may be the correct answer. Review the various types of valvular repair procedures if you had difficulty with this question.

Level of Cognitive Ability: Comprehension
Client Needs: Physiological Integrity
Integrated Concept/Process: Nursing Process/Planning
Content Area: Adult Health/Cardiovascular

Reference:
Phipps, W., Monahan., F., Sands, J. (2003) *Medical surgical nursing: health and illness perspectives* (7th ed.). St. Louis: Mosby, p. 743.

---

492. An LPN has been assigned to the care of a client in the diuretic phase of renal failure. The nurse reviews the plan of care developed by the RN and monitors for signs of which of the following in the client?

1 Hypocalcemia and hyperkalemia
2 Hypermagnesemia and hyperkalemia
3 Hypernatremia and hypokalemia
4 Hyponatremia and hypokalemia

Answer: 4
Rationale: In the diuretic phase of acute renal failure, the client loses large amounts of fluid, accompanied by losses of sodium and potassium, because of the kidney's inability to properly concentrate urine. The nurses monitors the client for these electrolyte imbalances, as well as for signs of dehydration.

Test-Taking Strategy: Use the process of elimination and note the key words *diuretic phase*. In the diuretic phase, you would expect losses of both fluids and electrolytes. The only option that addresses *hypo* in the entire option is option 4. Review the clinical manifestations that occur in the diuretic phase of renal failure if you had difficulty with this question.

Level of Cognitive Ability: Application
Client Needs: Physiological Integrity
Integrated Concept/Process: Nursing Process/Data Collection
Content Area: Adult Health/Renal

Reference:
Black, J., Hawks, J., & Keene, A. (2001). *Medical-surgical nursing: clinical management for positive outcomes* (6th ed.). Philadelphia: W.B. Saunders, p. 877.

---

493. A client with chronic renal failure (CRF) has a protein restriction in the diet. The nurse avoids giving the client which of the following sources of incomplete protein in the diet?

1 Nuts
2 Eggs
3 Milk
4 Fish

Answer: 1
Rationale: The client whose diet has a protein restriction should be careful to ensure that the proteins eaten are complete proteins with the highest biologic value. Foods such as meat, fish, milk, and eggs are complete proteins, which are optimal for the client with CRF. Nuts are an incomplete protein.

Test-Taking Strategy: Use the process of elimination. Note the key word *avoids* and focus on the issue: a source of an incomplete protein. Use knowledge of basic nutritional principles and knowledge about foods that are complete and incomplete proteins to answer this question. Review these nutritional concepts if you had difficulty with this question.

Level of Cognitive Ability: Application
Client Needs: Physiological Integrity
Integrated Concept/Process: Nursing Process/Implementation
Content Area: Adult Health/Renal

Reference:
Williams, S. (2001). *Basic nutrition & diet therapy* (11th ed.). St. Louis: Mosby, p. 48.

---

494. A nurse looks at the clock and notes that a client is due in hydrotherapy for a burn dressing change in 30 minutes. The nurse plans to do which of the following next in the care of this client?
1 Immediately place the client on NPO status
2 Administer a narcotic analgesic that was last given 6 hours ago
3 Gather dressing supplies to send with the client to hydrotherapy
4 Get out a robe and slippers for the client

Answer: 2
Rationale: The client should receive pain medication approximately 20 minutes before a burn dressing change. This helps the client to tolerate an otherwise painful procedure. The client does not need to be NPO for this procedure. Dressing supplies are not sent with the client because they are normally available in the hydrotherapy area. A robe and slippers are given to the client for transport but are not indicated 30 minutes ahead of time.

Test-Taking Strategy: Note the key word *next*. Use Maslow's Hierarchy of Needs theory and the ability to sequence nursing activities in terms of time to answer this question. Thinking about the procedure to be done and noting the client's diagnosis directs you to option 2. Review care of the client scheduled for hydrotherapy if you had difficulty with this question.

Level of Cognitive Ability: Application
Client Needs: Physiological Integrity
Integrated Concept/Process: Nursing Process/Planning
Content Area: Adult Health/Integumentary

Reference:
Lewis, S., Heitkemper, M., & Dirksen, S. (2000). *Medical-surgical nursing: assessment and management of clinical problems* (5th ed.). St. Louis: Mosby, p. 530.

---

495. A client is complaining of skin irritation from the edges of a cast applied the previous day. The skin edges are pink and irritated. The nurse plans to do which of the following as a corrective action?
1 Use a hair dryer set on cool high setting to soothe the irritation
2 Petal the edges of the cast with tape
3 Massage the skin at the rim of the cast
4 Shake a small amount of powder under the cast rim

Answer: 2
Rationale: The nurse should petal the edges of the cast with tape to minimize skin irritation. A hair dryer is used on a cool low setting if a nonplaster cast becomes wet, or if the client's skin itches under a cast. Massaging the skin does not alleviate the problem. Powder should not be shaken under the cast because it could clump, become moist, and cause skin breakdown.

Test-Taking Strategy: Begin to answer this question by determining the cause of the client's skin irritation. Because the question tells you that the cast edges are the cause, you can then systematically eliminate each of the incorrect options. Also note the relationship between the words *skin edges are pink and irritated* in the question and the words in option 2. Review the principles of cast care if you had difficulty with this question.

Level of Cognitive Ability: Application

Client Needs: Physiological Integrity
Integrated Concept/Process: Nursing Process/Planning
Content Area: Adult Health/Musculoskeletal

Reference:
Lewis, S., Heitkemper, M., & Dirksen, S. (2000). *Medical-surgical nursing: assessment and management of clinical problems* (5th ed.). St. Louis: Mosby, p. 1772.

---

496. A client with a diagnosis of Guillain-Barré syndrome is being admitted to the hospital. The client's chief complaint is an ascending paralysis that has reached the level of the waist. The nurse is asked to prepare for the admission of the client. The nurse plans to have which of the following items available for emergency use?
1 Cardiac monitor and intubation tray
2 Blood pressure cuff and flashlight
3 Nebulizer and pulse oximeter
4 Flashlight and incentive spirometer

Answer: 1
Rationale: The client with Guillain-Barré syndrome is at risk for respiratory failure because of ascending paralysis. An intubation tray should be available for use. Another complication of this syndrome is cardiac dysrhythmia, which necessitates the use of cardiac monitoring. Although some of the items in options 2, 3, and 4 may be used in the routine care of the client, they are not needed for emergency use.

Test-Taking Strategy: Use the process of elimination and note the key words *emergency use.* This tells you that the correct answer is an option that contains equipment that is not routinely used in providing care. With this in mind, eliminate options 2 and 4 first. From the remaining options, recalling the complications of this syndrome directs you to option 1. Review nursing care measures for the client with Guillain-Barré syndrome if you had difficulty with this question.

Level of Cognitive Ability: Comprehension
Client Needs: Physiological Integrity
Integrated Concept/Process: Nursing Process/Planning
Content Area: Adult Health/Neurological

Reference:
Black, J., Hawks, J., & Keene, A. (2001). *Medical-surgical nursing: clinical management for positive outcomes* (6th ed.). Philadelphia: W.B. Saunders, p. 2016.

---

497. A nurse responds to a call bell and finds a client lying on the floor after a fall. The nurse suspects that the client's arm may be broken. Which of the following actions is the highest priority of the nurse before moving the client?
1 Tell the client that there will be no permanent damage
2 Immobilize the arm
3 Take the vital signs
4 Call the radiology department

Answer: 2
Rationale: When a fracture is suspected, it is imperative that the area be splinted and immobilized before the client is moved. Emergency help should be called for if the client is external to a hospital, and a physician should be called if the client is hospitalized. The nurse should remain with the client and provide realistic reassurance. The client should not be told that there will be no permanent damage.

Test-Taking Strategy: Use the process of elimination and note the key words *highest priority.* Eliminate option 4 because the physician will order radiology films. Option 1 is eliminated next because the nurse does not make a statement that provides false reassurance. When considering the remaining options, focus on the situation in the question. Immobilizing the limb is imperative for the client's safety, which makes it a better choice than taking vital signs. Review care of the client with a suspected extremity fracture if you had difficulty with this question.

Level of Cognitive Ability: Application
Client Needs: Physiological Integrity
Integrated Concept/Process: Nursing Process/Implementation
Content Area: Adult Health/Musculoskeletal

Reference:
Black, J., Hawks, J., & Keene, A. (2001). *Medical-surgical nursing: clinical management for positive outcomes* (6th ed.). Philadelphia: W.B. Saunders, p. 591.

---

498. A nurse is preparing a client for surgery. Which of the following is a component of the plan of care?
1   Be sure that the prescribed preoperative studies are performed
2   Report any increases in blood pressure on the day of surgery to the physician
3   Verify that the client has remained NPO for 24 hours before surgery
4   Instruct the client to avoid oral hygiene on the morning of surgery

Answer: 1
Rationale: The nurse should be sure that preoperative studies prescribed were performed. If any abnormal findings are noted, the nurse should alert the registered nurse, who in turn should notify the physician. Some increase in both blood pressure and pulse is common because of client anxiety about surgery. The client usually has a restriction of food and fluids for 8 hours before surgery, not 24 hours. Oral hygiene is allowed preoperatively, but the client should not swallow any water.

Test-Taking Strategy: Read the options carefully and use the process of elimination to answer the question. Recalling that surgery can produce anxiety in the client assists in eliminating option 2. Option 4 can be eliminated next because there is no reason to avoid oral hygiene as long as the client does not swallow any water. Careful reading of option 3 assists in eliminating this option and directs you to option 1. Review general preoperative care if you had difficulty with this question.

Level of Cognitive Ability: Application
Client Needs: Physiological Integrity
Integrated Concept/Process: Nursing Process/Planning
Content Area: Fundamental Skills

Reference:
deWit, S. (2001). *Fundamental concepts and skills for nursing.* Philadelphia: W.B. Saunders, p. 754.

---

499. A nurse has been told to institute aneurysm precautions for a client with a cerebral aneurysm. Which of the following items does the nurse plan for this client?
1   Instruct the client not to strain with bowel movements
2   Allow the client to read and watch television
3   Allow ambulation in the room only
4   Encourage the client to take his or her own daily bath

Answer: 1
Rationale: Aneurysm precautions include placing the client on bed rest in a quiet setting. Lights are kept dim to minimize environmental stimulation. Any activity that increases the blood pressure (BP) or impedes venous return from the brain is prohibited, such as pushing, pulling, sneezing, coughing, or straining. The nurse provides all physical care to minimize increases in BP. For the same reason, visitors, radio, television, and reading materials are prohibited or limited. Stimulants such as caffeine and nicotine are prohibited; decaffeinated coffee or tea may be used.

Test-Taking Strategy: To answer this question you must understand that a global principle in aneurysm precautions is to limit the amount of stimulation (in any form) that the client receives, and to prevent increased intracranial pressure (ICP). With this in mind, you eliminate options 3 and 4 first. From the remaining options, recall that straining can increase ICP, so it is appropriate to tell the client not to do so. Review the components of aneurysm precautions if you had difficulty with this question.

Level of Cognitive Ability: Application
Client Needs: Physiological Integrity
Integrated Concept/Process: Nursing Process/Planning
Content Area: Adult Health/Neurological

Reference:
Black, J., Hawks, J., & Keene, A. (2001). *Medical-surgical nursing: clinical management for positive outcomes* (6th ed.). Philadelphia: W.B. Saunders, p. 1942.

---

500. When the LPN is changing the back dressing of a client who has had a lumbar laminectomy, the nurse observes bulging at the incision site. The LPN takes which of the following most important actions?

1. Notifies the RN
2. Places a soft, multilayer absorbent dressing on the site
3. Tries to express fluid from the incision site
4. Applies a clear transparent dressing

Answer: 1

Rationale: After laminectomy or diskectomy, bulging at the incision site could indicate hematoma formation or cerebrospinal fluid leak. This must be reported to the RN, who then contacts the surgeon. The LPN should not try to express the fluid, because this could disrupt the incision and possibly introduce pathogens. A dressing should be replaced as part of routine nursing practice, but the most important action is notification of the RN about this complication.

Test-Taking Strategy: Use the process of elimination and note the key words *most important*. Recalling that bulging at the incisional site indicates a complication of surgery directs you to option 1. Review the complications associated with this surgical procedure if you had difficulty with this question.

Level of Cognitive Ability: Application
Client Needs: Physiological Integrity
Integrated Concept/Process: Nursing Process/Implementation
Content Area: Adult Health/Neurological

Reference:
Lewis, S., Heitkemper, M., & Dirksen, S. (2000). *Medical-surgical nursing: assessment and management of clinical problems* (5th ed.). St. Louis: Mosby, p. 1808.

---

501. A client who has had a spinal cord injury is wheelchair-bound. The nurse plans to obtain which of the following most effective pressure relief devices to place in the seat of the client's wheelchair?

1. Egg crate pad
2. Gel pad
3. Soft pillow
4. Air ring

Answer: 2

Rationale: The client who is wheelchair-bound is at risk for skin breakdown under bony prominences and benefits greatly from special pressure-relief devices such as a gel pad. The other items listed in the options are useful for some clients in selected situations, but do not disperse pressure the way that this special device does.

Test-Taking Strategy: Use the process of elimination and note the key words *most effective*. Visualize each of these items to assist in directing you to the correct option. Review the effects and use of these pressure relief devices if you had difficulty with this question.

Level of Cognitive Ability: Application
Client Needs: Physiological Integrity
Integrated Concept/Process: Nursing Process/Planning
Content Area: Fundamental Skills

Reference:
Lewis, S., Heitkemper, M., & Dirksen, S. (2000). *Medical-surgical nursing: assessment and management of clinical problems* (5th ed.). St. Louis: Mosby, p. 1725.

---

502. A client is seen in the ambulatory care clinic with a complaint of *feeling something in my eye*. The nurse is asked to prepare for ocular irrigation and obtains which of the following solutions to be used as an irrigant?
  1   Proparacaine hydrochloride (Ophthaine)
  2   Fluorescein
  3   Sterile normal saline (0.9%)
  4   Sterile water

Answer: 3
Rationale: Ocular irrigation is performed using sterile normal saline because it is an isotonic solution. Fluorescein is used to visualize a corneal abrasion secondary to injury. Proparacaine hydrochloride is used as a topical anesthetic before the irrigation is performed.

Test-Taking Strategy: Use the process of elimination and note the key word *irrigant*. Recalling that normal saline is an isotonic solution assists in directing you to the correct option. Review the procedure for eye irrigation if you had difficulty with this question.

Level of Cognitive Ability: Application
Client Needs: Physiological Integrity
Integrated Concept/Process: Nursing Process/Planning
Content Area: Adult Health/Eye

Reference:
Lewis, S., Heitkemper, M., & Dirksen, S. (2000). *Medical-surgical nursing: assessment and management of clinical problems* (5th ed.). St. Louis: Mosby, p. 452.

---

503. A client who has had an application of a right arm cast for a fractured humerus complains of pain at the wrist when the arm is passively moved. The nurse first:
  1   Checks for paresthesias and paralysis of the right arm
  2   Checks for similar symptoms on the left arm
  3   Medicates with an additional dose of a narcotic
  4   Calls the physician

Answer: 1
Rationale: Compartment syndrome is a complication for the client who has trauma to the extremities and application of a cast. Pain in the compartment may occur with passive movement, rather than at the site of injury. Additional symptoms to check for include paresthesias, paralysis, and excessive edema. Medication at this time without further data collection is not a safe nursing action. The nurse reports the findings to the registered nurse, who then calls the physician. Calling the physician without additional data is not the first action.

Test-Taking Strategy: Use the process of elimination. Note the key word *first*. Eliminate option 3 first as an unsafe action. Eliminate option 2 next because it is an irrelevant action in this situation. Discriminate between options 1 and 4 by reasoning that a single piece of datum is not usually reported to the physician without additional data being gathered. Option 1 addresses data collection specific to the client's condition. Review complications associated with a cast if you had difficulty with this question.

Level of Cognitive Ability: Application
Client Needs: Physiological Integrity
Integrated Concept/Process: Nursing Process/Implementation
Content Area: Adult Health/Musculoskeletal

Reference:
Lewis, S., Heitkemper, M., & Dirksen, S. (2000). *Medical-surgical nursing: assessment and management of clinical problems* (5th ed.). St. Louis: Mosby, p. 1786.

504. A client who had intracranial surgery has a decreasing pulse rate with an increasing blood pressure. The nurse avoids which of the following activities until the client is stabilized?
1. Elevating the head of the bed to 30 degrees
2. Suctioning
3. Keeping the neck midline
4. Carefully monitoring fluid intake

Answer: 2

Rationale: The client is showing signs of increasing intracranial pressure (ICP). The nurse avoids activities that further increase the ICP, such as suctioning the client. The nurse positions the head of the bed at 30 degrees and keeps the neck midline to promote venous drainage from the cranium. The nurse carefully monitors fluid intake to prevent fluid overload.

Test-Taking Strategy: Use the process of elimination and note the key word *avoids*. Note that the client is exhibiting signs of increased ICP and recall the preventive measures. Therefore the nurse avoids suctioning because it will increase intracranial pressure. This directs you to option 2. Review care of the client after intracranial surgery if you had difficulty with this question.

Level of Cognitive Ability: Application
Client Needs: Physiological Integrity
Integrated Concept/Process: Nursing Process/Implementation
Content Area: Adult Health/Neurological

Reference:
Ignatavicius, D., & Workman, M. (2002). *Medical-surgical nursing: critical thinking for collaborative care* (4th ed.). Philadelphia: W.B. Saunders, p. 997.

---

505. A nurse is preparing to feed a client with dysphagia. The nurse plans to do which of the following to assist the client with swallowing?
1. Place the equivalent of 30 mL of food on the fork
2. Place the food on the tip of the tongue
3. Use water to help the client swallow food in the mouth
4. Provide foods that have a soft consistency

Answer: 4

Rationale: No more than a standard amount of food should be placed on the feeding utensil, which is roughly the equivalent of 15 mL. Food should be placed on the posterior part of the tongue to aid in swallowing. Foods are provided that have a soft consistency. Liquids are thickened and are given separate from solid foods to prevent choking.

Test-Taking Strategy: Use the process of elimination. Noting the key word *dysphagia* and recalling that this indicates that the client has difficulty with swallowing directs you to option 4. Review care of the client with dysphagia if you had difficulty with this question.

Level of Cognitive Ability: Application
Client Needs: Physiological Integrity
Integrated Concept/Process: Nursing Process/Planning
Content Area: Adult Health/Neurological

Reference:
Ignatavicius, D., & Workman, M. (2002). *Medical-surgical nursing: critical thinking for collaborative care* (4th ed.). Philadelphia: W.B. Saunders, p. 987.

---

506. A client is experiencing a sleep pattern disturbance. The nurse plans to do which of the following to best help the client obtain sufficient rest?
1. Adjust the number of pillows, lights, and noise to the client's preference

Answer: 1

Rationale: An environment that is conducive to sleep is one that simulates the client's natural environment, including number of pillows, bedcovers, light, temperature, and noise. The nurse should plan to be flexible in care delivery times to allow the client rest periods as needed. Sedative medications are used as necessary, and ideally are limited to three times per week. The client

2 Institute a rigid time frame for delivery of nursing care

3 Use maximum doses of sedative medication at bedtime

4 Allow at least 60 minutes of uninterrupted sleep at a time

needs at least 90 minutes without interruption to complete one sleep cycle.

Test-Taking Strategy: Use the process of elimination. The key words in the question are *best* and *sufficient rest.* Eliminate options 2 and 3 first because they contain the words *rigid* and *maximum,* respectively. Knowing that a full sleep cycle is 90 minutes long helps you to choose option 1 over option 4. Review measures to promote sleep if you had difficulty with this question.

Level of Cognitive Ability: Application
Client Needs: Physiological Integrity
Integrated Concept/Process: Nursing Process/Planning
Content Area: Fundamental Skills

Reference:
Ackley, B., & Ladwig, G. (2002). *Nursing diagnosis handbook: a guide to planning care* (5th ed.). St. Louis: Mosby, p. 692.

---

507. A client with a closed-head injury has fluid leaking from the ear. The nurse should first:
1 Irrigate the ear canal gently
2 Test the drainage for glucose
3 Test the drainage for pH
4 Notify the physician

Answer: 2
Rationale: The client with a closed head injury may have leakage of cerebrospinal fluid (CSF) from the nose or ear. The nurse first determines whether the fluid tests positive for glucose, indicating that it is indeed CSF. The nurse then notifies the RN, who then notifies the physician. The ear is not irrigated because of the risk of infection. Testing of pH is not indicated.

Test-Taking Strategy: Not the key words *closed-head injury.* Recall that this client is at risk for CSF leakage and the appropriate method of determining the presence of CSF. With this in mind, you eliminate options 1 and 3. From the remaining options, noting the key word *first* directs you to option 2. Review care of the client with a closed-head injury if you had difficulty with this question.

Level of Cognitive Ability: Application
Client Needs: Physiological Integrity
Integrated Concept/Process: Nursing Process/Implementation
Content Area: Adult Health/Neurological

Reference:
Ignatavicius, D., & Workman, M. (2002). *Medical-surgical nursing: critical thinking for collaborative care* (4th ed.). Philadelphia: W.B. Saunders, p. 995.

---

508. A nurse is assisting in caring for a client after a craniectomy. The nurse is told that the client's incision is supratentorial. How should the nurse position the client?
1 Head of the bed flat
2 Head of the bed elevated 90 degrees
3 Head of the bed elevated 30 degrees
4 Lying on the operative side

Answer: 3
Rationale: Craniectomy involves removal of a portion of the client's cranium; therefore lying on the operative side is contraindicated because the bony protection of the skull has been removed. The head of the bed should be elevated 30 degrees to promote optimal venous drainage while maintaining arterial perfusion to the brain.

Test-Taking Strategy: Use the process of elimination and recall the impact of craniectomy on client positioning, as well as the concepts related to the general positioning of the client with a neurological problem. Note the key word *supratentorial*. Remember, *supra* means up. This assists in eliminating options 1 and 4. Visualize the positions in the remaining two options. Option 3 provides more client comfort than option 2. Option 3 also does not potentially interfere with arterial circulation to the brain. If this question was difficult, review care of the client after craniectomy.

Level of Cognitive Ability: Application
Client Needs: Physiological Integrity
Integrated Concept/Process: Nursing Process/Implementation
Content Area: Adult Health/Neurological

Reference:
Ignatavicius, D., & Workman, M. (2002). *Medical-surgical nursing: critical thinking for collaborative care* (4th ed.). Philadelphia: W.B. Saunders, p. 1004.

---

509. A previously healthy client with a long leg cast is on prescribed bed rest. The nurse plans to institute which of the following general measures in client care?
1   Check neurovascular status every 8 hours
2   Reposition every 4 to 6 hours
3   Request a low fiber diet
4   Increase fluids to 3 L per day

Answer: 4
Rationale: Routine measures for the immobile client who has had application of a long leg cast include checking the neurovascular status ever hour to every 1 to 4 hours (depending on time since application), repositioning every 2 to 4 hours, and providing a diet high in fiber and fluids (to prevent constipation).

Test-Taking Strategy: Use the process of elimination. The key words in this question are *previously healthy, cast,* and *bed rest.* Knowledge of basic care measures for the immobile client assists you to eliminate options 2 and 3. Recalling the concepts related to cast care, data collection, and time frames assists in eliminating option 1. Review nursing measures for cast care if you had difficulty with this question.

Level of Cognitive Ability: Application
Client Needs: Physiological Integrity
Integrated Concept/Process: Nursing Process/Planning
Content Area: Adult Health/Musculoskeletal

Reference:
Ignatavicius, D., & Workman, M. (2002). *Medical-surgical nursing: critical thinking for collaborative care* (4th ed.). Philadelphia: W.B. Saunders, p. 940.

---

510. A client with a long leg cast is afraid of wetting the top of the cast while urinating. The nurse best plans to keep the cast dry by doing which of the following?
1   Requesting an order for a Foley catheter
2   Petaling the edges of the cast
3   Using a trapeze when placing the client on a bedpan
4   Tucking a plastic material (such as food wrap) around the area before toileting

Answer: 4
Rationale: A waterproof material such as plastic food wrap is very useful in preventing cast material from becoming wet during urination. Using a trapeze aids in proper positioning but does not necessarily prevent spillage or wetting during urination. Petaling cast edges prevents skin irritation, but does not affect wetting the cast. Foley catheter insertion carries a risk of infection and is not recommended unless needed for other reasons.

Test-Taking Strategy: Use the process of elimination and focus on the issue, preventing wetting of the cast during urination. Eliminate option 1 first using principles of infection control. Eliminate option 2 next because it does not address the issue. From the remaining options, select option 4 because it most directly prevents the problem of getting the cast wet. Review care of the client with a cast if you had difficulty with this question.

Level of Cognitive Ability: Application
Client Needs: Physiological Integrity
Integrated Concept/Process: Nursing Process/Planning
Content Area: Adult Health/Musculoskeletal

Reference:
Lewis, S., Heitkemper, M., & Dirksen, S. (2000). *Medical-surgical nursing: assessment and management of clinical problems* (5th ed.). St. Louis: Mosby, p. 1782.

---

511. A nurse is caring for a client with skeletal traction requiring pin care who has moderate amounts of crusty drainage at the pin sites. The nurse avoids doing which of the following during the procedure?
1 Using sterile solution and applicators
2 Pouring the sterile cleaning solution into a sterile bowl
3 Using one cotton-tipped applicator per pin site
4 Moistening any 2 × 2 inch sponges stuck to the site with a sterile solution before removal

Answer: 3
Rationale: The use of sterile supplies and technique is critical to preventing infection in the client with skeletal pins in place. The solution, swabs, and containers must all be checked for sterility. Each applicator is swabbed on the site once and thrown away. Pin sites with sufficient drainage may require the use of several individual swabs. Any gauze sponges that are stuck to the site are moistened with sterile saline or water before removal. This prevents the sponges from having a local debriding effect.

Test-Taking Strategy: Use the process of elimination and note the key word *avoids*. Note that options 1, 2, and 4 all indicate the use of sterile supplies. This directs you to option 3 as the measure to avoid. Review pin site care if you had difficulty with this question.

Level of Cognitive Ability: Application
Client Needs: Physiological Integrity
Integrated Concept/Process: Nursing Process/Implementation
Content Area: Adult Health/Musculoskeletal

Reference:
Lewis, S., Heitkemper, M., & Dirksen, S. (2000). *Medical-surgical nursing: assessment and management of clinical problems* (5th ed.). St. Louis: Mosby, p. 1773.

---

512. A client has been placed in skeletal leg traction. The nurse avoids which of the following as part of routine care?
1 Keeping all ropes in the center of the pulley tract
2 Repositioning the client from side to side
3 Having the client push up in bed using the unaffected foot
4 Inspecting bony prominences

Answer: 2
Rationale: The client in skeletal traction is kept in the supine position. Minor position changes are made only briefly to expedite delivery of basic nursing care. All parts of the traction set-up are regularly checked for integrity. Bony prominences are inspected as part of diligent, ongoing skin care. The client is allowed to push with the unaffected foot to aid in repositioning.

Test-Taking Strategy: Use the process of elimination. Note the key word *avoids*. Visualize the client in skeletal leg traction and try to imagine providing care to this client. This assists in directing you to the correct option. Review the principles of care related to traction if you had difficulty with this question.

Level of Cognitive Ability: Application
Client Needs: Physiological Integrity

Integrated Concept/Process: Nursing Process/Implementation
Content Area: Adult Health/Musculoskeletal

Reference:
Lewis, S., Heitkemper, M., & Dirksen, S. (2000). *Medical-surgical nursing: assessment and management of clinical problems* (5th ed.). St. Louis: Mosby, p. 1774.

---

513. A client is being discharged to go home but requires ongoing chest pulmonary therapy (CPT). The LPN is asked to reinforce instructions about this procedure. The LPN incorporates which of the following items when reinforcing the instructions to the family about how to correctly do this procedure?

1   Perform the procedure within 1 hour after a meal
2   Position the client so the head and chest are elevated
3   Expect that the respiratory status will worsen during the procedure
4   Continue the therapy up to the prescribed ideal time if tolerated

Answer: 4

Rationale: CPT should be avoided for 2 hours after meals and for 1 hour after a liquid meal to avoid vomiting after mealtime. The head and chest are placed in the proper position prescribed for the client; this position incorporates having the head and chest lower than the rest of the body, if tolerated. The client's respiratory status should be monitored and the procedure modified if the respiratory status worsens. The therapy is performed to the ideal time, usually 15 minutes, as long as it is tolerated by the client.

Test-Taking Strategy: Use the process of elimination. Recalling that CPT utilizes the principles of gravity assists in eliminating options 1 and 2. Option 3 does not offer protection for the client's airway and is therefore eliminated next. Review the procedure for CPT if you had difficulty with this question.

Level of Cognitive Ability: Application
Client Needs: Physiological Integrity
Integrated Concept/Process: Teaching/Learning
Content Area: Adult Health/Respiratory

Reference:
Perry, A., & Potter, P., (2002). *Clinical nursing skills & techniques* (5th ed.). St. Louis: Mosby, pp. 347-349.

---

514. A nurse is assigned to care for a client with a history of asthma. In the event that the client experiences an asthma attack, the nurse should do which of the following first?

1   Place the client in a high-Fowler's position
2   Obtain a set of vital signs
3   Obtain an IV cannula for starting an IV line
4   Prepare to administer oxygen at 21%

Answer: 1

Rationale: The initial nursing action is to place the client in a position that aids in breathing, which is sitting bolt upright or in a high-Fowler's position. Other nursing actions follow in rapid sequence and include monitoring vital signs and administering bronchodilators and oxygen (but at levels of 2 to 5 liters per minute or 24% to 28% by Ventimask). Insertion of an IV line and ongoing monitoring of respiratory status also are indicated.

Test-Taking Strategy: Use the process of elimination and note the key word *first*. Eliminate option 4 first because oxygen at 21% is ambient air, not supplemental oxygen. Option 2 is not the best first choice when a client is in respiratory distress; therefore eliminate this option. The correct option protects the client's airway, which guides you to choose option 1 instead of option 3. Review care of the client experiencing an asthma attack if you had difficulty with this question.

Level of Cognitive Ability: Application
Client Needs: Physiological Integrity
Integrated Concept/Process: Nursing Process/Implementation
Content Area: Adult Health/Respiratory

Reference:
Black, J., Hawks, J., & Keene, A. (2001). *Medical-surgical nursing: clinical management for positive outcomes* (6th ed.). Philadelphia: W.B. Saunders, p. 1690.

---

515. A client has just undergone intermaxillary fixation (jaw wiring). The nurse assigned to assist in caring for the client plans to avoid which of the following immediately after return to the surgical nursing unit?

1 Elevating the head of the bed to a 45-degree angle
2 Applying moist heat to the jaws for comfort
3 Keeping wire cutters or scissors at the bedside
4 Performing oral suctioning

Answer: 2

Rationale: The client who has had intermaxillary fixation has limited movement of the mouth and is at risk of aspiration. Performing oral suctioning and elevating the head of the bed after recovery from anesthesia promotes maintenance of a patent airway. The presence of wire cutters or scissors at the bedside is also indicated in case the client experiences respiratory obstruction from vomiting or other causes. The nurse should verify with the physician the circumstances under which the wires may be cut. Ice is applied to the jaws for 30 minutes each hour for the first 12 hours postoperatively to reduce swelling.

Test-Taking Strategy: Use the process of elimination and note the key word *avoid.* Recalling that heat promotes swelling directs you to option 2. Also note that each of the other options promotes airway maintenance. Review postoperative care after intermaxillary fixation if you had difficulty with this question.

Level of Cognitive Ability: Application
Client Needs: Physiological Integrity
Integrated Concept/Process: Nursing Process/Planning
Content Area: Adult Health/Respiratory

Reference:
Black, J., Hawks, J., & Keene, A. (2001). *Medical-surgical nursing: clinical management for positive outcomes* (6th ed.). Philadelphia: W.B. Saunders, p. 1327.

---

516. A client is to undergo renal arteriography to rule out renal pathology. As an essential element of care, the nurse asks the client about a history of:

1 Frequent antibiotic use
2 Long-term diuretic therapy
3 Allergy to shellfish or iodine
4 Familial renal disease

Answer: 3

Rationale: The client undergoing any type of arteriography should be questioned about allergy to shellfish, seafood, or iodine. This is essential to identify potential allergic reaction to contrast dye, which may be used in some diagnostic tests. The other items also are useful as part of the data collection but are not as critical as the allergy determination.

Test-Taking Strategy: Use the process of elimination and note the key word *essential.* This implies that more than one or all options may be correct. However, one of them is of highest priority. Option 4 can be eliminated first as the least pertinent to current care. Because the question indicates that arteriography is planned, the items are evaluated against their potential connection to this test. Thus you should eliminate all options except option 3, which is directly related to the test. Review preprocedural care for arteriography if you had difficulty with this question.

Level of Cognitive Ability: Application
Client Needs: Physiological Integrity
Integrated Concept/Process: Nursing Process/Data Collection
Content Area: Adult Health/Renal

Reference:
Black, J., Hawks, J., & Keene, A. (2001). *Medical-surgical nursing: clinical management for positive outcomes* (6th ed.). Philadelphia: W.B. Saunders, pp. 198; 759.

---

517. A nurse is planning to implement a bladder retraining program for the client who has incontinence. Which of the following interventions is contraindicated as the nurse develops this plan?
1   Limit the oral fluid intake of the client
2   Teach pelvic muscle strengthening exercises
3   Ensure accessibility to a toilet
4   Adhere strictly to scheduled toileting times

Answer: 1
Rationale: For a bladder retraining program to be successful, several components must be in place. The client should learn and practice pelvic muscle strengthening exercises to promote bladder emptying. The nurse should ensure accessibility to bathroom facilities and adhere strictly to the toileting schedule. Limiting fluid intake is contraindicated. Adequate fluid intake is necessary to produce enough urine to stimulate micturition.

Test-Taking Strategy: Use the process of elimination. Note the key word *contraindicated*. Because options 3 and 4 are most obviously correct, these are eliminated according to the wording of the question. From the remaining options, it is necessary to know that sufficient fluid is necessary to cause bladder filling and proper stimulation of the micturition reflex. Knowing this allows you to select option 1 as the intervention that is contraindicated. Review the components for a bladder retraining program if you had difficulty with this question.

Level of Cognitive Ability: Application
Client Needs: Physiological Integrity
Integrated Concept/Process: Nursing Process/Planning
Content Area: Adult Health/Renal

Reference:
Black, J., Hawks, J., & Keene, A. (2001). *Medical-surgical nursing: clinical management for positive outcomes* (6th ed.). Philadelphia: W.B. Saunders, p. 838.

---

518. A client has been prescribed phenazopyridine hydrochloride (Pyridium) after a urological procedure. Which of the following should the nurse plan to include when reinforcing medication instructions to the client?
1   The medication exerts an antimicrobial effect
2   The urine may have a reddish-orange discoloration that may stain clothing
3   The medication provides an antibacterial effect
4   The medication must taken on an empty stomach

Answer: 2
Rationale: Phenazopyridine is a urinary tract analgesic with no antimicrobial or antibacterial properties. It is used to relieve the frequency, burning, or dysuria that follows urological procedures or accompanies infection. The medication is usually taken for 2 days or until symptoms have resolved, and then is discontinued. Any accompanying antibiotics are continued until finished. Phenazopyridine stains clothing and bedclothes an orange-red color that is permanent. For this reason, clients are advised to wear sanitary napkins to protect undergarments. The medication should be taken with food to avoid gastrointestinal upset.

Test-Taking Strategy: Use the process of elimination. Eliminate options 1 and 3 first because they are similar. From the remaining options, eliminate option 4 because of the absolute word *must*. Review this medication if you had difficulty with this question.

Level of Cognitive Ability: Application
Client Needs: Physiological Integrity
Integrated Concept/Process: Nursing Process/Planning
Content Area: Pharmacology

Reference:
Hodgson, B., & Kizior, R. (2003). *Saunders nursing drug handbook 2003.* Philadelphia: W.B. Saunders, p. 880.

---

519. A client has a cuffed tracheostomy tube and is being weaned from its use. The nurse assisting in caring for the client checks for which critical occurrence before plugging the client's tracheostomy?

1   The airway is totally free of secretions
2   The cuff is fully deflated
3   The oxygen saturation is at least 99%
4   The respiratory rate is 16 breaths per minute

Answer: 2

Rationale: The cuff must be deflated before plugging a cuffed tracheostomy tube. Otherwise, the client cannot ventilate around the tube and could suffer respiratory arrest. Other correct nursing actions include suctioning the airway to promote ventilation and monitoring adequacy of oxygen saturation. (Baseline may vary slightly depending on the client.) A respiratory rate of 16 is within the normal range and is not a critical observation in this situation.

Test-Taking Strategy: Use the process of elimination. The question asks for a *critical observation* before plugging the tracheostomy. Options 3 and 4 indicate good respiratory status, but these values or results may not be realistic for every client and are not "critical." Likewise, it is hard to assure that the airway is "totally" free of secretions. The best option is the tracheostomy cuff, which should be fully deflated. Review care of the client with a tracheostomy if you had difficulty with this question.

Level of Cognitive Ability: Analysis
Client Needs: Physiological Integrity
Integrated Concept/Process: Nursing Process/Evaluation
Content Area: Adult Health/Respiratory

Reference:
Black, J., Hawks, J., & Keene, A. (2001). *Medical-surgical nursing: clinical management for positive outcomes* (6th ed.). Philadelphia: W.B. Saunders, p. 1653.

---

520. A nurse is preparing to give a client a dose of iron dextran (INFeD) by the intramuscular route. The nurse should plan to:

1   Use a 5/8-inch, 25-gauge needle to administer the medication
2   Administer the medication into the deltoid muscle in the arm
3   Inject the medication deeply using a Z-track technique
4   Avoid changing the needle between drawing up the medication and injection

Answer: 3

Rationale: Iron dextran may permanently stain subcutaneous tissue. For this reason, the medication is administered using Z-track technique deep into the upper outer quadrant of the buttock. It is never given in the arm or in other exposed areas. An intramuscular (2- to 3-inch), 19- or 20-gauge needle is used. The needle is changed after drawing up the medication and before administration to minimize subcutaneous staining.

Test-Taking Strategy: Use the process of elimination and note the key words *intramuscular route.* This assists in eliminating options 1 and 2. Remembering that iron stains assists in eliminating option 4. Review the procedure for administering iron dextran if you had difficulty with this question.

Level of Cognitive Ability: Application
Client Needs: Physiological Integrity
Integrated Concept/Process: Nursing Process/Planning
Content Area: Pharmacology

Reference:
Lehne, R. (2001). *Pharmacology for nursing care* (4th ed.). Philadelphia: W.B. Saunders, p. 594.

FILL-IN-THE-BLANK

A nurse is measuring the vital signs of a client who sustained a head injury and is experiencing increased intracranial pressure (ICP). The client's respirations have a variable rate and the cycle of respirations begins shallowly with an increase in depth to hyperventilation, and then decrease in depth to apnea. The cycle then repeats itself. The nurse documents that the client is exhibiting what type of respirations?
Answer: _____

Answer: Cheyne-Stokes
Rationale: The client with increased intracranial pressure may exhibit Cheyne-Stokes respirations. This type of respirations has a variable rate. The cycle of respirations begins shallowly and then increases in depth to hyperventilation, followed by a decrease in depth to apnea. The cycle then repeats itself.

Test-Taking Strategy: Focus on the description of the respiratory pattern in the question. This description and noting that the client has a diagnosis of increased ICP will assist in identifying the respiratory pattern. Review this type of respiratory pattern if you had difficulty with this question.

Level of Cognitive Ability: Analysis
Client Needs: Physiological Integrity
Integrated Concept/Process: Nursing Process/Data Collection
Content Area: Adult Health/Neurological

Reference:
Linton, A. & Maebius, N. (2003). Introduction to medical-surgical nursing (3rd ed.). Philadelphia: W.B. Saunders, p. 456.

MULTIPLE RESPONSE – SELECT ALL THAT APPLY

A nurse is assisting in developing a plan of care for a client at risk for seizures. Select all interventions to include in the plan if the client experiences a seizure.
____ Place an oral airway between the client's teeth
____ Call a code blue
____ Remove any objects that could cause harm away from the client
____ Place the client in a supine position
____ Note the time the seizure began and how it progressed
____ Restrain the client's extremities
____ Monitor and document postseizure status

Answers:
____ Remove any objects that could cause harm away from the client
____ Note the time the seizure began and how it progressed
____ Monitor and document postseizure status

Rationale: In the event of a seizure the nurse would remove any objects that could cause harm away from the client. The nurse would turn the client to the side and note the time the seizure began and how it progressed. It is not necessary to call a code blue. The nurse would call a medical emergency if a generalized tonic-clonic seizure lasts more than 4 minutes or if seizures occur in rapid succession. The client's extremities are not restrained and the nurse would not place anything between the client's teeth during a seizure.

Test-Taking Strategy: Use the process of elimination and focus on the issue: a client experiencing a seizure. Recalling that maintaining a patent airway and that the client should be protected from injury will assist in identifying the interventions to manage a seizure. Review these interventions if you had difficulty with this question.

Level of Cognitive Ability: Application
Client Needs: Physiological Integrity

Integrated Concept/Process: Nursing Process/Planning
Content Area: Adult Health/Neurological

Reference:
Linton, A. & Maebius, N. (2003). *Introduction to medical-surgical nursing* (3rd ed.). Philadelphia: W.B. Saunders, p. 387.

REFERENCES

Ackley, B., & Ladwig, G. (2002). *Nursing diagnosis handbook: a guide to planning care* (5th ed.). St. Louis: Mosby.

Bauer, B., & Hill, S. (2000). *Mental health nursing.* Philadelphia: W.B. Saunders.

Black, J., Hawks, J., & Keene, A. (2001). *Medical-surgical nursing: clinical management for positive outcomes* (6th ed.). Philadelphia: W.B. Saunders.

Burroughs, A., & Leifer, G. (2002). *Maternity nursing* (8th ed.). Philadelphia: W.B. Saunders.

Chernecky, C., & Berger, B. (2001). *Laboratory tests and diagnostic procedures* (3rd ed.). Philadelphia: W.B. Saunders.

Clark S., Queener, S., & Karb, V. (2002). *Pharmacologic basis of nursing practice* (6th ed.). St. Louis: Mosby.

deWit, S. (2001). *Fundamental concepts and skills for nursing.* Philadelphia: W.B. Saunders.

Ebersole, P., & Hess, P. (2001). *Geriatric nursing & healthy aging.* St. Louis: Mosby.

Gutierrez, K., & Queener, S. (2003). *Pharmacology for nursing practice.* St. Louis: Mosby.

Ignatavicius, D., & Workman, M. (2002). *Medical-surgical nursing: critical thinking for collaborative care* (4th ed.). Philadelphia: W.B. Saunders.

Johnson, M., Bulechek, G., Dochterman, J., Maas, M., & Moorhead, S. (2001). *Nursing diagnoses, outcomes, and interventions.* St. Louis: Mosby.

Lehne, R. (2001). *Pharmacology for nursing care* (4th ed.). Philadelphia: W.B. Saunders.

Lewis, S., Heitkemper, M., & Dirksen, S. (2000). *Medical-surgical nursing: assessment and management of clinical problems* (5th ed.). St. Louis: Mosby.

Lewis, S., Heitkemper, M., & Dirksen, S. (2004). *Medical-surgical nursing: assessment and management of clinical problems* (6th ed.). St. Louis: Mosby.

Linton, A., & Maebias, N. (2003). *Introduction to medical surgical nursing* (3rd ed.). Philadelphia: W. B. Saunders.

McKinney, E., Ashwill, J., Murray, S., James, S., Gorrie, T., & Droske, S. (2000). *Maternal-child nursing.* Philadelphia: W.B. Saunders.

Murray, S., McKinney, E., & Gorrie, T. (2002). *Foundations of maternal-newborn nursing* (3rd ed.). Philadelphia: W.B. Saunders.

Perry, A., & Potter, P. (2002). *Clinical nursing skills & techniques* (5th ed.). St. Louis: Mosby.

Phipps, W., Monahan, F., Sands, J. (2003). *Medical-surgical nursing: health and illness perspectives* (7th ed.). St. Louis: Mosby.

Potter, P., & Perry, A. (2001). *Fundamentals of nursing* (5th ed.). St. Louis: Mosby.

Schulte, E., Price, D., & Gwin, J. (2001). *Thompson's pediatric nursing* (8th ed.). Philadelphia: W.B. Saunders.

Varcarolis, E. (2002). *Foundations of psychiatric mental health nursing* (4th ed.). Philadelphia: W.B. Saunders.

Williams, S. (2001) *Basic nutrition & diet therapy* (11th ed.). St. Louis: Mosby.

Wong, D., & Hockenberry-Eaton, M. (2001). *Wong's essentials of pediatric nursing* (6th ed.). St. Louis: Mosby.

Integrated Concepts and Processes

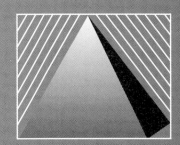

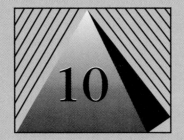

Integrated Concepts and Processes and the NCLEX-PN Test Plan

INTEGRATED CONCEPTS AND PROCESSES

In the new Test Plan implemented in April 2002, the National Council of State Boards of Nursing has identified a test plan framework based on Client Needs. This framework was selected based on the analysis of the findings in a practice analysis study of newly licensed practical and vocational nurses in the United States. This study identified the nursing activities performed by these nurses in relation to the frequency of their performance, their impact on maintaining client safety, and the settings in which they were performed. The National Council of State Boards of Nursing identifies four major categories of Client Needs. The Client Needs categories, which include Safe, Effective Care Environment; Health Promotion and Maintenance; Psychosocial Integrity; and Physiological Integrity are described in Chapter 5.

The 2002 NCLEX-PN Test Plan also identifies six concepts and processes that are fundamental to the practice of nursing. These concepts and processes are integrated throughout the four major categories of Client Needs. The Test Plan for NCLEX-PN identifies these components as Integrated Concepts and Processes. The Integrated Concepts and Processes include Clinical Problem Solving Process (Nursing Process); Caring; Communication and Documentation; Cultural Awareness; Self-Care; and Teaching and Learning (Box 10-1).

CLINICAL PROBLEM-SOLVING PROCESS (NURSING PROCESS)

The Clinical Problem-Solving Process (Nursing Process) provides a scientific approach for delivering care to clients. The steps of this process include Data Collection, Planning, Implementation, and Evaluation (Box 10-2).

Data Collection

Data collection is the first step of the nursing process. In the process of data collection, the nurse participates in a systematic method of establishing a database about the client. This step of the nursing process includes gathering information relative to the client, communicating information gained in data collection, and contributing to the formulation of nursing diagnoses. The database provides the foundation for the remaining steps of the nursing process.

Data collection begins with the first contact with the client. During all successive contacts, the nurse continues to collect information that is significant and relevant to the needs of the client. With each contact, the nurse uses all of the senses to gather data about the client.

During the process of data collection, the nurse collects data about the client from a variety of sources. The client is the primary source of data. Family members or significant others are secondary sources of data, and these sources may supplement or verify information provided by the client. Data may also be obtained from other health care team members and from the client's current and prior health records.

The information collected by the nurse includes both subjective and objective data. Subjective data includes the information that the client states and is based on the client's opinion. Objective data are the observable, measurable pieces of information about the client. Objective data include measurements such as vital signs or laboratory findings, and information obtained from observation of the client. Objective data also include clinical manifestations such as the signs and symptoms of an illness or disease.

In the process of data collection, the nurse is responsible for recognizing significant findings in the client, determining the need for additional information,

---

BOX 10-1

Integrated Concepts and Processes

Clinical Problem-Solving Process (Nursing Process)
Caring
Communication and Documentation
Cultural Awareness
Self-Care
Teaching and Learning

BOX 10-2

Clinical Problem-Solving Process (Nursing Process)

Data Collection
Planning
Implementation
Evaluation

---

reporting findings to the registered nurse (RN) or other relevant health care team members, and documenting findings thoroughly and accurately.

The nurse contributes to the formulation of nursing diagnoses by assisting in organizing relevant health care data and by assisting in determining significant relationships between data and client needs, problems, or both.

On NCLEX-PN, remember that data collection is the first step in the nursing process. When answering these type of questions, focus on the data in the question and select the option that addresses a data collection action. Also, use skills of prioritizing and the ABCs—airway, breathing, and circulation—to answer the question (Box 10-3).

Planning

Planning is the second step of the nursing process. In this step, the nurse provides input into plan development, participates in setting goals for meeting the client's needs, and participates in designing strategies to achieve these goals.

In the planning phase, the nurse assists in the formulation of the goals of care by participating in the identification of nursing interventions to achieve goals, and by communicating client needs that may require alteration of the goals of care. The nurse takes the nursing diagnosis written by the RN and states it as a nursing problem in objective, specific terms. The nurse then sets goals, lists interventions, and lists data collection. When evidence of a new client problem emerges, the nurse collects data about the problem, collaborates with the RN,

and the RN formulates a new nursing diagnosis. Setting priorities assists the nurse to organize and plan care that solves the most urgent problems. The client should be included in identifying the priorities of care. Priorities may change as the client's level of wellness changes. The most important problems, those that are potentially life threatening, must be taken care of immediately.

Once priorities are established, the client and nurse mutually decide on the expected goals. A goal must be set for each priority or client need. The selected goals serve as a guide for individualizing the care of the client. The goals must be client-centered, measurable, realistic, time referenced, and determined by the client and nurse together. Unless criteria for the goals have been predetermined, it is difficult to know whether the goal is achieved and the problem is resolved.

The nurse assists in the development of the plan of care by collaborating with the client and health care team members in selecting nursing interventions that will achieve the goals, and by planning for client safety, comfort, and maintenance of optimal functioning. The nurse participates in identifying health or social resources available to the client and family, and collaborates with other health care team members when planning the delivery of care. The nurse should communicate client needs, review the plan of care with the RN, and document the plan of care thoroughly and accurately.

When answering questions on NCLEX-PN, remember that this is a nursing examination, and the answer to the question most likely involves something that is included in the nursing care plan, rather than the

---

BOX 10-3

Nursing Process: Data Collection

A child with hemophilia is brought into the emergency room after being hit on the neck with a baseball. The nurse immediately checks the child for:
1   Spontaneous hematuria
2   Airway obstruction
3   Headache and slurred speech
4   Factor VIII deficiency

Answer: 2
Rationale: Trauma to the neck may cause bleeding into the tissues of the neck, which may compromise the airway. Though hematuria is a symptom of hemophilia, it is not associated with neck injury. Headache and slurred speech are associated with head trauma. Factor VIII deficiency is not a symptom of hemophilia but rather a common form of the disease. Use the ABCs—airway, breathing, and circulation—to answer this question. Airway is always a first priority!

BOX 10-4

Nursing Process: Planning

A nurse is caring for a hospitalized client with dementia who has a nursing diagnosis of Self-Care Deficit. The nurse assists in planning for which most appropriate goal for this client?

1. Client will be oriented to place by the time of discharge
2. Client will correctly identify objects in his or her room by the time of discharge
3. Client will be free of hallucinations
4. Client will feed self with cueing within 24 hours

Answer: 4
Rationale: Option 4 identifies a goal that is directly related to the client's ability to care for self. Options 1, 2, and 3 are not related to the nursing diagnosis of Self-Care Deficit. Remember, based on Maslow's Hierarchy of Needs theory, physiological needs take precedence. Option 4 is the only option that addresses a physiological need.

---

medical plan. Also, remember that actual problems are usually more important than potential or at-risk problems and that physiological needs are usually the priority (Box 10-4).

Implementation

Implementation is the third step of the Nursing Process that includes initiating and completing nursing actions required to accomplish the defined goals. This step is the action phase that involves assisting with organizing and managing client care, providing care to achieve established goals of care, and communicating nursing interventions.

The nurse assists in organizing and managing the client's care by implementing the established plan of care and by participating in client care conferences. The nurse is responsible for using safe and appropriate techniques and precautionary and preventive interventions when providing care to a client. The nurse is also responsible for instituting nursing interventions if adverse responses occur, initiating lifesaving interventions for emergency situations, and providing an environment conducive to the attainment of goals of care.

This step of the nursing process also includes the role of providing care based on the client's needs, preferences, or both; encouraging the client to follow the prescribed treatment plan; and assisting the client to maintain optimal functioning. Additionally, the process of implementation includes monitoring client care administered by unlicensed nursing personnel and reinforcing teaching on principles, procedures, and techniques required for the maintenance and promotion of health.

The implementation step concludes when the nurse's actions are completed and these actions, including their effects and the client's response, are communicated to the relevant members of the health care team.

NCLEX-PN is an examination about nursing, so focus on the nursing action rather than the medical action unless the question is asking what prescribed medical action is anticipated (Box 10-5).

Evaluation

Evaluation is the fourth step of the nursing process. Evaluation is a way of measuring client progress toward meeting goals. Although evaluation is the final step of the nursing process, it is an ongoing and integral component of each step. The process of data collection is reviewed to determine whether sufficient information was obtained, and whether the information obtained was specific and appropriate. The plan and expected outcomes are examined to determine if they are realistic, achievable, time-referenced, measurable, and effective. Interventions

---

BOX 10-5

Nursing Process: Implementation

A client with heart failure is receiving furosemide (Lasix) and digoxin (Lanoxin) daily. When the nurse enters the room to administer the morning doses, the client complains of anorexia, nausea, and ocular disturbances. The nurse should do which of the following first?

1. Administer the medications
2. Give the digoxin only
3. Check the morning serum potassium level
4. Check the morning serum digoxin level

Answer: 4
Rationale: The nurse should check the result of the digoxin level that was drawn because the symptoms are compatible with digitalis toxicity. Because a low potassium level may contribute to digitalis toxicity, checking the serum potassium level may give useful additive information, but the digoxin level is checked first. The digoxin should be withheld until the level is known. Noting the key word *first* will assist in determining that the nurse's action is to further investigate the cause of the client's complaints.

are examined to determine their effectiveness in achieving the expected outcomes.

Because evaluation is an ongoing process, it is vital to all steps of the nursing process. It is the continuous process of comparing actual outcomes with expected outcomes of care, and it provides the means for determining the need to modify the plan of care. Inherent in this step of the nursing process are the communication of evaluation findings and the process of documenting and reporting the client's response to treatment and care, and the effectiveness of teaching to relevant members of the health care team.

Evaluation type questions on NCLEX-PN may be written to address a client's response to treatment measures or to determine a client's understanding of the prescribed treatment measures (Box 10-6).

CARING

Caring is the essence of nursing and is basic to any helping relationship. Caring is central to every encounter that a nurse may have with a client. Through caring, the nurse humanizes the client. Treating the client with respect and dignity is a true expression of caring. In the technological environment of health care, emphasizing the client's individuality counteracts any potential process of depersonalization. Caring is an Integrated Concept and Process of the Test Plan for NCLEX-PN so this concept is nuclear to all Client Needs components of the test plan. The National Council of State Boards of Nursing describes caring as the interaction of the nurse and client in an atmosphere of mutual respect and trust, and that in this collaborative environment, the nurse provides support and compassion to help achieve desired outcomes.

In NCLEX-PN, the concept of caring is primary. It is easy to become involved with looking at a question from a technological viewpoint. The concept of caring should be addressed when reading a test question and when selecting an option. Always address the client's

feelings and provide support. Remember, this examination is all about nursing, and that Nursing is Caring (Box 10-7)!

COMMUNICATION AND DOCUMENTATION

The process of communication occurs as a nurse interacts either verbally or nonverbally with a client. Therapeutic communication techniques are key to an effective nurse-client relationship. Communication-type test questions are integrated throughout the NCLEX-PN test plan and may address a client situation in any health care setting. The National Council of State Boards of Nursing describes communication and documentation as the verbal, the nonverbal, or both types of interactions between the client, significant others, and members of the health care team, and the events and activities associated with client care as validated through a written or electronic record that reflects standards of practice and accountability into the provision of care.

When answering a question on NCLEX-PN, use of a communication tool indicates a correct option, and the use of a communication block indicates an incorrect option. In addition, some communication type questions may focus on psychosocial issues or issues related to client anxiety, fears, or concerns. In communication-type questions, always focus on the client's feelings FIRST. If an option reflects the client's feelings, anxiety, or concerns, select that option.

Documentation is a critical component of a nurse's responsibility. The process of documentation serves many purposes and provides a comprehensive representation of the client's health status and the care given by all members of the health care team. There are many methods for documenting, but the responsibilities surrounding this practice remains the same.

When answering a question on NCLEX-PN related to documenting, consider the ethical and legal responsibilities related to documentation, and the specific guidelines related to both narrative and computerized documentation systems (Box 10-8).

BOX 10-6

Nursing Process: Evaluation

A nurse employed in a clinic gathers data from a child with a diagnosis of celiac disease. Which of these findings would best indicate that a gluten-free diet is being maintained and has been effective?

1   The child is free of diarrhea
2   The child is free of bloody stools
3   The child tolerates dietary wheat and rye
4   The child has a balanced fluid and electrolyte status as noted on the laboratory results

Answer: 1

Rationale: This question addresses the child's response to prescribed dietary measures for celiac disease. Watery diarrhea is a frequent clinical manifestation of celiac disease. The absence of diarrhea indicates effective treatment. The grains of wheat and rye contain gluten and are not allowed. A balance in fluids and electrolytes does not necessarily demonstrate improved status of celiac disease. Remember, an evaluation type question addresses a client's response to a treatment measure.

BOX 10-7

Caring

A female client and her infant have undergone testing for human immunodeficiency virus (HIV) and both clients were found to be positive. The news is devastating and the mother is crying. The most appropriate intervention at this time is to:

1 Call an HIV counselor and make an appointment for them
2 Describe the progressive stages and treatments for HIV
3 Examine with the mother how she got HIV
4 Listen quietly while the mother talks and cries

Answer: 4

Rationale: This client has just received devastating news and should have someone present with her as she begins to cope with this issue. The nurse should sit and actively listen while the mother talks and cries. Calling an HIV counselor may be helpful, but it is not what the client needs at this time. The other options are not appropriate for this stage of coping with the news that both she and the infant are HIV-positive. Remember to address the client's feelings and to support the client. The nurse should sit and listen and provide support because this is the most caring response.

CULTURAL AWARENESS

Cultural awareness is a concept and process that is fundamental to the practice of nursing. Often, nurses care for clients who come from ethnic, cultural, and religious backgrounds that differ from their own. Awareness of and sensitivity to the unique health and illness beliefs and practices are essential in the delivery of safe and effective care. Acknowledgment and acceptance of cultural differences with a nonjudgmental attitude is essential in providing culturally sensitive care.

The National Council of State Boards of Nursing describes cultural awareness as the knowledge of and the sensitivity to the beliefs and values of the client and nurse, and the integration of such awareness in the provision of nursing care. The belief underlying the NCLEX-PN Test Plan is that people are unique individuals and define their own systems of daily living, which reflects their values, motives, and lifestyles. On NCLEX-PN, look for data in the question that relates to the issue of cultural awareness (Box 10-9).

BOX 10-8

Communication and Documentation

COMMUNICATION

A client says to the nurse, "I'm going to die and I wish my family would stop hoping for a cure! I get so angry when they carry on like this! After all, I'm the one who's dying." The most therapeutic response by the nurse is:

1 "You're feeling angry that your family continues to hope for you to be cured?"
2 "I think we should talk more about your anger at your family."
3 "Well, it sounds like you're being pretty pessimistic. After all, years ago people died of pneumonia."
4 "Have you shared your feelings with your family?"

Answer: 1

Rationale: Reflection is the therapeutic communication technique that redirects the client's feelings back to validate what the client is saying. Option 1 uses the therapeutic technique of reflection. In option 2, the nurse attempts to use focusing, but the attempt to discuss central issues seems premature. In option 3, the nurse makes a judgment and is nontherapeutic. In option 4, the nurse is attempting to assess the client's ability to openly discuss feelings with family members. Although this may be appropriate at some point, the timing is somewhat premature and closes off facilitation of the client's feelings. Remember, the use of a communication tool indicates a correct option.

DOCUMENTATION

A nurse hears a client calling out for help. The nurse hurries down the hallway to the client's room and finds a client lying on the floor. The nurse checks the client thoroughly and assists the client back to bed. The nurse notifies the registered nurse of the incident and completes an incident report. Which of the following would the nurse document on the incident report?

1 The client was found lying on the floor
2 The client climbed over the side rails
3 The client fell out of bed
4 The client became restless and tried to get out of bed

Answer: 1

Rationale: The incident report should contain the client's name, age, and diagnosis. It should contain a factual description of the incident, any injuries experienced by those involved, and the outcome of the situation. Option 1 is the only option that describes the facts as observed by the nurse. Options 2, 3, and 4 are interpretations of the situation and are not factual data as observed by the nurse. Remember to focus on factual information when documenting and avoid including interpretations.

BOX 10-9

CULTURAL AWARENESS

A nurse is reinforcing discharge instructions to a Chinese client about prescribed dietary modifications. During the teaching session, the client continuously turns away from the nurse. Which nursing action is most appropriate?
1. Continue with the instructions, verifying client understanding
2. Tell the client about the importance of the instructions for the maintenance of health care
3. Walk around the client so that the nurse continuously faces the client
4. Give the client a dietary booklet and return later to continue with the instructions

Answer: 1
Rationale: Most Chinese people maintain a formal distance with others, which is a form of respect. Chinese people may be uncomfortable with face-to-face communications, especially when there is direct eye contact. If the client turns away from the nurse during a conversation, the most appropriate action is to continue with the conversation. Walking around to the client so that the nurse faces the client is in direct conflict with the cultural practice. Telling the client about the importance of the instructions for the maintenance of health care may be viewed as degrading. The client may view returning later to continue with the explanation as a rude gesture. Remember, awareness of and sensitivity to the unique health and illness beliefs and practices is essential in the delivery of safe and effective care.

SELF-CARE

The ability to care for oneself promotes an overall sense of well-being in the client. When a client's health is compromised, it is necessary for the nurse to provide the needed care to the client. Whenever possible, or as soon as the client is able, the nurse should promote the client's ability to perform self-care. When promoting independence in the client, the nurse should provide information to the client about safety measures related to personal needs, prescribed treatment measures, and medication administration. Nursing care involves promoting growth and development throughout the life span, promoting self-care, and providing support systems and the measures related to the prevention and early treatment of disease. The nurse is instrumental as a teacher in promoting self-care through client and family teaching and by assisting with facilitating the coordination of support services for the client and family.

The National Council of State Boards of Nursing describes self-care as the practice of assisting the client to meet their own health care needs, including maintenance of health, restoration of function, or both.

When answering questions on NCLEX-PN, remember to promote independence in the client. Use concepts related to growth and development when selecting an answer (Box 10-10).

TEACHING AND LEARNING

Client and family education is a primary nursing responsibility. The National Council of State Boards of Nursing describes this concept as facilitating the acquisition of knowledge, skills, and attitudes that lead to a change in behavior.

The principles related to the teaching and learning process are used when the nurse functions in the role of a teacher. The nurse should remember that determining the client's readiness and the client's

---

BOX 10-10

Self-Care

A 9-year-old child has recently been diagnosed with type 1 diabetes mellitus. The nurse is assisting in planning for home care with the child and his family. The nurse suggests that an age-appropriate activity for this child for health maintenance is:
1. Independently self-administer insulin
2. Make independent decisions about sliding scale coverage of insulin
3. Have an adult assist in self-administration of insulin and glucose monitoring
4. Administer insulin drawn up by an adult

Answer: 1
Rationale: School-aged children have the cognitive and motor skills to independently administer insulin with adult supervision. Developmentally, they do not yet have the maturity to make situational decisions without adult validation. Options 3 and 4 suppress the maximum level of independence appropriate to the level of this child. Remember, use concepts related to growth and development when selecting an answer.

BOX 10-11

Teaching and Learning

A nurse reinforces instructions to a client about administering nitroglycerin ointment (Nitro-Bid). The nurse determines that the client is using correct technique when applying the ointment if the client:
1. Applies additional ointment if chest pain occurs
2. Applies the ointment directly to the skin, then rubs the ointment into the skin
3. Applies the ointment to a nonhairy area of the body
4. Washes the ointment off when bathing and reapplies after the bath

Answer: 3

Rationale: Nitroglycerin ointment is used on a scheduled basis and is not prescribed specifically for the occurrence of chest pain. The ointment is not rubbed into the skin. It is reapplied only as directed. The correct client action (option 3) indicates knowledge about administering the prescribed medication.

---

motivation to learn is the initial step in the teaching and learning process.

When answering a question on NCLEX-PN related to the teaching and learning process, use the principles related to Teaching and Learning Theory. If a test question addresses client education, remember that client motivation and client readiness to learn is the FIRST priority (Box 10-11).

REFERENCES

deWit, S. (2001). *Fundamental concepts and skills for nursing.* Philadelphia: W.B. Saunders.

Hodgson, B., & Kizior, R. (2003). *Saunders nursing drug handbook 2003.* Philadelphia: W.B. Saunders.

National Council of State Boards of Nursing (eds.) (2001). *Test Plan for the National Council Licensure Examination for Practical/Vocational Nurses.* Chicago: Author.

National Council of State Boards of Nursing (eds.) (2000). *The NCLEX Process: Serving as an Anchor for the NCLEX Examination.* Chicago: Author.

National Council of State Boards of Nursing. Web site: http://www.ncsbn.org

Potter, P., & Perry, A. (2001). *Fundamentals of nursing* (5th ed.). St. Louis: Mosby.

Riley, J. (2000). *Communication in nursing* (4th ed.). St. Louis: Mosby.

Smith, J., Crawford, L., & Gawel, S. (2000). *Linking the NCLEX-PN national licensure examination to practice: 2000 practice analysis of newly licensed practical/vocational nurses in the United States.* Chicago: National Council of State Boards of Nursing.

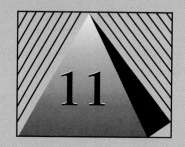

Integrated Concepts and Processes

CLINICAL PROBLEM-SOLVING PROCESS (NURSING PROCESS)

Nursing Process: Data Collection

1. A nurse reviews the record of a client receiving external radiation therapy and notes documentation of a skin finding noted as moist desquamation. The nurse expects to note which of the following on assessment of the client's skin?
 1. Reddened skin
 2. A rash
 3. Weeping of the skin
 4. Dermatitis

Answer: 3
Rationale: Moist desquamation occurs when the basal cells of the skin are destroyed. The dermal level is exposed, which results in the leakage of serum. Reddened skin, a rash, and dermatitis may occur with external radiation but is not described as a moist desquamation.

Test-Taking Strategy: Use the process of elimination. Noting the key word *moist* will direct you to option 3. Options 1, 2, and 4 are eliminated because they are similar and describe a dry rather than a moist skin alteration. Review the signs associated with a moist desquamation if you had difficulty with this question.

Level of Cognitive Ability: Comprehension
Client Needs: Physiological Integrity
Integrated Concept/Process: Nursing Process/Data Collection
Content Area: Adult Health/Oncology

Reference:
Black, J., Hawks, J., & Keene, A. (2001). *Medical-surgical nursing: clinical management for positive outcomes* (6th ed.). Philadelphia: W.B. Saunders, p. 1310.

---

2. A nurse is assisting in collecting data from a pregnant client with a history of cardiac disease and is checking the client for venous congestion. The nurse checks which of the following body areas knowing that venous congestion is most commonly noted in this area?
 1. Vulva
 2. Fingers of the hands
 3. Around the eyes
 4. Around the abdomen

Answer: 1
Rationale: Assessment of the cardiovascular system includes observation for venous congestion that can develop into varicosities. Venous congestion is most commonly noted in the legs, vulva, or rectum. It would be difficult to check for the presence of edema in the abdominal area of a client who is pregnant. Although edema may be noted in the fingers and around the eyes, edema in these areas would not be directly associated with venous congestion.

Test-Taking Strategy: Use the process of elimination. Focusing on the key words *venous congestion* will direct you to option 1. Review data collection techniques of the cardiovascular system in a pregnant client if you had difficulty with this question.

Level of Cognitive Ability: Application
Client Needs: Physiological Integrity
Integrated Concept/Process: Nursing Process/Data Collection
Content Area: Maternity

Reference:
Murray, S., McKinney, E. & Gorrie, T. (2002). *Foundations of maternal-newborn nursing* (3rd ed.). Philadelphia: W.B. Saunders, p. 143.

---

3. A client who has been receiving long-term diuretic therapy is admitted to the hospital with a diagnosis of dehydration (fluid volume deficit). The nurse would check the client for which sign or symptom that correlates with this fluid imbalance?
1. Increased blood pressure
2. Decreased pulse
3. Decreased central venous pressure (CVP)
4. Bibasilar crackles

Answer: 3
Rationale: A client with dehydration has a low CVP. The normal CVP is between 4 and 11 mm H_2O. Other findings that occur with fluid volume deficit (dehydration) are increased pulse and respirations, weight loss, poor skin turgor, dry mucous membranes, decreased urine output, concentrated urine with increased specific gravity, increased hematocrit, and altered level of consciousness. The signs in options 1, 2, and 4 occur with fluid volume excess.

Test-Taking Strategy: Use the process of elimination focusing on the client's diagnosis. Remember that central venous pressure reflects the pressure under which blood is returned to the right atrium, and that pressure (volume) decreases with a fluid volume deficit. If you had difficulty with this question, review the signs and symptoms of fluid volume deficit.

Level of Cognitive Ability: Comprehension
Client Needs: Physiological Integrity
Integrated Concept/Process: Nursing Process/Data Collection
Content Area: Fundamental Skills

Reference:
Ignatavicius, D., & Workman, M. (2002). *Medical-surgical nursing: critical thinking for collaborative care* (4th ed.). Philadelphia: W.B. Saunders, p. 163.

---

4. A nurse is assisting in preparing a plan of care for a child with Reye's syndrome. The nurse prioritizes the nursing interventions included in the plan and monitors for:
1. Signs of increased intracranial pressure (ICP)
2. The presence of protein in the urine
3. Signs of a bacterial infection
4. Signs of hyperglycemia

Answer: 1
Rationale: Intracranial pressure, encephalopathy, and hepatic dysfunction can occur in Reye's syndrome. Protein is not present in the urine. Reye's syndrome is related to a history of viral infections and hypoglycemia is a manifestation of this disease.

Test-Taking Strategy: Use the process of elimination and focus on the diagnosis. Note the key word *prioritizes*. Recalling that increased ICP is a major concern in Reye's syndrome will direct you to option 1. If you had difficulty with this question, review the care to the child with Reye's syndrome.

Level of Cognitive Ability: Application
Client Needs: Physiological Integrity
Integrated Concept/Process: Nursing Process/Data Collection
Content Area: Child Health

Reference:
Wong, D., & Hockenberry-Eaton, M. (2001). *Wong's essentials of pediatric nursing* (6th ed.). St. Louis: Mosby, p. 1096.

---

5. A nurse reads the chart of a client who was seen by the physician and notes that the physician has documented that the client has Lyme disease stage III. When collecting data from the client, which of the following clinical manifestations would the nurse expect to note?
1. A generalized skin rash
2. A cardiac dysrhythmia
3. Enlarged and inflamed joints
4. Palpitations

Answer: 3
Rationale: Stage III develops within a month to several months after the initial infection. It is characterized by arthritic symptoms, such as arthralgias and enlarged or inflamed joints, which can persist for several years after the initial infection. Cardiac and neurological dysfunction occurs in stage II. A rash occurs in stage I.

Test-Taking Strategy: Use the process of elimination. Eliminate options 2 and 4 first because they are both cardiac related. Recalling that a rash occurs in stage I will direct you to option 3. If you had difficulty with this question, review the clinical manifestations associated with Lyme disease.

Level of Cognitive Ability: Comprehension
Client Needs: Physiological Integrity
Integrated Concept/Process: Nursing Process/Data Collection
Content Area: Adult Health/Integumentary

Reference:
Black, J., Hawks, J., & Keene, A. (2001). *Medical-surgical nursing: clinical management for positive outcomes* (6th ed.). Philadelphia: W.B. Saunders, p. 1829.

---

6. A female client with narcolepsy has been prescribed dextroamphetamine (Dexedrine). The client complains to the nurse that she cannot sleep well anymore at night and does not want to take the medication any longer. The nurse asks the client if the medication is taken at which of the following appropriate times?
1. At least 6 hours before bedtime
2. 2 hours before bedtime
3. Before a bedtime snack
4. Just before going to sleep

Answer: 1
Rationale: Dextroamphetamine is a central nervous system (CNS) stimulant that acts by releasing norepinephrine from nerve endings. The client should take the medication at least 6 hours before going to bed at night to prevent disturbances with sleep.

Test-Taking Strategy: Use the process of elimination. Evaluate each of the options in terms of how far removed the scheduled dose is from the client's bedtime. Recalling that this medication causes CNS stimulation and interferes with sleep will direct you to option 1. Review this medication if you had difficulty with this question.

Level of Cognitive Ability: Application
Client Needs: Physiological Integrity
Integrated Concept/Process: Nursing Process/Data Collection
Content Area: Pharmacology

Reference:
Hodgson, B., & Kizior, R. (2003). *Saunders nursing drug handbook 2003.* Philadelphia: W.B. Saunders, p. 331.

---

7. A nurse is monitoring the level of consciousness in a child with a head injury and documents that the child is obtunded. Based on this documentation, which of the following observations did the nurse make?

Answer: 4
Rationale: If the child is obtunded, the child sleeps unless aroused and once aroused has limited interaction with the environment. Option 1 describes disorientation. Option 2 describes confusion. Option 3 describes stupor.

1. The child is unable to recognize place or person
2. The child is unable to think clearly and rapidly
3. The child requires considerable stimulation for arousal
4. The child sleeps unless aroused and once aroused has limited interaction with the environment

Test-Taking Strategy: Use the process of elimination noting the key word *obtunded*. Knowledge about the standard terms used to identify level of consciousness will direct you to option 4. If you are unfamiliar with monitoring the level of consciousness, review this content.

Level of Cognitive Ability: Comprehension
Client Needs: Physiological Integrity
Integrated Concept/Process: Nursing Process/Data Collection
Content Area: Child Health

Reference:
Wong, D., & Hockenberry-Eaton, M. (2001). *Wong's essentials of pediatric nursing* (6th ed.). St. Louis: Mosby, p. 1063.

---

8. A nurse is monitoring a client with Addison's disease for signs of hyperkalemia. The nurse expects to note which of the following if hyperkalemia is present?
1. Polyuria
2. Dry mucous membranes
3. Cardiac dysrhythmias
4. Prolonged bleeding time

Answer: 3
Rationale: The inadequate production of aldosterone in Addison's disease causes inadequate excretion of potassium and results in hyperkalemia. The clinical manifestations of hyperkalemia are the result of altered nerve transmission. The most harmful consequence of hyperkalemia is its effect on cardiac function. Options 1, 2, and 4 are not manifestations associated with Addison's disease or hyperkalemia.

Test-Taking Strategy: Use the process of elimination. Recalling the effects of hyperkalemia will direct you to option 3. If you had difficulty with this question, review the pathophysiology associated with Addison's disease and the effects of hyperkalemia.

Level of Cognitive Ability: Comprehension
Client Needs: Physiological Integrity
Integrated Concept/Process: Nursing Process/Data Collection
Content Area: Adult Health/Endocrine

Reference:
Black, J., Hawks, J., & Keene, A. (2001). *Medical-surgical nursing: clinical management for positive outcomes* (6th ed.). Philadelphia: W.B. Saunders, p. 1124.

---

9. A client goes into respiratory distress and an arterial blood gas (ABG) is drawn from the radial artery. The nurse assists in performing the Allen test before the ABGs to determine the adequacy of the:
1. Femoral circulation
2. Brachial circulation
3. Carotid circulation
4. Ulnar circulation

Answer: 4
Rationale: Before radial puncture for obtaining an arterial specimen for ABGs, an Allen test should be performed to determine adequate ulnar circulation. Failure to assess collateral circulation could result in severe ischemic injury to the hand, should damage to the radial artery occur with arterial puncture. The other options are incorrect.

Test-Taking Strategy: Use the process of elimination and note the key words *radial artery*. Using knowledge of anatomy of the cardiovascular system, eliminate options 1, 2, and 3. Review the purpose and procedure of the Allen test if you had difficulty with this question.

Level of Cognitive Ability: Application
Client Needs: Physiological Integrity

Integrated Concept/Process: Nursing Process/Data Collection
Content Area: Fundamental Skills

Reference:
Lewis, S., Heitkemper, M., & Dirksen, S. (2000). *Medical-surgical nursing: assessment and management of clinical problems* (5th ed.). St. Louis: Mosby, p. 1920.

---

10. A pregnant client with diabetes mellitus arrives at the health care clinic for a follow-up visit. In this client, the nurse most importantly monitors:
1. Urine for glucose and ketones
2. Blood pressure, pulse, and respirations
3. Urine for specific gravity
4. For the presence of edema

Answer: 1
Rationale: The nurse monitors the pregnant client with diabetes mellitus for glucose and ketones in the urine at each prenatal visit because the physiological changes of pregnancy can drastically alter insulin requirements. Assessment of blood pressure, pulse, respirations, urine for specific gravity, and the presence of edema are more related to the client with pregnancy-induced hypertension.

Test-Taking Strategy: Use the process of elimination focusing on the client's diagnosis. The only option that specifically addresses diabetes mellitus is option 1. If you had difficulty with this question, review prenatal care of the client with diabetes mellitus.

Level of Cognitive Ability: Application
Client Needs: Physiological Integrity
Integrated Concept/Process: Nursing Process/Data Collection
Content Area: Maternity

Reference:
Lowdermilk, D., Perry, S., & Bobak, I. (2000). *Maternity & women's health care* (7th ed.). St. Louis: Mosby, p. 872.

---

11. A nurse is caring for a client at home who is in a body cast. The nurse is collecting data from the client about the psychosocial adjustment of the client to the cast. During data collection, the nurse would most appropriately check:
1. The type of transportation available for follow-up care
2. The ability to perform activities of daily living
3. The need for sensory stimulation
4. The amount of home care support available

Answer: 3
Rationale: A psychosocial assessment of the client who is immobilized would most appropriately include the need for sensory stimulation. This assessment should also include such factors as body image, past and present coping skills, and the coping methods used during the period of immobilization. Although transportation, home care support, and the ability to perform activities of daily living are components of an assessment, they are not as specifically related to psychosocial adjustment as is the need for sensory stimulation.

Test-Taking Strategy: Use the process of elimination and focus on the key words *psychosocial* and *most appropriately*. Option 2 can be eliminated first because it relates to physiological integrity rather than psychosocial integrity. Next eliminate options 1 and 4 because they are more closely related to physical supports than psychosocial needs of the client. Review the components of a psychosocial assessment if you had difficulty with this question.

Level of Cognitive Ability: Analysis
Client Needs: Psychosocial Integrity
Integrated Concept/Process: Nursing Process/Data Collection
Content Area: Adult Health/Musculoskeletal

Reference:
Ignatavicius, D., & Workman, M. (2002). *Medical-surgical nursing: critical thinking for collaborative care* (4th ed.). Philadelphia: W.B. Saunders, p. 1131.

---

12. A nurse is caring for a client with acquired immunodeficiency syndrome (AIDS). Which finding noted in the client indicates the presence of an opportunistic respiratory infection?
1. White plaques located on the oral mucosa
2. Fever, exertional dyspnea, and nonproductive cough
3. Ophthalmic nerve involvement causing blindness
4. Colitis and ulcerated perirectal lesions

Answer: 2

Rationale: Fever, exertional dyspnea, and a nonproductive cough are signs of pneumocystis pneumonia, a common, life-threatening opportunistic infection afflicting those with AIDS. Options 1, 3, and 4 are not associated with a respiratory infection. Option 1 describes the fungal infection oral candidiasis (*Candida albicans*) called thrush. Option 3 describes the viral infection, herpes zoster (shingles), when it has spread to involve the ophthalmic nerve. Option 4 describes herpes simplex, which occurs in homosexual men.

Test-Taking Strategy: Use the process of elimination and focus on the issue: respiratory infection. Option 2 is the only option that identifies symptoms related to the respiratory system. Review the signs of respiratory infection if you had difficulty with this question.

Level of Cognitive Ability: Analysis
Client Needs: Physiological Integrity
Integrated Concept/Process: Nursing Process/Data Collection
Content Area: Adult Health/Immune

Reference:
Ignatavicius, D., & Workman, M. (2002). *Medical-surgical nursing: critical thinking for collaborative care* (4th ed.). Philadelphia: W.B. Saunders, p. 373.

---

13. An adult client seeks treatment in a clinic for complaints of a left earache, nausea, and a full feeling in the left ear. The client has an elevated temperature. The nurse first questions the client about:
1. A history of a recent brain abscess
2. A history of a recent upper respiratory infection (URI)
3. Whether acetaminophen (Tylenol) relieves the pain
4. Whether hearing is magnified in that ear

Answer: 2

Rationale: Otitis media in the adult is typically one-sided and presents as an acute process with earache, nausea and possible vomiting, fever, and fullness in the ear. The client may complain of diminished hearing in that ear. The nurse takes a client history first to determine whether the client has had a recent URI. It is unnecessary to question the client about a brain abscess. The nurse may ask the client if anything relieves the pain, but ear infection pain is usually not relieved until antibiotic therapy is initiated.

Test-Taking Strategy: Use the process of elimination. Note the key word *first*. Recalling the relationship between a URI and otitis media will direct you to option 2. Review otitis media, if you had difficulty with this question.

Level of Cognitive Ability: Analysis
Client Needs: Physiological Integrity
Integrated Concept/Process: Nursing Process/Data Collection
Content Area: Adult Health/Ear

Reference:
Black, J., Hawks, J., & Keene, A. (2001). *Medical-surgical nursing: clinical management for positive outcomes* (6th ed.). Philadelphia: W.B. Saunders, p. 1842.

14. A nurse is caring for an older client at home who has urinary incontinence and is very disturbed by the incontinent episodes. The nurse checks the client's home situation to determine environmental barriers to normal voiding. The nurse determines that which of the following items may be contributing to the client's problem?
 1. Presence of hand railings in the bathroom
 2. Having one bathroom on each floor of the home
 3. Night light present in the hall between the bedroom and bathroom
 4. Bathroom located on the second floor, bedroom on the first floor

Answer: 4

Rationale: Having a bathroom on the second floor and the bedroom on the first floor may pose a problem for the elderly client with incontinence. The need to negotiate the stairs and the distance may interfere with reaching the bathroom in a timely fashion. It is more helpful to the incontinent client to have a bathroom on the same floor as the bedroom, or to have a commode rented for use. The presence of night lights and hand railings are helpful to the client in reaching the bathroom quickly and safely.

Test-Taking Strategy: Use the process of elimination. Focus on the issue, an environmental barrier to normal voiding. Note that options 1, 2, and 3 are similar in that they all are helpful and safe. Review measures that promote normal voiding if you had difficulty with this question.

Level of Cognitive Ability: Comprehension
Client Needs: Health Promotion and Maintenance
Integrated Concept/Process: Nursing Process/Data Collection
Content Area: Fundamental Skills

Reference:
Black, J., Hawks, J., & Keene, A. (2001). *Medical-surgical nursing: clinical management for positive outcomes* (6th ed.). Philadelphia: W.B. Saunders, p. 833.

---

15. A nurse is assisting in preparing to administer continuous IV fluid replacement to a client with a diagnosis of dehydration. Which of the following is essential for the nurse to check before initiating the IV fluid?
 1. Usual sleep patterns
 2. Ability to ambulate
 3. Body weight
 4. Intake and output

Answer: 3

Rationale: Body weight is an accurate indicator of fluid status. As a client is hydrated with IV fluids, the nurse monitors for increasing body weight. Accurate body weight is a better measurement of gains and losses than intake and output records. An IV should not greatly alter sleep patterns, and clients will still be able to ambulate with a peripheral IV site.

Test-Taking Strategy: Use the process of elimination. Focusing on the client's diagnosis will direct you to option 3. Remember, body weight is an accurate measurement of gains and losses. Review care to the dehydrated client if you had difficulty with this question.

Level of Cognitive Ability: Application
Client Needs: Physiological Integrity
Integrated Concept/Process: Nursing Process/Data Collection
Content Area: Fundamental Skills

Reference:
Potter, P., & Perry, A. (2001). *Fundamentals of nursing* (5th ed.). St. Louis: Mosby, p. 1218.

---

16. A client is scheduled for an angiography using a radiopaque dye. The nurse checks which most critical item before the procedure?

Answer: 4

Rationale: This procedure requires a signed informed consent because it involves injection of a radiopaque dye into the blood vessel. Although options 1, 2, and 3 are components of the

1. Intake and output
2. Vital signs
3. Height and weight
4. Allergy to iodine or shellfish

preprocedure assessment, the risk of allergic reaction and possible anaphylaxis is most critical.

Test-Taking Strategy: Use the process of elimination noting the key words *most critical*. Recalling the risk of anaphylaxis related to the dye will direct you to option 4. If you had difficulty with this question, review preprocedure care for angiography.

Level of Cognitive Ability: Application
Client Needs: Physiological Integrity
Integrated Concept/Process: Nursing Process/Data Collection
Content Area: Adult Health/Neurological

Reference:
Ignatavicius, D., & Workman, M. (2002). *Medical-surgical nursing: critical thinking for collaborative care* (4th ed.). Philadelphia: W.B. Saunders, p. 641.

---

17. A nurse is assisting in performing a cardiovascular assessment on a client. Which of the following items would the nurse check to obtain the best information about the client's left-sided heart function?
1. Status of breath sounds
2. Presence of peripheral edema
3. Presence of jugular vein distention
4. Presence of hepatojugular reflux

Answer: 1
Rationale: The client with heart failure may present different symptoms depending on whether the right or the left side of the heart is failing. Peripheral edema, jugular vein distention, and hepatojugular reflux are all signs of right-sided heart function. The status of breath sounds provides information about left-sided heart function.

Test-Taking Strategy: Use the process of elimination and focus on the issue: the status of left-sided heart function. Remember *left* and *lungs*. Options 2, 3, and 4 reflect right-sided heart failure. Review the signs of right and left-sided heart failure if you had difficulty with this question.

Level of Cognitive Ability: Analysis
Client Needs: Physiological Integrity
Integrated Concept/Process: Nursing Process/Data Collection
Content Area: Adult Health/Cardiovascular

Reference:
Ignatavicius, D., & Workman, M. (2002). *Medical-surgical nursing: critical thinking for collaborative care* (4th ed.). Philadelphia: W.B. Saunders, p. 701.

---

18. A nurse is obtaining a history on a client admitted to the hospital with a thrombotic cerebrovascular accident (CVA). The nurse collects data from the client knowing that before the CVA, the client most likely experienced:
1. Transient hemiplegia and loss of speech
2. Throbbing headaches
3. Unexplained episodes of loss of consciousness
4. No symptoms at all

Answer: 1
Rationale: Cerebral thrombosis does not occur suddenly. In the few hours or days preceding a thrombotic CVA, the client may experience a transient loss of speech, hemiplegia, or paresthesias on one side of the body. Other signs and symptoms of thrombotic CVA vary but may include dizziness, cognitive changes, or seizures. Headache is rare and loss of consciousness is not likely to occur.

Test-Taking Strategy: Use the process of elimination. Option 4 is eliminated first. From the remaining options, focus on the type of stroke addressed in the question to direct you to option 1. If you had difficulty with this question, review the signs and symptoms of a thrombotic CVA.

Level of Cognitive Ability: Analysis
Client Needs: Physiological Integrity
Integrated Concept/Process: Nursing Process/Data Collection
Content Area: Adult Health/Neurological

Reference:
Ignatavicius, D., & Workman, M. (2002). *Medical-surgical nursing: critical thinking for collaborative care* (4th ed.). Philadelphia: W.B. Saunders, p. 974.

---

19. A client in a long-term care facility has had a series of gastrointestinal (GI) diagnostic tests including an upper GI series and endoscopies. On return to the long-term care facility, the priority nursing assessment should focus on:
1. Level of consciousness
2. Activity tolerance
3. Hydration and nutrition status
4. Comfort level

Answer: 3
Rationale: Many of the diagnostic studies to identify GI disorders require that the GI tract be cleaned (usually with laxatives and enemas) before testing. In addition, the client is most often NPO before and during the testing period. Because the studies may be done over a period exceeding 24 hours, the client may become dehydrated, malnourished, or both. Although options 1, 2, and 4 may be a component of the assessment, option 3 is the priority.

Test-Taking Strategy: Note the key words *priority nursing assessment.* Use Maslow's Hierarchy of Needs theory to direct you to option 3. Review care to the client after diagnostic GI tests if you had difficulty with this question.

Level of Cognitive Ability: Application
Client Needs: Physiological Integrity
Integrated Concept/Process: Nursing Process/Data Collection
Content Area: Adult Health/Gastrointestinal

Reference:
Ignatavicius, D., & Workman, M. (2002). *Medical-surgical nursing: critical thinking for collaborative care* (4th ed.). Philadelphia: W.B. Saunders, p. 1172.

---

20. A nurse is monitoring a client for the vegetative signs of depression. The nurse checks for these signs by determining the client's:
1. Ability to think, concentrate, and make decisions
2. Appetite, weight, sleep patterns, and psychomotor activity
3. Level of self-esteem
4. Level of suicidal ideation

Answer: 2
Rationale: The vegetative signs of depression are changes in physiological functioning during depression. These include appetite, weight, sleep patterns, and psychomotor activity. Options 1, 3, and 4 represent psychological assessment categories.

Test-Taking Strategy: Use the process of elimination. Recalling that the vegetative signs of depression refer to physiological changes directs you to option 2. Review the characteristics of depression if you had difficulty with this question.

Level of Cognitive Ability: Application
Client Needs: Physiological Integrity
Integrated Concept/Process: Nursing Process/Data Collection
Content Area: Mental Health

Reference:
Bauer, B. & Hill, S. (2000). *Mental health nursing.* Philadelphia: W.B. Saunders, p.102.

21. A nurse is caring for a client diagnosed with cirrhosis of the liver. The client is receiving spironolactone (Aldactone) 50 mg PO daily. Which of the following would indicate to the nurse that the client is experiencing a side effect related to the medication?
  1. Hypokalemia
  2. Hyperkalemia
  3. Constipation
  4. Dry skin

Answer: 2
Rationale: Spironolactone is a potassium-sparing diuretic. Side effects include hyperkalemia, dehydration, hyponatremia, and lethargy. Although the concern with most diuretics is hypokalemia, this medication is potassium-sparing, which means that the concern with the administration of this medication is hyperkalemia. Additional side effects include nausea, vomiting, cramping, diarrhea, headache, ataxia, drowsiness, confusion, and fever.

Test-Taking Strategy: Use the process of elimination. Recalling that this medication is potassium-sparing will direct you to option 2. If you had difficulty with this question, review those medications in the classification of potassium-sparing diuretics.

Level of Cognitive Ability: Analysis
Client Needs: Physiological Integrity
Integrated Concept/Process: Nursing Process/Data Collection
Content Area: Pharmacology

Reference:
Hodgson, B., & Kizior, R. (2003). *Saunders nursing drug handbook 2003.* Philadelphia: W.B. Saunders, p. 1028.

22. A nurse is preparing a woman in labor for an amniotomy. The nurse would check which priority data before the procedure?
  1. Maternal blood pressure
  2. Maternal heart rate
  3. Fetal heart rate
  4. Fetal scalp sampling

Answer: 3
Rationale: Fetal well-being must be confirmed before and after amniotomy. Fetal heart rate should be checked by Doppler or by the application of an external fetal monitor. Although maternal vital signs may be assessed, fetal heart rate is the priority. A fetal scalp sampling cannot be done when the membranes are intact.

Test-Taking Strategy: Use the process of elimination and note the key word *priority*. Eliminate option 4 first, knowing that a fetal scalp sampling cannot be done before an amniotomy. Eliminate options 1 and 2 next, noting that they are both similar and address maternal vital signs. Option 3 addresses fetal well-being. Review preprocedure care for amniotomy if you had difficulty with this question.

Level of Cognitive Ability: Application
Client Needs: Physiological Integrity
Integrated Concept/Process: Nursing Process/Data Collection
Content Area: Maternity

Reference:
Lowdermilk, D., Perry, S., & Bobak, I. (2000). *Maternity & women's health care* (7th ed.). St. Louis: Mosby, p. 995.

23. A nurse is assisting in monitoring a client receiving an oxytocin (Pitocin) infusion for the induction of labor. The nurse would suspect water intoxication if which of the following were noted?

Answer: 3
Rationale: During an oxytocin infusion, the woman is monitored closely for water intoxication. Signs of water intoxication include tachycardia, cardiac dysrhythmias, shortness of breath, nausea, and vomiting.

1. Bradycardia
2. Lethargy
3. Tachycardia
4. Fatigue

Test-Taking Strategy: Use the process of elimination. Focus on the issue of the question: water intoxication. Think about the physiological response that occurs when fluid overload exists to direct you to option 3. Review the signs of water intoxication if you had difficulty with this question.

Level of Cognitive Ability: Analysis
Client Needs: Physiological Integrity
Integrated Concept/Process: Nursing Process/Data Collection
Content Area: Maternity

Reference:
Lowdermilk, D., Perry, S., & Bobak, I. (2000). *Maternity & women's health care* (7th ed.). St. Louis: Mosby, p. 572.

---

24. A nurse in a well baby clinic is collecting data about the motor development of a 15-month-old child. Which of the following is the highest level of development that the nurse would expect to observe in this child?
1. The child builds a tower of two blocks
2. The child opens a door knob
3. The child unzips a large zipper
4. The child puts on simple clothes independently

Answer: 1
Rationale: At age 15 months, the nurse would expect that the child could build a tower of two blocks. A 24-month-old would be able to open a door knob and unzip a large zipper. At age 30 months, the child would be able to put on simple clothes independently.

Test-Taking Strategy: Use the process of elimination. Note the age of the child and the key words *highest level of development*. Visualize each of the motor skills presented in the options to assist in selecting the correct option. Review these developmental milestones if you had difficulty with this question.

Level of Cognitive Ability: Comprehension
Client Needs: Health Promotion and Maintenance
Integrated Concept/Process: Nursing Process/Data Collection
Content Area: Child Health

Reference:
Wong, D., & Hockenberry-Eaton, M. (2001). *Wong's essentials of pediatric nursing* (6th ed.). St. Louis: Mosby, p. 135.

---

25. A nurse is admitting a child with a diagnosis of irritable bowel syndrome to the hospital. Which of the following data would the nurse expect to obtain when collecting data about the child?
1. Reports of frothy diarrhea
2. Reports of profuse, watery diarrhea and vomiting
3. Reports of foul-smelling ribbon stools
4. Reports of diffuse abdominal pain unrelated to meals or activity

Answer: 4
Rationale: Irritable bowel syndrome causes diffuse abdominal pain unrelated to meals or activity. Alternating constipation and diarrhea with the presence of undigested food and mucus in the stools may also be noted. Option 1 is a clinical manifestation of lactose intolerance. Option 2 is a clinical manifestation of celiac disease. Option 3 is a clinical manifestation of Hirschsprung's disease.

Test-Taking Strategy: Use the process of elimination and focus on the child's diagnosis. Noting the name of the syndrome will direct you to option 4 because you would expect abdominal pain in such a disorder. Review the clinical manifestations associated with this disorder if you had difficulty with this question.

Level of Cognitive Ability: Comprehension
Client Needs: Physiological Integrity
Integrated Concept/Process: Nursing Process/Data Collection
Content Area: Child Health

Reference:
McKinney, E., Ashwill, J., Murray, S. et al. (2002). *Maternal-child nursing.* Philadelphia: W.B. Saunders, p. 1128.

---

26. A nurse is caring for a child diagnosed with rubeola (measles). The nurse notes that the physician has documented the presence Koplik spots. Based on this documentation, which of the following would the nurse expect to note in the child?

1. Petechiae spots that are reddish and pinpoint on the soft palate
2. Whitish vesicles located across the chest
3. Small, blue white spots with a red base found on the buccal mucosa
4. Pinpoint petechiae noted on both legs

Answer: 3

Rationale: Koplik spots appear approximately 2 days before the appearance of the rash. These are small, blue white spots with a red base found on the buccal mucosa. The spots last approximately 3 days, after which time they slough off. Options 1, 2, and 4 are incorrect.

Test-Taking Strategy: Knowledge about the characteristics associated with rubeola and the characteristics of Koplik spots is necessary to answer this question. If you are unfamiliar with these characteristics, review this content.

Level of Cognitive Ability: Comprehension
Client Needs: Physiological Integrity
Integrated Concept/Process: Nursing Process/Data Collection
Content Area: Child Health

Reference:
Wong, D., & Hockenberry-Eaton, M. (2001). *Wong's essentials of pediatric nursing* (6th ed.). St. Louis: Mosby, p. 460.

---

27. A child is hospitalized with a diagnosis of nephrotic syndrome. Which of the following assessment findings would the nurse expect to note in the child?

1. Weight loss
2. Excitability
3. Abdominal pain
4. Constipation

Answer: 3

Rationale: Clinical manifestation associated with nephrotic syndrome include edema, anorexia, fatigue, and abdominal pain from the presence of extra fluid in the peritoneal cavity. Diarrhea resulting from edema of the bowel occurs and may cause decreased absorption of nutrients. Increased weight and a normal blood pressure are most likely noted.

Test-Taking Strategy: Use the process of elimination. Recalling that edema is a clinical manifestation associated with nephrotic syndrome will direct you to option 3. If you had difficulty with this question or are unfamiliar with the clinical manifestations associated with this disorder, review this content.

Level of Cognitive Ability: Analysis
Client Needs: Physiological Integrity
Integrated Concept/Process: Nursing Process/Data Collection
Content Area: Child Health

Reference:
Wong, D., & Hockenberry-Eaton, M. (2001). *Wong's essentials of pediatric nursing* (6th ed.). St. Louis: Mosby, p. 1043.

---

28. A nurse is caring for a full-term infant whose bilirubin level is reported to be 14 mg/dL at 16 hours of age. The nurse determines this level to be indicative of:

Answer: 4

Rationale: Total bilirubin levels that rise above 12 mg/dL within 24 hours of birth are considered pathological. Pathological jaundice is of concern because of its association with kernicterus. Breast milk jaundice is usually associated with insufficient intake

1. Physiological jaundice
2. Breast milk jaundice
3. True breast milk jaundice
4. Pathological jaundice

because of infant sleepiness, poor suck, or nursing on an infrequent schedule. Insufficient intake prevents the infant from receiving enough colostrum, which acts like a natural laxative and facilitates the passage of meconium stools that contain high levels of bilirubin. The cause of true breast milk jaundice is different from inadequate intake. The exact cause is not known but seems to be the combination of several factors that cause the bilirubin level to rise.

Test Taking Strategy: Knowledge of the different types of jaundice and the acceptable bilirubin levels is needed to answer this question. Review the types of jaundice in a newborn if you had difficulty with this question.

Level of Cognitive Ability: Analysis
Client Needs: Physiological Integrity
Integrated Concept/Process: Nursing Process/Data Collection
Content Area: Maternity

Reference:
Burroughs, A., & Leifer, G. (2002). *Maternity nursing* (8th ed.). Philadelphia: W.B. Saunders, p. 280.

---

29. A nurse is assigned to care for a child with a basilar skull fracture. The nurse reviews the child's record and notes that the physician has documented the presence of Battle sign. Which of the following would the nurse expect to note in the child?
1. Bruising behind the ear
2. Edematous periorbital area
3. Bruised periorbital area
4. Presence of epistaxis

Answer: 1
Rationale: The most serious type of skull fracture is a basilar skull fracture. Two classic findings associated with this type of skull fracture are Battle's sign and raccoon eyes. Battle sign is the presence of bruising or ecchymosis behind the ear caused by leaking of blood into the mastoid sinuses. Raccoon eyes occur as a result of blood leaking into the frontal sinus and cause an edematous and bruised periorbital area.

Test-Taking Strategy: Use the process of elimination. Eliminate options 2 and 3 first because they are similar. From the remaining options, recalling the description of Battle's sign will direct you to option 1. If you are unfamiliar with this sign and its description review this content.

Level of Cognitive Ability: Comprehension
Client Needs: Physiological Integrity
Integrated Concept/Process: Nursing Process/Data Collection
Content Area: Child Health

Reference:
Wong, D., & Hockenberry-Eaton, M. (2001). *Wong's essentials of pediatric nursing* (6th ed.). St. Louis: Mosby, p. 246.

---

30. A mother brings a child to the health care clinic. The child has been complaining of severe headaches and has been vomiting. The child has a high fever and the nurse notes the presence of nuchal rigidity in the child. The nurse suspects a possible diagnosis of bacterial meningitis and checks the

Answer: 1
Rationale: Kernig's sign is the inability of the child to extend the legs fully when lying supine. Brudzinski's sign is flexion of the hips when the neck is flexed from a supine position. Both of these signs are frequently present in bacterial meningitis. Nuchal rigidity is also present in bacterial meningitis and occurs when pain prevents the child from touching the chin to the chest. Homan's

child for the presence of Kernig's sign. Which of the following findings would indicate the presence of this sign?

1. Inability of the child to extend the legs fully when lying supine
2. Flexion of the hips when the neck is flexed from a lying position
3. Pain when the chin is pulled down to the chest
4. Calf pain when the foot is dorsiflexed

sign is elicited when pain occurs in the calf region when the foot is dorsiflexed. Homan's sign is present in thrombophlebitis.

Test-Taking Strategy: Use the process of elimination focusing on the child's possible diagnosis. Option 4 is eliminated first because this is an assessment test for the presence of thrombophlebitis, not meningitis. Next eliminate option 3 because this option identifies the presence of nuchal rigidity. From the remaining options, it is necessary to be able to distinguish between Kernig's sign and Brudzinski's signs. If you had difficulty with this question, review the assessment findings in meningitis.

Level of Cognitive Ability: Comprehension
Client Needs: Physiological Integrity
Integrated Concept/Process: Nursing Process/Data Collection
Content Area: Child Health

Reference:
Wong, D., & Hockenberry-Eaton, M. (2001). Wong's essentials of pediatric nursing (6th ed.). St. Louis: Mosby, p. 1093.

Nursing Process: Planning

1. A nurse is caring for a client who is receiving total parenteral nutrition (TPN). The nurse plans which nursing intervention to prevent infection in the client?
   1. Using strict aseptic technique for intravenous site dressing changes
   2. Monitoring the serum blood urea nitrogen daily
   3. Weighing the client daily
   4. Encouraging increased fluid intake

Answer: 1
Rationale: Strict aseptic technique is vital during dressing changes because the IV catheter can serve as a direct entry for microorganisms. Options 2, 3, and 4 are not measures that will prevent infection.

Test-Taking Strategy: Use the process of elimination. Note the relationship between *infection* in the question, and *aseptic* in the correct option. Additionally, the only option that will prevent infection is option 1. If you had difficulty with this question, review care to a client receiving TPN.

Level of Cognitive Ability: Application
Client Needs: Safe, Effective Care Environment
Integrated Concept/Process: Nursing Process/Planning
Content Area: Fundamental Skills

Reference:
Ignatavicius, D., & Workman, M. (2002). *Medical-surgical nursing: critical thinking for collaborative care* (4th ed.). Philadelphia: W.B. Saunders, p. 208.

---

2. A nurse develops a plan of care for a client with a spica cast that covers a lower extremity. When planning for bowel elimination needs, the nurse includes which of the following in the plan of care?
   1. Use a fracture pan for bowel elimination
   2. Use a regular bedpan to prevent spilling of contents in the bed

Answer: 1
Rationale: A fracture pan is designed for use in clients with body or leg casts. A client with a spica cast (body cast) that covers a lower extremity cannot bend at the hips to sit up. Therefore a regular bedpan and a commode would be inappropriate. Daily enemas are not a part of routine care.

Test-Taking Strategy: Focus on the key words *covers a lower extremity*. Use the process of elimination noting the key word *fracture* in

3. Use a bedside commode for all elimination needs
4. Administer an enema daily

the correct option. Review care to the client with a spica cast if you had difficulty with this question.

Level of Cognitive Ability: Application
Client Needs: Physiological Integrity
Integrated Concept/Process: Nursing Process/Planning
Content Area: Fundamental Skills

Reference:
Potter, P., & Perry, A. (2001). *Fundamentals of nursing* (5th ed.). St. Louis: Mosby, p. 1459.

---

3. A nurse is caring for a postpartum client with thromboembolitic disorder. When planning care to prevent the complication of pulmonary embolism, the nurse prepares specifically to:
   1. Monitor anticoagulant therapy as prescribed
   2. Check the breath sounds frequently
   3. Enforce strict bed rest
   4. Monitor vital signs frequently

Answer: 1
Rationale: The purpose of anticoagulant therapy to treat thromboembolitic disorder is to prevent the clot from moving to another area, thus preventing pulmonary embolism. Although options 2, 3, and 4 may be implemented for a client with thromboembolitic disorder, option 1 will specifically prevent pulmonary embolism.

Test-Taking Strategy: Focus on the issue, prevent the complication of pulmonary embolism. Note the key word *specifically* in the stem of the question. Anticoagulant therapy is the only intervention listed that will prevent the clot from traveling to the pulmonary circulation. Review interventions for the client with thromboembolitic disorder that will prevent pulmonary embolism if you had difficulty with this question.

Level of Cognitive Ability: Application
Client Needs: Physiological Integrity
Integrated Concept/Process: Nursing Process/Planning
Content Area: Maternity

Reference:
Murray, S., McKinney, E., & Gorrie, T. (2002). *Foundations of maternal-newborn nursing* (3rd ed.). Philadelphia: W.B. Saunders, p. 787.

---

4. After reviewing a client's serum electrolytes, the physician states that the client would benefit most from an isotonic IV solution. The nurse plans care anticipating that the order will indicate that which of the following solutions will be administered?
   1   0.45% normal saline
   2   5% dextrose in water
   3   10% dextrose in water
   4   5% dextrose in 0.9% normal saline

Answer: 2
Rationale: 5% dextrose in water is an isotonic solution. Another example of an isotonic solution is 0.9% normal saline; 0.45% normal saline is a hypotonic solution; 10% dextrose in water and 5% dextrose in 0.9% normal saline are hypertonic solutions.

Test-Taking Strategy: To answer this question accurately, you must be familiar with the tonicity of various IV solutions. Note the key word *isotonic* and recall that 5% dextrose in water and 0.9% normal saline are isotonic. If this question was difficult, review the tonicity of IV fluids.

Level of Cognitive Ability: Analysis
Client Needs: Physiological Integrity
Integrated Concept/Process: Nursing Process/Planning
Content Area: Fundamental Skills

Reference:

Ignatavicius, D., & Workman, M. (2002). *Medical-surgical nursing: critical thinking for collaborative care* (4th ed.). Philadelphia: W.B. Saunders, p. 166.

---

5. A nurse is assisting with admitting a client to the hospital who recently had a bilateral adrenalectomy. Which of the following interventions is essential for the nurse to suggest to include in the client's plan of care?
  1. Prevent social isolation
  2. Discuss changes in body image
  3. Consider occupational therapy
  4. Avoid stress-producing situations and procedures

Answer: 4
Rationale: Adrenalectomy can lead to adrenal insufficiency. Adrenal hormones are essential in maintaining homeostasis in response to stressors. Options 1, 2, and 3 are not essential interventions specific to this client's problem.

Test-Taking Strategy: Note the key word *essential* in the stem of the question. This indicates the need to prioritize. Remember that according to Maslow's Hierarchy of Needs theory, physiological needs come first. The stress reaction involves physiological processes. Review the postoperative effects after an adrenalectomy if you had difficulty with this question.

Level of Cognitive Ability: Application
Client Needs: Physiological Integrity
Integrated Concept/Process: Nursing Process/Planning
Content Area: Adult Health/Endocrine

Reference:

Black, J., Hawks, J., & Keene, A. (2001). *Medical-surgical nursing: clinical management for positive outcomes* (6th ed.). Philadelphia: W.B. Saunders, p. 1131.

---

6. A perinatal client is admitted to the obstetric unit during an exacerbation of a heart condition. When planning for the nutritional requirements of the client, the nurse would consult with the dietitian to ensure which of the following?
  1. A low-calorie diet to ensure absence of weight gain
  2. A diet low in fluids and fiber to decrease blood volume
  3. A diet high in fluids and fiber to decrease constipation
  4. Unlimited sodium intake to increase circulating blood volume

Answer: 3
Rationale: Constipation can cause the client to use the Valsalva maneuver. This maneuver can cause blood to rush to the heart and overload the cardiac system. A low-calorie diet is not recommended during pregnancy. Diets low in fluid and fiber can cause a decrease in blood volume that can deprive the fetus of nutrients. Therefore adequate fluid intake and high-fiber foods are important. Sodium should be restricted to some degree as prescribed by the physician because this will cause an overload to the circulating blood volume and contribute to cardiac complications.

Test-Taking Strategy: Use the process of elimination. Think about the physiology of the cardiac system, the maternal and fetal needs, and the factors that increase the workload on the heart to answer the question. If you had difficulty with this question, review nursing measures for the pregnant client with cardiac disease.

Level of Cognitive Ability: Application
Client Needs: Physiological Integrity
Integrated Concept/Process: Nursing Process/Planning
Content Area: Maternity

Reference:

Murray, S., McKinney, E., & Gorrie, T. (2002). *Foundations of maternal-newborn nursing* (3rd ed.). Philadelphia: W.B. Saunders, pp. 713-714.

7. A nurse is assisting in developing a plan of care for a client with a hip spica cast. In the planning, the nurse includes measures to limit complications of prolonged immobility. The nurse includes which essential item in the plan to prevent this complication?
1. Provide a daily fluid intake of 1000 mL
2. Monitor for signs of low serum calcium
3. Maintain the client in a supine position
4. Limit the intake of milk and milk products

Answer: 4

Rationale: Daily fluid intake should be 2000 mL or greater a day. The nurse should monitor for signs and symptoms of hypercalcemia, such as nausea, vomiting, polydipsia, polyuria, and lethargy. A supine position increases urinary stasis; therefore it should be limited or avoided. Limiting milk and milk products is the best measure.

Test-Taking Strategy: Use the process of elimination. Focus on the issue: a complication of prolonged immobility. Option 3 should be eliminated immediately because it refers to maintaining an immobile client in one position. Eliminate option 1 next noting the amount of fluid in this option. From the remaining options, recalling the effect of the movement of calcium into the blood from the bones will direct you to option 4. If you had difficulty with this question review the complications of immobility.

Level of Cognitive Ability: Application
Client Needs: Physiological Integrity
Integrated Concept/Process: Nursing Process/Planning
Content Area: Adult Health/Musculoskeletal

Reference:
Ignatavicius, D., & Workman, M. (2002). *Medical-surgical nursing: critical thinking for collaborative care* (4th ed.). Philadelphia: W.B. Saunders, pp. 188-189.

8. A nurse determines that a Mantoux tuberculin skin test is positive. To most accurately diagnose tuberculosis (TB), the nurse plans to consult with the registered nurse to follow up the skin test with a:
1. Chest x-ray
2. A computed tomography scan of the chest
3. Sputum culture
4. Complete blood cell count

Answer: 3

Rationale: Although the findings on chest x-ray examination are important, it is not possible to make a diagnosis of TB solely on the basis of this examination because other diseases can mimic the appearance of TB. The bacteriological demonstration of tubercle bacilli is essential for establishing a diagnosis. Microscopic examination of sputum for acid-fast bacilli is usually the first bacteriological evidence of the presence of tubercle bacilli. Options 2 and 4 will not diagnosis TB.

Test-Taking Strategy: Use the process of elimination. Note the key words *most accurately diagnose tuberculosis*. Recalling that the presence of tubercle bacilli indicates TB will direct you to option 3. Review the tests used in diagnosing tuberculosis if you had difficulty with this question.

Level of Cognitive Ability: Application
Client Needs: Physiological Integrity
Integrated Concept/Process: Nursing Process/Planning
Content Area: Adult Health/Respiratory

Reference:
Ignatavicius, D., & Workman, M. (2002). *Medical-surgical nursing: critical thinking for collaborative care* (4th ed.). Philadelphia: W.B. Saunders, pp. 585-586.

9. A nurse is assisting in preparing a plan of care for a client with Meniere's disease who is experiencing severe vertigo. Which

Answer: 2

Rationale: The nurse instructs the client to make slow head movements to prevent worsening of the vertigo. Dietary changes such

nursing intervention would the nurse suggest to include in the plan of care to assist the client in controlling the vertigo?

1. Encourage the client to increase daily fluid intake
2. Encourage the client to avoid sudden head movements
3. Instruct the client to cut down on cigarette smoking
4. Instruct the client to increase sodium in the diet

as salt and fluid restrictions that reduce the amount of endolymphatic fluid are sometimes prescribed. Clients are advised to stop smoking because of its vasoconstrictive effects.

Test-Taking Strategy: Use the process of elimination. Identify the issue of the question, severe vertigo. Note the relationship between vertigo and the correct option, which states to avoid sudden head movements. Recalling that salt and fluid restrictions are sometimes prescribed will also assist in eliminating options 1 and 4. Noting the words *cut down* in option 3 will assist in eliminating this option. If you had difficulty with this question, review measures that will reduce vertigo in the client with Meniere's disease.

Level of Cognitive Ability: Application
Client Needs: Health Promotion and Maintenance
Integrated Concept/Process: Nursing Process/Planning
Content Area: Adult Health/Ear

Reference:
Black, J., Hawks, J., & Keene, A. (2001). *Medical-surgical nursing: clinical management for positive outcomes* (6th ed.). Philadelphia: W.B. Saunders, p.1848.

---

10. An 18-year-old woman is admitted to a mental health unit with the diagnosis of anorexia nervosa. The nurse assists in planning care knowing that health promotion should focus on:
    1. Helping the client identify and examine dysfunctional thoughts and beliefs
    2. Emphasizing social interaction with clients who are withdrawn
    3. Providing a supportive environment
    4. Examining intrapsychic conflicts and past issues

Answer: 1
Rationale: Health promotion focuses on helping clients identify and examine dysfunctional thoughts as well as identify and examine values and beliefs that maintain these thoughts. Providing a supportive environment is important but is not as primary as option 1 in this client. Emphasizing social interaction is not appropriate at this time. Examining intrapsychic conflicts and past issues is not directly related to the client's problem.

Test-Taking Strategy: Use the process of elimination focusing on the issue of health promotion. Option 1 is the only option that is specifically client centered. This option also focuses on data collection, the first step of the nursing process. Review care to the client with anorexia nervosa if you had difficulty with this question.

Level of Cognitive Ability: Application
Client Needs: Health Promotion and Maintenance
Integrated Concept/Process: Nursing Process/Planning
Content Area: Mental Health

Reference:
Bauer, B., & Hill, S. (2000). *Mental health nursing.* Philadelphia: W.B. Saunders, p.175.

---

11. A nurse is assisting in preparing discharge plans for a client who has attempted suicide. The nurse suggests to include which of the following in the plan?
    1. Weekly follow-up appointments
    2. Contracts and immediate available crisis resources

Answer: 2
Rationale: Crisis times may occur between appointments. Contracts facilitate clients feeling responsibility for keeping a promise. This gives the client control. Family and friends cannot always be present. Providing phone numbers will not ensure available and immediate crisis resources.

3. Encouraging family and friends to always be present

4. Providing phone numbers for the hospital and physician

Test-Taking Strategy: Use the process of elimination. Focus on the issue, the availability of immediate resources for the client. Eliminate option 3 first because this is unrealistic. Options 1 and 4 will not necessarily provide immediate resources. Also, note the word *immediate* in the correct option. Review discharge plans for the client who attempted suicide if you had difficulty with this question.

Level of Cognitive Ability: Application
Client Needs: Psychosocial Integrity
Integrated Concept/Process: Nursing Process/Planning
Content Area: Mental Health

Reference:
Bauer, B., & Hill, S. (2000). *Mental health nursing.* Philadelphia: W.B. Saunders, p.195.

---

12. A nurse is assisting in developing a plan of care for a newborn infant diagnosed with bilateral club feet. The nurse includes instructions in the plan to tell the parents that:

1. Genetic testing is wise for future pregnancies, as other children born to this couple may also be affected

2. If casting is needed, it will begin at birth and continue for 12 weeks, then the condition will be reevaluated

3. Surgery performed immediately after birth has been found to be most effective in achieving a complete recovery

4. The regimen of manipulation and casting is effective in all cases of bilateral club feet

Answer: 2
Rationale: Casting should begin at birth and continue for at least 12 weeks or until maximum correction is achieved. At this time, corrective shoes may provide support to maintain alignment or surgery can be performed. Surgery is usually delayed until age 4 to 12 months. Options 3 and 4 are inaccurate. Option 1 does not address the issue of the question.

Test-Taking Strategy: Use the process of elimination. Focus on the issue: parental instructions for the child with bilateral club feet. Eliminate option 1 because this is not the time to discuss the future. Eliminate option 3 because of the word *immediately.* From the remaining options, note that option 2 provides accurate information and that option 4 contains the absolute word *all.* Review the treatment plan for bilateral club feet if you had difficulty with this question.

Level of Cognitive Ability: Application
Client Needs: Health Promotion and Maintenance
Integrated Concept/Process: Nursing Process/Planning
Content Area: Child Health

Reference:
Wong, D., & Hockenberry-Eaton, M. (2001). *Wong's essentials of pediatric nursing* (6th ed.). St. Louis: Mosby, p. 1225.

---

13. A nurse is planning to assist with obtaining a set of arterial blood gases on a client. In addition to sending the specimen to the laboratory immediately, the nurse plans to provide which of the following items to optimally maintain the integrity of the specimen?

1. A syringe containing a preservative

2. A syringe containing a preservative and a bag of ice

Answer: 4
Rationale: The arterial blood gas sample is obtained using a heparinized syringe. The sample of blood is placed on ice and sent to the laboratory immediately. A preservative is not used.

Test-Taking Strategy: Use the process of elimination. Specific knowledge about this procedure is needed to answer this question. If you are unfamiliar with this procedure, review this content.

Level of Cognitive Ability: Application
Client Needs: Physiological Integrity

3.   A heparinized syringe and a preservative

4.   A heparinized syringe and a bag of ice

Integrated Concept/Process: Nursing Process/Planning
Content Area: Adult Health/Respiratory

Reference:
Black, J., Hawks, J., & Keene, A. (2001). *Medical-surgical nursing: clinical management for positive outcomes* (6th ed.). Philadelphia: W.B. Saunders, p. 1641.

---

14.   A client is experiencing diabetes insipidus secondary to cranial surgery. The nurse who is assisting in caring for the client plans to implement which of these anticipated therapies?

1.   Fluid restriction
2.   IV replacement of fluid losses
3.   Increased sodium intake
4.   Administering diuretics

Answer: 2
Rationale: The client with diabetes insipidus excretes large amounts of extremely dilute urine. This usually occurs as a result of decreased synthesis or release of antidiuretic hormone in conditions such as head injury, surgery near the hypothalamus, or increased intracranial pressure. Corrective measures include allowing ample oral fluid intake, administering IV fluid as needed to replace sensible and insensible losses, and administering vasopressin (Pitressin). Sodium is not administered because the serum sodium level is usually high, as is the serum osmolality. Option 4 is incorrect.

Test-Taking Strategy: Use the process of elimination. Focus on the client's diagnosis recalling that a large fluid loss is the problem in this client. This will assist in eliminating options 1 and 4. From the remaining options, recalling that the serum sodium level is already elevated in this disorder, or knowing that fluid replacement is the most direct form of therapy for fluid loss, will direct you to option 2. Review the treatment for diabetes insipidus if you had difficulty with this question.

Level of Cognitive Ability: Analysis
Client Needs: Physiological Integrity
Integrated Concept/Process: Nursing Process/Planning
Content Area: Adult Health/Neurological

Reference:
Black, J., Hawks, J., & Keene, A. (2001). *Medical-surgical nursing: clinical management for positive outcomes* (6th ed.). Philadelphia: W.B. Saunders, p. 1144.

---

15.   A nurse is assisting in planning care for a child with an infectious and communicable disease. The nurse determines that the primary goal is that the:

1.   Child will experience only minor complications
2.   Child will not spread the infection to others
3.   Public health department will be notified
4.   Child will experience only mild discomfort

Answer: 2
Rationale: The primary goal is to prevent the spread of the disease to others. The child should experience no complications. Although the health department may need to be notified at some point, it is not the most important primary goal. It is also important to prevent discomfort as much as possible.

Test-Taking Strategy: Use the process of elimination. Note the key words *primary goal.* Recognize the relationship between *infectious and communicable disease* in the question and *infection* in the correct option. Review goals of care for the child with an infectious and communicable disease if you had difficulty with this question.

Level of Cognitive Ability: Analysis
Client Needs: Health Promotion and Maintenance
Integrated Concept/Process: Nursing Process/Planning
Content Area: Child Health

Reference:
Wong, D., & Hockenberry-Eaton, M. (2001). *Wong's essentials of pediatric nursing* (6th ed.). St. Louis: Mosby, p. 457.

---

16. A nurse is preparing to care for an infant with pertussis. In planning care, the nurse addresses which most critical problem first?
1. Ineffective airway clearance
2. Fluid volume excess
3. Sleep pattern disturbance
4. High risk for infection

Answer: 1

Rationale: The most important problem relates to adequate air exchange. Because of the copious, thick secretions that occur with pertussis and the small airways of an infant, air exchange is critical. A fluid volume deficit is more likely to occur in this infant because of the thick secretions and vomiting. Sleep patterns may be disturbed because of the coughing, but they are not the most critical issue. Infection is an important consideration, but airway is the priority.

Test-Taking Strategy: Use the process of elimination and the ABCs—airway, breathing, and circulation. Airway is always the most critical concern. This should direct you to option 1. Review care to the infant with pertussis if you had difficulty with this question.

Level of Cognitive Ability: Application
Client Needs: Physiological Integrity
Integrated Concept/Process: Nursing Process/Planning
Content Area: Child Health

Reference:
Wong, D., & Hockenberry-Eaton, M. (2001). *Wong's essentials of pediatric nursing* (6th ed.). St. Louis: Mosby, p.461.

---

17. A nurse is assisting in planning care for an infant who has pyloric stenosis. To most effectively meet the infant's preoperative needs, the nurse includes which of the following in the plan of care?
1. Monitor the IV infusion, intake and output, and weight
2. Provide small frequent feedings of glucose, water, and electrolytes
3. Administer enemas until returns are clear
4. Provide the mother privacy to breast-feed every 2 hours

Answer: 1

Rationale: Important preoperative nursing responsibilities include monitoring the IV infusion, intake and output, and weight, and obtaining urine specific gravity measurements. In addition, weighing the infant's diapers provides information about output. The infant is kept NPO preoperatively unless the physician prescribes a thickened formula. Enemas until clear would further compromise the fluid volume status.

Test-Taking Strategy: Use the process of elimination, noting the key word *preoperative*. Eliminate options 2 and 4 because the infant should be NPO in the preoperative period. Eliminate option 3 because enemas would further compromise the fluid balance status. Review preoperative care of the infant with pyloric stenosis if you had difficulty with this question.

Level of Cognitive Ability: Application
Client Needs: Physiological Integrity
Integrated Concept/Process: Nursing Process/Planning
Content Area: Child Health

Reference:
Wong, D., & Hockenberry-Eaton, M. (2001). *Wong's essentials of pediatric nursing* (6th ed.). St. Louis: Mosby, p. 922.

18. A client who was a victim of a gun shot incident states, "I feel like I am losing my mind. I keep hearing the gunshots and seeing my friend lying on the ground." The nurse most appropriately plans strategies to formulate a therapeutic relationship that will include:
1. Asking the psychiatrist to order an antianxiety medication
2. Encouraging the client to talk about the incident and feelings related to it
3. Encouraging the client to think about how lucky he or she is to be alive
4. Teaching the client relaxation techniques

Answer: 2
Rationale: In developing a therapeutic relationship, it is important to acknowledge and validate the client's feelings. Although teaching the client relaxation techniques may be helpful at some point, this process is not related to the issue of the question. Options 1 and 3 are nontherapeutic techniques and do not promote a therapeutic relationship.

Test-Taking Strategy: Use therapeutic communication techniques. Eliminate options 1 and 3 because they do not encourage further discussion about the client's feelings. Teaching the client how to relax may be helpful at some point but not in the beginning of the therapeutic relationship. Remember to address the client's feelings. Review therapeutic communication techniques if you had difficulty with this question.

Level of Cognitive Ability: Application
Client Needs: Psychosocial Integrity
Integrated Concept/Process: Nursing Process/Planning
Content Area: Mental Health

Reference:
Varcarolis, E. (2002). *Foundations of psychiatric mental health nursing* (4th ed.). Philadelphia: W.B. Saunders, p. 260.

19. A nurse is caring for a hospitalized child with a diagnosis of rheumatic fever (RF) who has developed carditis. The mother asks the nurse to explain the meaning of carditis. The nurse plans to respond knowing that which of the following most appropriately describes this complication of RF?
1. Tender painful joints, especially in the elbows, knees, ankles, and wrists
2. Inflammation of all parts of the heart, primarily the mitral valve
3. Involuntary movements affecting the legs, arms, and face
4. Red skin lesions that start as flat or slightly raised macules usually over the truck and that spread peripherally

Answer: 2
Rationale: Carditis is the inflammation of the heart, primarily the mitral valve, and is a complication of RF. Option 1 describes polyarthritis. Option 3 describes chorea. Option 4 describes erythema marginatum.

Test-Taking Strategy: Use the process of elimination. Note the relationship between the word *carditis* in the question and *heart* in the correct option. If you are unfamiliar with this complication that is associated with rheumatic fever, review this content.

Level of Cognitive Ability: Application
Client Needs: Physiological Integrity
Integrated Concept/Process: Nursing Process/Planning
Content Area: Child Health

Reference:
Wong, D., & Hockenberry-Eaton, M. (2001). *Wong's essentials of pediatric nursing* (6th ed.). St. Louis: Mosby, p. 966.

20. A nurse receives a telephone call from the emergency room and is told that a 7-month-old infant with febrile seizures will be admitted to the pediatric unit. In planning care for the admission of the infant, the nurse would anticipate the need for which of the following?
1. A padded tongue blade taped to the head of the bed

Answer: 4
Rationale: A padded tongue blade should never be used; in fact, nothing should be placed in a client's mouth during a seizure. During a seizure, the infant should be placed in a side-lying position but should not be restrained. Suctioning may be necessary during a seizure to remove secretions that obstruct the airway. It is not necessary to place a code cart at the bedside, but a cart should be readily available in the nursing unit.

2. A code cart at the bedside
3. Restraints at the bedside
4. Suction equipment at the bedside

Test-Taking Strategy: Use the process of elimination and the ABCs—airway, breathing, and circulation—to answer the question. Option 4 is the only option that specifically relates to airway. Review nursing interventions for an infant with seizures if you had difficulty with this question.

Level of Cognitive Ability: Application
Client Needs: Physiological Integrity
Integrated Concept/Process: Nursing Process/Planning
Content Area: Child Health

Reference:
Wong, D., & Hockenberry-Eaton, M. (2001). *Wong's essentials of pediatric nursing* (6th ed.). St. Louis: Mosby, p. 763.

---

21. A 10-month-old infant is hospitalized for respiratory syncytial virus (RSV), and the nurse assists in developing a plan of care for the infant. Based on the developmental stage of the infant, the nurse suggests to include which of the following in the plan of care?
1. Wash hands, wear a mask when caring for the child, and keep the child as quiet as possible
2. Follow the home feeding schedule and allow the infant to be held only when the parents visit
3. Restrain the infant with a total body restraint to prevent any tubes from being dislodged
4. Provide a consistent routine, as well as touching, rocking, and cuddling, throughout the hospitalization

Answer: 4
Rationale: A 10-month-old infant is in the trust versus mistrust stage of psychosocial development (Erikson) and in the sensorimotor period of cognitive development (Piaget). RSV is not airborne (mask is not required) and is usually transmitted by the hands. Touching and holding the infant only when the parents visit will not provide adequate stimulation and interpersonal contact for the infant. Total body restraint is unnecessary and an incorrect action. Hospitalization may have an adverse effect. A consistent routine accompanied by touching, rocking, and cuddling will help the child to develop trust and provide sensory stimulation.

Test-Taking Strategy: Note the age and diagnosis of the infant. Focusing on the key words *developmental stage of the infant* will direct you to option 4. Review the psychosocial needs of an infant if you had difficulty with this question.

Level of Cognitive Ability: Application
Client Needs: Physiological Integrity
Integrated Concept/Process: Nursing Process/Planning
Content Area: Child Health

Reference:
Wong, D., & Hockenberry-Eaton, M. (2001). *Wong's essentials of pediatric nursing* (6th ed.). St. Louis: Mosby, p. 842.

---

22. A nurse is told that a child with a diagnosis of Reye's syndrome is being admitted to the hospital. The nurse assists in developing a plan of care for the child and suggests to include which priority nursing action in the plan?
1. Provide a quiet environment with low dimmed lighting
2. Monitor for hearing loss
3. Monitor intake and output (I&O)
4. Position the child supine

Answer: 1
Rationale: Cerebral edema is a progressive part of the disease process in Reye's syndrome. A major component of care for a child with Reye's syndrome is to maintain effective cerebral perfusion and control intracranial pressure. Decreasing stimuli in the environment would decrease the stress on the cerebral tissue and neuron responses. Hearing loss does not occur in this disorder. Although monitoring I&O may be a component of the plan, it is not the priority. The child should be in a head elevated position to decrease the progression of cerebral edema and promote drainage of cerebrospinal fluid.

Test-Taking Strategy: Use the process of elimination. Note the key words *priority nursing action*. Recalling that increased intracranial pressure is a concern will direct you to option 1. If you had difficulty with this question, review the priorities in the plan of care for the child with Reye's syndrome.

Level of Cognitive Ability: Application
Client Needs: Physiological Integrity
Integrated Concept/Process: Nursing Process/Planning
Content Area: Child Health

Reference:
Wong, D., & Hockenberry-Eaton, M. (2001). *Wong's essentials of pediatric nursing* (6th ed.). St. Louis: Mosby, p. 1096.

---

23. A nursing student is preparing to conduct a clinical conference about cerebral palsy. Which of the following characteristics related to this disorder will the student plan to include in the discussion?
1. Cerebral palsy is a chronic disability characterized by a difficulty in controlling muscles
2. Cerebral palsy is an infectious disease of the central nervous system
3. Cerebral palsy is an inflammation of the brain as a result of a viral illness
4. Cerebral palsy is a congenital condition that results in moderate to severe retardation

Answer: 1
Rationale: Cerebral palsy is a chronic disability characterized by a difficulty in controlling muscles because of an abnormality in the extrapyramidal or pyramidal motor system. Meningitis is an infectious process of the central nervous system. Encephalitis is an inflammation of the brain that occurs as a result of viral illness or central nervous system infections. Down syndrome is an example of a congenital condition that results in moderate to severe retardation.

Test-Taking Strategy: Use the process of elimination. Eliminate options 2 and 3 first, noting that they are similar and basically state the same thing. From the remaining options, note the relationship between *palsy* in the question and *muscles* in the correct option. If you had difficulty with this question, review the characteristics associated with cerebral palsy.

Level of Cognitive Ability: Application
Client Needs: Physiological Integrity
Integrated Concept/Process: Nursing Process/Planning
Content Area: Child Health

Reference:
Wong, D., & Hockenberry-Eaton, M. (2001). *Wong's essentials of pediatric nursing* (6th ed.). St. Louis: Mosby, p. 1247.

---

24. A nursing student is asked to conduct a clinical conference about autism. The student plans to include in the discussion that the primary characteristic associated with autism is:
1. The consistent imitation of others actions
2. Normal social play
3. Lack of social interaction and awareness
4. Normal verbal communication

Answer: 3
Rationale: Autism is a severe developmental disorder that begins in infancy or toddlerhood. A primary characteristic is lack of social interaction and awareness. Social behaviors in autism include lack of or abnormal imitations of others' actions and the lack of or abnormal social play. Additional characteristics include lack of or impaired verbal communication and marked abnormal nonverbal communication.

Test-Taking Strategy: Use the process of elimination. Eliminate options 2 and 4 first because they address normal behaviors. From the remaining options, recalling that the autistic child lacks social interaction and awareness will direct you to option 3. If you had difficulty with this question, review the characteristics associated with autism.

Level of Cognitive Ability: Application
Client Needs: Psychosocial Integrity
Integrated Concept/Process: Nursing Process/Planning
Content Area: Child Health

Reference:
Wong, D., & Hockenberry-Eaton, M. (2001). *Wong's essentials of pediatric nursing* (6th ed.). St. Louis: Mosby, p. 408.

---

25. A nurse is assisting in developing a plan of care for the child returning from the operating room after a tonsillectomy. The nurse avoids placing which intervention in the plan of care?
1. Offer clear cool liquids when awake
2. Eliminate milk or milk products from the diet
3. Monitor for bleeding from the surgical site
4. Suction whenever necessary

Answer: 4
Rationale: After tonsillectomy, suction equipment should be available, but suctioning is not performed unless there is an airway obstruction. Clear cool liquids are encouraged. Milk and milk products are avoided initially because they coat the throat, causing the child to clear their throat, thus increasing the risk of bleeding. Option 3 is an important intervention after any type of surgery.

Test-Taking Strategy: Use the process of elimination noting the key word *avoids*. Eliminate option 3 first because this is an expected general nursing procedure. From the remaining options, thinking about the anatomical location of the surgery will direct you to option 4. Suctioning after tonsillectomy will disrupt the integrity of the surgical site and can cause bleeding. Review postoperative care after tonsillectomy if you had difficulty with this question.

Level of Cognitive Ability: Application
Client Needs: Physiological Integrity
Integrated Concept/Process: Nursing Process/Planning
Content Area: Child Health

Reference:
Schulte, E. Price, D., & Gwin, J. (2001). *Thompson's pediatric nursing* (8th ed.). Philadelphia: W.B. Saunders, p. 220.

---

26. A nurse is assisting in preparing a plan of care for a child being admitted to the hospital with a diagnosis of congestive heart failure (CHF). The nurse avoids including which of the following in the plan?
1. Limiting the time the child is allowed to bottle-feed
2. Elevating the head of the bed
3. Waking the child for feeding to ensure adequate nutrition
4. Providing oxygen during stressful periods

Answer: 3
Rationale: Measures that will decrease the workload on the heart include limiting the time the child is allowed to bottle-feed or breastfeed, elevating the head of the bed, allowing for uninterrupted rest periods, and providing oxygen during stressful periods.

Test-Taking Strategy: Use the process of elimination. Note the key word *avoids* in the stem of the question. Review each option carefully recalling that the goal for a child with CHF is to decrease the workload on the heart. Option 3 is the only option that will not provide this measure. If you are unfamiliar with the measures associated with caring for the child with CHF, review this content.

Level of Cognitive Ability: Application
Client Needs: Physiological Integrity

Integrated Concept/Process: Nursing Process/Planning
Content Area: Child Health

Reference:
Schulte, E. Price, D., & Gwin, J. (2001). *Thompson's pediatric nursing* (8th ed.). Philadelphia: W.B. Saunders, p. 88.

---

27. A nurse is assisting in preparing a plan of care for a child with leukemia who is scheduled to receive chemotherapy. Which of the following nursing interventions will be included in the plan of care?
1. Monitor rectal temperatures every 4 hours
2. Monitor mouth and anus each shift for signs of breakdown
3. Provide meticulous mouth care several times daily using an alcohol-based mouthwash and a toothbrush
4. Encourage the child to consume fresh fruits and vegetables to maintain nutritional status

Answer: 2
Rationale: When the child is receiving chemotherapy, the nurse should avoid taking rectal temperatures. Oral temperatures are also avoided if mouth ulcers are present. Axillary temperatures should be done to prevent alterations in skin integrity. Meticulous mouth care should be performed; the nurse should use a soft-bristled toothbrush but avoid use of alcohol-based mouthwash. The nurse should assess the mouth and anus each shift for ulcers, erythema, or breakdown. Bland, nonirritating foods and liquids should be provided to the child. Fresh fruits and vegetables should be avoided because they can harbor organisms. Chemotherapy can cause neutropenia, and the child should be maintained on a low-bacteria diet if the white blood cell count is low.

Test-Taking Strategy: Use the process of elimination reading each option carefully. Thinking about the side effects that can occur with chemotherapy will direct you to option 2. If you had difficulty with this question, review these important nursing measures.

Level of Cognitive Ability: Application
Client Needs: Physiological Integrity
Integrated Concept/Process: Nursing Process/Planning
Content Area: Child Health

Reference:
Schulte, E. Price, D., & Gwin, J. (2001). *Thompson's pediatric nursing* (8th ed.). Philadelphia: W.B. Saunders, p. 232.

---

28. A nurse is assisting in preparing to admit a client from the postanesthesia care unit who has had microvascular decompression of the trigeminal nerve. The nurse plans to ensure that which of the following equipment is at the bedside when the client arrives?
1. Flashlight and pulse oximeter
2. Padded bed rails and pulse oximeter
3. Padded bed rails and suction equipment
4. Blood pressure cuff and cardiac monitor

Answer: 1
Rationale: Postoperative care of the client having microvascular decompression of the trigeminal nerve is the same as for the client undergoing craniotomy. This client requires hourly neurological assessment, as well as monitoring of cardiovascular and respiratory status. Cardiac monitoring and padded bed rails are not indicated unless there is a special need based on a client history of cardiac disease or seizures, respectively. Suctioning is done cautiously and only when necessary after craniotomy to avoid increasing intracranial pressure.

Test-Taking Strategy: Use the process of elimination, focusing on the data in the question. The client is not necessarily at risk for postoperative seizures, so options 2 and 3 are eliminated first. Knowing that the procedure is done by craniotomy enables you to recall that neurological assessment is needed, which helps you choose option 1 from the remaining options. A flashlight would be necessary to perform a neurological assessment. Review care to the client after this procedure if you had difficulty with this question.

Level of Cognitive Ability: Application
Client Needs: Physiological Integrity
Integrated Concept/Process: Nursing Process/Planning
Content Area: Adult Health/Neurological

Reference:
Black, J., Hawks, J., & Keene, A. (2001). *Medical-surgical nursing: clinical management for positive outcomes* (6th ed.). Philadelphia: W.B. Saunders, p. 1927.

---

29. A nurse is receiving a client in transfer from the emergency room who has a diagnosis of Guillain-Barré syndrome. The client's chief complaint is an ascending paralysis that has reached the level of the waist. The nurse plans to have which of the following items available for emergency use?
1. Intubation tray
2. Flashlight
3. Nebulizer
4. Incentive spirometer

Answer: 1
Rationale: The client with Guillain-Barré syndrome is at risk for respiratory failure because of ascending paralysis. An intubation tray should be available for emergency use. Another complication of this syndrome is cardiac dysrhythmias, which necessitates the need for cardiac monitoring.

Test-Taking Strategy: Use the process of elimination. Note the key words *emergency use.* This tells you that the correct answer will be an option that contains the piece of equipment that is not routinely used in providing care. With this in mind, eliminate options 2, 3, and 4. Review nursing care measures for the client with Guillain-Barré syndrome if you had difficulty with this question.

Level of Cognitive Ability: Application
Client Needs: Physiological Integrity
Integrated Concept/Process: Nursing Process/Planning
Content Area: Adult Health/Neurological

Reference:
Black, J., Hawks, J., & Keene, A. (2001). *Medical-surgical nursing: clinical management for positive outcomes* (6th ed.). Philadelphia: W.B. Saunders, p. 2016.

---

30. A nurse is informed that a newborn infant whose mother is Rh negative will be admitted to the nursery. In planning care for the infant's arrival, the priority nursing action would be to:
1. Obtain the necessary equipment from the blood bank needed for an exchange transfusion
2. Call the maintenance department and ask for a phototherapy unit to be brought to the nursery
3. Obtain the newborn infant's blood type and direct Coombs' test results from the laboratory
4. Obtain a vial of vitamin K from the pharmacy and prepare to administer an injection to prevent isoimmunization

Answer: 3
Rationale: To further plan for the newborn infant's care, the infant's blood type and direct Coombs' test must be known. Umbilical cord blood is taken at the time of delivery to determine blood type, Rh factor, and antibody titer (direct Coombs' test) of the newborn infant. The nurse should plan to obtain these results from the laboratory. Options 1 and 2 are inappropriate at this time and additional data are needed to determine if these actions are needed. Option 4 is incorrect because vitamin K is given to prevent hemorrhagic disease of the newborn infant.

Test-Taking Strategy: Use the process of elimination and focus on the issue: the mother is Rh negative. Note the relationship between the issue of the question and option 3. Also note that option 3 is the only option that addresses data collection. Review Rh incompatibilities if you had difficulty with this question.

Level of Cognitive Ability: Application
Client Needs: Physiological Integrity
Integrated Concept/Process: Nursing Process/Planning
Content Area: Maternity

Reference:
Murray, S., McKinney, E., & Gorrie, T. (2002). *Foundations of maternal-newborn nursing* (3rd ed.). Philadelphia: W.B. Saunders, p. 694.

Nursing Process: Implementation

1. A nurse is preparing to administer a feeding to a client receiving enteral nutrition through a nasogastric tube. What is the priority nursing action before administering the feeding?
1. Measuring intake and output
2. Weighing the client
3. Adding blue food coloring to the formula
4. Determining tube placement

Answer: 4

Rationale: Initiating a tube feeding before determining tube placement can lead to serious complications such as aspiration. Options 1 and 2 are part of the total plan of care for a client on enteral feedings. Option 3 is instituted for a client who has been identified as a high risk for aspiration. Option 4 is the priority nursing action.

Test-Taking Strategy: Use the ABCs—airway, breathing, and circulation—and the nursing process to answer the question. Option 4 relates to data collection and to the risk of aspiration. If you had difficulty with this question, review nursing interventions when initiating a tube feeding.

Level of Cognitive Ability: Application
Client Needs: Physiological Integrity
Integrated Concept/Process: Nursing Process/Implementation
Content Area: Fundamental Skills

Reference:
Lewis, S., Heitkemper, M., & Dirksen, S. (2000). *Medical-surgical nursing: assessment and management of clinical problems* (5th ed.). St. Louis: Mosby, p. 1058.

2. A nurse teaches a client with a rib fracture to cough and deep breathe. The client resists directions by the nurse because of the pain. The nurse most appropriately:
1. Continues to give the client gentle encouragement to do so
2. Requests that a nerve block be performed to deaden the pain
3. Explains in detail the potential complications from lack of coughing and deep breathing
4. Premedicates the client and assists the client to splint the area during these exercises

Answer: 4

Rationale: Shallow respirations that occur with rib fracture predispose the client to developing atelectasis and pneumonia. It is essential that the client perform coughing and deep breathing to prevent these complications. The nurse accomplishes this most effectively by premedicating the client with pain medication and assisting the client with splinting during the exercises.

Test-Taking Strategy: Use the process of elimination noting the key words *most appropriately*. Options 2 and 3 are likely to be the most extreme or unrealistic options, respectively, and should be eliminated first. From the remaining options, premedication and assistance are more likely to be effective than continued gentle encouragement. Review care to the client with rib fracture if you had difficulty with this question.

Level of Cognitive Ability: Application
Client Needs: Physiological Integrity
Integrated Concept/Process: Nursing Process/Implementation
Content Area: Adult Health/Respiratory

Reference:
Ignatavicius, D., & Workman, M. (2002). *Medical-surgical nursing: critical thinking for collaborative care* (4th ed.). Philadelphia: W.B. Saunders, p. 612.

3. An older client who has been in traction for several days is becoming disoriented. The best intervention to deal with the disorientation is to:
1. Go along with the disorientation to not upset the client
2. Let the family reorient the client
3. Order laboratory tests to check for imbalances
4. Use environmental clues such as calendars and clocks along with gentle corrective reminders to reorient the client

Answer: 4

Rationale: An inactive older person may become disoriented because of a lack of sensory stimulation. The family can help with orientation, but it is the nurse's responsibility to help reorient the client. This client is in traction so the client's understanding and cooperation is essential to the treatment. Therefore the disorientation cannot be ignored. Ordering laboratory tests is outside the scope of practice for a nurse.

Test-Taking Strategy: Note the key word *best*. Use the process of elimination. Options 1 and 3 can be eliminated first because they do not directly deal with the issue of disorientation. From the remaining options, select option 4 because it is the nurse's responsibility to care for the client. Review nursing measures for the disoriented client if you had difficulty with this question.

Level of Cognitive Ability: Application
Client Needs: Psychosocial Integrity
Integrated Concept/Process: Nursing Process/Implementation
Content Area: Fundamental Skills

Reference:
Lewis, S., Heitkemper, M., & Dirksen, S. (2000). *Medical-surgical nursing: assessment and management of clinical problems* (5th ed.). St. Louis: Mosby, p. 1790.

4. A nurse is caring for a 14-year-old child who is hospitalized and placed in Crutchfield traction. The child is having difficulty adjusting to the length of the hospital confinement. Which nursing action would be most appropriate to meet the child's needs?
1. Allow the child to have his or her hair dyed if the parent agrees
2. Allow the child to play loud music in the hospital room
3. Let the child wear own clothing when friends visit
4. Allow the child to keep the shades closed and the room darkened at all times

Answer: 3

Rationale: Adolescents need to identify with peers and belong to a group. They like to dress like the group and wear similar hairstyles. The hospitalized child should be allowed to wear his or her own clothing to feel a sense of belonging to the group. Because Crutchfield traction uses skeletal pins, hair dye is not appropriate. Loud music may disturb others in the hospital. The child's request for a darkened room is indicative of a possible problem with depression that may need further evaluation and intervention.

Test-Taking Strategy: Use the process of elimination and focus on the issues: Crutchfield traction and a 14-year-old child. Knowledge about Crutchfield traction and its limitations, and knowledge of growth and development concepts, will direct you to option 3. Review growth and development and care to the child in traction if you had difficulty with this question.

Level of Cognitive Ability: Application
Client Needs: Psychosocial integrity
Integrated Concept/Process: Nursing Process/Implementation
Content Area: Child Health

Reference:
Potter, P., & Perry, A. (2001). *Fundamentals of nursing* (5th ed.). St. Louis: Mosby, pp. 213; 216.

5. A nurse is told that a client in leg traction will be admitted to the nursing unit. The nurse prepares for the arrival and obtains

Answer: 2

Rationale: A trapeze is essential to allow the client to lift straight up while being moved so the amount of pull exerted on the

which of the following items that will be essential for helping the client move in bed while in the leg traction?
1. An electric bed
2. A bed trapeze
3. Extra pillows
4. A foot board

limb in traction is not altered. An electric bed or manual bed can be used for traction but neither specifically assists the client to move in bed. A foot board and extra pillows do not facilitate moving.

Test-Taking Strategy: Note the key words *essential* and *move in bed.* Attempt to visualize the items in the options focusing on the issue: helping the client move in bed. Using the process of elimination will direct you to option 2. Review care to the client in traction if you had difficulty with this question.

Level of Cognitive Ability: Application
Client Needs: Physiological Integrity
Integrated Concept/Process: Nursing Process/Implementation
Content Area: Adult Health/Musculoskeletal

Reference:
Black, J., Hawks, J., & Keene, A. (2001). *Medical-surgical nursing: clinical management for positive outcomes* (6th ed.). Philadelphia: W.B. Saunders, p. 610.

---

6. A physician's order reads: tobramycin sulfate (Nebcin), 7.5 mg intramuscular BID. The medication label reads: 10 mg/mL. The nurse prepares how many milliliters to administer one dose?
1. 0.25 mL
2. 0.50 mL
3. 0.75 mL
4. 1.33 mL

Answer: 3
Rationale: Use the formula for calculating a medication dose.

Formula:

$$\frac{\text{Desired}}{\text{Available}} \times \text{Volume} = \text{mL per dose}$$

$$\frac{7.5 \text{ mg}}{10 \text{ mg}} \times 1.0 \text{ mL} = 0.75 \text{ mL}$$

Test-Taking Strategy: Identify the key components of the question and what the question is asking. In this case, the question asks for the mL per dose. Use the formula to determine the correct dosage. Review the formula for calculating a medication dose if you had difficulty with this question.

Level of Cognitive Ability: Application
Client Needs: Physiological Integrity
Integrated Concept and Process: Nursing Process/Implementation
Content Area: Fundamental Skills

Reference:
Kee, J., & Marshall, S. (2000). *Clinical calculations: with applications to general and specialty areas* (4th ed.). Philadelphia: W.B. Saunders, p. 78.

---

7. A nurse is collecting data from a client in the second trimester of pregnancy. The nurse notes that the fetal heart rate (FHR) is 100 beats per minute. Which of the following nursing actions would be most appropriate?

Answer: 3
Rationale: The fetal heart rate should be between 120 to 160 beats per minute during pregnancy. A fetal heart rate of 100 beats per minute would require that the RN be notified and the client be further evaluated. Options 1, 2 and 4 are inaccurate nursing actions.

1. Document the findings
2. Inform the mother that the FHR is normal and everything is fine
3. Notify the RN
4. Instruct the mother to return to the clinic in 1 week for reevaluation of the fetal heart rate

Test-Taking Strategy: Use the process of elimination. Knowing that the limits for the fetal heart rate are between 120 and 160 beats per minute will direct you to option 3. If you had difficulty with this question, review the normal findings in the pregnant client.

Level of Cognitive Ability: Application
Client Needs: Physiological Integrity
Integrated Concept/Process: Nursing Process/Implementation
Content Area: Maternity

Reference:
Murray, S., McKinney, E., & Gorrie, T. (2002). *Foundations of maternal-newborn nursing* (3rd ed.). Philadelphia: W.B. Saunders, p. 978.

---

8. A client is admitted to the hospital with a leaking cerebral aneurysm and is scheduled for surgery. The nurse implements which of the following during the preoperative period?
   1. Encourages the client to be up at least twice a day
   2. Allows the client to ambulate to the bathroom
   3. Obtains a bedside commode for the client's use
   4. Places the client on strict bed rest

Answer: 4
Rationale: The client's activity is kept at a minimum to prevent Valsalva maneuver. Clients often hold their breath and strain while pulling up to get out of bed. This exertion may cause a rise in blood pressure, which increases bleeding. Clients who have bleeding aneurysms in any vessel will have activity curtailed.

Test-Taking Strategy: Use the process of elimination, focusing on the client's diagnosis and the key words *preoperative period.* Eliminate options 1, 2, and 3 because they are similar and they all involve out-of-bed activity. If you had difficulty with this question, review aneurysm precautions.

Level of Cognitive Ability: Application
Client Needs: Physiological Integrity
Integrated Concept/Process: Nursing Process/Implementation
Content Area: Adult Health/Neurological

Reference:
Ignatavicius, D., & Workman, M. (2002). *Medical-surgical nursing: critical thinking for collaborative care* (4th ed.). Philadelphia: W.B. Saunders, pp. 985-986.

---

9. A physician calls a nurse to obtain the daily laboratory results of a client receiving total parenteral nutrition (TPN). Which of the following laboratory results would the nurse obtain from the client's record that would provide the most valuable information about the client's status related to the TPN?
   1. Serum electrolyte levels
   2. Arterial blood gas levels
   3. White blood cell count (WBC)
   4. Complete blood cell count (CBC)

Answer: 1
Rationale: TPN solutions contain amino acid and dextrose solutions, with electrolyte and trace elements added. The physician uses the electrolyte values to determine whether changes are needed in the composition of the TPN solutions that will be administered during the next 24 hours. This prevents the client from developing electrolyte imbalance. Options 2, 3, and 4 are not directly related to the client's status relative to TPN.

Test-Taking Strategy: Use the process of elimination. Eliminate options 3 and 4 first because a CBC includes a WBC count. From the remaining options, focusing on the issue and considering the composition of TPN solutions will direct you to option 1. If you had difficulty with this question, review the composition of TPN.

Level of Cognitive Ability: Application
Client Needs: Physiological Integrity

Integrated Concept/Process: Nursing Process/Implementation
Content Area: Fundamental Skills

Reference:
Black, J., Hawks, J., & Keene, A. (2001). *Medical-surgical nursing: clinical management for positive outcomes* (6th ed.). Philadelphia: W.B. Saunders, p. 668.

---

10. A client who has episodes of bronchospasm and a history of tachydysrhythmias is admitted to the hospital. The nurse reviews the physician's orders and questions the RN about which medication, if prescribed by the physician?
1. Metaproterenol (Alupent)
2. Albuterol (Proventil)
3. Epinephrine (Primatene Mist)
4. Salmeterol (Serevent)

Answer: 3
Rationale: A client with a history of tachydysrhythmias should not be given bronchodilators that contain catecholamines, such as epinephrine and isoproterenol hydrochloride (Isuprel). Other sympathomimetics that are noncatecholamines should be used instead. These include metaproterenol, albuterol, and salmeterol.

Test-Taking Strategy: Focus on the client's diagnosis: tachydysrhythmias. Use the process of elimination. Recalling that epinephrine is a catecholamine will direct you to this option. Review the effects of epinephrine if you had difficulty with this question.

Level of Cognitive Ability: Analysis
Client Needs: Physiological Integrity
Integrated Concept/Process: Nursing Process/Implementation
Content Area: Pharmacology

Reference:
Hodgson, B., & Kizior, R. (2003). *Saunders nursing drug handbook 2003.* Philadelphia: W.B. Saunders, p. 401.

---

11. A client has a compulsive bed making ritual in which the client makes and remakes a bed numerous times. The client often misses breakfast and some of the morning activities because of the ritual. Which of the following nursing actions would be most helpful?
1. Verbalize tactful, mild disapproval of the behavior
2. Help the client to make the bed so that the task can be finished quicker
3. Discuss the ridiculousness of the behavior
4. Offer reflective feedback, such as, "I see you have made your bed several times."

Answer: 4
Rationale: Verbalizing disapproval would increase the client's anxiety and reinforce the need to perform the ritual. Helping with the ritual is nontherapeutic and also reinforces the behavior. The client is usually aware of the irrationality (or ridiculousness) of the behavior. Reflective feedback acknowledges the client's behavior.

Test-Taking Strategy: Use the process of elimination. Recalling that the purpose of the ritual is to relieve anxiety would assist in eliminating options 1 and 3 because these actions would increase the anxiety. Eliminate option 2 because there is no therapeutic value in participating in the ritual. Review the appropriate interventions for the client with compulsive behavior if you had difficulty with this question.

Level of Cognitive Ability: Application
Client Needs: Psychosocial Integrity
Integrated Concept/Process: Nursing Process/Implementation
Content Area: Mental Health

Reference:
Varcarolis, E. (2002). *Foundations of psychiatric mental health nursing* (4th ed.). Philadelphia: W.B. Saunders, p. 351.

12. An older client who has undergone internal fixation after fracturing a left hip has developed a reddened left heel. The nurse obtains which of the following as a priority item to manage this problem?
   1. Bed cradle
   2. Sheepskin
   3. Trapeze
   4. Draw sheet

Answer: 2

Rationale: The reddened heel results from pressure of the foot against the mattress. The nurse obtains a sheepskin, heel protectors, or an alternating pressure mattress. The bed cradle is unnecessary in managing this problem. A draw sheet and trapeze are of general use for this client but are not specific in dealing with the reddened heel.

Test-Taking Strategy: Use the process of elimination. Note the issue of the question: a reddened left heel. Eliminate option 1 first as an unnecessary measure. Eliminate options 3 and 4 next, because although they are generally helpful in aiding the client's mobility, they are not related to the issue of the question. Option 2 addresses the problem stated in the question. Review measures that prevent skin breakdown in the immobile client if you had difficulty with this question.

Level of Cognitive Ability: Application
Client Needs: Physiological Integrity
Integrated Concept/Process: Nursing Process/Implementation
Content Area: Adult Health/Musculoskeletal

Reference:
Black, J., Hawks, J., & Keene, A. (2001). *Medical-surgical nursing: clinical management for positive outcomes* (6th ed.). Philadelphia: W.B. Saunders, p. 1295.

13. A nurse is caring for an infant after pyloromyotomy performed to treat hypertrophic pyloric stenosis. The nurse places the infant in which position following surgery?
   1. Flat on the unoperative side
   2. Flat on the operative side
   3. Prone with the head of the bed elevated
   4. Supine with the head of the bed elevated

Answer: 3

Rationale: After pyloromyotomy, the head of the bed is elevated and the infant is placed prone to reduce the risk of aspiration. Options 1, 2, and 4 are incorrect positions after this type of surgery.

Test-Taking Strategy: Consider the anatomical location of the surgical procedure and the risks associated with the procedure to answer the question. Visualize each of the positions identified in the options. Keeping in mind that aspiration is a major concern will direct you to option 3. Review nursing care measures after pyloromyotomy if you had difficulty with this question.

Level of Cognitive Ability: Application
Client Needs: Physiological Integrity
Integrated Concept/Process: Nursing Process/Implementation
Content Area: Child Health

Reference:
Schulte, E. Price, D., & Gwin, J. (2001). *Thompson's pediatric nursing* (8th ed.). Philadelphia: W.B. Saunders, p. 136.

14. A mother of a child with mumps calls the health care clinic to tell the nurse that the child has been very lethargic and has been vomiting. The nurse most appropriately tells the mother:
   1. To continue to monitor the child
   2. That lethargy and vomiting are normal manifestations of mumps

Answer: 3

Rationale: Mumps generally affect the salivary glands but can also affect multiple organs. The most common complication is septic meningitis, with the virus being identified in the cerebrospinal fluid. Common signs include nuchal rigidity, lethargy, and vomiting. The child should be seen by the physician.

3. To bring the child to the clinic to be seen by the physician
4. That as long as there is no fever there is nothing to be concerned about

Test-Taking Strategy: Use the process of elimination. Focus on the signs and symptoms presented in the question. Recalling that meningitis is a complication of mumps will direct you to option 3. Review the complications of mumps and the associated clinical manifestations if you had difficulty with this question.

Level of Cognitive Ability: Application
Client Needs: Physiological Integrity
Integrated Concept/Process: Nursing Process/Implementation
Content Area: Child Health

Reference:
Schulte, E. Price, D., & Gwin, J. (2001). *Thompson's pediatric nursing* (8th ed.). Philadelphia: W.B. Saunders, p. 245.

---

15. A nurse is reviewing the physician's orders for a child admitted to the hospital with vasoocclusive pain crisis from sickle cell anemia. The nurse questions the registered nurse about which prescribed order?
1. Intravenous fluids
2. Supplemental oxygen
3. Bed rest
4. Meperidine hydrochloride (Demerol) for pain

Answer: 4
Rationale: Meperidine hydrochloride is contraindicated for ongoing pain management because of the increased risk of seizures associated with the use of the medication. Management for severe pain generally includes the use of strong narcotic analgesics such as morphine sulfate or hydromorphone (Dilaudid). These medications are usually most effective when given as a continuous infusion or at regular intervals around the clock. Options 1, 2, and 3 are appropriate prescriptions for treating vasoocclusive pain crisis.

Test-Taking Strategy: Use the process of elimination. Note the issue: questioning an order. Recalling that oxygen, fluids, and bed rest are components of care will direct you to option 4. Review care to a child with sickle cell anemia, if you had difficulty with this question

Level of Cognitive Ability: Application
Client Needs: Physiological Integrity
Integrated Concept/Process: Nursing Process/Implementation
Content Area: Child Health

Reference:
Schulte, E. Price, D., & Gwin, J. (2001). *Thompson's pediatric nursing* (8th ed.). Philadelphia: W.B. Saunders, p. 132.

---

16. A nurse is caring for an infant with laryngomalacia (congenital laryngeal stridor). Which of the following positions would the nurse place the infant to decrease the incidence of stridor?
1. Supine
2. Supine with the neck flexed
3. Prone
4. Prone with the neck hyperextended

Answer: 4
Rationale: The prone position with the neck hyperextended improves the child's breathing. Options 1, 2, and 3 are not appropriate positions.

Test-Taking Strategy: Use the process of elimination noting the key words *decrease the incidence of stridor.* Visualize each of the positions identified in the options to assist in directing you to option 4. If you had difficulty with this question, review this content.

Level of Cognitive Ability: Application
Client Needs: Physiological Integrity

Integrated Concept/Process: Nursing Process/Implementation
Content Area: Child Health

Reference:
Schulte, E. Price, D., & Gwin, J. (2001). *Thompson's pediatric nursing* (8th ed.). Philadelphia: W.B. Saunders, p. 183.

---

17. A nurse in the newborn nursery prepares to admit a newborn infant with spina bifida, meningomyelocele type. Which of the following is the priority nursing action in the immediate plan of care for this infant?
   1. Monitor blood pressure
   2. Monitor specific gravity of the urine
   3. Inspect the anterior fontanel for bulging
   4. Monitor temperature

Answer: 3
Rationale: Increased intracranial pressure is a complication associated with spina bifida. A sign of intracranial pressure in the newborn infant with spina bifida is a bulging or tough anterior fontanel. The newborn infant is at risk for infection before the surgical procedure and closure of the gibbus, and monitoring the temperature is an important intervention; however, inspecting the anterior fontanel for bulging is the immediate priority. A normal saline dressing is placed over the affected site to maintain moisture of the gibbus and its contents. This prevents tearing or breakdown of skin integrity at the site. Blood pressure is difficult to check during the newborn period, and it is not the best indicator of infection or a potential complication. Urine concentration is not well developed in the newborn stage of development.

Test-Taking Strategy: Use the process of elimination focusing on the key words *priority nursing action*. Eliminate options 1 and 2 first because blood pressure and specific gravity are not as reliable an indicator of changes in the newborn status as they would be for an older child. From the remaining options, focusing on the key words will direct you to option 3. Review care to the infant with spina bifida if you had difficulty with this question.

Level of Cognitive Ability: Application
Client Needs: Physiological Integrity
Integrated Concept/Process: Nursing Process/Implementation
Content Area: Child Health

Reference:
Schulte, E. Price, D., & Gwin, J. (2001). *Thompson's pediatric nursing* (8th ed.). Philadelphia: W.B. Saunders, p. 82.

---

18. When collecting data on a child, a nurse notes that the child's genitals are swollen. The nurse suspects that the child is being sexually abused. Which action by the nurse is most appropriate?
   1. Document the child's physical findings
   2. Report the case in which the abuse is suspected
   3. Refer the family to appropriate support groups
   4. Assist the family in identifying resources and support systems

Answer: 2
Rationale: The primary legal responsibility of the nurse when child abuse is suspected is to report the case. All 50 states require health care professionals to report all cases of suspected abuse. Although documentation of findings, assisting the family, and referring the family to appropriate resources and support groups are important, the primary legal responsibility is to report the case.

Test-Taking Strategy: In addition to the many implications associated with child abuse, recall that abuse is a crime. Keeping this in mind will direct you to option 2. If you had difficulty with this question, review the responsibilities of the nurse when child abuse is suspected.

Level of Cognitive Ability: Application

Client Needs: Psychosocial Integrity
Integrated Concept/Process: Nursing Process/Implementation
Content Area: Child Health

Reference:
Wong, D., & Hockenberry-Eaton, M. (2001). *Wong's essentials of pediatric nursing* (6th ed.). St. Louis: Mosby, p. 486.

---

19. A nurse is caring for an infant with a diagnosis of encephalocele located in the occipital area. Which of the following items would the nurse use to assist in positioning the child to avoid pressure on the encephalocele?
1. Sheepskin
2. Foam half donut
3. Feather pillows
4. Sandbags

Answer: 2
Rationale: The infant is positioned to avoid pressure on the lesion. If the encephalocele is in the occipital area, a foam half donut may be useful in positioning to prevent this pressure. A sheepskin, feather pillow, or sandbag will not protect the encephalocele from pressure.

Test-Taking Strategy: Note the key word *occipital* and use the process of elimination. Note the similarities in options 1, 3, and 4 in that they would require the head to remain flat and therefore would not protect the lesion. If you have difficulty with this question, review nursing care associated with a child with an encephalocele.

Level of Cognitive Ability: Application
Client Needs: Physiological Integrity
Integrated Concept/Process: Nursing Process/Implementation
Content Area: Child Health

Reference:
Wong, D., & Hockenberry-Eaton, M. (2001). *Wong's essentials of pediatric nursing* (6th ed.). St. Louis: Mosby, p. 1254.

---

20. A nurse is caring for a child with a head injury. When reviewing the record, the nurse notes that the physician has documented decorticate posturing. During care of the child, the nurse notes extension of the upper extremities and internal rotation of the upper arm and wrist. The nurse also notes that the lower extremities are extended with some internal rotation noted at the knees and feet. Based on these findings, which of the following is the appropriate nursing action?
1. Document the findings
2. Continue to monitor for posturing of the child
3. Attempt to flex the child's lower extremities
4. Notify the RN

Answer: 4
Rationale: Decorticate posturing refers to flexion of the upper extremities and extension of the lower extremities. Plantar flexion of the feet may also be observed. Decerebrate posturing involves extension of the upper extremities with internal rotation of the upper arm and wrist. The lower extremities will extend with some internal rotation noted at the knees and feet. The progression from decorticate to decerebrate posturing usually indicates deteriorating neurological function and warrants RN notification; the RN will then contact the physician.

Test-Taking Strategy: Focus on the data in the question and use knowledge about the findings associated with decerebrate and decorticate positioning. It is also necessary to know the neurological findings that indicate deterioration in the condition of the neurological status in the child. If you had difficulty with this question or are unfamiliar with these findings, review this content.

Level of Cognitive Ability: Application
Client Needs: Physiological Integrity
Integrated Concept/Process: Nursing Process/Implementation
Content Area: Child Health

Reference:
Wong, D., & Hockenberry-Eaton, M. (2001). *Wong's essentials of pediatric nursing* (6th ed.). St. Louis: Mosby, p. 1066.

21. A child with a diagnosis of hepatitis B is being cared for at home. The mother of the child calls the health care clinic and tells the nurse that the jaundice seems to be worsening. Which of the following responses to the mother would be most appropriate?
1. "The hepatitis may be spreading."
2. "You should bring the child to the health care clinic to see the physician."
3. "The jaundice may appear to get worse before it resolves."
4. "It is necessary to isolate the child from the others."

Answer: 3
Rationale: The parents should be instructed that jaundice may appear to get worse before it resolves. The parents of a child with hepatitis should also be taught the danger signs that could indicate a worsening of the child's condition, specifically changes in neurological status, bleeding, and fluid retention.

Test-Taking Strategy: Use the process of elimination and knowledge about the physiology associated with hepatitis to answer this question. Knowing that the jaundice worsens before it resolves will direct you to the correct option. If you had difficulty with this question, review the instructions to the parents of a child with hepatitis.

Level of Cognitive Ability: Application
Client Needs: Physiological Integrity
Integrated Concept/Process: Nursing Process/Implementation
Content Area: Child Health

Reference:
Wong, D., & Hockenberry-Eaton, M. (2001). *Wong's essentials of pediatric nursing* (6th ed.). St. Louis: Mosby, p. 907.

22. A nurse is preparing to suction a tracheotomy on an infant. The nurse obtains the equipment for the procedure and turns the suction to which of the following settings?
1. 40 mmHg
2. 90 mmHg
3. 110 mmHg
4. 120 mmHg

Answer: 2
Rationale: The suctioning procedure for pediatric clients varies from that used in adults; suctioning in infants and children requires the use of a smaller suction catheter and lower suction settings. Suction settings should range from 60 to 100 mmHg for infants and children and 40 to 60 mmHg for preterm infants.

Test-Taking Strategy: Use the process of elimination, noting the key word *infant*. Recalling the procedure that is used in an adult will direct you to option 2. If you are unfamiliar with this procedure, review this content.

Level of Cognitive Ability: Application
Client Needs: Physiological Integrity
Integrated Concept/Process: Nursing Process/Implementation
Content Area: Child Health

Reference:
Perry, A., & Potter, P. (2002). *Clinical nursing skills & techniques* (5th ed.). St. Louis: Mosby, p. 371.

23. A nurse is caring for a client who begins to experience seizure activity while in bed. The nurse determines that this particular client is at risk of aspiration. Which of the following actions by the

Answer: 4
Rationale: Positioning the client on one side with the head flexed forward allows the tongue to fall forward and facilitates drainage of secretions, which could help prevent aspiration. The nurse would also remove restrictive clothing and the pillow, and raise

nurse would be most helpful to prevent this from occurring?

1. Loosen restrictive clothing
2. Remove the pillow and raise the padded side rails
3. Raise the head of the bed
4. Position the client on the side if possible, with the head flexed forward

the padded side rails, but these actions would not decrease the risk of aspiration. Rather, they are general safety measures to use during seizure activity. The nurse would not raise the head of the bed.

Test-Taking Strategy: Use the process of elimination. Note that the key words *aspiration, most helpful,* and *prevent.* Visualizing the effect that each of the options would have on airway and aspiration will direct you to option 4. Review care to the client with seizures who is at risk for aspiration if you had difficulty with this question.

Level of Cognitive Ability: Application
Client Needs: Physiological Integrity
Integrated Concept/Process: Nursing Process/Implementation
Content Area: Adult Health/Neurological

Reference:
Black, J., Hawks, J., & Keene, A. (2001). *Medical-surgical nursing: clinical management for positive outcomes* (6th ed.). Philadelphia: W.B. Saunders, p. 2277.

---

24. A client with a cerebrovascular accident has episodes of coughing while swallowing liquids. The client has developed a temperature of 101° F, oxygen saturation of 91% (down from 98% previously), slight confusion, and noticeable dyspnea. The nurse would take which of the following most appropriate actions?

1. Administer a bronchodilator ordered on a PRN basis
2. Administer an acetaminophen (Tylenol) suppository
3. Encourage the client to cough and deep breathe
4. Notify the RN

Answer: 4
Rationale: The client is exhibiting clinical signs and symptoms of aspiration, which include fever, dyspnea, decreased arterial oxygen levels, and confusion. Other symptoms that occur with this complication are difficulty in managing own saliva, or coughing or choking while eating. Because the client has developed a complication requiring medical intervention, the most appropriate action is to notify the RN who will then intervene.

Test-Taking Strategy: Use the process of elimination. Focusing on the data in the question will indicate that aspiration has most likely occurred. Eliminate options 1, 2, and 3 because these actions will not assist in alleviating this life-threatening condition. Review the findings in the client who is aspirating and the appropriate nursing interventions if you had difficulty with this question.

Level of Cognitive Ability: Application
Client Needs: Physiological Integrity
Integrated Concept/Process: Nursing Process/Implementation
Content Area: Adult Health/Neurological

Reference:
Black, J., Hawks, J., & Keene, A. (2001). *Medical-surgical nursing: clinical management for positive outcomes* (6th ed.). Philadelphia: W.B. Saunders, p. 1953.

---

25. A nurse is providing care to a client after a bone biopsy. Which of the following actions would the nurse take as part of aftercare for this procedure?

1. Keep the area in a dependent position
2. Monitor vitals signs once per day

Answer: 3
Rationale: Nursing care after bone biopsy includes monitoring the site for swelling, bleeding, or hematoma formation. The biopsy site is elevated for 24 hours to reduce edema. The vital signs are monitored every 4 hours for 24 hours. The client usually requires mild analgesics; more severe pain usually indicates that complications are arising.

3. Monitor the site for swelling, bleeding, or hematoma formation
4. Administer intramuscular narcotic analgesics

Test-Taking Strategy: Use the process of elimination. Begin to answer this question by recalling that the client must have periodic assessments after this procedure. With this in mind, eliminate option 2 because the time frame is too infrequent. Knowing that the procedure is done under local anesthesia helps you to eliminate option 4 next. From the remaining options, recalling the principles related to circulation and positioning will direct you to option 3. Review care of a client after bone biopsy if you had difficulty with this question.

Level of Cognitive Ability: Application
Client Needs: Physiological Integrity
Integrated Concept/Process: Nursing Process/Implementation
Content Area: Adult Health/Musculoskeletal

Reference:
Black, J., Hawks, J., & Keene, A. (2001). *Medical-surgical nursing: clinical management for positive outcomes* (6th ed.). Philadelphia: W.B. Saunders, p. 548.

---

26. A nurse is caring for the client who will have an arthrogram using a contrast medium. Which of the following actions by the nurse is the highest priority?
1. Determining the presence of client allergies
2. Telling the client that the extremity will be moved around during the procedure
3. Asking if the client has any last minute questions
4. Telling the client to try to move the bowels before leaving the unit

Answer: 1
Rationale: Because of the risk of allergy to contrast medium, the nurse places highest priority on determining whether the client has an allergy to iodine or shellfish. The nurse also reinforces information about the test and reminds the client about the need to remain still during the procedure. There is no special need to ensure that the bowel is empty before the procedure, but it is helpful to have the client void before the procedure for comfort.

Test-Taking Strategy: Use the process of elimination noting the key words *contrast medium* and *highest priority*. Recalling the risk associated with the administration of contrast medium will direct you to option 1. Review preprocedure care for an arthrogram if you had difficulty with this question.

Level of Cognitive Ability: Application
Client Needs: Physiological Integrity
Integrated Concept/Process: Nursing Process/Implementation
Content Area: Adult Health/Musculoskeletal

Reference:
Black, J., Hawks, J., & Keene, A. (2001). *Medical-surgical nursing: clinical management for positive outcomes* (6th ed.). Philadelphia: W.B. Saunders, p. 546.

---

27. A nurse responds to a call bell and finds a client lying on the floor after a fall. The nurse suspects that the client's arm may be broken. Which action would the nurse take as the highest priority before moving the client?
1. Tell the client that everything will be fine
2. Immobilize the arm
3. Take a set of vital signs
4. Call the radiology department

Answer: 2
Rationale: When a fracture is suspected, it is imperative that the area is splinted before the client is moved. The nurse should remain with the client and provide realistic reassurance. The client would not be told that everything will be fine. The physician will order radiology films. Vital signs would be taken, but this is not the highest priority in this situation.

Test-Taking Strategy: Use the process of elimination, noting the key words *highest priority*. Eliminate option 4 because the physician will order radiology films. Option 1 is eliminated next because the nurse does not make statements to the client that could provide false reassurance. From the remaining options, noting that a fracture is suspected will direct you to option 2. Review care to the client with a suspected extremity fracture if you had difficulty with this question.

Level of Cognitive Ability: Application
Client Needs: Physiological Integrity
Integrated Concept/Process: Nursing Process/Implementation
Content Area: Adult Health/Musculoskeletal

Reference:
Black, J., Hawks, J., & Keene, A. (2001). *Medical-surgical nursing: clinical management for positive outcomes* (6th ed.). Philadelphia: W.B. Saunders, p. 590.

---

28. A nurse in the postpartum unit checks the temperature of a client who delivered a healthy newborn infant 4 hours previously. The mother's temperature is 100.8° F. The nurse provides oral hydration to the mother and encourages fluid intake. Four hours later the nurse rechecks the temperature and notes that it is still 100.8° F. Which of the following is the most appropriate nursing intervention?
1. Notify the RN
2. Continue hydration and recheck the temperature four hours later
3. Document the temperature
4. Increase the IV fluids

Answer: 1
Rationale: A temperature of greater than 100.4° F in two consecutive readings is considered febrile, and the RN should be notified. The RN will then contact the physician. Options 2, 3, and 4 are inappropriate actions at this time.

Test-Taking Strategy: Use the process of elimination. Option 4 can be eliminated first because this action requires a physician order. From the remaining options, noting that the temperature has remained unchanged after nursing intervention should provide you with the clue that further intervention is necessary and direct you to option 1. Review normal and abnormal findings in the postpartum period if you had difficulty with this question.

Level of Cognitive Ability: Application
Client Needs: Physiological Integrity
Integrated Concept/Process: Nursing Process/Implementation
Content Area: Maternity

Reference:
Lowdermilk, D., Perry, S., & Bobak, I. (2000). *Maternity & women's health care* (7th ed.). St. Louis: Mosby, p. 1032.

---

29. A nurse is checking the fundus in a postpartum woman. The nurse notes that the uterus is soft and spongy. Which of the following nursing actions is most appropriate initially?
1. Massage the fundus gently until firm
2. Document fundal position, and consistency and height
3. Encourage the mother to ambulate
4. Notify the RN

Answer: 1
Rationale: If the fundus is boggy (soft) it should be massaged gently until firm by the nurse, who observes for increased bleeding or clots. Option 3 is an inappropriate action at this time. The nurse should document fundal position, consistency and height, the need to perform fundal massage, and the client's response to the intervention. The RN is notified and will contact the physician if uterine massage is not helpful. The initial action, however, is stated in option 1.

Test-Taking Strategy: Use the process of elimination. Note the key words *most appropriate initially*. Recognize the relationship between the data in the question (soft and spongy) and the data in the correct option (massage the fundus gently until firm). Review nursing interventions related to this occurrence if you had difficulty with this question.

Level of Cognitive Ability: Application
Client Needs: Physiological Integrity
Integrated Concept/Process: Nursing Process/Implementation
Content Area: Maternity

Reference:
Lowdermilk, D., Perry, S., & Bobak, I. (2000). *Maternity & women's health care* (7th ed.). St. Louis: Mosby, p. 593.

---

30. A primipara is being evaluated in the clinic during her second trimester of pregnancy. The nurse checks the fetal heart rate (FHR) and notes that it is 190 beats per minute. The most appropriate nursing action would be to:
1. Document the finding
2. Consult with the registered nurse
3. Tell the client that the FHR is normal
4. Recheck the FHR with the client in the standing position

Answer: 2
Rationale: The fetal heart rate should be 120 to 160 beats per minute throughout pregnancy. In this situation, the FHR is elevated from the normal range, and the nurse should most appropriately consult with the RN who will then contact the physician. The FHR would be documented, but option 2 is the most appropriate action. The nurse would not tell the client that the FHR is normal because this is not accurate information. Option 4 is an inappropriate action.

Test-Taking Strategy: Use the process of elimination. Note the key words *most appropriate* in the stem of the question. Recalling that the normal FHR is 120 to 160 beats per minute will direct you to option 2. If you had difficulty with this question, review the normal FHR.

Level of Cognitive Ability: Application
Client Needs: Physiological Integrity
Integrated Concept/Process: Nursing Process/Implementation
Content Area: Maternity

Reference:
Murray, S., McKinney, E., & Gorrie, T. (2002). *Foundations of maternal-newborn nursing* (3rd ed.). Philadelphia: W.B. Saunders, p. 978.

Nursing Process: Evaluation

1. A nurse has been encouraging the intake of oral fluids in the laboring woman to improve hydration. Which of the following indicates a successful outcome of this action?
1. A urine specific gravity of 1.020
2. Continued leaking of amniotic fluid during labor
3. Blood pressure of 150/90 mmHg
4. Ketones in the urine

Answer: 1
Rationale: Urine specific gravity measures the concentration of the urine. During the first stage of labor, the renal system has a tendency to concentrate urine. Labor and birth require hydration and caloric intake to replenish energy expenditure and promote efficient uterine function. An elevated blood pressure and ketones in the urine are not expected outcomes related to labor and hydration. Once membranes are ruptured, it is expected that amniotic fluid may continue to leak.

Test-Taking Strategy: Use the process of elimination, focusing on the issue: a successful outcome related to oral intake. Recalling the relationship of oral intake to urine concentration will direct you to option 1. Review the importance of hydration in the woman in labor if you had difficulty with this question.

Level of Cognitive Ability: Comprehension
Client Needs: Health Promotion and Maintenance

Integrated Concept/Process: Nursing Process/Evaluation
Content Area: Maternity

Reference:
Chernecky, C., & Berger, B. (2001). *Laboratory and diagnostic procedure* (3rd ed.). Philadelphia: W.B. Saunders, p. 949.

---

2. A postpartum client has a nursing diagnosis of Risk for Infection. A goal has been developed that states, "The client will not develop an infection during her hospital stay." Which of the following data would support that the goal has been met?
1. Presence of chills
2. Abdominal tenderness
3. Absence of fever
4. Loss of appetite

Answer: 3

Rationale: Fever is the first indication of an infection. Chills, abdominal tenderness, and loss of appetite also indicate the presence of an infection. Therefore the absence of a fever indicates that an infection is not present.

Test-Taking Strategy: Use the process of elimination, noting the key words *that the goal has been met*. The question is asking for a means of evaluating the effectiveness of a goal that relates to infection. Options 1, 2, and 4 would indicate that the goal had not been met. Review the signs of postpartum infection if you had difficulty with this question.

Level of Cognitive Ability: Comprehension
Client Needs: Physiological Integrity
Integrated Concept/Process: Nursing Process/Evaluation
Content Area: Maternity

Reference:
Murray, S., McKinney, E., & Gorrie, T. (2002). *Foundations of maternal-newborn nursing* (3rd ed.). Philadelphia: W.B. Saunders, p. 853.

---

3. A nurse is monitoring the nutritional status of the client receiving enteral nutrition because of dysphagia resulting from a head injury. The nurse monitors which of the following to best determine the effectiveness of the tube feedings for this client?
1. Calorie count
2. Daily intake and output
3. Daily weight
4. Serum protein level

Answer: 3

Rationale: The most accurate measurement of the effectiveness of nutritional management of the client is through monitoring of daily weight. This should be done at the same time (preferably early morning), in the same clothes, and using the same scale. Options 1, 2, and 4 assist in measuring nutrition and hydration status. However, the effectiveness of the diet is measured by maintenance of body weight.

Test-Taking Strategy: Use the process of elimination. Note the key word *effectiveness*. This tells you that the correct option is an outcome. With this in mind, eliminate options 1 and 2 first because these are tools the nurse uses to measure nutrition and fluid status. Eliminate option 4 next because it reflects only one component of the diet, namely protein. If you had difficulty with this question, review the methods of monitoring nutritional status.

Level of Cognitive Ability: Application
Client Needs: Physiological Integrity
Integrated Concept/Process: Nursing Process/Evaluation
Content Area: Fundamental Skills

Reference:
Lewis, S., Heitkemper, M., & Dirksen, S. (2000). *Medical-surgical nursing: assessment and management of clinical problems* (5th ed.). St. Louis: Mosby, p. 1056.

4. An adult client with a critically high potassium level has received sodium polystyrene sulfonate (Kayexalate). The nurse evaluates that the medication was most effective if the client's repeat serum potassium level is:
   1. 6.2 mEq/L
   2. 5.8 mEq/L
   3. 5.4 mEq/L
   4. 4.9 mEq/L

Answer: 4
Rationale: The normal serum potassium level in the adult is 3.5 to 5.1 mEq/L. Option 4 is the only option reflecting a value that has dropped down into the normal range. Options 1, 2, and 3 identify elevated potassium levels.

Test-Taking Strategy: Use the process of elimination. Note the key words *critically high*. You would expect that this medication is administered to lower the potassium level. Recalling the normal serum potassium level will direct you to option 4. If this question was difficult, review the expected effects of this medication and the normal potassium level.

Level of Cognitive Ability: Comprehension
Client Needs: Physiological Integrity
Integrated Concept/Process: Nursing Process/Evaluation
Content Area: Fundamental Skills

Reference:
Hodgson, B., & Kizior, R. (2003). *Saunders nursing drug handbook 2003.* Philadelphia: W.B. Saunders, p. 1022.

---

5. A nurse is caring for a client who has a nasogastric tube (NG) in place and connected to suction after abdominal surgery. Which observation by the nurse indicates most reliably that the tube is functioning properly?
   1. The suction gauge reads low intermittent suction
   2. The distal end of the NG tube is pinned to the client's gown
   3. The client indicates that pain is a 3 on a 1-to-10 scale
   4. The client denies nausea and has 250 mL of fluid in the suction collection container

Answer: 4
Rationale: A NG tube connected to suction is used postoperatively to decompress and rest the bowel. The gastrointestinal tract lacks peristaltic activity because of manipulation during surgery. Although the nurse makes pertinent observations of the tube to ensure it is secure and connected to suction properly, the client is assessed for the effect. The client should not experience symptoms of ileus (nausea and vomiting) if the tube is functioning properly. A pain indicator of 3 is an expected finding in a postoperative client.

Test-Taking Strategy: Use the process of elimination. Focus on the issue: the tube is functioning properly. Recalling the purpose of the NG tube in a postoperative client will direct you to option 4. Review care to the client with a NG tube if you had difficulty with this question.

Level of Cognitive Ability: Comprehension
Client Needs: Physiological Integrity
Integrated Concept/Process: Nursing Process/Evaluation
Content Area: Adult Health/Gastrointestinal

Reference:
Ignatavicius, D., & Workman, M. (2002). *Medical-surgical nursing: critical thinking for collaborative care* (4th ed.). Philadelphia: W.B. Saunders, p. 1210.

---

6. A nurse has instructed a client about a low-sodium diet. The nurse evaluates that the client understands the information if the client selects which of the following dairy products as appropriate for use?
   1. Yogurt
   2. American cheese

Answer: 3
Rationale: The client on a low-sodium diet should be taught that any foods that derive from animal sources contain physiological saline and are therefore higher in sodium than many foods from plant sources. Powdered milk is often manufactured to be lower in sodium, so is the best dairy choice of those presented in the options for clients on a low-sodium diet.

3. Powdered milk
4. Whole milk

Test-Taking Strategy: Use the process of elimination. Note that options 1, 2, and 4 are similar because they are directly derived from animal sources. Review sodium-restricted diets if you had difficulty with this question.

Level of Cognitive Ability: Comprehension
Client Needs: Health Promotion and Maintenance
Integrated Concept/Process: Nursing Process/Evaluation
Content Area: Adult Health/Cardiovascular

Reference:
Williams, S. (2001) *Basic nutrition & diet therapy* (11th ed.). St. Louis: Mosby, p. 365.

---

7. A nurse who is caring for a client with Graves' disease notes a nursing diagnosis of "Imbalanced Nutrition: less than body requirements related to the effects of the hypercatabolic state" in the care plan. Which of the following would indicate a successful outcome for this diagnosis?
1. The client maintains his or her normal weight or gradually gains weight if it is below normal
2. The client demonstrates knowledge about the need to consume a diet high in fat and low in protein
3. The client verbalizes the need to avoid snacking between meals
4. The client discusses the relationship between meal time and the blood glucose level

Answer: 1
Rationale: Graves' disease causes a state of chronic nutritional and caloric deficiency as a result of the metabolic effects of excessive T3 and T4. Clinical manifestations are weight loss and increased appetite. It is therefore a nutritional goal that the client will not lose additional weight and will gradually return to the ideal body weight if necessary. To accomplish this, the client must be encouraged to eat frequent high-calorie, high-protein, and high-carbohydrate meals and snacks. The relationship between meal-time and the blood glucose level is unrelated to the issue.

Test-Taking Strategy: Use the process of elimination, focusing on the key words *hypercatabolic state*. Option 2 and 3 would not be beneficial for a client in a hypercatabolic state. Option 4 can be eliminated because discussing the fluctuation in the blood glucose level will not assist a client who is hypercatabolic. If you had difficulty with this question, review altered nutrition and Graves' disease.

Level of Cognitive Ability: Analysis
Client Needs: Health Promotion and Maintenance
Integrated Concept/Process: Nursing Process/Evaluation
Content Area: Adult Health/Endocrine

Reference:
Ignatavicius, D., & Workman, M. (2002). *Medical-surgical nursing: critical thinking for collaborative care* (4th ed.). Philadelphia: W.B. Saunders, p. 1426.

---

8. A nurse is reviewing a plan of care for a client who is in traction and notes a nursing diagnosis of Self-Care Deficit. The nurse evaluates the plan of care and determines that which of the following observations indicates a successful outcome?
1. The client allows the nurse to complete the care on a daily basis
2. The client allows the family to assist in the care
3. The client refuses care
4. The client assists in self-care as much as possible

Answer: 4
Rationale: A successful outcome for the nursing diagnosis of Self-Care Deficit is for the client to do as much of the self-care as possible. The nurse should promote independence in the client and allow the client to perform as much self-care as is optimal, considering the client's condition. The nurse would determine that the outcome is unsuccessful if the client refused care or allows others to handle the care.

Test-Taking Strategy: Use the process of elimination. Focus on the key words *successful outcome*. Option 3 can be eliminated first. Note that options 1 and 2 are similar because they indicate relying on others to perform care. Review successful outcomes related to the nursing diagnosis of Self-Care Deficit if you had difficulty with this question.

Level of Cognitive Ability: Analysis
Client Needs: Health Promotion and Maintenance
Integrated Concept/Process: Nursing Process/Evaluation
Content Area: Adult Health/Musculoskeletal

Reference:
Ignatavicius, D., & Workman, M. (2002). *Medical-surgical: critical thinking for collaborative care* (4th ed.). Philadelphia: W.B. Saunders, p. 128.

---

9. A nurse instructs a parent about the appropriate actions to take when the toddler has a temper tantrum. Which statement by the parent indicates a successful outcome of the instructions?
   1. "I will send my child to a room alone for 10 minutes after every tantrum."
   2. "I will reward my child with candy at the end of each day without a tantrum."
   3. "I will give frequent reminders that only bad children have tantrums."
   4. "I will ignore the tantrums as long as there is no physical danger."

Answer: 4
Rationale: Ignoring a negative attention-seeking behavior is considered the best way to extinguish it, provided the child is safe from injury. Option 1 gives attention to the tantrum. Providing candy for rewards is unhealthy and unlikely to be effective at the end of a day. Option 3 is untrue and negative.

Test-Taking Strategy: Use the process of elimination. Recalling that ignoring a tantrum is the best way to extinguish it will direct you to option 4. If you had difficulty with this question, review interventions for the child that has temper tantrums.

Level of Cognitive Ability: Comprehension
Client Needs: Health Promotion and Maintenance
Integrated Concept/Process: Nursing Process/Evaluation
Content Area: Child Health

Reference:
Wong, D., & Hockenberry-Eaton, M. (2001). *Wong's essentials of pediatric nursing* (6th ed.). St. Louis: Mosby, p. 423.

---

10. A nurse is caring for a client in seclusion. The nurse determines that it is safe for the client to come out of seclusion when the nurse hears the client say which of the following?
   1. "I am no longer a threat to myself or others."
   2. "I need to use the rest room right away."
   3. "I'd like to go back to my room and be alone for a while."
   4. "I can't breathe in here. The walls are closing in on me."

Answer: 1
Rationale: Option 1 indicates that the client may be safely removed from seclusion. The client in seclusion must be assessed at regular intervals (usually every 15 to 30 minutes) for physical needs, safety, and comfort. Option 2 indicates a physical need that could be met with a urinal, bedpan, or commode. It does not indicate that the client has calmed down enough to leave the seclusion room. Option 3 could be an attempt to manipulate the nurse; it gives no indication that the client will control himself or herself when alone in the room. Option 4 could be handled by supportive communication or a PRN medication, if indicated. It does not necessitate discontinuing seclusion.

Test-Taking Strategy: Use the process of elimination. Focus on the issue of the question: removing a client from seclusion. Recalling the purpose and the use of seclusion will direct you to option 1. Review seclusion procedure if you had difficulty with this question.

Level of Cognitive Ability: Comprehension
Client Needs: Psychosocial Integrity

Integrated Concept/Process: Nursing Process/Evaluation
Content Area: Mental Health

Reference:
Varcarolis, E. (2002). *Foundations of psychiatric mental health nursing* (4th ed.). Philadelphia: W.B. Saunders, p. 509.

---

11. A client has had a laryngectomy for throat cancer and has started oral intake. The nurse evaluates that the client has tolerated the first stage of dietary advancement if the client takes which of the following types of diet without aspiration or choking?
  1. Bland
  2. Clear liquids
  3. Full liquids
  4. Semisolid foods

Answer: 4
Rationale: Oral intake after laryngectomy is started with semisolid foods. Once the client can manage this type of food, liquids may be introduced. Thin liquids are not given until the risk of aspiration is negligible. A bland diet is not appropriate. The client may not be able to tolerate the texture of some of the solid foods that would be included in a bland diet.

Test-Taking Strategy: Use the process of elimination. Eliminate options 2 and 3 first, recalling that a client with swallowing difficulty will be unable to manage liquids. From the remaining options, recall that a bland diet provides no control over the consistency or texture of the food. Review dietary measures for a client after laryngectomy if you had difficulty with this question.

Level of Cognitive Ability: Analysis
Client Needs: Physiological Integrity
Integrated Concept/Process: Nursing Process/Evaluation
Content Area: Adult Health/Oncology

Reference:
Ignatavicius, D., & Workman, M. (2002). *Medical-surgical nursing: critical thinking for collaborative care* (4th ed.). Philadelphia: W.B. Saunders, p. 524.

---

12. An older male client, who is a victim of elder abuse, and his family have been seen in the counseling center weekly for the past month. Which of the following statements, if made by the abusive family member, would indicate that he or she has learned more positive coping skills?
  1. "I will be more careful to make sure that my father's needs are 100% met."
  2. "I am so sorry and embarrassed that the abusive event occurred. It won't happen again."
  3. "I feel better equipped to care for my father now that I know where to turn if I need assistance."
  4. "Now that my father is moving into my home, I will have to stop drinking alcohol."

Answer: 3
Rationale: Elder abuse sometimes results when family members are expected to care for their aging parents. This care can cause the family to become overextended, frustrated, or financially depleted. Knowing where to turn in the community for assistance in caring for an aging family member can bring the much needed relief. Using these alternatives is a positive alternative coping skill for many families. Options 1, 2, and 4 are statements of good faith or promises, which may or may not be kept in the future.

Test-Taking Strategy: Focus on the issue, a positive coping skill, and use the process of elimination. Only option 3 identifies a means of coping with the issues, and outlines a definitive plan for handling the pressure associated with the father's care. Review the concepts related to elder abuse if you had difficulty with this question.

Level of Cognitive Ability: Analysis
Client Needs: Psychosocial Integrity
Integrated Concept/Process: Nursing Process/Evaluation
Content Area: Mental Health

Reference:
Varcarolis, E. (2002). *Foundations of psychiatric mental health nursing* (4th ed.). Philadelphia: W.B. Saunders, p. 709.

13. A nurse is caring for a 24-hour-old term infant who had a confirmed episode of hypoglycemia at 1 hour of age. Which of the following observations by the nurse would indicate the need for further evaluation?
1. Blood glucose level of 40 mg/dL before the last feeding
2. High-pitched cry, eating 10 to 15 mL of formula per feeding
3. Weight loss of 4 ounces and dry, peeling skin
4. Breastfeeding for 20 minutes or greater, strong sucking

Answer: 2

Rationale: At 24 hours of age, a term infant should be able to consume at least 1 ounce of formula per feeding. A high-pitched cry is indicative of neurological involvement. Blood glucose levels are acceptable at 40 mg/dL in the first few days of life. Weight loss during the first few days of life and dry, peeling skin are normal findings for term infants. Breast feeding for 20 minutes with a strong suck is an excellent finding. Hypoglycemia causes central nervous system symptoms (high-pitched cry) and weakness, which makes the infant unable to eat enough for growth.

Test-Taking Strategy: Use the process of elimination noting the key words *need for further evaluation.* Eliminate options 1, 3, and 4 because these are normal findings. Also, the words *high-pitched cry* should direct you to option 2. If you had difficulty with this question, review normal newborn findings and the indications of hypoglycemia.

Level of Cognitive Ability: Analysis
Client Needs: Physiological Integrity
Integrated Concept/Process: Nursing Process/Evaluation
Content Area: Maternity

References:
Burroughs, A., & Leifer, G. (2002). *Maternity nursing* (8th ed.). Philadelphia: W.B. Saunders, p. 290.

14. A nurse is caring for a client diagnosed with tuberculosis. The client is receiving rifampin (Rifadin) 600 mg PO daily. Which of the following would indicate to the nurse that the client is experiencing an adverse reaction?
1. A white blood cell count of 6000/μL
2. An alkaline phosphatase of 25 units/dL
3. A sedimentation rate of 15 mm/hr
4. A total bilirubin of 0.5 mg/dL

Answer: 2

Rationale: Adverse reactions or toxic effects of rifampin include hepatotoxicity, hepatitis, blood dyscrasias, Stevens-Johnson syndrome, and antibiotic-related colitis. The nurse monitors for increased liver enzymes, bilirubin, blood urea nitrogen, and uric acid because elevations indicate an adverse reaction. A normal white blood cell count is 4500 to 11,000/μL. The normal sedimentation rate is 0 to 30 mm/hr. The normal total bilirubin level is less than 1.5 mg/dL. The normal alkaline phosphatase is 4.5 to 13 King-Armstrong units/dL.

Test-Taking Strategy: Use the process of elimination. Knowing that the medication is metabolized in the liver will assist in eliminating options 1 and 3 because these laboratory studies are not directly related to assessing liver function. From the remaining options, knowledge of normal laboratory values will direct you to option 2. If you are unfamiliar with this medication or these laboratory values, review this content.

Level of Cognitive Ability: Analysis
Client Needs: Physiological Integrity
Integrated Concept/Process: Nursing Process/Evaluation
Content Area: Pharmacology

Reference:
Hodgson, B., & Kizior, R. (2003). *Saunders nursing drug handbook 2003.* Philadelphia: W.B. Saunders, p. 977.

15. A nurse is assisting in caring for a woman in labor who is receiving oxytocin (Pitocin) by IV infusion. The nurse monitors the client, knowing that which of the following indicates an adequate contraction pattern?
1. Three to five contractions in 10 minutes, with resultant cervical dilation
2. One contraction per minute, with resultant cervical dilation
3. Four contractions every 5 minutes, with resultant cervical dilation
4. One contraction every 10 minutes, without resultant cervical dilation

Answer: 1
Rationale: The preferred oxytocin dosage is the minimal amount necessary to maintain an adequate contraction pattern characterized by three to five contractions in a 10-minute period, with resultant cervical dilation. If contractions are more frequent than every 2 minutes, contraction quality may be decreased.

Test-Taking Strategy: Use the process of elimination. Focusing on the issue, an adequate contraction pattern, will assist in eliminating option 4. Next, eliminate options 2 and 3 because they are similar. If you had difficulty with this question, review the expected effects of this medication.

Level of Cognitive Ability: Analysis
Client Needs: Physiological Integrity
Integrated Concept/Process: Nursing Process/Evaluation
Content Area: Maternity

Reference:
Lowdermilk, D., Perry, S., & Bobak, I. (2000). *Maternity & women's health care* (7th ed.). St. Louis: Mosby, p. 572.

---

16. A nurse is assigned to care for a preschooler who has a diagnosis of scarlet fever and is on bed rest. What data obtained by the nurse would indicate that the child is coping with the illness and bed rest?
1. The child is coloring and drawing pictures in a notebook
2. The mother keeps providing new activities for the child to do
3. The child insists that the mother stay in the room
4. The child sucks the thumb whenever the child does not get what is asked for

Answer: 1
Rationale: According to Piaget, play is the best way for preschoolers to understand and adjust to life's experiences. They are able to use pencils and crayons. They can draw stick figures and other rudimentary things. A child with scarlet fever needs quiet play, and drawing will provide that. Options 2, 3, and 4 do not address positive coping mechanisms.

Test-Taking Strategy: Think about the developmental level of preschoolers. Note the issue: determining if the child is coping with the disease and bed rest. Option 1 is a positive coping mechanism for preschoolers. Options 2, 3, and 4 do not address positive coping mechanisms. Review the expected developmental level of a preschooler and the effects of bed rest on the child if you had difficulty with this question.

Level of Cognitive Ability: Comprehension
Client Needs: Psychosocial integrity
Integrated Concept/Process: Nursing Process/Evaluation
Content Area: Child Health

Reference:
Wong, D., & Hockenberry-Eaton, M. (2001). *Wong's essentials of pediatric nursing* (6th ed.). St. Louis: Mosby, p. 449.

---

17. A client has just taken a dose of trimethobenzamide (Tigan). The nurse evaluates that the medication has been effective if the client states relief of:
1. Heartburn
2. Constipation

Answer: 3
Rationale: Trimethobenzamide is an antiemetic agent that is used in the treatment of nausea and vomiting. The medication is not used to treat heartburn, constipation, or abdominal pain.

3. Nausea and vomiting
4. Abdominal pain

Test-Taking Strategy: Use the process of elimination. Recalling that this medication is an antiemetic will direct you to option 3. Review the action of this medication if you had difficulty with this question.

Level of Cognitive Ability: Analysis
Client Needs: Physiological Integrity
Integrated Concept/Process: Nursing Process/Evaluation
Content Area: Pharmacology

Reference:
Hodgson, B., & Kizior, R. (2003). *Saunders nursing drug handbook 2003.* Philadelphia: W.B. Saunders, p. 1130.

---

18. A nurse is reinforcing instructions to the mother of a child with a diagnosis of strabismus of the left eye. The nurse reviews the procedure for patching the child. The nurse determines that the mother understands the procedure if the mother makes which statement?
1. "I will place the patch on the right eye."
2. "I will place the patch on both eyes."
3. "I will place the patch on the left eye."
4. "I will alternate the patch from the right to the left eye every hour."

Answer: 1
Rationale: Patching may be used in the treatment of strabismus to strengthen the weak eye. In this treatment, the good eye is patched. This encourages the child to use the weaker eye. It is most successful when done during the preschool years. The schedule for patching is individualized and prescribed by the ophthalmologist.

Test-Taking Strategy: Use the process of elimination. Remembering that this condition is a lazy eye will direct you to the correct option. It makes sense to patch the unaffected eye to strengthen the muscles in the affected eye. Review the procedure for patching if you had difficulty with this question.

Level of Cognitive Ability: Comprehension
Client Needs: Physiological Integrity
Integrated Concept/Process: Nursing Process/Evaluation
Content Area: Child Health

Reference:
Wong, D., & Hockenberry-Eaton, M. (2001). *Wong's essentials of pediatric nursing* (6th ed.). St. Louis: Mosby, p. 170.

---

19. A nurse is monitoring a client with pregnancy-induced hypertension (PIH) who was admitted to the hospital 48 hours previously. Which of the following data obtained would indicate that the condition has not yet resolved?
1. Blood pressure reading at prenatal baseline
2. Urinary output is increased
3. Client complaints of blurred vision
4. Presence of trace urinary protein

Answer: 3
Rationale: Client complaints of headache or blurred vision indicate a worsening of the condition and warrant immediate further evaluation. Options 1, 2, and 4 are all signs that the pregnancy-induced hypertension is being resolved.

Test-Taking Strategy: Use the process of elimination. Note the key words *has not yet resolved.* This indicates that you need to look for the option that identifies a symptom of PIH. Options 1 and 2 can be eliminated first because they are normal findings. From the remaining options, note that option 4 contains the word *trace* and is the more normal finding of these two options. If you had difficulty with this question, review the clinical manifestations associated with PIH.

Level of Cognitive Ability: Analysis
Client Needs: Physiological Integrity

Integrated Concept/Process: Nursing Process/Evaluation
Content Area: Maternity

Reference:
Murray, S., McKinney, E., & Gorrie, T. (2002). *Foundations of maternal-newborn nursing* (3rd ed.). Philadelphia: W.B. Saunders, p. 631.

20. A client has begun medication therapy with betaxolol (Kerlone). The nurse would evaluate that the client is experiencing the intended effects of therapy if which of the following is noted?
1. Weight gain of 5 pounds
2. Pulse rate increased from 58 to 74 beats per minute
3. Blood pressure decreased from 142/94 mmHg to 128/82 mmHg
4. Edema present at 3+

Answer: 3
Rationale: Betaxolol is a beta–adrenergic-blocking agent used to lower blood pressure, relieve angina, or eliminate dysrhythmias. Side effects include bradycardia and symptoms of congestive heart failure, such as weight gain and increased edema.

Test-Taking Strategy: Use the process of elimination. Note that the question asks for the *intended effect* of the medication. Remember that beta–adrenergic-blocking agents end with the suffix *olol*. Recalling the action of the medication will direct you to option 3. Review the intended effects of this medication if you had difficulty with this question.

Level of Cognitive Ability: Analysis
Client Needs: Physiological Integrity
Integrated Concept/Process: Nursing Process/Evaluation
Content Area: Pharmacology

Reference:
Hodgson, B., & Kizior, R. (2003). *Saunders nursing drug handbook 2003.* Philadelphia: W.B. Saunders, p. 120.

21. A nurse has taught a client taking a xanthine bronchodilator about beverages to avoid. The nurse evaluates that the client understands the information if the client chooses which of the following beverages from the dietary menu?
1. Chocolate milk
2. Cranberry juice
3. Coffee
4. Cola

Answer: 2
Rationale: Cola, coffee, and chocolate contain xanthine and should be avoided by the client taking a xanthine bronchodilator. This could lead to an increased incidence of cardiovascular and central nervous system side effects that can occur with the use of these type of bronchodilators.

Test-Taking Strategy: Use the process of elimination. Note the similarity between options 1, 3, and 4 in that they all contain some form of stimulant. Review dietary measures for a client taking a xanthine bronchodilator if the question was difficult.

Level of Cognitive Ability: Analysis
Client Needs: Health Promotion and Maintenance
Integrated Concept/Process: Nursing Process/Evaluation
Content Area: Pharmacology

Reference:
Black, J., Hawks, J., & Keene, A. (2001). *Medical-surgical nursing: clinical management for positive outcomes* (6th ed.). Philadelphia: W.B. Saunders, p. 1691.

22. A client is started on tolbutamide (Orinase) once daily. The nurse observes for which of the following intended effects of this medication?

Answer: 2
Rationale: Tolbutamide is an oral hypoglycemic agent that is taken in the morning. It is not used to decrease blood pressure, enhance weight loss, or treat infection.

1. Decreased blood pressure
2. Decreased blood glucose
3. Weight loss
4. Resolution of infection

Test-Taking Strategy: Use the process of elimination. Note the key words *intended effects*. Recalling that this medication is an oral hypoglycemic will direct you to option 2. Review the action of this medication if you had difficulty with this question.

Level of Cognitive Ability: Analysis
Client Needs: Physiological Integrity
Integrated Concept/Process: Nursing Process/Evaluation
Content Area: Pharmacology

Reference:
Hodgson, B., & Kizior, R. (2003). *Saunders nursing drug handbook 2003.* Philadelphia: W.B. Saunders, p. 1099.

---

23. A mother of a 2 1/2 year-old child is discussing dental care with the nurse. Which of the following statements made by the mother would indicate that more teaching would be needed?
    1. "Aged-cheese is a good snack instead of sweets for a young child."
    2. "I took the child for the first dental examination right after his second birthday."
    3. "It is not necessary to teach proper dental care to a toddler. Their baby teeth just fall out anyway."
    4. "I have my child brush his teeth with clear water, because he sometimes shallows the toothpaste."

Answer: 3
Rationale: Option 3 identifies that the mother does not understand the proper measures to ensure part of proper dental care. Options 1, 2, and 4 are appropriate statements that reflect an understanding of proper dental care for the child.

Test-Taking Strategy: Note the key words *more teaching would be needed*. Use the process of elimination also noting the words *not necessary* in the correct option. If you had difficulty with this question, review the proper dental health care measures for a child.

Level of Cognitive Ability: Comprehension
Client Needs: Health Promotion and Maintenance
Integrated Concept/Process: Nursing Process/Evaluation
Content Area: Child Health

Reference:
Wong, D., & Hockenberry-Eaton, M. (2001). *Wong's essentials of pediatric nursing* (6th ed.). St. Louis: Mosby, p. 450.

---

24. A client has received a dose of a PRN medication called loperamide (Imodium). The nurse evaluates the client after administration to see if the client has relief of:
    1. Constipation
    2. Diarrhea
    3. Tarry stools
    4. Abdominal pain

Answer: 2
Rationale: Loperamide is an antidiarrheal agent. It is commonly administered after loose stools. It is used in the management of acute diarrhea and also in chronic diarrhea, such as with inflammatory bowel disease. It can also be used to reduce the volume of drainage from an ileostomy.

Test-Taking Strategy: Use the process of elimination. Recalling that this medication is an antidiarrheal agent will direct you to option 2. Review the purpose of this medication if you had difficulty with this question.

Level of Cognitive Ability: Analysis
Client Needs: Physiological Integrity
Integrated Concept/Process: Nursing Process/Evaluation
Content Area: Pharmacology

Reference:
Hodgson, B., & Kizior, R. (2003). *Saunders nursing drug handbook 2003.* Philadelphia: W.B. Saunders, p. 675.

25. A nurse has reinforced instructions to a client with chronic renal failure about reducing pruritus from uremia. The nurse evaluates that the client needs further information if the client states he or she will use which of the following items for skin care?

1. Mild soap
2. Oil in the bath water
3. Astringent facial cleansing pads
4. Lanolin-based lotion

Answer: 3

Rationale: The client with chronic renal failure often has dry skin, accompanied by itching (pruritus) from uremia. The client should use mild soaps, lotions, and bath water oils to reduce dryness without increasing skin irritation. Products that contain perfumes or alcohol increase dryness and pruritus and should be avoided.

Test-Taking Strategy: Use the process of elimination. Note the key words *needs further information*. Options 2 and 4 are similar and should be eliminated. From the remaining options, select option 3 knowing that the client should avoid using irritating products on the skin. Review the skin care measures for pruritus if you had difficulty with this question.

Level of Cognitive Ability: Comprehension
Client Needs: Health Promotion and Maintenance
Integrated Concept/Process: Nursing Process/Evaluation
Content Area: Adult Health/Renal

Reference:
Black, J., Hawks, J., & Keene, A. (2001). *Medical-surgical nursing: clinical management for positive outcomes* (6th ed.). Philadelphia: W.B. Saunders, p. 1286.

26. A client has been given a prescription for a course of azithromycin (Zithromax). The nurse evaluates that the medication is having the intended effect if which of the following is noted?

1. Signs and symptoms of infection are relieved
2. Pain is relieved
3. Joint discomfort is reduced
4. Blood pressure is lower

Answer: 1

Rationale: Azithromycin is a macrolide antibiotic, which is used to treat infection. It is not ordered for the treatment of pain, joint discomfort, or blood pressure.

Test-Taking Strategy: Use the process of elimination. Eliminate options 2 and 3 first because they are similar. From the remaining options, recalling the action of this medication will direct you to option 1. Review the action and purpose of azithromycin if you had difficulty with this question.

Level of Cognitive Ability: Analysis
Client Needs: Physiological Integrity
Integrated Concept/Process: Nursing Process/Evaluation
Content Area: Pharmacology

Reference:
Hodgson, B., & Kizior, R. (2003). *Saunders nursing drug handbook 2003.* Philadelphia: W.B. Saunders, p. 98.

27. A nurse is assigned to care for a client with acquired immunodeficiency syndrome (AIDS) who is receiving amphotericin B (Fungizone) for a fungal respiratory infection. Which of the following would indicate an adverse reaction to the medication?

1. Hypocalcemia
2. Hypokalemia
3. Hypercalcemia
4. Hyperkalemia

Answer: 2

Rationale: Clients receiving amphotericin B may develop hypokalemia, which can be severe and lead to extreme muscle weakness and electrocardiogram changes. Distal renal tubular acidosis commonly occurs, contributing to the development of hypokalemia. High potassium levels do not occur. The medication does not cause calcium levels to fluctuate.

Test-Taking Strategy: Use the process of elimination. Knowledge that hypokalemia is an adverse reaction to amphotericin B is necessary to answer the question. Review this medication if you had difficulty with this question.

Level of Cognitive Ability: Analysis
Client Needs: Physiological Integrity
Integrated Concept/Process: Nursing Process/Evaluation
Content Area: Pharmacology

Reference:
Hodgson, B., & Kizior, R. (2003). *Saunders nursing drug handbook 2003.* Philadelphia: W.B. Saunders, p. 60.

---

28. A client is seen in the health care clinic, and a diagnosis of conjunctivitis is made. The nurse provides instructions to the client about care of the disorder while at home. Which of the following statements if made by the client indicates a need for further instruction?
1. "I do not need to be concerned about spreading this infection to others in my family."
2. "I should apply a warm compress before instilling antibiotic drops if purulent discharge is present in my eye."
3. "I should perform a saline eye irrigation before instilling the antibiotic drops into my eye if purulent discharge is present."
4. "I can use an ophthalmic analgesic ointment at night time if I have eye discomfort."

Answer: 1
Rationale: Conjunctivitis is highly contagious. Antibiotic drops are usually administered four times a day. When purulent discharge is present, saline eye irrigations or eye applications of warm compresses may be necessary before instilling the medication. Ophthalmic analgesic ointment or drops may be instilled, especially at bedtime because discomfort becomes more noticeable when the eyelids are closed.

Test-Taking Strategy: Use the process of elimination noting the key words *need for further instruction.* Knowing that this disorder is considered highly contagious will direct you to option 1. If you have difficulty with this question, review management of the client with this disorder.

Level of Cognitive Ability: Comprehension
Client Needs: Health Promotion and Maintenance
Integrated Concept/Process: Nursing Process/Evaluation
Content Area: Adult Health/Eye

Reference:
Black, J., Hawks, J., & Keene, A. (2001). *Medical-surgical nursing: clinical management for positive outcomes* (6th ed.). Philadelphia: W.B. Saunders, p. 1827.

---

29. A nurse reviews the nursing care plan of a hospitalized child who is immobilized because of skeletal traction. The nurse notes a nursing diagnosis of Risk for Delayed Growth and Development related to immobilization and hospitalization. Which of the following evaluative statements indicates a positive outcome for the child?
1. The fracture heals without complications
2. The child displays age-appropriate developmental behaviors
3. The caregivers verbalize safe and effective home care
4. The child maintains normal joint and muscle integrity

Answer: 2
Rationale: Regression and inappropriate developmental behaviors may be displayed in response to immobilization and hospitalization. With individualized care planning, a positive outcome of age-appropriate behavior can be achieved. Options 1, 3, and 4 are appropriate evaluative statements for an immobilized child but do not directly address the nursing diagnosis, Risk for Delayed Growth and Development.

Test-Taking Strategy: Focus on the issue Risk for Delayed Growth and Development. Use the process of elimination. Recalling that Delayed Growth and Development is the state in which an individual is not performing age-appropriate tasks will direct you to option 2. All options are evaluative statements, but only option 2 addresses this nursing diagnosis. Review the defining characteristics and the appropriate outcomes for this nursing diagnosis if you had difficulty with this question.

Level of Cognitive Ability: Analysis
Client Needs: Health Promotion and Maintenance
Integrated Concept/Process: Nursing Process/Evaluation
Content Area: Child Health

Reference:
Wong, D., & Hockenberry-Eaton, M. (2001). *Wong's essentials of pediatric nursing* (6th ed.). St. Louis: Mosby, p. 423.

---

30. A nurse is evaluating the effects of care for the client with nephrotic syndrome. The nurse determines that the client showed the least amount of improvement if which of the following information was obtained serially during 2 days of care?
1. Initial weight 208 pounds, down to 203 pounds
2. Daily intake and output record of 2100 mL intake and 1900 mL output, and 2000 mL intake and 2900 mL output
3. Blood pressure 160/90 mmHg, down to 140/80 mmHg
4. Serum albumin 1.9 g/dL, up to 2.0 g/dL

Answer: 4
Rationale: The goal of therapy in nephrotic syndrome is to heal the leaking glomerular membrane. This would then control edema by stopping the loss of protein in the urine. Fluid balance and albumin levels are monitored to determine effectiveness of therapy. Option 1 (weight loss) represents a loss of fluid that slightly exceeds 2 liters and represents a significant improvement. Option 2 represents a total fluid loss of 700 mL over the 2 days, which is also helpful. Option 3 shows improvement because both systolic and diastolic blood pressures are lower. The least amount of improvement is in the serum albumin level, as the normal albumin level is 3.5 to 5.0 g/dL.

Test-Taking Strategy: Use the process of elimination noting the key words *least amount of improvement*. Option 1 illustrates the greatest improvement and is eliminated first. Option 2 is also a significant improvement and is eliminated next. From the remaining options, noting that the blood pressure has reentered the normal range will direct you to option 4. Review care to the client with nephrotic syndrome if you had difficulty with this question.

Level of Cognitive Ability: Analysis
Client Needs: Physiological Integrity
Integrated Concept/Process: Nursing Process/Evaluation
Content Area: Adult Health/Renal

Reference:
Black, J., Hawks, J., & Keene, A. (2001). *Medical-surgical nursing: clinical management for positive outcomes* (6th ed.). Philadelphia: W.B. Saunders, p. 863.

Caring

1. A woman comes into the emergency room in a severe state of anxiety after a car accident. The most important nursing intervention at this time would be to:
1. Remain with the client
2. Put the client in a quiet room
3. Teach the client deep breathing
4. Encourage the client to talk about her feelings and concerns

Answer: 1
Rationale: If the client with severe anxiety is left alone, she may feel abandoned and become overwhelmed. Placing the client in a quiet room is also indicated, but the nurse must stay with the client. It is not possible to teach the client deep breathing or relaxation exercises until the anxiety decreases. Encouraging the client to discuss concerns and feelings would not take place until the anxiety has decreased.

Test-Taking Strategy: Use the process of elimination. Note the key words *severe state of anxiety*. Because the anxiety state is *severe*, eliminate options 3 and 4. From the remaining options, consider the words *most important* in the stem of the question. This should direct you to option 1. Review care to the client with severe anxiety if you had difficulty with this question.

Level of Cognitive Ability: Application
Client Needs: Psychosocial Integrity
Integrated Concept/Process: Caring
Content Area: Mental Health

Reference:
Varcarolis, E. (2002). *Foundations of psychiatric mental health nursing* (4th ed.). Philadelphia: W.B. Saunders, p. 284.

---

2. A nurse had been caring for a client who died a few minutes ago. The nurse reflects on the care given to the client. Which of the following statements supports the nurse's belief that the client died with dignity?
   1. The family thanks the nurse and states that the client was not in pain and was peaceful at the end
   2. The physician recognizes that all the orders were carried out and there were no questions
   3. A new nurse states it is difficult to give that kind of care to a dying client
   4. The nurse gave increasing doses of pain medication to keep the client well sedated

Answer: 1
Rationale: The family response is an external perception and is extremely important. Families derive a great deal of comfort knowing their loved one received the best care possible. Option 1 provides external validation that the client received comprehensive, quality care. Option 2 focuses on physician's orders rather than client care. Option 3 focuses on the feelings of a new nurse who may be expressing his or her own anxiety. Option 4 reflects on only one aspect of caring for a dying client.

Test-Taking Strategy: Use the process of elimination and focus on the issue: the client died with dignity. The only option that addresses this issue is option 1. Review the concepts related to death and dying if you had difficulty with this question.

Level of Cognitive Ability: Comprehension
Client Needs: Psychosocial Integrity
Integrated Concept/Process: Caring
Content Area: Fundamental Skills

Reference:
Black, J., Hawks, J., & Keene, A. (2001). *Medical-surgical nursing: clinical management for positive outcomes* (6th ed.). Philadelphia: W.B. Saunders, p. 457.

---

3. The family of a client with Parkinson's disease tells the nurse that the client is having difficulty adjusting to the disorder and that they do not know what to do to help. The nurse advises the family that which of the following would be most therapeutic in assisting the client to cope with the disease?
   1. Encourage and praise client efforts to exercise and perform activities of daily living (ADLs)
   2. Cluster activities at the end of the day when the client is restless and bored
   3. Plan only a few activities for the client during the day
   4. Assist the client with ADLs as much as possible

Answer: 1
Rationale: The client with Parkinson's disease has a tendency to become withdrawn and depressed, which can be limited by encouraging the client to be an active participant in own care. The family should also give the client encouragement and praise for perseverance in these efforts. The family should plan activities intermittently throughout the day to inhibit daytime sleeping and boredom.

Test-Taking Strategy: Use the process of elimination. Eliminate option 2 first because clustering activities at one time will tire the client. Eliminate option 3 next because of the use of the absolute word *only*. From the remaining options, recalling that the client should be an active participant in own care will direct you to option 1. Review therapeutic techniques for the client with Parkinson's disease to assist with adjustment to the disease if you had difficulty with this question.

Level of Cognitive Ability: Application
Client Needs: Psychosocial Integrity
Integrated Concept/Process: Caring
Content Area: Adult Health/Neurological

Reference:
Black, J., Hawks, J., & Keene, A. (2001). *Medical-surgical nursing: clinical management for positive outcomes* (6th ed.). Philadelphia: W.B. Saunders, p. 2020.

---

4. A nurse is assisting in caring for a group of homeless people in a certain area of a city. In planning for the potential needs of this group, what is the most immediate concern?
  1. Peer support through structured groups
  2. Setting up a 24-hour crisis center and hot line
  3. Meeting the basic needs to ensure that adequate food, shelter, and clothing are available
  4. Finding affordable housing for the group

Answer: 3
Rationale: The question asks about the immediate concern. The immediate concern is always attending to peoples basic needs of food, shelter, and clothing. Options 1, 2, and 4 are other activities that may be carried out at a later time.

Test-Taking Strategy: Use Maslow's Hierarchy of Needs theory to answer the question. Option 3 addresses basic physiological needs. Although options 1, 2, and 4 are also appropriate actions, option 3 is the immediate concern. Review the needs of the homeless population if you had difficulty with this question.

Level of Cognitive Ability: Analysis
Client Needs: Physiological Integrity
Integrated Concept/Process: Caring
Content Area: Mental Health

Reference:
Varcarolis, E. (2002). *Foundations of psychiatric mental health nursing* (4th ed.). Philadelphia: W.B. Saunders, p. 792.

---

5. During the transition period of labor, the nurse notes that a client is having difficulty concentrating on her breathing technique. Her coach anxiously states that he just doesn't know how to help her. The most appropriate intervention would be to:
  1. Keep them informed about the labor process and events using positive terms
  2. Tell them that during the transitional period no interventions are effective
  3. Relieve the coach of the responsibilities because he doesn't know how to help
  4. Provide pharmacological interventions so that the client doesn't have to concentrate

Answer: 1
Rationale: During the transition period of active labor, the client and support system must be kept informed of appropriate information. When the client and support system are kept informed, they can better take part in the labor process and remain in control. Option 2 is incorrect. Options 3 and 4 are inappropriate.

Test-Taking Strategy: Use the process of elimination, noting the key words *most appropriate*. In addition, using therapeutic communication techniques and noting the word *positive* will assist in directing you to option 1. Review care to the client during the transition period of labor if you had difficulty with this question.

Level of Cognitive Ability: Application
Client Needs: Psychosocial Integrity
Integrated Concept/Process: Caring
Content Area: Maternity

Reference:
Burroughs, A., & Leifer, G. (2002). *Maternity nursing* (8th ed.). Philadelphia: W.B. Saunders, p. 67.

6. While talking to a prenatal client about her dietary and alcohol drinking habits, the nurse observes that the client has difficulty concentrating and appears agitated. The nurse should proceed with the conversation using which guideline?
1. Discussion of possible consequences of drinking alcohol during pregnancy should be avoided
2. Women respond negatively to a hopeful message of the potential benefits of drinking cessation during pregnancy
3. A nonjudgmental approach may help to gain maternal trust
4. Provoking maternal guilt may help a woman recognize her problem and seek support services

Answer: 3
Rationale: The potential effects of alcohol abuse during pregnancy for both the mother and fetus have been well documented. The nurse who expresses genuine concern with suspected abusers may motivate positive behavioral changes during the prenatal period. The maternal behaviors of lack of concentration and agitation are frequently seen in childbearing women abusing alcohol. Options 1, 2, and 4 are inappropriate guidelines for the nurse to follow in this situation, and they do not address a caring approach.

Test-Taking Strategy: Use therapeutic communication techniques and the process of elimination. Remember that it is important to display a caring and nonjudgmental attitude. Review therapeutic communication techniques if you had difficulty with this question.

Level of Cognitive Ability: Application
Clients Needs: Psychosocial Integrity
Integrated Concept/Process: Caring
Content Area: Maternity

Reference:
Lowdermilk, D., Perry, S., & Bobak, I. (2000). *Maternity & women's health care* (7th ed.). St. Louis: Mosby, p. 945.

---

7. A client who was drinking alcohol and fell asleep while driving a car was injured in an automobile accident. The client's only daughter, who was a passenger in the car, was killed instantly. In report, the nurse is told that the client is upset and withdrawn. When caring for the client, what is the most appropriate nursing action initially?
1. Let the client have some time alone to grieve over the loss
2. Tell the client that the injury and the daughter's death was a result of alcohol abuse and refer the client for counseling
3. Request medication to assist the client in coping with the loss
4. Reflect back to the client that he or she appears upset

Answer: 4
Rationale: The nurse should encourage the client to express feelings. Reflection statements tend to elicit deeper awareness of feelings. In addition, option 4 validates the perception that the client is upset. Option 2 is inappropriate and is a block to communication. Options 1 and 3 address interventions before assessing the situation.

Test-Taking Strategy: Note the key words *most appropriate* and *initially*. Use therapeutic communication techniques and the process of elimination. Select the option that encourages the client to express his or her feelings and talk more. Remember to always address the client's feelings. Review therapeutic communication techniques if you had difficulty with this question.

Level of Cognitive Ability: Application
Client Needs: Psychosocial Integrity
Integrated Concept/Process: Caring
Content Area: Mental Health

Reference:
Varcarolis, E. (2002). *Foundations of psychiatric mental health nursing* (4th ed.). Philadelphia: W.B. Saunders, p. 354.

---

8. A nurse employed in the emergency room is assigned to care for an older client who has been identified as a victim of physical abuse. In planning care for this client, the nurse's priority is focused on:

Answer: 4
Rationale: Whenever the abused client remains in the abusive environment, priority must be placed on determining whether the person is in any immediate danger. If so, emergency action must be taken to remove them from the abusing situation.

1. Referring the abusing family member for treatment
2. Adhering to the mandatory abuse reporting laws
3. Encouraging the client to file charges against the abuser
4. Removing the client from any immediate danger

Options 1 and 2 may be appropriate interventions but are not the priority. Option 3 is not an appropriate intervention at this time and may produce increased fear and anxiety in the client.

Test-Taking Strategy: Use the process of elimination and eliminate option 3 first, knowing that this action may produce increased fear and anxiety in the client. Use Maslow's Hierarchy of Needs theory to select from the remaining options, remembering that if a physiological need is not present, safety is the priority. This guide should direct you to option 4, the only option that directly addresses client safety. Review the principles related to caring for the abused client if you had difficulty with this question.

Level of Cognitive Ability: Application
Client Needs: Safe, Effective Care Environment
Integrated Concept/Process: Caring
Content Area: Mental Health

Reference:
Varcarolis, E. (2002). *Foundations of psychiatric mental health nursing* (4th ed.). Philadelphia: W.B. Saunders, p. 709.

---

9. A nurse is working with older residents involved in a recent flood. Many of the residents were emotionally despondent and refused to leave their homes for days. In planning for the rescue and relocation of these older residents, what is the first item that the nurse should consider?
   1. Attending to the emotional needs of older residents
   2. Attending to the nutritional status and basic needs of older residents
   3. Contacting older residents' families
   4. Arranging for ambulance transportation for older residents

Answer: 2
Rationale: The question asks about the first thing that the nurse needs to consider. The most important intervention is to attend to peoples basic needs of food, shelter, and clothing. Options 1, 3, and 4 are other activities that may or may not be needed at a later date.

Test-Taking Strategy: Use Maslow's Hierarchy of Needs theory to answer the question. Option 2 addresses basic physiological needs. Although options 1, 3, and 4 may be appropriate actions at a later time, option 2 is the immediate concern. Review care to clients experiencing crisis if you had difficulty with this question.

Level of Cognitive Ability: Application
Client Needs: Physiological Integrity
Integrated Concept/Process: Caring
Content Area: Mental Health

Reference:
Varcarolis, E. (2002). *Foundations of psychiatric mental health nursing* (4th ed.). Philadelphia: W.B. Saunders, p. 633.

---

10. A nurse is assisting in planning care for a suicidal client. To provide a caring, therapeutic environment, which of the following is included in the nursing care plan?
    1. Placing the client in a private room to ensure privacy and confidentiality
    2. Establishing a therapeutic relationship and conveying unconditional positive regard

Answer: 2
Rationale: The establishment of a therapeutic relationship with the suicidal client increases feelings of acceptance. Although the suicidal behavior and thinking of the client is unacceptable, the use of unconditional positive regard acknowledges the client in a human-to-human context and increases the client's sense of self-worth. The client would not be placed in a private room because this is an unsafe action and may intensify the client's feelings of worthlessness. Placing the client in charge of the morning chess game is a premature intervention that can overwhelm and

3. Placing the client in charge of a meaningful unit activity such as the morning chess tournament

4. Maintaining a distance of 12 inches at all times to ensure the client that control will be provided

cause the client to fail. This can reinforce the client's feelings of worthlessness. Distances of 18 inches or less between two individuals constitute intimate space. Invasion of this space may be misinterpreted by the client and increase the client's tension and feelings of helplessness.

Test-Taking Strategy: Use the process of elimination. Eliminate option 1 because isolation (private room) is not a safe and therapeutic intervention. Option 3 may produce feelings of worthlessness. Eliminate option 4 because a distance of 12 inches is restrictive. Option 2 is the only option that addresses a caring and therapeutic environment. Review care to the suicidal client if you had difficulty with this question.

Level of Cognitive Ability: Application
Client Needs: Safe, Effective Care Environment
Integrated Concept/Process: Caring
Content Area: Mental Health

Reference:
Varcarolis, E. (2002). *Foundations of psychiatric mental health nursing* (4th ed.). Philadelphia: W.B. Saunders, p. 639.

---

11. A client has died, and the nurse asks a family member about the funeral arrangements. The family member refuses to discuss the issue. The nurse's most appropriate action is to:
    1. Provide information needed for decision making
    2. Assess the risk of self-harm and refer the family member to a mental health professional
    3. Demonstrate acceptance of the family member's feelings
    4. Remain with the family member without discussing funeral arrangements

Answer: 4
Rationale: The family member is exhibiting the first stage of grief, which is denial. Option 1 may be an appropriate intervention for the bargaining stage. Option 2 may be an appropriate intervention for depression. Option 3 is an appropriate intervention for the acceptance or reorganization and restitution stage.

Test-Taking Strategy: Note the key words *most appropriate action.* Use therapeutic communication techniques. Eliminate options 1 and 2 because they do not address the issue of the question. From the remaining options, noting the key words *refuses to discuss the issue* will direct you to option 4. Acceptance of feelings is important but in this situation, remaining with the family member is most appropriate. Review the grieving process and therapeutic communication techniques if you had difficulty with this question.

Level of Cognitive Ability: Application
Client Needs: Psychosocial Integrity
Integrated Concept/Process: Caring
Content Area: Fundamental Skills

Reference:
Varcarolis, E. (2002). *Foundations of psychiatric mental health nursing* (4th ed.). Philadelphia: W.B. Saunders, p. 839.

---

12. A 39-year-old man just learned that his 36-year-old wife has an incurable cancer and is expected to live for not more than a few weeks. The nurse explores the client's feelings and identifies which of these

Answer: 3
Rationale: The expression of anger is known to be a normal response to impending loss, and the anger may be directed toward the self, the dying person, God or other spiritual being, or the caregivers. Options 1 and 2 indicate possibly rash and unilateral

responses by the husband as indicative of effective individual coping?

1. He states that he will not allow his wife to come home to die
2. He immediately arranges for their three teen-aged children to live with relatives in another state
3. He expresses his anger at God and the physicians for allowing this to happen
4. He refuses to visit his wife in the hospital or to discuss her illness

decisions made by the husband, without taking into consideration anyone else's feelings. There is evidence of denial in option 4, as he refuses to visit or discuss his wife's illness. The only option that indicates effective individual coping by the husband is option 3.

Test-Taking Strategy: Use the process of elimination. Note the key words *effective individual coping.* Knowledge of the stages of grief associated with loss will easily direct you to option 3. Review effective coping mechanisms if you had difficulty with this question.

Level of Cognitive Ability: Analysis
Client Needs: Psychosocial Integrity
Integrated Concept/Process: Caring
Content Area: Fundamental Skills

Reference:
Harkreader, H. (2000). *Fundamentals of nursing: caring and clinical judgment.* Philadelphia: W.B. Saunders, p. 1366.

---

13. A nurse is providing care to a Cuban-American client who is terminally ill. Numerous family members are present most of the time, and many of the family members are very emotional. The most appropriate nursing action is to:
    1. Restrict the number of family members visiting at one time
    2. Inform the family that emotional outbursts are to be avoided
    3. Request permission to move the client to a private room and allow the family members to visit
    4. Contact the physician to speak to the family members about their behaviors

Answer: 3
Rationale: In the Cuban-American culture, loud crying and other physical manifestations of grief are considered socially acceptable. Of the options provided, option 3 is the only option that identifies a culturally sensitive and caring approach on the part of the nurse. Options 1, 2, and 4 are inappropriate nursing interventions.

Test-Taking Strategy: Focus on the client(s) of the question, who are the family members of a Cuban-American client. Use the process of elimination, recalling the characteristics of this culture and the importance of cultural sensitivity. This will easily direct you to option 3. If you had difficulty with this question, review the characteristics of this culture.

Level of Cognitive Ability: Application
Client Needs: Psychosocial Integrity
Integrated Concept/Process: Caring
Content Area: Fundamental Skills

Reference:
Potter, P., & Perry, A. (2001). *Fundamentals of nursing* (5th ed.). St. Louis: Mosby, p. 115.

---

14. A nurse is caring for an older client who has been recently admitted from home to a long-term care facility. The client has a diagnosis of end-stage renal cancer. The nurse recognizes that the resident is coping with many losses. The best way to address the client's psychosocial needs is to:
    1. Provide total care to the client
    2. Medicate the client for pain every four hours as prescribed

Answer: 3
Rationale: Clients admitted from home into a long-term care facility are dealing with losses in control over their environment, independence, and privacy. Providing total care does not facilitate independence. Medicating for pain will keep the client comfortable, but this does not address psychosocial needs. Sitting with the client to allow the client to express feelings is the best way to address psychosocial needs. Participation in daily social activities will not meet the special psychosocial needs of this client.

3. Sit with the client to allow the client to verbalize feelings

4. Encourage the client to participate in daily social activities

Test-Taking Strategy: Use the process of elimination. Focus on the key words, *psychosocial needs.* Eliminate options 1 and 2 first because these options deal with physiological needs. From the remaining options, recalling that the client's feelings should be addressed first will direct you to option 3. Review care to the client experiencing loss if you had difficulty with this question.

Level of Cognitive Ability: Application
Client Needs: Psychosocial Integrity
Integrated Concept/Process: Caring
Content Area: Fundamental Skills

Reference:
Potter, P., & Perry, A. (2001). *Fundamentals of nursing* (5th ed.). St. Louis: Mosby, pp. 614-615.

---

15. A client with diabetes mellitus is told that amputation of the leg is necessary to sustain life. The client is very upset and states to the nurse, "This is all the doctor's fault! I have done everything that the doctor has asked me to do!" The nurse interprets the client's statement as:

1. An expected coping mechanism
2. A need to notify the hospital lawyer
3. An expression of guilt on the part of the client
4. An ineffective coping mechanism

Answer: 1
Rationale: The expression of anger is known to be a normal response to impending loss, and the anger may be directed toward self, God or other spiritual being, or caregivers. The nurse should be aware of the effective and ineffective coping mechanisms that can occur in a client when loss is anticipated. Notifying the hospital lawyer is inappropriate. Guilt may or may not be a component of the client's feelings, and the information in the question does not provide an indication that guilt is present.

Test-Taking Strategy: Focus on the data provided in the question. Note that options 1 and 4 address coping mechanisms. This may provide you with the clue that one of these may be the correct option. Noting that the client is blaming the doctor and knowledge of the stages of grief associated with loss will direct you to option 1. Review these stages and expected client expressions if you had difficulty with this question.

Level of Cognitive Ability: Analysis
Client Needs: Psychosocial Integrity
Integrated Concept/Process: Caring
Content Area: Fundamental Skills

Reference:
Potter, P., & Perry, A. (2001). *Fundamentals of nursing* (5th ed.). St. Louis: Mosby, pp. 616-617.

---

16. A nurse has been caring for a terminally ill client whose death is imminent. The nurse has developed a close relationship with the family of the client. Which of the following nursing interventions will the nurse avoid in dealing with the family during this difficult time?

1. Making the decisions for the family during the difficult moments
2. Encouraging family discussion of feelings

Answer: 1
Rationale: Maintaining effective and open communication among family members affected by death and grief is of utmost importance. The nurse should maintain and enhance communication as well as preserve the family's sense of self-direction and control. Option 2 is likely to enhance communication. Option 3 is also an effective intervention because spiritual practices give meaning to life and have an impact on how people react to crisis. Option 4 is also an effective technique, and the family needs to know that someone will be there that is supportive and nonjudgmental. Option 1 removes autonomy and decision making from

3. Facilitating the use of spiritual practices identified by the family

4. Accepting the family's expressions of anger

the family at a time when they are already experiencing feelings of loss of control. This is an ineffective intervention that can impair communication.

Test-Taking Strategy: Note the key word *avoid* in the stem of the question. Use the process of elimination focusing on therapeutic communication techniques. This will direct you to option 1. Review therapeutic techniques for individuals in crisis if you had difficulty with this question.

Level of Cognitive Ability: Application
Client Needs: Psychosocial Integrity
Integrated Concept/Process: Caring
Content Area: Fundamental Skills

Reference:
Potter, P., & Perry, A. (2001). *Fundamentals of nursing* (5th ed.). St. Louis: Mosby, p. 617.

---

17. A client brought to the emergency room is dead on arrival (DOA). The family of the client tells the physician that the client had terminal cancer. The emergency room physician examines the client and asks the nurse to contact the medical examiner about an autopsy. The family of the client tells the nurse that they do not want an autopsy performed. Which of the following responses to the family is most appropriate?

1. "It is required by federal law. Why don't we talk about it, and why don't you tell me how you feel?"

2. "The decision is made by the medical examiner."

3. "I will contact the medical examiner regarding your request."

4. "An autopsy is mandatory for any client who is DOA."

Answer: 3
Rationale: An autopsy is required by state law in certain circumstances, including the sudden death of a client and a death that occurs under suspicious circumstances. It is not a requirement by federal law. It is not mandatory that every client who is DOA have an autopsy. If a family requests not to have an autopsy performed on a family member, then the nurse should contact the medical examiner about the request.

Test-Taking Strategy: Use the process of elimination. Note the key words *most appropriate*. Use knowledge about the laws and issues surrounding autopsy and therapeutic communication techniques to answer the question. Eliminate options 1 and 4 because these statements are not accurate. From the remaining options, option 3 is the most therapeutic and caring response to the family. Review the issues and laws surrounding autopsy if you had difficulty with this question.

Level of Cognitive Ability: Application
Client Needs: Safe, Effective Care Environment
Integrated Concept/Process: Caring
Content Area: Fundamental Skills

Reference:
Potter, P., & Perry, A. (2001). *Fundamentals of nursing* (5th ed.). St. Louis: Mosby, p. 436.

---

18. An older client with coronary artery disease is scheduled for hospital discharge and lives alone. The client states, "I don't know how I'll be able to remember all these instructions and take care of myself once I get home." The nurse should plan which of the following actions to assist the client?

1. Ask an out-of-town relative to stay with the client for a day or so

Answer: 4
Rationale: With earlier hospital discharge, clients are returning home with greater acuity of problems than before, and they may require support from a home health agency until they are independent in functioning. Option 3 does nothing to actively assist the client, and option 2 is not realistic in the current health care environment. Although option 1 is a viable option, it does not ensure the client continued care until the client is able to independently manage his or her own care.

2. Ask the physician to delay the discharge until the client is better able to manage self-care

3. Suggest that the social worker follow up with a telephone call after discharge to ensure the client is progressing

4. Suggest that the physician be asked for a referral to a home health agency for nursing and home health aide support

Test-Taking Strategy: Focus on the issue of the question and the client's concern. Use the process of elimination, noting that option 4 is the only action that will ensure that the client has the necessary assistance until independence is achieved. Review the concepts related to home care support if you had difficulty with this question.

Level of Cognitive Ability: Application
Client Needs: Safe, Effective Care Environment
Integrated Concept/Process: Caring
Content Area: Fundamental Skills

Reference:
Potter, P., & Perry, A. (2001). *Fundamentals of nursing* (5th ed.). St. Louis: Mosby, p. 32.

---

19. A nurse is interacting with the family of a client who is unconscious as a result of a head injury. Which of the following approaches would the nurse use to help the family cope with this situation?
1. Enforce adherence to visiting hours to ensure the client's rest
2. Encourage the family not to "give in" to their feelings of grief
3. Discourage the family from touching the client
4. Explain equipment and procedures on an ongoing basis

Answer: 4
Rationale: Families often need assistance to cope with the sudden severe illness of a loved one. The nurse should explain all equipment, treatments, and procedures, and supplement or reinforce information given by the physician. Family members should be encouraged to touch and speak to the client and to become involved in the client's care in some way if they are comfortable doing so. The nurse should allow the family to stay with the client whenever possible. The nurse also encourages the family members to eat properly and to obtain enough sleep to maintain their strength.

Test-Taking Strategy: Use the process of elimination and therapeutic basic communication techniques to answer this question. Each of the incorrect options places distance between the family and the client. Review therapeutic techniques that assist the family to deal with a sudden illness if you had difficulty with this question.

Level of Cognitive Ability: Application
Client Needs: Psychosocial Integrity
Integrated Concept/Process: Caring
Content Area: Adult Health/Neurological

Reference:
Phipps, W., Monahan, F., Sands, J. et al (2003). *Medical surgical nursing: health and illness perspectives* (7th ed.). St. Louis: Mosby, p. 1325.

---

20. A nurse is collecting data from a client being admitted to the hospital. The client has right-sided weakness, aphasia, and urinary incontinence. One of the client's family members states, "If this is a stroke, it's the kiss of death." The nurse's best response would be:
1. "Wait until the doctor gets here to think like that."
2. "A stroke is not the kiss of death."
3. "You feel as if your parent is dying?"
4. "These symptoms may be reversible."

Answer: 3
Rationale: Option 3 allows the family member to verbalize and begin to cope and adapt to what is happening. By restating what was said, the nurse is able to clarify the family member's feelings and begin to offer information that will help to ease some of the fears that they may face at the moment. Options 1 and 2 offer disapproval and put the family member's feeling on hold. Option 4 provides false hope at this point.

Test-Taking Strategy: Use therapeutic communication techniques. Option 3 is the only option that addresses the family member's feelings. Review therapeutic communication techniques if you had difficulty with this question.

Cognitive Level of Ability: Application
Client Needs: Psychosocial Integrity
Integrated Concept/Process: Caring
Content Area: Fundamental Skills

Reference:
Potter, P., & Perry, A. (2001). *Fundamentals of nursing* (5th ed.). St. Louis: Mosby, p. 459.

Communication And Documentation

1. A nurse is trying to determine the client's adjustment to a new diagnosis of coronary heart disease before discharge from the hospital. Of the following questions, which one would the nurse ask to elicit the most useful response by the client in determining adjustment?
  1. "Do you have anyone at home to help with housework and shopping?"
  2. "How do you feel about the lifestyle changes you are planning to make?"
  3. "Do you understand the use of your new medications?"
  4. "Are you going to book your follow-up physician visit?"

Answer: 2
Rationale: All questions relate to aspects of post-hospital care, but only option 2 explores the client's feelings about adjustment to the disease. Options 1, 3, and 4 do not address the client's feelings related to adjustment to the disease.

Test-Taking Strategy: Use therapeutic communication techniques. Open-ended questions explore the client's reactions or feelings to a particular situation. Closed-ended responses generally elicit a "yes" or "no" response exclusively. All of the incorrect options are closed-ended responses. Review therapeutic communication techniques if you had difficulty with this question.

Level of Cognitive Ability: Application
Client Needs: Health Promotion and Maintenance
Integrated Concept/Process: Communication and Documentation
Content Area: Fundamental Skills

Reference:
Potter, P., & Perry, A. (2001). *Fundamentals of nursing* (5th ed.). St. Louis: Mosby, p. 459.

2. A female client with a long leg cast has been using crutches to ambulate for 1 week. She comes to the clinic with complaints of pain, fatigue, and frustration with crutch walking. She states, "I feel like I have a crippled leg." Which of the following responses by the nurse is most appropriate?
  1. "I know how you feel, I had to use crutches before, too."
  2. "Just remember, you'll be done with the crutches in another month."
  3. "Why don't you take a couple of days off work and rest."
  4. "Tell me what is bothersome for you."

Answer: 4
Rationale: Option 4 is the therapeutic communication technique of clarification and validation and indicates that the nurse is dealing with the client's problem from the client's perspective. Option 1 devalues the client's feelings and thus blocks communication. Option 2 provides false reassurances because the client may not be finished using the crutches in another month. In addition, option 2 does not focus on the present problem. Option 3 gives advice and is a communication block.

Test-Taking Strategy: Use therapeutic communication techniques. Option 4 is the only response that encourages communication. Review therapeutic communication techniques if you had difficulty with this question.

Level of Cognitive Ability: Application
Client Needs: Psychosocial Integrity

Integrated Concept/Process: Communication and Documentation
Content Area: Adult Health/Musculoskeletal

Reference:
Potter, P., & Perry, A. (2001). *Fundamentals of nursing* (5th ed.). St. Louis: Mosby, p. 459.

---

3. An 18-year-old client is being discharged from the hospital after surgery and will need to ambulate with a cane for the next 6 months. The nurse asks the client which question that will provide data about the psychosocial status of the client about the use of the cane?
1. "How do you feel about having to ambulate with a cane for the next 6 months?"
2. "Do you have any questions about how to ambulate with the cane?"
3. "Time will pass quickly, don't you think?"
4. "You are not worried about what your friends will think, are you?"

Answer: 1
Rationale: How a client feels is an important part of the psychosocial assessment. Option 2 deals with a physical issue. Option 3 gives an opinion. Option 4 can be intimidating to the client. Additionally, options 2, 3, and 4 are closed-ended responses and are barriers to effective communication.

Test-Taking Strategy: Use therapeutic communication techniques. Avoid responses that include communication blocks. Eliminate options 2, 3, and 4 because they are closed-ended responses and are blocks to communication. Remember to address the client's feelings first. Review therapeutic communication techniques if you had difficulty with this question.

Level of Cognitive Ability: Application
Client Needs: Psychosocial Integrity
Integrated Concept/Process: Communication and Documentation
Content Area: Fundamental Skills

Reference:
Potter, P., & Perry, A. (2001). *Fundamentals of nursing* (5th ed.). St. Louis: Mosby, p. 459.

---

4. A client will be self-administering an anticoagulant subcutaneously at home and says to the nurse, " I'm not sure I will be able to take this medication at home." Which of the following statements by the nurse is the most appropriate?
1. "What are your concerns about taking this medication at home?"
2. "Don't worry. Your doctor knows what's best for you."
3. "You'll be fine once you get used to giving your own shots."
4. "Maybe your wife can give you your shot."

Answer: 1
Rationale: Option 1 restates the client's concern and provides the opportunity to verbalize. Options 2 and 3 show false reassurance, which invalidates the client's concern. Option 4 offers advice without knowing what the client's concerns really are.

Test-Taking Strategy: Use therapeutic communication techniques to answer this question. Remembering to focus on the client's feelings will direct you to option 1. Review therapeutic communication techniques if you had difficulty with this question.

Level of Cognitive Ability: Application
Client Needs: Psychosocial Integrity
Integrated Concept/Process: Communication and Documentation
Content Area: Fundamental Skills

Reference:
Potter, P., & Perry, A. (2001). *Fundamentals of nursing* (5th ed.). St. Louis: Mosby, p. 459.

---

5. A client is diagnosed with thrombophlebitis of the left leg. The nurse documents in the nursing care plan that

Answer: 2
Rationale: Elevation of the affected leg facilitates blood flow by the force of gravity and also decreases venous pressure, which in turn

the client should be placed on bed rest with:

1. The left leg kept flat
2. Elevation of the left leg
3. The left leg in a dependent position
4. Bathroom privileges

relieves edema and pain. Bed rest is indicated to prevent emboli and pressure fluctuations in the venous system that occur with walking. Thus the nurse documents to elevate the left leg. Options 1, 3, and 4 are inappropriate positions and will not facilitate blood flow.

Test-Taking Strategy: Use the process of elimination. Focus on the client's diagnosis and think about the principles related to gravity flow and edema to answer the question. If you had difficulty with this question, review nursing care for a client with a venous disorder.

Level of Cognitive Ability: Application
Client Needs: Physiological Integrity
Integrated Concept/Process: Communication and Documentation
Content Area: Fundamental Skills

Reference:
Black, J., Hawks, J., & Keene, A. (2001). *Medical-surgical nursing: clinical management for positive outcomes* (6th ed.). Philadelphia: W.B. Saunders, p. 1423.

---

6. A female client who is experiencing disordered thinking about food being poisoned is admitted to the mental health unit. The nurse uses which communication technique to encourage the client to eat dinner?
   1. Open-ended questions and silence
   2. Offering opinions about the need to eat
   3. Verbalizing reasons that the client may not choose to eat
   4. Focusing on self-disclosure of own food preferences

Answer: 1
Rationale: Open-ended questions and silence are strategies used to encourage a client to discuss the problem in a descriptive manner. Options 2 and 3 are not helpful to the client because they do not encourage the client to express feelings. Option 4 is not a client-centered intervention.

Test-Taking Strategy: Use the process of elimination and therapeutic communication techniques. Eliminate options 2 and 3 first because they do not support client expression of feelings. Eliminate option 4 next because it is not a client-centered response. Review therapeutic communication techniques if you had difficulty with this question.

Level of Cognitive Ability: Application
Client Needs: Physiological Integrity
Integrated Concept/Process: Communication and Documentation
Content Area: Mental Health

Reference:
Varcarolis, E. (2002). *Foundations of psychiatric mental health nursing* (4th ed.). Philadelphia: W.B. Saunders, p. 253.

---

7. A pregnant client reports that the prescribed iron supplement is causing nausea, constipation, and heartburn and that she plans to stop the medication. The nurse's best response is:
   1. "Your baby needs that iron, you can't stop taking it."
   2. "These gastric reactions are most intense during initial therapy and become less bothersome with continued use."

Answer: 2
Rationale: It is most important that pregnant clients receive iron supplements because of the extra demands placed on maternal circulation by the fetus. Option 2 offers needed information to the client and addresses the issues that are bothersome. Options 1 and 3 show disapproval of the client's feelings. Option 4 places the client's issue of the side effects on hold.

Test-Taking Strategy: Use therapeutic communication techniques. Remembering to focus on the client's feeling and concerns will

3.   "Do not stop taking your medication without talking to the doctor."

4.   "In time you will get used to the side effects."

direct you to option 2. Review these techniques if you had difficulty with this question.

Level of Cognitive Ability: Application
Client Needs: Psychosocial Integrity
Integrated Concept/Process: Communication and Documentation
Content Area: Fundamental Skills

Reference:
Potter, P., & Perry, A. (2001). *Fundamentals of nursing* (5th ed.). St. Louis: Mosby, p. 459.

---

8.   A client with type 2 diabetes mellitus was recently hospitalized for hyperglycemic hyperosmolar nonketotic syndrome (HHNS). Upon discharge from the hospital, the client expresses concern about the recurrence of HHNS. Which statement by the nurse is the most therapeutic?

1.   Don't worry, your family will help you."

2.   "I'm sure this won't happen again."

3.   "You have concerns about the treatment for your condition?"

4.   "I think you might need to go to a nursing home."

Answer: 3
Rationale: The nurse should provide time and listen to the client's concerns. In option 3, the nurse is attempting to clarify the client's feelings. Options 1 and 2 provide inappropriate false reassurance. In addition, the nurse does not tell the client not to worry. Option 4 is not an appropriate nursing response. It disregards the client's concerns and gives advice.

Test-Taking Strategy: Use therapeutic communication techniques. Remembering to always address the client's feelings will direct you to option 3. Review these therapeutic techniques if you had difficulty with this question.

Level of Cognitive Ability: Application
Client Needs: Psychosocial Integrity
Integrated Concept/Process: Communication and Documentation
Content Area: Adult Health/Endocrine

Reference:
Potter, P., & Perry, A. (2001). *Fundamentals of nursing* (5th ed.). St. Louis: Mosby, p. 459.

---

9.   The husband of a client who has a Sengstaken-Blakemore tube states to the nurse, "I thought having this tube down her nose the first time would convince my wife to quit drinking." The most appropriate response by the nurse is:

1.   "Alcoholism is a disease that affects the whole family."

2.   "You sound frustrated in dealing with your wife's drinking problem."

3.   "Have you discussed this subject at the support group meetings?"

4.   "I think you are a good person to stay with your wife."

Answer: 2
Rationale: In option 2, the nurse uses the therapeutic communication techniques of clarifying and focusing in assisting the client (the spouse) to express feelings concerning the wife's chronic illness. Stereotyping (option 1), changing the subject (option 3), and showing approval (option 4) are nontherapeutic techniques and block communication.

Test-Taking Strategy: Use therapeutic communication techniques. Remembering to always address the client's feelings will direct you to option 2. Review these therapeutic techniques if you had difficulty with this question.

Level of Cognitive Ability: Application
Client Needs: Psychosocial Integrity
Integrated Concept/Process: Communication and Documentation
Content Area: Adult Health/Gastrointestinal

Reference:
Potter, P., & Perry, A. (2001). Fundamentals of nursing (5th ed.). St. Louis: Mosby, p. 459.

10. A nurse has an order to institute aneurysm precautions for a client with a cerebral aneurysm. Which of the following items would the nurse document on the plan of care for this client?

1. Instruct the client not to strain with bowel movements
2. Allow the client to read and watch television
3. Limit out of bed activities to twice daily
4. Encourage the client to take his or her own daily bath

Answer: 1

Rationale: Aneurysm precautions include placing the client on bed rest in a quiet setting. Lights are kept dim to minimize environmental stimulation. Any activity that increases the blood pressure (BP) or impedes venous return from the brain is prohibited, such as pushing, pulling, sneezing, coughing, or straining. The nurse provides all physical care to minimize increases in the BP. For the same reason, visitors, radio, television, and reading materials are prohibited or limited. Stimulants such as caffeine and nicotine are prohibited. The nurse documents that the client is instructed to avoid straining with bowel movements.

Test-Taking Strategy: Use the process of elimination. Recall that the components of aneurysm precautions are to limit the amount of stimulation (in any form) that the client receives and to prevent increased intracranial pressure (ICP). With this in mind, eliminate options 3 and 4 first. From the remaining options, recall that straining can increase ICP, so it is appropriate to tell the client not to do so. Review the components of aneurysm precautions if you had difficulty with this question.

Level of Cognitive Ability: Application
Client Needs: Physiological Integrity
Integrated Concept/Process: Communication and Documentation
Content Area: Adult Health/Neurological

Reference:
Black, J., Hawks, J., & Keene, A. (2001). *Medical-surgical nursing: clinical management for positive outcomes* (6th ed.). Philadelphia: W.B. Saunders, p. 1944.

11. A client with myasthenia gravis is having difficulty with the motor aspects of speech. The client has difficulty forming words and the voice has a nasal tone. The nurse would use which of the following communication strategies when working with this client?

1. Repeat what the client said to verify the message
2. Encourage the client to speak quickly
3. Nod continuously while the client is speaking
4. Engage the client in lengthy discussions to strengthen the voice

Answer: 1

Rationale: The client has speech that is nasal in tone and dysarthritic as a result of cranial nerve involvement of the muscles governing speech. The nurse listens attentively and verbally verifies what the client has said. Other helpful techniques are to ask questions requiring a yes or no response, and to develop alternative communication methods (letter board, picture board, pen and paper, flash cards). Encouraging the client to speak quickly is inappropriate and counterproductive. Continuous nodding may be distracting and is unnecessary. Lengthy discussions will tire the client rather than strengthen the voice.

Test-Taking Strategy: Use the process of elimination and basic principles of communication techniques to answer this question. This will direct you to option 1. If this question was difficult, review this disorder and effective communication strategies.

Level of Cognitive Ability: Application
Client Needs: Physiological Integrity
Integrated Concept/Process: Communication and Documentation
Content Area: Adult Health/Neurological

Reference:
Black, J., Hawks, J., & Keene, A. (2001). *Medical-surgical nursing: clinical management for positive outcomes* (6th ed.). Philadelphia: W.B. Saunders, p. 2021.

12. A nurse is planning a dietary regimen with an anemic client. The client states, "My iron pills will have to do. I can't afford to buy any of that fancy food." The nurse's best response is:

1. "Ground beef is not very expensive right now."
2. "This is very important, so pay attention."
3. "Would you like for me to check into some other options for you?"
4. "Why don't you ask your family for help?"

Answer: 3

Rationale: Option 3 validates the concern that the client has with income. The nurse offers help in a nonthreatening manner that will allow the client to accept or decline. Options 1 and 2 block further communication by placing the client's issues on hold. Option 4 is requesting an explanation and uses the word *why?*

Test-Taking Strategy: Use therapeutic communication techniques to answer the question. Note that option 3 is the only option that addresses the client's concern. Remember to always focus on the client's concerns. Review these techniques if you had difficulty with this question.

Level of Cognitive Ability: Application
Client Needs: Psychosocial Integrity
Integrated Concept/Process: Communication and Documentation
Content Area: Fundamental Skills

Reference:
Potter, P., & Perry, A. (2001). *Fundamentals of nursing* (5th ed.). St. Louis: Mosby, p. 459.

---

13. A nurse is observing a nursing assistant talking to a client who is hearing impaired. The nurse would intervene if which of the following were performed by the nursing assistant during communication with the client?

1. The nursing assistant is facing the client when speaking
2. The nursing assistant is speaking clearly to the client
3. The nursing assistant is speaking directly into the impaired ear
4. The nursing assistant is speaking in a normal tone of voice

Answer: 3

Rationale: When communicating with a hearing-impaired client, the nurse should speak in a normal tone to the client and should not shout. The nurse should talk directly to the client while facing the client and speak clearly. If the client does not seem to understand what is said, the nurse should express the statement differently. Moving closer to the client and toward the better ear may facilitate communication, but the nurse should avoid talking directly into the impaired ear.

Test-Taking Strategy: Use the process of elimination, noting the key words *the nurse would intervene*. Knowledge about effective communication techniques for the hearing impaired will direct you to option 3. If you had difficulty with this question, review these therapeutic communication techniques.

Level of Cognitive Ability: Comprehension
Client Needs: Safe, Effective Care Environment
Integrated Concept/Process: Communication and Documentation
Content Area: Adult Health/Ear

Reference:
Potter, P., & Perry, A. (2001). *Fundamentals of nursing* (5th ed.). St. Louis: Mosby, p. 1651.

---

14. A nurse is assigned to care for a client diagnosed with catatonic stupor. When the nurse enters the client's room, the client is found lying on the bed with the body pulled into a fetal position. The most appropriate nursing action is to:

1. Leave the client alone and continue with providing care to other clients

Answer: 3

Rationale: Clients who are withdrawn may be immobile and mute and require consistent, repeated approaches. Intervention includes establishment of interpersonal contact. Communication with withdrawn clients requires much patience from the nurse. The nurse facilitates communication with the client by sitting in silence, asking open-ended questions, and pausing to provide opportunities for the client to respond. The client would not be

2. Take the client into the dayroom to be with other clients

3. Sit beside the client in silence and occasionally ask open-ended questions

4. Ask the client direct questions to encourage talking

left alone. Asking direct questions to the client is not therapeutic. It is not appropriate at this time to place the client in a public place such as a dayroom.

Test-Taking Strategy: Use the process of elimination. Eliminate option 1 because you would not leave the client alone. Eliminate option 2 because it is not appropriate to place the client in a public place. Eliminate option 4 because asking direct questions of this client is not therapeutic. Option 3 is the best action because it provides client supervision and communication with the client. Review care to the client with catatonic stupor if you had difficulty with this question.

Level of Cognitive Ability: Application
Client Needs: Psychosocial Integrity
Integrated Concept/Process: Communication and Documentation
Content Area: Mental Health

Reference:
Varcarolis, E. (2002). *Foundations of psychiatric mental health nursing* (4th ed.). Philadelphia: W.B. Saunders, p. 534.

---

15. A nurse is developing a plan of care for an older client and includes strategies that will facilitate effective communication. The nurse would include which strategy to accomplish this goal?

1. Use an authoritarian approach

2. Use active listening

3. React enthusiastically during the conversation

4. React only to the facts during conversation

Answer: 2
Rationale: For effective communication, the nurse uses active listening and creates an environment in which the client feels comfortable expressing feelings. An authoritarian approach is directive and not permissive and will not create an environment for verbal exchange from the client. Reacting only to the facts is an example of inactive listening. Reacting enthusiastically is not the most effective strategy.

Test-Taking Strategy: Use the process of elimination and therapeutic communication techniques. This will direct you to option 2. If you had difficulty with this question or are unfamiliar with these techniques, review this content.

Level of Cognitive Ability: Application
Client Needs: Psychosocial Integrity
Integrated Concept/Process: Communication and Documentation
Content Area: Fundamental Skills

Reference:
Potter, P., & Perry, A. (2001). *Fundamentals of nursing* (5th ed.). St. Louis: Mosby, p. 459.

---

16. A nurse has made an error in documenting vital signs on a client and obtains the client's record to correct the error. The nurse corrects the error by:

1. Using whiteout

2. Erasing the error

3. Documenting a late entry

4. Drawing one line through the error, and initialing and dating the line

Answer: 4
Rationale: If a nurse makes an error in documenting in the client's record, the nurse should follow agency policies to correct the error. This includes drawing one line through the error, initialing and dating the line, and then providing the correct information. Erasing data from the client's record and the use of whiteout are prohibited. A late entry is used to document additional information not remembered at the initial time of documentation.

Test-Taking Strategy: Use the process of elimination and principles related to documentation. Recalling that alterations to a client's record is avoided will eliminate options 1 and 2. From the remaining options, focusing on the issue of the question will direct you to option 4. Review the principles related to documentation if you had difficulty with this question.

Level of Cognitive Ability: Application
Client Needs: Safe, Effective Care Environment
Integrated Concept/Process: Communication and Documentation
Content Area: Fundamental Skills

Reference:
Potter, P., & Perry, A. (2001). *Fundamentals of nursing* (5th ed.). St. Louis: Mosby, p. 504.

---

17. A client with hyperparathyroidism talks to the nurse about the dietary changes prescribed by the physician. The client states, "I guess I'll never be able to eat ice cream and yogurt, again." The nurse most appropriately responds by stating:
1. "There are lots of other foods you can eat."
2. "Ice cream has too much fat content, anyway."
3. "You don't think you will be able to eat them at all?"
4. "Why do you say that?"

Answer: 3
Rationale: Treatment for clients with hyperparathyroidism includes a low-calcium diet. Ice cream and yogurt are high in calcium and should be restricted. The nurse should respond by rephrasing the client's statement. Options 1, 2, and 4 are examples of communication blocks, such as giving advice and requesting an explanation.

Test-Taking Strategy: Use therapeutic communication techniques to answer the question. Options 1, 2, and 4 are communication blocks. Option 3 seeks to validate what the nurse heard to determine if additional instruction is needed. Review therapeutic communication techniques if you had difficulty with this question.

Level of Cognitive Ability: Application
Client Needs: Psychosocial Integrity
Integrated Concept/Process: Communication and Documentation
Content Area: Fundamental Skills

Reference:
Lewis, S., Heitkemper, M., & Dirksen, S. (2000). *Medical-surgical nursing: assessment and management of clinical problems* (5th ed.). St. Louis: Mosby, p. 1415.

---

18. A client diagnosed with angina pectoris appears to be very anxious and states, " So I had a heart attack, right?" Which of the following is the best response for the nurse to make?
1. "No, and we will see to it that you do not have a heart attack."
2. "Yes, this is why you are here."
3. "No, but the doctor wants to monitor you and control or eliminate your pain."
4. "Yes, but there is minimal damage to your heart."

Answer: 3
Rationale: Angina pectoris occurs as a result of an inadequate blood supply to the myocardium. A myocardial infarction refers to a heart attack. Option 1 provides false reassurance. Neither the nurse nor the physician can guarantee that a heart attack will not occur.

Test-Taking Strategy: Use therapeutic communication techniques and knowledge about the definition of angina pectoris to eliminate options 2 and 4. From the remaining options, eliminate option 1 because it provides false reassurance. Review the pathophysiology associated with angina pectoris and therapeutic communication techniques if you had difficulty with this question.

Level of Cognitive Ability: Application

Client Needs: Psychosocial Integrity
Integrated Concept/Process: Communication and Documentation
Content Area: Adult Health/Cardiovascular

Reference:
Black, J., Hawks, J., & Keene, A. (2001). *Medical-surgical nursing: clinical management for positive outcomes* (6th ed.). Philadelphia: W.B. Saunders, p. 1448.

---

19. A nurse is caring for a hospitalized client with a diagnosis of depression who is silent and not communicating. The nurse develops a plan of care and incorporates strategies for communicating with the client. Which of the following statements would be most appropriate for the nurse to make when caring for the client?
    1. "Can you tell me how you are feeling today?"
    2. "Do you feel like talking today?"
    3. "You are wearing your new shoes."
    4. "Can you tell me how you slept last night?"

Answer: 3
Rationale: When a depressed client is mute or silent, the nurse should use the communication technique of making observations. A statement such as "you are wearing your new shoes" is an appropriate statement to make to the client. When the client is not ready to talk, direct questions (options 1, 2, and 4) can cause anxiety. Pointing to commonalties in the environment draws the client into and reinforces reality.

Test-Taking Strategy: Use therapeutic communication techniques and note the client's diagnosis. Eliminate options 1, 2, and 4 because they are similar. These options are direct questions requiring a response from the client. Review communication techniques for the depressed client if you had difficulty with this question.

Level of Cognitive Ability: Application
Client Needs: Psychosocial Integrity
Integrated Concept/Process: Communication and Documentation
Content Area: Mental Health

Reference:
Varcarolis, E. (2002). *Foundations of psychiatric mental health nursing* (4th ed.). Philadelphia: W.B. Saunders, p. 465.

---

20. A nurse is caring for a client with delirium who states, "Look at the spiders on the wall." Which of the following nursing responses is most appropriate?
    1. "I can see the spiders on the wall, but they are not going to hurt you."
    2. "Would you like me to kill the spiders for you?"
    3. "I know you are frightened, but I do not see spiders on the wall."
    4. "You're having a hallucination; there are no spiders in this room at all."

Answer: 3
Rationale: When hallucinations are present, the nurse should reinforce reality with the client. In option 3, the nurse addresses the client's feelings and reinforces reality. Options 1 and 2 do not reinforce reality. Option 4 reinforces reality but does not address the client's feelings.

Test-Taking Strategy: Use therapeutic communication techniques. Eliminate options 1 and 2 because they reinforce the client's hallucination. Eliminate option 4 because although it reinforces reality, it diminishes the importance of the client's feelings. Review therapeutic communication techniques for the client experiencing altered thought processes if you had difficulty with this question.

Level of Cognitive Ability: Application
Client Needs: Psychosocial Integrity
Integrated Concept/Process: Communication and Documentation
Content Area: Mental Health

Reference:
Varcarolis, E. (2002). *Foundations of psychiatric mental health nursing* (4th ed.). Philadelphia: W.B. Saunders, p. 581.

Cultural Awareness

1. A nurse is developing a plan of care for a hospitalized Asian-American client. The nurse avoids including which of the following in the plan of care?

   1. Maintain physical space with the client

   2. Limit eye contact

   3. Clarify responses to questions

   4. Provide light touch to the head for comfort

Answer: 4

Rationale: Avoiding physical closeness, limiting eye contact, avoiding hand gestures, and clarifying responses to questions are all a component of the plan of care for an Asian-American client. In the Asian-American-culture, the head is considered to be sacred; therefore touching someone on the head is disrespectful. Remember, in this culture, touch the client's head only when necessary, and inform the client before doing so.

Test-Taking Strategy: Use the process of elimination noting the key word *avoids*. Eliminate options 1 and 2 because they are similar in that they both address avoiding contact. Eliminate option 3 because it is a therapeutic communication technique. If you had difficulty with this question, review the beliefs associated with this culture.

Level of Cognitive Ability: Application
Client Needs: Psychosocial Integrity
Integrated Concept/Process: Cultural Awareness
Content Area: Fundamental Skills

Reference:
Potter, P., & Perry, A. (2001). *Fundamentals of nursing* (5th ed.). St. Louis: Mosby, p. 130.

---

2. A nurse consults with a nutritionist about the dietary preferences of an Asian-American client. Which of the following foods would most appropriately be included in the dietary plan?

   1. Red meat

   2. Rice

   3. Fried foods

   4. Chili

Answer: 2

Rationale: Asian-Americans food preferences include raw fish, rice, and soy sauce. African-American food preferences include pork, greens, rice, and fried foods. Hispanic Americans prefer beans, fried foods, spicy foods, chili, and carbonated beverages. European Americans prefer carbohydrates and red meat.

Test-Taking Strategy: Use the process of elimination. Correlate rice with Asian Americans. This may assist when answering other questions similar to this one. If you had difficulty with this question, review the food preferences associated with the Asian-American culture.

Level of Cognitive Ability: Application
Client Needs: Physiological Integrity
Integrated Concept/Process: Cultural Awareness
Content Area: Fundamental Skills

Reference:
Williams, S. (2001). *Basic nutrition & diet therapy* (11th ed.). St. Louis: Mosby, p. 258.

---

3. An European-American client maintains eye contact with the nurse during a conversation about the preoperative teaching

Answer: 4

Rationale: In the European-American culture, eye contact is viewed as indicating trustworthiness. Eye contact is considered

plan. The nurse interprets this nonverbal communication as:

1. Rudeness
2. Arrogance
3. Indicating uneasiness
4. Indicating trustworthiness

rude in Asian-American culture. Arrogance and uneasiness are incorrect interpretations of this nonverbal communication in the European-American client.

Test-Taking Strategy: Use the process of elimination, noting that options 1, 2, and 3 are similar because they indicate a negative response. Option 4 is the only option indicating positivity. If you had difficulty with this question, review the communication practices of the European-American culture.

Level of Cognitive Ability: Comprehension
Client Needs: Psychosocial Integrity
Integrated Concept/Process: Cultural Awareness
Content Area: Fundamental Skills

Reference:
Potter, P., & Perry, A. (2001). *Fundamentals of nursing* (5th ed.). St. Louis: Mosby, p. 451.

---

4. A nurse understands that becoming familiar with the cultural beliefs and practices of a childbearing woman may facilitate positive outcomes during pregnancy because:

1. All women are comfortable discussing sexual practices with their health care providers
2. Many women exist in traditional relationships with their sexual partners; thus discussing and making decisions about reproductive issues may be difficult for some
3. Most males from all cultures are knowledgeable about issues related to the spread of sexually transmitted diseases
4. Safe sex practices are common among couples 18 years and older in all cultures

Answer: 2
Rationale: The nurse providing care to women in their childbearing years must be familiar with the cultural framework within which the client lives and operates. Once this is achieved, appropriate communication techniques can be used to facilitate client care and to identify health-promotion educational strategies. Options 1, 3, and 4 generalize clients.

Test-Taking Strategy: Use the process of elimination. Eliminate options 1, 3, and 4 because of the word *all*. Additionally, these options identify situations that generalize childbearing clients. Review concepts related to cultural practices and differences if you had difficulty with this question.

Level of Cognitive Ability: Comprehension
Client Needs: Psychosocial Integrity
Integrated Concept/Process: Cultural Awareness
Content Area: Maternity

Reference:
McKinney, E., Ashwill, J., Murray, S. et al. (2000). *Maternal-child nursing.* Philadelphia: W.B. Saunders, p. 300.

---

5. A nurse calls the dietary department to obtain a dinner meal for an Italian-American client who was admitted to the hospital at 4:00 PM. The physician prescribed a diet "as tolerated." Considering the practices and preferences of the Italian-American, which of the following foods would the nurse request for the meal?

1. Bread and pasta
2. Blue cornmeal
3. Kosher foods
4. Rice

Answer: 1
Rationale: Food preferences of Italian-Americans include bread and pasta, cheese, meats, poultry and fish. Native-American preferences include blue cornmeal, fish, game, fruits, and berries. Asian-Americans prefer rice and raw fish. Dietary kosher laws are adhered to by members of the Jewish community.

Test-Taking Strategy: Use the process of elimination. Remember that kosher foods are important to the Jewish population, blue cornmeal with Native Americans, and rice with Asian Americans. Review food preferences of the various cultures if you had difficulty with this question.

Level of Cognitive Ability: Application
Client Needs: Psychosocial Integrity
Integrated Concept/Process: Cultural Awareness
Content Area: Fundamental Skills

Reference:
Williams, S. (2001). *Basic nutrition & diet therapy* (11th ed.). St. Louis: Mosby, p. 259.

---

6. A Hispanic-American mother brings her child to the clinic for an examination. Which of the following would be most important during data collection of the child?
1. Avoiding eye contact
2. Touching the child during the examination
3. Avoiding speaking to the child
4. Using body language only

Answer: 2
Rationale: In the Hispanic-American culture, eye behavior is significant. The "evil eye" can be given to a child if a person looks at and admires a child without touching the child. Therefore touching the child during the examination is very important. Although avoiding eye contact indicates respect and attentiveness, this is not the most important intervention during data collection. Avoiding speaking to the child and using body language only are not therapeutic interventions.

Test-Taking Strategy: Use the process of elimination and note the key words *most important*. Eliminate options 3 and 4 first because they are similar. From the remaining options, select the intervention that is most therapeutic, which is touch. If you had difficulty with this question, review the characteristics associated with Hispanic Americans.

Level of Cognitive Ability: Application
Client Needs: Psychosocial Integrity
Integrated Concept/Process: Cultural Awareness
Content Area: Fundamental Skills

Reference:
Potter, P., & Perry, A. (2001). *Fundamentals of nursing* (5th ed.). St. Louis: Mosby, p. 127.

---

7. A nurse is caring for a Hispanic-American client admitted to the hospital with a diagnosis of diabetic ketoacidosis. Several family members are present. Which of the following behaviors, if displayed by the family members, would the nurse interpret as characteristic of this cultural group?
1. Dramatic body language
2. Consistently expressing negative feelings
3. Maintaining consistent eye contact with the nurse
4. Consistently confronting the nurse directly

Answer: 1
Rationale: Characteristics of the Hispanic-American culture include the use of dramatic body language, such as gestures or facial expressions, to express emotion or pain. Their belief is that direct confrontation is disrespectful, and the expression of negative feelings is impolite. Additionally, in this culture, avoiding direct eye contact indicates respect and attentiveness.

Test-Taking Strategy: Use the process of elimination and focus on the Hispanic-American culture. Recalling that dramatic body language is a characteristic of this culture will direct you to option 1. If you had difficulty with this question, review the beliefs of the Hispanic-American culture.

Level of Cognitive Ability: Comprehension
Client Needs: Psychosocial Integrity
Integrated Concept/Process: Cultural Awareness
Content Area: Fundamental Skills

Reference:
Potter, P., & Perry, A. (2001). *Fundamentals of nursing* (5th ed.). St. Louis: Mosby, p. 126.

8. A nurse assists to develop a plan of care for a Native-American client and considers the practices and preferences of the culture. In developing the plan, the nurse understands that which of the following is not a practice of this ethnic group?
  1. Religion and healing practices
  2. Touching the body of a dead family member
  3. Avoiding eye contact
  4. Use of healing practices

Answer: 2
Rationale: In the Native-American culture, touching a dead body is prohibited. The use of religion and healing practices is integrated into health care and illness practices. Eye contact is avoided because it is a sign of disrespect.

Test-Taking Strategy: Use the process of elimination, noting the key word *not*. Eliminate options 1 and 4 first because they are similar. Remembering that maintaining eye contact is a sign of disrespect will direct you to option 2. If you had difficulty with this question, review the traditional beliefs of the Native American.

Level of Cognitive Ability: Comprehension
Client Needs: Psychosocial Integrity
Integrated Concept/Process: Cultural Awareness
Content Area: Fundamental Skills

Reference:
Potter, P., & Perry, A. (2001). *Fundamentals of nursing* (5th ed.). St. Louis: Mosby, p. 132.

---

9. A nurse caring for an Orthodox Jewish client plans a diet that adheres to the practices of Judaism. The nurse avoids including which of the following in the diet plan?
  1. Fish with scales and fins
  2. Well-cooked meats
  3. Unleavened bread during Passover week
  4. Meat and milk eaten together

Answer: 4
Rationale: Dietary kosher laws must be adhered to by Orthodox Jews. Rare meats are prohibited. Fish that have scales and fins are allowed; however, any combination of meat and milk is prohibited. During Passover week, only unleavened bread is eaten.

Test-Taking Strategy: Use the process of elimination, noting the key word *avoids* in the stem of the question. Recalling the dietary practices in Judaism will direct you to option 4. If you had difficulty with the question, review the dietary practices of this cultural group.

Level of Cognitive Ability: Application
Client Needs: Psychosocial Integrity
Integrated Concept/Process: Cultural Awareness
Content Area: Fundamental Skills

Reference:
Potter, P., & Perry, A. (2001). *Fundamentals of nursing* (5th ed.). St. Louis: Mosby, p. 1347.

---

10. A nurse is caring for an African-American client. The nurse enters the room and after a greeting and introduction to the client, the nurse begins to describe the angiogram procedure scheduled for the next day. The client turns away from the nurse. Which of the following nursing actions is most appropriate?
  1. Continue with the explanation
  2. Ask the client if he or she can hear the nurse

Answer: 1
Rationale: In the African-American culture, direct eye contact is often viewed as being rude. If the client turns away from the nurse during a conversation, the most appropriate action is to continue with the conversation. Walking around to the client so that the nurse faces the client is in direct conflict with this cultural practice. Asking the client if he or she can hear the nurse or leaving the room and returning later to continue with the explanation may be viewed as a rude gesture by the client.

Test-Taking Strategy: Use the process of elimination and therapeutic communication techniques. Eliminate options 2 and 4 first

3. Walk around to the client so that the nurse faces the client
4. Leave the room and return later to continue with the explanation

because these are nontherapeutic actions. From the remaining options, option 1 is the most therapeutic. If you had difficulty with this question, review the communication practices of this cultural group.

Level of Cognitive Ability: Application
Client Needs: Psychosocial Integrity
Integrated Concept/Process: Cultural Awareness
Content Area: Fundamental Skills

Reference:
Potter, P., & Perry, A. (2001). *Fundamentals of nursing* (5th ed.). St. Louis: Mosby, p. 122.

---

11. A nurse caring for a Chinese-American client is reviewing the plan of care with the client. The client frequently nods the head during the review. The nurse interprets this behavior as that:
    1. The client agrees with the plan
    2. The client may not necessarily agree with the plan
    3. The client would like to hear more about the plan
    4. The client is very anxious

Answer: 2
Rationale: In the Chinese-American culture, head nodding does not necessarily mean that the client is in agreement with what is being presented, agrees with the plan, or is anxious. The nurse should be alert to nonverbal communication and validate the client's nonverbal communication.

Test-Taking Strategy: Focus on the issue of the question: interpreting nonverbal communication. Using the process of elimination and recalling the characteristics of this cultural group will direct you to option 2. Review the importance and meaning of nonverbal communication in the Chinese-American culture if you had difficulty with this question.

Level of Cognitive Ability: Comprehension
Client Needs: Psychosocial Integrity
Integrated Concept/Process: Cultural Awareness
Content Area: Fundamental Skills

Reference:
Potter, P., & Perry, A. (2001). *Fundamentals of nursing* (5th ed.). St. Louis: Mosby, p. 1348.

---

12. A nursing instructor is providing a session on cultural beliefs related to health and illness. After the session, the instructor asks a nursing student to describe the beliefs of an African American in regard to illness. Which of the following would be the most appropriate response by the student?
    1. "Illness is due to an imbalance between yin and yang."
    2. "Illness is a punishment for sins."
    3. "Illness is a disharmonious state that may be caused by demons and spirits."
    4. "Illness is due to lack of exercise."

Answer: 3
Rationale: In the African-American culture, illness is viewed as a disharmonious state that may be caused by demons and spirits. The goal of treatment, from the traditional African perspective, is to remove the harmful spirit from the body of the ill person. Asian Americans believe that illness is due to an imbalance between yin and yang, as well as to prolonged sitting or lying, or to overexertion. Hispanic Americans believe that illness occurs as a result of punishment for sins.

Test-Taking Strategy: Use the process of elimination. Focus on the issue, African-American health beliefs. Recalling the beliefs in this culture will direct you to option 3. If you had difficulty with the question, review the various beliefs of the African-American culture.

Level of Cognitive Ability: Comprehension
Client Needs: Psychosocial Integrity

Integrated Concept/Process: Cultural Awareness
Content Area: Fundamental Skills

Reference:
Potter, P., & Perry, A. (2001). *Fundamentals of nursing* (5th ed.). St. Louis: Mosby, p. 17.

---

13. A nurse is gathering admission data from an African-American client scheduled for a cataract removal and an intraocular lens implant. Which of the following questions would be inappropriate for the nurse to ask initially?
1. "Do you have any difficulty breathing?"
2. "Do you have a close family relationship?"
3. "Do you ever experience chest pain?"
4. "Do you frequently have episodes of headache?"

Answer: 2
Rationale: In the African-American culture, it is considered to be intrusive to ask personal questions on the initial contact or meeting. African Americans are highly verbal and express feelings openly to family or friends, but what transpires within the family is viewed as private. The psychosocial assessment would be the least priority during the initial admission assessment. Additionally, respiratory, cardiovascular, and neurological data are physiological and are the priority.

Test-Taking Strategy: Use Maslow's Hierarchy of Needs theory to answer the question. Note the key words *inappropriate* and *initially*. Options 1, 3, and 4 address physiological needs. Option 2 addresses the psychosocial need. Review the cultural beliefs of the African-American culture if you had difficulty with this question.

Level of Cognitive Ability: Application
Client Needs: Psychosocial Integrity
Integrated Concept/Process: Cultural Awareness
Content Area: Fundamental Skills

Reference:
Potter, P., & Perry, A. (2001). *Fundamentals of nursing* (5th ed.). St. Louis: Mosby, p. 1671.

---

14. A nurse is preparing to deliver a food tray to a client whose religion is Jewish. The nurse checks the food on the tray and notes that the client has received a roast beef dinner with whole milk as a beverage. Which of the following actions will the nurse take?
1. Deliver the food tray to the client
2. Call the dietary department and ask for a new meal tray
3. Replace the whole milk with fat free milk
4. Ask the dietary department to replace the roast beef with pork

Answer: 2
Rationale: In the Jewish religion, the dairy-meat combination is not acceptable. Pork and pork products are not allowed in the traditional Jewish religion. The only correct nursing action is to ask the dietary department to deliver a new meal tray.

Test-Taking Strategy: Use the process of elimination. Recalling that the dairy-meat combination is not acceptable in this religion will direct you to option 2. Review the dietary rules of this religious group if you had difficulty with this question.

Level of Cognitive Ability: Application
Client Needs: Psychosocial Integrity
Integrated Concept/Process: Cultural Awareness
Content Area: Fundamental Skills

Reference:
Potter, P., & Perry, A. (2001). *Fundamentals of nursing* (5th ed.). St. Louis: Mosby, p. 1348.

15. A nurse is planning to instruct a Mexican-American client about nutrition and dietary restrictions. When developing the plan, the nurse is aware that this ethnic group:
  1. Enjoys food that lacks color, flavor, and texture
  2. Primarily eats raw fish
  3. Enjoys eating red meat
  4. Views food as a primary form of socialization

Answer: 4

Rationale: Mexican foods are rich in color, flavor, texture, and spiciness. In the Mexican American culture, any occasion is seen as a time to celebrate with food and enjoy the companionship of family and friends. Because food is a primary form of socialization in the Mexican culture, Mexican-Americans may have difficulty adhering to a prescribed diet. Asian Americans eat raw fish, rice, and soy sauce. European Americans prefer carbohydrates and red meat.

Test-Taking Strategy: Use the process of elimination. Recalling the food practices and preferences and the meaning of food in the Mexican-American culture will direct you to option 4. If you had difficulty with this question, review the food preferences associated with this culture.

Level of Cognitive Ability: Comprehension
Client Needs: Psychosocial Integrity
Integrated Concept/Process: Cultural Awareness
Content Area: Fundamental Skills

Reference:
Potter, P., & Perry, A. (2001). *Fundamentals of nursing* (5th ed.). St. Louis: Mosby, p. 1348.

16. A nurse has volunteered to assist in providing health care instructions to a Native-American community group. The nurse plans instructions based on the common practices and rituals of this group, knowing that which of the following is not a common characteristic associated with this ethnic group?
  1. Corn is an important component of the diet
  2. Alcohol use is minimal
  3. Fried bread and mutton are prepared in lard
  4. Vitamin D deficiency is a concern

Answer: 2

Rationale: Native-American diets may be deficient in vitamin D because many individuals in this group suffer from lactose intolerance or do not drink milk. Corn is an important staple in the diet of the Navajo and other Native-American tribes. Fried bread and mutton are prepared in lard, and these dietary rituals have attributed to the increased risk of gallbladder disease in this population. Alcohol abuse is a concern, and many Native-American tribes exhibit high-risk behaviors related to alcohol abuse.

Test-Taking Strategy: Use the process of elimination. Note the key word *not* in the stem of the question. Recalling that alcohol abuse is a concern in this ethnic group will direct you to option 2. Review the common rituals and health care practices in this cultural group if you had difficulty with this question.

Level of Cognitive Ability: Comprehension
Client Needs: Psychosocial Integrity
Integrated Concept/Process: Cultural Awareness
Content Area: Fundamental Skills

Reference:
Potter, P., & Perry, A. (2001). *Fundamentals of nursing* (5th ed.). St. Louis: Mosby, p. 1348.

17. A nurse is assigned to collect admission data from a Mexican-American client. On initial meeting of the client, the nurse should plan to:
  1. Greet the client with a handshake
  2. Avoid touching the client

Answer: 1

Rationale: To demonstrate respect, compassion, and understanding, health care providers should greet Mexican-American clients with a handshake. On establishing rapport, care providers may further demonstrate approval and respect through touch, smiling, and affirmative nods of the head. Given the diversity of dialects

3. Avoid any affirmative nods during the conversations with the client

4. Smile and use humor throughout the entire admission assessment

and the nuances of language, culturally congruent use of humor is difficult to accomplish and therefore should be avoided.

Test-Taking Strategy: Use the process of elimination. Recalling the cultural communication patterns of the Mexican American will direct you to option 1. Review the characteristics of this cultural group if you had difficulty with this question.

Level of Cognitive Ability: Application
Client Needs: Psychosocial Integrity
Integrated Concept/Process: Cultural Awareness
Content Area: Fundamental Skills

Reference:
Potter, P., & Perry, A. (2001). *Fundamentals of nursing* (5th ed.). St. Louis: Mosby, p.240.

---

18. A nurse is developing a postoperative plan of care for a 40-year-old male Filipino client scheduled for an appendectomy. The nurse most appropriately includes in the plan of care to:

1. Inform the client the he will need to ask for pain medication when needed

2. Offer pain medication when nonverbal signs of discomfort are identified

3. Offer pain medication on a regular basis as prescribed

4. Allow the client to maintain control and request pain medication on his own

Answer: 3
Rationale: Filipinos view pain as part of living an honorable life. The client may appear stoic and be tolerant of a high degree of pain. The nurse should offer pain medication on a regular basis and in fact encourage pain relief interventions for the Filipino client who does not complain of pain, despite physiological indicators. Option 3 is the most appropriate intervention to include in the plan of care.

Test-Taking Strategy: Note the key words *most appropriately*. Use the process of elimination and eliminate options 1 and 4 first because they are similar. From the remaining options, recalling the cultural responses to pain in the Filipino client will direct you to option 3. If you had difficulty with this question, review the characteristics of this cultural group.

Level of Cognitive Ability: Application
Client Needs: Psychosocial Integrity
Integrated Concept/Process: Cultural Awareness
Content Area: Fundamental Skills

Reference:
Potter, P., & Perry, A. (2001). *Fundamentals of nursing* (5th ed.). St. Louis: Mosby, p. 1342.

---

19. A nurse is planning a menu with the hospital dietitian for a Chinese client. After the nurse collaborated with the dietitian, the meal plan is designed to include which of the following foods that are generally included in the diet of this cultural group?

1. Vegetables

2. Milk

3. A dessert high in sugar content

4. Large portions of meat

Answer: 1
Rationale: The Chinese diet is generally vegetarian. Native Chinese generally do not drink milk or eat milk products because of a genetic tendency for lactose intolerance. Most Chinese do not eat large portions of meat or desserts high in sugar content.

Test-Taking Strategy: Use the process of elimination. Recalling the food rituals related to the Chinese culture will direct you to option 1. If you had difficulty with this question review the dietary characteristics of this culture.

Level of Cognitive Ability: Application

Client Needs: Psychosocial Integrity
Integrated Concept/Process: Cultural Awareness
Content Area: Fundamental Skills

Reference:
Potter, P., & Perry, A. (2001). *Fundamentals of nursing* (5th ed.). St. Louis: Mosby, p. 971.

---

20. A nurse is preparing to examine a Hispanic child who was brought to the clinic by the mother. During data collection, the nurse avoids which of the following?
1. Asking the mother questions about the child
2. Admiring the child
3. Taking the child's temperature
4. Obtaining an interpreter if necessary

Answer: 2
Rationale: Hispanic clients may believe in the "evil eye." They believe that an individual becomes ill as a result of excessive admiration by another. Options 1 and 3 are appropriate interventions. It is appropriate for the nurse to obtain an interpreter if the child or mother does not speak the same language as the nurse.

Test-Taking Strategy: Use the process of elimination. Note the key word *avoids* in the stem of the question. Options 1 and 4 can be eliminated because these are therapeutic and appropriate interventions. Eliminate option 3 because there is no reason to avoid taking the child's temperature. If you had difficulty with this question review the cultural characteristics of the Hispanic population.

Level of Cognitive Ability: Application
Client Needs: Psychosocial Integrity
Integrated Concept/Process: Cultural Awareness
Content Area: Fundamental Skills

Reference:
Potter, P., & Perry, A. (2001). *Fundamentals of nursing* (5th ed.). St. Louis: Mosby, p. 127.

Self-Care

1. A nurse is checking a client's functional abilities and ability to perform activities of daily living (ADLs). The nurse focuses data collection on:
1. Self-care needs such as toileting, feeding, and ambulating
2. The normal everyday routine in the home
3. Ability to do light housework, heavy housework, and pay the bills
4. Ability to drive a car

Answer: 1
Rationale: ADLs refer to the client's ability to bathe, toilet, ambulate, dress, and feed himself or herself. The normal routine in the home is not a component of a functional assessment. The ability to do housework and drive a car relates to instrumental ADLs.

Test-Taking Strategy: Use the process of elimination, focusing on the issue ability to perform ADLs. Recalling that ADLs refer to self-care needs will direct you to option 1. Review the concepts of ADLs if you had difficulty with this question.

Level of Cognitive Ability: Application
Client Needs: Health Promotion and Maintenance
Integrated Concept/Process: Self-Care
Content Area: Fundamental Skills

Reference:
Potter, P., & Perry, A. (2001). *Fundamentals of nursing* (5th ed.). St. Louis: Mosby, p. 355.

2. A client with a short leg plaster cast complains of an intense itching under the cast, and the nurse provides instructions to the client about relief measures for the itching. Which statement by the client indicates an understanding of the measures to relieve the itching?

1. "I can use the blunt part of a ruler to scratch the area."

2. "I need to obtain assistance when placing an object into the cast for the itching."

3. "I can use a hair dryer on a cool setting and allow the air to blow into the cast."

4. "I can trickle small amounts of water down inside the cast."

Answer: 3

Rationale: Itching is a common complaint of clients with casts. Objects should not be put inside a cast because of the risk of scratching the skin and providing a point of entry for bacteria. A plaster cast can break down when wet. Therefore the best way to relieve itching is with blowing cool air inside the cast with a hair dryer.

Test-Taking Strategy: Use the process of elimination and eliminate options 1 and 2 first because they both involve the use of an object being placed inside the cast. Recalling that water can soften a plaster cast and cause maceration of the skin will direct you to option 3. Review client education about cast care if you had difficulty with this question.

Level of Cognitive Ability: Comprehension
Client Needs: Health Promotion and Maintenance
Integrated Concept/Process: Self-Care
Content Area: Adult Health/Musculoskeletal

Reference:
Black, J., Hawks, J., & Keene, A. (2001). *Medical-surgical nursing: clinical management for positive outcomes* (6th ed.). Philadelphia: W.B. Saunders, p. 602.

---

3. A nurse is planning to instruct a client with chronic vertigo about safety measures to prevent exacerbation of symptoms or injury. The nurse plans to teach the client that it is important to:

1. Drive at times when the client does not feel dizzy

2. Go to the bedroom and lie down when vertigo is experienced

3. Remove throw rugs and clutter in the home

4. Turn the head slowly when spoken to

Answer: 3

Rationale: The client with chronic vertigo should avoid driving and using public transportation. The sudden movements involved in each could precipitate an attack. To further prevent vertigo attacks, the client should change positions slowly and should turn the entire body, not just the head, when spoken to. If vertigo does occur, the client should immediately sit down or grasp the nearest piece of furniture. The client should remove clutter and throw rugs in the home because trying to regain balance after slipping could trigger the onset of vertigo.

Test-Taking Strategy: Use the process of elimination and focus on the issue: safety. Begin to answer this question by eliminating options 1 and 2 first because they put the client at greatest risk of injury secondary to vertigo. Choose option 3 instead of option 4 because it is the safer intervention of the remaining options. Review safety measures for the client with vertigo if you had difficulty with this question.

Level of Cognitive Ability: Application
Client Needs: Health Promotion and Maintenance
Integrated Concept/Process: Self-Care
Content Area: Adult Health/Ear

Reference:
Black, J., Hawks, J., & Keene, A. (2001). *Medical-surgical nursing: clinical management for positive outcomes* (6th ed.). Philadelphia: W.B. Saunders, p. 1799.

---

4. A nurse has reinforced instructions to a client who has been prescribed disulfiram (Antabuse). Which statement by the client

Answer: 1

Rationale: Clients who are taking disulfiram must be taught that substances containing alcohol can trigger an adverse reaction.

would indicate the need for further instructions?

1. "As long as I don't drink alcohol I'll be fine."
2. "I must be careful taking cold medicines."
3. "I'll have to check my aftershave lotion."
4. "I'll have to be more careful with the ingredients I use for cooking."

Sources of hidden alcohol include foods (soups, sauces, vinegars), medicine (cold medicine), mouthwashes, and skin preparations (alcohol rubs, aftershave lotions).

Test-Taking Strategy: Use the process of elimination and note the key words *need for further instructions*. Remember that disulfiram is used for clients who have alcoholism, and that any form of alcohol should be avoided with this medication. If you are unfamiliar with this medication and the health teaching that is indicated when this medication is prescribed, review this content.

Level of Cognitive Ability: Analysis
Client Needs: Health Promotion and Maintenance
Integrated Concept/Process: Self-Care
Content Area: Pharmacology

Reference:
Hodgson, B., & Kizior, R. (2003). *Saunders nursing drug handbook 2003.* Philadelphia: W.B. Saunders, p. 364.

---

5. A nurse has reinforced instructions to a client receiving external radiation therapy. Which of the following, if stated by the client, would indicate a need for further instructions about self-care related to the radiation therapy?

1. "I should avoid exposure to sunlight."
2. "I should wash my skin with a mild soap and pat dry."
3. "I should apply pressure on the radiated area to prevent bleeding."
4. "I should eat a high-protein diet."

Answer: 3
Rationale: The client should avoid pressure on the radiated area and should wear loose-fitting clothing. Options 1, 2, and 4 are accurate measures about radiation therapy.

Test-Taking Strategy: Use the process of elimination and note the key words *need for further instructions* in stem of the question. The word *pressure* in option 3 is an indication that this is an inappropriate measure. Review client teaching points related to skin care and radiation therapy if you had difficulty with this question.

Level of Cognitive Ability: Comprehension
Client Needs: Health Promotion and Maintenance
Integrated Concept/Process: Self-Care
Content Area: Adult Health/Oncology

Reference:
Black, J., Hawks, J., & Keene, A. (2001). *Medical-surgical nursing: clinical management for positive outcomes* (6th ed.). Philadelphia: W.B. Saunders, p. 395.

---

6. A female client tells a nurse that her skin is very dry and irritated. Which of the following products would the nurse suggest that the client apply to the dry skin?

1. Glycerin emollient
2. Aspercreme
3. Myoflex
4. Acetic acid solution

Answer: 1
Rationale: Glycerin is an emollient that is used for dry, cracked, and irritated skin. Aspercreme and Myoflex are used to treat muscular aches. Acetic acid solution is used for irrigating, cleansing, and packing wounds infected by *Pseudomonas aeruginosa.*

Test-Taking Strategy: Use the process of elimination. Noting the key words *skin is very dry and irritated* will direct you to option 1. Review these products if you had difficulty with this question.

Level of Cognitive Ability: Application
Client Needs: Health Promotion and Maintenance
Integrated Concept/Process: Self-Care
Content Area: Pharmacology

Reference:
Hodgson, B., & Kizior, R. (2003). *Saunders nursing drug handbook 2003.* Philadelphia: W.B. Saunders, p. 100.

---

7. A client being discharged from the mental health unit has a history of anxiety and command hallucinations to harm self or others. The nurse teaches the client about interventions for hallucinations and anxiety. The nurse determines that the client understands these measures when the client says:

1. "If I take my medication I won't be anxious."
2. "I can call my clinical specialist when I'm hallucinating so that I can talk about my feelings and plans and not hurt anyone."
3. "I can go to support group and talk about my feelings."
4. "If I get enough sleep and eat well, I won't get anxious and hear things."

Answer: 2

Rationale: There may be an increased risk for impulsive or aggressive behavior or both if a client is receiving command hallucinations to harm self or others. Talking about auditory hallucinations can interfere with subvocal muscular activity associated with a hallucination. Options 1, 3, and 4 are general interventions but are not specific to anxiety and hallucinations.

Test-Taking Strategy: Focus on the issue: anxiety and hallucinations. Options 1, 3, and 4 are all interventions that a client can do to aid wellness. However, option 2 is specific to the issue and indicates self-responsible commitment and control over personal behavior. Also, note the relationship between the words *hallucinations* in the question and *hallucinating* in the correct option. Review interventions for anxiety and hallucinations if you had difficulty with this question.

Level of Cognitive Ability: Comprehension
Client Needs: Health Promotion and Maintenance
Integrated Concept/Process: Self-Care
Content Area: Mental Health

Reference:
Varcarolis, E. (2002). *Foundations of psychiatric mental health nursing* (4th ed.). Philadelphia: W.B. Saunders, p. 579.

---

8. A nurse has provided instructions to a client about the testicular self-examination (TSE). Which of the following statements by the client indicates that the client needs further teaching about TSE?

1. "I feel the spermatic cord in back and going up."
2. "I know to report any small lumps."
3. "I examine myself after I take a warm shower."
4. "I examine myself every 2 months."

Answer: 4

Rationale: TSE should be performed every month. Small lumps or abnormalities should be reported. The spermatic cord finding in option 1 is normal. After a warm bath or shower the scrotum is relaxed, making it easier to perform TSE.

Test-Taking Strategy: Use the process of elimination. Remembering that breast-self examination needs to be performed monthly may assist in recalling that TSE is also performed monthly. If you had difficulty with this question, review the procedure for TSE.

Level of Cognitive Ability: Comprehension
Client Needs: Health Promotion and Maintenance
Integrated Concept/Process: Self-Care
Content Area: Adult Health/Oncology

Reference:
Black, J., Hawks, J., & Keene, A. (2001). *Medical-surgical nursing: clinical management for positive outcomes* (6th ed.). Philadelphia: W.B. Saunders, p. 41.

---

9. A male client who initially denied that he drank "2 six packs of beer a day" is being discharged from the hospital and is now willing to admit that he has a problem drinking. The client states he will "get some

Answer: 2

Rationale: Alcoholics Anonymous is a major self-help organization for the treatment of alcoholism. Option 1 is a group for families of alcoholics. Option 3 is for parents of children who abuse substances. Option 4 is for nicotine addicts.

help" to live a healthier lifestyle. The nurse plans for a meeting with a representative of which of the following groups to meet with the client before discharge?

1. Al Anon
2. Alcoholics Anonymous
3. Families Anonymous
4. Fresh Start

Test-Taking Strategy: Use the process of elimination. Note the relationship between *drinking* in the question and *Alcoholics* in the correct option. Review the purpose of specific support groups if you had difficulty with this question.

Level of Cognitive Ability: Application
Client Needs: Health Promotion and Maintenance
Integrated Concept/Process: Self-Care
Content Area: Mental Health

Reference:
Varcarolis, E. (2002). *Foundations of psychiatric mental health nursing* (4th ed.). Philadelphia: W.B. Saunders, p. 772.

---

10. A client with acquired immunodeficiency syndrome (AIDS) has a nursing diagnosis of fatigue. The nurse plans to teach the client which of the following strategies to conserve energy after discharge from the hospital?

1. Stand in the shower instead of taking a bath
2. Bathe before eating breakfast
3. Sit for as many activities as possible
4. Group all tasks to be performed early in the morning

Answer: 3
Rationale: The client is taught to conserve energy by sitting for as many activities as possible including dressing, shaving, preparing food, and ironing. The client should also sit in a shower chair instead of standing while bathing. The client should prioritize activities such as eating breakfast before bathing and should intersperse each major activity with a period of rest.

Test-Taking Strategy: Focus on the issue: to conserve energy. Think about the amount of exertion needed by the client to perform each of the activities in the options. Options 1 and 4 are obviously taxing for the client and are eliminated first. From the remaining options, recalling that bathing may take away energy that could be used for eating, which is not helpful, will direct you to the correct choice. Review measures that conserve energy if you had difficulty with this question.

Level of Cognitive Ability: Application
Client Needs: Health Promotion and Maintenance
Integrated Concept/Process: Self-Care
Content Area: Adult Health/Immune

Reference:
Black, J., Hawks, J., & Keene, A. (2001). *Medical-surgical nursing: clinical management for positive outcomes* (6th ed.). Philadelphia: W.B. Saunders, p. 2206.

---

11. A nurse has reinforced self-care activity instructions to a client after insertion of an automatic internal cardioverter-defibrillator (AICD). The nurse determines that further instruction is needed if the client makes which of the following statements?

1. "I should try to avoid doing strenuous things that would make my heart rate go up to or above the rate cutoff on the AICD."
2. "I should keep away from electromagnetic sources such as transformers,

Answer: 3
Rationale: Postdischarge instructions typically include avoiding tight clothing or belts over AICD insertion sites; rough contact with the AICD insertion site; electromagnetic fields from sources such as electrical transformers, radio/TV/radar transmitters, and metal detectors; and proximity to running motors of cars or boats. Clients must also alert physicians or dentists of the device because certain procedures such as diathermy, electrocautery, and magnetic resonance imaging may need to be avoided to prevent device malfunction. Clients should follow the specific advice of a physician about activities that are potentially hazardous to self or others, such as swimming, driving, or operating heavy equipment.

large electrical generators, and metal detectors, and not lean over running motors."

3. "I can perform activities such as swimming, driving, or operating heavy equipment as I need too."

4. "I need to avoid doing anything where there would be rough contact with the AICD insertion site."

Test-Taking Strategy: Use the process of elimination noting the key words *further instruction is needed.* Options 2 and 4 can be eliminated first because they are similar to standard postpacemaker insertion instructions. From the remaining options, noting the words *heavy equipment* in option 3 will direct you to this option. Review client teaching points for AICD if you had difficulty with this question.

Level of Cognitive Ability: Comprehension
Client Needs: Health Promotion and Maintenance
Integrated Concept/Process: Self-Care
Content Area: Adult Health/Cardiovascular

Reference:
Black, J., Hawks, J., & Keene, A. (2001). *Medical-surgical nursing: clinical management for positive outcomes* (6th ed.). Philadelphia: W.B. Saunders, p. 1570.

---

12. A perinatal client has been instructed about the prevention of genital tract infections. Which statement by the client indicates an understanding of these preventive measures?

1. "I should avoid the use of condoms."
2. "I can douche anytime I want."
3. "I can wear my tight fitting jeans."
4. "I should wear underwear with a cotton panel liner."

Answer: 4
Rationale: Condoms should be used to minimize the spread of genital tract infections. Wearing tight clothes irritates the genital area and does not allow for air circulation. Douching is to be avoided. Wearing items with a cotton panel liner allows for air movement in and around the genital area.

Test-Taking Strategy: Use the process of elimination noting the key words *indicates an understanding.* Options 1, 2, and 3 are all incorrect statements about client self-care. If you had difficulty with this question, review prevention measures associated with genital tract infections.

Level of Cognitive Ability: Comprehension
Client Needs: Health Promotion and Maintenance
Integrated Concept/Process: Self-Care
Content Area: Maternity

Reference:
McKinney, E., Ashwill, J., Murray, S. et al. (2000). *Maternal-child nursing.* Philadelphia: W.B. Saunders, p. 959.

---

13. A nurse has given a client information about the use of as-needed nitroglycerin sublingual tablets for chest pain. The nurse determines that the client understands how to self-administer the medication if the client stated to:

1. Avoid using the medication until chest pain actually begins and intensifies
2. Take acetylsalicylic acid (aspirin) to treat a headache that may occur with early use
3. Discard unused tablets 6 to 9 months after the bottle is opened
4. Keep the medication in a shirt pocket close to the body

Answer: 3
Rationale: Nitroglycerin may be self-administered sublingually 5 to 10 minutes before an activity that triggers chest pain. Tablets should be discarded 6 to 9 months after opening the bottle, and a new bottle of pills should be obtained from the pharmacy. Nitroglycerin is very unstable and is affected by heat and cold, so it should not be kept close to the body (warmth) in a shirt pocket; rather it should be kept in a jacket pocket or purse. Headache often occurs with early use and diminishes in time. Acetaminophen (Tylenol) may be used to treat headache.

Test-Taking Strategy: Use the process of elimination noting the key words *understands how to self-administer the medication.* Recalling that nitroglycerin loses its potency in 6 to 9 months will direct you to option 3. Review the client teaching points related to nitroglycerin if you had difficulty with this question.

Level of Cognitive Ability: Analysis
Client Needs: Health Promotion and Maintenance
Integrated Concept/Process: Self-Care
Content Area: Pharmacology

Reference:
Hodgson, B., & Kizior, R. (2003). *Saunders nursing drug handbook 2003.* Philadelphia: W.B. Saunders, p. 815.

---

14. A client with a cerebral vascular accident is prepared for discharge from the hospital. The physician has prescribed range-of-motion (ROM) exercises for the client's right side. In planning for the client's care, the nurse:
1. Considers the use of active, passive, or active-assisted exercises in the home
2. Implements ROM exercises to the point of pain for the client
3. Encourages the client to be dependent on a home health care nurse to complete the exercise program
4. Develops a schedule of ROM exercises every 2 hours while awake even if the client is fatigued

Answer: 1
Rationale: The nurse must consider all forms of ROM for the client. Even if the client has right hemiplegia, the client can assist in some of his or her own rehabilitative care. In addition, the goal is for the client to assume as much self-care and independence as possible. The nurse needs to plan care so that the client becomes self-reliant. Options 2 and 4 are incorrect from a physiological perspective.

Test-Taking Strategy: Use the process of elimination. Options 2 and 4 can be eliminated first because these actions can be harmful to the client. From the remaining options, recall that dependency is not in the best interest of a client's sense of health promotion, which eliminates option 3. Also, note that option 1 is the global option. Review basic knowledge related to ROM exercises and self-care if you had difficulty with this question.

Level of Cognitive Ability: Application
Client Needs: Health Promotion and Maintenance
Integrated Concept/Process: Self-Care
Content Area: Adult Health/Neurological

Reference:
Ignatavicius, D., & Workman, M. (2002). *Medical-surgical nursing: critical thinking for collaborative care* (4th ed.). Philadelphia: W.B. Saunders, p. 986.

---

15. A nurse plans to instruct a client with candidiasis (thrush) of the oral cavity about care for the disorder. The nurse avoids telling the client to:
1. Rinse the mouth four times daily with a commercial mouthwash
2. Eliminate spicy foods from the diet
3. Eliminate citrus juices and hot liquids from the diet
4. Eat foods that are liquid or pureed

Answer: 1
Rationale: Clients with thrush cannot tolerate commercial mouthwashes because the high alcohol concentration in these products can cause pain and discomfort to the lesions. A solution of warm water or mouthwash formulas without alcohol are better tolerated and may promote healing. A change in diet to liquid or pureed food often eases the discomfort of eating. The client should avoid spicy foods, citrus juice, and hot liquids.

Test-Taking Strategy: Use the process of elimination and note the key word *avoids*. Also, noting the words *commercial mouthwash* in option 1 should direct you to this option. Review the client teaching points related to candidiasis (thrush) if you had difficulty with this question.

Level of Cognitive Ability: Application
Client Needs: Health Promotion and Maintenance

Integrated Concept/Process: Self-Care
Content Area: Adult Health/Immune

Reference:
Black, J., Hawks, J., & Keene, A. (2001). *Medical-surgical nursing: clinical manage-ment for positive outcomes* (6th ed.). Philadelphia: W.B. Saunders, p. 1311.

---

16. A client with a history of hypertension has been prescribed triamterene (Dyrenium). The nurse determines that the client under-stands the impact of this medication on the diet if the client states to avoid which of the following fruits?
1. Apples
2. Pears
3. Bananas
4. Cranberries

Answer: 3
Rationale: Triamterene is a potassium-sparing diuretic and the client should avoid foods high in potassium. Fruits that are natu-rally higher in potassium include avocado, bananas, fresh oranges, mangoes, nectarines, papayas, and dried prunes.

Test-Taking Strategy: Use the process of elimination and note the key word *avoid*. Recall that triamterene is a potassium-sparing diuretic. Then identify the high potassium food. If you had diffi-culty with this question, review this medication and those food items high in potassium.

Level of Cognitive Ability: Comprehension
Client Needs: Health Promotion and Maintenance
Integrated Concept/Process: Self-Care
Content Area: Adult Health/Cardiovascular

References:
Hodgson, B., & Kizior, R. (2003). *Saunders nursing drug handbook 2003.* Philadelphia: W.B. Saunders, p. 1124; Williams, S. (2001) *Basic nutrition & diet therapy* (11th ed.). St. Louis: Mosby, p. 121.

---

17. Breathing exercises and postural drainage is prescribed for a child with cystic fibrosis (CF). A nurse plans to teach the child how to implement these procedures by telling the child to:
1. Perform the postural drainage, then the breathing exercises
2. Perform the breathing exercises, then the postural drainage
3. Schedule the procedures so they are 4 hours apart
4. Perform postural drainage in the morning and breathing exercises in the evening

Answer: 1
Rationale: Breathing exercises are recommended for the major-ity of children with CF, even for those with minimal pul-monary involvement. The exercises are usually performed twice daily, and they are preceded with postural drainage. The postural drainage will mobilize secretions, and the breathing exercises will then assist with expectoration. Exercises to assist with posture and to mobilize the thorax are included, such as swinging the arms and bending and twisting the trunk. The ultimate aim of these exercises is to establish a good habitual breathing pattern.

Test-Taking Strategy: Use the process of elimination. Recalling that postural drainage and breathing exercises are most effective when performed together will assist in eliminating options 3 and 4. Considering the effectiveness that each procedure will have on the mobilization of secretions will direct you to option 1 from the remaining options. Review these procedures if you had diffi-culty with this question.

Level of Cognitive Ability: Application
Client Needs: Health Promotion and Maintenance
Integrated Concept/Process: Self-Care
Content Area: Child Health

Reference:
Wong, D., & Hockenberry-Eaton, M. (2001). *Wong's essentials of pediatric nursing* (6th ed.). St. Louis: Mosby, p. 863.

---

18. A client with peptic ulcer disease (PUD) but no other significant medical history asks the nurse what to take for a headache that would not be irritating to the stomach and the rest of the gastrointestinal (GI) tract. The nurse tells the client to take:
1. Acetylsalicylic acid (aspirin)
2. Ibuprofen (Motrin)
3. Acetaminophen (Tylenol)
4. Naproxen (Aleve)

Answer: 3
Rationale: Acetaminophen is not irritating to the lining of the stomach and can be used safely by clients with PUD. Ibuprofen and naproxen are nonsteroidal antiinflammatory drugs (NSAIDs), which are typically irritating to the GI tract. These should be avoided by clients with a history of PUD. Aspirin is an analgesic that is highly irritating to the GI tract.

Test-Taking Strategy: Use the process of elimination. Eliminate options 2 and 4 first because they are similar and are both NSAIDs. From the remaining options, eliminate option 1 because it is irritating to the GI tract. Review the pathophysiology associated with PUD and these medications if you had difficulty with this question.

Level of Cognitive Ability: Application
Client Needs: Health Promotion and Maintenance
Integrated Concept/Process: Self-Care
Content Area: Adult Health/Gastrointestinal

Reference:
Hodgson, B., & Kizior, R. (2003). *Saunders nursing drug handbook 2003*. Philadelphia: W.B. Saunders, p. 1534.

---

19. A client is being discharged to go home after application of a plaster leg cast. The nurse would evaluate that the client understands proper care of the cast if the client states to:
1. Avoid getting the cast wet
2. Use the fingertips to lift and move the leg
3. Cover the casted leg with warm blankets
4. Use a padded coat hanger end to scratch under the cast

Answer: 1
Rationale: A plaster cast must remain dry to keep its strength. The cast should be handled using the palms of the hands, not the fingertips, until fully dry. Air should circulate freely around the cast to help it dry. The cast also gives off heat as it dries. The client should never scratch under the cast. A cool hair dryer may be used to relieve an itch.

Test-Taking Strategy: Use the process of elimination noting the key word *plaster*. Option 4 is dangerous to skin integrity and is eliminated first. Knowing that a wet cast can be dented with the fingertips, causing pressure underneath, helps to eliminate option 2. Recalling that the cast needs to dry eliminates option 3. Remember, plaster casts, once they have dried after application, should not become wet. Review home care instructions for a client with a plaster cast if you had difficulty with this question.

Level of Cognitive Ability: Comprehension
Client Needs: Health Promotion and Maintenance
Integrated Concept/Process: Self-Care
Content Area: Adult Health/Musculoskeletal

Reference:
Black, J., Hawks, J., & Keene, A. (2001). *Medical-surgical nursing: clinical management for positive outcomes* (6th ed.). Philadelphia: W.B. Saunders, p. 606.

20. A client is being discharged to go home while recovering from acute renal failure (ARF). The client indicates an understanding of the therapeutic dietary regimen if the client states to eat foods that are lower in:
1. Vitamins
2. Potassium
3. Carbohydrates
4. Fats

Answer: 2

Rationale: Most of the excretion of potassium and the control of potassium balance are normal functions of the kidneys. In the client with renal failure, potassium intake must be restricted as much as possible (30 to 50 mEq/day). The primary mechanism of potassium removal during ARF is dialysis. Options 1, 3, and 4 are not normally restricted in the client with ARF unless a secondary health problem warrants the need to do so.

Test-Taking Strategy: Use the process of elimination. Noting the diagnosis of the client will assist in answering the question. Recalling that potassium balance and excretion are controlled by the kidney will direct you to option 2. Review the therapeutic diet in the client with ARF if you had difficulty with this question.

Level of Cognitive Ability: Comprehension
Client Needs: Health Promotion and Maintenance
Integrated Concept/Process: Self-Care
Content Area: Adult Health/Renal

Reference:
Grodner, M., Anderson, S., & DeYoung, S. (2000). *Foundations and clinical applications of nutrition: a nursing approach.* St. Louis: Mosby, pp. 594-595.

Teaching and Learning

1. A nurse has given instructions on site care to a hemodialysis client who had an implantation of an arteriovenous (AV) fistula in the right arm. The nurse determines that the client needs further instructions if the client states to:
1. Avoid carrying heavy objects on the right arm
2. Sleep on the right side
3. Report an increased temperature, redness, or drainage at the site
4. Perform range-of-motion exercises routinely on the right arm

Answer: 2

Rationale: Routine instructions to the client with an AV fistula, graft, or shunt includes reporting signs and symptoms of infection, performing routine range-of-motion to the affected extremity, avoiding sleeping with the body weight on the extremity with the access site, and avoiding carrying heavy objects or compressing the extremity that has the access site.

Test-Taking Strategy: Use the process of elimination noting the key words *needs further instructions.* Recalling the importance of maintaining the patency of the AV fistula will direct you to option 2. Review home care instructions for a client with an AV fistula if you had difficulty with this question.

Level of Cognitive Ability: Comprehension
Client Needs: Health Promotion and Maintenance
Integrated Concept/Process: Teaching/Learning
Content Area: Adult Health/Renal

Reference:
Black, J., Hawks, J., & Keene, A. (2001). *Medical-surgical nursing: clinical management for positive outcomes* (6th ed.). Philadelphia: W.B. Saunders, p. 892.

2. A nurse has reinforced instructions to the parents of a child with glomerulonephritis. Which statement by a parent indicates a need for further instructions?

Answer: 1

Rationale: In the child with glomerulonephritis, fluid intake should be limited as prescribed. Children with fluid excess may develop pulmonary edema. A low-sodium diet is followed as

1. "I should encourage an increased intake of fluids."
2. "I should keep my child on a low-sodium diet."
3. "I should monitor the weight of my child."
4. "I should limit play activities to short periods."

prescribed because excessive sodium will increase fluid retention. Weight should be monitored to determine fluctuations in fluid status. The child may tire easily, so playtime should be limited to short periods and extended as the condition improves.

Test-Taking Strategy: Use the process of elimination and note the key words *need for further instructions.* Recalling that this disorder relates to an alteration in renal function will direct you to option 1. Review interventions for glomerulonephritis if you had difficulty with this question.

Level of Cognitive Ability: Comprehension
Client Needs: Health Promotion and Maintenance
Integrated Concept/Process: Teaching/Learning
Content Area: Child Health

Reference:
Wong, D., & Hockenberry-Eaton, M. (2001). *Wong's essentials of pediatric nursing* (6th ed.). St. Louis: Mosby, p. 1046.

---

3. A nurse is reinforcing medication instructions to a client receiving furosemide (Lasix). The nurse determines that further teaching is necessary if the client makes which of the following statements?
1. "I should avoid the use of salt substitutes."
2. "I should change positions slowly."
3. "I should talk to my physician about the use of alcohol."
4. "I should be careful not to get overheated in warm weather."

Answer: 1
Rationale: Furosemide is a potassium-losing diuretic, so there is no need to avoid high-potassium products such as a salt substitute. Orthostatic hypotension is a risk, and the client must use caution when changing positions and with exposure to warm weather. The client should discuss the use of alcohol with the physician.

Test-Taking Strategy: Use the process of elimination noting the key words *further teaching is necessary.* Recalling that furosemide is a potassium-losing diuretic, and that diuretic therapy can induce hypokalemia will direct you to option 1. Review this medication if you had difficulty with this question.

Level of Cognitive Ability: Analysis
Client Needs: Health Promotion and Maintenance
Integrated Concept/Process: Teaching/Learning
Content Area: Pharmacology

Reference:
Hodgson, B., & Kizior, R. (2003). *Saunders nursing drug handbook 2003.* Philadelphia: W.B. Saunders, p. 499.

---

4. A client has been prescribed a clonidine patch (Catapres TTS), and the nurse has reinforced instructions with the client on the use of the patch. The nurse determines that further instruction is needed if the nurse noted that the client:
1. Verbalized to leave the patch in place during bathing or showering
2. Verbalized to change the patch every 7 days

Answer: 3
Rationale: The clonidine patch should be applied to a hairless site on the torso or upper arm. It is changed every 7 days and is left in place when bathing or showering. The patch should not be trimmed because it will alter the medication dose. If it becomes slightly loose, it should be covered with an adhesive overlay from the medication package. If it becomes very loose or falls off, it should be replaced. The patch is discarded by folding it in half with the adhesive sides together.

3. Trimmed the patch because one edge was loose
4. Selected a hairless site on the torso for application

Test-Taking Strategy: Use the process of elimination noting the key words *further instruction is needed*. Noting the words *trimmed the patch* will direct you to this option because this client action would alter the medication dose. Review this medication if you had difficulty with this question.

Level of Cognitive Ability: Analysis
Client Needs: Health Promotion and Maintenance
Integrated Concept/Process: Teaching/Learning
Content Area: Pharmacology

Reference:
Hodgson, B., & Kizior, R. (2003). *Saunders nursing drug handbook 2003.* Philadelphia: W.B. Saunders, p. 262.

---

5. A client is being discharged from the hospital to go home and will be taking cholestyramine (Questran). The nurse determines that further teaching is needed if the client makes which of the following statements?
1. "I should mix the Questran with juice or applesauce."
2. "I should call my doctor immediately if I develop diarrhea."
3. "I should increase my fluid intake while taking this medication."
4. "I should take this medication with meals."

Answer: 2
Rationale: This medication should not be taken dry and can be mixed in water, juice, carbonated beverage, applesauce, or soup. Common side effects include constipation, nausea, indigestion, and flatulence. Increasing fluids will minimize the constipating effects of the medication. Questran must be administered with food to be effective. Diarrhea is not a concern, but severe constipation is.

Test-Taking Strategy: Use the process of elimination noting the key words *further teaching is needed*. Select option 2 because there are normally measures that can be taken for diarrhea rather than immediately calling the physician. Review this medication if you are unfamiliar with it.

Level of Cognitive Ability: Analysis
Client Needs: Health Promotion and Maintenance
Integrated Concept/Process: Teaching/Learning
Content Area: Pharmacology

Reference:
Hodgson, B., & Kizior, R. (2003). *Saunders nursing drug handbook 2003.* Philadelphia: W.B. Saunders, p. 235.

---

6. A nurse is preparing written medication instructions for a client receiving colestipol hydrochloride (Colestid). The nurse plans to include instructions about the need for the client to take which of the following to counteract unintended medication effects?
1. Vitamin D
2. All fat-soluble vitamins
3. B-complex vitamins
4. Vitamin C

Answer: 2
Rationale: Colestipol, a bile-sequestering agent, is used to lower blood cholesterol levels. However, the bile salts (rich in cholesterol) interfere with the absorption of the fat-soluble vitamins A, D, E, and K, as well as folic acid. With ongoing therapy, the client is at risk of deficiency of these vitamins and is counseled to take supplements of these vitamins.

Test-Taking Strategy: Use the process of elimination. Recalling that bile-sequestering agents interfere with the absorption of fat-soluble vitamins will assist in eliminating options 3 and 4. From the remaining options, select option 2 because it is the global option. Review client teaching points about this medication if you had difficulty with this question.

Level of Cognitive Ability: Application
Client Needs: Health Promotion and Maintenance
Integrated Concept/Process: Teaching/Learning
Content Area: Pharmacology

Reference:
Hodgson, B., & Kizior, R. (2003). *Saunders nursing drug handbook 2003.* Philadelphia: W.B. Saunders, p. 275.

---

7. A client with tuberculosis (TB) is preparing for discharge from the hospital. Which of the following client statements indicates that further teaching is necessary?
    1. "If I miss a dose of medication because of nausea, I just skip that dose and resume my regular schedule."
    2. "I need to eat foods that are high in iron, protein, and vitamin C."
    3. "I need to place used tissues in a plastic bag when I am home."
    4. "I will not need respiratory isolation when I am home."

Answer: 1
Rationale: Because of the resistant strains of tuberculosis, the nurse must emphasize that noncompliance with medication requirements could lead to an infection that is difficult to treat and may cause total drug resistance. Clients may prevent nausea related to the medications by taking the daily dose at bedtime. Antinausea medications may also prevent this symptom. Medication doses should not be skipped. Options 2, 3, and 4 are correct statements.

Test-Taking Strategy: Use the process of elimination noting the key words *further teaching is necessary*. General principles related to medication administration will direct you to option 1. Review medication therapy and its importance in TB if you had difficulty with this question.

Level of Cognitive Ability: Analysis
Client Needs: Health Promotion and Maintenance
Integrated Concept/Process: Teaching/Learning
Content Area: Pharmacology

Reference:
Black, J., Hawks, J., & Keene, A. (2001). *Medical-surgical nursing: clinical management for positive outcomes* (6th ed.). Philadelphia: W.B. Saunders, p. 1722.

---

8. A nurse is planning to teach a client who has recently been diagnosed with tuberculosis (TB) on how to prevent the spread of TB. Which of the following instructions would be least effective in preventing the spread of TB?
    1. Teach the client to cover the mouth when coughing
    2. Teach the client to sterilize dishes at home
    3. Teach the client to properly dispose of Kleenex
    4. Teach the client that close contacts should be tested for TB

Answer: 2
Rationale: Options 1, 3, and 4 would assist in breaking the chain of infection. Option 2 would not only be impractical, but there is no evidence to suggest that sterilizing dishes would break the chain of infection with pulmonary TB.

Test-Taking Strategy: Focus on the issue: to prevent the spread of TB. Use the process of elimination noting the key words *least effective*. Recalling the methods of transmission of TB will direct you to option 2. Review home care principles related to TB if you had difficulty with this question.

Level of Cognitive Ability: Application
Client Needs: Safe, Effective Care Environment
Integrated Concept/Process: Teaching/Learning
Content Area: Adult Health/Respiratory

Reference:
Black, J., Hawks, J., & Keene, A. (2001). *Medical-surgical nursing: clinical management for positive outcomes* (6th ed.). Philadelphia: W.B. Saunders, p. 345.

9. A client is being discharged to go home after abdominal surgery with a heparin lock (intermittent IV catheter) to receive a week of antibiotic IV therapy at home. When evaluating the discharge teaching, which of the following statements by the client indicates the need for further instruction?

  1. "I'll examine the IV site frequently."
  2. "If the IV site becomes wet or moist it can air dry."
  3. "Pain, redness, and swelling should be reported to the physician."
  4. "If the lock or catheter accidentally comes out, I'll apply pressure to the site."

Answer: 2

Rationale: Clients who will be at home with an IV site should be instructed on site assessment as well as complications to report to the physician. Clients should also know how to treat complications such as bleeding at the IV site. Clients should be aware that if the dressing is wet or soiled, it needs to be changed immediately to prevent infection.

Test-Taking Strategy: Using the process of elimination and principles related to asepsis will easily direct you to option 2. Review these principles if you had difficulty with this question.

Level of Cognitive Ability: Comprehension
Client Needs: Safe, Effective Care Environment
Integrated Concept/Process: Teaching/Learning
Content Area: Fundamental Skills

Reference:
Potter, P., & Perry, A. (2001). *Fundamentals of nursing* (5th ed.). St. Louis: Mosby, p. 1235.

---

10. A nurse reinforces instructions to a client with jaundice who is experiencing pruritus. The nurse avoids telling the client to:

  1. Wear loose cotton clothing
  2. Use tepid water for bathing
  3. Maintain a warm house temperature
  4. Take the prescribed antihistamines to relieve the itch

Answer: 3

Rationale: Pruritus is caused by the accumulation of bile salts in the skin and results from obstructed biliary excretion. Antihistamines may relieve the itching as will tepid water or emollient baths. The client should avoid the use of alkaline soap and wear loose, soft cotton clothing. The client is instructed to keep the house temperature cool.

Test-Taking Strategy: Use the process of elimination noting the key word *avoids*. Recalling that heat causes vasodilation will assist in answering this question. This principle should direct you to option 3 as the measure to avoid in the treatment of pruritus. If you had difficulty with this question, review the measures that assist in alleviating pruritus.

Level of Cognitive Ability: Application
Client Needs: Health Promotion and Maintenance
Integrated Concept/Process: Teaching/Learning
Content Area: Adult Health/Gastrointestinal

Reference:
Black, J., Hawks, J., & Keene, A. (2001). *Medical-surgical nursing: clinical management for positive outcomes* (6th ed.). Philadelphia: W.B. Saunders, p. 1286.

---

11. A nurse reinforces home care instructions to a client hospitalized for a transurethral resection of the prostate (TURP). Which statement by the client indicates the need for further instructions?

  1. "I should avoid strenuous activity for 4 to 6 weeks."
  2. "I should maintain a daily intake of 6 to 8 glasses of water daily."

Answer: 3

Rationale: The client should be advised to avoid strenuous activity for 4 to 6 weeks and to avoid lifting items weighing more than 20 pounds. The client should consume a daily intake of at least 6 to 8 glasses of nonalcoholic fluids to minimize clot formation. Straining during defecation is avoided to prevent bleeding. Prune juice is a satisfactory bowel stimulant.

n lift and push objects up to 30
nds in weight."
hould include prune juice in
iet."

Test-Taking Strategy: Use the process of elimination, noting the key words *need for further instructions*. Options 1 and 2 can be easily eliminated. Because of the anatomical location of the surgical procedure, it would be reasonable to think that constipation should be avoided; therefore eliminate option 4. Items weighing 30 pounds are excessive. Review TURP discharge teaching points if you had difficulty with this question.

Level of Cognitive Ability: Application
Client Needs: Health Promotion and Maintenance
Integrated Concept/Process: Teaching/Learning
Content Area: Adult Health/Renal

Reference:

Black, J., Hawks, J., & Keene, A. (2001). *Medical-surgical nursing: clinical management for positive outcomes* (6th ed.). Philadelphia: W.B. Saunders, p. 949.

---

12. A nurse is reinforcing home care instructions to a client who will be receiving IV therapy at home. The nurse teaches the client that the most important action to prevent an infection from the IV site is to:
    1. Check the IV site carefully every day for redness and edema
    2. Re-dress the IV site daily, cleansing it with alcohol
    3. Carefully wash hands with antibacterial soap before working with the IV site or equipment
    4. Change IV tubing and fluid containers daily

Answer: 3
Rationale: While assessment of the IV site is important, it will not actively prevent an infection. IV sites do not need to be re-dressed daily unless the dressing becomes soiled, wet, or loose. Whereas IV containers should be changed daily, tubing should be changed only every 48 to 72 hours, based on the Centers for Disease Control guidelines. It is extremely important for the client to understand the absolute necessity of hand washing before working with IV fluids.

Test-Taking Strategy: Use the process of elimination. Note the key words *most important* and focus on the issue, preventing infection. Remember, the top priority in infection prevention always includes proper hand washing technique. Review universal precautions and its role in preventing infection if you had difficulty with this question.

Level of Cognitive Ability: Application
Client Needs: Safe, Effective Care Environment
Integrated Concept/Process: Teaching/Learning
Content Area: Fundamental Skills

Reference:

Potter, P., & Perry, A. (2001). *Fundamentals of nursing* (5th ed.). St. Louis: Mosby, p. 1235.

---

13. A 64-year-old client is being treated for an atrial dysrhythmia with quinidine gluconate (Duraquin), and the nurse reinforces instructions to the client about the medication. Which statement by the client indicates that the instructions have been effective?
    1. "If I miss a dose, I take two doses of the medication at the next scheduled time."
    2. "If I miss a dose, I should call my doctor."

Answer: 4
Rationale: The client should be instructed not to take an extra dose. The client should be instructed to take the medication if remembered within 2 hours of the missed dose, or to omit the dose and then resume the normal schedule. Quinidine gluconate must be taken exactly as prescribed. There is no need to call the doctor.

Test-Taking Strategy: Use the process of elimination and general principles related to medication administration. Eliminate option 1 because this action is inaccurate and could cause toxic effects. There is no need to call the doctor unless toxic effects

3. "If I miss a dose, I should take the dose in the evening if I remember."

4. "If I miss a dose, I should take the next prescribed dose as usual."

occur; therefore eliminate option 2. From the remaining options, recalling that a missed dose can be taken within 2 hours if remembered will direct you to option 4. If you had difficulty with this question, review the basic principles associated with medication administration.

Level of Cognitive Ability: Comprehension
Client Needs: Health Promotion and Maintenance
Integrated Concept/Process: Teaching/Learning
Content Area: Pharmacology

Reference:
Hodgson, B., & Kizior, R. (2003). *Saunders nursing drug handbook 2003.* Philadelphia: W.B. Saunders, p. 956.

---

14. A client asks the nurse for a recommendation about how to prevent fires and burn injury. The nurse tells the client that the one single intervention that has been shown to decrease the risk of dying in a residential fire is:

1. The installation of a sprinkler system

2. Fire extinguishers placed in key areas such as the kitchen, near the furnace, and near the hot water heater

3. The use of operable smoke detectors

4. Installation of fire resistant drywall panels throughout the house

Answer: 3
Rationale: Early detection of smoke and, subsequently, immediate evacuation from the house have been shown to significantly impact mortality. The installation of a sprinkler system is expensive and not usually used in residential situations. Fire extinguishers are important to have in the kitchen for small fires, but they are unrealistic and dangerous to use to attempt to extinguish large fires. Although fire-resistant products may help slow down a blaze, fire-resistant products can eventually catch on fire.

Test-Taking Strategy: Use the process of elimination. Look for the health prevention measure that is simple to implement and will alert individuals of the need to evacuate a residence. This will direct you to option 3. If you had difficulty with this question, review fire safety.

Level of Cognitive Ability: Application
Client Needs: Safe, Effective Care Environment
Integrated Concept/Process: Teaching/Learning
Content Area: Fundamental Skills

Reference:
Potter, P., & Perry, A. (2001). *Fundamentals of nursing* (5th ed.). St. Louis: Mosby, p. 1021.

---

15. A client has had same-day surgery to insert a ventilating tube in the tympanic membrane. The nurse determines that the client understands the discharge instructions if the client states to:

1. Use a shower cap if taking a shower

2. Swim only with the head above water

3. Wash the hair quickly in 2 minutes or less

4. Avoid taking any medication for pain

Answer: 1
Rationale: After insertion of tubes in the tympanic membrane, it is important to avoid getting water in the ears. For this reason, swimming, showering, or washing the hair is avoided after surgery until the time frame designated for each is identified by the surgeon. A shower cap or ear plug may be used when showering, if allowed by the physician. The client should take medication as advised for postoperative discomfort.

Test-Taking Strategy: Use the process of elimination noting the key words *understands the discharge instructions.* Eliminate option 2 because of the absolute word *only* and option 3 because of the word *quickly.* From the remaining options, focusing on the anatomical location of the surgery will direct you to option 1.

Review client instructions after this type of surgery if you had difficulty with this question.

Level of Cognitive Ability: Comprehension
Client Needs: Health Promotion and Maintenance
Integrated Concept/Process: Teaching/Learning
Content Area: Adult Health/Ear

Reference:
Black, J., Hawks, J., & Keene, A. (2001). *Medical-surgical nursing: clinical management for positive outcomes* (6th ed.). Philadelphia: W.B. Saunders, p. 1846.

---

16. A nurse has completed diet teaching for a client on a low-sodium diet for the treatment of hypertension. The nurse determines that further teaching is necessary if the client makes which of these statements?
1. "This diet will help to lower my blood pressure."
2. "The reason I need to lower my salt intake is to reduce fluid retention."
3. "This diet is not a replacement for my antihypertensive medications."
4. "Frozen foods are lowest in sodium."

Answer: 4
Rationale: A low-sodium diet is used as an adjunct to antihypertensive medications for the treatment of hypertension. Sodium retains fluid, which leads to hypertension secondary to increased fluid volume. Frozen foods use salt as a preservative and should not be encouraged as part of a low-sodium diet.

Test-Taking Strategy: Note the key words *further teaching is necessary*. Use the process of elimination and eliminate options 1, 2, and 3 because these are accurate statements related to hypertension. If you had difficulty with this question, review the treatment of hypertension and foods high in sodium.

Level of Cognitive Ability: Comprehension
Client Needs: Health Promotion and Maintenance
Integrated Concept/Process: Teaching/Learning
Content Area: Adult Health/Cardiovascular

Reference:
Black, J., Hawks, J., & Keene, A. (2001). *Medical-surgical nursing: clinical management for positive outcomes* (6th ed.). Philadelphia: W.B. Saunders, p. 1388.

---

17. A nurse reinforces home care instructions for the parents of a child with generalized tonic-clonic seizures who is being treated with oral phenytoin (Dilantin). The nurse includes instructions about:
1. Monitoring the child's intake and output daily
2. Checking the child's blood pressure before the administration of the medication
3. Providing oral hygiene, especially care of the gums
4. Administering the medication 1 hour before food intake

Answer: 3
Rationale: Phenytoin causes gum bleeding and hyperplasia; therefore a soft toothbrush and gum massage should be instituted to diminish this complication and prevent trauma. Options 1 and 2 are incorrect because the intake and output, as well as the blood pressure, are not affected by this medication. Option 4 is incorrect because directions for administration of this medication includes to take with food to minimize gastrointestinal upset.

Test-Taking Strategy: Use the process of elimination. Correlate phenytoin with gum bleeding and hyperplasia. Also, note the word *oral* in the question and in the correct option. Review the side effects and the method of administration of this medication if you had difficulty with this question.

Level of Cognitive Ability: Application
Client Needs: Health Promotion and Maintenance
Integrated Concept/Process: Teaching/Learning
Content Area: Pharmacology

Reference:
Hodgson, B., & Kizior, R. (2003). *Saunders nursing drug handbook 2003.* Philadelphia: W.B. Saunders, p. 889.

---

18. A nurse notes that a pregnant client is at risk for toxoplasmosis. The nurse would teach the client which of the following to prevent exposure to this disease?
1. Wash hands only before meals
2. Eat raw meats
3. Avoid exposure to litter boxes used by cats
4. Use topical corticosteroid treatments prophylactically

Answer: 3
Rationale: Infected cats transmit toxoplasmosis through the feces. Handling litter boxes can transmit the disease to the pregnant client. Meats that are undercooked can harbor microorganisms that can cause infection. Hands should be washed frequently throughout the day. The use of topical corticosteroids will not prevent exposure to the disease.

Test-Taking Strategy: Use the process of elimination. Eliminate option 1 because of the absolute word *only*. Option 2 represents an extreme statement and can also be eliminated. Focusing on the key words *prevent exposure* will direct you to option 3. Review the causes of toxoplasmosis if you had difficulty with this question.

Level of Cognitive Ability: Application
Client Needs: Health Promotion and Maintenance
Integrated Concept/Process: Teaching/Learning
Content Area: Maternity

Reference:
Murray, S., McKinney, E., & Gorrie, T. (2002). *Foundations of maternal-newborn nursing* (3rd ed.). Philadelphia: W.B. Saunders, p. 728.

---

19. A nurse is instructing the mother of a child with cystic fibrosis (CF) about appropriate dietary measures. The nurse tells the mother that the child should consume a:
1. Low-calorie, low-fat diet
2. High-calorie, high-protein diet
3. Low-calorie, low-protein diet
4. High-calorie, restricted fat

Answer: 2
Rationale: Children with CF are managed with a high-calorie, high-protein diet. Pancreatic enzyme replacement therapy and fat-soluble vitamin supplements are administered. Fat restriction is not necessary.

Test-Taking Strategy: Use the process of elimination. Eliminate options 1 and 4 first because they are similar. Thinking about the pathophysiology related to CF will direct you to option 2 from the remaining options. If you are unfamiliar with the diet plan for the child with CF, review these measures.

Level of Cognitive Ability: Application
Client Needs: Physiological Integrity
Integrated Concept/Process: Teaching/Learning
Content Area: Child Health

Reference:
Wong, D., & Hockenberry-Eaton, M. (2001). *Wong's essentials of pediatric nursing* (6th ed.). St. Louis: Mosby, p. 864.

---

20. A nurse in the ambulatory care unit is reviewing the surgical instructions with a client who will be admitted for knee replacement surgery. The nurse informs the

Answer: 2
Rationale: It is best to determine crutch walking ability and instruct the client in the use of crutches before surgery because this task can be difficult to learn when the client is in pain

client that crutches will be needed for ambulation after surgery and that the client will be instructed in the use of the crutches:

1. At the time of discharge after surgery
2. Before surgery
3. On the second postoperative day
4. On the first postoperative day

postoperatively. Options 1, 3, and 4 are not the appropriate times to teach a client about crutch walking.

Test-Taking Strategy: Use the process of elimination. Note that options 1, 3, and 4 are similar because they all address the postoperative period. Review preoperative teaching principles if you had difficulty with this question.

Level of Cognitive Ability: Application
Client Needs: Health Promotion and Maintenance
Integrated Concept/Process: Teaching/Learning
Content Area: Adult Health/Musculoskeletal

Reference:
Black, J., Hawks, J., & Keene, A. (2001). *Medical-surgical nursing: clinical management for positive outcomes* (6th ed.). Philadelphia: W.B. Saunders, p. 564.

FILL-IN-THE-BLANK

A nurse tells a client that the physician prescribed ibuprofen (Advil) 0.4 Gm for mild pain. The client tells the nurse that the medication bottle states ibuprofen (Advil) 200 mg tablets and asks the nurse about the number of tablets to take. How many tablet(s) will the nurse instruct the client to take?
Answer: _____

Answer: 2 tablets
Rationale: Convert 0.4 Gm to mg. In the metric system, to convert larger to smaller multiply by 1000 or move the decimal 3 places to the right. Then, follow the following formula.

$$0.4 \text{ Gm} = 400 \text{ mg}$$

$$\frac{400 \text{ mg}}{200 \text{ mg}} \times 1 \text{ Tablet} = 2 \text{ tablets}$$

Test-Taking Strategy: Knowledge of the formula for the calculation of a medication is required to answer this question. Remember to convert grams to milligrams. Follow the formula and make sure that the calculated dose makes sense. If you had difficulty with this question, review conversions and calculations.

Level of Cognitive Ability: Application
Client Needs: Physiological Integrity
Integrated Concept/Process: Teaching/Learning
Content Area: Fundamental Skills

Reference:
Kee, J. & Marshall, S. (2000). *Clinical calculations: With applications to general and specialty areas* (4th ed.). Philadelphia: W.B. Saunders, p. 162.

MULTIPLE RESPONSE – SELECT ALL THAT APPLY

A nurse is monitoring a hospitalized client with diabetes mellitus for signs of hyperglycemia. Select all signs of hyperglycemia.
____ Hunger
____ Kussmaul's respirations

Answers:
____ Kussmaul's respirations
____ Excessive thirst
____ Increased urine output

_____ Sweating
_____ Excessive thirst
_____ Diaphoresis
_____ Increased urine output

Rationale: Signs of hyperglycemia include excessive thirst, fatigue, restlessness, confusion, weakness, Kussmaul's respirations, diuresis, and coma, when severe. If the client presents with these symptoms, the blood glucose level should be checked immediately. Hunger, sweating, and diaphoresis are signs of hypoglycemia.

Test-Taking Strategy: Focus on the issue, signs of hyperglycemia. Remember the 3 "Ps," polyuria, polydipsia, and polyphagia that is associated with hyperglycemia. Also, recall that in hyperglycemia, the rate and depth of respirations increase (Kussmaul's respirations). Review the signs of hyperglycemia if you had difficulty with this question.

Level of Cognitive Ability: Application
Client Needs: Physiological Integrity
Integrated Concept/Process: Nursing Process/Data Collection
Content Area: Adult Health/Endocrine

Reference:
Perry, A. & Potter, P. (2002). *Clinical nursing skills and techniques* (5th ed.). St. Louis: Mosby, p. 687.

REFERENCES

Black, J., Hawks, J., & Keene, A. (2001). *Medical-surgical nursing: clinical management for positive outcomes* (6th ed.). Philadelphia: W.B. Saunders.

Bauer, B., & Hill, S. (2000). *Mental health nursing.* Philadelphia: W.B. Saunders.

Burroughs, A., & Leifer, G. (2002). *Maternity nursing* (8th ed.). Philadelphia: W.B. Saunders.

Chernecky, C., & Berger, B. (2001). *Laboratory tests and diagnostic procedures* (3rd ed.). Philadelphia: W. B. Saunders.

Grodner, M., Anderson, S., & DeYoung, S. (2000). *Foundations and clinical applications of nutrition: a nursing approach.* St. Louis: Mosby.

Harkreader, H. (2000). *Fundamentals of nursing: caring and clinical judgment.* Philadelphia: W.B. Saunders.

Hodgson, B., & Kizior, R. (2003). *Saunders nursing drug handbook 2003.* Philadelphia: W.B. Saunders.

Ignatavicius, D., & Workman, M. (2002). *Medical-surgical nursing: critical thinking for collaborative care* (4th ed.). Philadelphia: W.B. Saunders.

Kee, J., & Marshall, S. (2000). *Clinical calculations: with applications to general and specialty areas* (4th ed.). Philadelphia: W.B. Saunders.

Lewis, S., Heitkemper, M., & Dirksen, S. (2000). *Medical-surgical nursing: assessment and management of clinical problems* (5th ed.). St. Louis: Mosby.

Lowdermilk, D., Perry, S., & Bobak, I. (2000). *Maternity & women's health care* (7th ed.). St. Louis: Mosby.

McKinney, E., Ashwill, J., Murray, S. et al. (2000). *Maternal-child nursing.* Philadelphia: W.B Saunders.

Murray, S., McKinney, E., & Gorrie, T. (2002). *Foundations of maternal-newborn nursing* (3rd ed.). Philadelphia: W.B. Saunders.

Perry, A., & Potter, P. (2002). *Clinical nursing skills and techniques* (5th ed.). St. Louis: Mosby.

Phipps, W., Monahan, F., Sands, J. et al. (2003). *Medical-surgical nursing: health and illness perspectives* (7th ed.). St Louis: Mosby.

Potter, P., & Perry, A. (2001). *Fundamentals of nursing* (5th ed.). St. Louis: Mosby.

Schulte, E., Price, D., & Gwin, J. (2001). *Thompson's pediatric nursing* (8th ed.). Philadelphia: W.B. Saunders.

Varcarolis, E. (2002). *Foundations of psychiatric mental health nursing* (4th ed.). Philadelphia: W.B. Saunders.

Williams, S. (2001). *Basic nutrition & diet therapy* (11th ed.). St. Louis: Mosby.

Wong, D., & Hockenberry-Eaton, M. (2001). *Wong's essentials of pediatric nursing* (6th ed.). St. Louis: Mosby.

Comprehensive Test

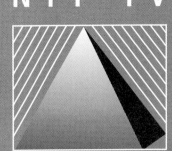

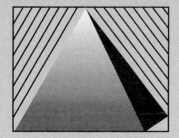

Comprehensive Test

1. A nurse is preparing to care for a client with a diagnosis of Meniere's disease. The nurse reviews the physician orders and expects to note that which of the following dietary measures is prescribed?

  1. Low-fiber diet with decreased fluids
  2. Low-sodium diet and fluid restriction
  3. Low-carbohydrate diet and the elimination of red meats
  4. Low-fat diet and restriction of citrus fruits

Answer: 2

Rationale: Dietary changes such as salt and fluid restrictions that reduce the amount of endolymphatic fluid is sometimes prescribed for clients with Meniere's disease. Options 1, 3, and 4 are not prescribed for this disorder.

Test-Taking Strategy: Use the process of elimination and focus on the client's diagnosis. Recalling that salt and fluid restrictions are sometimes necessary to reduce the amount of endolymphatic fluid will assist in directing you to option 2. Review the pathophysiology related to this condition and the treatment if you had difficulty with this question.

Level of Cognitive Ability: Analysis
Client Needs: Physiological Integrity
Integrated Concept/Process: Nursing Process/Planning
Content Area: Adult Health/Ear

Reference:
Black, J., Hawks, J., & Keene, A. (2001). *Medical-surgical nursing: clinical management for positive outcomes* (6th ed.). Philadelphia: W.B. Saunders, p. 1848.

---

2. A nurse is collecting data from a client who is taking prazosin (Minipress). Which of the following client statements would support the nursing diagnosis of noncompliance with medication therapy?

  1. "I don't understand why I have to keep taking the pills when my blood pressure is normal."
  2. "I can't see the numbers on the label to know how much salt is in food."
  3. "If I feel dizzy, I'll skip my dose for a few days."
  4. "If I have a cold, I'll shouldn't take any over-the-counter remedies without consulting my doctor."

Answer: 3

Rationale: Side effects of prazosin are dizziness and impotence. The client should be instructed to call the physician if these side effects occur. Holding (skipping) medication causes an abrupt rise in blood pressure. Option 1 indicates a knowledge deficit. Option 2 indicates a self-care deficit. Option 4 indicates client understanding regarding the medication.

Test-Taking Strategy: Use the process of elimination. Focus on the nursing diagnosis, noncompliance, to select the correct option. Noting the key words *I'll skip my dose* will direct you to option 3. Review the defining characteristics of noncompliance if you had difficulty with this question.

Level of Cognitive Ability: Analysis

Client Needs: Health Promotion and Maintenance
Integrated Concept/Process: Nursing Process/Data Collection
Content Area: Pharmacology

Reference:
Hodgson, B., & Kizior, R. (2003). *Saunders nursing drug handbook 2003.* Philadelphia: W.B. Saunders, p. 915.

---

3. A client with a history of self-managed peptic ulcer disease has frequently used excessive amounts of oral antacids. The nurse interprets that this client is most at risk for which acid-base disturbance?
1. Metabolic acidosis
2. Metabolic alkalosis
3. Respiratory alkalosis
4. Respiratory acidosis

Answer: 2
Rationale: Oral antacids commonly contain bicarbonate, or other alkaline components. These bind onto the hydrochloric acid in the stomach to neutralize the acid. Excessive use of oral antacids containing bicarbonate can cause a metabolic alkalosis over time. Options 1, 3, and 4 are incorrect.

Test-Taking Strategy: Use the process of elimination. Note that the question indicates that the problem is not respiratory in nature. With this in mind, eliminate options 3 and 4 first. Choose correctly from the remaining options knowing that the word *antacid* must work *against* acids. Review the causes of metabolic alkalosis if you had difficulty with the question.

Level of Cognitive Ability: Analysis
Client Needs: Physiological Integrity
Integrated Concept/Process: Nursing Process/Data Collection
Content Area: Fundamental Skills

Reference:
Ignatavicius, D., & Workman, M. (2002). *Medical-surgical nursing: critical thinking for collaborative care* (4th ed.). Philadelphia: W.B. Saunders, p. 230.

---

4. A nurse is collecting data from a 39-year-old Caucasian female client. The client has a blood pressure (BP) of 152/92 mmHg at rest, total cholesterol of 190 mg/dL, and a fasting blood glucose level of 114 mg/dL. The nurse would place priority on which risk factor for coronary artery disease (CAD) in this client?
1. Age
2. Hyperlipidemia
3. Hypertension
4. Glucose intolerance

Answer: 3
Rationale: Hypertension, cigarette smoking, and hyperlipidemia are major risk factors of CAD. Glucose intolerance, obesity, and response to stress are also contributing factors. Age greater than 40 years is a nonmodifiable risk factor. A cholesterol level of 190 mg/dL and a blood glucose level of 114 mg/dL are within the normal range. The nurse places priority on major risk factors that need modification.

Test-Taking Strategy: Use the process of elimination. Focus on the data in the question and note the key word *priority.* Note that the only abnormal value is the BP. This will direct you to option 3. Review the risk factors associated with CAD if you had difficulty with this question.

Level of Cognitive Ability: Analysis
Client Needs: Health Promotion and Maintenance
Integrated Concept/Process: Nursing Process/Data Collection
Content Area: Adult Health/Cardiovascular

Reference:
Ignatavicius, D., & Workman, M. (2002). *Medical-surgical nursing: critical thinking for collaborative care* (4th ed.). Philadelphia: W.B. Saunders, pp. 792, 812-813.

5. A nurse is caring for a client who has just returned to the nursing unit after an intravenous pyelogram (IVP). The nurse determines that which of the following is a priority in the postprocedure care of this client?
1. Encouraging increased intake of oral fluids
2. Ambulating the client in the hallway
3. Encouraging the client to try to void frequently
4. Maintaining the client on bed rest

Answer: 1
Rationale: After IVP the client should increase fluid intake to aid clearance of the dye used for the procedure. It is unnecessary to void frequently after the procedure. The client is usually allowed activity as tolerated, without any specific activity guidelines.

Test-Taking Strategy: Use the process of elimination and note the key word *priority*. Option 3 has no useful purpose and is eliminated first. From the remaining options, recall that there are no specific activity guidelines after this procedure. Also, recall that fluids are necessary to promote clearance of the dye from the client's system. Review this procedure if you had difficulty with this question.

Level of Cognitive Ability: Analysis
Client Needs: Physiological Integrity
Integrated Concept/Process: Nursing Process/Planning
Content Area: Adult Health/Renal

Reference:
Ignatavicius, D., & Workman, M. (2002). *Medical-surgical nursing: critical thinking for collaborative care* (4th ed.). Philadelphia: W.B. Saunders, p. 1609.

---

6. A client with advanced cirrhosis of the liver is not tolerating protein well, as evidenced by abnormal laboratory values. The nurse anticipates that which of the following medications will be prescribed for the client?
1. Lactulose (Chronulac)
2. Ethacrynic acid (Edecrin)
3. Folic acid (Folvite)
4. Thiamine (Vitamin B_1)

Answer: 1
Rationale: The client with cirrhosis has impaired ability to metabolize protein as a result of liver dysfunction. Administration of lactulose aids in the clearance of ammonia via the gastrointestinal (GI) tract. Ethacrynic acid is a diuretic. Folic acid and thiamine are vitamins, which may be used in clients with liver disease as supplemental therapy.

Test-Taking Strategy: Use the process of elimination. To answer this question correctly, it is necessary to know that ammonia levels are elevated with advanced liver disease, and that lactulose is a standard form of medication therapy for this condition. Review this disorder and the purpose of this medication if you had difficulty with this question.

Level of Cognitive Ability: Analysis
Client Needs: Physiological Integrity
Integrated Concept/Process: Nursing Process/Planning
Content Area: Pharmacology

Reference:
Hodgson, B., & Kizior, R. (2003). *Saunders nursing drug handbook 2003.* Philadelphia: W.B. Saunders, p. 638.

---

7. A nurse is caring for a child with renal disease and is analyzing the laboratory results. The nurse notes a sodium level of 148 mEq/L. Based on this finding, which clinical manifestation would the nurse expect to note in the child?

Answer: 3
Rationale: Hypernatremia occurs when the sodium level is greater that 145 mEq/L. Clinical manifestations include intense thirst, oliguria, agitation and restlessness, flushed skin, peripheral and pulmonary edema, dry sticky mucous membranes, and nausea and vomiting. Options 1, 2, and 4 are

1. Increased heart rate
2. Cold clammy skin
3. Dry, sticky mucous membranes
4. Lethargy

not associated with the clinical manifestations of hypernatremia.

Test-Taking Strategy: Use the process of elimination. First, determine that the sodium level is elevated and that the child is experiencing hypernatremia. Recalling the clinical manifestations associated with hypernatremia will direct you to option 3. Review the normal sodium level and clinical manifestations associated with an imbalance if you had difficulty with this question.

Level of Cognitive Ability: Analysis
Client Needs: Physiological Integrity
Integrated Concept/Process: Nursing Process/Data Collection
Content Area: Child Health

Reference:
McKinney, E., Ashwill, J., Murray, S. et al. (2000). *Maternal-child nursing:.* Philadelphia: W.B. Saunders, p. 1088.

---

8. A client is scheduled for a cardiac catheterization. Which of the following data, if noted in the client's health record, must the nurse report to the physician before the catheterization?
1. Allergy to meperidine hydrochloride (Demerol)
2. Allergy to shellfish
3. History of coronary artery disease (CAD)
4. History of hypertension

Answer: 2
Rationale: The dye used during the catheterization contains iodine, so any allergies to shellfish or iodine should be reported immediately to prevent allergic reactions. An allergy to meperidine hydrochloride is not specifically related to a cardiac catheterization, although it must be noted on the client's record. CAD may be the reason for performing the cardiac catheterization and hypertension is normally associated with CAD.

Test-Taking Strategy: Use the process of elimination and recall that an allergy to shellfish is significant with any procedure requiring the instillation of a dye. Review preprocedure care for a client scheduled for a cardiac catheterization if you had difficulty with this question.

Level of Cognitive Ability: Application
Client Needs: Safe, Effective Care Environment
Integrated Concept/Process: Nursing Process/Implementation
Content Area: Fundamental Skills

Reference:
Black, J., Hawks, J., & Keene, A. (2001). *Medical-surgical nursing: clinical management for positive outcomes* (6th ed.). Philadelphia: W.B. Saunders, p. 198.

---

9. A child was diagnosed with acute poststreptococcal glomerulonephritis and renal insufficiency is suspected. Which of the following laboratory results will the nurse expect to note?
1. An elevated white blood cell (WBC) count
2. Negative red blood cells in the urinalysis
3. Negative protein in the urinalysis
4. An elevated blood urea nitrogen (BUN) and creatinine

Answer: 4
Rationale: In poststreptococcal glomerulonephritis, a urinalysis reveals hematuria with red cell casts. Proteinuria is also present. If renal insufficiency occurs, the BUN and creatinine levels are elevated. The WBC is usually within normal limits and mild anemia is common.

Test-Taking Strategy: Use the process of elimination focusing on the child's diagnosis. Recalling that the BUN and creatinine are laboratory studies that relate to the renal system will direct you to option 4. Review the clinical manifestations associated with this disorder if you had difficulty with this question.

Level of Cognitive Ability: Analysis
Client Needs: Physiological Integrity
Integrated Concept/Process: Nursing Process/Data Collection
Content Area: Child Health

Reference:
Wong, D., & Hockenberry-Eaton, M. (2001). *Wong's essentials of pediatric nursing* (6th ed.). St. Louis: Mosby, p. 1046-1047.

---

10. An infant is brought to the health care clinic, and the mother tells the nurse that her infant has been vomiting after meals and that the vomiting is now becoming more frequent and forceful and the infant seems to be constipated. During data collection, the nurse notes visible peristaltic waves moving from left to right across the abdomen. Based on this finding, the nurse would suspect which of the following?
  1. Colic
  2. Intussusception
  3. Pyloric stenosis
  4. Congenital megacolon

Answer: 3
Rationale: In pyloric stenosis, the vomitus contains sour, undigested food, but no bile; the child is constipated; and visible peristaltic waves move from left to right across the abdomen. A movable, palpable, firm olive-shaped mass in the right upper quadrant may be noted. Crying during the evening hours, appearing to be in pain, but eating well and gaining weight are clinical manifestations of colic. An infant who suddenly becomes pale, cries out, and draws the legs up to the chest is demonstrating physical signs of intussusception. Ribbonlike stool, bile-stained emesis, absence of peristalsis, and abdominal distention are symptoms of congenital megacolon (Hirschsprung's disease).

Test-Taking Strategy: Use the process of elimination. Focus on the data provided in the question. Consider each condition presented in the options and think about the clinical manifestations of each. Recalling the manifestations associated with pyloric stenosis will direct you to option 3. If you are unfamiliar with this disorder review its clinical manifestations.

Level of Cognitive Ability: Analysis
Client Needs: Physiological Integrity
Integrated Concept/Process: Nursing Process/Data Collection
Content Area: Child Health

Reference:
Wong, D., & Hockenberry-Eaton, M. (2001). *Wong's essentials of pediatric nursing* (6th ed.). St. Louis: Mosby, p. 922.

---

11. A nurse is reviewing the laboratory analysis of cerebrospinal fluid (CSF) obtained during a lumbar puncture from a child suspected of having bacterial meningitis. Which of the following results would most likely confirm this diagnosis?
  1. Cloudy CSF with low protein and low glucose
  2. Cloudy CSF with high protein and low glucose
  3. Clear CSF with low protein and low glucose
  4. Decreased pressure, cloudy CSF with high protein

Answer: 2
Rationale: A diagnosis of meningitis is made after testing CSF obtained by lumbar puncture. In the case of bacterial meningitis, findings usually include increased pressure, cloudy CSF, high protein, and low glucose. Options 1, 3, and 4 are incorrect.

Test-Taking Strategy: Use the process of elimination. Eliminate options 3 and 4 first because clear CSF and decreased pressure are not likely to be found with an infectious process such as meningitis. From the remaining options, recalling that high protein indicates a possible diagnosis of meningitis will direct you to option 2. If you had difficulty with this question, review this diagnostic test.

Level of Cognitive Ability: Analysis
Client Needs: Physiological Integrity

Integrated Concept/Process: Nursing Process/Data Collection
Content Area: Child Health

Reference:
McKinney, E., Ashwill, J., Murray, S. et al. (2000). *maternal-child nursing*. Philadelphia: W.B. Saunders, p. 1468.

---

12. A mother brings her child to the health care clinic for a routine examination. The mother tells the nurse that the teacher has reported that the child appears to be day-dreaming and starring off into space. The teacher tells the mother that this occurs numerous times throughout the day. The rest of the day the child is alert and participates in classroom activity. The nurse reports the findings to the registered nurse and suspects that which of the following are occurring with this child?

   1. The child has attention deficit hyper-activity syndrome and is in need of medication
   2. The child probably has school phobia
   3. The child is experiencing absence seizures
   4. The child is showing signs of a behavioral problem

Answer: 3
Rationale: Absence seizures are a type of generalized seizure that was formally known as petit mal seizures. They consist of a sudden, brief (no longer than 30 seconds) arrest of the child's motor activities accompanied by a blank stare and loss of awareness. The child's posture is maintained at the end of the seizure. The child returns to activity that was in process as though nothing happened. A child with attention deficit hyperactivity syndrome becomes easily distracted, is fidgety, and has difficulty following directions. School phobia includes physical symptoms that usually occur at home and may prevent the child from attending school. Behavior problems would be noted by more overt symptoms than described in this question.

Test-Taking Strategy: Use the process of elimination focusing on the information provided in the question to direct you to option 3. If you are unfamiliar with the characteristics associated with absence seizures, review this content.

Level of Cognitive Ability: Analysis
Client Needs: Physiological Integrity
Integrated Concept/Process: Nursing Process/Data Collection
Content Area: Child Health

Reference:
Wong, D., & Hockenberry-Eaton, M. (2001). *Wong's essentials of pediatric nursing* (6th ed.). St. Louis: Mosby, p. 1099.

---

13. A mother of a 3-week-old infant arrives at the well baby clinic for a rescreening test for phenylketonuria (PKU). The nurse reviews the results of the serum phenylalanine levels and notes that the level is 1.0 mg/dL. The nurse determines this level as:

   1. Normal
   2. Elevated indicating PKU
   3. Inconclusive
   4. Requiring a repeat study

Answer: 1
Rationale: The normal PKU level is less the 2 mg/dL. With early postpartum discharge, screening is often performed at less than 2 days of age because of concern that the infant will be lost to follow-up evaluation. Infants should be rescreened by 14 days of age if the initial screen was done at 24 to 48 hours after delivery.

Test-Taking Strategy: Use the process of elimination and knowledge regarding the normal phenylalanine level. Recalling that the normal level is less the 2 mg/dL will direct you to option 1. Review this content if you are unfamiliar with this screening test.

Level of Cognitive Ability: Comprehension
Client Needs: Physiological Integrity
Integrated Concept/Process: Nursing Process/Data Collection
Content Area: Child Health

Reference:
Wong, D., & Hockenberry-Eaton, M. (2001). *Wong's essentials of pediatric nursing* (6th ed.). St. Louis: Mosby, p. 319.

14. A nurse is caring for a client with an intracranial aneurysm. The nurse determines that which of the following is related to dysfunction of cranial nerve III (oculomotor)?

1. Mild drowsiness
2. Less frequent spontaneous speech
3. Slight slurring of speech
4. Ptosis of the left eyelid

Answer: 4
Rationale: Ptosis of the eyelid is due to pressure on and dysfunction of cranial nerve III. Options 1, 2, and 3 identify early signs of a deteriorating level of consciousness.

Test-Taking Strategy: Use the process of elimination. Note the key words *cranial nerve III (oculomotor)*. Recalling the function of this nerve will direct you to option 4. Review the function of cranial nerve III if you had difficulty with this question.

Level of Cognitive Ability: Analysis
Client Needs: Physiological Integrity
Integrated Concept/Process: Nursing Process/Data Collection
Content Area: Adult Health/Neurological

Reference:
Black, J., Hawks, J., & Keene, A. (2001). *Medical-surgical nursing: clinical management for positive outcomes* (6th ed.). Philadelphia: W.B. Saunders, p. 1885.

---

15. A client with thrombotic cerebrovascular accident (CVA) experiences periods of emotional lability. The client alternately laughs and cries and intermittently becomes irritable and demanding. The nurse determines that this behavior indicates that:

1. The problem is likely to get worse before it gets better
2. The client is experiencing the usual sequelae of a CVA
3. The client is not adapting well to the disability
4. The client is experiencing side effects of prescribed anticoagulants

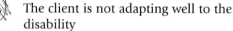

Answer: 2
Rationale: After CVA, the client often experiences periods of emotional lability, which is characterized by sudden bouts of laughing or crying, or by irritability, depression, confusion, or being demanding. This is a normal part of the clinical picture for the client with this health problem, although it may be difficult for health care personnel and family members to deal with. The other options are incorrect.

Test-Taking Strategy: Use the process of elimination. Eliminate options 1 and 4 first. Anticoagulants do not cause emotional lability, and there is no information in the question to support option 1. From the remaining options, recalling the emotional changes that accompany a CVA will direct you to option 2. Review the effects of a CVA if you had difficulty with this question.

Level of Cognitive Ability: Analysis
Client Needs: Psychosocial Integrity
Integrated Concept/Process: Nursing Process/Data Collection
Content Area: Adult Health/Neurological

Reference:
Black, J., Hawks, J., & Keene, A. (2001). *Medical-surgical nursing: clinical management for positive outcomes* (6th ed.). Philadelphia: W.B. Saunders, p. 1960.

---

16. A nurse is caring for a client with myasthenia gravis. The client is vomiting and complaining of abdominal cramps and diarrhea. The nurse also notes that the client is hypotensive and is experiencing facial muscle twitching. The nurse determines that these symptoms are compatible with:

1. Systemic infection
2. A reaction to plasmapheresis

Answer: 3
Rationale: Signs and symptoms of cholinergic crisis include nausea, vomiting, abdominal cramping, diarrhea, blurred vision, pallor, facial muscle twitching, pupillary myosis, and hypotension. Cholinergic crisis is due to overmedication with cholinergic (anticholinesterase) medications and is treated by withholding medications. Myasthenic crisis is an exacerbation of myasthenic symptoms caused by undermedication with anticholinesterase medications. There is no information in the question to support options 1, 2, and 4.

3. Cholinergic crisis
4. Myasthenic crisis

Test-Taking Strategy: Use the process of elimination. Note the client's diagnosis and think about the treatment for this disorder. Recalling the effects of cholinergic medications and focusing on the data in the question will direct you to option 3. Review the clinical manifestations associated with cholinergic crisis if you had difficulty with this question.

Level of Cognitive Ability: Analysis
Client Needs: Physiological Integrity
Integrated Concept/Process: Nursing Process/Data Collection
Content Area: Adult Health/Neurological

Reference:
Black, J., Hawks, J., & Keene, A. (2001). *Medical-surgical nursing: clinical management for positive outcomes* (6th ed.). Philadelphia: W.B. Saunders, p. 2022.

---

17. A nurse determines that health teaching regarding arteriosclerosis has been successful when the client describes the condition as:
1. Fatty plaques lining the arteries
2. Loss of elasticity of the veins
3. Hardening of the arteries
4. Loss of muscle mass around the heart

Answer: 3
Rationale: Arteriosclerosis is described as hardening of the arteries. Option 1 describes atherosclerosis, and options 2 and 4 are normal age-related changes in older individuals.

Test-Taking Strategy: Focusing on the word *arteriosclerosis* will assist in eliminating options 2 and 4. Recalling that *atherosclerosis* relates to fatty plaques will direct you to option 3. Review these disorders if you had difficulty with this question.

Level of Cognitive Ability: Comprehension
Client Needs: Health Promotion and Maintenance
Integrated Concept/Process: Teaching/Learning
Content Area: Fundamental Skills

Reference:
Ignatavicius, D., & Workman, M. (2002). *Medical surgical nursing: critical thinking for collaborative care* (4th ed.). Philadelphia: W. B. Saunders, p. 728.

---

18. A nurse is collecting data from a Hispanic client regarding medication history. The nurse understands that people from this cultural group:
1. Are offended if direct eye contact is made by the interviewer
2. Often use home remains in addition to prescription medications
3. Often defer all questions to the male members of the family
4. Do not permit blood transfusions

Answer: 2
Rationale: Hispanics commonly use a folk healer and home remedies. Options 1, 3, and 4 are not common in this culture.

Test-Taking Strategy: Knowledge regarding the cultural practices of the Hispanic population is required to answer this question. If you are unfamiliar with these cultural practices, review this content.

Level of Cognitive Ability: Comprehension
Client Needs: Psychosocial Integrity
Integrated Concept/Process: Cultural Awareness
Content Area: Fundamental Skills

Reference:
Potter, P., & Perry, A. (2001). *Fundamentals of nursing* (5th ed.). St. Louis: Mosby, pp. 126-128.

19. A client is admitted to the hospital with chest pain and a myocardial infarction is suspected. The nurse informs the client about the importance of notifying a staff member immediately if pain occurs, knowing that the most common reaction exhibited by clients with initial chest pain is:

1. Denial
2. Anger
3. Depression
4. Hostility

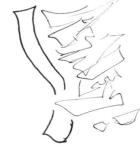

Answer: 1

Rationale: Most clients experiencing chest discomfort use rationalization and deny that they are experiencing pain. Anger, depression, and hostility may occur, but denial and rationalization are the most common reactions.

Test-Taking Strategy: Knowledge that denial is the most common defense mechanism exhibited by clients with chest pain is required to answer this question. Review the psychosocial impact related to chest pain and cardiac disease if you had difficulty with this question.

Level of Cognitive Ability: Comprehension
Client Needs: Psychosocial Integrity
Integrated Concept/Process: Nursing Process/Implementation
Content Area: Adult Health/Cardiovascular

Reference:
Black, J., Hawks, J., & Keene, A. (2001). *Medical-surgical nursing: clinical management for positive outcomes* (6th ed.). Philadelphia: W.B. Saunders, p. 1598.

---

20. A client diagnosed with angina is scheduled for an angioplasty. Which statement by the client indicates a need for further instruction?

1. "This test will clean out my arteries so that I can eat anything I choose."
2. "I should keep my leg with the dressing straight after the test."
3. "This procedure should help to make me pain free."
4. "I should follow suggested dietary restrictions and stop smoking."

Answer: 1

Rationale: Successful angioplasty may need to be repeated because of abrupt closure of the artery. Following recommended dietary and lifestyle changes assists in preventing further atherosclerosis and resultant angina. Options 2, 3, and 4 are correct statements to make after this procedure.

Test-Taking Strategy: Note the key words *a need for further instruction*. Use the process of elimination recalling that the client should follow recommended lifestyle changes to prevent further disease development. Review client instructions after this procedure if you had difficulty with this question.

Level of Cognitive Ability: Comprehension
Client Needs: Health Promotion and Maintenance
Integrated Concept/Process: Nursing Process/Evaluation
Content Area: Adult Health/Cardiovascular

Reference:
Black, J., Hawks, J., & Keene, A. (2001). *Medical-surgical nursing: clinical management for positive outcomes* (6th ed.). Philadelphia: W.B. Saunders, p. 1406.

---

21. A nurse is assigned to assist in caring for a client at risk for self-harm. The client says, "You won't have to worry about me much longer." The nurse interprets this statement as:

1. The expression of hopelessness
2. An expression of depression
3. An intention for self-mutilation
4. The intention of suicide

Answer: 4

Rationale: The client at risk for self-harm who says he or she will not be around much longer is expressing suicidal intent. An individual who is depressed is frequently suicidal. The individual with suicidal tendencies frequently does self-mutilating acts. However, the client's statement is a direct comment about the act.

Test-Taking Strategy: Use the process of elimination. Focusing on the client's statement will assist in directing you to option 4. Review the signs of suicide if you had difficulty with this question.

Level of Cognitive Ability: Comprehension
Client Needs: Psychosocial Integrity
Integrated Concept/Process: Nursing Process/Evaluation
Content Area: Mental Health

Reference:
Bauer, B., & Hill, S. (2000). *Mental health nursing.* Philadelphia: W.B. Saunders, pp. 195-196.

---

22. A nurse reviews home care management instructions with a client who was recently diagnosed with cirrhosis. Which client statement indicates a need for further education?

1. "I will take Tylenol if I get a headache."
2. "I will obtain adequate rest."
3. "I do not need to restrict fat in my diet."
4. "I should monitor my weight on a regular basis."

Answer: 1
Rationale: Acetaminophen (Tylenol) is avoided because it can cause fatal liver damage in the client with cirrhosis. Adequate rest and nutrition are important. Fat restriction is not necessary, and the diet should supply sufficient carbohydrates with a total daily intake of 2000 to 3000 calories. The client's weight should be monitored on a regular basis.

Test-Taking Strategy: Note the key words *need for further education.* Options 2 and 4 can be easily eliminated. Recalling that acetaminophen is hepatotoxic will assist in directing you to the correct option. Review medications that are restricted or are avoided in clients with cirrhosis if you had difficulty with this question.

Level of Cognitive Ability: Comprehension
Client Needs: Health Promotion and Maintenance
Integrated Concept/Process: Self-Care
Content Area: Adult Health/Gastrointestinal

Reference:
Ignatavicius, D., & Workman, M. (2002). *Medical-surgical nursing: critical thinking for collaborative care* (4th ed.). Philadelphia: W.B. Saunders, p. 1313.

---

23. A client who has a history of gout is also diagnosed with urolithiasis. The stones are determined to be of the uric acid type. The nurse gives the client instructions to avoid which food items?

1. Liver
2. Apples
3. Carrots
4. Milk

Answer: 1
Rationale: Foods containing high amounts of purines should be avoided in the client with uric acid stones. This includes limiting or avoiding organ meats, such as liver, brain, heart, kidney, and sweetbreads. Other foods to avoid include herring, sardines, anchovies, meat extracts, consommés, and gravies. Foods that are low in purines include all fruits, many vegetables, milk, cheese, eggs, refined cereals, sugars and sweets, coffee, tea, chocolate, and carbonated beverages.

Test-Taking Strategy: Note the key word *avoid.* To answer this question, begin by examining the options and classifying the types of food sources they represent. Options 2 and 3 represent foods that are grown, whereas options 1 and 4 represent foods that derive from animal sources. Because purines are end products of protein metabolism, eliminate options 2 and 3 first. From the remaining options, you would need to know that organ meats such as liver provide a greater quantity of protein than does milk. With this in mind, choose option 1 as the food to avoid. Review foods high in purine if you had difficulty with this question.

Level of Cognitive Ability: Application

Client Needs: Health Promotion and Maintenance
Integrated Concept/Process: Teaching/Learning
Content Area: Fundamental Skills

Reference:
Williams, S. (2001) *Basic nutrition & diet therapy* (11th ed.). St. Louis: Mosby, p. 415.

---

24. A client tells the nurse that the client gets dizzy and lightheaded with each use of the incentive spirometer. The nurse asks the client to demonstrate the use of the device, expecting that the client is:
1. Not forming a tight seal around the mouthpiece
2. Inhaling too slowly
3. Not resting adequately between breaths
4. Rebreathing exhaled air

Answer: 3
Rationale: If the client does not breathe normally between incentive spirometer breaths, hyperventilation and fatigue can result. Hyperventilation is the most common cause of respiratory alkalosis, which is characterized by light-headedness and dizziness.

Test-Taking Strategy: To answer this question easily, evaluate each of the possible options to see if they would be expected to cause dizziness or light-headedness in the client. Only option 3, not resting adequately between breaths, would result in hyperventilation and subsequent dizziness or light-headedness. Options 1 and 2 would result in ineffective use, and option 4 would result in mental cloudiness. Review the appropriate use of an incentive spirometer if you had difficulty with this question.

Level of Cognitive Ability: Comprehension
Client Needs: Health Promotion and Maintenance
Integrated Concept/Process: Nursing Process/Evaluation
Content Area: Adult Health/Respiratory

Reference:
Ignatavicius, D., & Workman, M. (2002). *Medical-surgical nursing: critical thinking for collaborative care* (4th ed.). Philadelphia: W.B. Saunders, pp. 251-252.

---

25. A nurse is participating in a health-screening clinic. The nurse interprets that which of the following clients has the greatest need for instruction to lower the risk of developing respiratory disease?
1. A 50-year-old smoker with cracked asbestos lining on basement pipes in the home
2. A 40-year-old smoker who works in a hospital
3. A 36-year-old who works with pesticides
4. A 25-year-old who does woodworking as a hobby

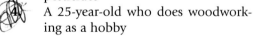

Answer: 1
Rationale: Smoking greatly enhances the client's risk of developing some form of respiratory disease. Other risk factors include exposure to harmful chemicals, airborne toxins, and dust or fumes. The client at greatest risk has two identified risk factors, one of which is smoking.

Test-Taking Strategy: Begin to answer this question by eliminating options 3 and 4 because the most harmful risk factor for the respiratory system is smoking. Select option 1 instead of option 2 because asbestos is toxic to the lungs if particles are inhaled. Also, option 1 identifies two risk factors, but the other options identify only one risk factor. Review the risk factors associated with respiratory disease if you had difficulty with this question.

Level of Cognitive Ability: Comprehension
Client Needs: Health Promotion and Maintenance
Integrated Concept/Process: Nursing Process/Data Collection
Content Area: Adult Health/Respiratory

Reference:
Black, J., Hawks, J., & Keene, A. (2001). *Medical-surgical nursing: clinical management for positive outcomes* (6th ed.). Philadelphia: W.B. Saunders, p. 1693.

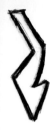

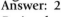

26. A female client is being discharged to home with an indwelling urinary catheter after surgical repair of a bladder that was injured as a result of trauma. The nurse concludes that the client understands the principles of catheter management if the client states to:

1. Cleanse the perineal area with soap and water once a day
2. Keep the drainage bag lower than the level of the bladder
3. Limit fluid intake so that the bag won't become full so quickly
4. Coil the tubing and place it under the thigh when sitting to avoid tugging on the bladder

Answer: 2
Rationale: The perineal area should be cleansed with soap and water twice a day and after each bowel movement. The drainage bag should be lower than the level of the bladder, and the tubing should be free of kinks and compression. Adequate fluid intake is necessary to prevent infection and to provide natural irrigation of the catheter from increased urine flow.

Test-Taking Strategy: Use the process of elimination. Option 4 is eliminated first because sitting on coiled tubing could cause compression and obstruct drainage. Eliminate option 3 next, knowing that increasing fluids is important. From the remaining options, noting that option 1 is insufficient in frequency would guide you to choose option 2 as correct. Option 2 is also correct because this action is consistent with principles of catheter management. Review these principles if you had difficulty with this question.

Level of Cognitive Ability: Comprehension
Client Needs: Safe, Effective Care Environment
Integrated Concept/Process: Self-Care
Content Area: Fundamental Skills

Reference:
Black, J., Hawks, J., & Keene, A. (2001). *Medical-surgical nursing: clinical management for positive outcomes* (6th ed.). Philadelphia: W.B. Saunders, p. 832.

---

27. A nurse is planning to reinforce instructions about caring for an ileal conduit with a client. The nurse plans to include which of the following items about ostomy care in discussions with the client?

1. Cut an opening in the faceplate of the appliance that is slightly smaller than the stoma
2. Plan to do appliance changes in the late evening hours
3. Limit fluids to minimize appliance odor caused by urine breakdown to ammonia
4. To cleanse the skin around the stoma, use mild soap and water; rinse and dry well

Answer: 4
Rationale: The skin around the stoma is cleansed at each appliance change using a mild, nonresidue soap and water. The skin is rinsed and then dried thoroughly. The appliance should be changed early in the morning when urine production is slowest because there is no fluid intake during sleep. The appliance is cut so that the opening is not more than 3 mm larger than the stoma. An opening smaller than the stoma prevents application of the appliance. Drinking fluids is encouraged to dilute the urine, thereby decreasing the incidence of odor.

Test-Taking Strategy: Use the process of elimination. Eliminate option 3 first. Limiting fluid intake will not limit ammonia odor; in fact; decreasing fluids will increase the concentration of the urine, making it stronger. Option 1 is eliminated next because an appliance cut in this way will be too small to fit over the stoma. From the remaining options, recalling that urine flow is slowest in the early morning from decreased intake during the night will direct you to option 4. Review these client teaching points if you had difficulty with this question.

Level of Cognitive Ability: Application
Client Needs: Health Promotion and Maintenance
Integrated Concept/Process: Nursing Process/Planning
Content Area: Adult Health/Renal

Reference:
Black, J., Hawks, J., & Keene, A. (2001). *Medical-surgical nursing: clinical management for positive outcomes* (6th ed.). Philadelphia: W.B. Saunders, p. 817.

28. A 24-year-old female with a familial history of heart disease presents to the physician's office asking to begin oral contraceptive therapy for birth control. The nurse would next inquire whether the client:

1. Has taken oral contraceptives before
2. Exercises regularly
3. Eats a low cholesterol diet
4. Is currently a smoker

Answer: 4

Rationale: Oral contraceptive use is a risk factor for heart disease, particularly when it is combined with cigarette smoking. Regular exercise and keeping total cholesterol levels under 200 mg/dL are general measures to decrease cardiovascular risk.

Test-Taking Strategy: Use the process of elimination. All options are partially correct because they relate either to cardiovascular disease risk factors or medication history. The question asks you to prioritize which option is most important by including the word *next* in the stem of the question. Use of oral contraceptives combined with smoking increases the risk of cardiovascular disease. Review these risks if you had difficulty with this question.

Level of Cognitive Ability: Comprehension
Client Needs: Health Promotion and Maintenance
Integrated Concept/Process: Nursing Process/Data Collection
Content Area: Adult Health/Cardiovascular

Reference:
Black, J., Hawks, J., & Keene, A. (2001). *Medical-surgical nursing: clinical management for positive outcomes* (6th ed.). Philadelphia: W.B. Saunders, p. 1448.

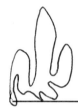

29. A nurse is implementing measures to maintain adequate peripheral tissue perfusion in a postcardiac surgery client. The nurse avoids which of the following while giving care to this client?

1. Range-of-motion (ROM) exercises to the feet
2. Application of compression stockings
3. Leg elevation while sitting in chair
4. Use of a knee gatch

Answer: 4

Rationale: After surgery, measures taken to prevent venous stasis include applying elastic stockings or leg wraps, using pneumatic compression boots, discouraging leg crossing, avoiding the use of a knee gatch or placing pillows in the popliteal area, and performing passive and active ROM. Leg elevation while sitting promotes venous drainage and helps prevent postoperative edema.

Test-Taking Strategy: Note the key word *avoids* and focus on the issue: maintaining adequate tissue perfusion. The use of a knee gatch is contraindicated because it puts pressure on blood vessels in the popliteal area, impeding venous return. Review these basic postoperative measures if you had difficulty with this question.

Level of Cognitive Ability: Application
Client Needs: Physiological Integrity
Integrated Concept/Process: Nursing Process/Implementation
Content Area: Adult Health/Cardiovascular

Reference:
Potter, P., & Perry, A. (2001). *Fundamentals of nursing* (5th ed.). St. Louis: Mosby, p. 1711.

30. The clinic nurse is instructing a client in the third trimester of pregnancy about measures to relieve heartburn. Which of the following instructions would the nurse provide to the client?

1. Eat fatty foods only once a day in the morning

Answer: 3

Rationale: Measures to relieve heartburn include small frequent meals and avoiding fatty fried foods, coffee, and cigarettes. Mild antacids can be used if they do not contain aspirin or sodium. Frequent sips of milk, hot tea, or water are helpful. Gum is also helpful for the relief of heartburn.

2. Avoid milk and hot tea
3. Chew gum
4. Use antacids that contain sodium

Test-Taking Strategy: Use the process of elimination. Eliminate option 4 first because sodium leads to edema and should be avoided. Eliminate option 1 next because fatty and fried foods should be avoided. Knowledge that milk and hot tea can be soothing to the gastrointestinal tract will assist in eliminating option 2 and direct you to option 3 as the answer to this question. Review the measures that will reduce heartburn if you had difficulty with this question.

Level of Cognitive Ability: Application
Client Needs: Health Promotion and Maintenance
Integrated Concept/Process: Teaching/Learning
Content Area: Maternity

Reference:
Murray, S., McKinney, E., & Gorrie, T. (2002). *Foundations of maternal-newborn nursing* (3rd ed.). Philadelphia: W.B. Saunders, p. 126.

---

31. A nurse is reinforcing instructions about home care to the parents of a 3-year-old child hospitalized with hemophilia. Which of the following would not be a component of the teaching plan?
1. The child should not be left unattended
2. Pad table corners in the home
3. Remove household items that can tip over
4. Avoid immunizations and dental hygiene

Answer: 4
Rationale: The nurse should stress the importance of immunizations, dental hygiene, and routine well-child care. Options 1, 2, and 3 are appropriate. The parents are also instructed in measures to implement in the event of blunt trauma, especially trauma involving the joints, and to apply prolonged pressure to superficial wounds until bleeding has stopped.

Test-Taking Strategy: Note the key word *not*. Recalling that bleeding is a concern in this disorder will assist in eliminating options 1, 2, and 3, which include measures of protection and safety for the child. Review care to the child with hemophilia if you had difficulty with this question.

Level of Cognitive Ability: Application
Client Needs: Health Promotion and Maintenance
Integrated Concept/Process: Teaching/Learning
Content Area: Child Health

Reference:
Wong, D., & Hockenberry-Eaton, M. (2001). *Wong's essentials of pediatric nursing* (6th ed.). St. Louis: Mosby, pp. 365-367; 997.

---

32. A nurse reinforces instructions to a client taking clorazepate (Tranxene) for management of an anxiety disorder. Which of the following instructions would the nurse provide to the client?
1. Drowsiness is a side effect that usually disappears with continued therapy
2. If dizziness occurs, call the physician
3. Smoking increases the effectiveness of the medication
4. If gastrointestinal (GI) disturbances occur, discontinue the medication

Answer: 1
Rationale: The client should be instructed to change positions slowly—from lying to sitting and before standing—if dizziness occurs. Smoking reduces medication effectiveness. GI disturbance is an occasional side effect, and the medication can be given with food if this occurs.

Test-Taking Strategy: Use the process of elimination. Eliminate option 4 first because the client should not be instructed to discontinue medication. Eliminate option 2 next because episodes of dizziness commonly occur with antianxiety medications, and the client should be told about interventions to alleviate the dizziness. From the remaining options, select option 1 because drowsiness is commonly associated with antianxiety medications and normally disappears with continued therapy. Review this medication if you had difficulty with this question.

Level of Cognitive Ability: Application
Client Needs: Health Promotion and Maintenance
Integrated Concept/Process: Nursing Process/Implementation
Content Area: Pharmacology

Reference:
Hodgson, B., & Kizior, R. (2003). *Saunders nursing drug handbook 2003.* Philadelphia: W.B. Saunders, p. 265.

---

33. A client with chlamydial infection has received instructions on self-care and prevention of further infection. The nurse evaluates that the client needs further reinforcement if the client states to:
   1. Reduce the chance of reinfection by limiting the number of sexual partners
   2. Use latex condoms to prevent disease transmission
   3. Return to the clinic as requested for a follow-up culture
   4. Use antibiotics prophylactically to prevent symptoms of chlamydia

Answer: 4
Rationale: Antibiotics are not taken prophylactically to prevent chlamydia. The risk of reinfection can be reduced by limiting the number of sexual partners and by the use of condoms. In some instances, follow-up culture is requested in 4 to 7 days to confirm a cure.

Test-Taking Strategy: Note the key words *needs further reinforcement.* Options 1 and 2 are correct and are therefore eliminated first. Knowing the basic principles of antibiotic therapy directs you to option 4 because antibiotics are not used intermittently at will for prophylaxis of this infection. Review measures to prevent chlamydial infection if you had difficulty with this question.

Level of Cognitive Ability: Comprehension
Client Needs: Health Promotion and Maintenance
Integrated Concept/Process: Self-Care
Content Area: Fundamental Skills

Reference:
Black, J., Hawks, J., & Keene, A. (2001). *Medical-surgical nursing: clinical management for positive outcomes* (6th ed.). Philadelphia: W.B. Saunders, p. 1044.

---

34. A nurse in the physician's office is reviewing the results of a client's phenytoin (Dilantin) level drawn that morning. The nurse determines that the client had a therapeutic drug level if the client's result was:
   1. 3 µg/mL
   2. 8 µg/mL
   3. 15 µg/mL
   4. 24 µg/mL

Answer: 3
Rationale: The therapeutic range for serum phenytoin levels is 10 to 20 µg/mL in clients with normal serum albumin levels and renal function. A level below this range indicates that the client is not receiving sufficient medication and is at risk for seizure activity. The medication dose should be adjusted upward. A level above this range indicates that the client is entering the toxic range and is at risk for toxic side effects of the medication. In this case, the dose should be decreased.

Test-Taking Strategy: To answer this question accurately, you should know the therapeutic drug level for phenytoin. Review this information if you had difficulty with this question.

Level of Cognitive Ability: Comprehension
Client Needs: Physiological Integrity
Integrated Concept/Process: Nursing Process/Evaluation
Content Area: Pharmacology

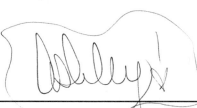

Reference:
Hodgson, B., & Kizior, R. (2003). *Saunders nursing drug handbook 2003.* Philadelphia: W.B. Saunders, p. 892.

---

35. A nurse is planning to teach dietary measures to promote fracture healing to a client with a fractured leg in a long leg cast. Which of the following suggestions would be least helpful to the client?
1. Follow a high-fat diet
2. Follow a well-balanced diet
3. Make sure to increase dietary fiber
4. Drink extra amounts of fluids

Answer: 1
Rationale: Clients who are casted have some degree of decreased mobility and should optimize nutrition to aid in healing. This can be accomplished by increasing intake of dietary fiber, drinking extra fluids, and following a well-balanced diet.

Test-Taking Strategy: Note the key words *least helpful*. Concepts that are useful in answering this question relate to wound healing and decreased mobility. Knowing that wound healing requires balanced nutrition helps eliminate option 2. With decreased mobility there is a risk of constipation, so the client needs increased fluid and dietary fiber. Therefore option 1 is the correct answer. Remember, the question asks for the item that will be *least* helpful. Review dietary measures to promote healing if you had difficulty with this question.

Level of Cognitive Ability: Application
Client Needs: Health Promotion and Maintenance
Integrated Concept/Process: Nursing Process/Implementation
Content Area: Adult Health/Musculoskeletal

Reference:
Williams, S. (2001). *Basic nutrition & diet therapy.* (11th ed.). St. Louis: Mosby, p. 421.

---

36. A nurse is caring for a client with a cerebrovascular accident (CVA) who has unilateral neglect. The nurse reinforces instructions to the family regarding home care. Which of the following would be included in the nurse's instructions?
1. Place personal items directly in front of the client
 2. Assist the client from the affected side
3. Assist the client from the unaffected side
4. Discourage the client from scanning the environment

Answer: 2
Rationale: Unilateral neglect is a pattern of lack of awareness of body parts such as paralyzed arms or legs. Personal items are placed on the unaffected side initially, but thereafter the client's attention is focused to the affected side. The client is assisted from the affected side. Cue the client to scan the entire environment.

Test-Taking Strategy: Use the process of elimination and focus on the key words *unilateral neglect*. Understanding the physiological alteration that occurs in unilateral neglect will assist in directing you to option 2. Review interventions associated with unilateral neglect if you had difficulty with this question.

Level of Cognitive Ability: Application
Client Needs: Safe, Effective Care Environment
Integrated Concept/Process: Teaching/Learning
Content Area: Adult Health/Neurological

Reference:
Black, J., Hawks, J., & Keene, A. (2001). *Medical-surgical nursing: clinical management for positive outcomes* (6th ed.). Philadelphia: W.B. Saunders, p. 1977.

37. A nurse has reinforced discharge instructions with a client who has had surgery for lung cancer. The nurse evaluates that the client has not understood all of the essential elements of home management if the client verbalizes to:

   1. Sit up and lean forward to breathe more easily
   2. Deal with any increases in pain independently
   3. Avoid exposure to crowds
   4. Call the physician for increased temperature or shortness of breath

Answer: 2

Rationale: Health teaching includes using positions that facilitate respiration such as sitting up and leaning forward, avoiding exposure to crowds or persons with respiratory infections, and reporting signs and symptoms of respiratory infection or an increase in pain.

Test-Taking Strategy: Use the process of elimination. Note the key words *client has not understood*. Recalling that the client should report signs of infection, difficulty breathing, and increased pain will direct you to option 2. Review client teaching points after lung surgery if you had difficulty with this question.

Level of Cognitive Ability: Comprehension
Client Needs: Health Promotion and Maintenance
Integrated Concept/Process: Nursing Process/Evaluation
Content Area: Adult Health/Oncology

Reference:
Black, J., Hawks, J., & Keene, A. (2001). *Medical-surgical nursing: clinical management for positive outcomes* (6th ed.). Philadelphia: W.B. Saunders, p. 466.

---

38. A nurse has assisted in providing an educational session to members of the local community about breast self-examination (BSE). Which of the following client statements indicates a need for further education?

   1. "I should perform the BSE when I have my period."
   2. "It is easiest to perform when I am in the shower when my hands are soapy."
   3. "I should perform this BSE every month."
   4. "I'll use the finger pads of my three middle fingers to feel for lumps and thickening."

Answer: 1

Rationale: The best time to perform BSE is after the monthly period when the breasts are not tender and swollen. Options 2, 3, and 4 identify accurate information regarding this important examination.

Test-Taking Strategy: Use the process of elimination. Note the key words *need for further education*. Recalling that the breasts are tender and swollen during menses will direct you to option 1. Review this procedure if you had difficulty with this question.

Level of Cognitive Ability: Comprehension
Client Needs: Health Promotion and Maintenance
Integrated Concept/Process: Self-Care
Content Area: Adult Health/Oncology

Reference:
Black, J., Hawks, J., & Keene, A. (2001). *Medical-surgical nursing: clinical management for positive outcomes* (6th ed.). Philadelphia: W.B. Saunders, pp. 41-42.

---

39. A nurse has given the client with a non-plaster (fiberglass) leg cast instructions on cast care at home. The nurse would evaluate that the client needs further instruction if the client makes which of the following statements?

   1. "I should avoid walking on wet, slippery floors."
   2. "It's OK to wipe dirt off the top of the cast with a damp cloth."
   3. "I'm not supposed to scratch the skin underneath the cast."

Answer: 4

Rationale: Client instructions should include avoiding walking on wet, slippery floors to prevent falls. Surface soil on a cast may be removed with a damp cloth. If the cast gets wet, it can be dried with a hair dryer set to a cool setting to prevent skin breakdown. If the skin under the cast itches, cool air from a hair dryer may be used for relief. The client should never scratch under a cast because of the risk of skin breakdown and ulcer formation.

Test-Taking Strategy: Use the process of elimination. Note the key words *needs further instruction*. Noting the word *hottest* in option 4 will direct you to this option. It may be helpful to remember

4. "If the cast gets wet, I can dry it with a hair dryer turned to the hottest setting."

never to use a hair dryer on a cast, or on the skin under any cast, with the dryer set at the hottest setting. Only cool settings are used to prevent burns. Review care to the client with a cast if you had difficulty with this question.

Level of Cognitive Ability: Comprehension
Client Needs: Health Promotion and Maintenance
Integrated Concept/Process: Nursing Process/Evaluation
Content Area: Adult Health/Musculoskeletal

Reference:
Black, J., Hawks, J., & Keene, A. (2001). *Medical-surgical nursing: clinical management for positive outcomes* (6th ed.). Philadelphia: W.B. Saunders, p. 603.

---

40. A nurse has completed reinforcing instructions on diet and fluid restriction with a client with chronic renal failure. The nurse would evaluate that the client best understands the information presented if the client selected which of the following desserts from the dietary menu?
1. Angel food cake
2. Ice cream
3. Sherbet
4. Jell-O

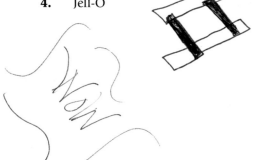

Answer: 1
Rationale: Dietary fluid includes anything that is liquid at room temperature, such as ice cream, sherbet, and Jell-O. With clients on a fluid-restricted diet, it is helpful to avoid "hidden" fluids to whatever extent is possible. This allows the client more fluid for drinking, which can help alleviate thirst.

Test-Taking Strategy: Use the process of elimination and remember that options that are similar are not likely to be correct. Evaluation of each of the options indicates that there is a greater amount of fluid in each of the incorrect options. In addition, these items are fluid at room temperature and therefore must be counted as fluid in the daily allotment. Review diet and fluid restrictions for the client with renal failure if you had difficulty with this question.

Level of Cognitive Ability: Comprehension
Client Needs: Health Promotion and Maintenance
Integrated Concept/Process: Self-Care
Content Area: Adult Health/Renal

Reference:
Lewis, S., Heitkemper, M., & Dirksen, S. (2000). *Medical-surgical nursing: assessment and management of clinical problems* (5th ed.). St. Louis: Mosby, p. 1314.

---

41. A nurse is planning to teach a client with a leg cast how to stand on crutches. The nurse plans to tell the client to place the crutches:
1. 3 inches to the front and side of the client's toes
2. 8 inches to the front and side of the client's toes
3. 15 inches to the front and side of the client's toes
4. 20 inches to the front and side of the client's toes

Answer: 2
Rationale: The classic tripod position is taught to the client before giving instructions on gait. The crutches are placed anywhere from 6 to 10 inches in front and to the side of the client, depending on the client's body size. This provides a wide enough base of support to the client and improves balance.

Test-Taking Strategy: Use the process of elimination. Three inches (option 1) and 20 inches (option 4) seem excessively short and long, respectively. These two options should be eliminated first. From the remaining options, 8 inches seems more in keeping with the normal length of a stride than 15 inches for someone wearing a cast. Review this procedure if you had difficulty with this question.

Level of Cognitive Ability: Application

Client Needs: Health Promotion and Maintenance
Integrated Concept/Process: Teaching/Learning
Content Area: Adult Health/Musculoskeletal

Reference:
Potter, P., & Perry, A. (2001). *Fundamentals of nursing* (5th ed.). St. Louis: Mosby, p. 1008.

---

42. A nurse is reinforcing instructions to a client who is beginning therapy with digoxin (Lanoxin). The nurse would teach the client to:
  1. Monitor blood pressure once a week
  2. Measure weight each morning before breakfast
  3. Take the pulse daily
  4. Have electrolyte levels drawn weekly

Answer: 3
Rationale: Clients taking digoxin should take the pulse each day and notify the physician if the heart rate drops below 60 beats per minute or exceeds 100 beats per minute. Options 1, 2, and 4 are not necessary.

Test-Taking Strategy: Use the process of elimination. Digoxin is not an antihypertensive medication, so eliminate option 1 first. The client may need to weigh daily for the condition requiring digoxin therapy, but it is not absolutely necessary for safe use of the medication. Weekly electrolyte levels are excessive, which leaves option 3, a "golden rule" of digoxin therapy. Review this medication if you had difficulty with this question.

Level of Cognitive Ability: Application
Client Needs: Health Promotion and Maintenance
Integrated Concept/Process: Teaching/Learning
Content Area: Pharmacology

Reference:
Hodgson, B., & Kizior, R. (2003). *Saunders nursing drug handbook 2003.* Philadelphia: W.B. Saunders, p. 348.

---

43. Cyclophosphamide (Cytoxan) is prescribed for a client with breast cancer. The nurse reinforces instructions to the client about the medication. Which of the following client statements indicates a need for further education?
  1. "I should avoid contact with anyone who recently had a live virus vaccine."
  2. "If I lose my hair, it will grow back."
  3. "If I develop a sore throat, I should notify the physician."
  4. "I should limit my fluid intake while taking this medication."

Answer: 4
Rationale: Hemorrhagic cystitis is an adverse reaction associated with this medication. The client should be instructed to consume copious amounts of fluid during therapy. Avoiding contact with persons who recently had a live virus vaccine is important because cyclophosphamide produces immunosuppression, placing the client at risk for infection. Hair will grow back, although it may have a different color and texture. A sore throat may be an indication of an infection and should be reported to the physician.

Test-Taking Strategy: Use the process of elimination. Note the key words *need for further education.* Recalling that this medication causes hemorrhagic cystitis and that fluids are important will assist in directing you to the correct option. Review the adverse effects of this medication if you had difficulty with this question.

Level of Cognitive Ability: Comprehension
Client Needs: Health Promotion and Maintenance
Integrated Concept/Process: Nursing Process/Evaluation
Content Area: Pharmacology

Reference:
Hodgson, B., & Kizior, R. (2003). *Saunders nursing drug handbook 2003.* Philadelphia: W.B. Saunders, p. 290.

44. A nurse reinforces instructions to a client with osteoarthritis who will be taking indomethacin (Indocin). Which of the following client statements indicates that further teaching is necessary?
1. "I can take a pill whenever I need to for pain."
2. "I should call the doctor if I notice a rash."
3. "I'll balance rest periods and moderate activity."
4. "I'll watch for any swollen feet or fingers or any gastric distress."

Answer: 1

Rationale: In osteoarthritis, a noninflammatory disorder of the movable joints, pain is aggravated by joint motion, weight bearing, and weather changes. The disease course is described as slow and progressive with no periods of remission or exacerbation. Rest and exercise should be balanced. When pain occurs, the client should limit movement. A rash should be reported because it could indicate hypersensitivity to the medication. The client should be instructed to monitor for swelling and gastric distress, which this medication can cause.

Test-Taking Strategy: Use the process of elimination. Noting the key words *further teaching is necessary* should direct you to option 1 because clients should not be instructed to take medication for pain whenever needed. Guidelines regarding time frames for medication should be provided. Review this medication if you had difficulty with this question.

Level of Cognitive Ability: Comprehension
Client Needs: Health Promotion and Maintenance
Integrated Concept/Process: Nursing Process/Evaluation
Content Area: Pharmacology

Reference:
Hodgson, B., & Kizior, R. (2003). *Saunders nursing drug handbook 2003.* Philadelphia: W.B. Saunders, p. 586.

45. A nurse has reinforced instructions on site care to a hemodialysis client who had implantation of a right arm arteriovenous (AV) fistula. The nurse evaluates that the client needs further information if the client states to:
1. Avoid carrying heavy objects on the right arm
2. Sleep on the right side
3. Report increased temperature, redness, or drainage at the site
4. Perform range-of-motion exercises routinely on the right arm

Answer: 2

Rationale: Routine instructions to the client with an AV fistula, graft, or shunt includes reporting signs and symptoms of infection, performing routine range of motion to the affected extremity, avoiding sleeping with the body weight on the limb with the access site, and avoiding carrying heavy objects or compressing the extremity that has the access site.

Test-Taking Strategy: Note the key words *needs further information*. Knowing that options 3 and 4 are part of routine care allows you to eliminate them first as possible answers. To choose correctly between options 1 and 2, it is necessary to understand the adverse effects of pressure on the patency of the access site. Review these home care instructions if you had difficulty with this question.

Level of Cognitive Ability: Comprehension
Client Needs: Health Promotion and Maintenance
Integrated Concept/Process: Nursing Process/Evaluation
Content Area: Adult Health/Renal

Reference:
Lewis, S., Heitkemper, M., & Dirksen, S. (2000). *Medical-surgical nursing: assessment and management of clinical problems* (5th ed.). St. Louis: Mosby, p. 1326.

46. A client with tuberculosis (TB) is preparing for discharge from the hospital. Which of the following statements indicates

Answer: 1

Rationale: With current resistant strains of tuberculosis, the nurse must emphasize that noncompliance regarding medication could

to the nurse that further teaching is necessary?

1. "If I miss a dose of medication because of nausea, I just skip that dose and resume my regular schedule."
2. "I should eat foods that are high in iron, protein, and vitamin C."
3. "I should place tissues in a plastic bag when I am home."
4. "I will not need respiratory isolation when I am home."

lead to an infection that is difficult to treat or has total drug resistance. Clients may prevent nausea related to the medications by taking the daily dose at bedtime. Antinausea medications may also prevent this symptom. Options 2, 3, and 4 are correct client statements.

Test-Taking Strategy: Note the key words *further teaching is necessary*. General principles related to medication administration should assist in directing you to option 1. Review medication therapy and its importance in TB if you had difficulty with this question.

Level of Cognitive Ability: Comprehension
Client Needs: Health Promotion and Maintenance
Integrated Concept/Process: Teaching/Learning
Content Area: Pharmacology

Reference:
Lewis, S., Heitkemper, M., & Dirksen, S. (2000). *Medical-surgical nursing: assessment and management of clinical problems* (5th ed.). St. Louis: Mosby, pp. 625; 628.

---

47. A nurse has given instructions to a client returning home after arthroscopy of the knee. The nurse determines that the client understands the instructions if the client states to:

1. Stay off the leg entirely for the rest of the day
2. Resume any type of activity the next day
3. Refrain from eating food for the remainder of the day
4. Report fever or site inflammation to the physician

Answer: 4
Rationale: After arthroscopy, the client can usually walk carefully on the leg once sensation has returned. The client is instructed to avoid strenuous exercise for at least a few days. The client may resume the usual diet. Signs and symptoms of infection should be reported to the physician.

Test-Taking Strategy: Use the process of elimination and general postoperative principles. Remember, the client is always taught signs and symptoms of infection to report to the physician. Review postprocedure instructions after arthroscopy if you had difficulty with this question.

Level of Cognitive Ability: Comprehension
Client Needs: Health Promotion and Maintenance
Integrated Concept/Process: Teaching/Learning
Content Area: Adult Health/Musculoskeletal

Reference:
Ignatavicius, D., & Workman, M. (2002). *Medical surgical nursing: critical thinking for collaborative care* (4th ed.). Philadelphia: W. B. Saunders, p. 1091.

---

48. A nurse is planning to teach a client with a below-the-knee amputation about skin care to prevent breakdown. Which of the following points would the nurse include in the teaching plan?

1. A stump sock must be worn at all times and changed twice a week
2. The residual limb is washed gently and dried every other day
3. The socket of the prosthesis is washed with a bactericidal agent daily

Answer: 4
Rationale: A stump sock must be worn at all times to absorb perspiration and is changed daily. The residual limb is washed, dried, and inspected for breakdown twice each day. The socket of the prosthesis is cleansed with a mild soap and rinsed and dried carefully each day. A bactericidal agent would not be used.

Test-Taking Strategy: Use the process of elimination. Recall that the residual limb is cared for twice a day. With this in mind, you can eliminate options 1 and 2. From the remaining options, recalling that a mild soap is used to wash the prosthesis will direct

4. The socket of the prosthesis must be dried carefully before using it

you to option 4. Review these teaching points if you had difficulty with this question.

Level of Cognitive Ability: Application
Client Needs: Health Promotion and Maintenance
Integrated Concept/Process: Self-Care
Content Area: Adult Health/Musculoskeletal

Reference:
Lewis, S., Heitkemper, M., & Dirksen, S. (2000). *Medical-surgical nursing: assessment and management of clinical problems* (5th ed.). St. Louis: Mosby, p. 1801.

---

49. A nurse has taught the principles of foot care to a client with diabetes mellitus. The nurse evaluates that the client understood the information if the client states to:
1. Apply lotion to dry skin areas between each of the toes
2. Wear shoes that are closed at the heel and toe
3. Cut the toenails down to the cuticle
4. Put a hot water bottle on the feet if they become cold

Answer: 2
Rationale: The client should wear shoes that are closed at the heel and toe to prevent injury to the feet. The client should avoid other potential sources of injury to the feet. Application of direct heat to the feet could cause burns, and application of lotion between the toes could cause skin breakdown. Toenails should be cut straight across at the level of the contour of the toe. Other general foot care measures include inspecting the feet daily, cleaning them with mild soap, rinsing and drying them well, and using lanolin-based lotions, except between the toes.

Test-Taking Strategy: Use the process of elimination. Recalling concerns related to skin integrity in a client with diabetes mellitus will direct you to option 2. Review diabetic foot care if you had difficulty with this question.

Level of Cognitive Ability: Comprehension
Client Needs: Health Promotion and Maintenance
Integrated Concept/Process: Nursing Process/Evaluation
Content Area: Adult Health/Endocrine

Reference:
Lewis, S., Heitkemper, M., & Dirksen, S. (2000). *Medical-surgical nursing: assessment and management of clinical problems* (5th ed.). St. Louis: Mosby, p. 1399.

---

50. A nurse is teaching a client with cholecystitis about foods that must be eliminated from the diet. The nurse would teach the client that which of the following foods will not aggravate the condition?
1. Fried chicken
2. French fries
3. Baked fish
4. Donuts

Answer: 3
Rationale: The client with cholecystitis should decrease overall intake of dietary fat. Foods that should be avoided include sauces and gravies, fatty meats, fried foods, products made with cream, and heavy desserts. The correct answer is baked fish, which is low in fat.

Test-Taking Strategy: Use the process of elimination, recalling that clients with cholecystitis should decrease fat intake. This will direct you to option 3. Review food items high in fat if you had difficulty with this question.

Level of Cognitive Ability: Application
Client Needs: Health Promotion and Maintenance
Integrated Concept/Process: Self-Care
Content Area: Adult Health/Gastrointestinal

Reference:
Ignatavicius, D., & Workman, M. (2002). *Medical-surgical nursing: critical thinking for collaborative care* (4th ed.). Philadelphia: W.B. Saunders, p. 1335.

---

51. The nurse has taught a client newly diagnosed with diabetes mellitus about blood glucose monitoring. The nurse would evaluate that the client understands the information if the client states to report blood glucose levels that exceed:

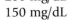

1. 350 mg/dL
2. 250 mg/dL
3. 200 mg/dL
4. 150 mg/dL

Answer: 2
Rationale: It is standard practice to teach the client to report blood glucose levels that exceed 250 mg/dL unless otherwise instructed by the physician. The values in options 3 and 4 are too low, and the value in option 1 is too high.

Test-Taking Strategy: Knowledge regarding the aspects of client teaching for blood glucose monitoring is needed to answer this question correctly. Review these teaching points if you had difficulty with this question.

Level of Cognitive Ability: Comprehension
Client Needs: Health Promotion and Maintenance
Integrated Concept/Process: Nursing Process/Evaluation
Content Area: Adult Health/Endocrine

Reference:
Lewis, S., Heitkemper, M., & Dirksen, S. (2000). *Medical-surgical nursing: assessment and management of clinical problems* (5th ed.). St. Louis: Mosby, p. 1384.

---

52. A client with hyperaldosteronism has undergone unilateral adrenalectomy. The nurse includes which of the following items in postoperative teaching?

1. The client is likely to experience hypertension
2. Diuretics must be taken for life
3. Glucocorticoids will be needed temporarily
4. The client needs to adhere strictly to a low-sodium diet

Answer: 3
Rationale: The client who has undergone unilateral adrenalectomy must take replacement corticosteroids for up to 2 years after surgery. This allows the remaining gland to resume function after being suppressed by the excessive hormone production of the diseased gland. Diuretics and a low-sodium diet are used in the preoperative period to manage hypertension. Once surgery has been performed, these measures are no longer required.

Test-Taking Strategy: Use the process of elimination and focus on the anatomical location of the surgery. Noting the key word *unilateral* will assist in directing you to option 3. Glucocorticoids are needed only temporarily with unilateral adrenalectomy. Review postoperative care after this surgery if you had difficulty with this question.

Level of Cognitive Ability: Application
Client Needs: Health Promotion and Maintenance
Integrated Concept/Process: Teaching/Learning
Content Area: Adult Health/Endocrine

Reference:
Lewis, S., Heitkemper, M., & Dirksen, S. (2000). *Medical-surgical nursing: assessment and management of clinical problems* (5th ed.). St. Louis: Mosby, p. 1441.

---

53. A client is being discharged to go home after subtotal gastrectomy. The nurse teaches the client to do which of the following to minimize the risk of dumping syndrome?

Answer: 3
Rationale: To minimize dumping syndrome after gastric surgery, the client should avoid taking liquids with meals. The client should also avoid high-carbohydrate food sources. The client should lie down for at least 30 minutes after eating, eat small frequent meals,

1. Eat highly concentrated carbohydrate foods
2. Eat only two large meals a day
3. Avoid drinking liquids during a meal
4. Sit up for 1 hour after eating

and sit semirecumbent while eating. Antispasmodic medications may be prescribed as needed to delay gastric emptying.

Test-Taking Strategy: Use the process of elimination. Noting the name of the disorder and recalling the pathophysiology associated with dumping syndrome will assist in directing you to the correct option. Review these client teaching points if you had difficulty with this question.

Level of Cognitive Ability: Application
Client Needs: Health Promotion and Maintenance
Integrated Concept/Process: Teaching/Learning
Content Area: Adult Health/Gastrointestinal

Reference:
Ignatavicius, D., & Workman, M. (2002). *Medical-surgical nursing: critical thinking for collaborative care* (4th ed.). Philadelphia: W.B. Saunders, p. 1233.

---

54. A client with an ileostomy is experiencing stools that contain too much liquid. The nurse would instruct the client to eliminate which of the following foods from the diet to thicken the stool?
1. Bran
2. Low-fat cheese
3. Pasta
4. Boiled rice

Answer: 1
Rationale: Ileostomy output is liquid by nature. Addition or elimination of various foods can help thicken or loosen this liquid drainage. Foods that help thicken the stool of the client with an ileostomy include pasta, boiled rice, and low-fat cheese. Foods that are high in dietary fiber, such as bran, increase output of watery stool by increasing propulsion of food through the bowel. High-fiber foods should be limited if there is a need to thicken the stool.

Test-Taking Strategy: Use the process of elimination. Recalling that high-fiber foods can aggravate watery stools will direct you to option 1. Review this dietary information if you had difficulty with this question.

Level of Cognitive Ability: Application
Client Needs: Health Promotion and Maintenance
Integrated Concept/Process: Teaching/Learning
Content Area: Adult Health/Gastrointestinal

Reference:
Ignatavicius, D., & Workman, M. (2002). *Medical-surgical nursing: critical thinking for collaborative care* (4th ed.). Philadelphia: W.B. Saunders, p. 1282.

---

55. A client is being discharged to home from the hospital after an episode of acute pancreatitis. The nurse would teach the client to call the physician if pain returns, which would be located in the:
1. Epigastric area and radiating to the umbilicus
2. Left lower quadrant and radiating to the hip
3. Epigastric area and radiating to the back

Answer: 3
Rationale: The nurse teaches the client to report recurrence of pain experienced with pancreatitis. This pain is often severe and unrelenting, is located in the epigastric region, and radiates to the back. The other options are incorrect.

Test-Taking Strategy: Use the process of elimination. Because the pain radiates to the back, it is a little easier to distinguish this pain from other gastrointestinal (GI) disorders. Consider the anatomical location of the pancreas to assist in directing you to the correct option. Review the signs and symptoms of acute pancreatitis if you had difficulty with this question.

4. Left lower quadrant and radiating to the groin

Level of Cognitive Ability: Application
Client Needs: Health Promotion and Maintenance
Integrated Concept/Process: Teaching/Learning
Content Area: Adult Health/Gastrointestinal

Reference:
Ignatavicius, D., & Workman, M. (2002). *Medical-surgical nursing: critical thinking for collaborative care* (4th ed.). Philadelphia: W.B. Saunders, p. 1341.

---

56. A client with a psychotic disorder has been taking haloperidol (Haldol). After 6 weeks of therapy, the client returns to the health care clinic for follow-up evaluation. The nurse documents a therapeutic response when the nurse notes:

1. A tense facial expression
2. An inability to concentrate
3. A well-groomed and neat appearance
4. An increase in muscle strength

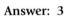

Answer: 3
Rationale: Haloperidol is an antipsychotic. The nurse evaluates for a therapeutic response by noting the client's interest in surroundings, improvement in self-care, increased ability to concentrate, and a relaxed facial expression.

Test-Taking Strategy: Use the process of elimination and note the key word *therapeutic* in the question. This should assist in eliminating options 1 and 2 because they do not indicate a positive response. Knowledge that haloperidol is an antipsychotic medication should assist in directing you to option 3 from the remaining options. Review the expected therapeutic response of this medication if you had difficulty with this question.

Level of Cognitive Ability: Analysis
Client Needs: Psychosocial Integrity
Integrated Concept/Process: Nursing Process/Evaluation
Content Area: Mental Health

Reference:
Hodgson, B., & Kizior, R. (2003). *Saunders nursing drug handbook 2003.* Philadelphia: W.B. Saunders, p. 540.

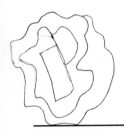

---

57. A client with chronic airflow limitation (CAL) gets particularly upset and agitated when episodes of dyspnea occur and the client feels unable to breathe. The nurse plans care, understanding that which of the following problems most appropriately relates to the client's complaints?

1. Ineffective coping measures
2. Fear
3. Lack of knowledge about breathing techniques
4. Loneliness

Answer: 2
Rationale: Fear is the most appropriate problem because breathlessness and dyspnea are upsetting the client. The other three problems listed may be appropriate for some clients with CAL, but no information in the question makes them appropriate responses here.

Test-Taking Strategy: Use the process of elimination. Note the key words *most appropriately* in the question and focus on the data in the question. The only problem that relates to dyspnea and the client's feeling unable to breathe is fear. Review the psychosocial problems associated with dyspnea and breathlessness if you had difficulty with this question.

Level of Cognitive Ability: Analysis
Client Needs: Psychosocial Integrity
Integrated Concept/Process: Nursing Process/Data Collection
Content Area: Adult Health/Respiratory

Reference:
Black, J., Hawks, J., & Keene, A. (2001). *Medical-surgical nursing: clinical management for positive outcomes* (6th ed.). Philadelphia: W.B. Saunders, p. 1700.

58. A nurse is reinforcing instructions on self-management of peritoneal dialysis at home. The nurse advises the client to avoid which of the following as part of self-care?
1. Take own vital signs daily
2. Monitor own weight daily
3. Use a strong adhesive tape to anchor the catheter dressing
4. Use meticulous aseptic technique for dialysate bag changes

Answer: 3
Rationale: The client is at risk for impairment of skin integrity because of the presence of the catheter, exposure to moisture, and irritation from tape and cleansing solutions. The client should be instructed to use paper or nonallergenic tape to prevent skin irritation and breakdown. It is proper procedure for the client to use aseptic technique and to self-monitor vital signs and weight on a daily basis.

Test Taking Strategy: Use the process of elimination. Note the key word *avoid*. Eliminate options 1 and 2 first because it is important for the client to monitor vital signs and weight each day. To choose correctly between options 3 and 4, remember that meticulous aseptic technique is used to prevent the occurrence of peritonitis, and that the skin should be protected from maceration through use of a variety of techniques. Review these home care instructions if you had difficulty with this question.

Level of Cognitive Ability: Application
Client Needs: Health Promotion and Maintenance
Integrated Concept/Process: Teaching/Learning
Content Area: Adult Health/Renal

Reference:
Black, J., Hawks, J., & Keene, A. (2001). *Medical-surgical nursing: clinical management for positive outcomes* (6th ed.). Philadelphia: W.B. Saunders, p. 891.

---

59. A nurse is providing dietary instructions to a client diagnosed with anemia. Which of the following food items suggested to the client would provide the highest source of iron?
1. Liver
2. Eggs
3. Oranges
4. Broccoli

Answer: 1
Rationale: A client with anemia should be taught the basics of good nutrition and encouraged to consume a diet high in protein, iron, and vitamins. The nurse should encourage the client to consume foods cooked in iron pots and to ingest foods such as liver, which has the highest source of iron of the foods identified in the options. Other foods that may provide high sources of iron include oysters, lean meats, kidney beans, whole-wheat bread, kale, spinach, egg yolks, turnip tops, beet greens, carrots, apricots, and raisins.

Test-Taking Strategy: Knowledge about food items high in iron is necessary to answer this question. Review these basic nutritional concepts if you had difficulty choosing the correct answer.

Level of Cognitive Ability: Comprehension
Client Needs: Health Promotion and Maintenance
Integrated Concept/Process: Teaching/Learning
Content Area: Fundamental skills

Reference:
Williams, S. (2001) *Basic nutrition & diet therapy* (11th ed.). St. Louis: Mosby, p. 131.

---

60. A client has an impaired corneal reflex on the right side after a head injury. The nurse instructs the client to use which of the following measures to best protect the eye?

Answer: 2
Rationale: With loss of the corneal (blink) reflex, the client is at risk for a dry eye and corneal abrasion if foreign matter comes in contact with the eye. Use of sterile saline drops helps keep the eyes lubricated. An eye patch would have to be used carefully

1. Wipe the inside of the lower eyelid with a cotton ball twice a day
2. Use sterile saline drops every few hours to keep the eye moist
3. Wear an eye patch
4. Tape the eye shut during the day

because corneal abrasion could result if the cornea comes in contact with the patch. Introduction of a foreign object (a cotton ball) inside the lower eyelid also risks corneal abrasion. Taping the eye shut could impair the client's vision, putting the client at risk for another injury, such as a fall.

Test-Taking Strategy: The best way to answer this question is from the viewpoint of potential trauma to the client. Note that the question includes the word *best*. Recalling the risk related to loss of corneal reflex will direct you to option 2. Review care to the client with an impaired corneal reflex if you had difficulty with this question.

Level of Cognitive Ability: Application
Client Needs: Health Promotion and Maintenance
Integrated Concept/Process: Self-Care
Content Area: Adult Health/Neurological

Reference:
Black, J., Hawks, J., & Keene, A. (2001). *Medical-surgical nursing: clinical management for positive outcomes* (6th ed.). Philadelphia: W.B. Saunders, p. 1976.

---

61. A nurse is teaching the family of a disoriented client with a neurological problem about providing an environment that minimizes confusion. The nurse tells the family to avoid which of the following in the home environment?
1. Using simple, clear directions
2. Providing sensory cues
3. Encouraging multiple visitors at one time
4. Keeping a stable environment

Answer: 3
Rationale: Clients with confusion from neurological dysfunction respond best to a stable environment, which is limited in the amount and types of sensory input. The family can provide sensory cues and give clear, simple directions in a positive manner. Confusion and agitation are reduced when environmental stimuli (television and multiple visitors) are minimized and when personal articles are visible to the client.

Test-Taking Strategy: Use the process of elimination. The key word in the question, *avoid*, guides you to look for an option that is an incorrect action by the family. The client who is confused can handle a limited amount of information at one time, which makes option 3 the correct answer. Review care to the disoriented client if you had difficulty with this question.

Level of Cognitive Ability: Application
Client Needs: Psychosocial Integrity
Integrated Concept/Process: Teaching/Learning
Content Area: Adult Health/Neurological

Reference:
Lewis, S., Heitkemper, M., & Dirksen, S. (2000). *Medical-surgical nursing: assessment and management of clinical problems* (5th ed.). St. Louis: Mosby, p. 55.

---

62. A nurse in the prenatal clinic is assisting in checking the deep tendon reflexes of a pregnant client. Which of the following accurately describes this data collection procedure?
1. The nurse places one hand under the knee to raise it slightly off the bed

Answer: 1
Rationale: To evaluate the deep tendon reflexes, the client's lower leg is exposed and one hand is placed under the knee to raise it slightly off the bed. A percussion hammer is used to strike the patellar tendon just below the patella. The normal response is extension and thrusting of the foot upward. Options 2, 3, and 4 are incorrect.

and uses a percussion hammer to strike the patellar tendon
2. The nurse places one hand under the client's knee and bends the knee slightly, places the other hand on the ball of the foot, encourages the woman to relax the foot, and sharply dorsiflexes the foot
3. The nurse places one hand under the client's upper arm to raise it slightly and uses a percussion hammer to strike the elbow tendon
4. The nurse uses a percussion hammer to strike the ankle tendon just above the Achilles tendon

Test-Taking Strategy: Use the process of elimination and knowledge about assessment of deep tendon reflexes to answer this question. Attempting to visualize this procedure will direct you to option 1. Review this data collection technique if you had difficulty with this question.

Level of Cognitive Ability: Comprehension
Client Needs: Health Promotion and Maintenance
Integrated Concept/Process: Nursing Process/Data Collection
Content Area: Maternity

Reference:
Murray, S., McKinney, E., & Gorrie, T. (2002). *Foundations of maternal-newborn nursing* (3rd ed.). Philadelphia: W.B. Saunders, p. 687.

---

63. A pregnant client is seen in the prenatal clinic and is complaining of constipation. The client is in the third trimester. Which of the following self-care measures would the nurse include in the teaching plan for the client?
    1. Decreasing daily fluid intake
    2. Decreasing whole grains in the diet
    3. Decreasing roughage in the diet
    4. Maintaining regular exercise

Answer: 4
Rationale: Constipation may result from slowing of peristalsis caused by increased levels of progesterone, displacement of the intestines by the expanding uterus, lack of activity, and inadequate fluid intake. Self-care measures for constipation include increasing daily intake of fluid, whole grains, and roughage, as well as exercising regularly.

Test-Taking Strategy: Use the process of elimination and basic concepts related to prevention of constipation to direct you to option 4. Review self-care measures to prevent constipation if you had difficulty with this question.

Level of Cognitive Ability: Application
Client Needs: Health Promotion and Maintenance
Integrated Concept/Process: Self-Care
Content Area: Maternity

Reference:
Murray, S., McKinney, E., & Gorrie, T. (2002). *Foundations of maternal-newborn nursing* (3rd ed.). Philadelphia: W.B. Saunders, p. 149.

---

64. A nurse is evaluating the mother-infant bonding process during the postpartum period. A maladaptive interaction would be indicated if the mother:
    1. Expressed discomfort with the role of motherhood
    2. Encouraged the nurse to feed the baby because she continues to be too tired
    3. Showed that she was willing to learn how to care for the cord
    4. Talked to the baby

Answer: 2
Rationale: A sign of maternal potential complications concerning psychosocial needs includes refusal to interact with or care for the infant. Options 3 and 4 identify situations in which the mother plans to or is demonstrating interaction with the infant. Expressing discomfort with the role of motherhood is not maladaptive.

Test-Taking Strategy: Focus on the issue of the question, *a maladaptive interaction.* Use the process of elimination, noting that only in option 2 does the mother avoid interaction with the infant. Review the signs of maladaptive behavior if you had difficulty with this question.

Level of Cognitive Ability: Comprehension
Client Needs: Psychosocial Integrity

Integrated Concept/Process: Nursing Process/Data Collection
Content Area: Maternity

Reference:
McKinney, E., Ashwill, J., Murray, S. et al. (2000). *Maternal-child nursing.* Philadelphia: W.B. Saunders, p. 498.

---

65. A nurse is caring for a client in active labor. Natural, soothing techniques that the nurse plans to use during active labor to assist the client to effectively manage the labor process include:
1. Isolation and distraction
2. Counterpressure and effleurage
3. Pharmacological interventions
4. Panting and pushing

Answer: 2
Rationale: Human touch produces positive effects during labor. Women appreciate gentle touching by support members. Options 1, 3, and 4 do not provide natural or soothing methods for addressing the processes encountered during labor.

Test-Taking Strategy: Use the process of elimination. Noting the key words *natural, soothing techniques* will assist in eliminating options 1, 3, and 4. Review care of the client during active labor and techniques that are soothing if you had difficulty with this question.

Level of Cognitive Ability: Application
Client Needs: Psychosocial Integrity
Integrated Concept/Process: Nursing Process/Planning
Content Area: Maternity

Reference:
Burroughs, A., & Leifer, G. (2002). *Maternity nursing* (8th ed.). Philadelphia: W.B. Saunders, p. 124.

---

66. Ice packs to the perineum are prescribed for a postpartum client. The nurse understands that the purpose of the ice packs are to:
1. Reduce the edema and numb the tissue
2. Promote healing and provide comfort
3. Reduce infection and stimulate peristalsis
4. Cleanse the perineum and prevent hemorrhoids

Answer: 1
Rationale: Ice is used during the first 24 hours postpartum to reduce edema and numb the tissue. Warm, moist heat (such as a sitz bath) is used after the first 24 hours postpartum to provide comfort, cleanse, promote healing, and reduce the incidence of infection.

Test-Taking Strategy: Use the process of elimination. Recalling the principles related to heat and cold will direct you to option 1. Review the effects of heat and cold if you had difficulty with this question.

Level of Cognitive Ability: Comprehension
Client Needs: Physiological Integrity
Integrated Concept/Process: Nursing Process/Implementation
Content Area: Maternity

Reference:
McKinney, E., Ashwill, J., Murray, S. et al. (2000). *Maternal-child nursing.* Philadelphia: W.B. Saunders, pp. 491-492.

---

67. An antenatal client who has experienced two episodes of bleeding as a result of a borderline placenta previa will be discharged to go home, and the nurse is

Answer: 3
Rationale: Daily monitoring of fetal movements is a reliable indicator of fetal health. The procedure is easy to learn and noninvasive and also allows self-care and reporting, which is a major goal

planning the discharge instructions. The nurse is aware that there is a potential for fetal distress if bleeding recurs. Which of the following should the nurse include in the instructions to help the client identify fetal distress?

1. Teach the father to listen to the fetal heart tones daily
2. Make a referral to a home health agency for weekly ultrasound examinations
3. Give the mother instructions for performing daily fetal movement counts and assist her to practice
4. Teach the father to measure the abdominal girth and fundal height of the client each morning

of health maintenance. Weekly ultrasound examinations are not necessary. Options 1 and 4 are assessments that should be performed by a health care professional.

Test-Taking Strategy: Use the process of elimination and focus on the issue: an intervention that can be performed by the mother. This will direct you to option 3. Options 1, 2, and 4 are interventions that should be performed by a health care professional. Review fetal movement counts if you had difficulty with this question.

Level of Cognitive Ability: Application
Client Needs: Health Promotion and Maintenance
Integrated Concept/Process: Teaching/Learning
Content Area: Maternity

Reference:
McKinney, E., Ashwill, J., Murray, S. et al. (2000). *Maternal-child nursing.* Philadelphia: W.B. Saunders, pp. 638-639.

---

68. A nurse is assigned to care for a postpartum client. When collecting data about the new mother's parental anxieties, which of the following suggests a potential problem with maternal-newborn attachment?

1. "Why did this baby have to inherit my family's ugly toes?"
2. "I feel really tired right now."
3. "He has his Daddy's deep blue eyes."
4. "I am so happy I feel like crying."

Answer: 1
Rationale: Negative statements about the newborn's features or gender may interfere with the mother's ability to bond with and care for the infant. Positive statements and identification with family members help the mother identify with the infant, promoting attachment. Fatigue is an expected response in the postpartum period and may cause the mother to request the staff to assume care of the infant temporarily; however, after a period of rest, she should begin to assume care for the infant.

Test-Taking Strategy: Note the key words *a potential problem with maternal attachment.* Use the process of elimination, seeking the option that identifies a potential problem. Option 1 is a negative comment about the newborn. Review the indicators of altered maternal-newborn attachment if you had difficulty with this question.

Level of Cognitive Ability: Comprehension
Client Needs: Psychosocial Integrity
Integrated Concept/Process: Nursing Process/Data Collection
Content Area: Maternity

Reference:
McKinney, E., Ashwill, J., Murray, S. et al. (2000). *Maternal-child nursing.* Philadelphia: W.B. Saunders, p. 498.

---

69. A nurse is monitoring an adolescent client for signs of depression. To recognize depression in the client, the nurse understands that normal adolescents:

1. Spend a lot of time in self-reflection, so depression is normal
2. Enjoy the unkempt look and do not care about their appearance

Answer: 4
Rationale: It is not normal for an adolescent to become depressed. Adolescents are concerned about body image and their appearance. Being moody and acting out a lot is not normal adolescent behavior. Adolescents enjoy staying up late.

Test-Taking Strategy: Knowledge regarding normal adolescent behaviors is necessary to answer this question. Use this knowledge

3. Are moody and act out a lot
4. Enjoy staying up late

and the concepts related to growth and development to assist in identifying the correct option. Review these concepts if you had difficulty with this question.

Level of Cognitive Ability: Comprehension
Client Needs: Psychosocial Integrity
Integrated Concept/Process: Nursing Process/Data Collection
Content Area: Child Health

Reference:
Schulte, E. Price, D., & Gwin, J. (2001). *Thompson's pediatric nursing* (8th ed.). Philadelphia: W.B. Saunders, pp. 314; 342.

---

70. A male client has been told he has hepatitis C and that the possibility of developing a chronic carrier state or liver cancer is very high. The client says to the nurse, "Am I going to die from this?" The most appropriate nursing response is:
1. "If you take good care of yourself and follow your doctor's orders, everything will be OK."
2. "Here is a pamphlet on hepatitis C that explains the complications and prognosis."
3. "You seem very upset. What did your doctor tell you about these possibilities?"
4. "Would you like to speak to a chaplain about your concern, to get your affairs in order?"

Answer: 3
Rationale: The client's psychosocial needs are best met when the nurse focuses the conversation on how the client is feeling, and attempts to encourage self-exploration and continued conversation. Option 1 is giving false reassurance. Option 2 places the client's concern on hold. Option 4 directs the client's concern to another health care team member when it primarily should be addressed by the nurse.

Test-Taking Strategy: Use therapeutic communication techniques to answer the question. Options 1, 2, and 4 are communication blocks. Option 3 addresses the client's concern. Review therapeutic communication techniques if you had difficulty with this question.

Level of Cognitive Ability: Application
Client Needs: Psychosocial Integrity
Integrated Concept/Process: Communication and Documentation
Content Area: Fundamental Skills

Reference:
Potter, P., & Perry, A. (2001). *Fundamentals of nursing* (5th ed.). St. Louis: Mosby, p. 459.

---

71. A nurse is employed in a long-term care facility. To facilitate effective communication with an older client, the nurse:
1. Uses an authoritarian approach
2. Uses active listening
3. Reacts only to nonverbal cues in the client's conversation
4. Listens only for facts in the client's conversation

Answer: 2
Rationale: For effective communication, the nurse uses active listening and creates an environment in which the client feels comfortable expressing feelings. An authoritarian approach is directive and not permissive and does not create an environment for verbal exchange. Reacting only to nonverbal cues and listening only for facts are examples of inactive listening.

Test-Taking Strategy: Note the key word *effective*. Use the process of elimination and knowledge regarding therapeutic communication skills. Eliminate options 3 and 4 first because of the word *only*. Next, eliminate option 1 knowing that it is nontherapeutic. Review therapeutic communication techniques if you had difficulty with this question.

Level of Cognitive Ability: Application
Client Needs: Psychosocial Integrity

Integrated Concept/Process: Communication and Documentation
Content Area: Fundamental Skills

Reference:
Lueckenotte, A. (2002). *Gerontologic nursing* (2nd ed.). St. Louis: Mosby, p. 143.

---

72. A nurse employed in a long-term care facility is observing for signs of depression in an older client. The nurse monitors for:
  1. Change in appetite and social withdrawal
  2. Change in appetite and gait disturbances
  3. Change in behavior and impaired judgment
  4. Delusions and disorganized thought processes

Answer: 1
Rationale: Changes in appetite or sleep patterns and social withdrawal are signs of depression. Gait disturbances are not a sign of depression. The depressed client may exhibit a change in behavior, but judgment is not normally impaired. Impaired judgment is more indicative of a dementia. Option 4 describes symptoms seen in delirium.

Test-Taking Strategy: Use the process of elimination. Focus on the issue of the question and note the similarity between the word *depression* in the question and *social withdrawal* in the correct option. Review signs of depression in the older client if you had difficulty with this question.

Level of Cognitive Ability: Application
Client Needs: Psychosocial Integrity
Integrated Concept/Process: Nursing Process/Data Collection
Content Area: Mental Health

Reference:
Lueckenotte, A. (2002). *Gerontologic nursing* (2nd ed.). St. Louis: Mosby, p. 66.

---

73. A nurse is assisting in the development of a plan of care for a client with a diagnosis of advanced stage Alzheimer's disease. To address the client's needs associated with memory deficits, the nurse will avoid:
  1. Adhering to the client's normal routine
  2. Keeping calendars, clocks, and pictures in view of the client
  3. Using pictures to label drawer contents
  4. Leaving the client alone

Answer: 4
Rationale: Memory impairment in advanced Alzheimer's disease is marked by loss of recent memory, loss of long-term memory, and forgetfulness of routines. Options 1, 2, and 3 are interventions that would be helpful to the client. The client should not be left alone when the disease is advanced and all memory areas are impaired.

Test-Taking Strategy: Note the key words *advanced* and *avoid*. Use the process of elimination noting that options 1, 2, and 3 would be helpful to the client. Review care to the client with Alzheimer's disease if you had difficulty with this question.

Level of Cognitive Ability: Application
Client Needs: Psychosocial Integrity
Integrated Concept/Process: Nursing Process/Planning
Content Area: Mental Health

Reference:
Lueckenotte, A. (2002). *Gerontologic nursing* (2nd ed.). St. Louis: Mosby, p. 638.

---

74. A nurse is employed in a long-term care facility. The nurse determines that an older client may be having suicidal thoughts when the client:

Answer: 3
Rationale: Giving away possessions of personal importance is a sign of potential suicide. Social withdrawal and the inability to make or carry through with decisions are signs of depression, not

1. Withdraws from social activities
2. Is unable to act on decisions
3. Gives away possessions of personal importance
4. Becomes dependent on alcohol

potential suicide. Although there is an increased risk of suicide in older alcoholics, alcohol dependency itself is not an indicator of suicidal ideation.

Test-Taking Strategy: Knowledge about the signs related to the potential for suicide is necessary to answer the question. Review these signs if you had difficulty with this question.

Level of Cognitive Ability: Comprehension
Client Needs: Psychosocial Integrity
Integrated Concept/Process: Nursing Process/Data Collection
Content Area: Mental Health

Reference:
Lueckenotte, A. (2002). *Gerontologic nursing* (2nd ed.). St. Louis: Mosby, p. 264.

---

75. A male client with diabetes mellitus who takes NPH insulin daily tells the nurse that mealtimes are not important and that he eats whenever it is convenient. It is important for the nurse to explain that mealtimes:

1. Must be at approximately the same time each day to maintain a stable blood glucose level
2. Can be varied as long as the time of insulin administration is also varied
3. Are not important as long as the client monitors the blood glucose regularly
4. Are not important as long as snack foods are readily available

Answer: 1
Rationale: Insulin should be given at approximately the same time each day. Likewise, meals should be eaten at approximately the same time each day to establish regular patterns of glucose availability. Options 2, 3, and 4 are incorrect.

Test-Taking Strategy: Use the process of elimination and note the issue of the question: the importance of mealtimes. Options 2, 3, and 4 can be eliminated because they imply that the time of meals is not important. Only option 1 stresses the importance of maintaining a regular mealtime pattern. Review the importance of diet in a client with diabetes mellitus if you had difficult with this question.

Level of Cognitive Ability: Application
Client Needs: Psychosocial Integrity
Integrated Concept/Process: Teaching/Learning
Content Area: Adult Health/Endocrine

Reference:
Lewis, S., Heitkemper, M., & Dirksen, S. (2000). *Medical-surgical nursing: assessment and management of clinical problems* (5th ed.). St. Louis: Mosby, pp. 1372-1373.

---

76. A client with acquired immunodeficiency syndrome (AIDS) shares with the nurse feelings of social isolation and loneliness since the diagnosis was made. The nurse suggests which of the following strategies as the most useful way to decrease the client's loneliness?

1. Using the Internet to facilitate communication while maintaining isolation
2. Using television and newspapers to maintain a feeling of being "in touch" with the world
3. Contacting any of the support groups available in the local region for clients with AIDS

Answer: 3
Rationale: The nurse encourages the client to maintain social contact and support, and assists the client in reducing barriers to social contact. This can include suggesting the use of community resources and support groups. Options 1 and 2 do not decrease the client's physical isolation and loneliness, and they maintain distance between the client and others. There is no information in the question to indicate loss of contact with the family, and the logistics of distance make this an unlikely solution to the client's feelings of isolation.

Test-Taking Strategy: Use the process of elimination focusing on the data provided in the question. Eliminate options 1 and 2 first because they will not decrease the client's physical isolation and loneliness. These options maintain a measure of distance between

4. Reinstituting contact with the client's family, who live in a distant city

the client and others. From the remaining options, select option 3 because there is no information in the question to indicate loss of contact with the family. Review interventions that decrease isolation and loneliness if you had difficulty with this question.

Level of Cognitive Ability: Application
Client Needs: Psychosocial Integrity
Integrated Concept/Process: Nursing Process/Implementation
Content Area: Mental Health

Reference:
Ignatavicius, D., & Workman, M. (2002). *Medical surgical nursing: critical thinking for collaborative care* (4th ed.). Philadelphia: W. B. Saunders, p. 386.

---

77. A client is being discharged from the hospital on warfarin sodium (Coumadin), and the nurse reinforces teaching about the medication. Which of the following statements indicates that the client understands the teaching provided?
  1. "I'll stop my medication if I see bruising."
  2. "Stiff joints are common when taking this medication."
  3. "This medication will prevent me from having a stroke."
  4. "If I notice blood-tinged urine, I will call the doctor immediately."

Answer: 4
Rationale: Warfarin sodium is an anticoagulant used for long-term prophylaxis to prevent thrombosis. Clients must receive detailed instructions about the signs of bleeding. Hematuria is a sign of bleeding that the client must report to the physician. Medication should not be stopped without physician approval. Stiff joints are not associated with warfarin sodium. Warfarin sodium will not prevent a stroke.

Test-Taking Strategy: Use the process of elimination and knowledge about this medication to answer the question. Recalling that bleeding is an adverse effect of the medication will direct you to option 4. Review the adverse effects of this medication that require physician notification if you had difficulty with this question.

Level of Cognitive Ability: Comprehension
Client Needs: Health Promotion and Maintenance
Integrated Concept/Process: Teaching/Learning
Content Area: Pharmacology

Reference:
Hodgson, B., & Kizior, R. (2003). *Saunders nursing drug handbook 2003.* Philadelphia: W.B. Saunders, p. 1168.

---

78. A client is prescribed a liquid iron preparation that has the potential to stain the teeth. The nurse would advise the client to:
  1. Brush the teeth before and after drinking the iron
  2. Dilute the iron in juice, drink it through a straw, and rinse the mouth afterwards
  3. Dilute more than the amount of iron prescribed to obtain the correct dosage
  4. Take the iron undiluted if the client has dentures

Answer: 2
Rationale: Liquid iron preparations stain the teeth. The best advice for the client who needs liquid iron is to dilute the iron in juice or water, drink it through a straw, and rinse the mouth well after taking. Brushing the teeth before taking the liquid iron would not be beneficial.

Test-Taking Strategy: Use the process of elimination. Eliminate options 1 and 4 first as the least likely options. Eliminate option 3 because an exact dose can be maintained by diluting only the amount prescribed. Review the procedure for the administration of oral iron if you had difficulty with this question.

Level of Cognitive Ability: Application
Client Needs: Health Promotion and Maintenance
Integrated Concept/Process: Teaching/Learning
Content Area: Pharmacology

Reference:
Lehne, R. (2001). *Pharmacology for nursing care* (4th ed.). Philadelphia: W.B. Saunders, p. 600.

79. A nurse is monitoring a client for complications after thyroidectomy. The nurse notes that the client's voice is very hoarse. The client is concerned about the hoarseness and asks the nurse about it. Which of the following responses would be most appropriate?

1. "Hoarseness and a weak voice may indicate permanent damage to the nerves."
2. "This complication is expected."
3. "This problem is temporary and will probably subside in a few days."
4. "It is best not to talk until the problem is further evaluated."

Answer: 3

Rationale: Temporary hoarseness and a weak voice may occur if there has been unilateral injury to the laryngeal nerve during surgery. If hoarseness or a weak voice is present, the client is reassured that the problem will probably subside in a few days. Unnecessary talking is discouraged to minimize hoarseness. Options 1, 2, and 4 are incorrect.

Test-Taking Strategy: Use therapeutic communication techniques to help you eliminate options 1 and 4. Although option 2 is basically correct, option 3 is most appropriate to assist in alleviating the client's concern. Review complications after thyroidectomy if you had difficulty with this question.

Level of Cognitive Ability: Application
Client Needs: Psychosocial Integrity
Integrated Concept/Process: Communication and Documentation
Content Area: Adult Health/Endocrine

Reference:
Lewis, S., Heitkemper, M., & Dirksen, S. (2000). *Medical-surgical nursing: assessment and management of clinical problems* (5th ed.). St. Louis: Mosby, p. 1422.

80. A client is seen in the health care clinic for complaints of pruritus. Diagnostic studies revealed that the pruritus is not caused by a physiological process. The nurse prepares instructions for the client to assist in reducing the problem and tells the client to:

1. Use a dehumidifier in the home
2. Ensure that the temperature in the home is high, especially during the winter months
3. Use a cool-mist vaporizer, especially during the winter months
4. Avoid the use of skin moisturizers after a bath

Answer: 3

Rationale: Itching can be a symptom of systemic disease, such as severe liver or renal disease. It can also follow medication hypersensitivity or blood reactions, and it may occur in older clients as a result of dry skin. Heat and low humidity also induce pruritis. During the winter months, using a moisturizer and increasing room humidity with a cool-mist vaporizer are advantageous.

Test-Taking Strategy: Use the process of elimination. Option 4 can be eliminated first because basic principles related to skin care include application of moisturizers to the skin. Next eliminate option 2, knowing that heat can aggravate pruritis. Read the remaining two options carefully, noting the word *dehumidifier* in option 1. A dehumidifier would remove moisture from the environment, causing a *dry* environment. This would not be helpful to the client with pruritis. Review teaching points for the client with pruritis if you had difficulty with this question.

Level of Cognitive Ability: Application
Client Needs: Health Promotion and Maintenance
Integrated Concept/Process: Teaching/Learning
Content Area: Adult Health/Integumentary

Reference:
Ignatavicius, D., & Workman, M. (2002). *Medical surgical nursing: critical thinking for collaborative care* (4th ed.). Philadelphia: W. B. Saunders, p. 1515.

81. A nurse has reinforced discharge instructions to a client after intermaxillary fixation for a fractured jaw. Which of the following client statements would indicate a need for further instruction?

1. "I should carry a wire cutter with me at all times."
2. "I should avoid carbonated beverages and alcohol."
3. "I can expect some weight loss while my jaws are wired."
4. "Swimming is a good exercise for me during this time."

Answer: 4

Rationale: Water-related activities such as swimming should be avoided. In an emergency, the airway cannot be cleared of water rapidly when jaws are wired, and there is an increased risk of drowning. The client should be instructed how to prepare a high-calorie, high-protein liquid diet, and liquid multivitamins may also be helpful. The client should avoid carbonated beverages and alcohol because carbonated beverages fizz in the back of the throat and can interfere with the airway, and alcohol can cause nausea and vomiting when combined with analgesics. A 10-pound weight loss is not uncommon while the jaws are wired.

Test-Taking Strategy: Use the process of elimination. Note the key words *need for further instruction*. Thinking about the anatomical location of this surgical procedure and the importance of maintaining a patent airway will assist in directing you to the correct option. Review client teaching points after this type of surgery if you had difficulty with this question.

Level of Cognitive Ability: Comprehension
Client Needs: Health Promotion and Maintenance
Integrated Concept/Process: Teaching/Learning
Content Area: Adult Health/Musculoskeletal

Reference:
Lewis, S., Heitkemper, M., & Dirksen, S. (2000). *Medical-surgical nursing: assessment and management of clinical problems* (5th ed.). St. Louis: Mosby, p. 1088.

82. A nurse is caring for a hospitalized school-aged child. The nurse determines that the most appropriate play activity for the child is:

1. Playing with a push-pull toy
2. Playing "peek-a-boo"
3. Hand-sewing a picture
4. Listening to music

Answer: 3

Rationale: In a school-aged child, play becomes organized with more direction. Option 3 is most appropriate for this age group. Push-pull toys are appropriate for toddlers. Option 2 is most appropriate for an infant. Option 4 is most appropriate for an adolescent.

Test-Taking Strategy: Noting the age group of the child and thinking about the related developmental stage will help you answer the question. Option 2 can be eliminated because this activity is most appropriate for an infant. Next, eliminate option 4 knowing that this activity is most appropriate for an adolescent. From the remaining options, recalling that in the school-aged child play activities become organized with more direction will help direct you to option 3. Review age-related activities and toys if you had difficulty with this question.

Level of Cognitive Ability: Comprehension
Client Needs: Health Promotion and Maintenance
Integrated Concept/Process: Nursing Process/Planning
Content Area: Child Health

Reference:
McKinney, E., Ashwill, J., Murray, S. et al. (2000). *Maternal-child nursing*. Philadelphia: W.B. Saunders, p. 132.

83. A nurse has taught a family how to communicate more effectively with a hearing-impaired client. The nurse evaluates that the family has incorporated the suggestions if the nurse observed which of the following behaviors by the family?
   1. Using appropriate hand motions with communication
   2. Shouting at the client to enhance hearing
   3. Speaking while standing behind the client
   4. Eating and drinking while talking to the client

Answer: 1
Rationale: Communication with a hearing-impaired client is enhanced by using appropriate hand signals while voicing words. Use of normal clear speech, not shouting, is most effective because shouting increases the frequency of the sounds, which makes the words harder to hear. Other helpful behaviors include speaking while positioned in front of the client, keeping hands away from the mouth while talking, having minimal distractions, and repeating and validating communication as needed.

Test-Taking Strategy: Use the process of elimination. Eliminate option 2 first because of the word *shouting*. From the remaining options, recall that a loss of hearing may be partially compensated for by sight. With this in mind, eliminate options 3 and 4. Review measures to communicate effectively with the hearing impaired if you had difficulty with this question.

Level of Cognitive Ability: Comprehension
Client Needs: Psychosocial Integrity
Integrated Concept/Process: Communication and Documentation
Content Area: Adult Health/Ear

Reference:
Lewis, S., Heitkemper, M., & Dirksen, S. (2000). *Medical-surgical nursing: assessment and management of clinical problems* (5th ed.). St. Louis: Mosby, p. 478.

---

84. A nurse is reinforcing discharge instructions to a client with peptic ulcer disease. The nurse would tell the client to take which over-the-counter medication for mild nonulcer pain?
   1. Aspirin (acetylsalicylic acid, ASA)
   2. Acetaminophen (Tylenol)
   3. Ibuprofen (Motrin)
   4. Diphenhydramine (Benadryl)

Answer: 2
Rationale: Acetaminophen is the only medication listed in the options that is a pain reliever that will not cause gastric irritation. Options 1 and 3 are pain relievers, but they irritate the gastric mucosa, which is contraindicated in clients with peptic ulcer disease. Option 4 is an antihistamine, not a pain reliever.

Test-Taking Strategy: Use the process of elimination. Recalling that the client with peptic ulcer disease should avoid items that are irritating to the gastric mucosa, and that aspirin and nonsteroidal antiinflammatory medication are irritants will assist in eliminating options 1 and 3. Focusing on the issue, medication for mild nonulcer pain, will assist in eliminating option 4. Review care to the client with peptic ulcer disease if you had difficulty with this question.

Level of Cognitive Ability: Application
Client Needs: Health Promotion and Maintenance
Integrated Concept/Process: Self-Care
Content Area: Pharmacology

Reference:
Black, J., Hawks, J., & Keene, A. (2001). *Medical-surgical nursing: clinical management for positive outcomes* (6th ed.). Philadelphia: W.B. Saunders, p. 718.

85. A nurse assigned to care for a postpartum client will promote parental-infant bonding by instructing the parents to:
1. Avoid talking to the infant
2. Allow the nursing staff to assume the infant care while in the hospital so they may rest
3. Hold and cuddle the infant closely
4. Allow the infant to sleep in the parental bed between the parents

Answer: 3
Rationale: Holding the infant close and feeling the warmth initiates a positive experience for the mother. It is self-quieting and consoles the infant. Talking to the infant and participating in infant care are other method of promoting parental-infant attachment. Infants should not be allowed to sleep between sleeping parents, not only because of the danger of suffocation but also because the couple will require meaningful rest and time to be alone as a couple.

Test-Taking Strategy: Focus on the issue, to promote parental-infant bonding. Use the process of elimination, recalling that holding and cuddling the infant initiates a positive experience. Review this content area if you had difficulty with this question.

Level of Cognitive Ability: Application
Client Needs: Psychosocial Integrity
Integrated Concept/Process: Teaching/Learning
Content Area: Maternity

Reference:
McKinney, E., Ashwill, J., Murray, S. et al. (2000). *Maternal-child nursing.* Philadelphia: W.B. Saunders, p. 498.

FILL-IN-THE-BLANK

A nurse is preparing to administer captopril (Capoten), an angiotensin-converting enzyme (ACE) inhibitor. Prior to administering the medication, the nurse would check which most important vital sign in the client?
Answer: _____

Answer: Blood pressure
Rationale: ACE inhibitors are potent antihypertensive medications. A baseline blood pressure is needed for comparison to evaluate the effectiveness of this therapy.

Test-Taking Strategy: Recalling that ACE inhibitors are most often used to treat hypertension will assist in answering this question. If you are unfamiliar with this action of these medications, review this content.

Level of Cognitive Ability: Application
Client Needs: Physiological Integrity
Integrated Concept/Process: Nursing Process/Data Collection
Content Area: Pharmacology

Reference:
Hodgson, B. & Kizior, R. (2003). *Saunders nursing drug handbook 2003.* Philadelphia: W.B. Saunders, p. 167.

MULTIPLE RESPONSE – SELECT ALL THAT APPLY

A nurse is reviewing the records of several hospitalized clients to identify the clients who are a candidate for receiving total parenteral

Answers:
___   Client with severe anorexia nervosa
___   Client with malabsorption syndrome

nutrition (TPN). Select all clients who would be a candidate for TPN.

___ Client scheduled for cholecystectomy
___ Client with severe anorexia nervosa
___ Client with uncomplicated gastroenteritis
___ Client with malabsorption syndrome
___ Client scheduled for appendectomy
___ Client with congestive heart failure
___ Client with pneumonia
___ Client receiving chemotherapy that has severe vomiting and diarrhea
___ Client with a severe burn injury
___ Client with diabetes mellitus that has an ulcer on the right ankle
___ Client receiving chemotherapy that has severe vomiting and diarrhea
___ Client with a severe burn injury

Rationale: TPN is indicated when the gastrointestinal (GI) tract is severely dysfunctional or nonfunctional, if the client had multiple GI surgeries, GI trauma, severe intolerance to enteral feedings, or intestinal obstructions, or when the bowel needs to rest for healing. Such conditions include acquired immunodeficiency syndrome (AIDS), cancer, malnutrition, burns, chronic vomiting and diarrhea, diverticulitis, malnutrition, hypermetabolic states such as sepsis, inflammatory bowel disease, pancreatitis, or severe anorexia nervosa.

Test-Taking Strategy: Thinking about the purpose and the components of TPN will assist in identifying the clients that are candidates for this form of nutrition. Review the indications for TPN if you had difficulty with this question.

Level of Cognitive Ability: Analysis
Client Needs: Physiological Integrity
Integrated Concept/Process: Nursing Process/Data Collection
Content Area: Adult Health/Gastrointestinal

Reference:
Linton, A. & Maebius, N. (2003). *Introduction to medical-surgical nursing* (3rd ed.). Philadelphia: W.B. Saunders, p. 93.

REFERENCES

Black, J., Hawks, J., & Keene, A. (2001). *Medical-surgical nursing: clinical management for positive outcomes* (6th ed.). Philadelphia: W.B. Saunders.

Bauer, B., & Hill, S. (2000). *Mental health nursing.* Philadelphia: W.B. Saunders.

Burroughs, A., & Leifer, G. (2002). *Maternity nursing* (8th ed.). Philadelphia: W.B. Saunders.

Chernecky, C., & Berger, B. (2001). *Laboratory tests and diagnostic procedures* (3rd ed.). Philadelphia: W.B. Saunders.

Ebersole, P., & Hess, P. (2001). *Geriatric nursing & healthy aging.* St. Louis: Mosby.

Hodgson, B., & Kizior, R. (2003). *Saunders nursing drug handbook 2003.* Philadelphia: W.B. Saunders.

Ignatavicius, D., & Workman, M. (2002). *Medical-surgical nursing: critical thinking for collaborative care* (4th ed.). Philadelphia: W.B. Saunders.

Lehne, R. (2001). *Pharmacology for nursing care* (4th ed.). Philadelphia: W.B. Saunders.

Lewis, S., Heitkemper, M., & Dirksen, S. (2000). *Medical-surgical nursing: assessment and management of clinical problems* (5th ed.). St. Louis: Mosby.

Linton, A., & Mackins, N. (2003). *Introduction to medical-surgical nursing* (3rd ed.). Philadelphia: W. B. Saunders.

Lueckenotte, A. (2002). *Gerontologic nursing* (2nd ed.). St. Louis: Mosby.

McKinney, E., Ashwill, J., Murray, S. et al. (2000). *Maternal-child nursing.* Philadelphia: W.B. Saunders.

Murray, S., McKinney, E., & Gorrie, T. (2002). *Foundations of maternal-newborn nursing* (3rd ed.). Philadelphia: W.B. Saunders.

Potter, P., & Perry, A. (2001). *Fundamentals of nursing* (5th ed.). St. Louis: Mosby.

Schulte, E. Price, D., & Gwin, J. (2001). *Thompson's pediatric nursing* (8th ed.). Philadelphia: W.B. Saunders.

Williams, S. (2001) *Basic nutrition & diet therapy* (11th ed.). St. Louis: Mosby.

Wong, D., & Hockenberry-Eaton, M. (2001). *Wong's essentials of pediatric nursing* (6th ed.). St. Louis: Mosby.

6/10